DAILY VALUES FOR FOOD LABELS

The Daily Values are standard values developed by the Food and Drug Administration (FDA) for use on food labels. In creating the Daily Values, the FDA first established two sets of reference values. The first set, the Reference Daily Intakes (RDI), are for protein, vitamins, and minerals and reflect average allowances based on the RDA. The second set, the Daily Reference Values (DRV), are for nutrients and food components, such as fat and fiber, that do not have an established RDA but do have important relationships with health. Together, the RDI and DRV make up the Daily Values used on food labels (Chapter 1 provides more details).

Reference Daily Intakes (RDI)

NUTRIENT	AMOUNT
Protein[a]	50 g
Thiamin	1.5 mg
Riboflavin	1.7 mg
Niacin	20 mg NE
Biotin	300 µg
Pantothenic Acid	10 mg
Vitamin B_6	2 mg
Folate	400 µg
Vitamin B_{12}	6 µg
Vitamin C	60 mg
Vitamin A[b]	5000 IU
Vitamin D [b]	400 IU
Vitamin E [b]	30 IU
Calcium	1000 mg
Iron	18 mg
Zinc	15 mg
Iodine	150 µg
Copper	2 mg

Daily Reference Values (DRV)

FOOD COMPONENT	DRV	CALCULATION
Fat	65 g	30% of kcalories
Saturated fat	20 g	10% of kcalories
Cholesterol	300 mg	Same regardless of kcalories
Carbohydrate (total)	300 g	60% of kcalories
Fiber	25 g	11.5 g per 1000 kcalories
Protein	50 g	10% of kcalories
Sodium	2400 mg	Same regardless of kcalories
Potassium	3500 mg	Same regardless of kcalories

Note: The DRV were established for adults and children over 4 years old. The values for energy-yielding nutrients are based on 2000 kcalories a day.

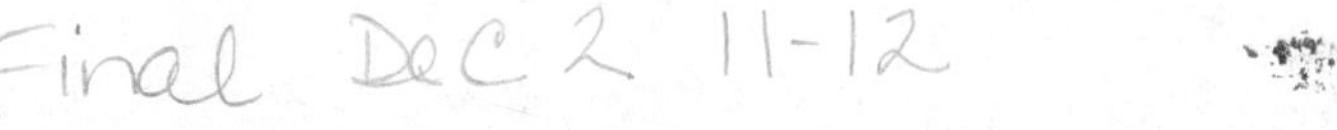

Nutrition for Health and Health Care

ELEANOR N. WHITNEY
CORINNE B. CATALDO
LINDA K. DeBRUYNE
SHARON R. ROLFES

WEST PUBLISHING COMPANY
Minneapolis/St. Paul New York Los Angeles San Francisco

Copyediting: Patricia A. Lewis
Text Design: Gary Hespenheide, Hespenheide Design
Illustration: Greg Gambino, J/B Woolsey and Associates
Dummy Artist: David Farr, ImageSmythe, Inc.
Composition: Parkwood Composition
Index: Barbara Farabaugh
Cover Image: Shirley Engen

West's Commitment to the Environment

In 1906, West Publishing Company began recycling materials left over from the production of books. This began a tradition of efficient and responsible use of resources. Today, up to 95 percent of our legal books and 70 percent of our college and school texts are printed on recycled, acid-free stock. West also recycles nearly 22 million pounds of scrap paper annually—the equivalent of 181,717 trees. Since the 1960s, West has devised ways to capture and recycle waste inks, solvents, oils, and vapors created in the printing process. We also recycle plastics of all kinds, wood, glass, corrugated cardboard, and batteries, and have eliminated the use of Styrofoam book packaging. We at West are proud of the longevity and the scope of our commitment to the environment.

Production, Prepress, Printing and Binding by West Publishing Company.

TEXT IS PRINTED ON 10% POST CONSUMER RECYCLED PAPER

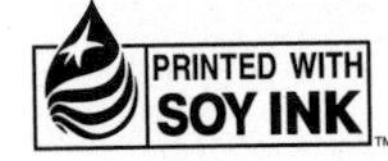

British Library Cataloguing-in-Publication Data. A catalogue record for this book is available from the British Library.

Printed in the United States of America

02 01 00 99 98 97 96 8 7 6 5 4 3 2 1

Library of Congress Cataloging-in-Publication Data

Whitney, Eleanor Noss.
Nutrition for health and health care/Eleanor N. Whitney [et al.].
p. cm.
Includes bibliographical references and index.
ISBN 0-314-04449-3
1. Nutrition. 2. Nutritionally induced diseases. 3. Diet therapy.
I. Whitney, Eleanor Noss.
QP143.N89 1995
612.3—dc20 95-3813
CIP

PHOTO CREDITS

1 Shirley Engen; **2** © Michael Newman/PhotoEdit; **10** © Myrleen Ferguson Cate/PhotoEdit; **12** Thomas Harm and Tom Peterson/Quest Photographic Inc.; **13** © H. Abernathy/H. Armstrong Roberts; **14, 15** Thomas Harm and Tom Peterson/Quest Photographic Inc.; **19** Courtesy of the FDA;

(continued after index)

DEDICATION

To the memory of my parents, Edith Tyler Noss, and Henry H.B. Noss, who supported me with love, discipline, and pride. **Ellie**

To my sister, Stephanie Balog, with faith and love to support you on your journey. **Corkie**

To my lifelong friend Lee, with love and appreciation for the time, energy, strength, and devotion you've given my family for so many years. **Linda**

To my Favorite Aunt Helen, with much love. **Sharon**

ABOUT THE AUTHORS

Eleanor Noss Whitney, Ph.D., R.D., received her B.A. in biology from Radcliffe College in 1960 and her Ph.D. in biology with an emphasis in genetics from Washington University, St. Louis, in 1970. Formerly an associate professor at the Florida State University, she now devotes full time to research, writing, and consulting on nutrition, health, and the environment. Her textbooks include *Nutrition: Concepts and Controversies, Nutrition and Diet Therapy, Life Choices,* and *The Fitness Triad,* among others. She is president of Nutrition and Health Associates, an information resource center in Tallahassee.

Corinne Balog Cataldo, M.M.Sc., R.D., C.N.S.D., received her B.S. in community health nutrition from Georgia State University in 1976 and her M.M.Sc. in clinical dietetics from Emory University in 1979. She has worked in private practice in Atlanta, as a clinical dietitian and metabolic support nutritionist at Georgia Baptist Medical Center in Atlanta, as a faculty member and dietetic internship coordinator at Emory University, and as a nutritionist with the Infant Formula Council. She has made numerous presentations, and in addition to this book, she has written a manual on tube feeding and the books *Nutrition and Diet Therapy: Principles and Practice* and *Understanding Clinical Nutrition.* She is a certified nutrition support dietitian and continues to do consulting work.

Linda Kelly DeBruyne, M.S., R.D., received her B.S. in 1980 and her M.S. in 1982 in nutrition and food science at the Florida State University. She serves on the board of directors of Nutrition and Health Associates, an information resource center in Tallahassee, Florida, where her specialty areas are fitness and life cycle nutrition. Her other textbooks include *Nutrition and Diet Therapy, Making Life Choices, Life Span Nutrition: Conception through Life,* and *The Fitness Triad: Motivation, Training, and Nutrition.* As a consultant for a group of Tallahassee pediatricians, she teaches infant nutrition classes to parents.

Sharon Rady Rolfes, M.S., R.D., received her B.S. in psychology and criminology in 1974 and her M.S. in nutrition and food science in 1982 at the Florida State University. She is a founding member of Nutrition and Health Associates, an information resource center that maintains an ongoing bibliographic data base of research on 1000 nutrition-related topics. Her other textbooks include *Understanding Nutrition, Understanding Normal and Clinical Nutrition,* and *Life Span Nutrition: Conception through Life.* In addition to writing, she is currently serving on the National Faculty Advisory Committee for a nutrition telecourse being developed by the Dallas County Community College District. She has also served as a nutrition consultant for the Florida House of Representatives, the Florida Department of Education Comprehensive School Health Programs, and interactive media science projects funded by the National Science Foundation and developed by the Florida State University.

CONTENTS IN BRIEF

CONTENTS

CHAPTER 9

CHAPTER 10

CHAPTER 11

PART TWO: Nutrition in Health Care

CHAPTER 12

CHAPTER 13

Self-Studies appear at the ends of the Chapters of Part One:

Case Studies appear throughout the Chapters of Parts Two and Three:

"How to" features are listed after the index

PREFACE

Welcome to the world of nutrition! We, the authors of this book, find it a rewarding and fascinating field. Our study of nutrition has not only enabled us to help others but has also enriched our own lives and personal health.

This book is intended to take you swiftly and efficiently through the basics of nutrition for the healthy individual, and then through the elements of clinical nutrition for the health care professional. Although primarily written for nurses and home health care workers, this book can also serve as a useful resource for anyone interested in nutrition, from homemakers to physicians.

Part One deals with how nutrition supports health: how to select foods and prepare meals that will maintain appropriate weight and meet the nutrient needs of normal, healthy adults and their families. Part Two moves into the health care setting and introduces the concept of nutrition assessment, the detective work that uncovers how well people's nutrient needs are being met. It then goes on to show how nutrition care plans are developed to meet those needs at different stages of the life cycle from pregnancy and infancy through old age. Part Three delves into the impacts on nutrition of diseases and disorders and explains how diet therapy supports life and promotes recovery.

The book offers many aids to learning and cues to the practical application of nutrition knowledge. Definitions of nutrition terms appear in the margins of the text where the terms first appear and also in a master glossary at the end of the book. "How-To" boxes in many chapters train readers in gaining the skills needed to calculate energy and nutrient needs in various settings, and to help clients work out ways to meet those needs when discomfort and disease make it difficult to do so. Study questions at the ends of the chapters guide readers in reviewing chapter material, and clinical application questions ask readers to synthesize what they have learned and solve clinical problems. Self-Studies in the chapters of Part One offer readers the opportunity to evaluate nutrition aspects of their own diets, and Case Studies in the chapters of Parts Two and Three provide practice in applying nutrition knowledge to individual clients' situations.

Each chapter is followed by a Nutrition in Practice section that explores a special aspect of clinical nutrition: a specialty area such as nutrition and dental health; new developments in research; or facets of practice such as the ways the health team delivers nutrition care. Finally, the appendixes support the book with a wealth of useful information on the nutrient contents of foods, U.S. and Canadian nutrient intake recommendations, food exchange systems, resources for further information, nutrition formulas, hospital menus, and aids to calculation.

Nutrition is a pleasing subject because it enhances health. We are grateful for the opportunity to offer you this information. We hope you will not only benefit from it, but also enjoy it.

Ellie Whitney
Corinne Cataldo
Linda DeBruyne
Sharon Rolfes

ACKNOWLEDGMENTS

We have been supported by the work of many fine people during the preparation of this book. Sabrina McGriff, Casy Sizer, Mary Ann Rivecchio, and Sally Lorch helped with many aspects of manuscript preparation. Betty Hands and Bob Geltz have created a superbly accurate food composition appendix. Our editors are the finest we could ask for: Peter Marshall, Angela Vroom, Kara ZumBahlen, and Sharon Kavanagh. John Woolsey and his staff have provided top quality art throughout, and Shirley Engen has created beautiful paintings for our chapter-opener pages. Reviewers have offered thoughtful, constructive criticism.

Our families and friends have encouraged us when the work became demanding and difficult. We are grateful to you all.

REVIEWERS

REVIEWERS OF *NUTRITION FOR HEALTH AND HEALTH CARE*

Connie S. Austin, RN, MA.Ed, MSN
Azusa Pacific University

Elaine Brown, BSN, MSN
Big Bend Community College

Janet Z. Burson, Ed.D, RD, LD
University of Southern Maine

Betty Clamp, MS, RD
Ohlone College

Kathryn Daughton, BSN, MA.Ed
Ashville Technical College

Lois Ellis, CRNA, Ed.D
Indiana Wesleyan University

Denise Garner, MS, RD
York College of Pennsylvania

Mary Jo Gerlach, RN, MSN
Medical College of Georgia—Athens

Alida Herling
Normandale Community College

Regina Jennette, RN, MSN
West Virginia Northern Community College

Joanne Lisk, RN, MSN
Alcorn State University

Isabelle Mosig, BSN, M.Ed
Hahnemann University

Carmen Nochera, Ph.D, LN-D
Grand Valley State University

Nancy Shaw, CNS, CHE
Southeast Louisiana University

Sue Tanner, RN, MS, CNS
Alvin Community College

Mary A. Weaver, RN, SNT, M.Ed
Daytona Beach Community College

Diane Wilson, Ed.D, RD
Medical University of South Carolina

1

Perspectives on Nutrition

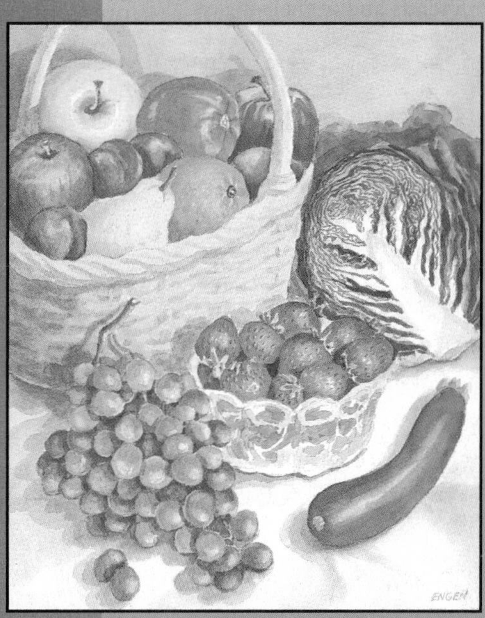

CONTENTS

You are a collection of molecules that move. All these moving parts are arranged in patterns of extraordinary complexity and order—cells, tissues, and organs. Although the arrangement remains constant, the parts are continually changing, using nutrients and energy derived from nutrients. To maintain your "self," therefore, you must continuously replace the *pieces* you lose and replenish the *energy* you burn.

The pieces you are made of and your energy come from the nutrients contained in the food you eat. The science of nutrition is the study of the nutrients in food and the body's handling of these nutrients.

science of nutrition: the study of nutrients in foods and of their ingestion, digestion, absorption, transport, metabolism, interaction, storage, and excretion. A broader definition includes the study of the environment and of human behavior as it relates to these processes.

Most people know that the nutrients in food nourish the body and promote health. Nevertheless, most people choose foods for reasons other than their nutrient contributions. Food choices are personal and not always sensible, and to a great extent, they resist change. Before undertaking diet planning, the planner must understand the dynamics of food choices, because people will alter their eating habits only if their preferences are honored.

Food Choices

Why do you choose the particular foods you do? Several reasons come to mind, but nutrition would be only one of them and would not necessarily be at the top of many people's lists. Even people who claim to choose foods primarily for nutrition's sake will admit that other factors also influence their food choices. They may *know how* to prepare nutritious meals, but that doesn't mean they actually *eat* such meals all the time. Instead, people's food choices tend to be powerfully influenced by a variety of personal factors.[1]

Preference Why do you like certain foods? One reason, of course, is your preference for certain tastes. Some tastes are widely liked, such as the sweetness of sugar and the zest of salt.

Associations People also like foods with which they have happy associations—foods eaten in the midst of warm family gatherings on traditional holidays or given to them as children by someone who loved them. By the same token, people can attach intense and unalterable dislikes to foods that they ate when they were sick or that were forced on them when they weren't hungry.

Habit Sometimes habit dictates people's food choices. You eat a sandwich for lunch or drink orange juice at breakfast simply because you have always done so. Your parents may have taught you to like and dislike certain foods for reasons of their own without even being aware of it.

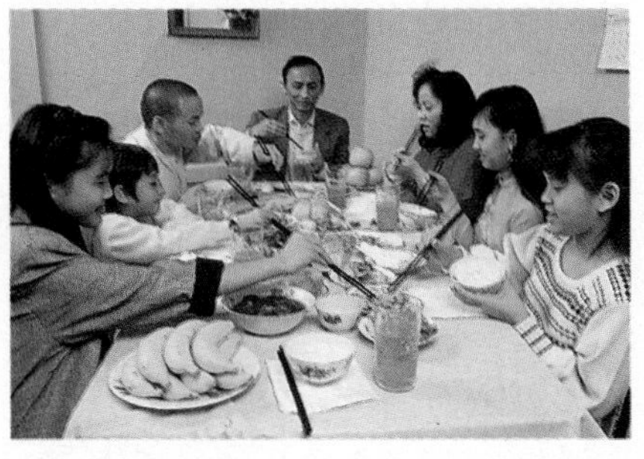

Ethnic meals and family gatherings nourish the spirit as well as the body.

Ethnic Heritage and Tradition Every country, and every region of a country, has its own typical foods and ways of combining them into meals. North America includes people from many different cultural and ethnic backgrounds. The foodways of this continent reflect this intermingling of cultures. Many foods with ethnic origins are familiar features on North American menus: tacos, egg rolls, lasagna, and gyros, to name a few. Still others, such as pizza, spaghetti, and croissants, are integral in the "American diet." North American regional cuisines like Cajun and TexMex blend the traditions of several cultures. Table 1–1 presents profiles of selected ethnic diets, together with comments on their nutrition merits and drawbacks.

ethnic diets: foodways and cuisines typical of national origins, races, cultural heritages, or geographic locations.

Values People's values, environmental ethics, religious beliefs, and political views also influence their food choices. By choosing to eat some foods or avoid others, people make statements about themselves that reflect their values. For example, people may select only foods that come in containers that can be reused or recycled. Some people choose only those brands of canned tuna fish that state "dolphin safe" on the label, meaning that dolphins were not killed when the tuna were netted. (Nutrition in Practice 11 elaborates further on ways the environment relates to food choices.) Religion also influences many people's food choices. Jewish law sets forth an extensive set of dietary rules. Many Christians forgo meat during Lent, the period prior to Easter. Other faiths prohibit some dietary practices and promote others. Diet planners can promote people's use of sound nutrition practices only if they respect and honor such values.

Social Pressure Social pressure is another powerful influence on people's food choices. How can you refuse when your friends are going out for pizza or ice cream? Such pressure operates in all circles and across all cultural lines. It is often considered rude to refuse food or drink being shared by a group or offered by a host. Often you become accepted as a member of a social gathering only when you "break bread" with the other members.

Emotional Comfort Some people eat in response to emotional stimuli—for example, to relieve boredom or depression or to calm anxiety. A lonely person may choose to eat rather than to call a friend and risk rejection. A person who has returned home from an exciting evening out may unwind with a late-night snack. Eating in response to emotions can easily lead to overeating and obesity, but may be appropriate at times. For example, sharing food at times of bereavement serves both the giver's need to provide comfort and the receiver's need to be cared for and to interact with others.

Availability, Convenience, and Economy The influence of these factors on people's food selections is clear. You cannot eat foods if they are not available, if you cannot prepare them, or if you cannot afford them. Convenience plays a major role in many people's food selections today. The demand for foods that are ready to eat or can be easily prepared in a microwave oven demonstrates this influence.[2]

Image Sometimes people associate foods with ideals of body image, and these ideals influence their food choices. The fashion and movie industries, not the medical community, have defined what people believe to be the ideal body—sometimes an excessively thin body for women, or

Table 1–1
Characteristics of Selected Ethnic Diets

STAPLE FOODS	STRENGTHS OF THE DIET	WEAKNESSES OF THE DIET
Hispanic Americans from Cuba, Haiti, Puerto Rico		
Include: ▸ Steamed white rice; wheat breads. ▸ Starchy vegetables (beans, cassavas, yuccas); plantains; green peppers; tomatoes; garlic. ▸ Dried, salted fish, chicken; pork. ▸ Lard; olive oil; sugar; jams and jellies; sweet pastries; sugared fruit juices; coffee. *Exclude:* ▸ Green, leafy vegetables. ▸ Milk as a beverage for adults. ▸ Fish other than dried and salted.	Provides adequate protein, many other nutrients, and fiber	May provide too much fat, especially animal fat; may lack calcium
Hispanic Americans from Mexico, Central America		
Include: ▸ Steamed rice, corn products such as tortillas. ▸ Many varieties of beans; chili peppers; tomatoes; mangoes; prickly pear fruit; potatoes. ▸ Meat and sausages; fish; poultry; eggs. ▸ Lard; chocolate and coffee drinks; cakes; pastries. *Exclude:* ▸ Green, leafy vegetables; yellow vegetables. ▸ Milk as a beverage for adults.	Most nutrients can be obtained	Is high in kcalories and fat, especially saturated fat, and high in sugar
Black Americans from West Indies, Central or South America and Recent African Immigrants		
Include: ▸ Millet, corn, wheat, rice, or barley. ▸ Starchy roots such as cassavas, yams; plantains; bananas; coconuts; peanuts; fresh fruits; hot peppers; tomatoes; onions; okra. ▸ Palm oil; fruit wine; tea; coffee; honey; molasses. *Exclude:* ▸ Milk and milk products (meat and fish limited use).	Is low in fat and salt; is high in fiber	Is low in calcium, iron, and vitamin B_{12}; is potentially low in protein, depending on availability of foods
Southern Black Americans from West Africa (Many Generations in United States)		
Include: ▸ Rice; hominy grits; biscuits; cornmeal and cornbread. ▸ Legumes; potatoes; onions; tomatoes; hot peppers; green leafy vegetables, okra; sweet potatoes; squashes; corn; cabbage; melons; peaches. ▸ Smoked pork; meats and poultry; fish; thick stews. ▸ Pecans; butter, shortening, and lard; sugar; bread puddings, pies, and sweets. *Exclude:* ▸ Milk and milk products. ▸ Yeast breads.	Provides ample nutrients of meat	Provides excess protein; is high in kcalories; provides excess fat, especially saturated fat; is high in salt; is low in calcium
Chinese Americans from China (Diets Sometimes Vary With Region)		
Include: ▸ Rice and rice gruel; wheat noodles; soy bean noodles. ▸ Corn; vegetables from the cabbage family; squashes; cucumbers; eggplant; leafy vegetables; various shoots (bamboo, mung, and soy); sweet potatoes; radishes; onions; peas and pods; mushrooms; roots; local vegetables; pickled vegetables; sea vegetables; plums; peaches; tangerines; kumquats; other citrus fruits; litchis; longans; mangoes; papayas; pomegranates. ▸ Soybean products (tofu and soy milk); meat; fish with bones; poultry; seafood. ▸ Soup or tea as beverage; soy sauce; sugar. *Exclude:* ▸ Milk and most milk products.	Is low in fat; is high in fiber and many nutrients	Depending on availability of protein-rich foods, protein and iron may be low; high in salt

Table 1–1 *(continued)*

STAPLE FOODS	STRENGTHS OF THE DIET	WEAKNESSES OF THE DIET
Japanese Americans from Japan *Include:* ▶ Rice. ▶ Vegetables (including pickled and sea); fruits; salads. ▶ Soy (miso, tofu, bean paste); fish with bones; seafood ▶ Sugars as seasoning; ginseng; soy sauce. *Exclude:* ▶ Milk and milk products.	Provides abundant nutrients with little fat	Is high in salt
Korean American from South Korea *Include:* ▶ Rice; noodles. ▶ Leafy vegetables; kimchi (hot pickled cabbage); sea vegetables; hot peppers; seasonal fruits; mushrooms. ▶ Small fish with bones; grilled beef; chicken; squid, octopus, and lobster; mussels; eggs. ▶ Lard and vegetable fat for frying; seasame oil; nuts and seeds; ginger; sugar as seasoning. *Exclude:* ▶ Milk and milk products.	Provides adequate protein	Is high in fat; monotonous in winter (kimchi is served at each meal, to the exclusion of other vegetables); without the traditional small fish with bones, calcium can be lacking
Vietnamese Americans from Vietnam *Include:* ▶ Rice, rice noodles; french bread and croissants. ▶ Hot peppers; curries of asparagus and potatoes; salads; tropical fruits and vegetables; lemons and limes. ▶ Small portions of poultry; eggs; fish pâtés; nuoc nam (a strong, fermented fish sauce). ▶ Sweets, candies, sweetened drinks; coffee; tea; butter. *Exclude:* ▶ Milk and milk products.	Provides adequate protein and vitamins	Can be low in iron or calcium
Native Americans *Include:* ▶ *Southeast:* corn; cornmeal; coontie (flour from a palmlike plant); fried breads; pumpkins; squashes; papayas; alligator, snake, wild hog, duck, fish, and shellfish. ▶ *Northeast:* blueberries; cranberries; beans; corn; pumpkins; fish; lobster; wild game; maple syrup. ▶ *Midwest:* bison; beans; corn; melons; squashes; tomatoes. ▶ *Southwest:* corn (many varieties); beans; squash; pumpkins; chili peppers; melons; pinenuts; cactus. ▶ *Northwest:* salmon; caviar; other fish; otter; seal; elk; whale; bear; other game; wild fruits, nuts, and greens. *Exclude:* ▶ Milk and milk products.	Varies with region; may provide adequate protein and fiber	Varies with region; may be low in calcium
Italian Americans from Italy *Include:* ▶ *Northern Italy:* egg-based, ribbon-shaped pastas; cheese; cream; butter; meat; eggs. ▶ *Southern Italy:* wheat pastas; artichokes, eggplants, peppers, and tomatoes; beans; olive oil.	Provides adequate protein and most nutrients	Varies with region; can be high in fat

an excessively muscular body for men. Both men and women seek "beautiful bodies," and in doing so, they select or avoid foods that they believe will improve or impair their physical appearance. Such intentions are rational when based on sound nutrition and fitness knowledge, but when based on faddism or carried to extremes, they undermine good health.

Medical Conditions Sometimes medical conditions and the medications used to treat the conditions limit which foods a person can select. The second half of this text discusses diets modified for different medical conditions.

Nutrition No matter what dietary tradition you follow, you have no guarantee of diet adequacy. Since sound nutrition promotes health and longevity, it is in every person's own best interest to know how to obtain optimal nourishment. Consumers today cite nutrition as a primary concern in making food choices, yet the foods they choose do not always reflect this concern; they need to know more about the nutrients in food.[3]

The Nutrients

Almost any food you eat is composed of dozens or even hundreds of different kinds of materials—atoms and molecules too small to see with even the most powerful microscope. A food such as spinach, for example, is composed mostly of water (95 percent), and most of its solid materials are organic compounds—carbohydrate, fat (properly called *lipid*), and protein. If you could remove these materials, you would find a tiny residue of minerals, vitamins, and other items. The nutrients in spinach are of six types: water, carbohydrate, fat, protein, vitamins, and minerals. Some of the other materials in spinach, such as the pigments and some minerals, are not nutrients. The body can make some nutrients for itself, at least in limited quantities, but it cannot make them all, and it makes some in insufficient quantities to meet its needs. Therefore the body must obtain many nutrients from foods. The nutrients that foods must supply are called *essential nutrients.*

nutrient: a substance obtained from food and used in the body to promote growth, maintenance, or repair.

The six classes of nutrients are water, carbohydrate, fat, protein, vitamins, and minerals.

essential nutrients: nutrients the body must obtain from food because it cannot make them for itself in sufficient quantity to meet physiological needs.

organic: carbon containing. The four organic nutrients are carbohydrate, fat, protein, and vitamins.

Metabolism, the set of processes by which nutrients are rearranged into body structures or broken down to yield energy, is described in Chapter 6.

energy-yielding nutrients: the fuel nutrients, those that yield energy the body can use.

Three Energy Nutrients Four of the six classes of nutrients (carbohydrate, fat, protein, and vitamins) are organic. During metabolism, three of these four (carbohydrate, fat, and protein) provide energy the body can use. These energy-yielding nutrients continually replenish the energy you spend daily. Without them you would soon die. Carbohydrate and fat are the major energy-yielding nutrients. Protein becomes a major fuel only when other fuels are unavailable.

Vitamins, Minerals, and Water Vitamins are organic but do not provide energy to the body. They facilitate the release of energy from the other three organic nutrients. In contrast, minerals and water are inorganic nutrients. Minerals yield no energy in the human body, but like vitamins, they help to regulate the release of energy. As for water, it is the medium in which all of the body's processes take place.

kCalories: Measures of Energy The amount of energy the energy-yielding nutrients release can be measured in calories (or more properly, kilocalories, or kcalories). kCalories are not constituents of foods; they are a measure of the energy in foods. It is as incorrect to refer to the kcalories in a food as it is to refer to the inches in a person. It is correct to refer to the *energy* in a food and to the *height* of a person. The energy in a food depends on how much carbohydrate, fat, and protein the food contains.

Carbohydrate yields 4 kcalories of energy from each gram, and so does protein. Fat yields 9 kcalories per gram. If you know how many grams of each nutrient a food contains, you can derive the number of kcalories potentially available from the food. Simply multiply the carbohydrate grams times 4, the protein grams times 4, and the fat grams times 9, and add the results together (see the accompanying box).

Energy Nutrients in Foods Practically all foods contain mixtures of the energy-yielding nutrients, although foods are sometimes classified by their predominant nutrient. Thus, to speak of meat as "a protein" or of bread as "a carbohydrate" is inaccurate. Each is rich in a particular nutrient, but a protein-rich food such as beef contains a lot of fat along with protein, and a carbohydrate-rich food such as cornbread also contains fat (corn oil) and protein. Only a few foods are exceptions to this rule, the common ones being sugar (which is pure carbohydrate) and oil (which is pure fat).

kcalorie: a unit by which energy is measured. Most people speak of these units simply as calories, but on paper the word calorie is prefaced by a k for kilocalorie. We use kcalories and kcal throughout this book.

Food energy can also be measured in kilojoules (kJ). One kcalorie equals 4.2 kJ. The kilojoule is the international unit of energy.

Energy Storage in the Body If your body doesn't use the energy-yielding nutrients to fuel metabolic and physical activities, it rearranges them into storage compounds, primarily body fat, and puts them away for later use. Thus, if you take in more energy than you expend, whether from carbohydrate, fat, or protein, the result is usually a gain of body fat. Too much meat (a protein-rich food) is just as fattening as too many potatoes (a carbohydrate-rich food), depending on the total energy in each.

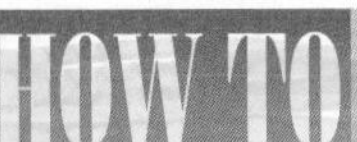

Calculate the Energy in a Food

The following example shows how to calculate the energy available from 1 slice of bread that has 1 teaspoon of butter on it. From food tables such as Appendix A in this book, you can determine that this food contains 15 grams carbohydrate, 2 grams protein, and 5 grams fat:

$$15 \text{ g carbohydrate} \times 4 \text{ kcal/g} = 60 \text{ kcal.}$$
$$2 \text{ g protein} \times 4 \text{ kcal/g} = 8 \text{ kcal.}$$
$$5 \text{ g fat} \times 9 \text{ kcal/g} = 45 \text{ kcal.}$$
$$\text{Total} = 113 \text{ kcal.}$$

Alcohol, Not a Nutrient When taken in excess of energy need, alcohol, too, is converted to body fat and stored. The body derives energy from alcohol at the rate of 7 kcalories per gram. Alcohol is not a nutrient, however, because it contributes nothing to the body's growth, maintenance, or repair. When alcohol contributes too much energy to a person's diet, the harm it does extends far beyond the making of body fat. Nutrition in Practice 8 discusses alcohol's effects on nutrition.

Nutrition Guidelines

To nourish yourself optimally, you need to eat foods that provide adequate amounts of essential nutrients and energy. To know how to choose appropriate foods, you need to know your own nutrient and energy needs, as well as the quantity of nutrients the foods contain.

Recommended Nutrient Intakes

Nutrient intake recommendations all have the same objective—to offer a rough guideline for dietary adequacy. This discussion focuses on the Recommended Dietary Allowances (RDA) of the United States as an example of recommended intakes; Canadian and other standards are in Appendix B.

Recommended Dietary Allowances (RDA): daily recommended intakes of selected nutrients considered adequate to meet the nutrient needs of practically all healthy people in the United States (see the inside front cover).

Various nations and international groups have published different sets of standards similar to the RDA. The Canadian equivalent is called the **RNI,** or **Recommended Nutrient Intakes** for Canadians. Among the most widely used recommendations is a set developed by two international groups, the Food and Agricultural Organization and the World Health Organization (the FAO/WHO recommendations). See Appendix B for all of these.

The RDA The main RDA table includes recommendations for protein, eleven vitamins, and seven minerals. A second RDA table specifies energy needs for people of different ages. A third table presents tentative recommendations for two more vitamins and eight more minerals. The main table is used and referred to so often that it is presented on the inside front cover of this book; the other RDA tables are in Appendix B.

Limits of the RDA The RDA have been much misunderstood. One person, on first learning of their existence, was outraged: "You mean Uncle Sam tells me that I must eat exactly 46 grams of protein every day?" This is not the intention of the committee on RDA, and the RDA are not laws, just recommendations. The following facts will help put the RDA in perspective.

- The RDA are published by the government, but the study group that determines them is composed of highly qualified scientists selected by the National Academy of Sciences.
- The RDA are based on available scientific evidence to the greatest extent possible; they are periodically reviewed and revised.
- The RDA are not minimum requirements. R stands for *recommended,* not for *required.* They are allowances, and except for energy (see Figures 1-1 and 1-2), they are generous. Even so, they do not necessarily cover every individual for every nutrient.
- The RDA are estimates of the needs of healthy persons only. Medical problems alter nutrient needs.
- The RDA take into account the differences among individuals and define a range within which most healthy persons' intakes of nutrients

requirement: the amount of a nutrient that will just prevent the development of specific deficiency signs; a theoretical value impossible to state for everyone. (In contrast, the RDA are generous allowances that include a safety factor to provide for individual variability.)

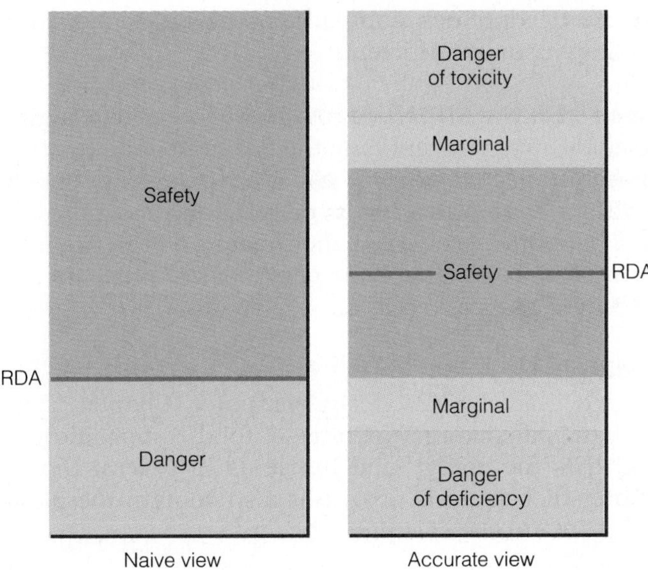

Figure 1–1
Naive versus Accurate View of Nutrient Needs
The RDA for a given nutrient represents a point within a range of appropriate and reasonable intakes that lies between toxicity and deficiency. The recommendation is high enough to provide reserves in times of short-term dietary inadequacies, but not so high as to approach toxicity. Nutrient intakes above or below this range might be equally harmful.

probably should fall. Individuals whose needs are higher than the average are included within this range.

- Separate recommendations are made for different sets of people: men, women, pregnant women, children, and other groups. Children aged 4 to 6 are distinguished from men and women aged 19 to 24, for example. Each individual can look up the recommendations for his or her own age and sex group.

Uses of the RDA With the understanding that the RDA are approximate, flexible, and generous, they can be used as a yardstick, not to assess the adequacy of individual diets but to measure the adequacy of diets in entire populations, such as those of a certain school or community. Diets of individuals are often assessed by comparing them to the RDA because it is impractical, if not impossible, to determine any one

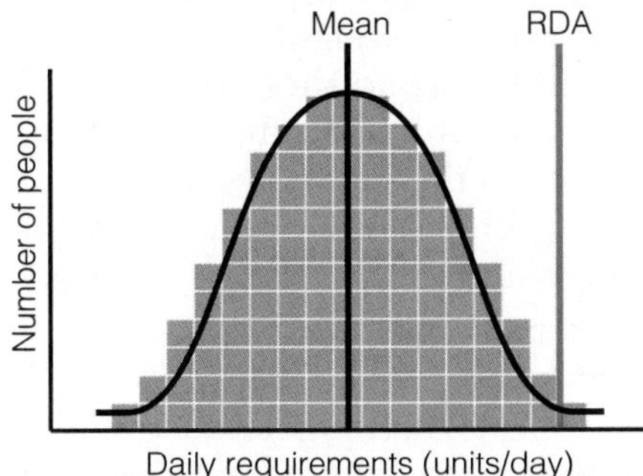

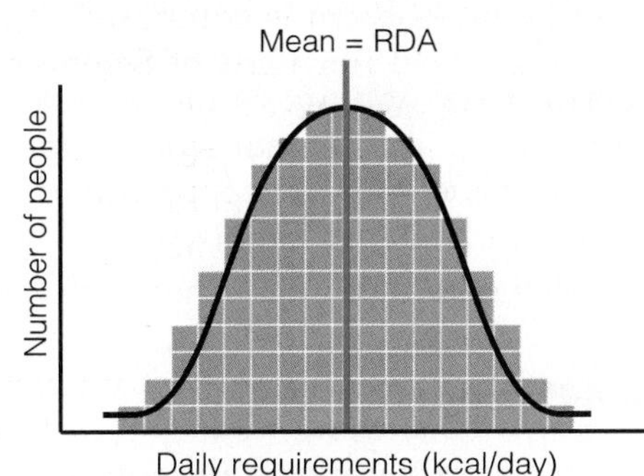

Figure 1–2
The Nutrient RDA and the Energy RDA

person's precise needs. Such comparisons provide a rough estimate of adequacy and are usually sufficient.

Tools Used with the RDA: Diet History To evaluate a diet, your own or someone else's, you need not only the RDA but also an accurate listing of the foods eaten over a period of time. An assessor uses a diet history form to obtain a record of the types of foods, with portion sizes, an individual eats (Chapter 12 provides a diet history form). Then the assessor adds up the nutrients and energy the person consumed and compares the totals with recommendations such as the RDA.

Diet Analysis Analyses of the energy and nutrients someone has consumed can be done by hand or by computer (Chapter 12 provides the details). For hand calculation, the table of food composition, Appendix A in this book, lists the energy and nutrients in several thousand foods. Many computer diet analysis programs also contain these data and can perform and print out the calculations.

Dietary Guidelines

Cholesterol is a member of the lipid family and receives attention in Chapter 3.

overnutrition: overconsumption of food energy or nutrients sufficient to cause disease or increased susceptibility to disease; a form of malnutrition.

undernutrition: underconsumption of food energy or nutrients severe enough to cause disease or increased susceptibility to disease; a form of malnutrition.

The RDA were developed to ensure *adequate* nutrient intakes, but they do little to protect people from *excess* intakes of fat, cholesterol, sugar, salt, and alcohol. Government authorities are now as much concerned about overnutrition as they once were about undernutrition. Research confirms that dietary excesses, especially of energy, fat, and alcohol, contribute to many diseases, including heart disease, cancer, diabetes, and liver disease.[4] Several sets of dietary recommendations have originated from the awareness that overnutrition contributes to disease.

Dietary Recommendations Many sets of dietary recommendations have been published in the United States with titles such as *dietary goals* or *dietary guidelines.* These sets of recommendations differ only a little from one another, and all emphasize prevention of overnutrition and disease. Table 1–2 summarizes the dietary recommendations from a report of the National Research Council (NRC) titled *Diet and Health: Implications for Reducing Chronic Disease Risk.*

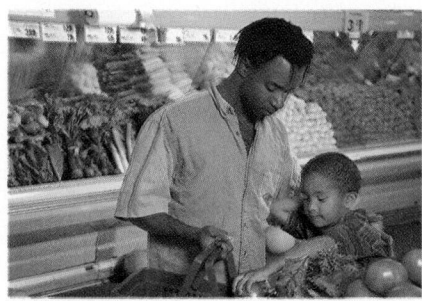

When people choose foods, they are selecting nutrients.

Weight Maintenance and Physical Activity The recommendations state not only what people should eat but also what they should avoid. In addition, the recommendations refer to weight maintenance and physical activity. Some people's diets are close to these recommendations, but the typical North American diet, which emphasizes meat, falls far short of the recommendations. So does the sedentary lifestyle of many North Americans who fail to meet even minimal guidelines for physical activity.

Diet-Planning Principles

How can people juggle the foods available to them to create a diet that supplies all the needed nutrients in the appropriate amounts for good

Table 1–2
***Diet and Health* Recommendations**

NUTRIENT AND ENERGY RECOMMENDATIONS	SUGGESTED FOOD CHOICES
Reduce total *fat* intake to 30% or less of kcalories. Reduce saturated fatty acid intake to less than 10% of kcalories and intake of cholesterol to less than 300 mg daily.	Reduce fat and cholesterol intake by substituting fish, poultry without skin, lean meats, and low-fat or nonfat dairy products for fatty meats and whole-milk products; by choosing more vegetables, fruits, cereals, and legumes; and by limiting fats, oils, egg yolks, and fried and other fatty foods.
Increase intake of starches and other *complex carbohydrates.*	Every day eat five or more servings of a combination of vegetables and fruits, especially green and yellow vegetables and citrus fruits, and six or more daily servings of a combination of breads, cereals, and legumes. The committee does not recommend increasing the intake of added sugars, because their consumption is strongly associated with dental caries.
Maintain *protein* intake at moderate levels.	Meet at least the RDA for protein; do not exceed twice the RDA.
Balance food intake and physical activity to maintain appropriate *body weight.*	
For those who drink *alcoholic beverages,* the committee recommends limiting consumption to the equivalent of less than 1 oz pure alcohol in a single day. Pregnant women should avoid alcoholic beverages.	The committee does not recommend alcohol consumption. One ounce of pure alcohol is the equivalent of two cans of beer, two small glasses of wine, or two average cocktails.
Limit total daily intake of *salt* (sodium chloride) to 6 g or less.	Limit the use of salt in cooking, and avoid adding it to food at the table. Salty, highly processed salty, salt-preserved, and salt-pickled foods should be consumed sparingly.
Maintain adequate *calcium* intake.	
Avoid taking dietary *supplements* in excess of the RDA in any one day.	
Maintain an optimal intake of *fluoride,* particularly during the years of primary and secondary tooth formation and growth.	

Source: Adapted from the National Academy of Sciences report *Diet and Health: Implications for Reducing Chronic Disease Risk,* (Washington, D.C.: National Academy Press, 1989).

health? The principle is simple enough: select a variety of foods that supply the nutrients your body needs. In practice, how do you do this? It helps to keep in mind six basic diet-planning principles, which are listed in the margin in alphabetical order for ease in remembering them.

Diet-planning principles:

- **A**dequacy.
- **B**alance.
- k**C**alorie control.
- Nutrient **D**ensity.
- **M**oderation.
- **V**ariety.

Adequacy The ideal of dietary adequacy has already been touched on. A diet that provides enough energy and enough of every nutrient to meet daily needs is adequate.

dietary adequacy: the characteristic of a diet that provides all the essential nutrients, fiber, and energy necessary to maintain health and body weight. Ideally, a diet will be more than just adequate; it will be optimal, providing an assortment and balance of nutrients and food energy that maintain a favorable body weight and the best possible state of health.

Balance As for dietary balance, the essential minerals calcium and iron illustrate its importance. Meats, fish, poultry, and legumes are rich in iron but are poor sources of calcium. Similarly, milk and milk products are rich in calcium but are poor sources of iron. In fact, milk (except breast milk) and milk products are so low in iron that overuse of these foods can actually lead to iron-deficiency anemia by displacing iron-rich

dietary balance: providing foods of a number of types in balance with one another such that foods rich in one nutrient do not crowd out foods that are rich in another nutrient.

foods from the diet. Yet milk is the single most nutritious food for infants and can be an important calcium source for people of all ages.

Use some meat and meat alternates for iron; use some milk and milk products for calcium. Save some space, too, for other foods, for a diet consisting only of milk and meat would be far from adequate. To obtain the other needed nutrients, you have to eat vegetables, fruits, grains, and other foods. In short, balance in the diet helps to ensure adequacy.

kcalorie control: management of food energy intake.

kCalorie Control While it takes thought and skill to design an adequate, balanced diet, incorporating kcalorie control presents an added challenge—to eat an adequate, balanced diet without overeating. (Energy balance and weight control are discussed in Chapter 9.)

nutrient density: a measure of the nutrients a food provides relative to the energy it provides. The more nutrients and the fewer kcalories, the higher the nutrient density.

moderation: providing enough, but not too much of a dietary constituent.

Nutrient Density To this end, the concept of nutrient density helps: seek out foods that deliver the highest nutrient values per kcalorie. For example, among foods containing calcium, a 1½-ounce portion of cheddar cheese and 1 cup of nonfat milk both provide about the same amount of calcium; but the cheese contributes twice as much food energy as the nonfat milk (see Appendix A). The nonfat milk, then, is more calcium dense: it offers the same amount of calcium for half the kcalories.

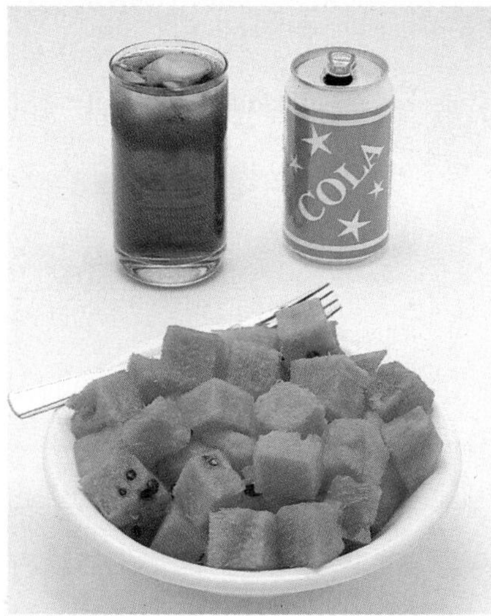

This cola and bowl of watermelon illustrate nutrient density. Each provides about 150 kcalories, but the watermelon offers a little protein, some vitamins, minerals, and fiber along with the energy; the cola beverage offers only "empty" kcalories. Watermelon, or any fruit for that matter, is more nutrient dense than cola beverages.

Moderate Sugar and Fat Intakes Moderation in diet planning refers to control of food constituents that are undesirable in excess—fat, sugar, and salt. Since fat and sugar add kcalories to foods, moderation in their use automatically helps with kcalorie control, too. Consider the example of the cheese and the milk once again. The nonfat milk not only offers the same amount of calcium at a lower food energy cost, but it also contains far less fat than the cheese. The cola and watermelon shown in the margin are another example: the cola contains only sugar, whereas the watermelon delivers many nutrients. People who exercise moderation in their sugar intakes will choose watermelon over cola and will meet their daily nutrient needs using fewer total kcalories. It all ties together: the most nutrient-dense foods are the best choices for the sake of both kcalorie control and moderation.

Moderate Salt Intakes Controlling salt intake might seem to require another approach: salt provides no kcalories, so added salt doesn't reduce the nutrient density of foods. Still, choosing nutrient-dense, low-fat, low-sugar foods does help keep your salt intake down. Why? The reason is that manufacturers usually add all three—salt, sugar, and fat—together when they dress up foods to make them tasty. Thus pursuing nutrient density helps keep your salt intake moderate. This recommendation may seem to be suggesting that you seek out mostly *unprocessed* foods. That is true in the sense that additions of sugar, salt, and fat are forms of processing. But other forms of food processing are beneficial, so wait until you've learned more about processing from Chapter 11 before attempting to generalize.

variety (dietary): using different foods to obtain the same nutrients on different occasions.

Variety Your diet can have all of the characteristics just described but still lack variety if you eat the same foods day after day. Vary your choices within each class of foods from day to day, for at least two reasons. First, different foods in the same group contain different arrays of nutrients. Among the fruits, for example, strawberries are especially rich in vitamin C, while peaches are rich in vitamin A. Thus variety helps ensure adequacy. Second, no food is guaranteed entirely free of constituents that in excess could harm you. (Contamination of foods is discussed in Chapter 11). By choosing strawberries today, peaches tomorrow, and watermelon the day after, you ensure that your total diet will have diluted concentrations of any contaminants that may be present in the foods available to you.

These diet-planning principles offer a framework of excellence to strive for in planning diets; they are dietary ideals. To plan a diet that achieves these ideals, the planner needs knowledge and skill. It helps to know what kinds of foods offer which nutrients and how many daily servings of the different foods are recommended.

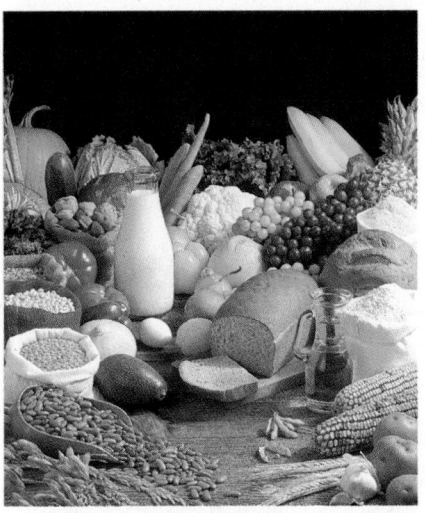

Variety helps to ensure an adequate and balanced diet.

Food Group Plans

About 40 vitamins and minerals are needed altogether. Each nutrient has its own unique pattern of distribution in foods. Although working all the nutrients into the meals you eat might seem quite a challenge, people all over the world obtain fine nutrition from an astonishing variety of diets.

Food Groups For many people, whether they know it or not, food group plans, such as the Four Food Group Plan they learned in school or the new Daily Food Guide, serve as the basis for planning adequate, balanced diets. Food group plans sort foods into clusters that make the same key nutrient contributions. For example, cheese and yogurt fall within the milk group because each is notable for calcium, riboflavin, and protein, as well as small amounts of other nutrients. Legumes are included in the meat, fish, and poultry group because these foods are notable for their protein, phosphorus, vitamin B_6, iron, and zinc.

Four Food Group Plan: the original and widely taught eating plan, developed to ensure dietary adequacy.

Daily Food Guide: a new plan for ensuring dietary adequacy that offers five categories of foods to choose from. (It treats vegetables and fruits as two separate groups.)

Miscellaneous Foods Food group plans exclude some foods from the main clusters because they make no notable nutrient contributions to people's intakes. These foods, called "miscellaneous" foods, are allowed in diet planning only as extras in small quantities once basic nutrient needs have been met by nutritious foods. Examples of miscellaneous foods are soft drinks, jams, salad dressings, and butter.

The Daily Food Guide Figure 1–3 presents the Daily Food Guide and includes the most notable nutrients within each food group, the number of servings recommended, the serving sizes, and the foods within each group categorized by nutrient density. Figure 1–3 also includes the Food Guide Pyramid, which presents the Daily Food Guide in pictorial form. The pyramid shape, with grains at the base, is designed to convey the idea that people should eat more grain foods than anything else—grains form the foundation of a sound diet. Fruits and vegetables share the next level of the pyramid, indicating that they, too, are prominent in the structure of a sound diet. Meats and milk are dense in protein and other nutrients, but can also contribute fat and kcalories. Their location just below the pyra-

Figure 1–3
The Daily Food Guide

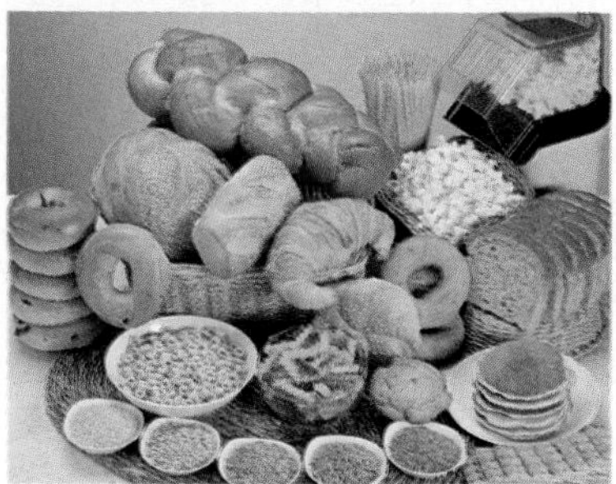

Breads, Cereals, and Other Grain Products

These foods are notable for their contributions of complex carbohydrates, riboflavin, thiamin, niacin, iron, protein, magnesium, and fiber.

6 to 11 servings per day.

Serving = 1 slice bread; 1/2 c cooked cereal, rice, or pasta; 1 oz ready-to-eat cereal; 1/2 bun, bagel, or English muffin; 1 small roll, biscuit, or muffin; 3 to 4 small or 2 large crackers.

◆ Whole grains (wheat, oats, barley, millet, rye, bulgur), enriched breads, rolls, tortillas, cereals, bagels, rice, pastas (macaroni, spaghetti), air-popped corn.

◆ Pancakes, muffins, cornbread, crackers, low-fat cookies, biscuits, presweetened cereals.

◆ Croissants, fried rice, granola.

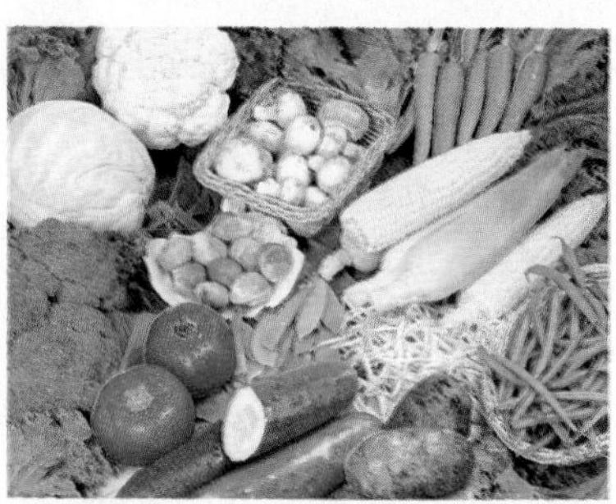

Vegetables

These foods are notable for their contributions of vitamin A, vitamin C, folate, potassium, magnesium, and fiber, and for their lack of fat and cholesterol.

3 to 5 servings per day (use dark green, leafy vegetables and legumes several times a week).

Serving = 1/2 c cooked or raw vegetables; 1 c leafy raw vegetables; 1/2 c cooked legumes; 3/4 c vegetable juice.

◆ Bean sprouts, broccoli, brussels sprouts, cabbage, carrots, cauliflower, cucumbers, green beans, green peas, leafy greens (spinach, mustard, and collard greens), legumes, lettuce, mushrooms, tomatoes, winter squash.

◆ Corn, potatoes, sweet potatoes.

◆ Avocados, french fries, olives, tempura vegetables.

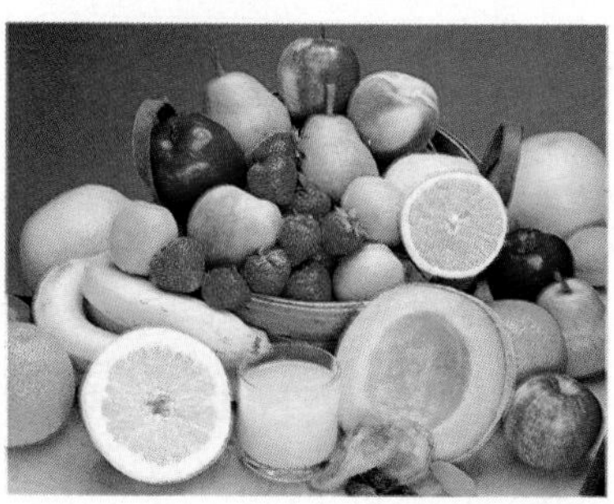

Fruits

These foods are notable for their contributions of vitamin A, vitamin C, potassium, and fiber, and for their lack of sodium, fat, and cholesterol.

2 to 4 servings per day.

Serving = typical portion (such as 1 medium apple, banana, or orange, 1/2 grapefruit, 1 melon wedge); 3/4 c juice; 1/2 c berries; 1/2 c diced, cooked, or canned fruit; 1/4 c dried fruit.

◆ Apricots, cantaloupe, grapefruit, oranges, orange juice, peaches, strawberries, apples, bananas, pears.

◆ Canned fruit.

◆ Dried fruit, coconut.

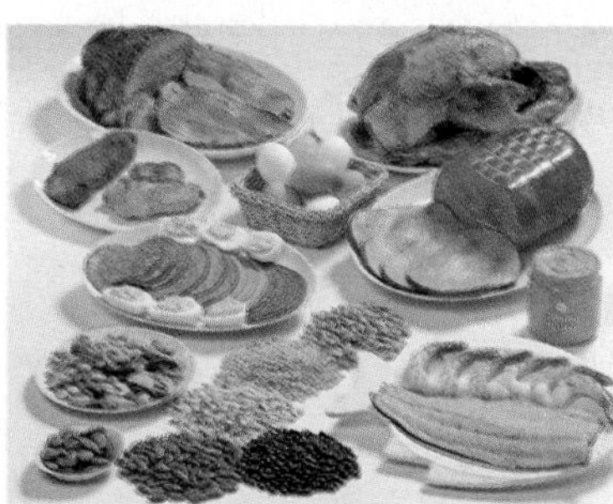

Meat, Poultry, Fish, and Alternates

These foods are notable for their contributions of protein, phosphorus, vitamin B_6, vitamin B_{12}, zinc, magnesium, iron, niacin, and thiamin.

2 to 3 servings per day.

Servings = 2 to 3 oz lean, cooked meat, poultry, or fish (total 5 to 7 oz per day); count 1 egg, 1/2 c cooked legumes, or 2 tbs peanut butter as 1 oz meat (or about 1/3 serving).

◆ Poultry, fish, lean meat (beef, lamb, pork, veal), legumes, egg whites.

◆ Fat-trimmed beef, lamb, pork; refried beans; egg yolks, tofu, tempeh.

◆ Hot dogs, luncheon meats, peanut butter, nuts, sausage, bacon, fried fish or poultry, duck.

Key:

◆ Foods generally highest in nutrient density (good first choice).

◆ Foods moderate in nutrient density (reasonable second choice).

◆ Foods lowest in nutrition density (limit selections).

Milk, Cheese, and Yogurt

These foods are notable for their contributions of calcium, riboflavin, protein, vitamin B_{12}, and, when fortified, vitamin D and vitamin A.

2 servings per day.

3 servings per day for teenagers and young adults, pregnant/lactating women, women past menopause.

4 servings per day for pregnant/lactating teenagers.

Serving = 1 c milk or yogurt; 2 oz process cheese food; 1 1/2 oz cheese.

♦ Nonfat and 1% low-fat milk (and nonfat products such as buttermilk, cottage cheese, cheese, yogurt); fortified soy milk.

♦ 2% low-fat milk (and low-fat products such as yogurt, cheese, cottage cheese); sherbet; ice milk.

♦ Whole milk (and whole-milk products such as cheese, yogurt, cottage cheese); cream; sour cream; cream cheese; custard; milkshakes; pudding; ice cream.

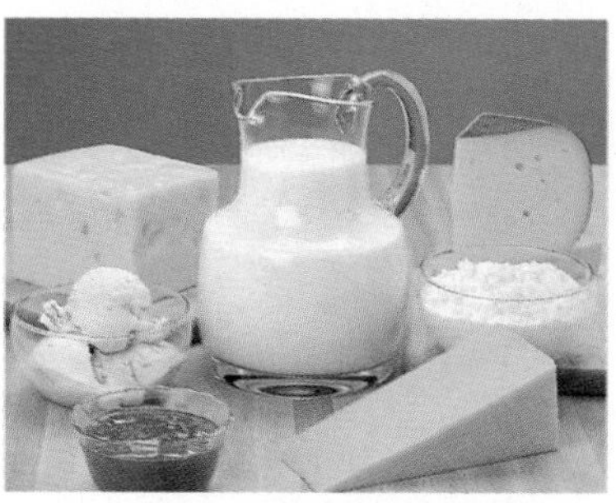

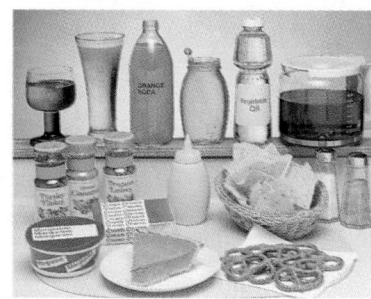

Miscellaneous Group

These foods are notable for their contributions of sugar, fat, salt, alcohol, and food energy. These foods are not in the pattern because they provide few nutrients. Note that some of the following items could be placed in more than one group or in a combination group. For example, potato chips are high in both salt and fat; doughnuts are high in both sugar and fat.

♦ Miscellaneous foods, not high in kcalories, include spices, herbs, coffee, tea, and diet soft drinks.

♦ Foods high in fat include margarine, salad dressings, oils, mayonnaise, cream, cream cheese, butter, gravy, and sauces.

♦ Foods high in salt include potato chips, corn chips, pretzels, pickles, olives, bouillon, prepared mustard, soy sauce, steak sauce, salt, and seasoned salt.

♦ Foods high in sugar include cake, pie, cookies, doughnuts, sweet rolls, candy, soft drinks, fruit drinks, jelly, syrup, gelatin, desserts, sugar, and honey.

♦ Alcoholic beverages include wine, beer, and liquor.

Note: Serve children at least the lower number of servings from each group, but in smaller amounts (for example, 1/4 to 1/3 cup rice). Children should receive the equivalent of 2 cups of milk each day, but again in smaller quantities per serving (for example: 4 half-cup portions). Pregnant women may require additional servings of fruits, vegetables, meats, and breads to meet their higher needs for energy, vitamins, and minerals.

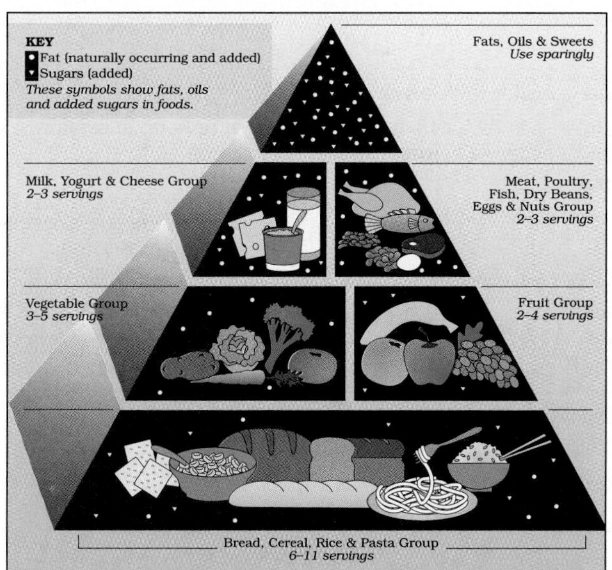

Food Guide Pyramid
A Guide to Daily Food Choices

The breadth of the base shows that grains (breads, cereals, rice, and pasta) deserve most emphasis in the diet. The tip is smallest: use fats, oils, and sweets sparingly.

mid's apex implies that servings must be limited. Fats, oils, and sweets occupy only a tiny triangle at the pyramid's apex, indicating they should be used sparingly.

Different Energy Intakes Possible People can control their food energy intakes while using the Daily Food Guide. The foods color-coded with green boxes are the highest in nutrient density; they contribute the most nutrients for the fewest kcalories. Those with yellow boxes are moderate in nutrient density; and those with red boxes are lowest in nutrient density. People who choose the smallest recommended number of servings, choose them all from the green-coded foods, and strictly limit foods from the miscellaneous group will obtain the needed nutrients at an energy intake of about 1600 kcalories. People who choose more servings or less nutrient-dense foods can easily boost their energy intakes. Depending on their energy needs, such choices might add to their body weight.

Flexible Food Choices The beauty of the Daily Food Guide is that it is simple and easy to learn. It may appear rigid, but it actually offers great flexibility once its intent is understood. For example, you can substitute cheese for milk because both supply the same nutrients (protein, calcium, and riboflavin) in about the same amounts. If you need to limit kcalories, choose nonfat milk; if you need to add kcalories, choose cheese. Legumes are alternative choices for meats, so vegetarians can adapt the pattern by using legumes in place of meat selections (see Table 1–3).

Table 1–3
Daily Food Guide for Vegetarians

FOOD GROUP	SUGGESTED DAILY SERVINGS	SERVING SIZES
Breads, cereals, and other grain products	6 or more	1 slice bread ½ bun, bagel, or English muffin ½ c cooked cereal, rice, or pasta 1 oz dry cereal
Vegetables	4 or more[a]	½ c cooked or 1 c raw
Fruits	3 or more	1 piece fresh fruit ¾ c fruit juice ½ c canned or cooked fruit
Legumes and other meat alternates	2 to 3	½ c cooked beans 4 oz tofu or tempeh 8 oz soy milk 2 tbs nuts or seeds (these tend to be high in fat, so use sparingly) 1 egg or 2 egg whites
Milk and milk products	2 to 3 servings[b]	1 c low-fat or nonfat milk 1 c low-fat or nonfat yogurt 1½ oz low-fat cheese

[a] Include 1 cup of dark green vegetables daily to help meet iron requirements.
[b] People who do not use milk or milk products: use soy milk fortified with calcium and vitamin B_{12}.

Source: Adapted with permission from The position of The American Dietetic Association: Vegetarian diets, *Journal of the American Dietetic Association* 93 (1993): 1318.

Planning Vegetarian Diets Making vegetarian diets adequate and balanced is not difficult, but does require skill. People adopt vegetarian diets for a variety of religious, ethical, social, or economic reasons, but to the diet planner all vegetarian diets present similar challenges. A few nutrients require careful attention if a vegetarian diet is to offer nutrition and health benefits to adults.[5] Nutrition in Practice 4 shows how to make vegetarian diets nutritious.

vegetarian diets: a general term used to describe diets that exclude meat, poultry, fish, or other animal-derived foods. The two main categories are *lacto-ovo vegetarian* and *vegan* diets.

lacto-ovo vegetarian diets: diets that include milk, cheese, and eggs (animal products) but exclude meat, fish, and poultry (animal flesh).

vegan diets: diets that exclude all animal products and include only plant foods; also known as **strict vegetarian diets.**

Nutrition Surveys

Researchers use nutrition surveys to determine which foods people are eating and, after calculating the nutrients in these foods, to assess people's nutritional health. One of the first nutrition surveys, taken before World War II, suggested that up to a third of the U.S. population might be eating poorly. Programs to correct nutrition problems have been evolving ever since.

U.S. Malnutrition During the 1970s, public awareness of the nutrition status of U.S. citizens reached a new high. The Senate's Poverty Subcommittee and the Select Committee on Nutrition and Human Needs held hearings, widely broadcast on national television, where witnesses described the plight of poor families unable to feed their children. Hunger in the United States became a controversial political issue and remains one today—some say the findings are exaggerated while others consider them a scandal and a national disgrace. The findings that originally generated the controversy arose from the Ten-State Survey conducted from 1968 to 1970. Other important nutrition surveys include the ongoing Health and Nutrition Examination Surveys (HANES) and the Nationwide Food Consumption Surveys (NFCS). These surveys have tended to confirm the impression that low-income groups in this country suffer from hunger and malnutrition. Nutrition in Practice 13 examines this problem more closely.

malnutrition: any condition caused by deficient or excess energy or nutrient intake or by an imbalance of nutrients. Nutrient or energy deficiencies are forms of *undernutrition;* nutrient or energy excesses are forms of *overnutrition.*

U.S. Obesity The most recent Nationwide Food Consumption Survey was conducted in 1987 and 1988.[6] One of its major conclusions was that many people are overweight and obese, not so much because they overeat, but because they are extraordinarily inactive. Inactivity makes it hard, especially for women, to eat the foods available, stay within the energy allowance that will maintain appropriate weight, and still meet needs for all nutrients. Indeed, most surveys that have assessed the nutrition status of families in the United States have revealed that obtaining the proper nutrients and sufficient physical activity to maintain weight while not overconsuming food energy are real concerns. Thus both undernutrition and overnutrition are problems in our society. In the interest of optimal health, everyone needs to choose foods intelligently.

Nutrition Labeling

Today consumers know more about the links between diet and disease than they ever did in the past, and they are demanding still more information on disease prevention.[7] Surveys show that many people rely on food labels to tell them which substances to avoid for health reasons and to provide them with information about nutrition.[8] The Nutrition Labeling and Education Act of 1990 revised the requirements for label information extensively to better accommodate consumers' nutrition and health needs. Most food labels must conform with all the new requirements.[9] Exceptions include plain coffee, tea, spices, and other foods contributing few nutrients; foods produced by small businesses; and foods prepared and sold in the same establishment.*

Information on Food Labels According to law, every food label must state the following:

- The common or usual name of the product.
- The name and address of the manufacturer, packer, or distributor.
- The net contents in terms of weight, measure, or count.

Then, the label must list in ordinary language the following:

- The ingredients, in descending order of predominance by weight.

In the past, a few foods such as mayonnaise and ice cream were exempt from the requirement to list their ingredients. Instead, manufacturers were held to strict standards called standards of identity that described the exact proportions of ingredients allowed in the products. Now all foods, including those with standards of identity, must list their ingredients on their labels.[10]

All labels must state at least this much. Even if they say no more, you can learn a lot about the nutritional value of a product from the ingredient list. Consider the following products:

- An orange powder that contains "sugar, citric acid, orange flavor. . . ."
- A juice that contains "water, tomato concentrate, concentrated juices of carrots, celery . . . ."

Knowing that the first ingredient named predominates by weight, you can tell that the first product is mostly sugar and that the second is mostly vegetable juice.

Information on Fresh Foods Voluntary labeling or point-of-purchase nutrition information is encouraged for the 20 most frequently eaten fresh fruits and vegetables.[11] Grocers often post nutrition-information placards or pamphlets near where the foods are on display.

For raw fish and for raw, single-ingredient meat and poultry products, producers who choose to provide nutrition information on labels must adhere to the requirements of the mandatory program. In other words, if a package of raw chicken breast carries a food label, it must provide the information required on all other food labels.

---

* Restaurants making "heart healthy" claims for menu items may be required to provide nutrient information for consumers.

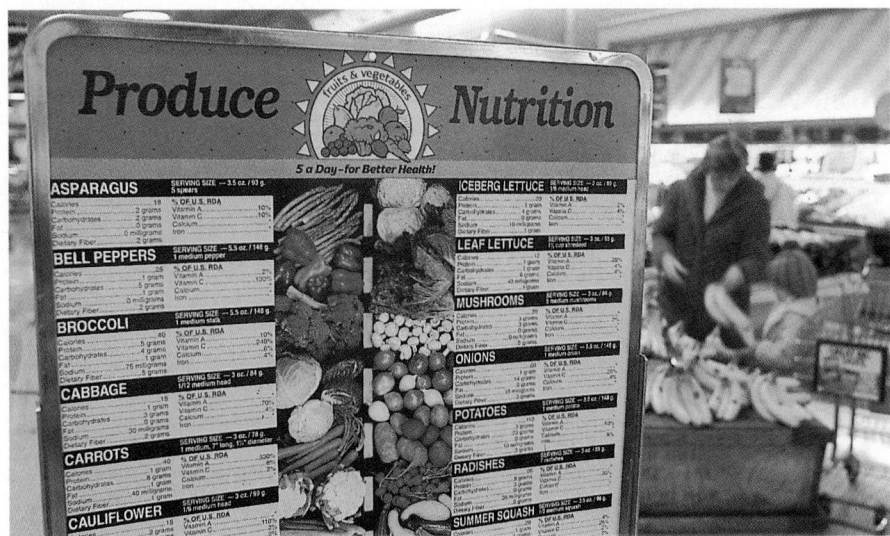

Posters in the produce department present nutrition information for nonpackaged items such as raw fruits and vegetables.

The New Nutrition Label To distinguish between a new label and an old one, look for the words "Nutrition Facts" on the new label's information panel. The old label says "Nutrition Information." The "Nutrition Facts" panel must provide:

- Standard serving size expressed in both common household and metric measures to allow comparison with other foods in the same category.
- Number of servings or portions per container.
- Total food energy (kcalories) per serving.
- Fat (grams) per serving with breakdown for saturated fat (grams) and cholesterol (milligrams).
- Sodium (milligrams) per serving.
- Total carbohydrate (grams) per serving.
- Fiber and sugars (grams) per serving.
- Total protein (grams) per serving.

In addition, for each of the nutrients just named plus vitamin A, vitamin C, calcium, and iron, amounts in a serving of the food must be expressed as percentages of the Daily Values for a person who requires 2000 kcalories per day.*

The Daily Values on Labels The Daily Values (inside front cover, right side) are a set of nutrient standards designed strictly for use on food labels. In creating Daily Values, the Food and Drug Administration (FDA) first established two sets of reference values. The first set, the Reference Daily Intakes (RDI), are for protein, vitamins, and minerals and reflect the 1968 RDA values for an adult with high nutrient needs. They represent

* The percent Daily Value for protein is not mandatory on all labels, but is required whenever a food makes a protein claim or is intended for consumption by children under four years old.[12]

Glossary of Label Terms

Daily Values: reference values developed by the FDA specifically for food labels. The Daily Values represent two sets of standards: Daily Reference Values (DRV) and Reference Daily Intakes (RDI).

Daily Reference Values (DRV): food labeling values for nutrients and food components (such as fat and fiber) that have important relationships with health but do not have an RDA value. The DRV derive from the NRC report on *Diet and Health.*

Reference Daily Intakes (RDI): food labeling values for protein, vitamins, and minerals; previously known as the U.S. RDA.

intakes to achieve; for example, the RDI for zinc is 15 milligrams—an amount to aim for daily. The RDI were previously called the U.S. RDA.*

The second set of reference values established by the FDA for labels is the Daily Reference Values (DRV). The DRV serve as food labeling values for nutrients and food components, such as fat and fiber, that do not have an established RDA but nevertheless have important relationships with health. The DRV are based on the National Research Council's *Diet and Health* recommendations. The accompanying glossary defines the terms used in nutrition labeling.

Labels on Different-Sized Packages A package's size helps determine how much information it must deliver. Large labels of 40 or more square inches must include all the information listed earlier and must also list the Daily Values for two people: one who consumes 2000 kcalories per day, and one who consumes 2500 kcalories per day. The label may also provide a reminder that a gram of carbohydrate or protein supplies 4 kcalories and that a gram of fat supplies 9 kcalories. The side panel of the box of cereal in Figure 1–4 provides all this information. Packages with labels smaller than 40 square inches, such as tuna cans, may omit the second set of Daily Values, but must deliver the other information listed earlier. The label on the can of chicken in Figure 1–5 shows a condensed label format. Tiny packages, such as a roll of mints, may provide only a phone number for consumers to call and obtain information.

One more factor helps to determine requirements for a label—the nutrients in the food. A food that contains insignificant amounts of more than half of the nutrients listed above may bear a simplified label that provides information only on the nutrients the food does contain.

Health Claims on Labels The FDA has set forth strict guidelines pertaining to claims about health on labels. Only foods that live up to their implied connection to health are permitted by law to bear health

* The U.S. RDA have been the labeling standard since 1975. Eventually, the U.S. RDA values may be replaced with a set that reflects more current RDA standards.

Table 1–4 *(continued)*

Low fat: containing 3 g or less fat per serving.

Low saturated fat: containing 1 g or less saturated fat per serving.

Percent fat free: may be used only if the product meets the definition of *low fat* or *fat-free*. Requires disclosure of grams fat per 100 g food.

Reduced or **less saturated fat:** containing 25% or less of the saturated fat in the comparison food *and* reduced by more than 1 g per serving.

Saturated fat free: containing less than 0.5 g of saturated fat and less than 0.5 g of *trans*-fatty acids.

OTHER TERMS

Free, without, no, zero: containing no amount or a trivial amount. *Calorie-free* means containing fewer than 5 kcalories per serving; *sugar-free* or *fat-free* means containing less than half a gram per serving.

Fresh: raw, unprocessed or minimally processed (blanched or irradiated) with no added preservatives.

Good source: provides 10 to 19% of the Daily Value of a given nutrient per serving.

High: Provides 20% or more of the Daily Value per serving.

Imitation food: this term must be used to describe a food intended to replace a standard food, if the replacement food lacks one or more nutrients provided by the original food. For example, imitation cheese for pizza lacks the calcium of real mozzarella cheese.

Less, fewer: provides 25% less of a nutrient or kcalories than a reference food. This may occur naturally or as a result of altering the food. For example, pretzels, which are usually low in fat, can claim to provide less fat than potato chips, a comparable food.

Light: this descriptor has three meanings on labels:

- A serving provides one-third fewer kcalories or half the fat of the regular product.
- A serving of a low-kcalorie, low-fat food provides half the sodium normally present.
- The product is light in color and texture; the label must make this intent clear, as in "light brown sugar."

More: contains at least 10% more of the Daily Value for a given nutrient than a comparable food. The nutrient may be added or may occur naturally.

Reduced: altered to provide 25% less per serving of something such as kcalories, fat, or sugar as compared to a "regular" product.

SODIUM TERMS

Low-sodium: contains 140 mg or less sodium per serving.

Very-low sodium: contains 35 mg or less sodium per serving.

[a]The word *lean* as part of the brand name (as in "Lean Supreme") indicates that the product contains fewer than 10 grams of fat per serving. *Lean* ground beef can contain up to 22.5 percent fat by weight.

Source: The new food label, *FDA Backgrounder,* 10 December 1992; Nutrition labeling of meat and poultry products, *FSIS Backgrounder,* January 1993.

Seven claims linking nutrients and food constituents to disease states are allowable under FDA guidelines. A statement on a label is allowed to refer to the following:

1. Calcium and osteoporosis. Foods that make this claim must be high in calcium.
2. Sodium and hypertension (high blood pressure). The food must be low in sodium.
3. Dietary fat and cancer. The food must be low in fat.
4. Dietary saturated fat, dietary cholesterol, and coronary heart disease. The food must be low in saturated fat, cholesterol, and fat.
5. Fiber-containing grain products, fruits, vegetables, and cancer. The food must be low in fat, and without added fiber, it must be a good source of dietary fiber.
6. Fruits, vegetables, and grain products that contain fiber, particularly soluble fiber, and risk of coronary heart disease. The food must be low in saturated fat, fat, and cholesterol. It must also contain at least 0.6 grams of soluble fiber (explained in Chapter 2) per serving.
7. Fruits and vegetables and cancer. The food must be low in fat, and without added nutrients, it must be a good source of fiber, vitamin A, or vitamin C.

These claims are allowed on food labels because they are well supported by the available scientific evidence. This means that whole milk, even though it is high in calcium, may not make a claim about osteoporosis because it contains too much saturated fat to qualify. Low-fat and nonfat milks, however, do qualify to bear the calcium and osteoporosis claim.

Those who design food labels must proceed carefully. For example, use of the word "healthy" in a name such as "Healthy Start" or the use of a heart-shaped logo may imply that a food is health promoting. Foods bearing such words or logos must not exceed limits set for fat, saturated fat, cholesterol, and sodium contents.

Consumers may wonder whether, if they eat only "healthy" foods, they are reducing their health risks. They may be, and that is all that a label is allowed to say: that a substance "may" or "might" reduce disease risks. This wording is tentative because science is still accumulating evidence concerning the roles of diet in disease. A claim must also state that the development of a disease rests on many factors. A permissible health claim reads like this: "Development of heart disease depends on many factors. A healthful diet low in saturated fat and cholesterol may lower blood cholesterol levels and may reduce the risk of heart disease." Health claims on labels are so carefully controlled that they can be an asset to consumers who would rather not worry about grams, percentages, and other mathematical stumbling blocks as they shop for foods.

The new food labels were designed to enhance consumers' knowledge about the foods they eat and how constituents in those foods impact health and the risk of disease. Interested consumers will find the new food labels fascinating reading.

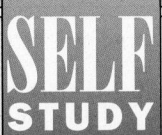

How Balanced Is Your Diet?

Our purpose in providing these exercises is to encourage you to study your own diet. Your reaction to them may be mixed. They will slow you down, and filling out all the forms can be tedious. Like your checkbook, they have to be done carefully, with frequent checking of arithmetic and clear handwriting so that they will be accurate and meaningful.

The benefits, however, may well outweigh the drawbacks. Most students who do these activities with thoughtful attention report that unlike a checkbook, they are intriguing, informative, and often reassuring. They are also rewarding—in direct proportion to your accuracy. They not only teach you about yourself but enable you to assess clients' diets once you are working in a health profession.

In this first Self-Study, make a record of your typical food intake, and analyze it for the nutrients it contains. You will use the results over and over again in succeeding Self-Studies, so invest time and effort now to achieve maximum accuracy. You can undertake this analysis before you have learned about the nutrients; having the results in front of you as you work will help make the reading meaningful.

1. Use three copies of Form 1, and record on them all the foods you eat for a three-day period. If, like most people, you eat differently on weekdays than on weekends, then you should probably record for two weekdays and one weekend day to get a true average, or record your food intake for a week. You will learn the most from these Self-Studies if you select days that are truly typical of your food intake and physical activity.

As you record each food, make careful note of the measure. Estimate the amount of the nearest ounce, quarter cup, tablespoon, or other common measure. In guessing at the sizes of meat portions, it helps to know that a piece of meat the size of the palm of your hand weighs about 3 or 4 ounces. If you are unable to estimate serving sizes in cups, tablespoons, or teaspoons, try measuring out servings in those proportions to see how they look. It also helps to know that a slice of cheese (like sliced American cheese) or a 1½-inch cube of cheese weighs about 1 ounce.

You may have to break down mixed dishes to their ingredients. Many mixed dishes, however, including soups, are listed in the miscellaneous section at the end of Appendix A. Other mixtures are simple to analyze. A ham and cheese sandwich, for example, can be listed as 2 slices of bread, 1 tablespoon of mayonnaise, 2 ounces of ham, 1 ounce of cheese, and so on. If you can't identify all the ingredients, just estimate the amounts of the major ones, like the beef, tomatoes, and potatoes in a beef-vegetable soup.

You will, of course, make errors in estimating amounts. In calculations of this kind, errors of up to 20 percent are expected and tolerated. Still, your rough approximation will enable you to compare your nutrient intakes with the recommended ones.

Do not record any nutrient supplements you take. It is important for you to discover whether your food choices alone deliver the nutrients you need. If they don't, you'll have the first clues to a solution, perhaps one that involves better food choices rather than supplements.

2. Using either a computer diet analysis program or Appendix A, calculate for each day your total intakes of kcalories, protein, fat, carbohydrate, calcium, iron, zinc, vitamin A, thiamin, riboflavin, niacin, folate, and vitamin C.

If a packaged food you have eaten does not appear in Appendix A, read the label on the package. If you eat a packaged food in which the nutrient amounts are listed on the label as "percent Daily Values," use the table on the inside front

(continued)

Self-Study (continued)

Form 1
Nutrient Intakes (Use One Form for Each Day)

Food	Approximate Measure or Weight	Energy[a] (kcal)	Prot[a] (g)	Carb[a] (g)	Fiber[a] (g)	Fat[a] (g)	Fat Breakdown			Chol[a] (mg)	Calcium[a] (mg)	Iron[b] (mg)	Magn[b] (mg)	Phos[b] (mg)	Sodium[b] (mg)	Zinc[b] (mg)	Vit A[a] (mg)	Thia[b] (RE)	Ribo[b] (mg)	Niac[b] (mg)	B_{12}[b] (mg)	Fol[a] (µg)	Vit C[b] (mg)
							Sat (g)	Mono (g)	Poly (g)														
Totals																							

[a] Compute these values to the nearest whole number..
[b] Compute these values to two decimal places.

Self-Study (continued)

cover of the text to convert to grams, milligrams, micrograms, or retinol equivalents. Suppose a food label states that a serving contains 25 percent of the Daily Value for iron, for example. The table shows that the Daily Value for iron is 18 milligrams. The food portion, therefore, contributes 25 percent of 18 milligrams, or 4.5 milligrams of iron.

For foods you eat in restaurants, at friends' houses, or elsewhere, ask the composition or use your ingenuity and make a guess. Use the most similar food you can find as a guide. For example, if you ate smoked cod (which is not listed in Appendix A), you would not be far off in using the values for smoked halibut. If you ate cream of celery soup, you might substitute the values for cream of mushroom soup.

Be careful in recording the nutrient amounts in odd-sized portions. For example, if you use 1/4 cup of milk, you will have to look up the nutrient values for a cup of milk and divide each one by 4. Also note the units in which the nutrients are measured:

- Energy is measured in kcalories (kcal).
- Protein, fat, carbohydrate, and fiber are measured in grams (g).
- Cholesterol, calcium, iron, magnesium, phosphorus, potassium, sodium, zinc, thiamin, riboflavin, niacin, vitamin B_6, and vitamin C are measured in milligrams (mg)—thousandths of a gram (0.001 g).
- Folate is measured in micrograms (µg)—thousandths of a milligram or millionths of a gram (0.001 mg or 0.000001 g). Thus 800 mg calcium is the same as 0.8 g calcium, and 400 µg folate is the same as 0.4 mg folate. Be sure to convert all calcium amounts to milligrams and all folate amounts to micrograms before adding them together and comparing them with standards.
- Vitamin A can be measured in international units (IU) or retinol equivalents (RE). Appendix A lists vitamin A in RE to ease comparison with the recommended intake, which is also in RE. If you eat a packaged food in which vitamin A is listed in IU on the label, be sure to convert to RE before calculating. (For more details, see Chapter 7.)

3. Now total the amount of each nutrient you've consumed for each day, and transfer your totals to Form 2. Form 2 provides a convenient means of deriving an average intake for each nutrient.
4. As a final step, transfer your average intakes to Form 3 for future reference. For comparison, enter the intakes recommended for a person of your age and sex, using either the RDA (on the inside front cover of the text) or the Recommended Nutrient Intakes for Canadians (in Appendix B), whichever you prefer. For cholesterol, carbohydrate, and fiber, use the Daily Values (inside front cover, right).

Suspend judgment about the adequacy of your intakes for the moment. You have much to learn about your individuality, the nutrients, and the recommendations before you can reach any reasonable conclusions.

5. Now, check your overall food intake for balance. You can get an indication of whether you are choosing a balanced selection of foods by using the Daily Food Selection Scorecard (Form 4—one copy for each day). How does your diet score by these criteria?
6. Another way to check your balance is to evaluate your diet using the guideline that about 58 percent of your kcalories should come from carbohydrate, about 12 percent from protein, and not more than 30 percent from fat. Use Form 5 to calculate these percentages. What percentage of the food energy you consume comes from protein? ___ percent. Fat? ___ percent. Carbohydrate? ___ percent. Is your diet balanced using these criteria?

As soon as you have perfected these skills on yourself, you can use them on clients to their benefit. In fact, dietitians use a similar approach in assessing a client's nutrient intake (see Chapter 12).

(continued)

Self-Study (continued)

Form 2
Average Daily Energy and Nutrient Intakes

Day	Energy (kcal)	Prot (g)	Carb (g)	Fiber (g)	Fat (g)	Fat Breakdown			Chol (mg)	Calcium (mg)	Iron (mg)	Magn (mg)	Phos (mg)	Sodium (mg)	Zinc (mg)	Vit A (mg)	Thia (RE)	Ribo (mg)	Niac (mg)	B_{12} (mg)	Fol (µg)	Vit C (mg)
						Sat (g)	Mono (g)	Poly (g)														
1																						
2																						
3																						
Total																						
Average daily intake (divide total by 3)																						

Form 3
Comparison with a Standard Intake

Day	Energy (kcal)	Prot (g)	Carb (g)	Fiber (g)	Fat (g)	Fat Breakdown			Chol (mg)	Calcium (mg)	Iron (mg)	Magn (mg)	Phos (mg)	Sodium (mg)	Zinc (mg)	Vit A (mg)	Thia (RE)	Ribo (mg)	Niac (mg)	B_{12} (mg)	Fol (µg)	Vit C (mg)
						Sat (g)	Mono (g)	Poly (g)														
Average daily intake (from Form 2)																						
Standard[a]																						
Intake as percentage of standard[b]																						

[a] Use the RDA tables (inside front cover, left, and Appendix B) or the Canadian standards in Appendix B, or in the case of fat, fiber, and cholesterol, the Daily Values (inside front cover, right). Alternatively for energy, use your calculation from Self-Study 6.

[b] For example, if your intake was 50 g and the standard for a person your age and sex was 46 g, you consumed $(50 \div 46) \times 100$, or 109% of the standard.

Self-Study (continued)

Form 4
Food Selection Scorecard

Record your day's food intake on a separate piece of paper (or review your record from Form 1). Assign each food you ate to its appropriate group and estimate the number of servings you ate (Figure 1-3 presents the foods found within each food group and serving sizes) Record the number of servings for each group in column 2. Then multiply that number by the points per serving to determine your score. You can earn up to 20 points for each of the five food groups.

FOOD GROUP AND RECOMMENDED INTAKE	NUMBER OF SERVINGS EATEN	YOUR SCORE
Breads and Cereals: 6 or more servings		
1 serving = 3.5 points	× 3.5 =	
Subtotal (no more than 20 points allowed)		
Vegetables: 3 or more servings		
1 serving vitamin A-rich dark green or deep yellow-orange vegetable (such as spinach, broccoli, carrots, squash = 10 points (no more than 10 points allowed—count additional servings as other vegetables below)	× 10 =	
1 serving other vegetables = 5 points	× 5 =	
Subtotal (no more than 20 points allowed)		
Fruits: 2 or more servings		
1 serving vitamin C-rich fruits (such as oranges, strawberries, watermelon) = 10 points (no more than 10 points allowed—count additional servings as other fruits below)	× 10 =	
1 serving other fruits = 10 points	× 10 =	
Subtotal (no more than 20 points allowed)		
Meats and Meat Alternates: 2 to 3 servings		
1 serving = 10 points	× 10 =	
Subtotal (no more than 20 points allowed		
Milk and Milk Products: 2 servings		
1 serving = 10 points	× 10 =	
Subtotal (no more than 20 points allowed)		
GRAND TOTAL (no more than 100 points allowed)		

The above foods are foundation foods. Additional foods are those that do not fit into any of the five food groups, but add flavor, interest, variety, and often kcalories. List additional foods:

(continued)

Self-Study (continued)

Form 5
Percentage of kCalories from Protein, Fat, and Carbohydrate

Average daily intakes from Form 2:

Protein: g/day × 4 kcal/g = (*P*)________ kcal/day.
Fat: g/day × 9 kcal/g = (*F*)________ kcal/day.
Carbohydrate: g/day × 4 kcal/g = (*C*)________ kcal/day.
Total kcal/day = (*T*)________ kcal/day.

Percentage of kcalories from protein: $\frac{(P)}{(T)} \times 100 =$ ________ % of total kcalories.

Percentage of kcalories from fat: $\frac{(F)}{(T)} \times 100 =$ ________ % of total kcalories.

Percentage of kcalories from carbohydrate: $\frac{(C)}{(T)} \times 100 =$ ________ % of total kcalories.

Note: The three percentages can total 99, 100, or 101, depending on the way figures were rounded off earlier.

If you used an alcoholic beverage, you have to add a line for kcalories from alcohol. To find out how many kcalories in the beverage were from alcohol, look the beverage up in Appendix A. Figure out how many kcalories were from carbohydrate (multiply carbohydrate grams times 4), fat (fat grams times 9), and protein (protein grams times 4). The remaining kcalories were from alcohol.

■ STUDY QUESTIONS ■

1. List five reasons why people choose the particular foods they do.
2. List the six classes of nutrients.
3. Name the energy-yielding nutrients.
4. Define the term *kcalorie.*
5. Describe how alcohol resembles nutrients, and then explain why it is, nevertheless, not considered a nutrient.
6. Explain the purpose of the RDA.
7. Identify the main purpose behind the dietary recommendations published in the United States.
8. List six diet-planning principles and explain the rationale for each.
9. Define the term *nutrient density* and explain why this concept is useful in diet planning.
10. Outline the Daily Food Guide and explain how it accomplishes the objectives of diet planning.
11. Describe a nutrition label. What can you learn from reading nutrition labels?

NUTRITION IN PRACTICE 1

Nutrition Professionals

With nutrition receiving so much attention in the popular press, it is easy to be overwhelmed with conflicting information. In fact, determining whether nutrition information is accurate may be one of your most challenging tasks. It should also be one of the most important, because nutrition affects both your professional and your personal life.

Everyone seems to be giving advice on nutrition. How can I tell whom to listen to?

Registered dietitians (R.D.'s) and nutrition professionals with advanced degrees (M.S., Ph.D.) are experts (see the accompanying glossary). These people are probably in the best position to answer your nutrition questions. On the other hand, "nutritionists" may be experts or quacks, depending on the state where they practice. Some states require people who use this title to meet strict standards; others do not, and a "nutritionist" may be any individual who claims a career connection with the nutrition field.

Other purveyors of nutrition information may also lack credentials. A health food store owner may be in the nutrition business simply because it is a lucrative market. Such a person may have a background in business or sales and no education in nutrition at all. Such a person is not qualified to provide nutrition information to customers. For accurate nutrition information, seek out a trained professional with a knowledge of nutrition—an expert in the field of dietetics.

What about other health care professionals?

All members of the health care team share responsibility for helping each client to achieve optimal health, but the registered dietitian (R.D.) remains the primary nutrition expert. Each of the other team members has a related specialty. Physicians, nurses, and dietetic technicians (D.T.R.'s) often assist dietitians in providing nutrition information and may help to administer direct nutrition care. Nurses play central roles in client care management and client relationships. Visiting nurses and home health care nurses may become intimately involved in clients' nutrition care at home, teaching them both theory and cooking techniques. Physical therapists can provide individualized exercise programs related to nutrition—for example, to help control obesity. Social workers may provide practical and emotional support.

What roles might these health professionals play in nutrition care?

Some of the responsibilities of the health care professional might be:

- Helping people understand why nutrition is important to them.
- Answering questions about food and diet.
- Explaining to clients how modified diets work.
- Collecting information about clients that may influence their nutrition health.

Glossary of Nutrition Experts

dietetic technician registered (D.T.R.): a professional who has earned an associate degree or higher; has completed a dietetic technician program approved by the American Dietetic Association (ADA); has passed a national registration exam; and assists in planning, implementing, and evaluating nutritional care.

dietetics: the practical application of nutrition, including the assessment of nutrition status, recommendation of appropriate diets, nutrition education, and the planning and serving of meals.

nutritionist: a person who specializes in the study of nutrition. Some nutritionists are registered dietitians, but others are self-described experts whose training may be minimal or nonexistent. Some states make the term meaningful by allowing it to apply only to people who have master's (M.S.) or doctoral (Ph.D.) degrees from institutions accredited to offer such degrees in nutrition or related fields.

registered dietitian (R.D.): a professional in dietetics with a bachelor's (B.S.) degree in nutrition or food science, a year's internship or the equivalent, and a passing score on the four-hour qualifying exam administered by the ADA or the Canadian Dietetic Association (CDA).

- Spotting clients at risk for poor nutrition status (see Chapters 12 and 13) and taking appropriate action.
- Recognizing when clients need more help with nutrition problems (in such cases, the problems should be referred to a dietitian or physician).

Health care professionals might routinely perform these nutrition-related tasks:

- Obtaining some information for diet histories.
- Weighing and measuring height.
- Feeding clients who cannot feed themselves.
- Recording what clients eat or drink.
- Observing clients' responses and reactions to foods.
- Helping clients mark menus.
- Monitoring weight changes.
- Monitoring food and drug interactions.
- Encouraging clients to eat.
- Assisting clients at home in planning their diets and managing their kitchen chores.
- Administering special feedings by tube (Chapter 22) or by vein (Chapter 23) for clients who cannot eat conventional foods.

As you can see, although the dietitian assumes the primary role as the nutrition expert on a health care team, other health care professionals play important roles in administering nutrition care.

■ NOTES ■

1. I. M. Parraga, Determinants of food consumption, *Journal of the American Dietetic Association* 90 (1990): 661–663.
2. C. Jackson, Today's food consumers: What they are looking for in a supermarket, *Cereal Foods World* 32 (1987): 417–419.
3. D. T. Farr, Consumer attitudes and the supermarket, *Cereal Foods World* 32 (1987): 413–415.
4. Diet, nutrition, and the prevention of chronic diseases: A report of the WHO Study Group on Diet, Nutrition, and Prevention of Noncommunicable Diseases, *Nutrition Reviews* 49 (1991): 291–301.
5. Position of the American Dietetic Association: Vegetarian diets, *Journal of the American Dietetic Association* 93 (1993): 1317-1319.
6. Federation of American Societies for Experimental Biology, Life Sciences Research Office, *Nutrition Monitoring in the United States: An Update Report on Nutrition Monitoring,* prepared for the U.S. Department of Health and Human Services (Washington, D.C.: Government Printing Office, 1989).
7. Parts of this discussion were adapted with permission from F. S. Sizer and E. N. Whitney, *Nutrition: Concepts and Controversies,* 6th ed. (St. Paul, Minn.: West Publishing Co., 1994).
8. U.S. Department of Health and Human Services, *A Consumer's Guide to Food Labels,* publication no. 88–2083 (Washington, D.C.: Government Printing Office, 1988); Food label importance, *FDA Consumer,* May 1990, p. 3.
9. J. E. Foulke, Cooking up the new food label, *FDA Consumer,* May 1993, pp. 33–38.
10. M. Segal, What's in a food? *FDA Consumer,* April 1993, pp. 14–18.
11. U.S. Department of Agriculture, Food Safety and Inspection Service, *FSIS Backgrounder,* January 1993, pp. 1–6.
12. E. C. Henley, Food and Drug Administration's proposed labeling rules for protein, *Journal of the American Dietetic Association* 92 (1992): 293–296.

2

Carbohydrates

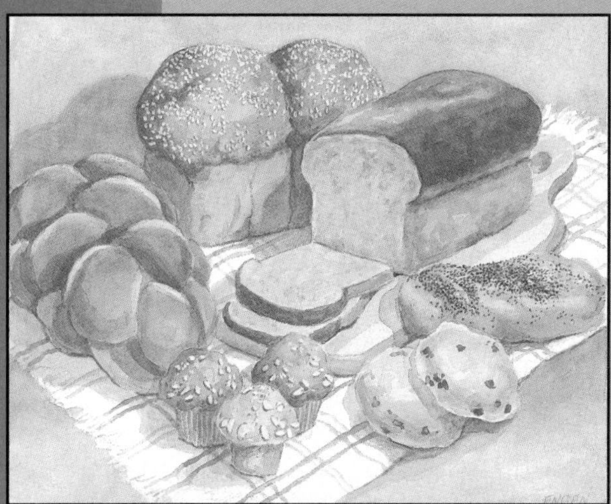

CONTENTS

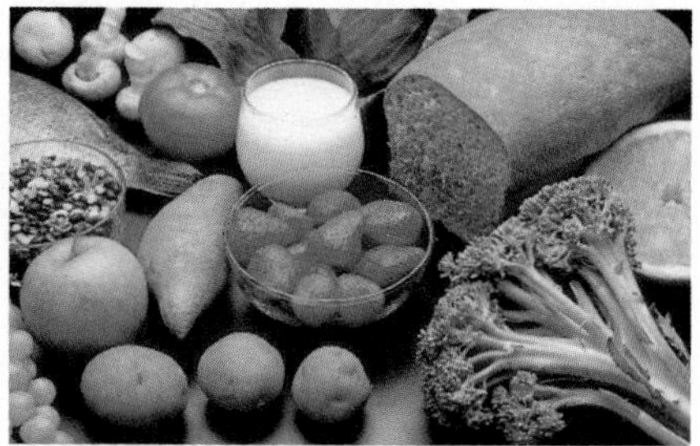

Carbohydrate-rich foods are found almost exclusively among the plants: milk is the only animal-derived food that is rich in carbohydrate.

carbohydrates: energy nutrients composed of monosaccharides.
carbo = carbon
hydrate = water

simple carbohydrates: the monosaccharides (glucose, fructose, and galactose) and the disaccharides (sucrose, lactose, and maltose); also called sugars.

complex carbohydrates: long chains of sugars arranged as starch or fiber; also called **polysaccharides.**

monosaccharide: a single sugar unit.

disaccharide: a pair of sugar units bonded together.

Most people would like to feel good all the time. No matter what each day may bring, the potential enjoyment available can be tremendous when a person's body and mind are tuned for it. The feeling of well-being that comes with energy, alertness, clear thinking, and confidence is so rewarding that if you know how to produce it, you will probably make the necessary effort. Part of the secret of feeling well is keeping your energy supply going with food. That means (from Chapter 1) choosing foods that contain the energy nutrients—carbohydrate and fat, primarily. But which to choose?

Carbohydrate is the preferred energy source for most of the body's functions. As long as carbohydrate is available, the human brain depends exclusively on it as an energy source. Athletes eat a "high-carb" diet to store as much muscle fuel as possible, and dietary recommendations urge people to eat carbohydrate-rich foods for better health. And where can you find carbohydrate-rich foods? Almost exclusively among the plants; milk is the only animal-derived food that contains significant amounts of carbohydrate.

Carbohydrate is the body's fuel of choice, fat is next. Fat, however, has disadvantages: it normally is not used as fuel by the brain and central nervous system, and diets high in fat are associated with many diseases. The other energy sources available to the body—protein and alcohol—offer no advantage as fuels. Protein is best left to serve its own diverse functions, as you will see in Chapter 4. Alcohol, of course, has well-known undesirable side effects.

The Chemist's View of Carbohydrates

Chemists divide the carbohydrates into two categories: simple and complex. The simple carbohydrates (sugars) are:

- Monosaccharides (single sugars).
- Disaccharides (double sugars).

White table sugar is one of the disaccharides. The complex carbohydrates (polysaccharides) are:

- Starch.
- Glycogen.
- Some fibers.

All of these carbohydrates are composed of the simple sugar glucose and other compounds that are much like glucose in composition and structure. Figure 2–1 shows the chemical structure of glucose.

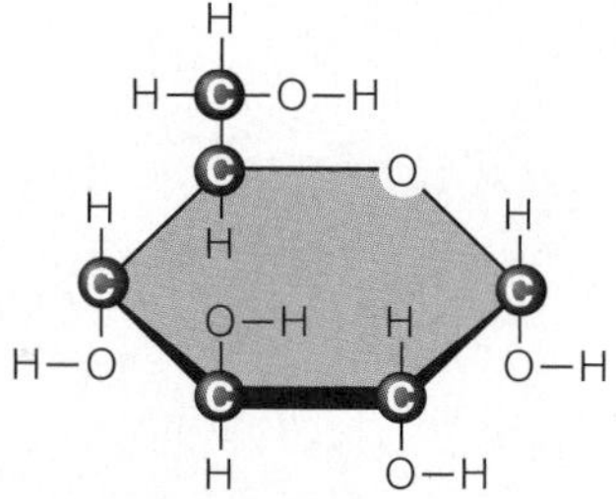

Figure 2–1
Chemical Structure of Glucose
On paper, the structure of glucose has to be drawn flat, but in nature the five carbons and oxygen are roughly in a plane, with "flags" of H, OH, and CH_2OH sticking out above and below it.

Monosaccharides (Single Sugars)

Three monosaccharides are important in nutrition: glucose, fructose, and galactose. Almost all the body's cells use glucose as their chief energy source. The body can obtain this glucose from all plant carbohydrates. Plants capture the sun's radiant energy and through the process of photosynthesis trap this energy in glucose. In the human body, the hormone insulin, among others, enables cells to take up glucose from the blood and so helps keep blood glucose constant (homeostasis).

Plants also make fructose, which is the sweetest of the sugars. It is abundant in fruits, honey, and saps. The body can convert fructose to glucose, or it can break fructose down to fragments and make fat from them. Glucose and fructose are the most common monosaccharides in nature. The third single sugar, galactose, appears in nature only as part of lactose, a disaccharide also known as milk sugar. Only during digestion is galactose freed as a single sugar.

glucose: a monosaccharide, the sugar common to all disaccharides and polysaccharides; also called blood sugar or dextrose.

insulin: a hormone secreted by the pancreas in response to high blood glucose; it promotes cellular glucose uptake and use or storage.

homeostasis: the maintenance of constant internal conditions (such as chemistry, temperature, and blood pressure) by the body's control systems.
homeo = the same
stasis = staying

fructose: a monosaccharide; sometimes known as fruit sugar. It is abundant in fruits, honey, and saps.
fruct = fruit

galactose: a monosaccharide; part of the disaccharide lactose.

sucrose: a disaccharide composed of glucose and fructose; commonly known as table sugar, beet sugar, or cane sugar.
sucro = sugar

Disaccharides (Double Sugars)

In disaccharides, pairs of single sugars are linked together. Lactose is an example of a disaccharide, and there are two others. All three have glucose as one of their single sugars. As Table 2–1 shows, the other monosaccharide is either another glucose (in maltose), or galactose (in lactose), or fructose (in sucrose). The shapes of the sugars in Table 2–1 reflect their chemical structures as drawn on paper.

Sucrose: Table Sugar Sucrose (table, or white, sugar) is the most familiar of the three disaccharides and is what people mean when they speak of "sugar." This sugar is usually obtained by refining the juice from sugar beets or sugarcane to provide the brown, white, and powdered sugars available in the supermarket, but it occurs naturally in many fruits and vegetables.

When you eat a food containing sucrose, enzymes in your digestive tract split the sucrose into its glucose and fructose components. Because the body can convert fructose to glucose, one molecule of sucrose can ultimately yield two molecules of glucose.

Honey versus Sugar People often ask: What is the difference between honey and white sugar? Is honey more nutritious? Honey, like white sugar, contains glucose and fructose. The difference is that in white sugar, the glucose and fructose are bonded together in pairs, whereas in honey some of them are paired and some are free single sugars. When you eat either white sugar or honey, though, your body breaks all of the sugars apart into single sugars. It ultimately makes no difference, then, whether you eat single sugars linked together, as in white sugar, or the same sugars unlinked, as in honey; they will end up as single sugars in

Table 2–1
The Major Sugars

MONOSACCHARIDES	DISACCHARIDES
Glucose	Sucrose (glucose + fructose)
Fructose	Lactose (glucose + galactose)
Galactose	Maltose (glucose + glucose)
(found only as part of lactose)	

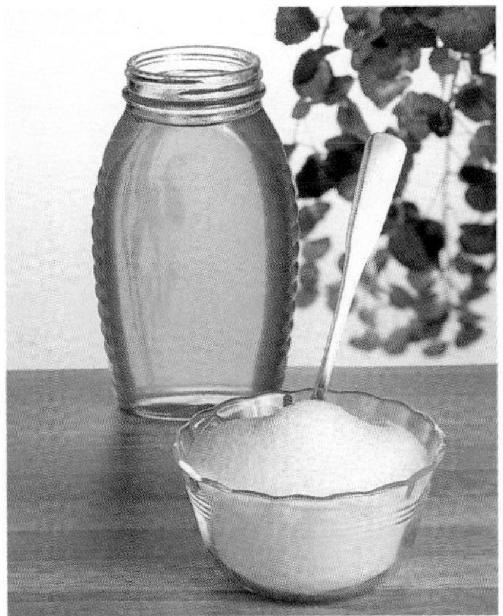

Honey, like sugar, contains glucose and fructose.

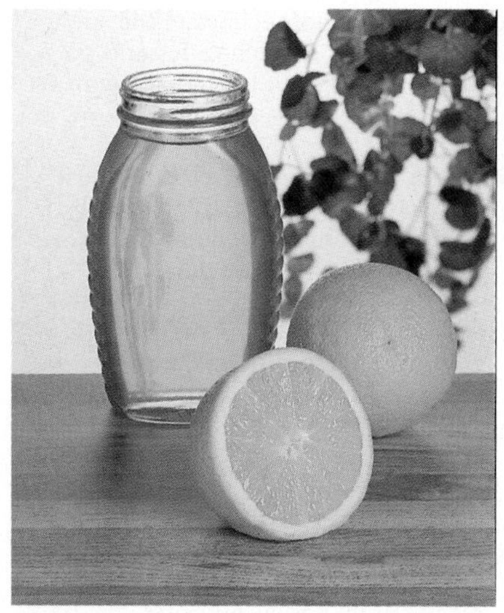

You receive the same sugars from an orange as from honey or sugar, but the packaging makes a big nutrition difference.

lactose: a disaccharide composed of glucose and galactose; commonly known as milk sugar.
lact = milk

your body. True, honey contains trace amounts of a few vitamins and minerals, but to say that honey is nutritious is misleading.

Fruits versus Sugar Some sugar sources are more nutritious than others, though. Consider a fruit such as an orange. You receive the same sugars and about the same energy from an orange as from a tablespoon of sugar or honey, but the packaging makes a big difference. The sugars of the orange are diluted in a large volume of fluid that contains valuable vitamins and minerals, and the flesh and skin of the orange are supported by fibers that also offer health benefits. A tablespoon of sugar or honey offers no such bonuses.

Cola Beverages and Sweets A cola beverage, containing many teaspoons of sugar, offers no advantages either. Table 2–2 shows sample nutrients supplied by some sugar sources; note the "0s" and "traces" by honey, sugar, and the cola beverage and the substantial numbers by the others. Sucrose is often the principal ingredient of carbonated beverages, candy, cakes, frostings, cookies, and other concentrated sweets, so they are often not nutritious.

Lactose: Milk Sugar Lactose is the principal carbohydrate of milk. Most human babies are born with the digestive enzymes necessary to split lactose into its two monosaccharide parts, glucose and galactose, so as to absorb it. Breast milk thus provides a simple, easily digested carbohydrate that meets a baby's energy needs; most formulas do too, because they are made from milk.

Lactose Intolerance Many people lose the ability to digest lactose after infancy. This condition, known as lactose intolerance, occurs in 70 to 100 percent of Native American, Asian, African, Mediterranean, and Middle Eastern people.[1] Lactose intolerance is not the same as milk aller-

Table 2–2
Sample Nutrients in Sugars and Other Foods

The indicated portion of any of these foods provides approximately 100 kcalories. Notice that for a similar number of kcalories, milk, legumes, fruits, and grains offer more of the other nutrients than do the sugars.

FOOD	PROTEIN (g)	CALCIUM (mg)	VITAMIN A (RE)
Sugar, white (2 tbs)	0	Trace	0
Cola beverage (1 c)	0	6	0
Honey, strained or extracted (1½ tbs)	Trace	2	0
Milk, 1% low-fat (1 c)	8	300	145
Kidney beans (½ c)	7	35	0
Apricots (6)	2	30	332
Bread, whole wheat (1½ slices)	3	48	Trace

gy, which is caused by an immune reaction to the protein in milk. Lactose intolerance is discussed further in Chapters 18 and 21, and milk allergy in Chapter 16.

Maltose The third disaccharide, maltose, is a plant sugar that consists of two glucose units. Maltose appears at only one stage in the life of a plant—when the plant is digesting its stored starch for energy and starting to sprout.

maltose: a disaccharide composed of two glucose units; sometimes known as malt sugar.

In summary, then, the major simple carbohydrates, or sugars, are the three single sugars and the three double sugars shown earlier in Table 2–1. Glucose, fructose, maltose, and sucrose come from plants; lactose and galactose from milk and milk products.

Starch and Glycogen (Energy-Yielding Polysaccharides)

Unlike the sugars, which contain the three monosaccharides—glucose, fructose, and galactose—in different combinations, the polysaccharides, starch and glycogen, are composed almost entirely of glucose. They differ from each other only in the nature of the bonds that link the glucose units together.

Starch Starch is a long, straight or branched chain of hundreds of glucose units linked together. These giant molecules are packed side by side in a rice grain or potato root—as many as a million per cubic inch of food. When you eat the plant, your body splits the starch into glucose units and uses the glucose for energy.

starch: a plant polysaccharide composed of glucose and digestible by human beings.

The short chains of glucose units that result from the breakdown of starch are known as **dextrins.** The word sometimes appears on food labels because dextrins can be used as thickening agents in foods.

Starchy Foods All starchy foods are plant foods. Grains are the richest food source of starch. Most human societies have a staple grain on which their people depend for much of their food energy: rice in Asia; wheat in Canada, the United States, and Europe; corn in much of Central and South America; and millet, rye, barley, and oats elsewhere. A second important source of starch is the legume (bean and pea) family. Legumes include peanuts and "dry" beans such as butter beans, kidney beans, "baked" beans, black-eyed peas (cowpeas), chickpeas (garbanzo beans), and soybeans. Root vegetables (tubers) such as potatoes and yams are a third major source of starch, and in many non-Western societies, they are the primary starch sources.

Grains, legumes, and tubers not only are rich in starch, but also contain abundant dietary fiber, protein, and other nutrients. When nutrition experts advise you to seek out carbohydrate-rich foods to meet most of your energy needs, these are the foods they are recommending. Grains, legumes, and tubers are excellent energy foods and sources of many nutrients.

Glycogen Glycogen molecules, which are also made of chains of glucose, are more highly branched than starch molecules. As starch stores energy for plants, glycogen stores energy for human beings and animals. Because glycogen does not occur in plants and is found in meats only to a limited extent, it is not important as a nutrient. Nevertheless, glycogen

glycogen (GLY-co-gen)**:** a polysaccharide composed of glucose, made and stored by liver and muscle tissues of human beings and animals as a storage form of glucose. Glycogen is not a significant food source of carbohydrate and is not counted as one of the complex carbohydrates in foods.

plays an important role in the body as a readily available source of glucose, especially during exercise.

Cellulose Cellulose is also composed of glucose units, but this polysaccharide is not classed as an energy-yielding carbohydrate because it is not digestible by human beings. It is classed as one of the nonnutritive fibers, discussed next.

The Fibers

fibers: a general term denoting in plant foods the polysaccharides cellulose, hemicellulose, pectins, gums, and mucilages, as well as the nonpolysaccharide lignins, that are not attacked by human digestive enzymes.

The fibers of plants are constituents of plant cell walls. Most fibers are polysaccharides—chains of sugars—just as starch is, but in fibers the sugar units are held together by bonds that human digestive enzymes cannot break. Figure 2–2 shows the difference between starch and cellulose. Fibers include the polysaccharides cellulose, hemicellulose, pectins, gums, and mucilages, as well as the nonpolysaccharide lignins.

Fibers in Foods Cellulose is the main constituent of plant cell walls, so it is found in all vegetables, fruits, and legumes. Hemicellulose is the main constituent of cereal fibers. Pectins are abundant in vegetables and fruits, especially citrus fruits and apples. The food industry uses pectins to thicken jelly and keep salad dressing from separating. Gums and mucilages have similar structures. They are used as additives or stabilizers by the food industry. Lignins are the tough, woody parts of plants. Few foods people eat contain much lignin.

Fibers in the Body Although cellulose and other fibers are not attacked by human enzymes, some fibers can be digested by bacteria in the human digestive tract and can yield some absorbable products. Food fibers therefore, can contribute some energy, depending on the extent to which they break down in the body. For the most part, the energy contribution of fibers is considered negligible, although it can be as high as 15 percent of a person's daily intake on a high-fiber diet.[2]

insoluble fibers: the tough, fibrous structures of fruits, vegetables, and grains; indigestible food components that do not dissolve in water.

soluble fibers: indigestible food components that readily dissolve in water and often impart gummy or gel-like characteristics to foods. An example is pectin from fruit, which is used to thicken jellies.

Soluble versus Insoluble Fibers Fibers are classified according to several characteristics, including their chemical structure, their digestibility by bacterial enzymes, and their solubility in water. Some fibers are insoluble, meaning that they do not dissolve readily in water; other fibers are soluble—they do dissolve in water. These distinctions influence the health effects of fibers, which are discussed in a later section.

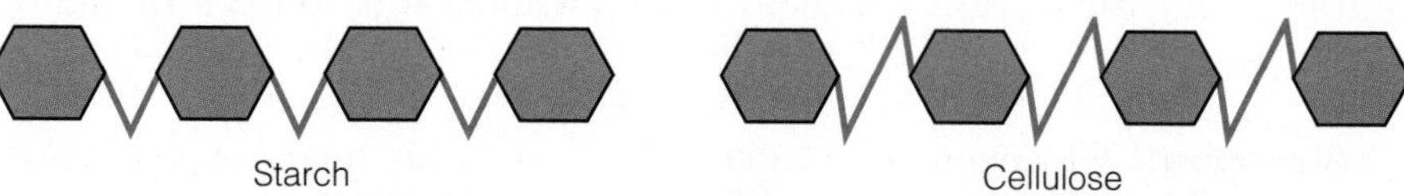

Figure 2–2
Starch and Cellulose Molecules Compared (Small Segments)
The bonds that link the glucose units together in cellulose are different from the bonds in starch (and glycogen). Human enzymes cannot digest cellulose.

Carbohydrates and Health

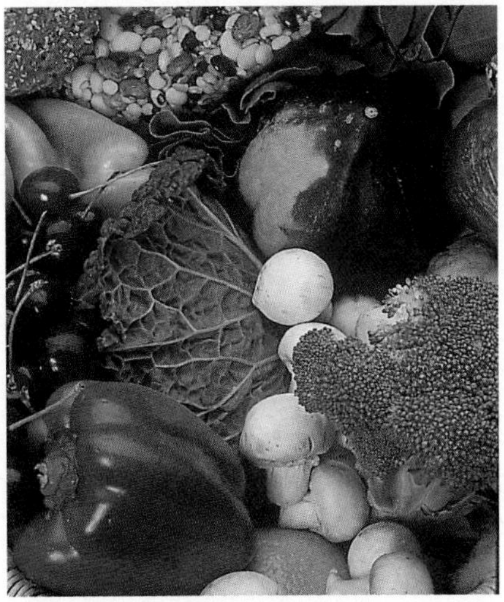

Starch and fiber-rich foods are the foods to emphasize.

Despite dietary recommendations that people should eat generous servings of complex carbohydrate–rich foods for their health, many people still believe that carbohydrate is the "fattening" component of foods. Gram for gram, carbohydrates contribute fewer kcalories to the body than dietary fat, so a diet of high-carbohydrate foods is likely to be *lower* in kcalories than a diet of high-fat foods.

Dietary recommendations state that carbohydrates should contribute 55 to 60 percent of the total daily energy intake. Concentrated sweets, however, should account for only 10 percent or less of total kcalories; starch-rich and fiber-rich foods such as vegetables, grains, legumes, and fruits should predominate. For most people this means that total carbohydrate intake should increase while sugar intake should decline. The sugars in vegetables, fruits, and milk are acceptable because they are accompanied by many nutrients. In contrast, concentrated sweets contribute many kcalories but relatively few nutrients, and so should be limited.

Sugars

Despite the recommendation that people limit their sugar intakes to 10 percent of total kcalories, people today actually obtain 11 to 20 percent of their total food energy from sugars.[3] This amounts to some 40 to 80 pounds of sugars a year. Recommendations that people reduce their consumption of concentrated sugars to 10 percent or less of total kcalories stem from widely published reports of research performed during the 1970s.[4] These reports implicated sugars (mainly sucrose) as a possible contributing factor in several diseases. Since then, many accusations have been made against the sugar sucrose, but the Food and Drug Administration and, more recently, the National Academy of Sciences have concluded that in the amounts people currently consume, sugar carries no proven health risk. Still, the controversy continues.[5] A brief description of accusations pertaining to sugar's effects on health may help clarify the issues. Most commonly, reports accuse sugar of causing (1) obesity, (2) diabetes, (3) heart disease, (4) hyperactivity and aggressive behavior in children, and (5) dental caries.

Sugar and Obesity On the first accusation—that sugar causes obesity—the facts are these. Population studies show that obesity rises as sugar consumption increases, but that sugar is not the sole cause. Whenever sugar intakes increase, usually fat and total energy intakes do, too. Simultaneously, physical activity declines. On the other hand, obesity also occurs where sugar intakes are low. In some instances, obese people eat less sugar than thin people.[6] Fat is more kcalorie dense than sugar and can easily contribute to obesity. Thus sugar can contribute to obesity, but does not, by itself, cause obesity.

Sugar and Diabetes On sugar's relation to diabetes, the evidence is conflicting and interesting. In many parts of the world, as sugar consumption has risen, a profound increase in the incidence of one type of diabetes (Type II) has occurred. Yet in other populations, no relationship has been found between diabetes and sugar consumption. Body fatness seems to be more related to diabetes than diet is: the majority of people with Type II diabetes are overweight or obese, and evidence shows that weight reduction helps prevent diabetes or relieve its symptoms. Thus the fairest conclusion is that *obesity* is a major factor causing Type II diabetes, and that sugar may be a causative factor only when it contributes to obesity. Chapter 25 discusses diabetes further.

Sugar and Heart Disease In relation to heart disease, fat, not sugar, is clearly the major dietary culprit in most cases (see Chapters 3 and 26). However, in a special subgroup of the population—"carbohydrate-sensitive" individuals—carbohydrate, including sugar, seems to worsen the risk of heart disease.* For most people, moderate sugar intakes do not influence the risk of heart disease.

Sugar and Behavior The accusation that sugar causes hyperactive or aggressive behavior in children stands unproven.[8] One group of researchers tested the effects of sugar on children already diagnosed as hyperactive.[9] The hyperactive children did become more distracted (paid less attention) than usual after eating a sugary breakfast, but did not behave more aggressively. Other studies have failed to demonstrate any consistent effect of sugar on behavior in either normal or hyperactive children. If sugar is related to behavior problems in children, it may be because sugary foods can take the place of nutrient-dense foods in children's diets, making nutrient deficiencies likely. Many different nutrient deficiencies adversely affect behavior. A lack of nutrients in children's diets, not sugar itself, can in some cases contribute to undesirable behavior.

Chapter 16 offers further discussion of children's nutrition.

Sugar and Dental Caries As to whether sugar causes dental caries, the evidence says yes. Any carbohydrate-containing food, including bread, bananas, or milk, as well as sugar, can support the bacterial growth in the mouth that produces the acid that eats away tooth enamel. Total sugar intake still plays a major role in caries incidence; populations with diets of more than 10 percent of kcalories from sugar have an unacceptable high incidence of dental caries.[10] Nutrition in Practice 2 discusses nutrition and dental health.

dental caries: the gradual decay and disintegration of a tooth.

Recommended Sugar Intakes In summary, moderate sugar intakes (5 to 10 percent of total kcalories) are not harmful—enough for pleasure, but not enough to displace more nutritious foods. Sugar is a delicious, concentrated source of food energy, but it contains no protein, vitamins, or minerals. Eaten in the place of nutrient- and fiber-rich foods, it makes malnutrition likely.

Recognizing Sugars People often fail to recognize sugar in all its forms, and so fail to realize how much they consume. To estimate how

*Carbohydrate-sensitive individuals respond to an oral carbohydrate challenge with abnormally high insulin secretion, but the insulin fails to stimulate glucose uptake. When carbohydrate-sensitive individuals eat sugar, high blood lipids result.[7]

much sugar you consume, treat all of the following concentrated sweets as equivalent to 1 teaspoon of white sugar:

- 1 teaspoon brown sugar, candy, jam, jelly, any corn sweetener, syrup, honey, molasses, or maple sugar.
- 1 tablespoon catsup.
- 1½ ounces carbonated soft drink (that's 8 teaspoons of sugar per 12-ounce can).

These portions of sugar all provide about the same number of kcalories. Some are closer to 10 kcalories (for example, 14 kcalories for molasses), while some are over 22 (22 kcalories for honey) so an average figure of 20 kcalories is an acceptable approximation. The accompanying glossary presents the multitude of names that denote sugar on food labels. The next section discusses sugar substitutes.

Glossary of Sugars

brown sugar: refined white sugar crystals to which manufacturers have added molasses syrup with natural flavor and color; 91 to 96 percent pure sucrose.
confectioner's sugar: finely powdered sucrose; 99.9 percent pure.
corn sweeteners: corn syrup and sugars derived from corn.
corn syrup: a syrup produced by the action of enzymes on cornstarch, containing mostly glucose. See also *high-fructose corn syrup (HFCS).*
dextrose: an older name for glucose.
fructose, galactose, glucose: already defined (p. 35).
granulated sugar: common table sugar, crystalline sucrose; 99.9 percent pure.
high-fructose corn syrup (HFCS): the predominant sweetener used in processed foods today. HFCS is mostly fructose; glucose makes up the balance.
honey: sugar (mostly sucrose) formed from nectar gathered by bees. An enzyme splits the sucrose into glucose and fructose. Composition and flavor vary, but honey always contains a mixture of sucrose, fructose, and glucose.
invert sugar: a mixture of glucose and fructose formed by splitting sucrose in a chemical process; sold only in liquid form, sweeter than sucrose. Invert sugar is used as an additive to help preserve food freshness and prevent shrinkage.
lactose: already defined (p. 36).
levulose: an older name for fructose.
maltose: already defined (p. 37).
maple sugar: a sugar (mostly sucrose) purified from concentrated sap of the sugar maple tree. Maple sugar is expensive compared with other sweeteners.
molasses: a thick brown syrup, left over from sugarcane juice during sugar refining. Blackstrap molasses contains iron, which comes from the machinery used to process it. This iron is not as well absorbed as the iron in meats and other foods.
natural sweeteners: a term used freely, without legal definition, to refer to any sugar or sweetener except refined sucrose.
raw sugar: the first crop of crystals harvested during sugar processing. Raw sugar cannot be sold in the United States because it contains too much filth (dirt, insect fragments, and the like). Sugar sold domestically as raw sugar has actually gone through about half of the refining steps.
sucrose: already defined (p. 35).
turbinado (ter-bih-NOD-oh) **sugar:** raw (brown) sugar from which the filth has been washed; legal to sell in the United States.
white sugar: pure sucrose, produced by dissolving, concentrating, and recrystallizing raw sugar.

Alternative Sweeteners: Sugar Alcohols

sugar alcohols: sugarlike compounds; like sugars, they are sweet to taste and yield 4 kcalories per gram. Examples are maltitol, mannitol, sorbitol, and xylitol.

nutritive sweeteners: sweeteners that yield energy, including both the sugars and the sugar alcohols.

People who want to limit their use of sugar may choose from two sets of alternative sweeteners: sugar alcohols and artificial sweeteners. The sugar alcohols are carbohydrates, and they yield about as much energy as sucrose: 4 kcalories per gram. They are therefore sometimes called nutritive sweeteners.

The sugar alcohols occur naturally in fruits. Mannitol, maltitol, and sorbitol are less sweet than sucrose, while xylitol is equivalent to sucrose in sweetness.[11] The body either absorbs the sugar alcohols more slowly or metabolizes them to glucose more slowly than most other sugars, but it does absorb and metabolize them. Side effects such as gas, abdominal discomfort, and diarrhea, however, make them less attractive than the artificial sweeteners.

The sugar alcohols offer a distinct advantage over sucrose when it comes to dental caries. Bacteria in the mouth metabolize sugar alcohols much more slowly than sucrose.[12] This in turn inhibits the production of acids that promote caries formation. Sugar alcohols are therefore less caries promoting than sugar is. They are valuable in chewing gums, breath mints, and other products that people keep in their mouths a while.

Alternative Sweeteners: Artificial Sweeteners

artificial sweeteners: noncarbohydrate, noncaloric synthetic sweetening agents; sometimes called **nonnutritive sweeteners.**

The artificial sweeteners are not carbohydrates. They yield virtually no energy in the amounts typically used and are sometimes called nonnutritive sweeteners. Like the sugar alcohols, artificial sweeteners make foods taste sweet without promoting tooth decay. The accompanying glossary offers details on six artificial sweeteners of interest.

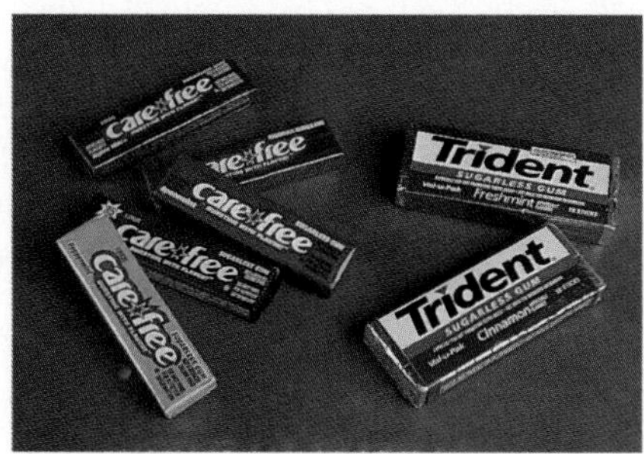

These chewing gums contain sugar alcohols, which are better than sugar for the teeth, but are not kcalorie-free.

Glossary of Artificial Sweeteners

acesulfame potassium: a low-kcalorie sweetener recently approved by the FDA; also known as acesulfame-K because K is the chemical symbol for potassium. Not approved in Canada.

alitame: a compound of two amino acids (alanine and aspartic acid) that is 2000 times sweeter than sucrose; FDA approval pending.

aspartame: a compound of two amino acids (phenylalanine and aspartic acid) that tastes like the sugar sucrose but is much sweeter. It provides about 4 kcalories per gram, as does protein, but because so little is used, it is virtually kcalorie-free. In powdered form it is sometimes mixed with lactose, however, so a 1-gram packet may contain 4 kcalories. It is used in both the United States and Canada.

cyclamate: a 0-kcalorie sweetener; FDA approval pending in the United States; available in Canada on grocery-store shelves but only as a tabletop sweetener, not as an additive.

saccharin: a 0-kcalorie sweetener used in the United States, but available in Canada only in pharmacies and only as a sweetener, not as an additive.

sucralose: a 0-kcalorie sweetener that is 600 times sweeter than sucrose; FDA approval pending in the United States; approved in Canada.

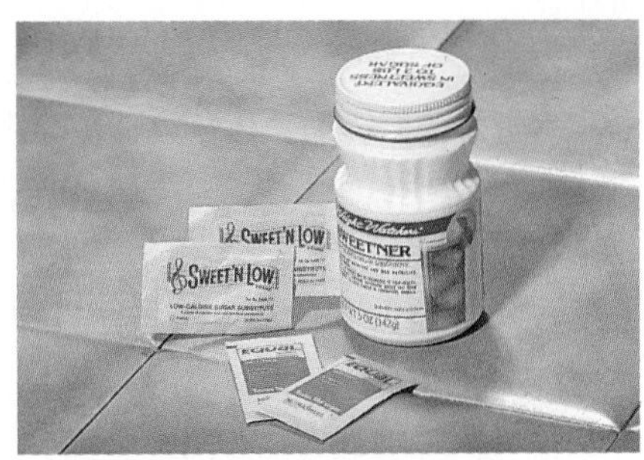

Artificial sweeteners offer the sweet taste of sugar without the kcalories.

Saccharin Saccharin has been used for more than 100 years in the United States and is currently used by more than 50 million people, mainly in soft drinks and as a tabletop sweetener. Questions about the safety of saccharin arose in 1977 when experiments suggested that it caused bladder tumors in second-generation rats fed high doses. The Food and Drug Administration (FDA) proposed banning saccharin as a result. Public outcry in favor of saccharin was so loud that Congress declared a moratorium on the ban, a moratorium that was repeatedly extended. In 1991, the FDA withdrew its proposal to ban saccharin.[13] The consumer warning, "use of this product may be hazardous to your health. This product contains saccharin, which has been determined to cause cancer in laboratory animals," is to remain on the label.

Does saccharin cause cancer? The largest population study to date, involving 9000 men and women, showed overall that saccharin use did not raise the risk of cancer. Among certain small groups of the population, however, such as those who both smoked heavily and used saccharin, the risk of bladder cancer was slightly greater. Other studies involving more than 5000 people with bladder cancer showed no association between bladder cancer and saccharin use.[14] Common sense dictates that consuming large amounts of saccharin is probably not safe, but at moderate intake levels, saccharin is currently assumed to be safe for most people.

Aspartame Aspartame is the active ingredient in NutraSweet, which is used in many commercially prepared foods, and in Equal, a tabletop sweetener. Aspartame was approved by the FDA in 1981 and currently dominates the world market for artificial sweeteners. Aspartame is one of the most studied of all food additives: extensive animal and human studies document its safety. Long-term consumption of aspartame is safe and is not associated with any adverse health effects.[15] Aspartame is approved for use in more than 90 countries.

The FDA's approval of aspartame is based on the assumption that no one will consume more than 50 milligrams per kilogram of body weight in a day. This maximum daily intake is indeed a lot: for a 128-pound person, it adds up to 83 packets of Equal or 14 soft drinks sweetened only with aspartame. Most people consume between 2 and 10 milligrams per kilogram of body weight per day.[16] Still, a child who drinks a quart of Kool-Aid sweetened with aspartame on a hot day, and who also has pudding, chewing gum, cereal, and other products sweetened with aspartame, takes in more than the FDA maximum level. Although this presents no proven hazard, it seems wise to offer children other foods so as not to exceed the limit.

Aspartame and PKU Although aspartame is considered safe for most people, individuals with the metabolic disorder phenylketonuria (PKU) are an exception. The labels of products that contain aspartame must include information for individuals with PKU. Aspartame contains the amino acid phenylalanine, and people with PKU cannot dispose of it efficiently. Adults with PKU can use some pure aspartame, but children with PKU need to get all their phenylalanine from nutrient-rich foods such as milk and meat (see Nutrition in Practice 25).

Acesulfame Potassium The FDA approved acesulfame potassium (acesulfame-K) in 1988 after reviewing more than 90 safety studies, conducted over 15 years. Some consumer groups believe that acesulfame-K causes tumors in rats and should not have been approved by the FDA. The FDA counters that the tumors were not caused by the sweetener, but were typical of those routinely found in rats.

Marketed under the trade names Sunette and Sweet One, acesulfame-K is about as sweet as aspartame. It is used in chewing gum, beverages, instant coffee and tea, gelatins, and puddings, as well as for table use. Unlike aspartame, acesulfame-K holds up well during cooking.

Other Artificial Sweeteners FDA approval for three other sweeteners—cyclamate, alitame, and sucralose—is still pending. To date, no safety issues have been raised for alitame or sucralose. Cyclamate, on the other hand, has been battling safety issues for 50 years. Approved by the FDA in 1949, cyclamate was banned in 1970 because of evidence indicating that it caused bladder cancer in rats. In 1985, the National Academy of Sciences concluded that evidence to date indicated that cyclamate did not cause cancer in human beings, but warranted further studies. In Canada, cyclamate is restricted to use as a tabletop sweetener on the advice of a physician. In the United States, the FDA is currently reviewing a petition to reapprove the use of cyclamate.

Artificial Sweeteners and Weight Control Many people eat and drink products sweetened with artificial sweeteners to help them control weight. Does this work? Ironically, a few studies have reported that after consuming such products, people experience heightened feelings of hunger. Despite these reports, most studies find that artificial sweeteners do not heighten feelings of hunger, enhance food intake, or cause weight gain in people.[17] Consumers of artificial sweeteners who want to control their weight should be careful to use the sweeteners as a replacement for sugar, not in addition to sugar, in their diets. If a person who drinks a diet soda then overcompensates by eating a food that delivers many kcalories, certainly the use of low-kcalorie sweeteners will have no impact on body weight.

Recommendations For people who choose to use artificial sweeteners, the most important consideration is to use them in moderation. After all, almost every substance, even water, can be harmful in excess. The American Dietetic Association recommends that artificial sweeteners be used in moderation and only as part of a well-balanced diet.[18]

Complex Carbohydrates

The health benefits you can expect from a diet high in complex carbohydrate foods and low in concentrated sugar are many and wonderful. Such a diet is almost invariably low in fat; low in food energy; and high in fiber, vitamins, and minerals. All these factors working together can help reduce the risks of obesity, cancer, cardiovascular disease, diabetes, dental caries, and malnutrition.

It is difficult to sort out which complex carbohydrates contribute to which health benefits. Starch and fibers almost always occur together in foods (except refined foods), so it is hard to distinguish their effects. Some health effects appear to be especially closely associated with fibers, however, and these are discussed next.

Fibers

Fibers benefit health in many ways. Fibers are thought to play a beneficial role in the prevention or management of:

- *Weight control.* Fibrous foods contribute little energy and promote a feeling of fullness as they absorb water. In addition, soluble fibers in a meal slow the movement of food through the upper digestive tract, so that you feel fuller longer. A diet high in fiber-rich foods can promote weight loss if those foods displace concentrated fats and sweets.
- *Constipation, hemorrhoids, and diarrhea.* Fibers that both enlarge and soften stools (such as insoluble wheat bran) relieve constipation and hemorrhoids. Other fibers help to solidify watery stools.
- *Appendicitis.* Some fibers (again, such as wheat bran) help keep the contents of the intestinal tract moving easily. This action helps prevent compaction of the intestinal contents, which could obstruct the appendix and permit bacteria to invade and infect it.
- *Diverticulosis.* Fibers stimulate the muscles of the digestive tract so that they retain their health and tone. This prevents the muscles from becoming weak and the lining of the digestive tract from bulging out in places, as occurs in diverticulosis.
- *Colon cancer.* Some evidence suggests that high-fiber foods may reduce the risk of colon cancer.
- *Heart disease.* Soluble fibers bind cholesterol compounds and carry them out of the body with the feces, thus lowering the body's cholesterol concentration and possibly the risk of heart disease.[19] High-fiber foods may also lower blood cholesterol indirectly—by displacing fatty, cholesterol-raising foods from the diet.[20] Even when dietary fat intake is low, research shows that high intakes of soluble fiber (such as that in apples and oat bran) exert a separate and significant blood cholesterol-lowering effect.[21]
- *Diabetes.* Some fibers delay the passage of nutrients from the stomach to the small intestine. This delay slows glucose absorption, thus eliciting a moderate insulin response and a moderate rise in blood glucose (Chapter 25 provides more details on diabetes).

Even with all these advantages, carbohydrate in the form of raw fiber is not a wonder cure. In some cases it can be detrimental. When too much fiber is consumed, essential vitamins and minerals are bound to it and excreted with it without ever becoming available for the body to use. Also, consuming purified fiber such as cellulose may not confer the same health benefits as consuming cellulose from a food source such as whole grains.[22]

Carbohydrates in Foods

Grains, vegetables, fruits, and milk—these are the foods noted for the valuable energy-yielding carbohydrates they contain: starches and dilute sugars. Each class of foods makes its own typical carbohydrate contribution.

Breads, Other Grains, and Starchy Vegetables One slice of whole-wheat bread offers 15 grams (60 kcalories) of starch. Equivalent foods are other breads, cereals, potatoes, rice, pasta, corn, peas, limas and other beans (legumes), and many other grains, legumes, and starchy vegetables. One portion (about ½ cup) of any of these offers some 60 kcalories of starch. (A ½-cup portion of a nonstarchy vegetable such as carrots, squash, or greens contributes about 5 grams, 20 kcalories, of carbohydrate.)

Fruits A typical fruit portion, such as ½ cup of orange juice, also contains 15 grams (60 kcalories) of carbohydrate, but mostly as sugars, including the fruit sugar, fructose. Fruits vary in their water and fiber contents, and therefore their sugar concentrations vary as well.

Milk Products One cup of milk or the equivalent (1 cup of yogurt or buttermilk, ⅓ cup of dry milk powder, or ½ cup of evaporated milk) donates a generous 12 grams (about 50 kcalories) of carbohydrate. Milk products vary in fat content, though, and this is an important consideration in choosing among them. Chapter 3 provides the details.

Recommendations There is no RDA for carbohydrate, but there is a recommendation that 55 to 60 percent of total kcalories should come from carbohydrate. For people who eat about 1700 kcalories a day, this recommended intake translates to some 900 to 1000 kcalories from carbohydrate per day or, at 4 kcalories per gram, some 225 to 250 grams. Considering that most of this carbohydrate should be starch, not sugars, you can see that many servings of starchy foods are needed to meet this recommendation. For example, suppose you started with the smallest number of recommended servings from the Daily Food Guide in Chapter 1 (Figure 1–3) as a core: 6 grain products, 3 vegetables, 2 fruits, 2 milk, and 2 meat servings. You would need an additional 1½ to 2 servings of grains, vegetables, fruits, and milk to obtain the recommended carbohydrate.

Figure 2–3 offers an example of meals that provide about 1700 kcalories and 225 grams of carbohydrate from nutrient-dense, fiber-rich foods. The carbohydrate content of a diet can be determined by using a nutrient composition table such as that found in Appendix A or by using the exchange list system described in Nutrition in Practice 6.

Fibers in Foods Meals selected according to these guidelines deliver ample fiber, too. Most people in the United States do not eat this way, though, and their average fiber intakes are only a third to a half of the recommended 20 to 35 grams daily.[23] To obtain enough fiber, eat ample servings of whole foods, remembering this rule of thumb:

Figure 2–3
A Day's Meals that Offer 1700 kCalories and Meet the Carbohydrate Recommendation

Before heading off to classes, a student eats breakfast:
- 2 shredded wheat biscuits.
- 1 c 1% low-fat milk.
- ½ banana (sliced).

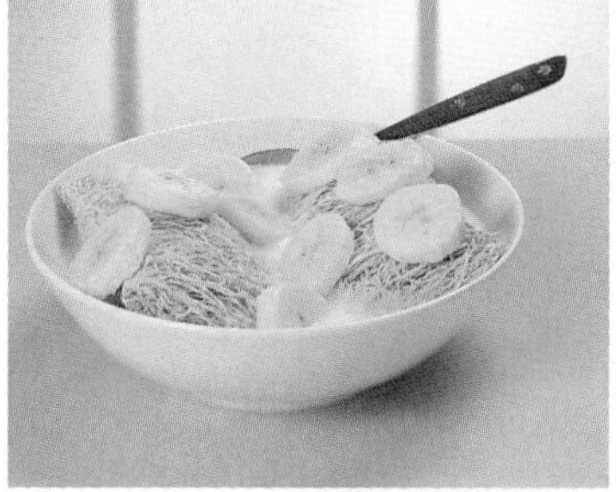

Then goes home for a quick lunch:
- 1 turkey sandwich on whole-wheat bread with mayonnaise and mustard.
- 1 c vegetable juice (canned).

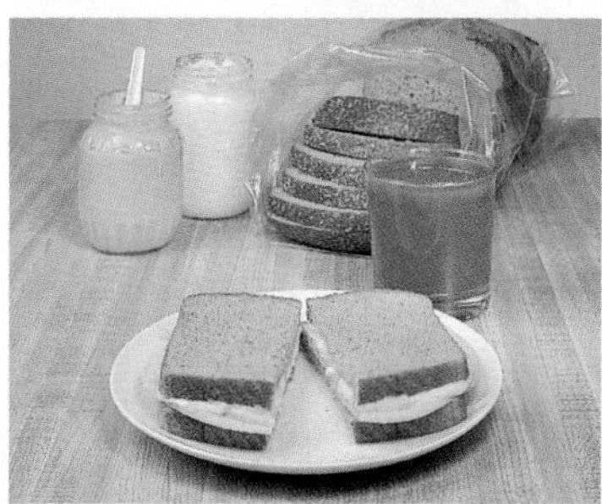

While studying that afternoon, the student eats a snack:
- 4 whole-wheat crackers.
- 1 oz cheddar cheese.
- 1 apple.

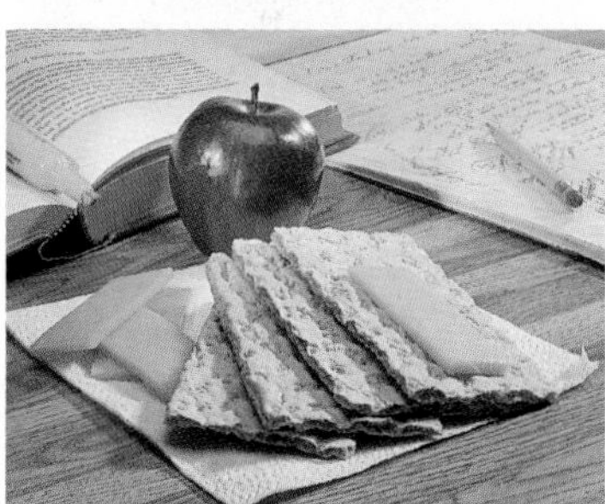

That night, the student makes dinner:
A salad made with:
- 1 c raw spinach leaves, shredded carrots, and sliced mushrooms.
- ⅓ c garbanzo beans.
- 5 lg olives.
- 1 tbs ranch salad dressing.

A dinner of:
- 1 c spaghetti with meat sauce.
- ½ c green beans.
- 2 tsp butter.

And, for dessert:
- 1¼ c strawberries (fresh).

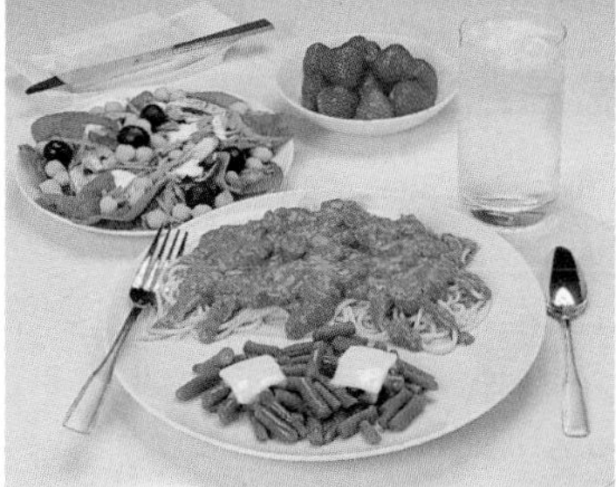

Later that evening, the student enjoys a bedtime snack:
- 3 graham crackers.
- 1 c 1% low-fat milk.

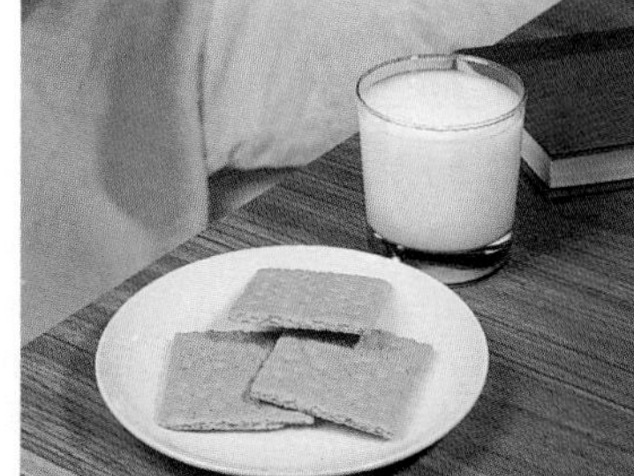

Total kcal: 1725
53% kcal from carbohydrate
29% kcal from fat
18% kcal from protein

- A serving of fruit, vegetable, or grain (bread or cereal) delivers 2 to 4 grams.
- A serving of legumes (½ to 1 cup) delivers about 8 grams.

Miscellaneous whole foods also add some fiber: you can get about 1 gram from ½ ounce of nuts, a tablespoon of peanut butter, a large pickle, or 5 olives. And on any day that you eat according to the Daily Food Guide (for example, the meals in Figure 2–3), you can assume your fiber intakes will be as follows:

4 servings vegetables × 3 g each	= 12 g.
3 servings fruits × 3 g each	= 9 g.
8 servings grains × 3 g each	= 24 g.
1 serving legumes × 8 g each	= 8 g.
Total	= 53 g.

Thus a day's meals based on the Daily Food Guide, such as those shown in Figure 2–3, not only meet carbohydrate recommendations, they provide abundant fiber, too.

Energy Nutrients in Perspective

An uninterrupted flow of energy is so vital to life that other functions are sometimes sacrificed to maintain it. For example, when a child is fed too little food, the food he or she does consume will be used for energy to keep the heart and lungs going, while growth comes to a standstill. To go totally without an energy supply, even for a few minutes, is to die. Over the course of evolution, the urgency of the need for energy has ensured that all creatures have developed ways of accumulating built-in reserves to protect themselves from being deprived of energy. One major provision against this sort of emergency is glycogen, the storage form of glucose. (The other is body fat, about which the next chapter says more.)

Glycogen Used for Energy When you do not eat carbohydrate, your body rapidly devours its glycogen stores. Stored glycogen can return glucose to the blood whenever the supply runs short, but the liver cells can store only limited amounts of glycogen. Once this supply is depleted, the body must turn to the other energy nutrients—fat and protein—to meet its energy needs.

Fat Used for Energy Unlike the liver cells, which can store only a limited amount of glycogen the body's fat cells can store virtually unlimited quantities of fat, so supplies almost never run out. Fat normally is used to meet two-thirds of the body's energy needs, and most tissues can use it as is. The brain and nerves, however, need their energy as glucose, and the body cannot convert fat to glucose. After a long period of glucose deprivation, brain and nerve cells develop the ability to derive about half of their energy from a special form of fat known as ketones, but they still require glucose as well. This means that people wanting to lose weight need to eat a certain minimum amount of carbohydrate to meet their energy needs even when they are limiting their food intakes. Chapter 9 offers guidelines for weight loss.

ketones (KEY-tones): acidic fat-related compounds formed from the incomplete breakdown of fat when carbohydrate is not available; technically known as *ketone bodies.*

Protein Used for Energy During a fast, when the available glycogen is gone and no carbohydrate is coming in from food, brain and nerve cells demand the glucose they need from the only available alternative source—protein. The body beings to dismantle its own muscles and other lean tissues to generate glucose. Only adequate dietary carbohydrate can prevent this use of protein for energy, and its action in doing so is known as the protein-sparing effect of carbohydrate.

protein-sparing effect: the effect of carbohydrate in providing energy that allows protein to be used for other purposes.

Ultimately, after half of the body protein is used, death occurs. Death from loss of lean body tissues will occur even in an obese person who fasts too long. It should be clear, then, that although carbohydrate is an ideal energy source, fat and sometimes protein are also extremely important in meeting energy demands.

SELF STUDY

How's Your Carbohydrate Intake?

From the forms you filled out for the Self-Study in Chapter 1, answer the following questions and complete Form 6.

1. How many grams of carbohydrate do you consume in an average day (from Form 2)? ______ grams
2. How many kcalories does this represent? ______ kcalories (Remember, 1 gram of carbohydrate contributes 4 kcalories.)
3. It is estimated that you should have at least 125 grams of carbohydrate in a day. How does your intake compare with this minimum? ______
4. What percentage of your total kcalories is contributed by carbohydrate (carbohydrate kcalories divided by total kcalories times 100—or use the answer you obtained on Form 5)? ______ percent
5. How does this figure compare with the recommendation stating that about 55 to 60 percent of the kcalories in your diet should come from carbohydrate? ______
6. Another dietary goal is that no more than 10 percent of total kcalories should come from refined and other processed sugars and foods high in such sugars. To assess your intake against this standard, sort the carbohydrate-containing food items you ate into three groups:

   - *Group A:* Foods containing complex carbohydrate (foods found among the bread, cereal, rice, and pasta group and the vegetable group) contributed ______ kcalories.
   - *Group B:* Nutritious foods containing simple carbohydrate (foods in the milk and fruit groups) contributed ______ kcalories.
   - *Group C:* Foods containing mostly concentrated simple carbohydrate (sugar, honey, molasses, syrup, jam, jelly, candy, cakes, doughnuts, sweet rolls, cola beverages, and so on) contributed ______ kcalories.

   Does your concentrated sugar intake (Group C) fall within the recommended maximum of 10 percent of total daily kcalories? ______ If not, what food choices account for the excess sugar? ______________________________

7. Estimate the number of pounds of sugar (concentrated simple carbohydrate) you eat in a year (1 pound = 454 grams):

   ______ kcalories from Group C ÷ 4 = ______ grams/day.

(continued)

Self-Study (continued)

______ grams/day × 365 days/year = ______ grams/year.

______ grams/year ÷ 454 grams/pound = ______ pounds/year.

How does your yearly sugar intake compare with the estimated U.S. and Canadian average of about 75 pounds per person per year? Comment on this. ______________________

When dietitians analyze a client's diet with respect to carbohydrate intake, they check for total carbohydrate, complex carbohydrate, sugar, and fiber. From this information, they can reinforce a client's current habits or make recommendations for changes.

Form 6
Carbohydrate and Sugar kCalories

Average daily carbohydrate intake: ________ grams

Total kcalories from carbohydrate: ________ kcalories (grams × 4)

Total kcalories from all sources: ________ kcalories

Total kcalories from carbohydrates should equal 55 to 60 % of total kcalories from all sources. Percentage of kcalories from carbohydrate: ________%

Breakdown of carbohydrate kcalories:

A. ________ complex

B. ________ nutritious simple

C. ________ concentrated simple

kCalories from concentrated simple sugars should equal 10% or less of total kcalories from all sources. Percentage of kcalories from concentrated simple sugars: ________%

■ STUDY QUESTIONS ■

1. What are the simple carbohydrates?
2. What are the complex carbohydrates?
3. What is the chief energy source of the body?
4. What is glycogen?
5. Name and describe the two types of alternative sweeteners.
6. What health benefits does a diet high in complex carbohydrates offer?
7. Describe some of the health benefits of fiber.
8. What is the "protein-sparing" effect of carbohydrate?

NUTRITION IN PRACTICE 2

Nutrition and Dental Health

The health value of eating complex carbohydrate-rich foods was emphasized throughout Chapter 2. These are sound nutrition practices that promote overall health, but unfortunately, they do not necessarily promote dental health. Nutrients in general support dental health in the same ways they support whole-body health, but carbohydrates in particular have to be handled in special ways to maximize dental health.

Nutrition plays a major role in facilitating the development of healthy teeth. Table 2–3 shows the effects of nutrient deficiencies on tooth development. The foods you eat and the times you eat them also play a major role in promoting or preventing dental caries—a pervasive health problem throughout the world.

What is dental caries?

Dental caries is an infectious oral disease that develops in the tooth enamel (see Figure 2–4). Caries develops when bacteria that reside in the plaque of teeth consume and metabolize carbohydrates, producing acids that attack the tooth enamel. Thus at least two main ingredients are required to make dental caries: bacteria and carbohydrates. In addition, factors such as heredity, nutrition status during early tooth development, dental hygiene practices, and fluoride intake influence a person's susceptibility to caries.

How do sugar and other carbohydrate-rich foods promote caries development?

The bacteria that promote dental caries thrive on food particles that contain carbohydrate. Both sugar and starch can support bacterial growth. Equally important is the length of time the food stays in the mouth, and this depends on how soon you brush your teeth after eating and how sticky the food is. The damage a food does relates to both the carbohydrate content and the food's stickiness. A sticky food, such as raisins or granola, causes more caries than a sugary food that is easily rinsed off, such as a sugary beverage.

You can eat sugar without inviting tooth decay if you remove it from your tooth surfaces promptly. A rule of thumb is that bacterial action is maximal in the first 20 minutes after the first contact. If immediate brushing is not possible, water or other beverages swished in the mouth after a meal can effectively rinse the teeth. Once-a-day flossing may also effectively control formation of caries, regardless of the carbohydrate content of the diet. Some people may never get caries because they have inherited resistance to them.

Can you rinse your mouth with your own saliva?

Yes, and some foods stimulate more saliva flow than others. Saliva protects against caries formation in several ways. It not only rinses the mouth, but also dilutes the caries-causing acid produced by bacteria, exerts antibacterial action, and provides protective minerals.[24] Foods that elicit saliva flow may therefore defend against caries formation, but not all of them are protective; foods that also liberate sugar may promote acid formation. Apples are an example: they stimulate saliva flow, but they also liberate sugar,

Table 2–3
Nutrient Deficiencies Affecting Tooth Development

NUTRIENT DEFICIENCY	EFFECT ON TOOTH DEVELOPMENT
Protein	Small, irregularly shaped teeth; delayed eruption; high caries susceptibility
Vitamin C	Disturbance of dentin formation
Vitamin A	Disturbance of enamel formation, delayed eruption
Vitamin D	Poor mineralization, pitting, striations
Calcium	Poor mineralization
Phosphorus	Poor mineralization
Magnesium	Enamel underdeveloped
Iron	High caries susceptibility
Zinc	High caries susceptibility
Fluoride	High caries susceptibility

Figure 2–4
A Tooth
The inner layer of dentin is bonelike material. The outer layer is enamel, which is harder than bone. Caries begin when acid dissolves the tooth's enamel.

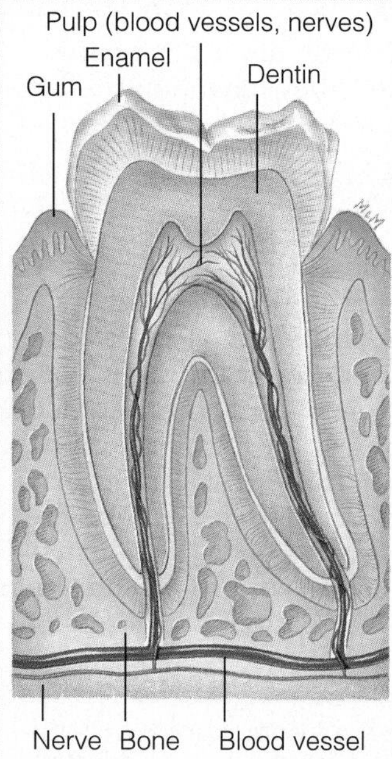

so they have both caries-preventing and caries-promoting effects. As you can see, many different factors influence caries development, making it difficult to predict exactly which foods are cariogenic.

Are any foods strictly caries preventing?

Yes. Some foods stimulate saliva flow and do not contribute to acid formation in the mouth: cheese is an example. Such foods are good choices to eat at the end of a meal. Cheese is a powerful saliva stimulant and does not promote acid formation, so it reduces the cariogenicity of a meal. Furthermore, the high calcium and phosphorus content of cheese contributes to dental health.

High-fiber foods are, in general, anticariogenic, especially if their carbohydrate content is low. For example, raw vegetables do not stick to the teeth, and because they require vigorous chewing, they stimulate saliva flow. Research indicates that cocoa products (including chocolate), coffee, tea, and beer all contain tannin, an acid that prevents caries formation.[25] Table 2–4 lists some dietary recommendations for controlling dental caries.

Besides foods, what other factors protect against dental caries development?

Research shows that when fluoride is added to the water supply, the children in the community have fewer dental caries than children who drink nonfluoridated water. In fact, water fluoridation is the most effective, least expensive way to provide dental care to everyone. The following recommendations will maximize protection against dental caries:

- Watch for hidden sugars in foods; use low-sugar or sugar-free products whenever possible.
- Restrict sweets to mealtimes.
- After you eat a meal or a between-meal snack, brush and

Table 2–4
Dietary Recommendations for Controlling Dental Caries

FOOD GROUP	LOW CARIOGENICITY (USE WHEN TEETH CANNOT BE BRUSHED IMMEDIATELY)	HIGH CARIOGENICITY (DO NOT USE UNLESS FOLLOWED BY PROMPT AND THOROUGH DENTAL HYGIENE)
Dairy	Milk, cheese, plain yogurt	Ice cream, ice milk, milkshakes, fruited yogurts, eggnog
Meats/meat alternates	Meat, fish, poultry, eggs, legumes	Peanut butter with added sugar, luncheon meats with added sugar, meats with sugared glazes
Fruits[a]	Fresh, packed in water or juice	Dried, packed in syrup, jams, jellies, preserves, fruit juices and drinks
Vegetables	Most vegetables	Candied sweet potatoes, glazed carrots
Breads/cereals[b]	Popcorn, soda crackers, toast, hard rolls, pretzels, corn chips, pizza	Cookies, sweet rolls, pies, cakes, cereals
Other	Sugarless gum, coffee or tea without sugar, nuts, red licorice[c]	Sugared soft drinks, candy, fudge, caramels, honey, sugars, syrups

[a]Tiny particles of bananas can get lodged between teeth and decompose, increasing risk of caries.
[b]Tiny particles of breads, crackers, and chips can also become lodged in teeth, promoting caries formation.
[c]Red licorice contains gylcyrrhizin, a flavoring that inhibits mineral loss.

floss, or at least, rinse with water.

- Limit the time that teeth are exposed to sticky foods.
- In any case, brush and floss at least once daily.
- Visit a dentist regularly.
- Drink fluoridated water; provide infants and children with fluoride supplements when such water is not available.
- Eat a balanced diet composed of a variety of foods that will maintain adequate nutrition status.
- Eat foods that are rich in calcium and phosphorus.
- Eat a variety of firm, fibrous foods that will stimulate saliva flow.

In summary, learning and practicing sound dental hygiene habits, as well as developing eating habits that are consistent with both dental health and nutritional health, will serve a person throughout life.

■ NOTES ■

1. E. Gudmand-Hoyer, The clinical significance of disaccharide maldigestion, *American Journal of Clinical Nutrition* (Supplement) 59 (1994): 735–741.
2. M. I. McBurney and L. U. Thompson, Dietary fiber and energy balance: Integration of the human ileostomy and in vitro fermentation models, *Animal Feed Science and Technology* 23 (1989): 261–275.
3. C. J. Lewis and coauthors, Nutrient intakes and body weights of persons consuming high and moderate levels of added sugars, *Journal of the American Dietetic Association* 92 (1992): 708–713.
4. B. Szepesi, Carbohydrates, in *Present Knowledge in Nutrition*, 6th ed., ed. M. L. Brown (Washington, D.C.: International Life Sciences Institute—Nutrition Foundation, 1990).
5. Food and Nutrition Board, National Research Council, Committee on Diet and Health, *Implications for Reducing Chronic Disease Risk* (Washington, D.C.: National Academy Press, 1989).
6. Lewis and coauthors, 1992.
7. G. M. Raven, Parma symposium: Current controversies in nutrition, *American Journal of Clinical Nutrition* 47 (1988): 1078–1082.
8. M. Kinsbourne, Sugar and the hyperactive child, *New England Journal of Medicine* 330 (1994): 355–356; M. L. Wolraich and coauthors, Effects of diets high in sucrose or aspartame on the behavior and cognitive performance of children, *New England Journal of Medicine* 330 (1994): 301–307.
9. E. H. Wender and M. V. Solanto, Effects of sugar on aggressive and inattentive behavior in children with Attention Deficit Disorder with Hyperactivity and normal children, *Pediatrics* 88 (1991): 960–966.
10. A. Sheilham, Why free sugar consumption should be below 15 kg per person per year in industrial countries: The dental evidence, *British Dental Journal* 171 (1991): 63–65.
11. W. L. Dills, Sugar alcohols as bulk sweeteners, *Annual Review of Nutrition* 9 (1989): 161–186.
12. Dills, 1989.
13. Withdrawal of certain pre-1986 proposed rules: final action, *Federal Register* 56 (1991): 67442; as cited in Position of the American Dietetic Association: Use of nutritive and nonnutritive sweeteners, *Journal of the American Dietetic Association* 93 (1993): 816–821.
14. Position of the American Dietetic Association: Use of nutritive and nonnutritive sweeteners, *Journal of the American Dietetic Association* 93 (1993): 816–821.
15. Position of the American Dietetic Association, 1993.
16. H. H. Butchko and F. N. Kotsonis, Acceptable daily intake vs actual intake: The aspartame example, *Journal of the American College of Nutrition* 10 (1991): 258–266.
17. B. J. Rolls, Effects of intense sweeteners on hunger, food intake, and body weight: A review, *American Journal of Clinical Nutrition* 53 (1991): 872–877; Position of the American Dietetic Association, 1993.
18. Position of the American Dietetic Association, 1993.
19. C. M. Ripsin and coauthors, Oat products and lipid lowering: A meta-analysis, *Journal of the American Medical Association* 267 (1992): 3317–3325.
20. J. F. Swain and coauthors, Comparison of the effects of oat bran and low-fiber wheat on serum lipoprotein levels and blood pressure, *New England Journal of Medicine* 322 (1990): 147–152.
21. D. J. A. Jenkins and coauthors, Effect on blood lipids of very high intakes of fiber in diets low in saturated fat and cholesterol, *New England Journal of Medicine* 329 (1993): 21–26; J. W. Anderson and coauthors, Prospective, randomized controlled comparison of the effects of low-fat plus high-fiber diets on serum lipid concentrations, *American Journal of Clinical Nutrition* 56

(1992): 887–894.
22. J. L. Slavin, Dietary fiber: Classification, chemical analyses, and food sources, *Journal of the American Dietetic Association* 87 (1987): 1164–1171.
23. Position of the American Dietetic Association: Health implications of dietary fiber, *Journal of the American Dietetic Association* 88 (1988): 216.
24. J. H. Shaw and E. A. Sweeney, Oral health, in *Nutritional Support of Medical Practice,* 2nd ed., eds. H. A. Schneider, C. E. Anderson, and D. B. Coursin (Philadelphia: Harper and Row, 1983), pp. 517–540.
25. University of California School of Dentistry, as cited in Dentists say sweet tooth isn't kiss of death for enamel, *Atlanta Constitution* March 21, 1991.

3

Lipids

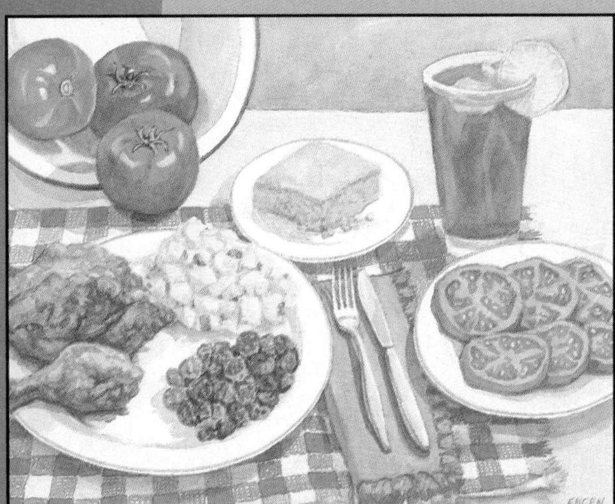

CONTENTS

You probably know that too much fat in the diet imposes health risks, but you may be surprised to learn that too little does, too. It is true, though, that people in the United States are more likely to eat too much fat than too little.

lipids: a family of compounds that includes triglycerides (fats and oils), phospholipids, and sterols.

Fat is a member of the class of compounds called lipids. The lipids in foods and in the human body include triglycerides (fats and oils), phospholipids, and sterols.

Energy from Fat Lipids perform many tasks in the body, but most importantly, they provide energy. A constant flow of energy is so vital to life that, in a pinch, any other function is sacrificed to maintain it. Chapter 2 described one safeguard against such an emergency—the stores of glycogen in the liver that provide glucose to the blood whenever the supply runs short. The body's stores of glycogen are limited, however. In contrast, the body's capacity to store fat for energy is virtually unlimited due to the fat-storing cells of the adipose tissue. Unlike most body cells, which can store only limited amounts of fat, the adipose, or fat, cells seem able to expand almost indefinitely. The more fat they store, the larger they grow. Figure 3–1 shows a fat cell. The fat stored in these cells supplies 60 percent of the body's ongoing energy needs during rest.[1] During exercise or prolonged periods of food deprivation, fat stores may make an even greater energy contribution.

adipose tissue: the body's fat, which consists of masses of fat-storing cells called adipose cells.

Roles of Body Fat In addition to supplying energy, fat serves other roles in the body. Natural oils in the skin provide a radiant complexion; in

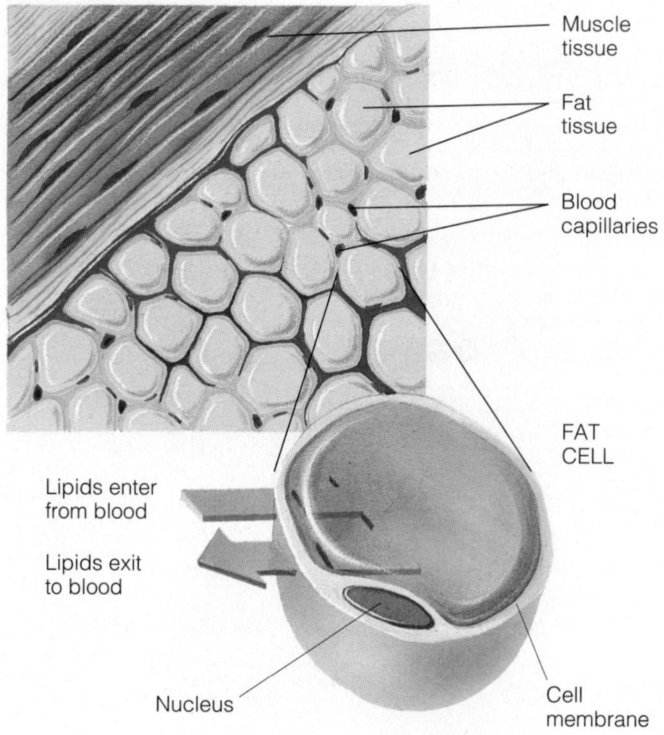

Figure 3–1
A Fat Cell
Within the fat cell, lipid is stored in a droplet. This droplet can greatly enlarge, and the fat cell membrane will grow to accommodate its swollen contents.

the scalp, they help nourish the hair and make it glossy. The layer of fat beneath the skin insulates the body from extremes of temperature. A pad of hard fat beneath each kidney protects it from being jarred and damaged, even during a motorcycle ride on a bumpy road. The soft fat in a woman's breasts protects her mammary glands from heat and cold and cushions them against shock. The fat that lies embedded in muscle tissue shares with muscle glycogen the task of providing energy when the muscles are active. The phospholipids and the sterol cholesterol are cell membrane constituents that help maintain the structure and health of all cells. Table 3–1 summarizes the major functions of fats in the body.

Table 3–1
The Functions of Fats in the Body

FATS IN THE BODY:
▸ Provide energy.
▸ Insulate the body against temperature extremes.
▸ Protect the body's vital organs from shock.
▸ Form the major material of cell membranes.

The Chemist's View of Lipids

The diverse and vital functions that lipids play in the body reveal why eating too little fat can be harmful. As mentioned earlier, though, too much fat in the diet seems to be the bigger problem for most people. To understand both the beneficial and harmful effects that fats exert on the body, a closer look at the structure and function of members of the lipid family is in order.

Triglycerides

When people talk about fat—for example, "I'm too fat" or "That meat is fatty"—they are usually referring to triglycerides. Among lipids, triglycerides predominate—both in the diet and in the body. The name *triglyceride* almost explains itself: three fatty acids (*tri*) attached to a glycerol "backbone." Figure 3–2 shows how three fatty acids combine with glycerol to make a triglyceride.

triglycerides: compounds composed of glycerol with three fatty acids attached.
tri = three
glyceride = a compound of glycerol

fatty acids: organic compounds composed of a chain of carbon atoms with hydrogens attached and an acid group at one end.

glycerol (GLISS-er-ol): a small compound related to carbohydrates that can form the backbone of triglycerides and phospholipids.

Fatty Acids

When energy from any energy-yielding nutrient is to be stored as fat, the nutrient is first broken into small fragments. Then the fragments are

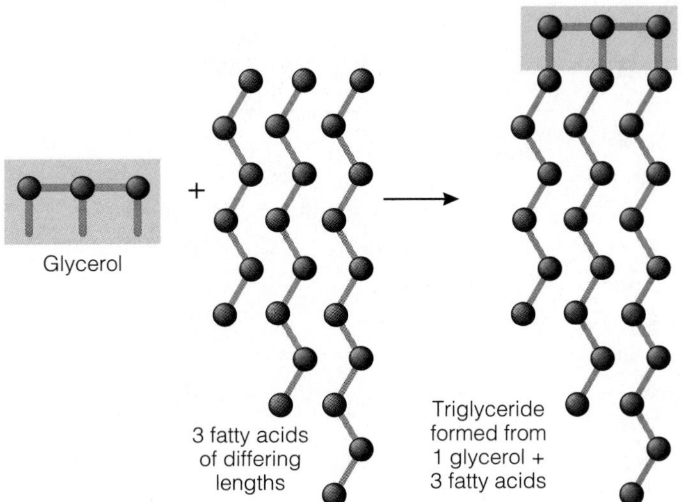

Figure 3–2
Triglyceride Formation
Glycerol, a small, water-soluble carbohydrate derivative, plus three fatty acids, equals a triglyceride.

linked together into chains known as fatty acids. The fatty acids are then packaged, three at a time, with glycerol to make triglycerides.

Chain Length and Saturation Fatty acids may differ from one another in two ways—in chain length and in degree of saturation. The chain length of a fatty acid affects the way it is absorbed (see Chapter 5). Saturation refers to its chemical structure—specifically, to the number of hydrogens the fatty acid chain is holding. If every available bond from the carbons is holding a hydrogen, the chain is called a saturated fatty acid, meaning that the chain is filled to capacity with hydrogen. The first zigzag structure in Figure 3–3 represents a saturated fatty acid.

saturated fatty acid: a fatty acid carrying the maximum possible number of hydrogen atoms (having no points of unsaturation). A saturated fat is a triglyceride that contains three saturated fatty acids.

unsaturated fatty acid: a fatty acid in which one or more points of unsaturation occur (includes monounsaturated and polyunsaturated fatty acids).

monounsaturated fatty acid: a fatty acid that has one point of unsaturation where hydrogens are missing, for example, oleic acid.

polyunsaturated fatty acid (PUFA): a fatty acid with two or more points of unsaturation. For example, linoleic acid has two such points, and linolenic acid has three. Thus a polyunsaturated *fat* is composed of triglycerides containing a high percentage of PUFA.

Unsaturated Fatty Acids In some fatty acids, especially those of plants and fish, hydrogens are missing in the fatty acid chains. The points where the hydrogens are missing are called points of unsaturation, and a chain containing such points is called an unsaturated fatty acid. If there is one point of unsaturation (as in oleic acid), the chain is monounsaturated. The second structure in Figure 3–3 is an example.

If there are *two* or more points of unsaturation, then the fatty acid is polyunsaturated (see the third structure in Figure 3–3). You sometimes see polyunsaturated fatty acids abbreviated on food labels as PUFA.

Hard and Soft Fat A triglyceride can contain any combination of fatty acids—long chain or short chain; saturated, monounsaturated, or polyunsaturated. Whether a fat is soft or hard depends on which fatty acids it contains. Fats that contain the shorter-chain or the more unsaturated fatty acids are softer and melt more readily (discussed later in this

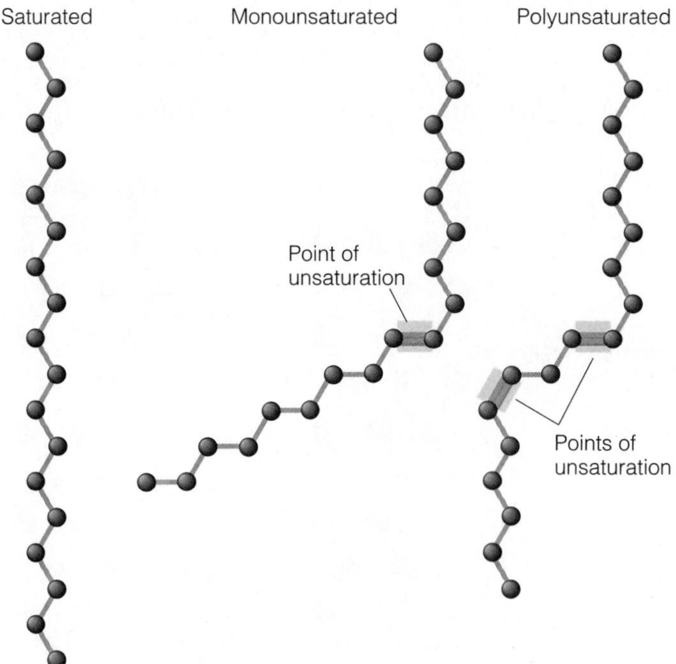

Figure 3–3
Three Fatty Acids
The more carbon atoms in a fatty acid, the longer its chain length. The more hydrogen atoms attached to those carbons, the more saturated the fatty acid.

chapter). Each animal species (including human beings) obeys its own genetic program and makes its own characteristic kinds of triglycerides; but fats in the diet can, within limits, affect the types of triglycerides made. For example, animals raised for food can be fed diets containing softer or harder fats to give their meat or other products softer or harder fat, whichever consumers demand. People, too, incorporate the fatty acids they eat into their own tissues.

Essential Fatty Acids The human body can synthesize all the fatty acids it needs from carbohydrate, fat, or protein except for two—linoleic and linolenic acid. Both are polyunsaturated fatty acids and cannot be made from other substances in the body. They must be obtained from food and are therefore called *essential* fatty acids. Linoleic and linolenic acid are found in small amounts in plant and fish oils, and the body readily stores them, making deficiencies unlikely. From both of these essential fatty acids, the body makes important hormonelike substances that regulate a wide range of body functions: blood pressure, clot formation, blood lipid concentration, the immune response, the inflammation response to injury, and many others.[2] These two essential nutrients also serve as structural components of cell membranes.

linoleic acid, linolenic acid: polyunsaturated fatty acids, essential for human beings.

essential fatty acids: fatty acids that the body requires but cannot make in amounts sufficient to meet its physiological need.

Linoleic Acid: An Omega-6 Fatty Acid Linoleic acid is an omega-6 fatty acid found in the seeds of plants and in the oils harvested from the seeds. Any diet that contains vegetable oils, seeds, nuts, and whole-grain foods provides enough linoleic acid to meet the body's needs. Researchers have long known and appreciated the importance of the omega-6 fatty acid family.

omega: the last letter of the Greek alphabet (Ω, sometimes replaced by the letter *w* or *n*), used by chemists to refer to the position of the last double bond in a fatty acid. In omega-6 fatty acids, the last double bond is six carbons back along the chain; in omega-3 fatty acids, it is three carbons back.

Linolenic Acid and Other Omega-3 Fatty Acids Linolenic acid belongs to a family of polyunsaturated fatty acids known as omega-3 fatty acids, a family that also includes EPA and DHA, seen on supplement labels. EPA and DHA are found primarily in fish oils. As mentioned, the human body cannot make linolenic acid, but given dietary linolenic acid, it can make EPA and DHA, although the process is slow.[3]

The importance of omega-3 fatty acids has only recently been recognized. During the 1980s, extensive worldwide research efforts began to unveil impressive roles for EPA and DHA in metabolism and disease prevention. DHA is one of the most abundant structural lipids in the brain, and both EPA and DHA are needed for normal brain development.[4] EPA and DHA are also especially active in the rods and cones of the retina of the eye.[5] Today researchers know that these omega-3 fatty acids are essential for normal growth and development and that they may play an important role in the prevention and treatment of heart disease, hypertension, arthritis, and cancer.[6]

omega-6 fatty acid: a polyunsaturated fatty acid with its endmost double bond six carbons back from the end of its carbon chain, long recognized as important in nutrition, Linoleic acid is an example.

omega-3 fatty acid: a polyunsaturated fatty acid with its endmost double bond three carbons back from the end of its carbon chain, relatively newly recognized as important in nutrition. Linolenic acid is an example.

DHA, EPA: omega-3 fatty acids made from linolenic acid. The full name for DHA is docosahexaenoic (DOE-cosa-HEXA-ee-NO-ick) acid. The full name for EPA is eicosapentaenoic (EYE-cosa-PENTA-ee-NO-ICK) acid.

Omega-3 Supplements Omega-3 fatty acid supplements are being aggressively marketed as a cure-all for many different diseases without regard for consumer safety. While some claims are based on research, confirmation that fish oil can prevent or treat heart disease, cancer, or other diseases in individuals or populations is lacking. Experts do agree that adding *fish* to the diet two or three times per week may be of benefit in preventing heart disease.[7] The idea that fish oil *supplements* are beneficial and safe in any amount is erroneous, however.

In the first place, the supplements themselves may carry hazards. They may contain toxic amounts of fat-soluble vitamins or pesticide residues. Even when the supplements are not toxic, they may have harmful effects on the body. One potential problem is that the supplement form may not function the same way as the form available directly from foods. Furthermore, omega-3 and omega-6 fatty acids compete for the same slots in the body. Consequently, taking supplements of one can easily induce a deficiency of the other. Still another drawback is that fish oil can also cause or aggravate illness by altering blood lipids or blood clotting. Finally, the quantities of omega-3 fatty acids in supplements vary widely from what the labels say they contain.

These fish provide at least 1 gram of omega-3 fatty acids, including EPA and DHA, in 100 grams of fish (about 3.5 ounces):

- Anchovy, European.
- Bluefish.
- Capelin conch.
- Herring.
- Mackerel.
- Mullet.
- Sablefish.
- Salmon, all varieties.
- Sturgeon.
- Trout, lake.
- Tuna, white albacore or bluefin (not canned light tuna).
- Whitefish, lake.

Eat Dark-Meat Fish Questions also remain about the appropriate amount of omega-3 fatty acids for a day's intake. While these questions await answers, the best way to increase your intake of omega-3 fatty acids is to eat several portions of fish each week, particularly the kinds listed in the margin. The darker flesh of fish has the highest fat content, and this is where most omega-3 fatty acids are found.

Phospholipids

Up to now, this discussion has focused on one of the three classes of lipids, the triglycerides (fats and oils), and their component parts, the fatty acids (see Table 3–2). The other two classes of lipids, the phospholipids and sterols, make up only 5 percent of the lipids in the diet, but they are nevertheless worthy of attention. Among the phospholipids, the lecithins are of particular interest.

phospholipids: one of the three main classes of lipids; these compounds are similar to triglycerides but have choline (or another compound) and a phosphorus-containing acid in place of one of the fatty acids.

lecithin: one of the phospholipids.

Structure of Phospholipids Like the triglycerides, the lecithins and some other phospholipids have a backbone of glycerol; they differ from

Table 3–2
The Major Lipids

TRIGLYCERIDES (FATS AND OILS)	PHOSPHOLIPIDS	STEROLS
Glycerol	Lecithin (example)	Cholesterol (example)
Fatty acids		
Saturated		
Monounsaturated		
Polyunsaturated		
Omega-6		
Omega-3		

the triglycerides in having only two fatty acids attached to them. In place of the third fatty acid is a molecule of choline or a similar compound. Lecithin is the best-known phospholipid.

Roles of Phospholipids Lecithins and other phospholipids are important constituents of cell membranes. They also act as emulsifiers, helping to keep other fats in solution in the blood and body fluids.

emulsifiers: substances that mix with both fat and water and that permanently disperse the fat in the water, forming an emulsion.

Phospholipids: Not Essential Lecithins periodically receive noisy attention in the popular press and are credited with great deeds. You may have heard that they are a major constituent of cell membranes (true), that the functioning of all cells depends on the integrity of the cell membranes (true), and that you must therefore purchase bottles of lecithin and give yourself daily doses (false). The body digests lecithins before it absorbs them, so the lecithins you eat do not reach the body tissues intact. Instead, the lecithins used for building cell membranes are made from scratch by the liver. In other words, the lecithins are not essential nutrients.

Before buying bottles of lecithin or any other wonder substance, ask yourself, "Do I really need this? What is the evidence that my body is likely to be deficient?"

Sterols

Sterols are large, complex molecules consisting of interconnected rings of carbon. Cholesterol is the most familiar sterol, but others, such as vitamin D and the sex hormones (for example, testosterone), are important, too.

sterols: one of the three main classes of lipids; sterols include cholesterol, vitamin D, and the sex hormones (such as testosterone).

Cholesterol Synthesis Like the lecithins, cholesterol can be made by the body, so it is not an essential nutrient. Your liver is manufacturing it now, as you read, at the rate of perhaps 50,000,000,000,000,000 molecules per second. The raw materials that the liver uses to make cholesterol can all be taken from glucose or saturated fatty acids. In other words, cholesterol can be made from either carbohydrate or fat. More than 90 percent of all the body's cholesterol ends up in the cells, where it performs vital structural and metabolic functions.

Cholesterol's Two Routes in the Body After being made, cholesterol either leaves the liver or is transformed there into related compounds such as vitamin D. Cholesterol leaves the liver by two routes:

1. It may be made into bile and pass into the intestine.
2. It may travel, via the bloodstream, to all the body's cells.

Cholesterol Recycled The bile that is made from cholesterol in the liver is released into the intestine to aid in the digestion and absorption of fat (see Chapter 5). After it does its job, some of the bile is reabsorbed, and some is excreted in the feces. Some of the cholesterol (as reabsorbed bile) is thus recycled—back to the liver, once again into bile, and back to the intestine again.

bile: a compound made by the liver from cholesterol and stored in the gallbladder. Bile prepares fat for digestion.

Cholesterol Excreted On its way around this cycle, during the time it spends out in the intestine, some of the bile can be trapped by certain kinds of dietary fibers or by some medications, which carry it out of the body in feces. The excretion of bile reduces the total amount of cholesterol remaining in the body.

Lipoproteins are made by both the intestine and the liver. Chapter 5 tells the story of lipid transport.

Cholesterol Transport Some cholesterol, packaged with other lipids and protein, leaves the liver via the arteries and is transported to the body tissues by the blood. The packages are called lipoproteins. As the lipoproteins travel through the body, tissues can extract lipids from them.

Fats and Health

cardiovascular disease (CVD): disease of the heart and blood vessels. The two most common forms of CVD are *atherosclerosis* and *hypertension* (Chapter 26).

Of all the dietary factors related to diseases prevalent in developed countries, fat is by far the most significant. Excessive intakes of dietary fat contribute to many diseases including obesity, diabetes, cancer, cardiovascular disease (CVD), and probably other diseases and disorders as well. Heart disease is the number one killer of adults in this country. In the interest of good health and disease prevention, the one change that most people should make in their diets is to limit their intakes of total fat. It is especially important to limit saturated fat and cholesterol.

Fats and Fatty Acids

The cholesterol that accumulates in arteries is manufactured largely from fragments derived from saturated fat. Most people realize that elevated blood cholesterol is an important risk factor for CVD. The higher the blood cholesterol, the greater the risk of heart disease. Most people may not realize, though, that cholesterol in *food* is not the main influential factor in raising *blood* cholesterol. It is total fat, especially saturated fat, that raises blood cholesterol. An extensive review of more than 200 studies of the effects of dietary fats on blood cholesterol revealed the same conclusions over and over again:

- Saturated fatty acids elevate blood cholesterol and are the main dietary determinants of blood cholesterol levels.*[8]

Less influential, but still significant, were the following factors:

- Polyunsaturated fatty acids lower blood cholesterol.
- Dietary cholesterol elevates blood cholesterol.

Saturated Fat and Blood Cholesterol In support of these conclusions, a recent study found that diets low in saturated fatty acids helped lower blood cholesterol in men.[9] Adding polyunsaturated fatty acids to the diet lowered blood cholesterol further. Probably, the researchers speculated, reducing dietary cholesterol would have reduced blood cholesterol still further. These results are consistent with population studies that

---

*It should be noted that not all saturated fatty acids have the same cholesterol-raising effect. For example, stearic acid, an 18-carbon fatty acid, does not raise blood cholesterol.

show that people who eat diets high in saturated fat are more likely to die from heart disease than those who eat the same diet, but also eat fish (rich in polyunsaturated fatty acids) a couple of times a week.[10]

Omega-3 Fatty Acids and Blood Cholesterol Of the polyunsaturated fatty acids, the omega-3 fatty acids appear to reduce blood cholesterol the most. This effect was first noticed when researchers learned that the Inuit peoples of Alaska and Greenland, despite high-energy, high-fat, high-cholesterol diets, enjoyed relative freedom from heart diseases—especially atherosclerosis. Analysis of the foods common in Inuit diets, which derive primarily from marine animals, revealed that they were rich in omega-3 fatty acids, particularly EPA and DHA. It is research findings such as these that have led the American Heart Association to recommend two to three fish meals a week.

Omega-3 Fatty Acids and Cancer Omega-3 fatty acids may also help to prevent cancer. High *fat* intakes appear to *promote* cancer, and animal studies suggest that the fatty acids most likely to promote cancer are polyunsaturated fatty acids from vegetable oils (mostly omega-6 fatty acids). In comparison, saturated fats have little or no effect, and polyunsaturated fats from fish oils (mostly omega-3 fatty acids) may delay cancer development, slow tumor growth rates, and reduce the size and number of tumors.[11]

Recommendations Dietary guidelines recommend that *total* fat intake should not exceed 30 percent of the day's total energy intake; 20 percent might be ideal. Saturated fats should contribute less than 10 percent; polyunsaturated fats should not exceed 10 percent; monounsaturates should provide the remaining 10 percent or so. Limiting dietary fat intake to 30 percent or less of total energy requires careful planning at every meal. According to research on people's food choices, people eat about 37 percent of their energy intakes as fat.[12] Even though this is less than in the recent past, it is more than at the turn of the century, when foods were less highly processed, and it is more than people need. Guidelines for cholesterol intake recommend less than 300 milligrams daily.[13] The next section tells why, and a later "How-to" box offers specific suggestions on putting these guidelines into practice.

Cholesterol

As discussed earlier, dietary cholesterol is less influential in raising blood cholesterol than is total dietary fat, especially saturated fat. Nevertheless, blood cholesterol does rise as more cholesterol is eaten, but the magnitude of the rise varies depending on people's cholesterol metabolism and on the amounts of dietary cholesterol they normally consume. It seems that the more cholesterol a person eats, the less sensitive the person's blood cholesterol is to changes in diet.[14] The typical American diet contains about 400 milligrams of cholesterol daily, a quantity large enough to help explain why changes in dietary cholesterol seem to have only a modest influence on blood cholesterol for many people. In contrast, when dietary cholesterol intakes are exceptionally low (below 160 milligrams per day), even small changes in cholesterol intake will influence blood cholesterol. When people reduce their intakes from 400 to 300 milligrams a day, blood cholesterol may decline by some 5 to 10 percent.

Fat Substitutes

As people learn more and more about the health consequences of high-fat diets, fat substitutes, also known as fat replacements or artificial fats, offer hope for the prevention and treatment of heart disease and obesity. Skeptics say that people will use fat substitutes the same way they use artificial sweeteners: in *addition* to fats, rather than *instead* of fats. Some research shows that when people use fat substitutes, they eat less fat but more sugar and starch, so that their energy intakes remain constant.[15]

Types of Fat Substitutes Food chemists have been working for decades on ways to reduce the fat in foods. Today shoppers are overwhelmed by the number of new fat-reduced products on grocery shelves. Fat-free bakery products, cheeses, frozen desserts, and many other products are available that taste rich but offer less than half a gram of fat in a serving. Products using traditional ingredients such as sugar, starch, nonfat milk, soluble fiber, or egg whites in place of fat are selling well.[16]

Some fat substitutes, made from substances already in the diet, are digested and used by the body in the same way as those original substances; examples are Simplesse and Stellar. Other fat substitutes, made from new substances, are indigestible and so contribute no food energy; examples are olestra and Oatrim.

Simplesse The Food and Drug Administration (FDA) declared Simplesse safe for use in ice cream and frozen desserts in 1990.[17] Simplesse is made from protein—either egg white or milk—which is processed into mistlike particles similar in consistency to fat. Because the components of Simplesse have long been used in foods, safety studies are not required. This fat substitute mimics the rich taste and texture of fat but cuts the kcalorie content by up to 80 percent. Since proteins coagulate at high temperatures, Simplesse cannot be used for frying or cooking, but can be used in ice creams, yogurts, salad dressings, mayonnaise, and butter.

Stellar Unlike Simplesse, the fat substitute Stellar can be heated. Stellar is a starch-based product that is derived from corn. Because Stellar is defined as a modified food starch and meets U.S. regulatory requirements, it is approved for use by food manufacturers. Stellar can replace the fat in a wide range of foods including margarine, salad dressings, ice cream, cheese products, meat products, soups, gravies, and sauces.

Olestra Olestra, which was formerly known as sucrose polyester (SPE), was invented in the late 1960s. It is a synthetic combination of sucrose and fatty acids that looks, feels, and tastes like food fat. Unlike other sucrose or fatty acids, though, olestra is indigestible; the body has no way to take it apart. Olestra can therefore be substituted for fats without adding kcalories or raising a person's blood lipids.

Olestra is currently awaiting FDA approval. Because olestra is considered a new structure and does not break down to its component parts during digestion, it must undergo stringent safety tests before approval. Research on animals and human beings seems to support the safety of olestra as a partial replacement for dietary fats and oils.

Oatrim Researchers at the U.S. Department of Agriculture (USDA) are testing a new extract of oats as a fat substitute.[18] The product, called Oatrim by the USDA researchers, is stable when heated and can be used as a fat substitute to reduce the energy content of foods such as frozen desserts, salad dressings, soups, and high-fiber baked goods. Researchers say Oatrim reduces the energy content of frozen desserts like ice cream by half. Unlike Simplesse or other fat substitutes, Oatrim retains the qualities of its fiber, so it lowers cholesterol not only by replacing saturated fat but also by providing fiber.

Do Fat Substitutes Work? Research has not yet shown that fat substitutes promote weight loss or lower blood lipid concentrations. If people use fat substitutes literally as substitutes for fat in their diets, then perhaps potential health benefits will be realized. Some experts are concerned, though, that people may feel at liberty to eat *more* high-fat foods by rationalizing that they obtain fat "credit" when they eat foods containing fat substitutes. Indeed, this seems to be the case with artificial sweeteners. Although consumption of sugar substitutes has risen since their introduction, sugar consumption has risen as well. Another concern is that people may become so carried away with eating foods containing fat substitutes that they will neglect to eat more nutrient-dense foods such as fresh fruits and vegetables. It seems that with fat substitutes, as with most things in life, moderation is the key to appropriate use.

Fats in Foods

Fats are important in foods as well as in the body. Many of the compounds that give foods their flavor and aroma are found in fats and oils. The delicious aromas associated with bacon, ham, and other meats, as well as with onions being fried, come from fats. Fats in foods also slow digestion, lending satiety to meals. People feel fuller longer after eating meals that include fat. Fats also make foods tender. Four vitamins—A, D, E, and K—are soluble in fat. When the fat is removed from a food, many of the fat-soluble compounds, including these vitamins, are also removed. Table 3–3 summarizes the roles of fats in foods.

satiety: the feeling of fullness or satisfaction that people feel after meals.

Table 3–3
The Functions of Fat in Foods

FATS IN FOODS:
▸ Contribute flavor and aroma. ▸ Provide satiety. ▸ Help make foods tender. ▸ Carry fat-soluble vitamins.

Fats are also an important part of most people's ethnic or national cuisines. Each culture has its own favorite food sources of fats and oils. In Canada, canola oil (also known as rapeseed oil) is widely used. In the Mediterranean area, Greeks, Italians, and Spaniards rely heavily on olive oil. Both canola oil and olive oil are rich sources of monounsaturated fatty acids. Asians use the polyunsaturated oil of soybeans. Jewish people traditionally employ chicken fat. Everywhere in North America, butter and margarine are widely used.

These cultural associations along with the very real pleasures fats contribute to meals help explain why fat consumption is so high. Nevertheless, reducing dietary fat is the single most important thing you can do for health; it is the top recommendation of almost every nutrition authority. The first step in reducing dietary fat is finding out where the fat is.

Finding the Fats in Foods

Most people recognize that butter, margarine, shortening, and oils contain only fat, and many consumers are aware of the high fat content of red meats. But many people are surprised to learn that an eighth of an avocado, one strip of bacon, or five small olives contain as much fat as a pat of butter (45 kcalories from fat). When you eat these foods, you are eating fat-rich foods.

The fats and the meats are two food groups that always contain fat, but two other food groups—the milk, cheese, and yogurt group and the breads—sometimes contain fat as well. Vegetables and fruits, if unprocessed, are virtually fat-free. Grains, too, in their natural state, contain little or no fat.

Hidden Fats in Foods Other foods that are significant contributors of fat include convenience foods, fried foods, lunch meats, and other prepared meats. The fat in these foods is sometimes referred to as invisible fat because it does not have the obvious appearance of fat. An ounce of lean meat or low-fat cheese supplies about half its kcalories from fat (28 kcalories from protein and 27 kcalories from fat). An ounce of a high-fat meat (such as bologna) or most cheeses supplies 72 percent of its energy from fat (28 kcalories from protein and 72 kcalories from fat). Two tablespoons of peanut butter supply 76 percent of their energy as fat (32 kcalories from protein and 140 kcalories from fat)! Thus foods that are usually thought of as protein-rich foods may actually contain more fat energy than protein energy. Note that the values for meat given here are for 1-ounce portions. An average serving of hamburger is usually 3 or 4 ounces. An average dinner steak may be 6 ounces or larger.

Remember that an ounce of meat is not an ounce of protein. An ounce (30 g) of lean meat contains 7 g protein and 3 g fat. The other 20 g are largely water with associated vitamins and minerals.

Surprisingly, abundant fat lurks even on salad bars; you can easily construct a plate of salad that delivers 50 percent of its energy as fat. Think about it: not only the salad dressings, but also the mixed salads—potato salad, macaroni salad, coleslaw, and marinated bean salads—are largely fat or oil. This is not to condemn salad bars, but only to remind you to choose your foods with an awareness of the fats they contain. As mentioned, along with the total fat in foods, people need to notice the saturated fat and cholesterol in foods.

Fats in Milk The fat in milk is about 62 percent saturated fat; the cholesterol content is 25 milligrams per cup for whole milk or 5 milligrams for nonfat milk. Thus choosing nonfat in place of whole milk reduces your intake of cholesterol as well as of saturated fat.

Fats in Meats, Eggs, and Fish The fats in meats and eggs are about half saturated. The fats in poultry and fish are more unsaturated than saturated, a healthier balance. The foods that contain the most cholesterol are eggs, organ meats such as liver and kidneys, and high-fat dairy products. Shellfish have been thought to contain high concentrations of cholesterol, but the findings on which this idea was based have been called into question. Shellfish contain sterols, but possibly not the kind that have metabolically negative effects, and they contain much less cholesterol than was thought in the past.

Cutting Fat Intake and Choosing Unsaturated Fats

Knowing which foods contain the most fat is the first step toward meeting the recommendation to reduce dietary fat in general and saturated fat in particular. As a general rule, a person who eats meat and wishes to reduce both saturated fat and cholesterol intake can accomplish these objectives by eating fewer high-fat meats and dairy foods, fewer eggs, and more poultry (without the skin), fish, and nonfat dairy products. A vegetarian who eats dairy products and eggs can shift to nonfat milk and low-fat cheeses and limit butter and egg intake. Vegetarians who omit animal-derived foods already eat a diet low in fat and consume no cholesterol because plant foods do not contain cholesterol. The box on page 70 offers strategies for lowering fat, food group by food group.

Fats and kCalories Removing fat from food also removes energy (see Figure 3–4 on the next page). A small pork chop with the fat trimmed to within a half-inch of the lean provides 275 kcalories; with the fat trimmed off completely, it supplies 165 kcalories. A baked potato with butter and sour cream (1 tablespoon each) has 350 kcalories; a plain baked potato has 220 kcalories. Indeed, the single most effective step you can take to reduce the energy value of a food is to eat it with less fat.

Remember, fat is a more concentrated energy source than the other energy nutrients: 1 g carbohydrate or protein = 4 kcal, but 1 g fat = 9 kcal.

Choosing Unsaturated Fats To the extent that a person does eat fats, those to choose are the unsaturated ones. The hardness of fats at room temperature is an indicator: the softer a fat is, the more unsaturated it is. Chicken fat is softer than pork fat, which is softer than beef tallow. Of the three, chicken fat is the more unsaturated, and beef tallow is the most saturated. Unsaturated fats melt more readily. Generally speaking, vegetable and fish oils are rich in polyunsaturates, olive oil and canola oil are rich in monounsaturates, and the harder fats—animal fats—are most saturated (see Figure 3–5 on page 69).

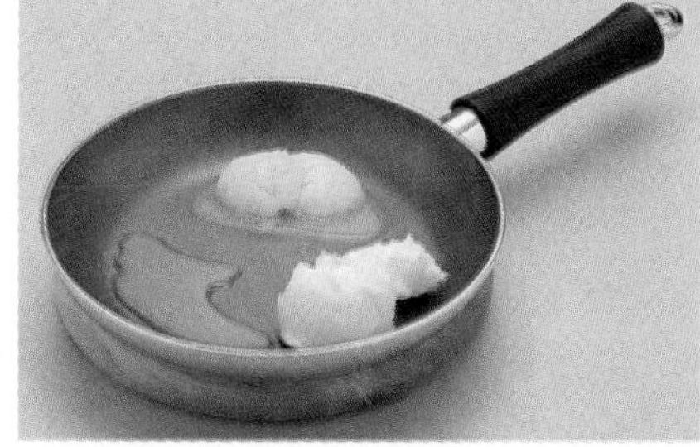

The more unsaturated a fat, the more liquid it is at room temperature. The more saturated a fat, the higher the temperature at which it melts.

Don't Overdo Fat Restriction Although it is very difficult to do, some people actually manage to eat too *little* fat—to their detriment. Among them are young women and men with eating disorders, described in Nutrition in Practice 9. As a practical guideline, it is wise to include the equivalent of at least a teaspoon of fat in every meal.

Cautions If you wish to make choices consistent with current recommendations, you should learn how to read food labels, limit fat in gen-

Figure 3–4
Food Fat and kCalories

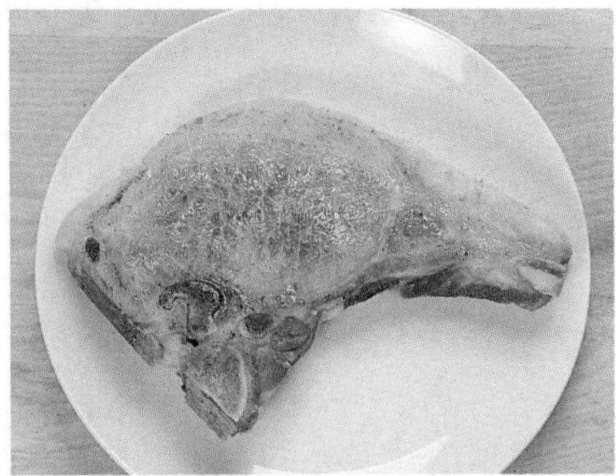
Pork chop with a half-inch of fat (275 kcal).

Potato with 1 tbs butter and 1 tbs sour cream (350 kcal).

Whole milk, 1 c (150 kcal).

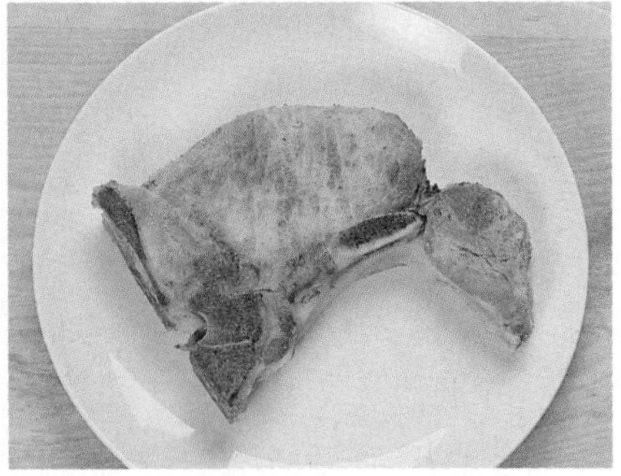

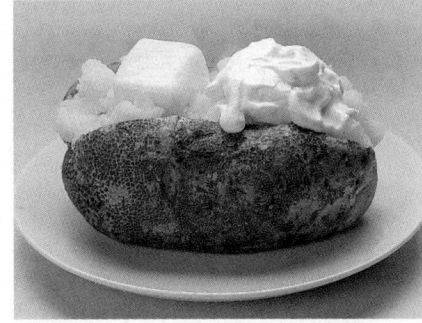
Pork chop with fat trimmed off (165 kcal).

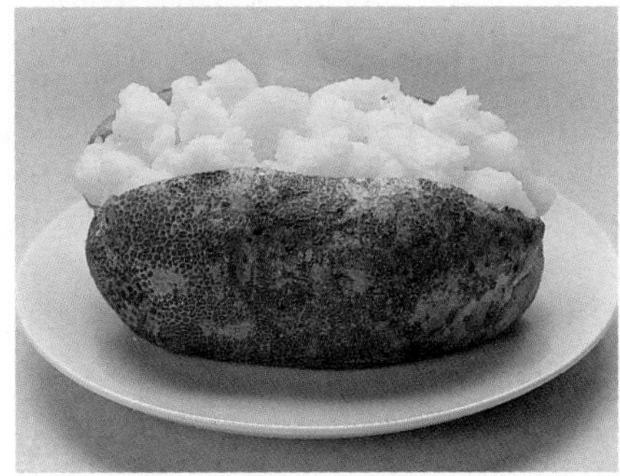
Plain potato (220 kcal).

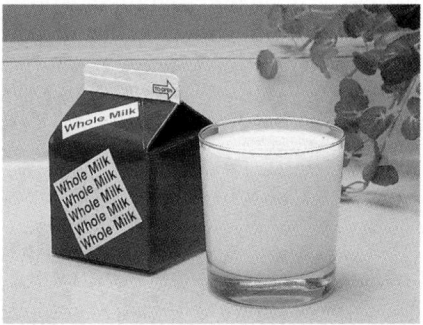

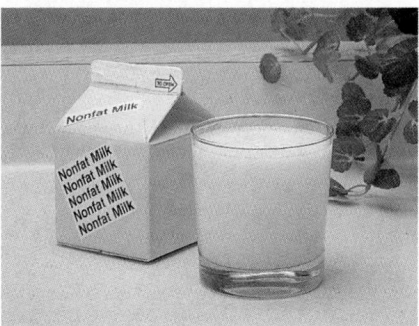

Nonfat milk, 1 c (90 kcal).

eral, and seek out the polyunsaturated and monounsaturated fats in preference to the saturated ones. But beware: vegetable fat or vegetable oil doesn't always mean unsaturated fat. Coconut oil and palm oil, for example, are often used in nondairy creamers, both are saturated fats, and both raise blood cholesterol.

hydrogenation: the process of adding hydrogen to unsaturated fat to make it more solid and resistant to chemical change.

Hydrogenated Fats Vegetable oils that are hydrogenated have lost their polyunsaturated character and the health benefits that go along with it. Food producers hydrogenate unsaturated fatty acids to prevent spoilage and make them harder—as when they hydrogenate corn oil to make spreadable margarine. The points of unsaturation in fatty acids are vulnerable to attack by oxygen, which makes them rancid.

***Trans*-Fatty Acids** When polyunsaturated oils are hydrogenated, the fatty acids not only become more saturated, but the hydrogenation process changes the shape of the molecules. In nature, most unsaturated fatty acids are *cis*-fatty acids—meaning that the hydrogens next to the double bonds are on the same side of the carbon chain. When hydrogenated, some of the fatty acids become *trans*-fatty acids—meaning that some of their hydrogens jump to the opposite side of the chain (see Figure 3–6).

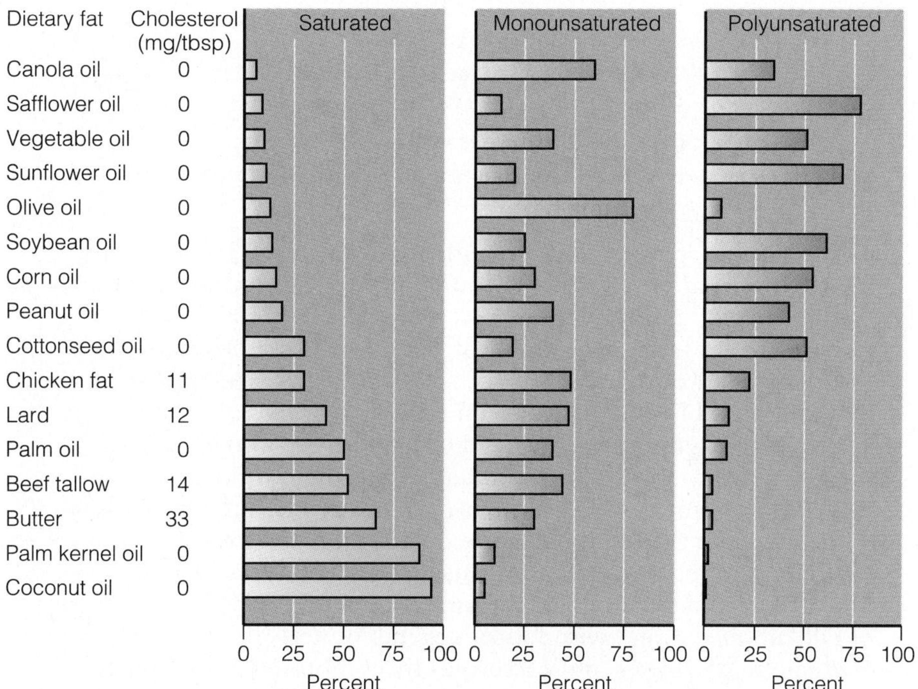

Figure 3–5
Comparison of Dietary Fats

Some preliminary evidence suggests that diets rich in *trans*-fatty acids (for example, diets using margarine instead of butter) raise blood cholesterol.[19] Reports in the media on this topic have raised consumer concerns about whether margarine is indeed a better option than butter for lowering the risk of heart disease. The American Heart Association states that because butter is rich in both saturated fat and cholesterol and because margarine is made from vegetable fat with no dietary cholesterol, margarine is still preferable to butter.[20] They further state that if consumers limit their fat intakes to 30 percent or less of total kcalories, they are not likely to ingest an excess of *trans*-fatty acids. The American Dietetic Association notes that *trans*-fatty acids provide only about 3 percent of total kcalories, whereas total fat accounts for about 36 percent of total kcalories. By limiting total fat, therefore, one can limit the health risks posed by all types of fat.[21]

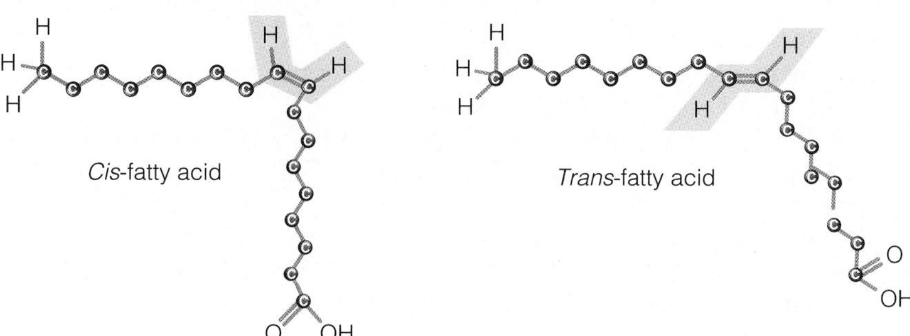

Figure 3–6
Cis- and Trans-Fatty Acids Compared

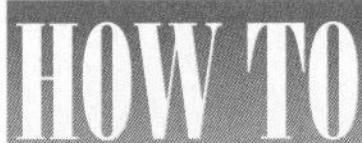

Lower Fat Intake—by Food Group

Fats can sneak into the diet in every food group. Inspect each group to discover where the fats are, and control them as follows.

Meat, Fish, and Poultry

- Choose fish, poultry, or lean cuts of pork or beef; look for cuts named *round* or *loin* (eye of round, top round, round tip, tenderloin, sirloin, and top loin).
- Trim the fat from pork and beef; remove the skin from poultry.
- Grill, roast, broil, bake, stir-fry, stew, or braise meats. (Don't fry.) When possible, place meat on a rack so that fat can drain.
- Use lean ground turkey instead of hamburger in recipes.
- Brown ground meats without added fat, then drain off fat.
- Refrigerate meat pan drippings and broth; when the broth solidifies, remove the fat and use the defatted broth in recipes.
- Select tuna packed in water; rinse oil-packed tuna with hot water to remove much of the fat.
- Fill kabob skewers with lots of vegetables and slivers of meat; create main dishes and casseroles by combining a little meat, fish, or poultry with a lot of pasta, rice, or vegetables.
- Make meatless spaghetti sauces and casseroles.
- Eat a meatless meal or two daily (use the milk and other food groups with care as suggested next).

Milk and Cheeses

- Drink nonfat and low-fat milk instead of whole milk.
- Use nonfat and low-fat cheeses (such as part-skim ricotta and low-fat mozzarella) instead of regular cheeses.
- Use nonfat or low-fat yogurt instead of sour cream.
- Use evaporated nonfat milk instead of cream.
- Enjoy nonfat frozen yogurt, sherbet, or ice milk instead of ice cream.

Fruits and Vegetables

- Use butter-flavored granules on vegetables instead of butter or margarine.
- Use nonfat yogurt or nonfat salad dressing instead of sour cream, cheese, mayonnaise, or other sauces on vegetables and in casseroles.
- Select nonfat or low-fat salad dressings, or use herbs, lemon juice, and spices instead of regular salad dressing.
- Add a little water to thick, bottled salad dressings to dilute the amount of fat each serving provides.
- Eat at least two vegetables (in addition to a salad) with dinner.
- Snack on raw vegetables or fruits instead of high-fat items like potato chips.
- Enjoy fruit for dessert.

How To (continued)

Breads and Cereals

- Use fruit butters or jellies instead of butter or margarine.
- Select breads, cereals, and crackers that are low in fat (for example, bagels instead of croissants).

Other Foods and Cooking Tips

- Use a nonstick pan or coat the pan lightly with cooking oil.
- Use egg substitutes in recipes instead of whole eggs or use 2 egg whites in place of each whole egg.
- Use half the margarine, butter, or oil called for in a recipe. (The minimum amount of fat for muffins, quick breads, and biscuits is 1 to 2 tbs per cup of flour; for cakes and cookies, 2 tbs per cup.)
- Select whipped butter, margarine, or cream cheese for use at the table; they contain half the kcalories of the regular types.
- Use wine, lemon juice, or broth instead of butter or margarine when cooking.
- Stir-fry in a small amount of oil; add moisture and flavor with broth, tomato juice, or wine.
- Use variety to enhance enjoyment of the meal: vary colors, textures, and temperatures—hot cooked versus cool raw foods—and use garnishes to complement the food.

Fats Used for Frying In the past, the fats used to fry foods were not a health concern. As research reveals more unhealthy links between saturated fats and heart disease and cancer, however, people are rightly concerned about the fats used to fry foods in restaurants. With fast foods becoming a major portion of many people's diets, it is important to know whether the fats are saturated. All fats have the same number of kcalories per gram, but the saturated fats have increased health risks associated with them. Some popular fast-food establishments continue to use beef tallow because it is economical, but some are beginning to take consumers' concerns into account. They are frying foods in polyunsaturated vegetable oils as well as offering low-fat alternatives to meats, such as raw-vegetable salads. Many movie theaters have switched from coconut oil to canola oil to prepare their popcorn, some are even trying air-popped popcorn. If consumers are concerned enough to voice their preferences, establishments will change the types of fats they use.

Chapters 2 and 3 have looked briefly at the two major energy fuels in the body—carbohydrate and fat. When used for energy, each has desirable characteristics. The glucose derived from carbohydrate is needed by the brain and nerve tissues and is easily used for energy in other cells. Fat is a particularly useful fuel because the body stores it efficiently and in generous amounts and can use it for energy if carbohydrate is not available. Chapter 4 looks at protein, a nutrient that can be used as fuel, but whose primary role is to provide machinery for getting things done.

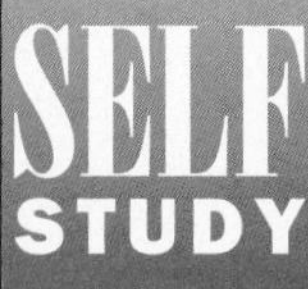

How's Your Fat Intake?

From the forms you filled out for the Self-Study in Chapter 1, answer the following questions:

1. How many grams of fat do you consume in an average day (from Form 2)? ___ grams. How many grams of saturated fat do you consume in an average day? ___ grams.
2. How many kcalories does this represent? (Remember, 1 gram of fat contributes 9 kcalories.) ___ kcalories from total fat and ___ kcalories from saturated fat.
3. What percentage of your total kcalories is contributed by fat (fat kcalories divided by total kcalories times 100—or use the answer you obtained on Form 5)? ___ percent from fat.
4. What percentage of your total kcalories is from saturated fat? ___ percent from saturated fat.
5. A dietary guideline says that fat should contribute no more than 30 percent of total kcalories and saturated fat no more than 10 percent. How does your fat intake compare with these recommendations? If it is higher, look over your food records. What specific foods could you cut down on or eliminate, and what foods could you add to your diet to bring your total fat intake into line?
6. You may not be aware of how much fat you are eating when you eat meat. Weigh your meat portions for a day or so; then calculate how much fat you derive from meat in a day (use Appendix A). To visualize this amount of fat, weigh out an equal amount from a bottle of oil, a can of cooking fat, or a tub of butter or margarine. Try the same demonstration with a fast-food meal that includes fried foods. How much fat do you eat in a day?

The connections between the overconsumption of fats and chronic diseases (obesity, diabetes, cancer, and cardiovascular disease) alert dietitians to carefully consider a client's fat intake. Using food intake data, dietitians determine the total amount of fat, the types of fat, and the total cholesterol intake. If fat intakes are excessive, dietitians recommend the same fat-cutting strategies recommended in this chapter.

In conducting the preceding Self-Study, imagine yourself to be a person with a high risk of one of the chronic diseases related to a high fat and saturated fat intake. Critique your diet on this basis and make realistic recommendations for change.

■ STUDY QUESTIONS ■

1. Name three classes of lipids found in the body and in foods.
2. What are some functions of fat in the body?
3. Describe the general structure of triglycerides.
4. What is the difference between a saturated and an unsaturated fatty acid?
5. Name the essential fatty acids.
6. What are the dietary recommendations regarding fat and cholesterol?
7. List some foods that are sources of "hidden fat."
8. List some of the ways you can reduce your intake of fat.

NUTRITION IN PRACTICE 3

Are Fat kCalories More Fattening?

Dietary recommendations to eat a diet low in fat and rich in complex carbohydrates originated almost two decades ago from the awareness that overnutrition (excess dietary fat and cholesterol) contributed to degenerative diseases such as heart disease and cancer. When following the recommendations resulted in weight loss, it was attributed to the effect of eating a greater bulk of fruits, vegetables, and whole grains, which satisfied the appetite sooner than foods high in fat, so that people ate fewer kcalories.

Today accumulating evidence offers new support for these not-so-new recommendations, but the long-held premise that a kcalorie is a kcalorie, regardless of its source, is losing ground. People seem to gain more body fat when they eat extra fat kcalories than when they eat extra carbohydrate kcalories. Researchers have been investigating whether fat in the diet may influence body fatness more than the diet's total kcalorie content.[22]

Where did this idea—that fat kcalories are more fattening—come from?

As often happens in science, researchers were testing a different question, whether a fat-rich diet could lead rats to overeat, when they stumbled onto this idea. The researchers found that rats became fatter on high-fat diets than on low-fat diets, even though the total *kcalories* in the diets were the same. Many years later, researchers began noticing similar results when studying human beings. In a classic study, men were *encouraged* to gain weight so that researchers could study the effects of a high-carbohydrate diet versus a high-fat diet on weight gain.[23] The researchers discovered that the men who overate the high-fat diet gained more weight more easily than the men who overate the high-carbohydrate diet, even though both groups were eating the same number of kcalories. In fact, the men eating the high-carbohydrate diet had difficulty gaining weight.

Well, that's an easy concept to grasp; if people eat a lot of fat, they gain a lot of fat, right?

So it seems, and population studies seem to bear this out. For example, since the turn of the century in the United States, the percentage of total kcalories from carbohydrate in the diet has steadily declined, while the percentage of kcalories from fat has risen. At the same time, obesity has become more prevalent. However, we can't quite conclude from such population data that it is the high fat intakes specifically that promote obesity. Such a conclusion would fail to recognize other significant factors. Total kcalorie intake has also risen, and physical activity levels have declined, so confirmation (based on population data) that a higher dietary fat intake causes obesity is lacking. Still other factors—smoking, alcohol consumption, eating patterns, metabolic differences, and genetics—further complicate the relationship between dietary fat and body fat.

Can't researchers study individuals, rather than whole populations, to answer this question?

Yes, and over and over again, the results of well-controlled studies of both men and women have shown a positive correlation between dietary fat and body fat and an inverse correlation between carbohydrate and body fat. In other words, the more carbohydrate people eat, the lower their body fat.[24]

Does the research offer any clues as to why fat kcalories seem to be more fattening than carbohydrate kcalories?

Research has begun to focus on the biochemical reasons for body fat buildup. What does the body do with fat and carbohydrate from a meal? Researchers gave men mixed meals of moderate energy value and found that their bodies used much of the carbohydrate for energy and converted much of the fat into body fat.[25]

Why do you suppose the body prefers to store fat over carbohydrate?

Probably because it costs less (in kcalories) to convert dietary fat to body fat. Converting dietary carbohydrate to body fat requires too much energy to make it worthwhile. The body is designed to conserve all possible energy at all opportunities.

So the bottom line is: the less fat you eat, the less fat you store—right?

Yes, more and more research shows that the amount of fat in the diet is an important factor in the body's fat storage.[26] One

researcher puts it this way, "The single most important thing you can do [to lose weight] is to get the fat out of [your] diet."[27]

■ NOTES ■

1. S. M. Hunt and J. L. Groff, *Advanced Nutrition and Human Metabolism* (St. Paul, Minn: West Publishing Co., 1990), pp. 405–423.
2. A. P. Simopoulos, Omega-3 fatty acids in health and disease and in growth and development, *American Journal of Clinical Nutrition* 54 (1991): 438–463.
3. A. P. Simopoulos, w-3 Fatty acids in growth and development and in health and disease, *Nutrition Today,* March/April 1988, pp. 10–19.
4. M. A. Crawford, The role of essential fatty acids in neural development: Implications for perinatal nutrition, *American Journal of Clinical Nutrition* 57 (1993): 703S–710S.
5. W. E. Connor, M. Neuringer, and S. Reisbick, Essential fatty acids: The importance of *n*-3 fatty acids in the retina and brain, *Nutrition Reviews,* April 1992, pp. 21–29.
6. Simopoulos, 1991.
7. Simopoulos, 1991.
8. D. M. Hegsted, Dietary fatty acids, serum cholesterol and coronary heart disease, in *Health Effects of Dietary Fatty Acids,* ed. G. J. Nelson (Champaign, Ill.: American Oil Chemists' Society, 1991), pp. 50–68.
9. A Nordoy and coauthors, Individual effects of dietary saturated fatty acids and fish oil on plasma lipids and lipoproteins in normal men, *American Journal of Clinical Nutrition* 57 (1993): 634–639.
10. M. L. Burr and coauthors, Effects of changes in fats, fish and fibre intakes on death and myocardial infarction: Diet and reinfarction trial (DART), *Lancet* 2 (1989): 757–761, as cited in Nordoy and coauthors, 1993.
11. Simopoulos, 1991; L. A. Sauer, R. T. Dauchy, and A. S. Hurtubise, Effects of omega-6 and omega-3 fatty acids on rate of H-thymidine incorporation in hepatoma, *FASEB Journal* 4 (1990): A508.
12. Federation of American Societies for Experimental Biology, Life Sciences Research Office, *Nutrition Monitoring in the United States: An Update Report on Nutrition Monitoring,* prepared for the U.S. Department of Health and Human Services (Washington, D.C.: Government Printing Office, 1989).
13. *National Cholesterol Education Program Report of the Expert Panel on Population Strategies for Blood Cholesterol Reduction* (Bethesda, Md.: National Heart, Lung, and Blood Institute, 1990), as cited in L. M. Smith-Schneider, M. J. Sigman-Grant, and P. M. Kris-Etherton, Dietary fat reduction strategies, *Journal of the American Dietetic Association* 92 (1992): 34–38.
14. P. N. Hopkins, Effects of dietary cholesterol on serum cholesterol: A meta-analysis and review, *American Journal of Clinical Nutrition* 55 (1992): 1060–1070.
15. R. W. Foltin and coauthors, Calorie compensation for lunches varying in fat and carbohydrate content by humans in a residential laboratory, *American Journal of Clinical Nutrition* 52 (1990): 969–980; B. J. Rolls and coauthors, Effects of olestra, a noncaloric fat substitute, on daily energy and fat intakes in lean men, *American Journal of Clinical Nutrition* 56 (1992): 84–92.
16. Position of the American Dietetic Association: Fat replacements, *Journal of the American Dietetic Association* 91 (1991): 1285–1288.
17. C. L. Rock and A. Coulston, Review: The new fat replacements, *Nutrition and the M.D.,* September 1990, p. 8.
18. Oatrim: New fat substitute (abstract), *Journal of the American Dietetic Association* 91 (1991): 738.
19. R. P. Mensink and M. B. Katan, Effect of dietary trans fatty acids on high-density and low-density lipoprotein cholesterol levels in healthy adults, *New England Journal of Medicine* 323 (1990): 439–440.
20. American Heart Association, Nutrition Advisory Committee, *News Release,* Trans fatty acids, May 13, 1994.
21. American Dietetic Association, *News Release,* Evidence inconclusive on trans fatty acids, May 16, 1994.
22. K. R. Westerterp, Food quotient, respiratory quotient, and energy balance, *American Journal of Clinical Nutrition* (supplement) 57 (1993): 759–765.
23. E. A. Sims and coauthors, Endocrine and metabolic effects of experimental obesity in man, *Recent Progress in Hormone Research* 29 (1973): 457–496, as cited in A. M. Dattilo, Dietary fat and its relationship to body weight, *Nutrition Today,* January/February 1992, pp. 13–19.
24. D. M. Dreon and coauthors, Dietary fat: carbohydrate ratio and obesity in middle-aged men, *American Journal of*

Clinical Nutrition 47 (1988): 995–1000; I. Romieu and coauthors, Energy intake and other determinants of relative weight, *American Journal of Clinical Nutrition* 47 (1988): 406–412; A. Tremblay and coauthors, Impact of dietary fat content and fat oxidation on energy intake in humans, *American Journal of Clinical Nutrition* 49 (1989): 799–805; W. C. Miller and coauthors, Diet composition, energy intake, and exercise in relation to body fat in men and women, *American Journal of Clinical Nutrition* 52 (1990): 426–430; T. E. Prewitt and coauthors, Changes in body weight, body composition, and energy intake in women fed high- and low-fat diets, *American Journal of Clinical Nutrition* 54 (1991): 304–310: Westerterp, 1993.

25. O. E. Owen and coauthors, Oxidative and nonoxidative macronutrient disposal in lean and obese men after mixed meals, *American Journal of Clinical Nutrition* 55 (1992): 630–636.
26. Miller and coauthors, 1990; C. N. Bouzer, A. Brasseur, and R. L. Atkinson, Dietary fat affects weight loss and adiposity during energy restriction in rats, *American Journal of Clinical Nutrition* 58 (1993): 846–852.
27. R. L. Atkinson, Role of diet in obesity treatment, an address at the North American Association for the Study of Obesity and Emory University School of Medicine conference Obesity Update: Pathophysiology, Clinical Consequences, and Therapeutic Options, Atlanta, Georgia, August 31–September 2, 1992.

4

Proteins and Amino Acids

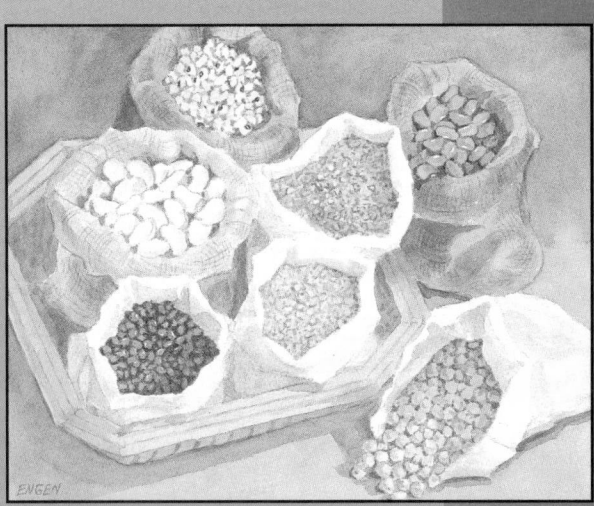

CONTENTS

People think of proteins as body-building nutrients, the material of strong muscles, and rightly so. No new living tissue can be built without them, for proteins are part of every cell, every bone, the blood, and every other tissue. Proteins constitute the cells' machinery—they do the cells' work. The energy to fuel that work comes from carbohydrate and fat.

The Chemist's View of Proteins

Proteins are chemical compounds that contain the same atoms as carbohydrate and lipid—carbon (C), hydrogen (H), and oxygen (O)—but proteins are different in that they also contain nitrogen (N) atoms. These nitrogen atoms give the name *amino* (nitrogen containing) to the amino acids that are the links in the chains we call proteins.

proteins: compounds composed of carbon, hydrogen, oxygen, *and* nitrogen atoms arranged into strands of amino acids. Some amino acids also contain sulfur atoms.

amino (a-MEEN-oh) **acids:** building blocks of protein; each has an amino group and an acid group attached to a central carbon, which also carries a distinctive side chain.
amino = containing nitrogen

dipeptide: two amino acids bonded together.
di = two
peptide = amino acid

tripeptide: three amino acids bonded together.
tri = three

polypeptide: many amino acids bonded together. *Many* refers to ten or more. An intermediate strand of between four and ten amino acids is an oligopeptide.
poly = many
oligo = few

The Structure of Proteins

All amino acids share a common chemical "backbone," and it is these backbones that are linked together to form proteins. Each amino acid also carries a side chain, which varies from one amino acid to another (see Figure 4–1). About 20 different amino acids may appear in proteins.* The side chains on amino acids are what make proteins so varied in comparison with either carbohydrates or lipids.

Protein Chains The 20 amino acids can be linked end-to-end in a virtually infinite variety of sequences to form proteins. When two amino acids bond together, the resulting structure is known as a dipeptide. Three amino acids bonded together form a tripeptide. As additional amino acids join the chain, the structure becomes a polypeptide. Most proteins are polypeptides that are 100 to 300 amino acids long.

Protein Shapes These polypeptide chains twist into complex shapes. Each amino acid has special characteristics that attract it to, or repel it from, other amino acids. Because of these interactions among their amino acids, polypeptide chains fold and intertwine into intricate

* Besides the 20 common amino acids, which can all be components of proteins, others occur individually (for example, ornithine). Chemists can make still others.

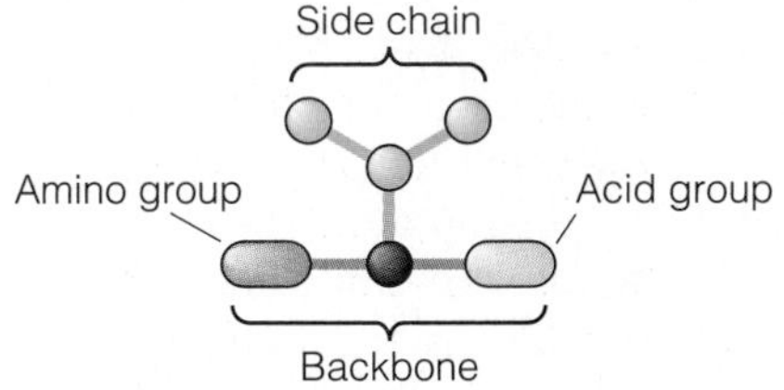

The "backbone" is the same for all amino acids. The nitrogen is in the amino group.

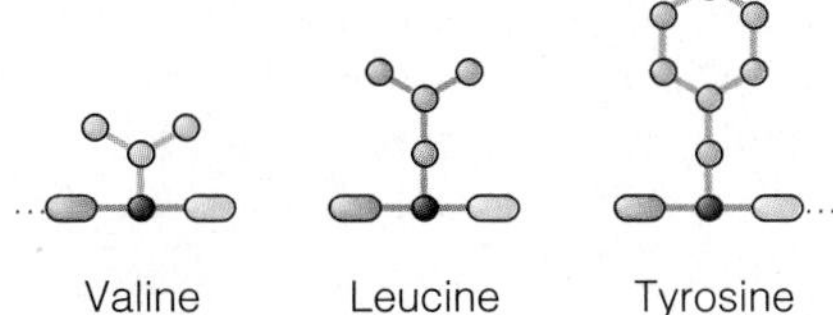

The side chain differs from one amino acid to the next.

Figure 4–1
Amino Acid Structure and Examples of Amino Acids

Figure 4–2
The Coiling and Folding of a Protein

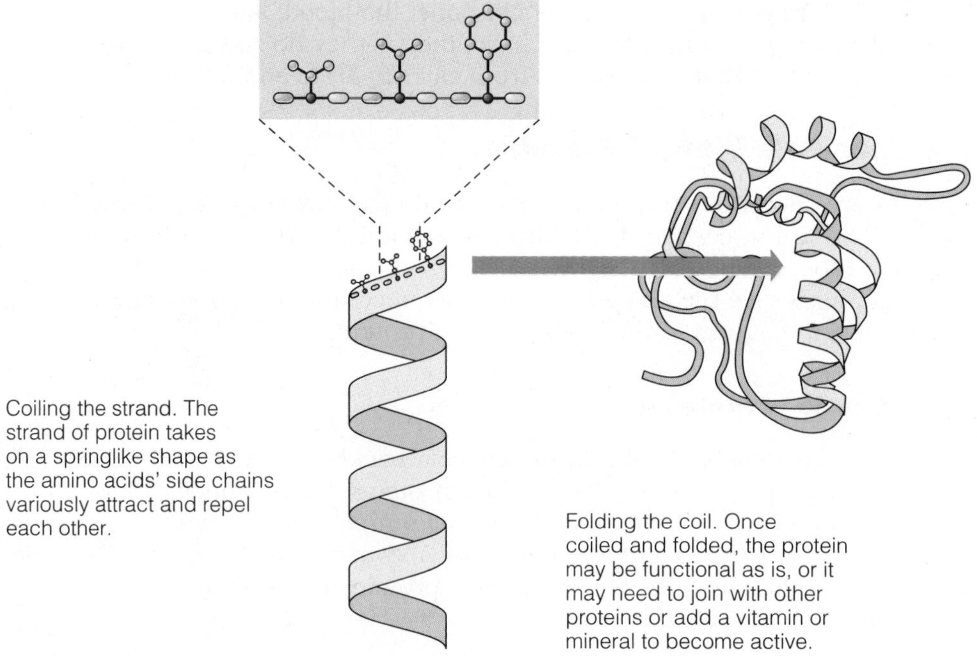

coils (see Figure 4–2). The amino acid sequence of a protein determines the specific way the chain will fold.

Coiling the strand. The strand of protein takes on a springlike shape as the amino acids' side chains variously attract and repel each other.
Folding the coil. Once coiled and folded, the protein may be functional as is, or it may need to join with other proteins or add a vitamin or mineral to become active.

Protein Functions The dramatically different shapes of proteins enable them to perform different tasks in the body. Some, such as hemoglobin in the blood (see Figure 4–3), are globular in shape; some are hollow balls that can carry and store materials within them; and some, such as those that form tendons, are more than ten times as long as they are wide, forming stiff, sturdy, rodlike structures.

essential amino acids: amino acids that the body cannot synthesize in amounts sufficient to meet physiological need. Also called *indispensable amino acids*. Nine amino acids are known to be essential for human adults:

- **histidine** (HISS-tuh-deen).
- **isoleucine** (eye-so-LOO-seen).
- **leucine** (LOO-seen).
- **lysine** (LYE-seen).
- **methionine** (meh-THIGH-oh-neen).
- **phenylalanine** (fen-il-AL-uh-neen).
- **threonine** (THREE-oh-neen).
- **tryptophan** (TRIP-toe-fane).
- **valine** (VAY-leen).

Essential Amino Acids

Proteins in foods do not provide body proteins directly, but rather supply the amino acids from which the body makes its own proteins. The body can make over half of the amino acids for itself; the protein in food does not need to supply these. But there are other amino acids that the body cannot make at all, and some that it cannot make fast enough to meet its needs. The proteins in foods must supply these amino acids to the body; they are therefore called the *essential* amino acids. Nine amino acids are essential. The distinction between essential and nonessential amino acids is not quite this clear-cut, however. For example, histidine has long been known to be an essential amino acid for infants, but only recently has it been added to the list of essential amino acids for adults.[1]

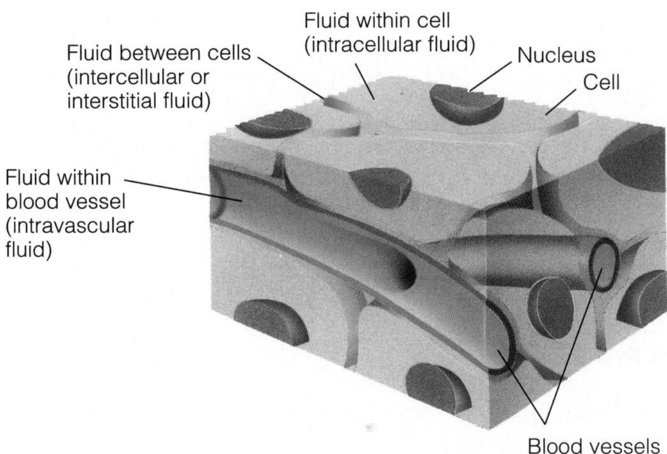

Figure 4–5
One Cell and Its Associated Fluids

Fluid Balance Proteins are able to help determine the distribution of fluids in living systems for two reasons: first, proteins cannot pass freely across the membranes that separate body compartments, and second, they are attracted to water. A cell that "wants" to keep a certain amount of water in its interior space can't move the water around directly, but it can manufacture proteins, and those proteins will hold water. Thus the cell can use proteins to help regulate the distribution of water indirectly. Similarly, the body makes proteins for the blood and the intercellular spaces. These proteins help maintain the fluid volume in those spaces.

Acid-Base Balance Proteins also help maintain the balance between acids and bases within the body's fluids. Normal body processes continually produce acids and bases, which must be carried by the blood to the kidneys and lungs for excretion. The blood must do this without upsetting its own acid-base balance. Blood pH is one of the most tightly controlled conditions in the body. If the blood becomes too acidic, the structure of vital proteins such as hemoglobin can be disrupted. When this happens, the proteins undergo denaturation, losing their shape and ability to function. A similar situation arises when the balance tips too far toward base. These imbalances are known as acidosis and alkalosis, respectively, and either can be fatal.

Proteins such as albumin in plasma help to prevent these imbalances from arising. In a sense, the proteins protect one another by gathering up extra acid (hydrogen) ions when there are too many in the surrounding medium and by releasing them when there are too few. By accepting and releasing hydrogen ions, proteins act as buffers, maintaining the acid-base balance of the blood and body fluids.

Antibodies and Hormones

Other major proteins in the blood—the antibodies—act against viruses, bacteria, and other disease agents. The antibodies work so efficiently that if a million bacterial cells are injected into the skin of a healthy person,

acids: compounds that release hydrogen ions in a solution.

bases: compounds that accept hydrogen ions in a solution.

acid-base balance: the balance maintained between acid and base concentrations in the blood and body fluids.

pH: the concentration of hydrogen ions. The lower the pH, the stronger the acid. Thus pH 2 is a strong acid; pH 6 is a weak acid; pH 7 is neutral; and a pH above 7 is alkaline.

denaturation (dee-nay-cher-AY-shun): the change in a protein's shape brought about by heat, acid, or other agents. Past a certain point, denaturation is irreversible.

acidosis: too much acid in the blood and body fluids.

alkalosis: too much base in the blood and body fluids.

buffers: compounds that can reversibly combine with hydrogen ions to help keep a solution's acidity or alkalinity constant.

antibodies: large proteins of the blood and body fluids, produced in response to invasion of the body by unfamiliar molecules (mostly proteins); antibodies inactivate the invaders and so protect the body. The invaders are called **antigens.**
anti = against.

Chapter 18 presents a discussion of the immune system.

hormones: chemical messengers. Hormones are secreted by a variety of glands in the body in response to altered conditions. Each travels to one or more target tissues or organs and elicits specific responses to restore normal conditions.

fewer than ten are likely to survive for five hours. This is why in a normal, healthy, individual, most diseases never have a chance to get started. Without sufficient protein, the body cannot maintain its resistance to disease.

The blood also carries messenger molecules known as hormones, and some of these are made of amino acids. (Recall that other hormones are sterols.) Among the hormones composed of amino acids are the thyroid hormones and insulin. Hormones have many profound effects, which will become evident in subsequent chapters.

Transport Proteins

Some of the body's proteins specialize in moving nutrients and other molecules into and out of cells. These transport proteins reside in cell membranes and act as "pumps," picking up compounds on one side of the membrane and depositing them on the other. In doing so, transport proteins enable cells to "decide" which substances to take up and which to release. Cells can switch the protein machinery of their membranes on or off in response to the body's needs. Often hormones do the switching, with marvelous precision.

Other transport proteins, not attached to membranes, move about in the body fluids, carrying nutrients and other molecules from one organ to another. The protein hemoglobin, which carries oxygen from the lungs to the body's cells, is a prime example. The lipoproteins transport lipids around the body. In addition, special proteins also carry vitamins and minerals.

Growth, Maintenance, and Repair

The body uses proteins to build all of its new tissues and to repair damaged tissues. The new tissues may be in an embryo, in a growing child, in new hair and nails, in an area healing after injury or surgery, or in new blood needed to replace blood lost for any reason. The protein collagen serves as the mending material of torn tissue, forming scars to hold the separated parts together.

Replacement and Growth Proteins help replace worn-out cells in everyone's body all the time. The millions of cells that line the intestinal tract live for only three days; they are constantly being shed and must be replaced. The cells of the skin die and rub off, and new ones grow from underneath.

Both inside and outside the body, then, cells constantly make and break down their proteins. When proteins break down, their component amino acids are liberated to join the general circulation. Some of these amino acids may be promptly recycled into other proteins; others may be stripped of their nitrogen and used for energy. By reusing amino acids to build proteins, however, the body conserves and recycles a valuable commodity.

People need to eat protein-rich foods every day to replace the protein they continuously lose. If the body is growing, it needs more protein than is necessary just for maintenance. Children end each day with more blood cells, more muscle cells, and more skin cells than they had at the beginning of the day. So protein is needed both for routine maintenance (replacement) and growth (addition).

Nitrogen Balance If the body maintains the same amount of protein in its tissues from day to day, it is in nitrogen balance. If the body adds protein, it is in positive nitrogen balance; if it loses protein, it is in negative nitrogen balance.

Normally, healthy adults are in nitrogen balance; that is, their nitrogen intakes equal their nitrogen outputs. Growing children and pregnant women are in positive nitrogen balance, because they are adding new blood, bone, and muscle cells to their bodies. People who are fasting or starving, such as those with anorexia nervosa, and people who are sick or in trauma, such as people with burns (see Chapter 19), are in negative nitrogen balance because they are being forced to use protein for energy.

nitrogen balance: the amount of nitrogen consumed (N in) as compared with the amount of nitrogen excreted (N out) in a given period of time. The laboratory scientist can estimate the protein in a sample of food, body tissue, or excreta by measuring the nitrogen in it.

Nitrogen equilibrium (zero nitrogen balance): N in = N out.
Positive nitrogen balance: N in > N out.
Negative nitrogen balance: N in < N out.

Energy

Even though amino acids are needed to do the work that only they can perform—build vital proteins—they will be sacrificed to provide energy and glucose if need be. Keeping energy and glucose available are among the body's highest priorities; without energy, cells die; without glucose, the brain and nervous system falter. When glucose or fatty acids are limited, then, cells are forced to use amino acids for energy and glucose. The body does not make a specialized storage form of protein as it does for carbohydrate and fat. Glucose is stored as glycogen, fat as triglycerides, but body protein is available only as the working and structural components of the tissues. When the need arises, the body dismantles its tissue proteins and uses them for energy.[3] Thus, over time, energy deprivation (starvation) always incurs wasting of lean body tissue as well as fat loss.

The list of protein functions discussed here and summarized in Table 4–1 is by no means exhaustive. Nevertheless, it does give you some sense of the immense variety of proteins and their importance in the body.

Protein and Health

In the short time that scientists have been studying nutrition, no nutrient has been more intensely scrutinized than protein. As you know by now, it is indispensable to life. And it should come as no surprise that protein deficiency can have devastating effects on people's health. But like the other nutrients, protein in excess can also be harmful; the end of this section discusses the consequences of protein excess.

Protein-Energy Malnutrition

When people are deprived of food and suffer an energy deficit, they degrade their own body protein for energy and indirectly suffer a protein deficiency, as well as an energy deficiency. Because protein and energy

Table 4–1
Summary of Functions of Proteins

- *Growth and maintenance.* Proteins serve as building materials for growth and repair of body tissues.
- *Enzymes.* Proteins facilitate needed chemical reactions.
- *Hormones.* Proteins regulate body processes. Some, but not all, hormones are made of protein.
- *Antibodies.* Proteins act against disease agents to fight diseases.
- *Fluid and electrolyte balance.* Proteins help to maintain the fluid and mineral composition of various body fluids.
- *Acid-base balance.* Proteins help maintain the acid-base balance of various body fluids by acting as buffers.
- *Energy.* Proteins provide some fuel for the body's energy needs.
- *Transportation.* Proteins help transport needed substances, such as lipids, minerals, and oxygen, around the body.
- *Structural components.* Proteins form integral parts of most body structures such as skin, tendons, ligaments, membranes, muscles, organs, and bones.

protein-energy malnutrition (PEM): a deficiency of protein and food energy; the world's most widespread malnutrition problem, including both marasmus and kwashiorkor.
mal = bad, poor

deprivation thus go hand in hand, public health officials have adopted an abbreviation for the overlapping pair: protein-energy malnutrition (PEM). PEM is the most widespread form of malnutrition in the world today, affecting over 500 million children.[4] Adults are not immune to PEM, however. PEM is prevalent in Africa, Central America, South America, the Near East, and the Far East. In the United States, impoverished people living on U.S. Indian reservations, in inner cities, and in rural areas have been diagnosed with PEM. Adult PEM has been recognized in people hospitalized with infections such as AIDS and tuberculosis and is almost invariably present in those suffering from the eating disorder anorexia nervosa. Growing numbers of homeless people in this country are at risk for PEM as well.[5] The consequences of PEM as a world malnutrition problem are considered here; the problems associated with PEM in the hospital are described in Chapter 18.

Of all population groups, children are most seriously affected by malnutrition. Children who are thin for their heights may be suffering from acute PEM (recent severe food restriction), whereas children who are short for their ages may have experienced chronic PEM (long-term food restriction). Stunted growth due to PEM is easy to overlook because a small child may look quite normal, but it may be the most common sign of malnutrition in the developing countries.

marasmus (ma-RAZZ-mus)**:** a disease related to PEM; marasmus results from severe deprivation, or impaired absorption, of protein, energy, vitamins, and minerals.

kwashiorkor (kwash-ee-OR-core or kwash-ee-or-CORE)**:** a disease related to PEM, but of uncertain cause.

Marasmus and Kwashiorkor—One Disease or Two? The long-held concept that the two forms of PEM—marasmus and kwashiorkor—are different diseases caused by different nutrient deficiencies has been challenged in recent years. Marasmus was thought to be caused by energy deficiency and kwashiorkor by protein deficiency. In reality, though, marasmus reflects inadequate food intake and therefore inadequate energy, protein, vitamins, and minerals as well. In addition, diets that are adequate in energy are rarely deficient in protein.[6] Some researchers now maintain that marasmus and kwashiorkor are two stages of the same disease.[7] Other researchers suggest that kwashiorkor develops when malnourished people eat moldy grains.[8] Researchers continue to question the exact causes of kwashiorkor, but clearly, protein deficiency is not the only factor involved. Most likely, dietary imbalances, multiple infections, parasitic diseases, and toxins together influence the development of kwashiorkor.[9]

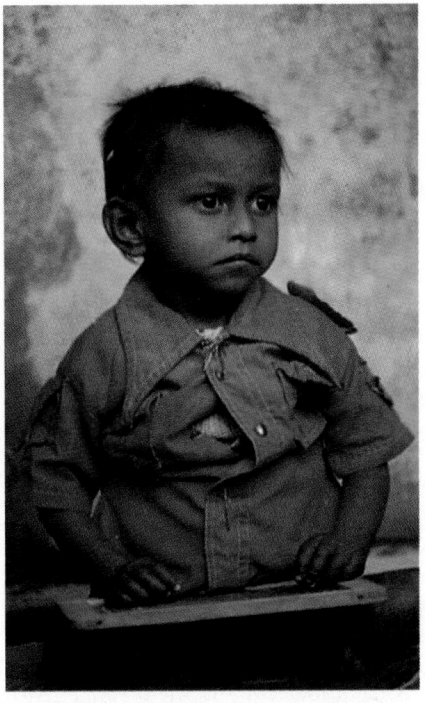

PEM affects millions of children worldwide.

Marasmus Marasmus occurs most commonly in children from 6 to 18 months of age in all the overpopulated urban slums of the world. Children in impoverished nations subsist on a weak cereal drink that supplies scant energy and protein of low quality: such food can barely sustain life, much less support growth. Consequently, marasmic children look like little old people—just skin and bones.

Without adequate nutrition, muscles, including the heart muscle, waste and weaken. Because the brain normally grows to almost its full adult size within the first two years of life, marasmus impairs brain development and learning ability. Reduced synthesis of key hormones leads to a metabolism so slow that the body temperature is subnormal. There is little or no fat under the skin to insulate against cold. Hospital workers find that the primary need of marasmic victims is to be wrapped up and kept warm.

The starving child faces this threat to life by engaging in as little activity as possible—not even crying for food. The body gathers all its forces to meet the crisis, so it cuts down on any expenditure of protein not needed for the heart, lungs, and brains to function. Growth ceases; the child is no larger at age four than at age two. Digestive enzymes are in short supply, the digestive tract lining deteriorates, and absorption fails. The child can't assimilate what little food is eaten.

Blood proteins, including hemoglobin, are no longer synthesized. Antibodies to fight off invading bacteria are degraded to provide amino acids for other uses, rendering the child vulnerable to infection. Then dysentery, an infection of the digestive tract, causes diarrhea, further depleting the body of nutrients. In the marasmic child, once infection has set in, kwashiorkor often follows.[10] The infection that occurs with malnutrition is responsible for two-thirds of the deaths in young children in developing countries.[11]

dysentery (DIS-en-terry)**:** an infection of the gastrointestinal tract caused by an amoeba or bacterium that gives rise to severe diarrhea.
dys = bad
entery = intestine

When two variables interact so that each increases the other, **synergism** (SIN-er-jiz-um) is said to be occurring. Malnutrition and infection are a deadly combination because they work in this way.
syn = with, together
ergism = work

If caught in time, a child's starvation may be reversed by careful nutrition therapy. (Chapter 18 describes the dangers of feeding people with PEM too rapidly.) The fluid balances are most critical. Diarrhea will have depleted the body's potassium and disturbed other electrolyte balances. Careful correction of fluid and electrolyte imbalances usually raises the blood pressure and strengthens the heart. After the first 24 to 48 hours, protein and energy may be given in small quantities, with gradually increasing intakes as tolerated.[12]

Kwashiorkor Kwashiorkor was originally a Ghanaian word meaning an "evil spirit that infects the first child when the second child is born." If you consider how kwashiorkor often develops, you can easily see how the Ghanaians arrived at this name for the disease. When a mother who has been nursing her first child bears a second child, she weans the first child and puts the second one on the breast. The first child, suddenly switched from nutrient-dense, protein-rich breast milk to a starchy, protein-poor gruel, soon begins to sicken and die. Kwashiorkor typically sets in at about the age of two. As mentioned earlier, some researchers believe that kwashiorkor and marasmus are two stages of the same disease. Some research indicates that marasmus represents the body's attempt to adapt to starvation, and that kwashiorkor develops when adaptation fails.

Some symptoms of kwashiorkor resemble those of marasmus, but without severe wasting of body fat. Proteins and hormones that previously maintained fluid balance diminish and fluid leaks out of the blood. The child's limbs and face become swollen with edema; the belly bulges with a fatty liver. The child's hair loses its color; the skin becomes patchy and scaly, sometimes with ulcers and sores that fail to heal.

edema (e-DEE-muh)**:** an accumulation of fluid. In kwashiorkor, hormonal imbalances lead to fluid imbalance. Water seeps out of the blood into the interstitial space and accumulates there.

fatty liver: an accumulation of fat in the liver. In PEM, fat accumulates in the liver because no protein is available to form the lipoproteins that normally escort fat molecules in the blood.

Experts assure us that we possess the knowledge, technology, and resources to end hunger. Programs that have involved the local people in the process of identifying the problem and devising its solution have met with some success. But until those who have the food, technology, and resources make fighting hunger a priority, the war on hunger will not be won.

Protein Excess

While many of the world's people struggle to obtain enough food and enough protein to survive, in the developed nations protein is so abundant that problems of protein excess are seen. Overconsumption of protein offers no benefits and may pose health risks. For example, protein-rich foods are often high-fat foods that contribute to obesity with its accompanying health risks. Some studies suggest a link between high-meat diets and colon cancer.[13] The higher a person's intake of protein-rich foods such as meat and milk, the more likely it is that fruits, vegetables, and grains will be crowded out, making the diet inadequate in other nutrients.

Some research suggests that diets high in protein promote calcium excretion, depleting the bones of their chief mineral. Diets high in *purified* protein dramatically increase calcium excretion. Calcium losses are smaller when high protein intakes are from natural whole foods, and when calcium intakes are high as well.[14] When high protein intakes are accompanied by low calcium intakes, as is typical of many women's diets in the United States, calcium losses incurred by excess protein may compromise bone health.[15] There are evidently no benefits to be gained by consuming a diet that derives more than 15 percent of its energy from protein. The *Diet and Health* recommendations (Table 1–2, Chapter 1) advise a moderate protein intake—one that falls between the RDA and twice the RDA.

Amino Acid Supplements Unnecessary In view of the high protein intakes of people in the United States and other developed nations, it is absurd that many people feel compelled to take protein and amino acid supplements. Popular reports that the amino acid tryptophan could relieve pain and cure depression and insomnia led to widespread public use. More than 1500 people who elected to take tryptophan developed an illness (EMS, short for *eosinophilia-myalgia syndrome*). EMS is characterized by severe muscle and joint pain, limb swelling, an elevated white blood cell count, extremely high fever, and, in at least 38 cases, death.[16] Some studies suggested that changes in procedures at a major Japanese tryptophan processing plant may have introduced contaminants that caused the disease. Later research suggests multiple factors are involved, and the exact causes of EMS remain uncertain. The Food and Drug Administration (FDA) issued a recall of all products containing tryptophan, except for specific medical formulas. If you own a bottle of tryptophan, throw it away. It is safer to derive your amino acids from protein-rich foods. The Dietary Supplement Act of 1992 proposed dietary supplement labeling rules based on the Nutrition Labeling and Education Act of 1990. The FDA's goal in issuing the supplement proposal is to assure consumers that health claims made on supplement labels are truthful.

Protein Recommendations

The committee that established the RDA states that a generous daily protein allowance for a healthy adult is 0.8 gram per kilogram (2.2 pounds) of appropriate or average body weight for height. The protein RDA is adjusted to cover additional needs for building new tissue and so is higher for infants, children, and pregnant and lactating women. (The protein needs of athletes are discussed in Chapter 10.) Protein RDA for people of average height at all ages are presented in the RDA table (inside front cover). If your height is not average, you can compute your own individualized RDA for protein (see the Self-Study that follows).

In setting the RDA, the committee assumes that the protein eaten will be of high quality, that it will be consumed together with adequate energy from carbohydrate and fat, and that other nutrients in the diet will be adequate. The committee also assumes that the RDA will be applied only to healthy individuals with no unusual alteration of protein metabolism. Most people in this country already eat this much protein, and more.

Protein in Foods

To make body protein, a cell must have all the needed amino acids available simultaneously. Therefore, the first important characteristic of protein in the diet of a healthy adult is that it should supply at least the 9 essential amino acids and enough nitrogen and energy for the synthesis of the other 11.

Complete Protein A protein that fits this description is called a complete protein. It contains all the essential amino acids in amounts adequate for human use; it may or may not contain all the others. Generally, proteins derived from animal foods (meats, fish, poultry, eggs, and milk) are complete, although gelatin is an exception. Proteins derived from plant foods (legumes, grains, and vegetables) vary more. Some plant

complete protein: a protein containing all the amino acids essential in human nutrition in amounts adequate for human use.

Table 4–2
Protein-Containing Foods

Milk, Cheese, and Yogurt

Each of the following provides about 8 grams of protein:[a]

- 1 cup of milk, buttermilk, or yogurt (choose low-fat or nonfat).
- 1 ounce of regular cheese (for example, cheddar or swiss).[b]
- ¼ cup of cottage cheese (choose low-fat or nonfat).

Meat, Poultry, Fish, and Alternates

Each of the following provides about 7 grams of protein:

- 1 ounce of meat, poultry, or fish (choose lean meats to limit fat intake).
- ½ cup of legumes (navy beans, pinto beans, black beans, lentils, soybeans, and other dried beans and peas).
- 1 egg.[b]
- ½ cup tofu (soybean curd).[b]
- 2 tablespoons of peanut butter.[b]
- 1 to 2 ounces of nuts or seeds.[b]

Breads, Cereals, and Other Grain Products

Each of the following provides about 3 grams of protein:

- 1 slice of bread.
- ½ cup of cooked rice, pasta, cereals, or other grain foods.

Vegetables

Each of the following provides about 2 grams of protein:

- ½ cup of cooked vegetables.
- 1 cup of raw vegetables.

[a] For reference, an adult might need from 40 to 100 grams of protein in a day.
[b] These are medium-fat or high-fat choices.

proteins are notoriously incomplete—for example, corn protein. Others are complete—for example, soy protein.[17] Using plant foods alone, the educated vegetarian can design a diet that is adequate in protein by choosing a variety of legumes, grains, and vegetables. (Vegetarian diets are discussed further in Nutrition in Practice 4.) Table 4–2 lists the protein contents of foods based on the food groups of the Daily Food Guide in Chapter 1.

Protein Digestibility and Quality Ideally, a protein should be not only complete, but easily digestible as well, so that sufficient numbers of amino acids reach the body's cells to permit them to make the proteins they need. Such a protein is called a high-quality protein. One of the finest proteins available by these standards is egg protein. Eggs are a highly valued protein source in developing nations where protein-rich foods are scarce.

high-quality protein: an easily digestible, complete protein.

Limiting Amino Acids Ideally, dietary protein supplies each amino acid in the amount needed for protein synthesis in the body. If one amino acid is supplied in an amount smaller than is needed, then the total amount of protein that can be synthesized will be limited. The body makes only complete proteins. (By analogy, suppose that a sign maker plans to make 100 identical signs saying "Left Turn Only." The sign maker needs 200 *L*s, 200 *N*s, 200 *T*s, and 100 of each of the other letters. If only 20 *L*s are available, only 10 signs can be made, even if all the other letters are available in unlimited quantities. Suppose further that the sign maker has no place to keep leftover letters—just as the body has no storage place for extra amino acids. If the sign maker doesn't get some additional *L*s right away, he will have to throw away all the other letters.)

limiting amino acid: the essential amino acid found in the shortest supply relative to the amounts needed for protein synthesis in the body. It limits the amount of protein the body can make.

Protein Sparing Dietary protein—no matter how high the quality—will not be used efficiently and will not support growth when energy from carbohydrate and fat is lacking. The body assigns top priority to meeting its energy need and, if necessary, will break down protein to meet this need. After stripping off and excreting the nitrogen from the amino acids, the body will use their carbon skeletons in much the same way it uses those from glucose or fat. A major reason why people must have ample carbohydrate and fat in the diet is to prevent this wasting of protein.

Reminder: Carbohydrate and fat allow amino acids to be used to build body proteins. This is known as the *protein-sparing effect* of carbohydrate and fat.

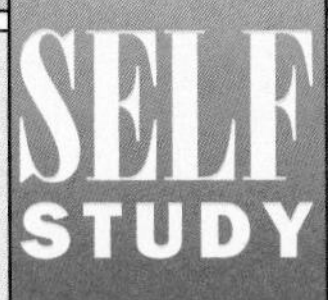

How's Your Protein Intake?

These exercises make use of the information you recorded on Forms 1 to 5.

1. How many grams of protein do you consume in a day? ___ grams
2. How many kcalories does this represent? (Remember, 1 gram of protein contributes 4 kcalories.) ___ kcalories
3. What percentage of your total kcalories is contributed by protein? ___ percent
4. Dietary guidelines suggest that protein should contribute about 10 to 15 percent of total kcalories. How does your protein intake compare with this recommendation? (Note: If you are on a kcalorie-restricted diet, a higher percentage of your kcalories should come from protein.) If your protein intake is out of line, what foods could you consume more or less of to bring it into line? ____________________

   ____
5. Compare your protein intake (from item 1) with the recommendation for an "average" person of your age and sex as shown in the RDA tables (inside front cover) or in the Canadian recommendations (Appendix B): ___ If you are not of average height or weight, figure your protein RDA:
   a. Look up the weight for a person your height (inside back cover). Assume this weight is "ideal" for you.
   b. Change pounds to kilograms: 2.2 pounds equal 1 kilogram.
   c. Multiply kilograms by 0.8 grams/kilogram.

   Example (for a medium-frame male 5 feet 10 inches tall):

   a. "Ideal" weight: about 150 pounds.
   b. 150 pounds x 1 kilogram/2.2 pounds = 68 kilograms (rounded off).
   c. 68 kilograms x 0.8 grams/kilogram = 54 grams protein (rounded off).
6. Compare your average daily protein intake with your RDA. About what percentage of that intake are you consuming each day? ___ percent. If you are "average" and healthy, the recommendation is probably generous for you, yet you may be eating more protein than that.

(continued)

Self-Study (continued)

If so, you may be spending protein prices for an energy nutrient. What substitutions could you make in your day's food choices that would enable you to derive the kcalories you need for energy from carbohydrate rather than from protein? ______________________

____

7. How many of your protein grams are from animal foods? ___ How many are from plant foods? ___ Assuming that the animal protein is of high quality, no more than 20 percent of your total protein intake need come from this source. Should you alter the ratio of plant to animal protein in your diet? ___ If you were to do so, what effect would this have on the total fat content of your diet? ______________________

____

PEM is a common finding among people in the hospital. The many negative effects of protein deficiency described in this chapter can help you to see why such a deficiency can be particularly dangerous at a time of severe illness (see Chapter 18). Dietitians assess protein status not only by checking protein intake but also by using anthropometric and biochemical measures. Chapter 13 describes these tests in detail.

STUDY QUESTIONS

1. Chemically, how does protein differ from carbohydrate and fat?
2. What is an essential amino acid?
3. What is an enzyme?
4. List and describe at least three main functions of proteins in the body.
5. How can kwashiorkor be distinguished from marasmus?
6. What is a complete protein?

NUTRITION IN PRACTICE 4

Vegetarian Diets

Eating patterns all along the continuum of dietary choices—from one end, where people eat no foods of animal origin, to the other end, where they eat generous quantities of meat every day—can support or compromise nutritional health. The quality of the diet depends not on whether it consists of all plant foods or centers on meat, but on whether the eater's food choices are based on sound nutrition principles—adequacy of nutrient intakes; balance and variety of foods chosen; appropriate energy intake; and moderation in intakes of substances such as fat, sodium, alcohol, and caffeine that are harmful in excess.

People choose to exclude meat and other animal-derived foods from their diets for various reasons—philosophies, health attitudes, or convenience. Some believe that vegetarianism is better for the environment; some, that it is healthier; and some, that it is less costly than the meat-eating alternative. Some just like it better. Whatever the reasons, vegetarians and health professionals who work with them should be aware of the nutrition and health implications of the vegetarian diet.

Because vegetarian diets vary in both the types and amounts of animal-derived foods they include, these differences must be considered when evaluating the health status of vegetarians. The glossary defines the various kinds of vegetarian diets.

I've been thinking about becoming a vegetarian, but I'm not sure vegetarian diets are nutritionally sound. Are they?

The American Dietetic Association takes the position that well-planned vegetarian diets offer nutrition and health benefits to adults in general.[18] Research suggests that meat-eating adults who switch to vegetarian diets reduce their risks of heart disease, hypertension, diabetes, and obesity.[19]

What should be my main concerns when planning a nutritionally sound vegetarian diet?

A vegetarian diet planner faces the same task as other diet planners—to plan to obtain a variety of foods that provide all the needed nutrients within an energy allowance that maintains a healthy body weight. The challenge is to do so using at least one less food group. Since all vegetarians omit meat, and some omit other animal-derived foods, protein, the nutrient that meat is famous for, merits some discussion here.

Yes, I've heard that vegetarian diets are low in protein. Is this true?

No, protein is not the problem it was once thought to be in vegetarian diets. People who include animal-derived foods such as milk and eggs in their diets need not worry at all about protein deficiency. Even for those who eat nothing but plant-derived foods, protein intakes are usually satisfactory as long as energy intakes are adequate and the protein sources varied.[20] A mixture of proteins from whole grains, legumes, seeds, nuts, and vegetables can provide adequate amounts of all the amino acids.

The idea persists that vegans must carefully combine their plant protein foods in order to

Glossary of Vegetarian Terms

complementary proteins: two or more proteins whose amino acid assortments complement each other in such a way that the essential amino acids missing from each are supplied by the other.

lacto-vegetarians: people who include milk or milk products, but exclude meat, poultry, fish, seafood, and eggs from their diets.

lacto-ovo vegetarians: people who include milk or milk products and eggs, but omit meat, fish, and poultry from their diets.

mutual supplementation: the strategy of combining two protein foods in a meal so that each food provides the essential amino acid(s) lacking in the other.

semivegetarians: people who include some, but not all, groups of animal-derived foods in their diets; they usually exclude meat and may occasionally include poultry, fish, and seafood; also called *partial vegetarians*.

vegans: people who exclude all animal-derived foods (including meat, poultry, fish, eggs, cheese, and milk) from their diet; also called *strict vegetarians* or *total vegetarians*.

obtain the full array of essential amino acids, but new knowledge indicates that this is not necessary. Plant foods can provide more than enough of all the essential amino acids and can sustain people in good health, as long as the diet supplies sufficient energy and does not include too many empty-kcalorie foods. It is true, however, that a meal delivers higher-quality protein when it combines two or more different individual plant protein sources, each of which supplies amino acids missing from the others. This strategy is called *mutual supplementation.* The protein foods that mutually supplement each other are called *complementary proteins.* Figure 4–6 shows combinations of plant proteins that provide higher-quality protein than the individual foods alone could supply.

What sorts of food energy intakes do vegetarian diets provide?

Researchers find that vegetarians as a group are closer to a healthy body weight than nonvegetarians. Since obesity impairs health in a number of ways, vegetarians therefore have a health advantage. Vegetarian diets tend to be high in complex carbohydrates and low in fat, characteristics that are consistent with current dietary recommendations aimed at reducing the incidence of obesity and other degenerative diseases in this country.

Not all vegetarians fit the average pattern, though. Obesity does threaten vegetarians who include milk, eggs, and cheese in their diets. They can easily consume both a high-fat diet and excess food energy, and so must be careful to select nonfat and low-fat dairy foods and to avoid relying too heavily on these foods in general.

In contrast, people who exclude all animal-derived foods (vegans) may have trouble obtaining *enough* food energy. This is especially true for children and pregnant and lactating women.[21] Vegan diets can fail to provide food energy sufficient to support the growth of a child within a bulk of food small enough for the child to eat.[22] Plant foods that are best suited to meeting energy needs in a small volume are cereals, legumes, and nuts; these foods should be emphasized in a vegan child's diet. Table 1–3 in

Figure 4–6
Nonmeat Mixtures That Provide High-Quality Protein
Vegetarians who eat no foods from animal sources select foods from two or more of these columns to create high-quality protein combinations:

Grains	Legumes	Seeds and Nuts	Vegetables
Oats	Peanuts	Cashews	Broccoli
Rice	Soy products	Nut butters	Cabbage
Whole-grain breads	Pinto beans	Sesame seeds	Peppers
Pasta	Black beans		Squash
			Spinach

Examples:

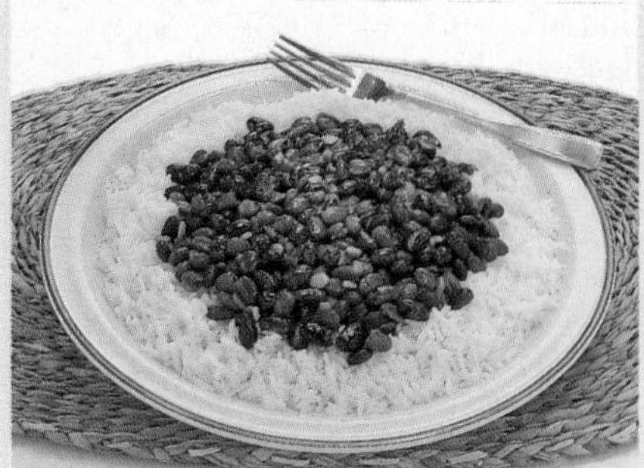
Black beans and rice, a favorite Hispanic combination.

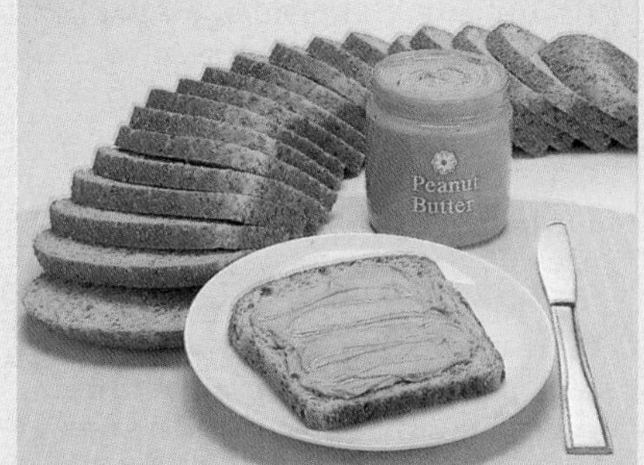

Peanut butter and wheat bread, a North American tradition.

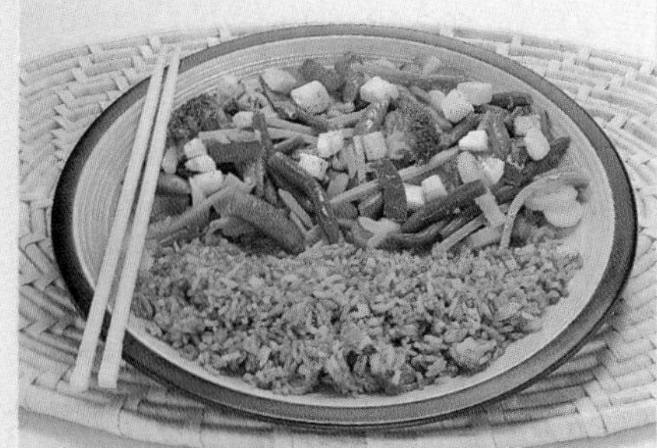
Tofu and stir-fried vegetables with rice, an Asian dish.

Chapter 1 offers a suggested daily food guide for vegetarians.

Tell me about vitamins and minerals. If I choose to eat a vegetarian diet, will I need to take vitamin supplements?

That depends on the kind of vegetarian diet you follow. The lacto-ovo vegetarian diet can be complete in all vitamins, but for the vegan, several vitamins may be a problem. One such vitamin is B_{12}. Because vitamin B_{12} occurs only in animal-derived foods, supplements are necessary to prevent deficiency. Women who have adhered to all-plant diets for many years are especially likely to have low vitamin B_{12} stores. Pregnant vegan women, whose needs for vitamin B_{12} are especially high, find it virtually impossible to maintain adequate vitamin B_{12} status without taking supplements or including a reliable food source of the nutrient.

A vitamin B_{12} deficiency can take a long time to develop in adults because up to four years' worth of the vitamin can be stored in the body. But when the deficiency sets in, it does severe damage to the nervous system (see Chapter 7). In infants, deficiencies set in more rapidly and so threaten their nervous systems early. All vegan mothers must be sure to take the appropriate supplements or to use vitamin B_{12}–fortified products.

What other vitamins do vegans need?

Another vitamin of concern is vitamin D. The milk drinker is protected, provided the milk is fortified with vitamin D, but there is no practical source of vitamin D in plant foods. Regular exposure to the sun will prevent a deficiency, but vegans who are homebound or live in a northern climate or smoggy city probably should take vitamin D supplements. Excesses of vitamin D are toxic, and one should not exceed the recommended daily amount of 5 micrograms.

Riboflavin, another vitamin often obtained from milk, is not a problem for the vegan who eats dark greens frequently in ample servings. The vegan who doesn't consume a lot of greens, however, may not meet riboflavin needs. Nutritional yeast is a rich source of riboflavin for the vegetarian.

So, on a vegan diet, vitamin B_{12}, vitamin D, and riboflavin can be problems if I'm not careful. What about minerals?

For *all* vegetarians, not just the vegan, two minerals may be of concern. These minerals are iron and zinc. Legumes are an important source of iron in the vegetarian diet. The iron in legumes, however, is not as absorbable as that in meat. In fact, people absorb three times as much iron from a meal that includes meat as from one that does not. Because vitamin C in fruits and vegetables can triple iron absorption from other foods eaten at the same meal, vegetarian meals should be rich in foods offering vitamin C.

Zinc may also be a problem nutrient for vegetarians. It is widespread in plant foods, but its availability may be hindered by the fibers and other binders found in fruits and vegetables. The zinc needs of vegetarians and the effects of mineral binders are subjects of intensive study at the present time. While research continues, vegetarians are advised to eat varied diets that include whole-grain breads well leavened with yeast, which improves the availability of their minerals.

What about calcium for the vegan?

Good thinking. Yes, of course calcium is of concern. The milk-drinking vegetarian is protected from deficiency, but the vegan must find other sources of calcium. Some good calcium sources are regular and ample servings of stone-ground meal, self-rising flour and meal, legumes, calcium-fortified soy milk, calcium-fortified orange juice, some nuts such as almonds, and certain seeds such as sesame seeds. The choices should be varied because binders in some of these foods may hinder absorption. The vegetarian is urged to use calcium-fortified soy milk in ample quantities regularly. This is especially important for children. Infant formula based on soy is fortified with calcium and can easily be used in cooking foods, even for adults.

It sounds as though I can do well with a vegetarian diet as long as I do a little planning. I could use some help with weight control. Are there any other health advantages to the vegetarian diet?

Yes. Vegetarian protein foods are often higher in fiber, richer in certain vitamins and minerals, and lower in fat than meats. Vegetarians can enjoy a nutritious diet very low in fat provided that they limit other high-fat foods such as butter, cream cheese, sour cream, and nuts. If vegetarians follow the guidelines presented here and plan carefully, they can support their health as well as, or perhaps better than, nonvegetarians.

Abundant evidence supports the idea that vegetarians may actually be healthier than meat eaters. Informed vegetarians are not only more likely to be at the desired weights for their heights,

but to have lower blood cholesterol levels, lower rates of certain kinds of cancer, better digestive function, and more. Even among people who are health conscious, generally vegetarians experience fewer deaths from cardiovascular disease than meat eaters do. Since vegetarians also often abstain from smoking and the consumption of alcohol, dietary practices alone probably do not account for all the aspects of improved health. Clearly, however, they contribute significantly to it.

■ NOTES ■

1. P. L. Pellett, Protein requirements in humans, *American Journal of Clinical Nutrition* 51 (1990): 723–727.
2. J. M. Lacey and D. W. Wilmore, Is glutamine a conditionally essential amino acid? *Nutrition Reviews* 48 (1990): 297–309; S. Mobrahan, Glutamine: A conditionally essential nutrient or another nutritional puzzle, *Nutrition Reviews* 50 (1992): 331–333.
3. V. R. Young and J. S. Marchini, Mechanisms and nutritional significance of metabolic responses to altered intakes of protein and amino acids, with reference to nutritional adaptation in humans, *American Journal of Clinical Nutrition* 51 (1990): 270–289.
4. M. C. Latham, Protein-energy malnutrition, in *Present Knowledge in Nutrition,* 6th ed., ed. M. L. Brown (Washington, D.C.: International Life Sciences Institute—Nutrition Foundation, 1990), pp. 39–46.
5. J. Wolgemuth and coauthors, Wasting malnutrition and inadequate nutrient intakes identified in a multiethnic homeless population, *Journal of the American Dietetic Association* 92 (1992): 834–839; E. Luder and coauthors, Health and nutrition survey in a group of urban homeless adults, *Journal of the American Dietetic Association* 90 (1990): 1387–1392.
6. C. Gopalan, The contribution of nutrition research to the control of undernutrition: The Indian experience, *Annual Review of Nutrition* 12 (1992): 1–17.
7. Goplan, 1992.
8. R. G. Hendrickse, Kwashiorkor: The hypothesis that incriminates aflatoxins, *Pediatrics* 88 (1991): 376–379.
9. D. B. Jelliffe and E. F. P. Jelliffe, Causation of kwashiorkor: Toward a multifactorial consensus, *Pediatrics* 90 (1992): 110–113.
10. L. Lewinter-Suskind and coauthors, The malnourished child, in *Textbook of Pediatric Nutrition,* 2nd ed., ed. R. M. Suskind and L. Lewinter-Suskind (New York: Raven Press, 1993), pp. 127–140.
11. R. K. Chandra, 1990 McCollum Award Lecture: Nutrition and immunity: Lessons from the past and new insights into the future, *American Journal of Clinical Nutrition* 53 (1991): 1087–1101.
12. Lewinter-Suskind and coauthors, 1993.
13. Pellett, 1990.
14. C. D. Arnold and S. D. Sanchez, The role of calcium in osteoporosis, *Annual Review of Nutrition* 10 (1990): 397–414.
15. R. P. Heaney, Protein intake and the calcium economy, *Journal of the American Dietetic Association* 93 (1993): 1259–1260.
16. D. Farley, Making sure hype doesn't overwhelm science, *FDA Consumer,* November 1993, pp. 9–13.
17. V. R. Young, Soy protein in relation to human protein and amino acid nutrition, *Journal of the American Dietetic Association* 91 (1991): 828–835.
18. Position of the American Dietetic Association: Vegetarian diets, *Journal of the American Dietetic Association* 93 (1993): 1317–1319.
19. T. C. Campbell and C. Junshi, Diet and chronic degenerative diseases: Perspectives from China, *American Journal of Clinical Nutrition* (Supplement) 59 (1994): 1153–1161; J. T. Dwyer, Health aspects of vegetarian diets, *American Journal of Clinical Nutrition* 48 (1988): 712–738.
20. Dwyer, 1988.
21. L. H. Allen and coauthors, The interactive effects of dietary quality on the growth and attained size of young Mexican children, *American Journal of Clinical Nutrition* 56 (1992): 353–364; T. Sanders and S. Reddy, Vegetarian diets and children, *American Journal of Clinical Nutrition* (supplement) 59 (1994): 1176–1181.
22. C. Jacobs and J. T. Dwyer, Vegetarian children: Appropriate and inappropriate diets, *American Journal of Clinical Nutrition* 48 (1988): 811–818.

5

Digestion and Absorption

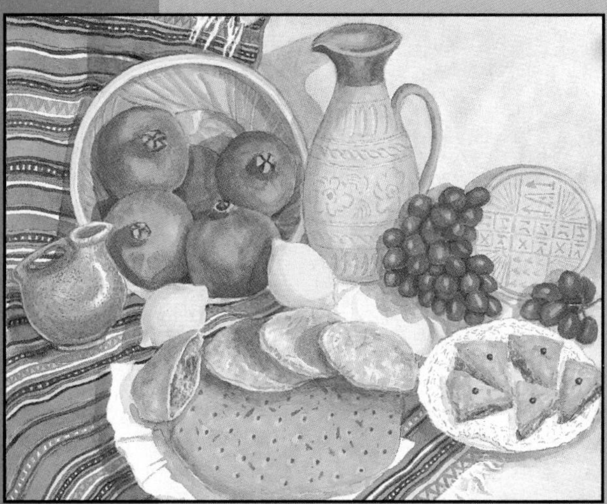

CONTENTS

Your body's ability to transform the foods you eat into the nutrients that fuel its work is quite remarkable. Yet most people probably give little, if any, thought to all the body does with food once it is eaten. This chapter offers you the opportunity to learn how the body digests, absorbs, and transports the nutrients, and how it excretes the unwanted substances in foods. The next chapter shows you how the body assimilates the nutrients once they have been absorbed and are traveling in the blood and lymph.

One of the beauties of the digestive tract is that it is selective. Materials that are nutritive for the body are broken down into particles that can be absorbed into the bloodstream. Most of the nonnutritive materials are left undigested and pass out the other end of the digestive tract.

Anatomy of the Digestive Tract

GI tract: the gastrointestinal tract or digestive tract; the principal organs are the stomach and intestines.
gastro = stomach

The gastrointestinal (GI) tract is a flexible muscular tube measuring about 26 feet in length from the mouth to the anus. Figure 5–1 on pp. 98–99 traces the path followed by food from one end to the other. The accompanying glossary defines GI anatomy terms. In a sense, the human body surrounds the GI tract. Only when a nutrient or other substance passes through the cells of the digestive tract wall does it actually enter the body.

The Digestive Organs

digestion: the process by which complex food particles are broken down to smaller absorbable particles.

The process of digestion begins in the mouth as you begin to chew. The teeth crush and soften foods, while saliva mixes with the food mass and moistens it for comfortable swallowing. Saliva also helps dissolve the food so that you can taste it; only particles in solution can react with taste buds.

bolus (BOH-lus)**:** the portion of food swallowed at one time.

Mouth to the Esophagus Once a mouthful of food has been swallowed, it is called a bolus. Each bolus first slides across your epiglottis, bypassing the entrance to your lungs. During each swallow, the epiglottis closes off your air passages so that you do not choke.

sphincter: a circular muscle surrounding, and able to close, a body opening.
sphincter = band (binder)

Esophagus to the Stomach Next, the bolus slides down the esophagus, which conducts it through the diaphragm to the stomach. The cardiac sphincter, a band of muscle surrounding the esophagus where it enters the stomach, closes behind the bolus so that it cannot slip back. The stomach retains the bolus for a while, adds juices to it (gastric juices are discussed on p. 104), and grinds it into a semiliquid mass called chyme. Then bit by bit, the stomach releases the chyme through another sphincter, the pyloric sphincter, which opens into the small intestine and then closes behind the chyme.

chyme (KIME)**:** the semiliquid mass of partly digested food expelled by the stomach into the duodenum.

The Small Intestine At the top of the small intestine, the chyme passes by an opening from the common bile duct. Through this opening, the gallbladder secretes fluids into the small intestine from outside the GI tract. The chyme travels on down the small intestine through its three segments—the duodenum, the jejunum, and the ileum—a total of 20 feet of tubing coiled within the abdomen.

The Colon (Large Intestine) Having traveled the length of the small intestine, the chyme passes through another sphincter, the ileocecal valve, into the beginning of the colon (large intestine) in the lower right-hand side of the abdomen. In the colon, the chyme travels up the right-hand side of the abdomen, across the front to the left-hand side, down to the

Glossary of GI Terms

These terms are listed in order from the beginning of the digestive tract to the end.

epiglottis (epp-ee-GLOT-tiss)**:** a cartilage structure in the throat that prevents fluid or food from entering the trachea when a person swallows.
epi = upon (over)
glottis = back of tongue

trachea (TRAKE-ee-uh)**:** the windpipe; the passageway from the mouth and nose to the lungs.

esophagus (e-SOFF-uh-gus)**:** the food pipe; the conduit from the mouth to the stomach.

cardiac sphincter (CARD-ee-ack SFINK-ter)**:** the sphincter muscle at the junction between the esophagus and the stomach.
cardiac = heart

pyloric (pie-LORE-ic) **sphincter:** the sphincter muscle separating the stomach from the small intestine (also called *pylorus* or *pyloric valve*).
pylorus = gatekeeper

gallbladder: the organ that stores and concentrates bile. When it receives the signal that fat is present in the duodenum, the gallbladder contracts and squirts bile through the bile duct into the duodenum.

pancreas: a gland that secretes enzymes and digestive juices into the duodenum. (This is its exocrine function; it also has the endocrine function of secreting insulin and other hormones into the blood.)

small intestine: a 20-foot length of small-diameter (1-inch) intestine that is the major site of digestion of food and absorption of nutrients.

duodenum (doo-oh-DEEN-um or doo-ODD-num)**:** the top portion of the small intestine (about "12 fingers' breadth" long, in ancient terminology).
duodecim = twelve

jejunum (je-JOON-um)**:** the first two-fifths of the small intestine beyond the duodenum.

ileum (ILL-ee-um)**:** the last segment of the small intestine.

ileocecal (ill-ee-oh-SEEK-ul) **valve:** the sphincter muscle separating the small and large intestines.

colon or **large intestine:** the last portion of the intestine, which absorbs water. Its main segments are the ascending colon, the transverse colon, the descending colon, and the sigmoid colon.
sigmoid = shaped like the letter S (*sigma* in Greek)

appendix: a narrow blind sac extending from the beginning of the colon; a vestigial organ with no known function.

rectum: the muscular terminal part of the GI tract extending from the sigmoid colon to the anus; the rectum stores waste prior to elimination.

anus (AY-nus)**:** the terminal sphincter muscle of the GI tract.

Figure 5–1
The Gastrointestinal Tract

FIBER	CARBOHYDRATE
Mouth The mechanical action of the mouth and teeth crushes and tears fiber in food and mixes it with saliva to moisten it for swallowing.	The salivary glands secrete a watery fluid into the mouth to moisten the food. The salivary enzyme amylase begins digestion: Starch $\xrightarrow{\text{amylase}}$ small polysaccharides, maltose.
Esophagus Fiber is unchanged.	Digestion of starch continues as swallowed food moves down the esophagus.
Stomach Fiber is unchanged.	Stomach acid and enzymes start to digest salivary enzymes, halting starch digestion. To a small extent, stomach acid hydrolyzes maltose and sucrose.
Small intestine Fiber is unchanged.	The pancreas produces enzymes and releases them through the pancreatic duct into the small intestine: Polysaccharides $\xrightarrow[\text{amylase}]{\text{pancreatic}}$ disaccharides. Then enzymes on the surfaces of the small intestinal cells break disaccharides into monosaccharides, and the cells absorb them: Maltose $\xrightarrow{\text{maltase}}$ glucose + glucose. Sucrose $\xrightarrow{\text{sucrase}}$ fructose + glucose. Lactose $\xrightarrow{\text{lactase}}$ galactose + glucose.
Colon (large intestine) Most fiber passes intact through the digestive tract to the colon. Here, bacterial enzymes digest some fiber: Some fiber $\xrightarrow[\text{enzymes}]{\text{bacterial}}$ fatty acids, gas. Fiber holds water; regulates bowel activity; and binds cholesterol and some minerals, carrying them out of the body as it is excreted with feces.	

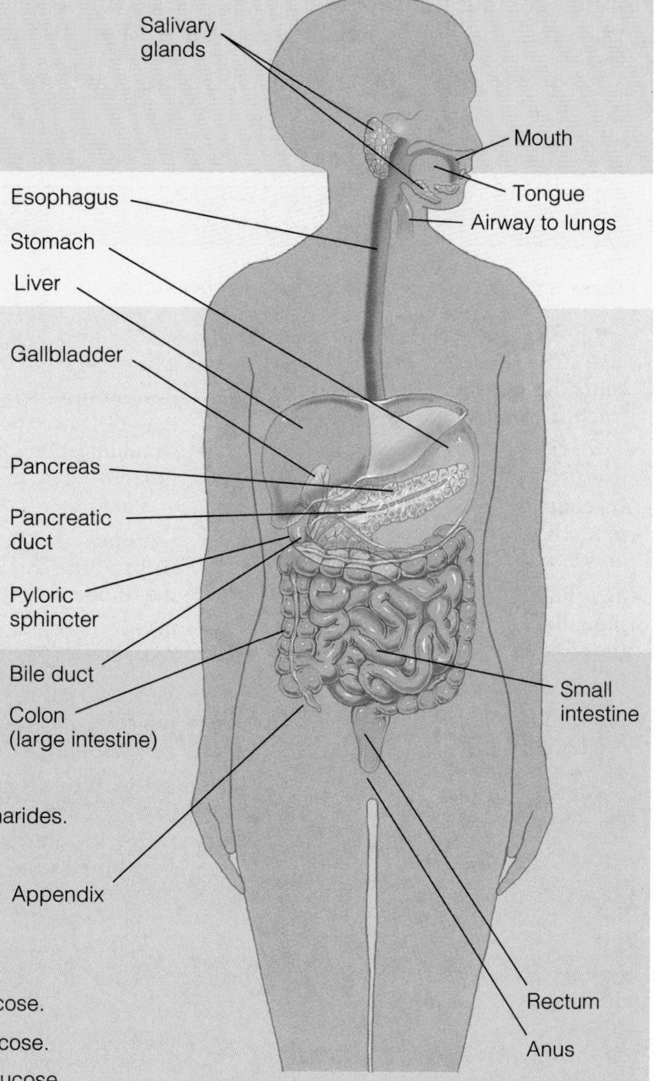

Salivary glands
Mouth
Tongue
Esophagus
Airway to lungs
Stomach
Liver
Gallbladder
Pancreas
Pancreatic duct
Pyloric sphincter
Bile duct
Small intestine
Colon (large intestine)
Appendix
Rectum
Anus

	FAT	PROTEIN	VITAMINS	MINERALS AND WATER
Mouth	Glands in the base of the tongue secrete a fat-digesting enzyme known as lingual lipase. Some hard fats begin to melt as they reach body temperature.	Chewing and crushing moisten protein-rich foods and mix them with saliva to be swallowed.	No action.	The salivary glands add water to disperse and carry food.
Esophagus	Fat is unchanged.	No action.	No action.	No action.
Stomach	The acid-stable lingual lipase splits one bond of triglycerides to produce diglycerides and fatty acids. The degree of hydrolysis is slight for most fats but may be appreciable for milk fats. The stomach's churning action mixes fat with water and acid. A gastric lipase accesses and hydrolyzes a very little fat.	Stomach acid uncoils protein strands and activates stomach enzymes: $\text{Protein} \xrightarrow[\text{HCl}]{\text{pepsin}} \text{smaller polypeptides.}$	Intrinsic factor (see Chapter 7) attaches to vitamin B_{12}.	Stomach acid (HCl) acts on iron to reduce it, making it more absorbable (see Chapter 8). The stomach secretes enough watery fluid to turn a moist, chewed mass of solid food into liquid chyme.
Small intestine	Bile flows in from the liver and gallbladder (via the common bile duct): $\text{Fat} \xrightarrow{\text{bile}} \text{emulsified fat.}$ Pancreatic lipase flows in from the pancreas (via the pancreatic duct): $\text{Emulsified fat} \xrightarrow[\text{lipase}]{\text{pancreatic}}$ monoglycerides, glycerol, fatty acids (absorbed).	Pancreatic and small intestinal enzymes split polypeptides further: $\text{Polypeptides} \xrightarrow[\text{and intestinal proteases}]{\text{pancreatic}}$ dipeptides, tripeptides, and amino acids. Then enzymes on the surface of the small intestinal cells hydrolyze these peptides, and the cells absorb them: $\text{Peptides} \xrightarrow[\text{dipeptidases and tripeptidases}]{\text{intestinal}} \text{amino acids (absorbed)}$	Bile emulsifies fat-soluble vitamins and aids in their absorption with other fats. Water-soluble vitamins are absorbed.	The small intestine, pancreas, and liver add enough fluid so that approximately 2 gallons are secreted into the intestine in a day. Many minerals are absorbed. Vitamin D aids in the absorption of calcium.
Colon	Some fat and cholesterol, trapped in fiber, exit in feces.		Bacteria produce vitamin K, which is absorbed.	More minerals and most of the water are absorbed.

Path of food:
- Mouth.
- Esophagus.
- Cardiac sphincter (or lower esophageal sphincter.
- Stomach.
- Pyloric sphincter.
- Duodenum (common bile duct enters here), jejunum, ileum.
- Ileocecal valve.
- Colon.
- Rectum.
- Anus.

lower left-hand side, and finally below the other folds of the intestines to the back side of the body above the rectum.

The Rectum During chyme's passage to the rectum, the colon withdraws water from it, leaving semisolid waste. The strong muscles of the rectum hold back this waste until it is time to defecate. Then the rectal muscles relax, and the last sphincter in the system, the anus, opens to allow the wastes to pass.

In summary, food follows the path shown in the margin. Considering all that happens on the way, the route is remarkably simple.

The Involuntary Muscles and the Glands

You are usually unaware of all the activity that goes on between the time you swallow and the time you defecate. As is the case with so much else that happens in the body, the muscles and glands of the digestive tract meet internal needs without your having to exert any conscious effort to get the work done.

People consciously chew and swallow, but even in the mouth there are some processes over which you have no control. The salivary glands secrete just enough saliva to moisten each mouthful of food so that it can pass easily down your esophagus.

gland: a cell or group of cells that secretes materials for special uses in the body. Glands may be *exocrine glands,* secreting their materials "out" (into the digestive tract or onto the surface of the skin) or *endocrine glands,* secreting their materials "in" (into the blood).
exo = outside
endo = inside
krine = to separate

gastric motility: spontaneous motion in the digestive tract accomplished by involuntary muscular contractions.

Gastric Motility Once you have swallowed, materials are moved through the rest of the GI tract by involuntary muscular contractions. This motion, known as gastric motility, consists of two types of movement, peristalsis and segmentation (see Figure 5–2). Peristalsis propels, or pushes; segmentation mixes, with more gradual pushing.

peristalsis: (peri-STALL-sis) successive waves of involuntary muscular contractions passing along the walls of the GI tract that push the contents along.
peri = around
stellein = wrap

Peristalsis Peristalsis begins when the bolus enters the esophagus. The entire GI tract is ringed with circular muscles that can squeeze it tightly. Surrounding these rings of muscle are longitudinal muscles. When the rings tighten and the long muscles relax, the tube is constricted. When the rings relax and the long muscles tighten, the tube bulges. These actions follow each other continuously and push the intestinal contents along. If you have ever watched a bolus of food pass along the body of a snake, you have a good picture of how these muscles work. The waves of contraction ripple through the GI tract at varying rates and intensities depending on the part of the GI tract and on whether food is present. Peristalsis, aided by the sphincter muscles that surround the tract at key places, keeps things moving along.

segmentation: a periodic squeezing or partitioning of the intestine by its circular muscles that both mixes and slowly pushes the contents along.

Segmentation The intestines not only push but also periodically squeeze their contents as if a string tied around the intestines were being pulled tight. This motion, called segmentation, forces the contents back a few inches, mixing them and promoting close contact with the digestive juices and the absorbing cells of the intestinal walls before letting them slowly move along again.

Figure 5–2
Peristalsis and Segmentation

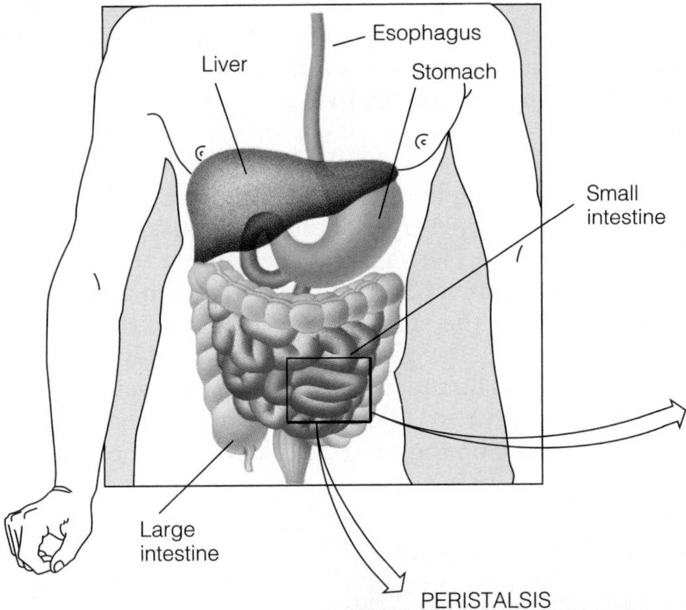

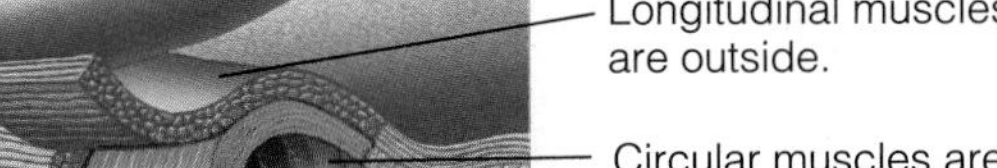

Longitudinal muscles are outside.

Circular muscles are on the inside.

The small intestine has two muscle layers that work together in peristalsis and segmentation.

PERISTALSIS

SEGMENTATON

The inner circular muscle layer contracts, tightening the tube and pushing the food forward in the intestine.

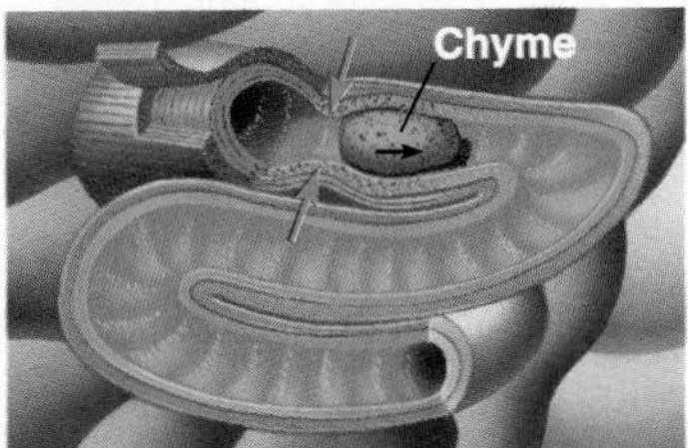

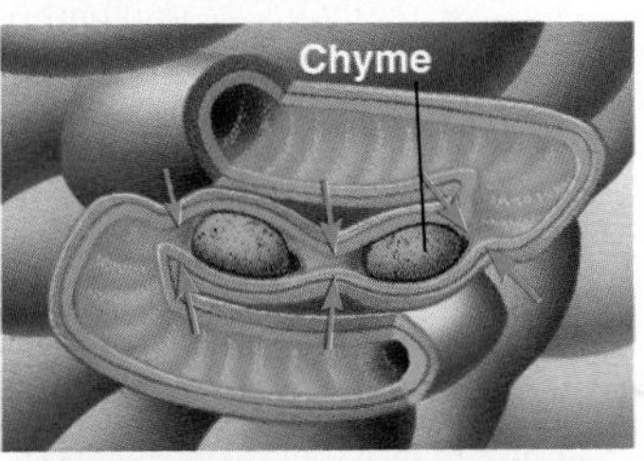

Simultaneous circular muscle contractions occur in food-containing sections of the intestine, creating segments within the intestine.

When the outer longitudinal muscles contract, the circular muscles relax and the intestinal tube is loose.

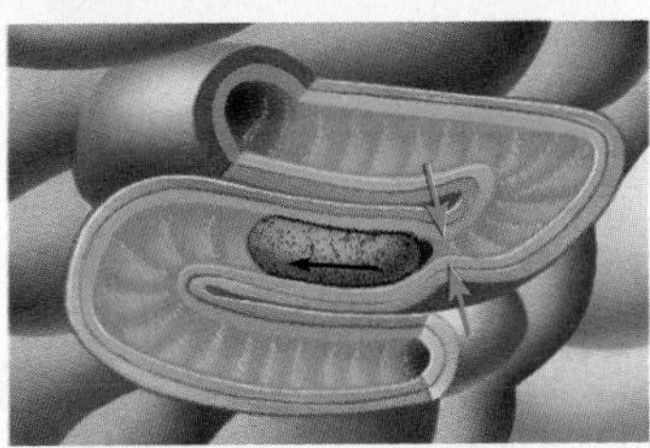

Muscles circling the middle of each segment contract and the first set of muscles relaxes. The chyme is broken up and mixed with digestive juices.

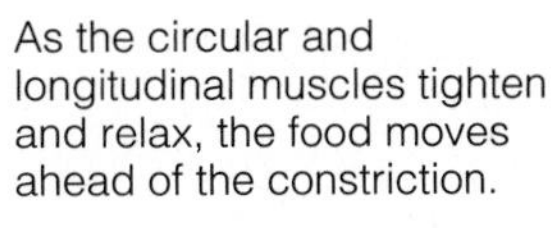

As the circular and longitudinal muscles tighten and relax, the food moves ahead of the constriction.

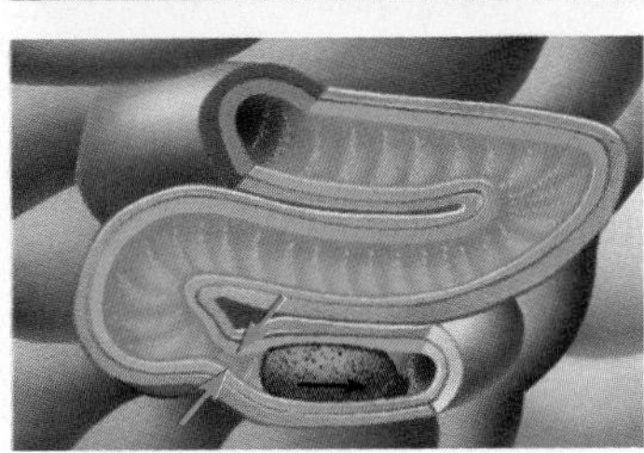

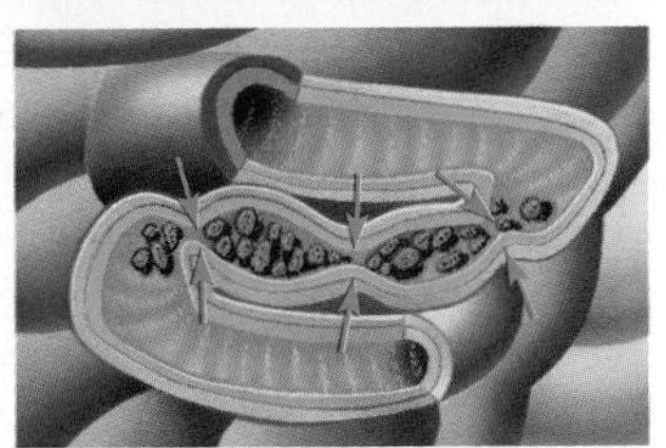

These alternating contractions, occuring 12 –16 times per minute, continue to mix the chyme and bring it into contact with the intestinal lining for absorption of nutrients.

Liquefying Process Besides forcing the intestinal contents along, the muscles of the GI tract help to liquefy them to chyme so that the digestive enzymes will have access to all their nutrients. The mouth initiates this liquefying process by chewing, adding saliva, and stirring with the tongue to reduce the food to a coarse mash suitable for swallowing. The stomach then further mixes and kneads the food.

Stomach Action The stomach has the thickest walls and strongest muscles of all the GI tract organs. In addition to the circular and longitudinal muscles, the stomach has a third layer of diagonal muscles that also alternately contract and relax (see Figure 5–3). These three sets of muscles work to force the chyme downward, but the pyloric sphincter usually remains tightly closed, so that the stomach's contents are thoroughly mixed and squeezed. Meanwhile, the gastric glands are adding juices. When the chyme is thoroughly liquefied, the pyloric sphincter opens briefly, about three times a minute, to allow small portions through. At this point, the intestinal contents no longer resemble food in the least.

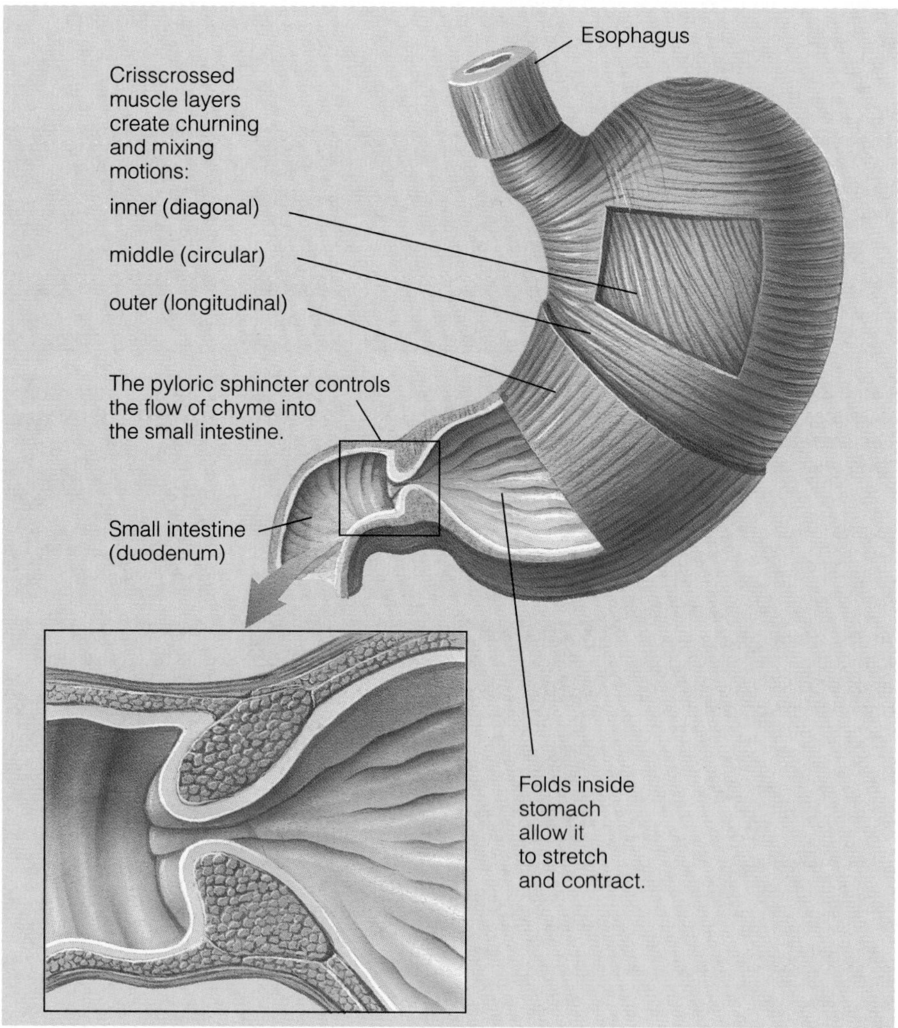
Esophagus
Crisscrossed muscle layers create churning and mixing motions:
inner (diagonal)
middle (circular)
outer (longitudinal)
The pyloric sphincter controls the flow of chyme into the small intestine.
Small intestine (duodenum)
Folds inside stomach allow it to stretch and contract.

Figure 5–3
Stomach Muscles
The stomach has three layers of muscles.

The Process of Digestion

One person eats nothing but vegetables, fruits, and nuts; another, nothing but meat, milk, and potatoes. How is it that both people wind up with essentially the same body composition? It all comes down to the fact that the body renders food—whatever it is to start with—into the basic units that make up carbohydrate, fat, and protein. The body absorbs these units and builds its tissues from them.

To digest food, five different body organs secrete digestive juices: the salivary glands, the stomach, the small intestine, the liver (via the gallbladder), and the pancreas. Each of the juices mixes with the food and promotes its breakdown into small units that can be absorbed into the body. The accompanying glossary defines some of the digestive glands and their juices.

Glossary of Digestive Glands and Their Juices

These terms are listed in order from the beginning of the digestive tract to the end.

salivary glands: exocrine glands that secrete saliva into the mouth.

saliva: the secretion of the salivary glands; the principal enzyme is salivary amylase.

amylase (AM-uh-lace)**:** an enzyme that splits amylose (a form of starch). Amylase is a carbohydrase. The ending *-ase* indicates an enzyme; the root tells what it digests. Other examples: protease, lipase.

gastric glands: exocrine glands in the stomach wall that secrete gastric juice into the stomach.
gastro = stomach

gastric juice: the digestive secretion of the gastric glands containing a mixture of water, hydrochloric acid, and enzymes. The principal enzymes are pepsin (acts on proteins) and lipase (acts on emulsified fats).

hydrochloric acid (HCl): an acid composed of hydrogen and chloride atoms. The gastric glands normally produce this acid.

mucus (MYOO-cuss)**:** a mucopolysaccharide (a relative of carbohydrate) secreted by cells of the stomach wall that protects the cells from exposure to digestive juices (and other destructive agents). The cellular lining of the stomach wall with its coat of mucus is known as the mucous membrane. (The noun is *mucus;* the adjective is *mucous.*)

pepsin: a protein-digesting enzyme (gastric protease) in the stomach. It circulates as a precursor, pepsinogen, and is converted to pepsin by the action of stomach acid.

intestinal juice: the secretion of the intestinal glands; contains enzymes for the digestion of carbohydrate and protein and a minor enzyme for fat digestion.

bile: an emulsifier that prepares fats and oils for digestion; made by the liver, stored in the gallbladder, and released into the small intestine when needed.

pancreatic (pank-ree-AT-ic) **juice:** the exocrine secretion of the pancreas, containing enzymes for the digestion of carbohydrate, fat, and protein. Juice flows from the pancreas into the small intestine through the pancreatic duct. The pancreas also has an endocrine function, the secretion of insulin and other hormones.

bicarbonate: an alkaline secretion of the pancreas; part of the pancreatic juice. (Bicarbonate also occurs widely in all cell fluids.)

Digestion in the Mouth

Digestion of carbohydrate begins in the mouth, where the salivary glands secrete saliva, which contains water, salts, and enzymes (including salivary amylase) that break the bonds in the chains of starch. Saliva also protects the tooth surfaces and linings of the mouth, esophagus, and stomach from attack by molecules that might harm them. The enzymes in the mouth do not affect the fats, proteins, vitamins, minerals, and fiber that are present in the foods people eat.

Digestion in the Stomach

Gastric juice is composed of water, enzymes, and hydrochloric acid. The acid is so strong that it burns the throat if it chances to reflux into the upper esophagus and mouth. The strong acidity of the stomach prevents bacterial growth and kills most bacteria that enter the body with food. You might expect that the stomach's acid would attack the stomach itself, but the cells of the stomach wall secrete mucus, a thick, slimy, white polysaccharide that coats the stomach's lining.

Digestive Activities The major digestive event in the stomach is the initial breakdown of proteins. Other than being crushed and mixed with saliva in the mouth, nothing happens to protein until it comes in contact with the gastric juices in the stomach. There, the acid helps to uncoil (denature) the protein's tangled strands so that the stomach enzymes can attack the bonds. Both the enzyme pepsin and the stomach acid itself act as catalysts in the process. Minor events are the digestion of some fat by a gastric lipase, the digestion of sucrose (to a very small extent) by the stomach acid, and the attachment of a protein carrier to vitamin B_{12}.

The stomach enzymes work efficiently in the stomach's strong acid, but salivary amylase, which is swallowed with food, does not work in acid this strong. Consequently, the digestion of starch gradually ceases as the acid penetrates the bolus. In fact, salivary amylase becomes just another protein to be digested. The amino acids in amylase end up being absorbed and recycled into other body proteins.

Antacids: Their Use and Misuse Note that the strong acidity of the stomach is a desirable condition, television commercials for antacids notwithstanding. In a person who overeats or who "inhales" food, the stomach is likely to react with such violence as to cause regurgitation (reverse peristalsis). When this happens, the stomach acid makes a bad taste in the mouth and the person may interpret this as "acid indigestion." Responding to television commercials, an overeater may take antacids to neutralize the stomach acid. But then the stomach will have to secrete more acid to enable the digestive enzymes to do their work. The consumer's stomach ends up with the same amount of acid but has had to work against the antacid to produce it.

Antacids are not designed to relieve the digestive discomfort of the hasty eater. Their proper use is to correct an abnormal condition, such as that of the person with ulcers, whose stomach or duodenal lining has been attacked by acid. To avoid falling into the same trap as our misguided consumer, hasty eaters should remember to chew food more thoroughly, eat it more slowly, and possibly eat less at a sitting.

Digestion in the Small and Large Intestines

By the time food leaves the stomach, digestion of all three energy-yielding nutrients has begun, but the process gains momentum in the small intestine. There, the pancreas, the liver, and intestine contribute additional digestive juices through the duct leading into the duodenum. These juices contain enzymes, bicarbonate, and bile.

Digestive Juices Pancreatic juice contributes enzymes that act on fats, proteins, and carbohydrates. Glands in the intestinal wall also secrete digestive enzymes. The pancreatic juice also contains sodium bicarbonate, which neutralizes the acidic chyme as it enters the small intestine. From this point on, the contents of the digestive tract are neutral or slightly alkaline. The enzymes of both the intestine and the pancreas work best in this environment.

Reminder: An emulsifier is a substance that mixes with both fat and water and that permanently disperses the fat in the water, forming an *emulsion.*

Bile Bile is secreted by the liver continuously and is concentrated and stored in the gallbladder. The gallbladder squirts bile into the duodenum whenever fat arrives there. Bile is not an enzyme but an emulsifier that brings fats into suspension in water (see Figure 5–4). After the fats are emulsified, enzymes can work on them, and they can be absorbed. Thanks to all these secretions, all three energy-yielding nutrients are digested in the small intestine.

Mayonnaise, made from vinegar and oil, would separate as other vinegar-and-oil salad dressings do if food chemists did not blend the vinegar and oil with a third ingredient—an emulsifier. The emulsifier mixes well with the fatty oil and the watery vinegar. In the case of mayonnaise, the emulsifier is lecithin from egg yolks.

The Rate of Digestion The rate of digestion of the energy nutrients depends upon the contents of the meal. If the meal is high in simple sugars, digestion proceeds fairly rapidly. On the other hand, if the meal is rich

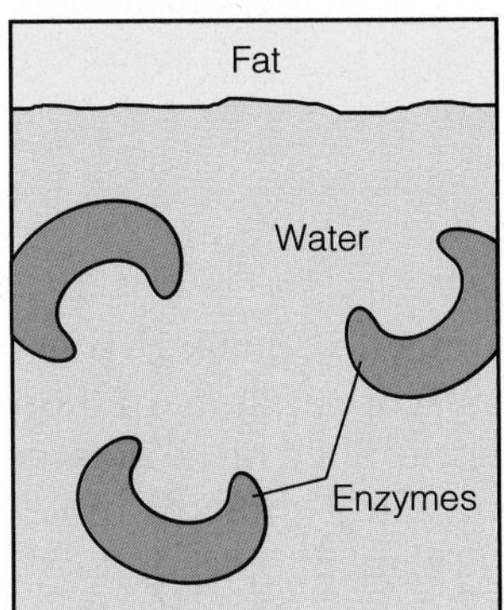

In the stomach, the fat and water are separate. The enzymes are in the water and can't get at the fat.

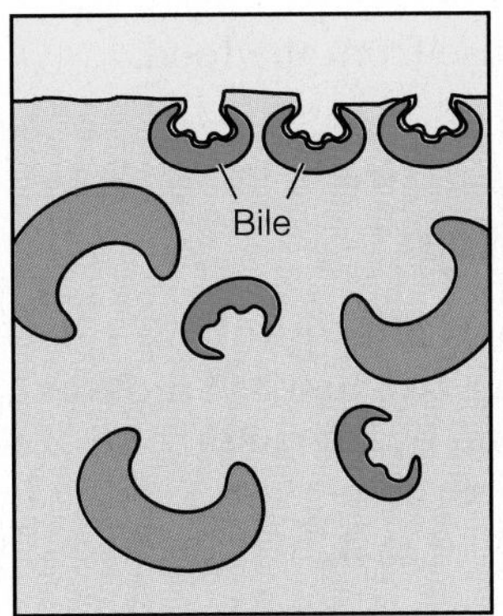

In the small intestine, bile (an emulsifier) arrives. Bile has an affinity for both fat and water and can therefore bring the fat into solution in the water.

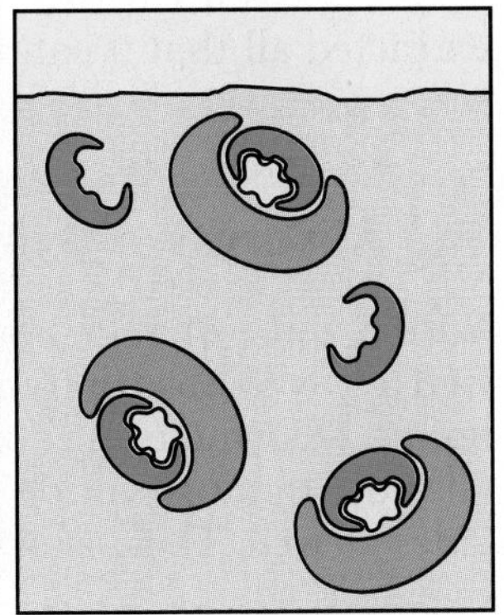

After emulsification, the fat is mixed in the water solution, so the enzymes have access to it.

Figure 5–4
The Action of Bile in Fat Digestion

Reminder: Satiety is the feeling of satisfaction and fullness that food brings.

in fat, digestion is slower. That fat slows digestion explains why fat increases the satiety value of a meal.

intestinal flora: the bacterial inhabitants of the GI tract.
flora = plant growth

Protective Factors The intestine also contains bacteria that produce a variety of vitamins, including biotin and vitamin K (although bacteria alone cannot meet the need for these vitamins). The GI bacteria also protect people from infections. Provided that the normal intestinal flora are thriving, infectious bacteria have a hard time getting established and launching an attack on the system. In addition, the small intestine and the entire GI tract manufacture and maintain a strong arsenal of defenses against foreign invaders. Several different types of defending cells are present there and confer specific immunity against intestinal diseases.

The Final Stage The story of how food is broken down into nutrients that can be absorbed is now nearly complete. The three energy-yielding nutrients—carbohydrate, fat, and protein—are disassembled to basic building blocks before they are absorbed. Most of the other nutrients—vitamins, minerals, and water—are absorbed as they are. Undigested residues, such as some fibers, are not absorbed but continue through the digestive tract, providing a semisolid mass that helps stimulate the muscles of the GI tract so that they will remain strong and perform peristalsis efficiently. Fiber also retains water, keeping the stools soft, and carries bile acids, sterols, and fat with it out of the body.

The process of absorbing the nutrients into the body is discussed in the next section. For the moment, let us assume that the digested nutrients simply disappear from the GI tract as they are ready. Virtually all are gone by the time the contents of the GI tract reach the end of the small intestine. Little remains but water, a few undissolved salts and body secretions, and undigested materials such as fiber. These enter the large intestine (colon).

In the colon, intestinal bacteria degrade some of the fiber to simpler compounds. The colon itself retrieves from its contents the materials that the body is designed to recycle—water and dissolved salts. The waste that is finally excreted has little or nothing of value left in it. The body has extracted all that it can use from the food.

The Absorptive System

Within three or four hours after you have eaten a meal, your body must find a way to absorb some two hundred thousand, million, million, million amino acid molecules one by one and comparable number of monosaccharide, monoglyceride, glycerol, fatty acid, vitamin, and mineral molecules as well. The absorptive system is ingeniously designed to accomplish this task.

The Small Intestine

The small intestine is a tube about 20 feet long and about an inch across, yet it provides a surface comparable in area to a quarter of a football field.

Nutrient molecules make contact with this surface and are absorbed. To remove these molecules rapidly and provide room for more to be absorbed, a rush of circulation continuously bathes the underside of the surface, washing away the absorbed nutrients and carrying them to the liver and other parts of the body.

Villi and Microvilli How does the intestine manage to provide such a large surface area? Its inner surface looks smooth, but viewed through a microscope, it turns out to be wrinkled into hundreds of folds. Each fold is covered with thousands of fingerlike projections called villi. The villi are as numerous as the hairs on velvet fabric. A single villus, magnified still more, turns out to be composed of several hundred cells, each covered with microscopic hairs called microvilli (see Figure 5–5 on p. 108).

The villi are in constant motion. Each villus is lined by a thin sheet of muscle so that it can wave, squirm, and wiggle like the tentacles of a sea anemone. Any nutrient molecule small enough to be absorbed is trapped among the microvilli and drawn into a cell beneath them. Some partially digested nutrients are caught in the microvilli, digested further by enzymes there, and then absorbed into the cells.

villi (VILL-ee or VILL-eye): fingerlike projections from the folds of the small intestine. The singular form is **villus.**
villus = shaggy hair

microvilli (MY-cro-VILL-ee or MY-cro-VILL-eye): tiny, hairlike projections on each cell of every villus that can trap nutrient particles and transport them into the cells. The singular form is **microvillus.**

Specialization in the Intestinal Tract As you can see, the intestinal tract is beautifully designed to perform its functions. A further refinement of the system is that the cells of successive portions of the tract are specialized to absorb different nutrients. The nutrients that are ready for absorption early on are absorbed near the top of the tract; those that take longer to be digested are absorbed further down. The rate at which the nutrients travel through the GI tract is finely adjusted to maximize their availability to the appropriate absorptive segment of the tract when they are ready. The lowly "gut" turns out to be one of the most elegantly designed organ systems in the body.

Release of Absorbed Nutrients

Once a molecule has entered a cell in a villus, the next step is to transmit it to a destination elsewhere in the body by way of the body's two transport systems—the bloodstream and the lymphatic system. As Figure 5–5 shows, both systems supply vessels to each villus. Through these vessels, the nutrients leave the cell and enter either the lymph or the blood. In either case, the nutrients end up in the blood, at least for a while. The water-soluble nutrients (including the smaller products of fat digestion) are released directly into the bloodstream by way of the capillaries, but the larger fats and the fat-soluble vitamins find access directly into the capillaries impossible because they are insoluble in water (and blood is mostly water). They require some packaging before they are released.

lymphatic system: a loosely organized system of vessels and ducts that conveys the products of digestion toward the heart.

lymph (LIMF): the body fluid found in lymphatic vessels; lymph consists of all the constituents of blood except red blood cells.

The intestinal cells assemble the monoglycerides and long-chain fatty acids into larger triglyceride molecules. These triglycerides, fat-soluble vitamins (when present), and other large lipids (cholesterol and the phospholipids) are then packaged for transport. They cluster together with special proteins to form chylomicrons, one kind of lipoprotein (lipoproteins are described beginning on p. 110). Finally, the cells release the chy-

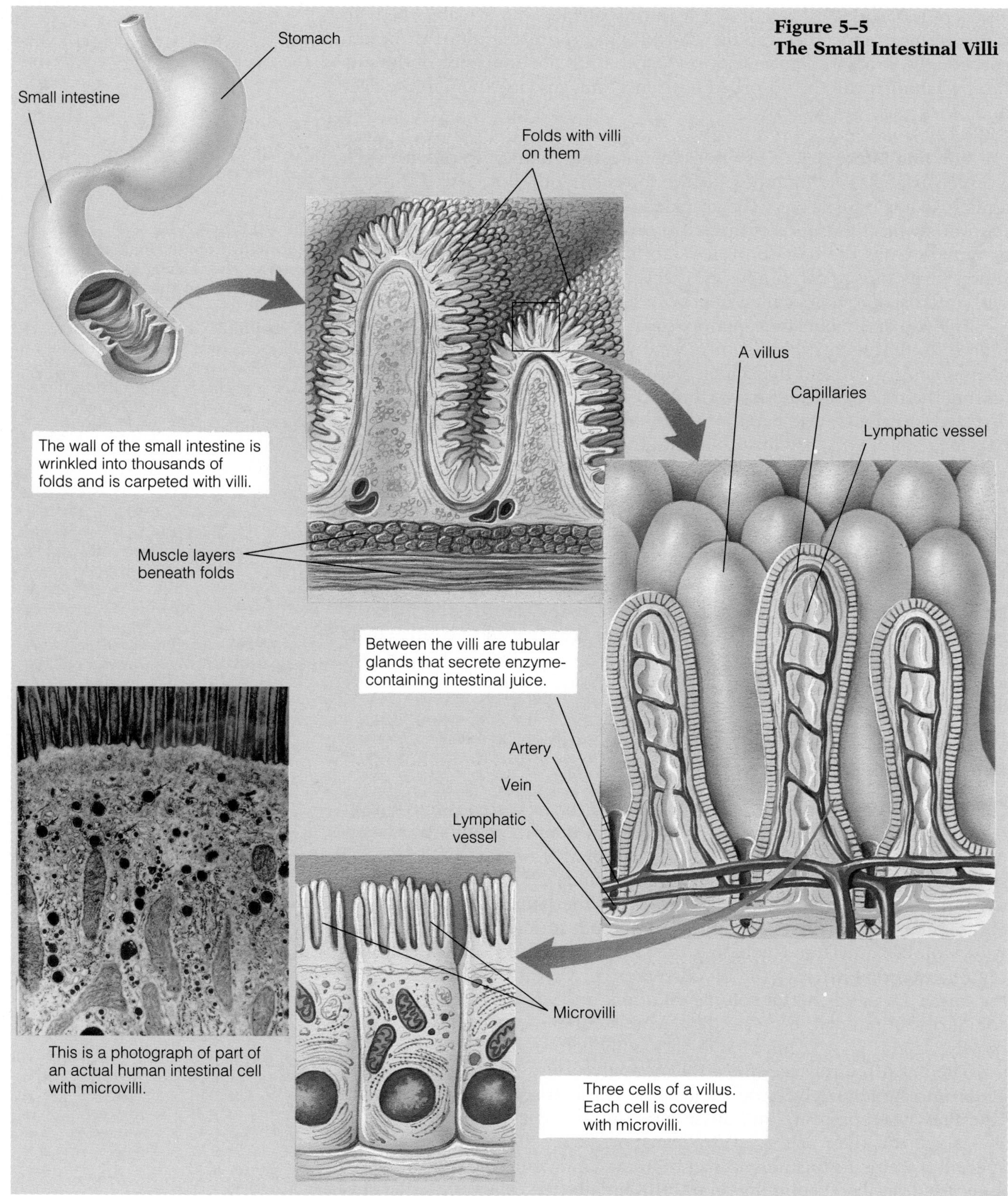
Stomach
Small intestine
Folds with villi on them
A villus
Capillaries
Lymphatic vessel
The wall of the small intestine is wrinkled into thousands of folds and is carpeted with villi.
Muscle layers beneath folds
Between the villi are tubular glands that secrete enzyme-containing intestinal juice.
Artery
Vein
Lymphatic vessel
Microvilli
This is a photograph of part of an actual human intestinal cell with microvilli.
Three cells of a villus. Each cell is covered with microvilli.

Figure 5–5
The Small Intestinal Villi

lomicrons into the lymphatic system. They can then glide through the lymph spaces until they arrive at a point of entry into the bloodstream near the heart.

chylomicrons (kye-lo-MY-crons): the lipoproteins that transport lipids from the intestinal cells into the body. The cells of the body remove the lipids they need from the chylomicrons, leaving chylomicron remnants to be picked up by the liver cells. The liver cells dismantle the chylomicron remnants and construct other lipoproteins for further transport of lipids.

Transport of Nutrients

Once a nutrient has entered the bloodstream or the lymphatic system, it may be transported to any part of the body and thus becomes available to any of the cells, from the tips of the toes to the roots of the hair. The circulatory systems are arranged to deliver nutrients wherever they are needed.

The Vascular System

The vascular or blood circulatory system is a closed system of vessels through which blood flows continuously in a figure eight, with the heart serving as a pump at the crossover point. On each loop of the figure eight, blood travels a simple route: heart to arteries to capillaries to veins to heart.

The routing of the blood through the digestive system is different, however. The blood is carried to the digestive system (as it is to all organs) by way of an artery, which (as in all organs) branches into capillaries to reach every cell. Blood leaving the digestive system, however, goes by way of a vein, not back to the heart, but to the liver. This vein *again* branches into capillaries so that every cell of the liver has access to the newly absorbed nutrients that the blood is carrying. Blood leaving the liver then returns to the heart by way of a vein. The route is heart to arteries to capillaries (in intestines) to vein to capillaries (in liver) to vein to heart.

An anatomist studying this system knows there must be a reason for this special arrangement. The liver is placed in the circulation at this point so that it will have the first chance at the materials absorbed from the GI tract. In fact, the liver is the body's major metabolic organ (see Figure 5–6 on p. 110). It must prepare the absorbed nutrients for use by the body, and it has many jobs to perform in this process. Furthermore, the liver stands as gatekeeper to waylay intruders that might otherwise harm the heart or brain. Chapter 24 offers more information about this noble organ.

artery: a vessel that carries blood away from the heart.

capillary (CAP-ill-ary): a small vessel that branches from an artery. Capillaries connect arteries to veins. Oxygen, nutrients, and waste materials are exchanged across capillary walls.

vein: a vessel that carries blood back to the heart.

The blood arriving at the intestines flows through the mesentery (MEZ-en-terry), a strong, flexible membrane that surrounds and supports the abdominal organs.
mes = middle

The vein that collects blood from the mesentery and conducts it to capillaries in the liver is the *portal vein.*
portal = gateway

The vein that collects blood from the liver capillaries and returns it to the heart is the *hepatic vein.*
hepat = liver

The artery that delivers oxygen-rich blood from the heart to the liver is the *hepatic artery.*

The Lymphatic System

The lymphatic system is a one-way route that fluids can travel to get from tissue spaces to the blood. The lymphatic system has no pump; instead, lymph is squeezed from one portion of the body to another like water in a sponge, as muscles contract and create pressure here and there. Ultimately, the lymph collects in a large duct behind the heart. This duct terminates in a vein that conducts the lymph into the heart. Thus, some materials from the GI tract enter the lymphatic system at first, then later enter the bloodstream.

The duct that conveys lymph toward the heart is the *thoracic* (thor-ASS-ic) *duct.* The *subclavian vein* connects this duct with the right upper chamber of the heart, providing a passageway by which lymph can be returned to the vascular system.

Figure 5–6
The Liver

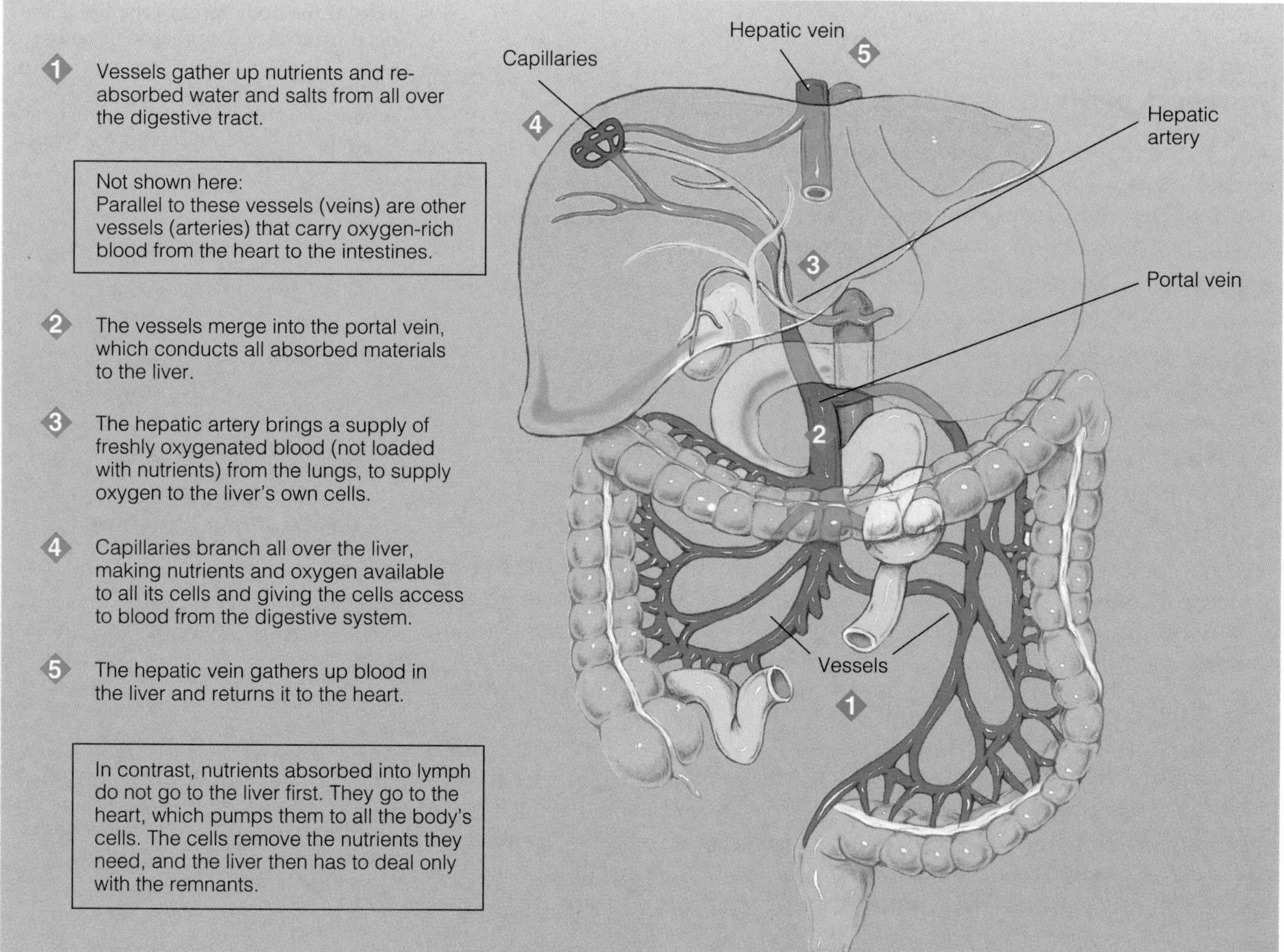

Hepatic vein
5
Capillaries
4
Hepatic artery
3
Portal vein
2
Vessels
1
1 Vessels gather up nutrients and reabsorbed water and salts from all over the digestive tract.
Not shown here:
Parallel to these vessels (veins) are other vessels (arteries) that carry oxygen-rich blood from the heart to the intestines.
2 The vessels merge into the portal vein, which conducts all absorbed materials to the liver.
3 The hepatic artery brings a supply of freshly oxygenated blood (not loaded with nutrients) from the lungs, to supply oxygen to the liver's own cells.
4 Capillaries branch all over the liver, making nutrients and oxygen available to all its cells and giving the cells access to blood from the digestive system.
5 The hepatic vein gathers up blood in the liver and returns it to the heart.
In contrast, nutrients absorbed into lymph do not go to the liver first. They go to the heart, which pumps them to all the body's cells. The cells remove the nutrients they need, and the liver then has to deal only with the remnants.

Transport of Lipids: Lipoproteins

Within the circulatory system, lipids always travel from place to place bundled with protein, that is, as lipoproteins. When physicians measure a person's blood lipid profile, they are interested not only in the types of fat present (such as triglycerides and cholesterol) but also in the types of lipoproteins that carry them. Figure 5–7 shows the relative sizes and composition of the lipoproteins.

VLDL (very-low-density lipoprotein)**:** the type of lipoprotein made primarily by liver cells to transport lipids to various tissues in the body; composed primarily of triglycerides.

VLDL, LDL, and HDL As mentioned earlier, chylomicrons transport newly absorbed (*diet-derived*) lipids from the intestinal cells to the rest of the body. As chylomicrons circulate through the body, cells remove their lipid contents, so they get smaller and smaller. The liver picks up and dismantles the chylomicron remnants and assembles new lipoproteins, which are known as very-low-density lipoproteins (VLDL). As the body's

Figure 5–7
The Lipoproteins

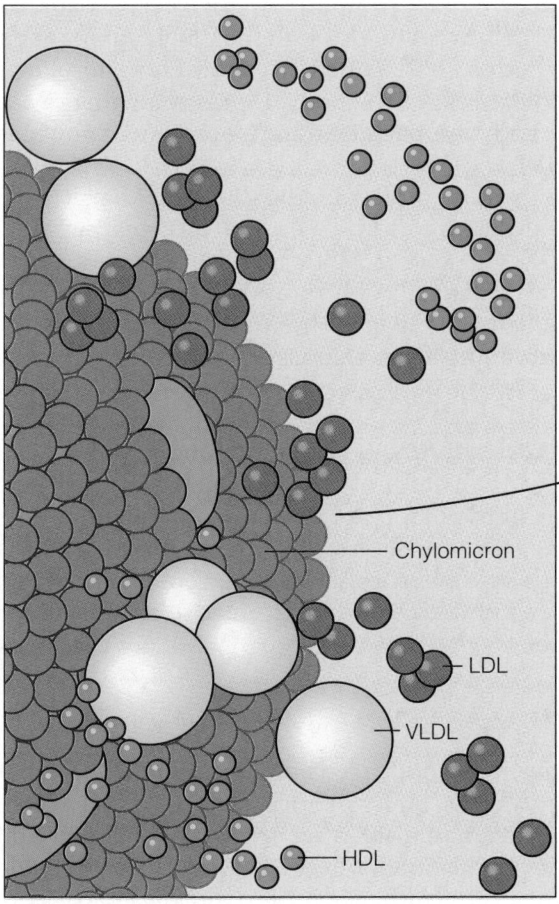

Chylomicron
LDL
VLDL
HDL

This solar system of lipoproteins shows their relative sizes. Notice how large the fat-filled chylomicron is compared with the others and how the others get progressively smaller as their proportion of fat declines and protein increases.

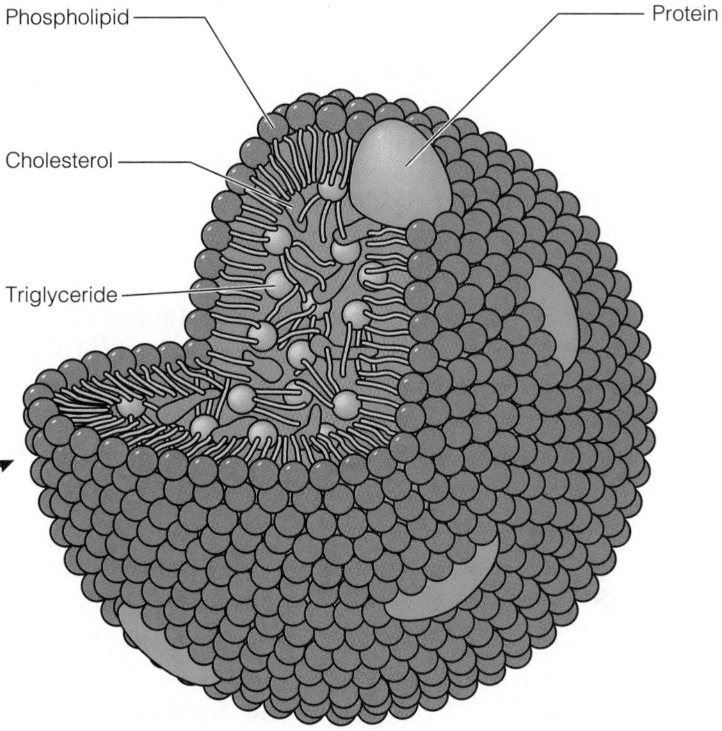

Phospholipid
Protein
Cholesterol
Triglyceride

A typical lipoprotein contains an interior of trigycerides and cholesterol surrounded by phospholipids. The phospholipids' fatty acid "tails" point toward the interior, where the lipids are. Proteins near the outer ends of the phospholipids cover the structure. This arrangement of hydrophobic molecules on the inside and hydrophilic molecules on the outside allows lipids to travel through the watery fluids of the blood.

Chylomicrons contain so little protein and so much triglyceride that they are the lowest in density.

Very-low-density lipoproteins (VLDL) are half triglycerides, accounting for their low density.

Low-density lipoproteins (LDL) are half cholesterol, accounting for their implication in heart disease.

High-density lipoproteins (HDL) are half protein, accounting for their high density.

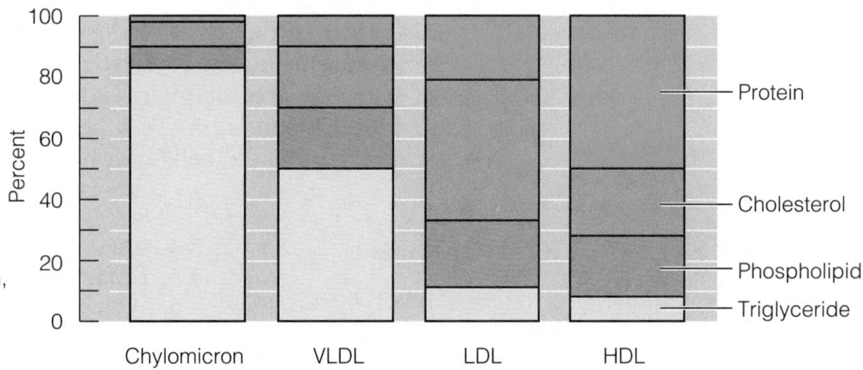

LDL (low-density lipoprotein)**:** the type of lipoprotein derived from VLDL as cells remove triglycerides from them. LDL carry cholesterol and triglycerides from the liver to the cells of the body and are composed primarily of cholesterol.

HDL (high-density lipoprotein)**:** the type of lipoprotein that transports cholesterol back to the liver from peripheral cells; composed primarily of protein.

cells remove triglycerides from the VLDL, the VLDL gather cholesterol from other lipoproteins in the blood and become low-density lipoproteins (LDL). This exchange explains why LDL contain few triglycerides but are loaded with cholesterol. The LDL circulate through the body making their contents available to all the body's cells. Thus LDL carry cholesterol and triglycerides *from* the liver to the rest of the body. Lipids returning *to* the liver from other parts of the body are packaged in lipoproteins known as high-density lipoproteins (HDL).

The more lipid in the lipoprotein molecule, the lower the density; the more protein, the higher the density. Both LDL and HDL carry lipids around in the blood, but LDL are larger, lighter, and more lipid filled; HDL are smaller, denser, and packaged with more protein. LDL deliver cholesterol and triglycerides from the liver to the tissues; HDL scavenge excess cholesterol and phospholipids from the tissues and return them to the liver for disposal.

Health Implications of LDL and HDL The distinction between LDL and HDL has implications for the health of the heart and blood vessels. Elevated LDL concentrations in the blood are associated with a high risk of heart attack, and elevated HDL concentrations are associated with a low risk.[1] This is why some people refer to LDL as "bad" cholesterol and HDL as "good" cholesterol. Lipoproteins and heart disease are discussed in Chapter 26.

The System at Its Best

The GI tract is the first organ in the body to deal with the nutrients that will ultimately maintain the health and nutrition status of the whole body. The intricate architecture of the GI tract makes it sensitive and responsive to conditions in its environment. One condition indispensable to its performance is its own good health. Such lifestyle factors as sleep, physical activity, state of mind, and nutrition affect GI tract health. For example, adequate sleep allows for repair and maintenance of tissue. Physical activity promotes healthy muscle tone and may protect against cancer of the colon.[2] Mental state profoundly affects digestion and absorption through the activity of nerves and hormones that help regulate these processes. A relaxed, peaceful attitude during a meal enhances digestion and absorption.[3]

Among the characteristics of meals that promote optimal absorption of nutrients are adequacy, balance, moderation, and variety, because every nutrient depends on every other. The nutrients all work together, and all are present in the cells of a healthy digestive tract.

■ STUDY QUESTIONS ■

1. Describe the path that food follows through the digestive tract once it is swallowed.
2. Describe peristalsis and segmentation.
3. List five digestive juices and the organs that secrete them.
4. What does bile do?
5. Name the two nutrient transport systems in the body.
6. Which nutrients enter the bloodstream directly? Which are first absorbed into the lymph?
7. What are chylomicrons?

NUTRITION IN PRACTICE 5

Common Digestive Problems

The facts of anatomy and physiology presented in Chapter 5 permit easy understanding of some common situations. Everyone, at one time or another, has to deal with various kinds of digestive distress. Short bouts of vomiting and diarrhea that do not seriously impair nutrition status are discussed here, together with ordinary constipation, belching, and gas. Later chapters deal with more serious causes and consequences of vomiting and diarrhea.

Please explain what causes vomiting, and when it is serious.

Vomiting can be a symptom of many different diseases or may arise in any situation that upsets the body's equilibrium, such as air or sea travel. For whatever reason, the waves of peristalsis reverse direction, and the contents of the stomach are propelled up through the esophagus to the mouth and expelled.

If vomiting continues long enough or is severe enough, the reverse peristalsis will carry not only the stomach contents but also the contents of the duodenum, with its green bile salts, into the stomach and then up the esophagus. Although unpleasant and wearying for the nauseated person, vomiting such as this is no cause for alarm. Vomiting is one of the body's adaptive mechanisms to rid itself of something irritating. The best advice is to rest and drink fluids (small amounts as tolerated) until the nausea subsides.

Vomiting can be serious, however, when large quantities of fluid are lost from the GI tract, causing dehydration. As Chapter 20 describes, prompt emergency care may be needed in those cases.

What are some cases in which vomiting requires medical attention?

In an infant, vomiting is likely to become serious early in its course, and a physician should be contacted soon after onset. Infants have more fluid between their body cells than adults do, so more fluid can move into the digestive tract and be lost from the body. Consequently, the body water of infants becomes depleted and fluid balance becomes upset earlier than in adults.

Self-induced vomiting, such as occurs in bulimia, also has serious consequences. (Bulimia is discussed in Nutrition in Practice 9.) Besides fluid and salt imbalances, repeated vomiting can irritate and infect the pharynx, esophagus, and salivary glands; erode the teeth; and cause dental caries. The esophagus or stomach may rupture or tear. Sometimes the eyes become red from pressure during vomiting. Bulimic behavior reflects underlying problems that require attention.

Projectile vomiting is also serious. The contents of the stomach are expelled with such force that they leave the mouth in a wide arc like a bullet leaving a gun. This type of vomiting requires immediate medical attention.

What about diarrhea? What should be done about it, and when is medical help needed?

The frequent, loose, watery stools of diarrhea indicate that the intestinal contents have moved too quickly through the intestines for fluid absorption to take place, or that water from the GI tract lining has been added to the food residue. Like vomiting, diarrhea can lead to considerable fluid and salt losses, but the acid-base composition of the fluids is different. Stomach fluids lost in vomiting are highly acidic; intestinal fluids lost in diarrhea are nearly neutral. When fluid losses require medical attention, correct replacement is crucial.

For short bouts of diarrhea, rest and drink fluids to replace losses. If diarrhea continues, call for help. For an infant, get help promptly, for diarrhea may quickly lead to dehydration so severe as to require emergency medical treatment.

What is constipation, and when does it require medical attention?

If a bowel movement is passed with difficulty, discomfort, or pain, then the person is constipated. Note, though, that the amount of time that has passed since the last bowel movement is irrelevant. Even if several days pass between bowel movements, so long as these movements take place without discomfort, the person is not constipated. No one needs to have daily movements, television commercials notwithstanding. No one absorbs "toxins" from unexcreted material that cause irritable behavior.

Constipation is generally not a cause for concern. Each person's GI tract responds to food in its own way, with its own rhythm.

Food is digested and its residue becomes ready for excretion in a predictable number of hours. Each GI tract thus has its own cycle, which depends on its owner's physical makeup, the type of food eaten, when it was eaten, and when the person makes time to defecate.

Often a person's own lifestyle may cause constipation. If a person receives the signal that says to defecate and ignores it, the signal may not return for several hours. In the meantime, water continues to be withdrawn from the fecal matter, so that when the person does defecate, the bowel movement is dry and hard.

Careful review of daily habits may reveal such a cause of constipation. Being too busy to respond to the defecation signal is a common complaint. A person's daily regimen may need to be revised, instituting regular eating and sleeping times that will allow time in the day's schedule to have a bowel movement when the body sends its signal. This may mean going to bed earlier in order to rise earlier, allowing ample time for a leisurely breakfast and a movement.

Another cause of constipation is the lack of physical activity.[4] In today's society many people drive cars or ride buses to work, stand at assembly lines or sit behind desks, and then sit in front of television sets in the evening. Increasing physical activity may require some rearrangement of one's lifestyle. People can work out in spas or health clubs, or more simply, they can park their cars a few blocks from the office and walk, or walk up several flights of stairs a day rather than taking the elevator. Such planning enables people to engage in activity that will improve the muscle tone, not just of the outer body, but also of the digestive tract.

Constipation usually reflects lifestyle habits, although in some cases it may be a side effect of medication or may reflect a medical problem such as tumors that are obstructing the passage of waste. If discomfort or distress is associated with passing fecal matter, a physician's help should be sought to rule out disease. Once this has been done, dietary or other measures for correction can be considered.

Does fiber, water, or prune juice help relieve ordinary constipation?

Yes to all three. The fibers in cereal products are especially helpful. In the GI tract, these fibers attract water, thus creating soft and bulky stools that stimulate bowel contractions to push the contents along. These contractions strengthen the intestinal muscles; the improved muscle tone and the water content of the stools not only aid elimination but also reduce pressure on the rectal veins, helping to prevent hemorrhoids.

Drinking plenty of water in conjunction with eating foods high in fiber supplies fluid for the fiber to take up. The resulting increased bulk physically stimulates the upper GI tract, promoting peristalsis throughout.

Prunes are not only high in fiber but also contain a laxative substance. If a morning defecation is desired, a person can drink prune juice at bedtime; if the evening is preferred, the person can drink prune juice with breakfast.

Another simple tactic that can help with some constipation is to add some fat to the diet. Fat summons bile into the duodenum, bile's salts draw water from the intestinal wall, and the water stimulates peristalsis and softens the fecal matter.

Is it ever necessary to take laxatives, enemas, or mineral oil for constipation?

The changes in diet or lifestyle just suggested should correct chronic constipation without the use of laxatives, enemas, or mineral oil, although television commercials often try to persuade people otherwise. One of the fallacies often perpetrated by television commercials is that one person's successful use of a product is a good recommendation for others to use that product.

As a matter of fact, even diet changes that relieve constipation for one person may increase the constipation of another. For instance, increasing fiber intake stimulates peristalsis and helps the person with a sluggish colon. Some people, though, have a spastic type of constipation, in which peristalsis promotes strong contractions that close off a segment of the colon and prevent passage. For these people, increasing fiber intake would be exactly the wrong thing to do.

A person who seems to need products such as laxatives should therefore seek a physician's opinion. Advice from friends may do more harm than good. Frequent use of laxatives and enemas can lead to dependency; can upset the body's fluid, salt, and mineral balances; and, in the case of mineral oil, can interfere with the absorption of fat-soluble vitamins. (Mineral oil dissolves the vitamins, but is not itself absorbed; instead, it leaves the body, carrying the vitamins with it.)

You promised to discuss belching and gas, too.

Many people complain of problems that they attribute to excessive gas. For some, belching is the complaint. Others blame intestinal gas for abdominal discomforts and embarrassment. Most people believe that the problems occur after they eat certain foods. This may be the case with intestinal gas, but belching results from swallowing air.

Everyone swallows a little air with every mouthful of food, but people who eat too fast may swallow too much air and then have to belch. Ill-fitting dentures, carbonated beverages, and chewing gum can also contribute to air swallowing and belching. Occasionally, belching can be a sign of a more serious disorder, such as gallbladder pain, colonic distress, or impending obstruction of a coronary blood vessel.

Little is known about intestinal gas, but techniques to collect gas directly from the abdomen have allowed researchers to gain some knowledge. While expelling gas can be a humiliating experience, it is quite normal. (People experiencing painful bloating from malabsorption diseases, however, require medical treatment.) Healthy people expel several hundred milliliters of gas several times a day. Almost all (99 percent) of the gases expelled—nitrogen, oxygen, hydrogen, methane, and carbon dioxide—are odorless. The remaining "volatile" gases are the infamous ones.

Foods that produce gas usually must be determined individually. Table 21-1, later in the book, lists some of the likely candidates. The most common offenders are foods rich in the carbohydrates—sugars, starches, and fibers. When partially digested carbohydrates reach the large intestine, bacteria digest them, giving off gas as a by-product. People can test foods suspected of forming gas by omitting them individually for a trial period and seeing if there is any improvement. The best advice seems to be to eat slowly, chew thoroughly, and relax while eating.

What about more serious digestive problems?

Some illnesses seriously affect the digestion and absorption of nutrients. Individuals with these disorders risk severe malnutrition and the diet must be altered to ensure health. The details of these disorders and their diet therapies are described in Chapter 18 through 29.

■ NOTES ■

1. NIH Consensus Conference, Triglyceride, high-density lipoprotein, and coronary heart disease, *Journal of the American Medical Association* 269 (1993): 505–510.
2. Committee on Diet and Health, Food and Nutrition Board, Calories: Total macronutrient intake, energy expenditure, and net energy stores, in *Diet and Health: Implications for Reducing Chronic Disease Risk* (Washington, D.C.: National Academy Press, 1989), pp. 139–158.
3. D. R. Morse and coauthors, Oral digestion of a complex-carbohydrate cereal: Effects of stress and relaxation on physiological and salivary measure, *American Journal of Clinical Nutrition* 49 (1989): 97–105.
4. R. S. Sandler, M. C. Jordan, and B. J. Shelton, Demographic and dietary determinants of constipation in the US population, *American Journal of Public Health* 80 (1990): 185–189.

6

Metabolism and Energy Balance

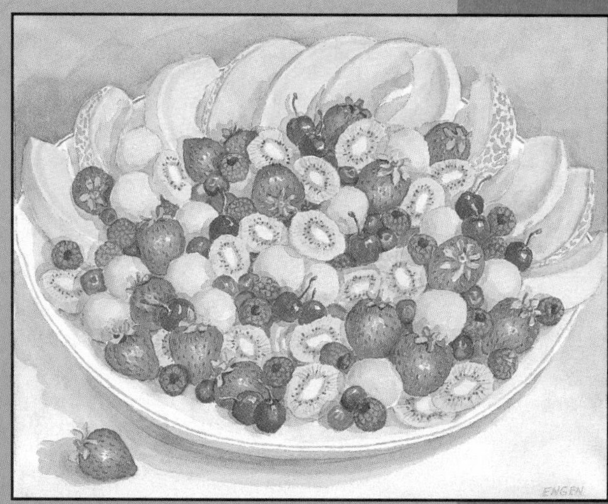

CONTENTS

metabolism: the sum total of all the chemical reactions that go on in living cells.
meta = among
bole = change

Every organ, every tissue, and every cell of the body engages in metabolism, the chemical reactions involved in breaking down compounds, making new compounds, and transporting compounds from place to place. Viewed from this perspective, the body is a giant chemical factory that works with astounding efficiency to produce a myriad of products and dispose of a myriad of wastes. All these processes are regulated by hormonal signals that coordinate supply and demand in much the same way as a superb communication system coordinates a smoothly functioning economy.

In disease, metabolic processes always become disturbed, and some diseases are caused by metabolic abnormalities. This chapter provides the normal background against which the disruptions caused by diseases can best be understood.

The Organs and Their Metabolic Roles

When everything in the body is functioning normally, every organ plays a metabolic role that serves the others. Metabolic reactions also consume or release energy and therefore affect body weight, with consequences for health.

The Principal Organs

Of particular concern are the digestive organs, the liver, the pancreas, the circulatory system, and the kidneys. Together, they perform much of the work of breaking down compounds, making new ones, transporting nutrients and oxygen throughout the body, and removing the waste products generated by the metabolic processes.

The Digestive Organs The digestive system has just received attention in Chapter 5. Notable among the digestive system's activities are the production of digestive juices and enzymes; the absorption of nutrients; the making of special "pumps" to absorb certain nutrients; the making of transport proteins to carry lipids and vitamins to other sites in the body; and in the lower digestive tract, the reabsorption of salts and fluids. The digestive system also possesses the body's most rapidly multiplying cells: when healthy, they replace themselves every few days. Disorders of the GI tract lead to failures to digest, absorb, and metabolize nutrients, as described in Chapters 20 and 21.

The Liver Nutrients absorbed into the bloodstream are conducted to the liver, as described in Chapter 5. The liver is one of the body's most active metabolic factories. It receives nutrients and metabolizes, packages, stores, or ships them out for use by other organs. It metabolizes and stores most vitamins and many minerals. It manufactures bile, which the body uses in emulsifying fat for digestion and absorption. It detoxifies drugs, prepares waste products for excretion, and participates in iron recycling and blood cell manufacture. It also makes clotting factors. When liver disorders disrupt metabolism, they profoundly affect both nutrition and general health status, as described in Chapter 24.

The Pancreas The pancreas contributes digestive juices to the GI tract, but also has another metabolic function: it produces insulin and other hormones that regulate the body's use of glucose. It is insulin that prompts cells to take glucose up and use it as fuel. Insulin also prompts liver cells in particular to store glucose as glycogen. The liver cells can later release glucose back into the blood as needed. Glucose is an indispensable fuel for brain and nerve cells and for red blood cells as well. Its availability is therefore crucial to normal nervous system activity and normal blood chemistry. The abnormalities associated with diabetes and hypoglycemia, described in Chapter 25, are the result of abnormalities in glucose metabolism.

The Heart and Blood Vessels The heart and blood vessels conduct blood with its cargo of nutrients and oxygen to all other body cells and carry wastes from them. Diseases of the heart and arteries therefore affect the health of the whole body. Metabolic reactions that affect the heart and blood vessels include, most importantly, the making and transport of lipoproteins, the carriers of cholesterol and other lipids from the liver to the tissues and back again. When lipoproteins deposit cholesterol in artery walls, the resulting disease causes high blood pressure and makes early death or disability from heart attacks and strokes likely. Chapter 26 is devoted to these conditions.

The Kidneys The kidneys are also active metabolic organs. Unceasingly, for 24 hours of every day, they filter waste products from the blood to be excreted in the urine and thereby maintain the blood's delicate chemical balances. The kidneys' cells also produce compounds that help to regulate blood pressure and convert a precursor compound to active vitamin D, thereby helping to maintain the bones. Disorders of the kidneys nearly always involve the heart and the skeleton; kidney disorders are the subject of Chapter 27.

Energy for Metabolic Work

The metabolic work that the body's cells do, like all work, requires energy, and food supplies that energy. Food in turn gets its energy from the sun, either directly (in the case of photosynthesizing plants) or indirectly (in the case of animals that eat plants). When chemical reactions in cells release stored energy from energy-yielding nutrients, that energy becomes available to do the cells' work.

Heat Energy and Body Temperature The cells of each organ conduct metabolic activities specific to that organ, but in addition, all cells must maintain themselves, and many must reproduce. To do this, they must have all the essential nutrients available to them: the energy nutrients, the vitamins, and the minerals, as well as water. As cells do their metabolic work, the chemical reactions involved release heat, and this heat keeps the body warm. It is by regulating the rates at which metabolic reactions release heat energy that the body maintains its constant normal temperature of 98.6° F.

Fast Metabolism, Fever, and Wasting During stress, metabolism speeds up. Fever sometimes develops. An accelerated metabolism signifies that fuels are being burned at a rate more rapid than normal; this may lead to wasting of body organs and loss of weight including loss of vital, lean tissue. Chapters 18 and 19 describe the metabolic consequences of severe stress, and in particular of severe infections, major surgery, and burns. Chapters 28 and 29 describe the metabolic consequences of the so-called wasting diseases, cancer and AIDS.

As this brief discussion has shown, metabolism occurs all through the body, all the time, and supports normal health. The remainder of this chapter delves into one aspect of metabolism—the metabolism of the energy nutrients and the resulting consequences of underweight and overweight.

The Body's Energy Metabolism

The body manages its energy supply with amazing precision. Consider, for example, that a consistent 1 percent error in energy intake can cause a person to become more than 200 pounds overweight in a lifetime. Yet most people maintain their weight within about a 10- to 20-pound range throughout their lives. How do they do this? How does the body manage excess energy? And how does it manage to do without food for prolonged periods—as when someone is starving or fasting? The answers to questions like these lie in an understanding of metabolism.

Energy metabolism is defined as the sum total of all the chemical reactions that manage energy nutrients in the body. Earlier chapters introduced the energy-yielding nutrients—carbohydrate, fat, and protein—and showed how they are broken down into basic units that are absorbed into the blood. Picking up from there, what becomes of these nutrients? The question is important because it provides insight into proper and improper ways to aid the body in maintaining or losing weight.

energy metabolism: all the reactions by which the body obtains and spends the energy from food or body stores.

Energy metabolism centers on four basic units:

- From carbohydrate: glucose.
- From lipids: glycerol.
- From lipids: fatty acids.
- From protein: amino acids.

Building Body Compounds

When the basic units of energy-yielding nutrients are not needed by the cells for energy, they can be used to build body compounds. The building up of body compounds is known as anabolism; this book represents anabolic reactions, wherever possible, by "up" arrows in chemical diagrams (such as those shown in Figure 6–1). Glucose units can be strung together to make glycogen chains. Glycerol and fatty acids can be assembled into triglycerides. Amino acids can be linked together to make proteins. These building reactions, in which simple compounds are put together to

anabolism (ann-ABB-o-lism)**:** reactions in which small molecules are put together to build larger ones. Anabolic reactions consume energy.
ana = up

Figure 6–1
Anabolic and Catabolic Reactions Compared

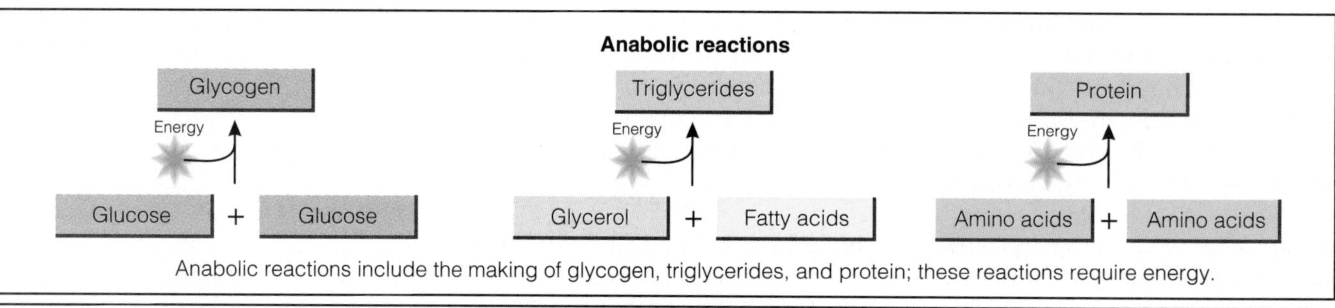

Anabolic reactions include the making of glycogen, triglycerides, and protein; these reactions require energy.

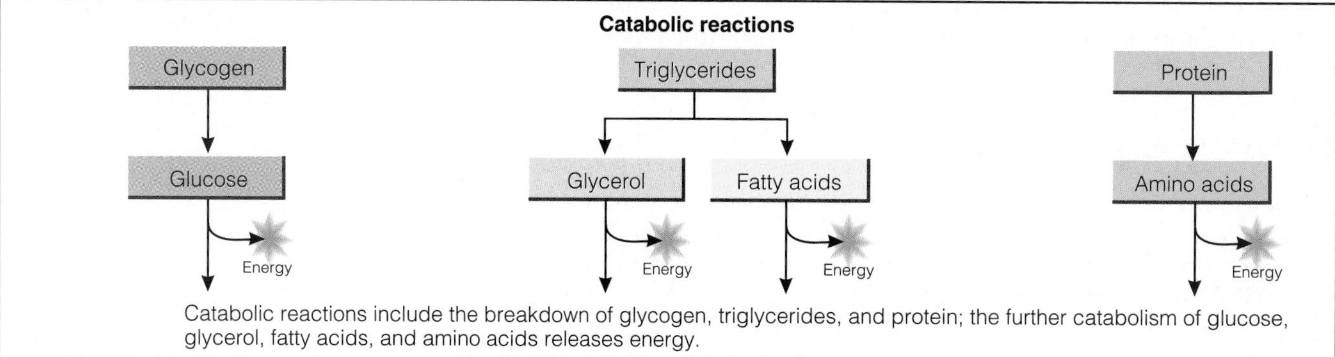

Catabolic reactions include the breakdown of glycogen, triglycerides, and protein; the further catabolism of glucose, glycerol, fatty acids, and amino acids releases energy.

form larger, more complex structures, involve doing work, and so require energy.

Breaking Down Nutrients for Energy

catabolism (ca-TAB-o-lism)**:** reactions in which large molecules are broken down to smaller ones. Catabolic reactions usually release energy.
kata = down

The breaking down of body compounds is known as catabolism; catabolic reactions usually release energy and are represented, wherever possible, by "down" arrows in chemical diagrams (see Figure 6–1). Glycogen can be broken down to glucose, triglycerides to fatty acids and glycerol, and protein to amino acids. When the body needs energy, it breaks any or all of the four basic units—glucose, fatty acids, glycerol, and amino acids—into even smaller units.

glycolysis (gligh-COLL-uh-sis)**:** the metabolic breakdown of glucose to pyruvate.
glyco = glucose
lysis = breakdown

pyruvate (PIE-roo-vate)**:** pyruvic acid, a 3-carbon compound derived from glucose, glycerol, and certain amino acids in metabolism. The term *pyruvate* means a salt of pyruvic acid.

Throughout this book, the ending *-ate* is used interchangeably with *-ic acid;* for our purposes they mean the same thing.

Glucose Breakdown Glucose breakdown occurs mostly via a pathway known as glycolysis. In glycolysis, glucose is first broken down to pyruvate. Pyruvate is then converted to a smaller compound, acetyl CoA. In a series of metabolic reactions called the tricarboxylic acid (TCA) cycle, acetyl CoA splits, and its energy is donated to storage compounds, used to do the body's work, or used to produce heat.

The following sequence is central to an understanding of metabolism:

Glucose $\leftrightarrow$ pyruvate $\rightarrow$ acetyl CoA $\rightarrow$ energy.

Notice the two-way arrow between glucose and pyruvate and the one-way arrows after pyruvate. They show that pyruvate can be reconverted to glucose but that acetyl CoA cannot. Any compound that can be converted to pyruvate can be used to make glucose. Any compound that is broken down to acetyl CoA cannot be used to make glucose. Fats cannot be converted to glucose, for the most part, because they consist mostly of triglycerides, which in turn consist mostly of fatty acids, which break down to acetyl CoA.

Fat Breakdown Because fatty acids are broken down to acetyl CoA, they cannot be used to make glucose. Glycerol is interconvertible with pyruvate and can yield glucose, but glycerol represents only about 5 percent of the weight of a triglyceride molecule. Thus fat is an inefficient source of glucose. About 95 percent of it cannot be converted to glucose at all; therefore fat, for the most part, cannot normally provide energy for the organs (brain and nervous system) that require glucose as fuel. This leaves the task of fueling the brain's activities mainly to protein and carbohydrate.

Amino Acid Breakdown Ideally, amino acids are used to maintain supplies of needed body proteins and will not be used for energy. If they are needed for energy, or if they are consumed in excess, they first undergo deamination, a reaction in which they are stripped of their nitrogen. The nitrogen can be used to make other compounds, including the nonessential amino acids, or it can be excreted. With nitrogen removed, about half of the amino acids can be converted to pyruvate and can therefore provide glucose. The other amino acids are converted to acetyl CoA directly or enter the TCA cycle at another point. Thus protein, unlike fat, is a fairly efficient source of glucose when carbohydrate is not available.

Figure 6–2 depicts the major metabolic pathways involving carbohydrates, fats, and amino acids. Note the central pathway from glucose to pyruvate to acetyl CoA to energy. Also note that all carbohydrates, some amino acids, and the glycerol from fat can be converted to pyruvate and then to glucose. Finally, note that the vast majority of fragments from fat can be used only for energy and not to make glucose. With these understandings, you can follow the events that lead to weight gain and weight loss.

CoA (coh-AY): a nickname for a small molecule that participates in metabolism. As pyruvate breaks down to the smaller compound acetic acid, a molecule of CoA is attached to it, making acetyl CoA (ASS-uh-teel or uh-SEET-ul co-AY).

The reactions by which the complete oxidation of acetyl CoA is accomplished are those of the TCA cycle, or Krebs cycle, and oxidative phsophorylation. The net result is that acetyl CoA splits, and some of its energy is made available for the body's use.

oxidation: a reaction in which electrons are removed from a molecule. Often, this occurs when a molecule reacts with oxygen, hence the name. Oxidation reactions usually result in the release of energy.

deamination: removal of the amino (NH_2) group from a compound such as an amino acid.

The principal nitrogen-excretion product of metabolism is **urea** (you-REE-uh).

The making of glucose from protein or fat is **gluconeogenesis** (gloo-co-nee-o-JEN-uh-sis). About 5% of fat (the glycerol portion of triglycerides) and about 50% of protein (the glycogenic amino acids) can be converted to glucose.
gluco, glyco = glucose
neo = new
genesis = making

The Body's Energy Budget

The average person takes in close to a million kcalories a year and expends more than 99 percent of them, maintaining a stable weight for years on end. In other words, the body's energy budget is balanced. Some people, however, eat too much and get fat; others eat too little and get thin. This section examines metabolism from the perspective of the energy budget, looking first at the two forms of unbalanced budgets, feasting and fasting, and then at a balanced budget.

The Economics of Feasting

Everyone knows that when you consume more energy than you expend, much of the excess is stored as body fat. Fat can be made from an excess

Figure 6–2
The Central Pathways of Energy Metabolism

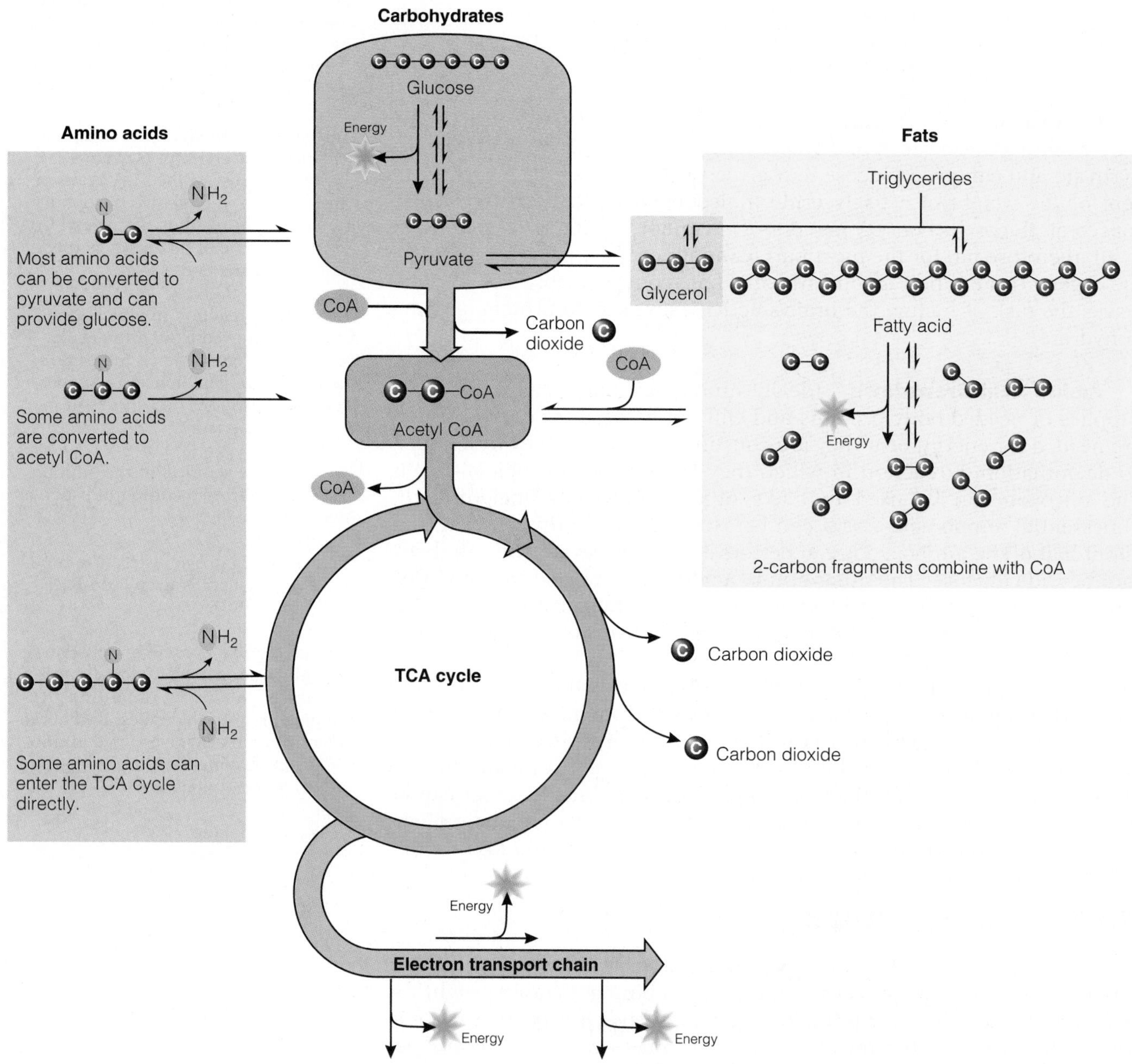

of any energy-yielding nutrient that you eat. Fat cells enlarge as they fill with fat, and the body's fat-storing capacity seems to be able to expand indefinitely, as Figure 6–3 shows.

Excess Carbohydrate Surplus carbohydrate (glucose) is first stored as glycogen, but the glycogen-storing cells have a limited capacity. Once

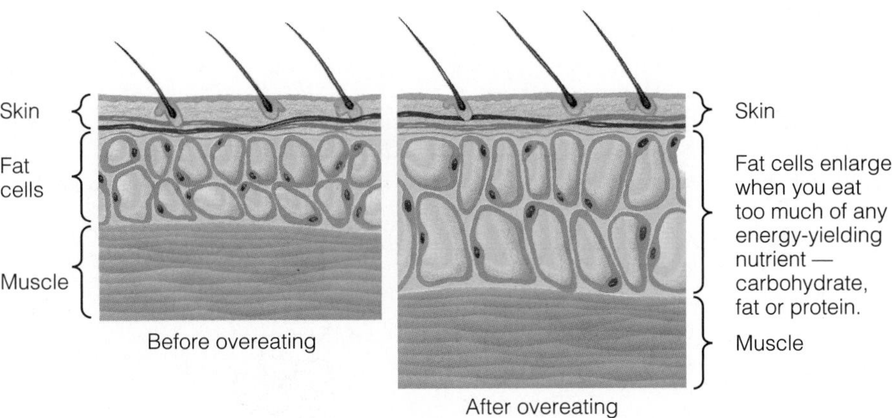
Skin
Fat cells
Muscle
Before overeating
After overeating
Skin
Fat cells enlarge when you eat too much of any energy-yielding nutrient — carbohydrate, fat or protein.
Muscle

Figure 6–3
Fat Cell Enlargement

glycogen stores are filled, any additional carbohydrate is routed to fat. Thus excess carbohydrate can contribute to obesity.

Excess Fat Surplus dietary fat contributes easily to the body's fat stores. During digestion and metabolism, fat may break down into fragments, such as acetyl CoA, but if the flow of these fragments is rapid enough to meet the body's need for energy, any excess fragments that are available will be stored as triglycerides in the fat cells.

Excess Protein Surplus protein may encounter the same fate. If not needed to build body protein or to meet energy needs, amino acids will lose their nitrogens and will be converted through the intermediates, pyruvate and acetyl CoA, to triglycerides. These, too, swell the fat cells and increase body weight. Figure 6–4 shows the metabolic events of feasting.

Alcohol Excess energy from alcohol is also stored as fat. In addition, alcohol has been shown to slow the body's use of fat for fuel, favoring even more fat storage.[1]

In summary, the following points deserve repeating:

- Energy from any food can make you fat if you eat enough of the food. Excess food energy is stored in the body as fat.
- Fat from food, as compared with carbohydrate and protein, is especially easy for the body to store in fat tissue.
- Alcohol both delivers kcalories and promotes fat storage.

The Economics of Fasting

When you consume less energy than you expend, you lose weight. The body spends energy all the time, because even when a person is asleep and totally relaxed, the cells of many organs are hard at work. In fact, this cellular work, which maintains all life processes without a person's awareness, represents about two-thirds of the total energy a person spends in a day. (The other one-third is the work that a person does during waking hours, using voluntary muscles.)

Figure 6–4
Feasting
When people overeat, they store energy.

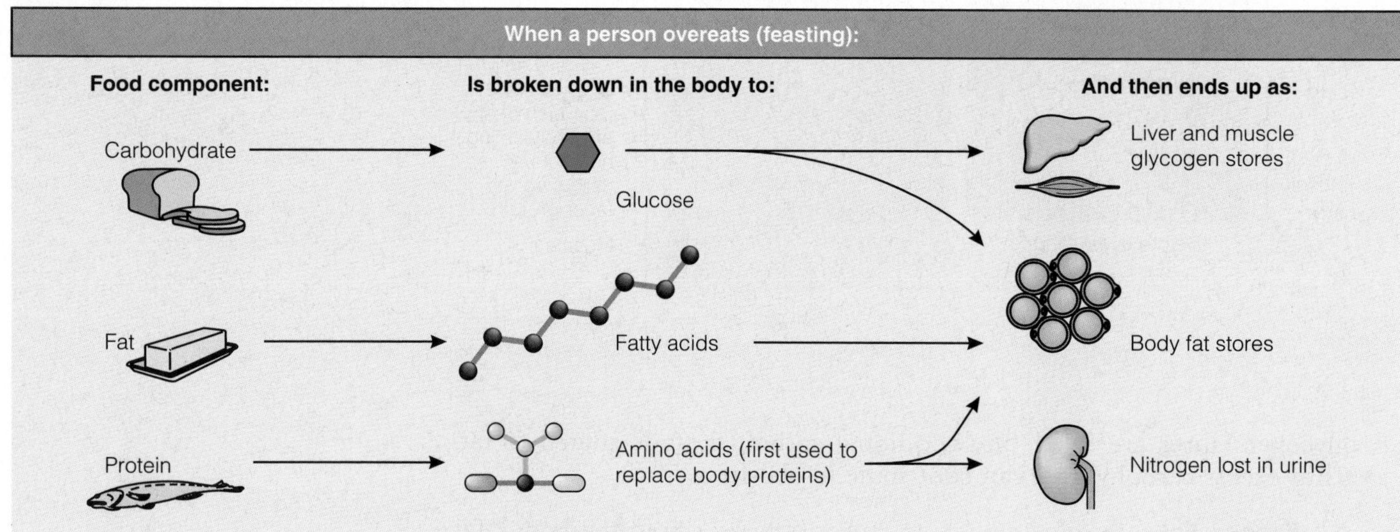

Energy Deficit The body's top priority is to meet the energy needs for this ongoing activity. Its normal way of doing so is by periodic refueling, that is, by eating, but when food is not available, the body uses other fuel sources from its own tissues. If people choose not to eat, we say they are fasting; if they have no choice (as in a famine), we say they are starving; but no metabolic difference exists between the two. In either case, the body is forced to switch to a wasting metabolism, drawing on its reserves of carbohydrate and fat and, within a day or so, on its vital protein tissues as well.

Glycogen Used First As a fast or period of starvation begins, glucose from the liver's stored glycogen and fatty acids from the body's stored fat both flow into cells to fuel their work. Several hours later, however, most of the glucose is used up—liver glycogen is exhausted. Low blood glucose concentrations serve as a signal to promote further fat breakdown.[2]

Glucose Needed for the Brain At this point, a few hours into a fast, most of the cells are depending on fatty acids to continue providing fuel. But the nervous system and brain cells cannot use fatty acids; they still need glucose. Even if other energy fuel is available, glucose has to be present to permit the brain's energy-metabolizing machinery to work. Normally, the nervous system (brain and nerves) consumes about two-thirds of the total glucose used each day—about 400 to 600 kcalories' worth.

Reminder: The liver releases glucose, and the fat cells release fat to fuel the body's cells, but the brain can use only glucose.

Protein Breakdown and Ketosis Because fat stores cannot provide the glucose needed by the brain, body protein tissues (such as liver and muscle) always break down to some extent during fasting. In the first few

Fasting = living on the body's fat and protein.

Figure 6–5
Fasting
When people are fasting, they draw on stored energy.

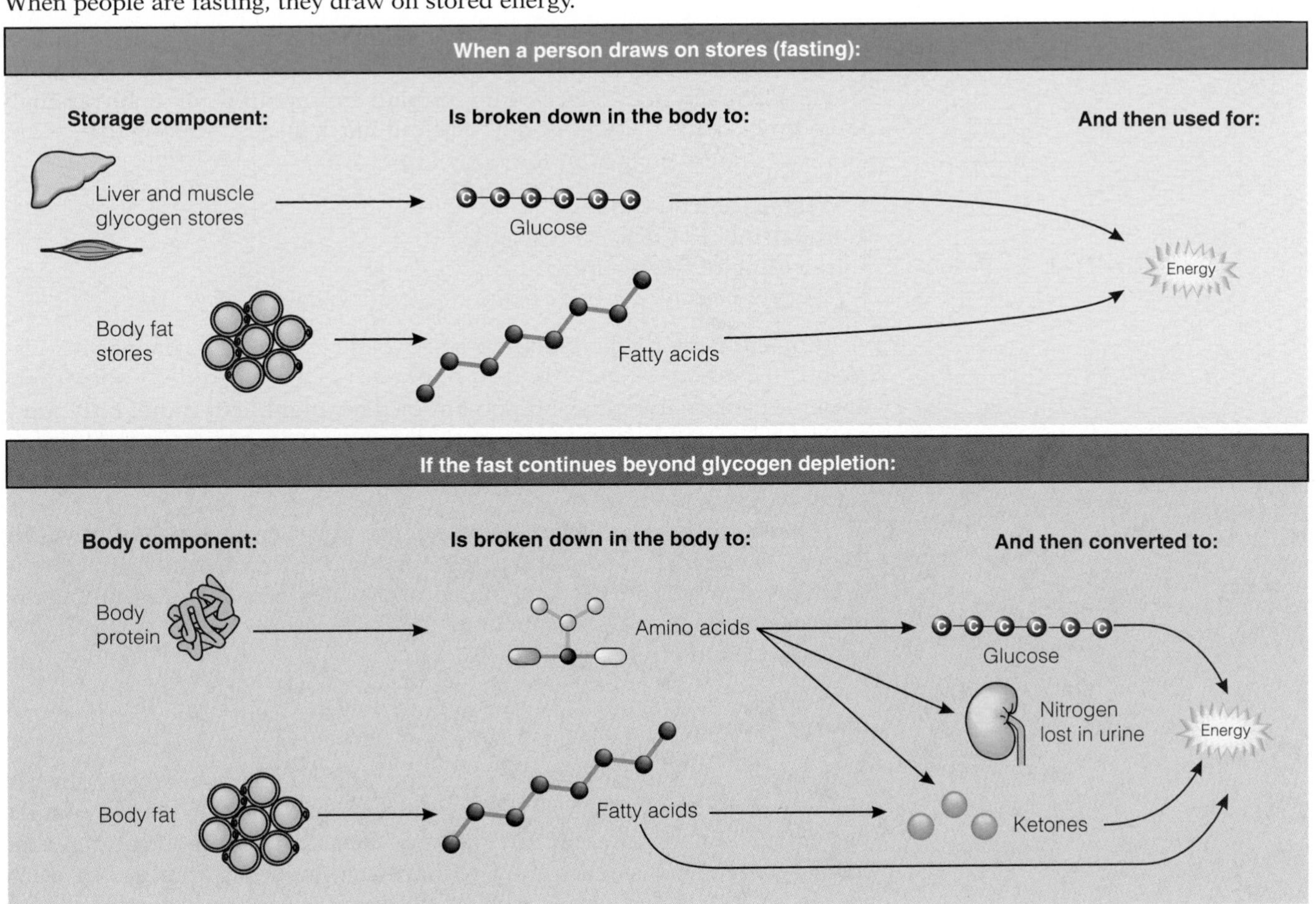

days of a fast, body protein provides about 90 percent of the needed glucose, and glycerol provides about 10 percent. If body protein loss were to continue at this rate, death would ensue within about three weeks. As the fast continues, however, the body finds a way to use its fat to fuel the brain. It adapts by condensing together acetyl CoA fragments derived from fatty acids to produce ketones, which can serve as fuel for some brain cells. Ketone production rises until, at the end of several weeks of fasting, it is meeting much of the nervous system's energy needs.[3] Still, many areas of the brain rely exclusively on glucose, and body protein continues to be sacrificed to produce it. Figure 6–5 shows the metabolic events that occur during fasting.

Slowed Metabolism As fasting continues and the body is shifting to partial dependence on ketones for energy, the body simultaneously reduces its energy output and conserves both its fat and lean tissue. Because of the slowed metabolism, the loss of fat falls to a bare minimum. Thus, although

In fasting, muscle and lean tissue give up protein to supply amino acids for conversion to glucose. This glucose, with ketones produced from fat, fuels the brain's activities.

Reminder: *Ketones* are acidic, fat-related compounds formed from the incomplete breakdown of fat when carbohydrate is not available. Small amounts of ketones are a normal part of the blood chemistry, but when their concentration rises, they spill into the urine. The combination of high blood ketones (*ketonemia*) and ketones in the urine (*ketonuria*) is termed *ketosis*.

weight loss during fasting may be quite dramatic, *fat* loss may actually be less than when at least some food is supplied.

Hazards of Fasting The body's adaptations to fasting are sufficient to maintain life for a long period. Mental alertness need not be diminished. Even physical energy may remain unimpaired for a surprisingly long time. Still, fasting is not without its hazards. Among the many changes that take place in the body are:

- Wasting of lean tissues.
- Impairment of disease resistance.
- Lowering of body temperature.
- Disturbances of the body's salt and water balance.

For the person who wants to lose weight, fasting is a dangerous way to go. The body's lean tissue continues to be degraded, sometimes amounting to as much as 50 percent of the weight lost. A diet only moderately restricted in energy can actually promote a greater rate of *weight* loss, a faster rate of *fat* loss, and the retention of more lean tissue than a severely restricted fast.[4]

Alterations similar to those in fasting are seen in low-carbohydrate dieting. Renewed food intake, especially of carbohydrate, results in dramatic changes in the body's salt and water balance, accounting for most of the wide swings in body weight seen in people on fasts or low-carbohydrate diets.

Energy Balance

If a person's weight is within the appropriate range for height and is not changing, the person has a balanced energy budget. Food energy intake has equaled energy expenditure, and so, deposits of fat made at one time have been compensated for by withdrawals made at another. In other words, the body uses fat as a savings account for energy. In the case of fat, though, unlike money, more is not better; there is an optimum.

A day's energy balance can be stated like this:

> Change in body fat stores (expressed in kcalories) equals the food energy taken in (kcalories) minus the energy spent on metabolic and other activities (kcalories).

More simply:

> Change in fat stores (kcalories) = energy in (kcalories) - energy out (kcalories).

Energy In and Energy Out You know about the "energy in" side of this equation. An apple gives you about 125 kcalories; a candy bar provides about 300 kcalories. On the "energy out" side, if you are physically active for an hour, you may spend 100, 300, or even 500 kcalories or more.

Energy Values of Foods Energy amounts for several hundred foods are listed in Appendix A. For weight-control purposes, though, it is perhaps more important to be aware of the fat contents of foods. Chapter 3 offered strategies for reducing fat intake, and the Nutrition in Practice at the end of this chapter introduces exchange lists to help diet planners keep track of the energy and fat in foods.

Energy Expenditures The body spends energy in two major ways: to fuel its basal metabolism and to fuel its voluntary activities. You can change your voluntary activities to spend more or less energy in a day, and over time you can also change your basal metabolism by building up your body's metabolically active lean tissue, as explained in Chapter 10.

basal metabolism: the energy needed to maintain life when a person is at complete rest after a 12-hour fast. Basal metabolism, sometimes called *basal metabolic rate (BMR),* is normally the largest part of a person's daily energy expenditure.

voluntary activities: the component of a person's daily energy expenditure that involves conscious and deliberate muscular work—walking, lifting, climbing, and other physical activities. Voluntary activities normally require less energy in a day than basal metabolism does.

Basal Metabolism The basal metabolism supports the work that goes on all the time without conscious awareness. The beating of the heart, the inhaling and exhaling of air, the maintenance of body temperature, and the sending of nerve and hormonal messages to direct these activities are the basal processes that maintain life.

Basal Metabolic Rate The basal metabolic rate (BMR) is the rate at which the body spends energy for these maintenance activities. This rate varies from person to person and may vary for a single individual with a change in circumstance or physical condition (see Table 6-1). For example, an infant's metabolic rate relative to body weight is much faster than an

Table 6–1
Factors That Affect BMR

FACTOR	EFFECT ON BMR
Age	In youth, the BMR is higher; age brings less lean body mass and slows the BMR.[a]
Height	In tall, thin people, the BMR is higher.[b]
Growth	In children and pregnant women, the BMR is higher.
Body composition	The more lean tissue, the higher the BMR. The more fat tissue, the lower the BMR.[c]
Fever	Fever raises the BMR.[d]
Stresses (including many diseases and certain drugs)	Stresses raise the BMR.
Environmental temperature	Both heat and cold raise the BMR.
Fasting/starvation	Fasting/starvation lowers the BMR.[e]
Malnutrition	Malnutrition lowers the BMR.
Thyroxine	The thyroid hormone thyroxine is a key BMR regulator; the more thyroxine produced, the higher the BMR.[f]

[a] The BMR begins to decrease in early adulthood (after growth and development cease) at a rate of about 2 percent/decade. A reduction in voluntary activity as well brings the total decline in energy expenditure to 5 percent/decade.

[b] If two people weigh the same, the taller, thinner person will have the faster metabolic rate, reflecting the greater skin surface, through which heat is lost by radiation, in proportion to the body's volume.

[c] In general, males tend to have a higher BMR than females due to their greater lean body mass.

[d] Fever raises BMR by 7 percent for each degree Fahrenheit.

[e] Prolonged starvation reduces the total amount of metabolically active lean tissue in the body, although the decline occurs sooner and to a greater extent than body losses alone can explain. More likely, the neural and hormonal changes that accompany fasting are responsible for changes in BMR.

[f] The thyroid gland releases hormones that travel to the cells and influence cellular metabolism. Thyroid hormone activity can speed up or slow down the rate of metabolism by as much as 50 percent.

HOW TO Estimate a Day's Energy Output

The calculation shown here exemplifies one way of calculating energy needs. Another way is often used in clinical practice: the BEE (basal energy expenditure) method, explained in Chapter 18, Table 18-3.

- *Basal metabolism.* Convert your body weight from pounds to kilograms. Then multiply by the factor 1.0 kcalorie per kilogram of body weight per hour for men (or 0.9 for women).[a] Then multiply by the 24 hours in a day. For example, for a 160-pound man:

1. Change pounds to kilograms:

   160 lb ÷ 2.2 lb/kg = 72.7 kg.

2. Multiply weight in kilograms by the BMR factor:

   72.7 kg x 1 kcal/kg/hr = 72.7 kcal/hr.

3. Multiply kcalories used in one hour by hours in a day:

   72.7 kcal/hr x 24 hr/day = 1744 kcal/day.

Energy for BMR equals 1744 kcalories per day.

- *Voluntary muscular activity.* To estimate the energy for your activities, determine from Table 6–2 the level of intensity that typifies your average daily activity. Then multiply your BMR by the corresponding activity factor. For example, if our 160-pound man engages in mostly light activity, his activity factor would be 1.6. Multiply this factor by his BMR kcalories:

  1.6 x 1744 kcal/day = 2790 kcal/day.

- *Total energy needs.* The result, 2790 kcalories/day, expresses his total daily energy needs.

Alternatively, total energy expenditure can be estimated in one step based on body weight as shown in the last column of Table 6–2. As an example, for a 160-pound man engaged in mostly light activity:

38 kcal/kg/day x 72.7 kg = 2762 kcal/day.

The difference between 2790 and 2762 is insignificant and acceptable. Either way, the man's total energy needs are about 2800 kcalories per day.

[a] Men's metabolic energy needs are assumed to be higher than women's because their hormones induce them to develop more lean tissue than do most women, and lean tissue burns more energy per hour.

adult's to support the infant's extraordinary growth rate. In general, BMR is fast in people with considerable lean body mass (growing children, pregnant women, and males). Thus one way to increase your BMR is to make endurance and strength-building activities regular habits, to maximize

Table 6–2
Estimating Daily Energy RDA at Various Levels of Physical Activity

LEVEL OF INTENSITY	TYPE OF ACTIVITY	ACTIVITY FACTOR (× BMR)	ENERGY EXPENDITURE (kcal/kg/day)
Very light	Seated and standing activities, painting trades, driving, laboratory work, typing, sewing, ironing, cooking, playing cards, playing a musical instrument		
Men		1.3	31
Women		1.3	30
Light	Walking on a level surface at 2.5 to 3 mph, garage work, electrical trades, carpentry, restaurant trades, housecleaning, child care, golf, sailing, table tennis		
Men		1.6	38
Women		1.5	35
Moderate	Walking 3.5 to 4 mph, weeding and hoeing, carrying a load, cycling, skiing, tennis, dancing		
Men		1.7	41
Women		1.6	37
Heavy	Walking with a load uphill, tree felling, heavy manual digging, basketball, climbing, football, soccer		
Men		2.1	50
Women		1.9	44
Exceptional	Athletes training in professional or world-class events		
Men		2.4	58
Women		2.2	51

Source: Reprinted with permission from *Recommended Daily Allowances:* 10th edition. Copyright 1989 by the National Academy of Sciences. Courtesy of the National Academy Press, Washington, D.C.

your body's lean tissue.[5] BMR is also fast in people who are tall and so have a large surface area for their weight, in people with fever or under stress, in people taking certain drugs, and in people with highly active thyroid glands. BMR is slowed down by loss of lean tissue and depression of thyroid hormone activity due to disease, inactivity, fasting, or malnutrition.

Basal Metabolic Needs Basal metabolic needs are surprisingly large. A person whose total energy needs are 2000 kcalories a day spends 1200 to 1400 of them to support basal metabolism. The accompanying box shows how to estimate your energy expenditure for basal metabolism, the first step in estimating total energy output for the day.

Energy for Activities The second step is to estimate the number of kcalories spent on voluntary activities. This depends on three factors: muscle mass, body weight, and activity. The larger the muscle mass required and the heavier the weight of the body part being moved, the more kcalories are spent. The activity's duration frequency, and intensity also influence energy costs—the longer, the more frequent, and the more intense the activity, the more kcalories spent. The energy spent on activities, added to the energy required for basal metabolism, equals the total energy you spend in a day (refer again to the accompanying box).

Energy to Manage Food One component of energy expenditure is not taken into account in the calculations in the box: the energy required for the body to manage food. When food is taken into the body, many cells that have been dormant begin to be active. The muscles that move the food through the intestinal tract speed up their rhythmic contractions; the cells that manufacture and secrete digestive juices begin their tasks. All these and other cells need extra energy as they come alive to participate in the digestion, absorption, and metabolism of food. This stimulation of cellular activity produces heat and is known as the thermic effect of food. The thermic effect of food is generally thought to represent about 10 percent of the total food energy taken in. For purposes of rough estimates, however, the thermic effect of food can be ignored; the 10 percent it might contribute to total energy output is smaller than the probable errors involved in estimating energy input from food or output for activities.

thermic effect of food: an estimation of the energy required to process food (digest, absorb, transport, metabolize, and store ingested nutrients).

In summary, the energy you spend in a day is about equal to the sum of two components—your basal metabolic energy and your activity energy. The Self-Study and accompany Form 7 take you through the steps for computing the range of total energy you spend in a day. This expenditure represents your approximate energy need, which you meet by eating food. If you eat more than this, you will store the excess energy in your body, mostly as fat. If you eat less than this, you will use up body tissue as fuel to make up the deficit.

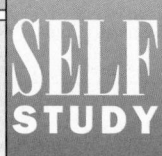

How Much Energy Do You Spend in a Day?

Use the box on p. 128 (How to Estimate a Day's Energy Output) to estimate the energy you spend in a day. Form 7 will help you record your calculations.

Form 7
Estimating Energy Output

BASAL METABOLISM

Step 1: My weight in pounds (___ lb) divided by 2.2 lb/kg equals my weight in kilograms: ___ kg.

Step 2: My weight in kilograms (___ kg) times 1.0 kcal/kg/hr for men or 0.9 kcal/kg/hr for women equals the number of kcalories I spend on basal metabolism in an hour: ___ kcal/hr.

Step 3: My energy expenditure per hour (___ kcal/hr) times the hours in a day (24) equals the number of kcalories I spend on basal metabolism in a day: ___ kcalories/day.

ACTIVITIES

MEN (do *one* of the following five calculations):

___ I am very lightly active, so my activity factor (see Table 6–2) is 1.3. Multiply this factor by your basal metabolic energy (step 3): 1.3 x ___ (BMR) = ___ kcal/day.

Your result, ___ kcal/day, expresses your total daily needs.

___ I am lightly active, so my activity factor (see Table 6–2) is 1.6. Multiply this factor by your basal metabolic energy (step 3): 1.6 x ___ (BMR) = kcal/day.

Self-Study (continued)

Your result, ___ kcal/day, expresses your total daily needs.

___ I am moderately active, so my activity factor (see Table 6–2) is 1.7. Multiply this factor by your basal metabolic energy (step 3): 1.7 x ___ (BMR) = ___ kcal/day.

Your result, ___ kcal/day, expresses your total daily needs.

___ I am very active (heavy activity) so my activity factor (see Table 6–2) is 2.1. Multiply this factor by your basal metabolic energy (step 3): 2.1 x ___ (BMR) = ___ kcal/day.

Your result, ___ kcal/day, expresses your total daily needs.

___ I am exceptionally active, so my activity factor (see Table 6–2) is 2.4. Multiply this factor by your basal metabolic energy (step 3): 2.4 x ___ (BMR) = ___ kcal/day.

Your result, ___ kcal/day, expresses your total daily needs.

WOMEN (do *one* of the following five calculations):

___ I am very lightly active, so my activity factor (see Table 6–2) is 1.3. Multiply this factor by your basal metabolism energy (step 3): 1.3 x ___ (BMR) = ___ kcal/day.

Your result, ___ kcal/day, expresses your total daily needs.

___ I am lightly active, so my activity factor (see Table 6–2) is 1.5. Multiply this factor by your basal metabolic energy (step 3): 1.5 x ___ (BMR) = ___ kcal/day.

Your result, ___ kcal/day, expresses your total daily needs.

___ I am moderately active, so my activity factor (see Table 6–2) is 1.6. Multiply this factor by your basal metabolic energy (step 3): 1.6 x ___ (BMR) = ___ kcal/day.

Your result, ___ kcal/day, expresses your total daily needs.

___ I am very active (heavy activity) so my activity factor (see Table 6–2) is 1.9. Multiply this factor by your basal metabolic energy (step 3): 1.9 x ___ (BMR) = ___ kcal/day.

Your result, ___ kcal/day, expresses your total daily needs.

__ I am exceptionally active, so my activity factor (see Table 6–2) is 2.2. Multiply this factor by your basal metabolic energy (step 3): 2.2 x ___ (BMR) = ___ kcal/day.

Your result, ___ kcal/day, expresses your total daily needs.

■ STUDY QUESTIONS ■

1. Elaborate on the statement that "Every cell in the body engages in metabolism."
2. What are the basic units of energy metabolism in the body?
3. Define metabolism, anabolism, and catabolism.
4. Why do body protein tissues break down during fasting?
5. Describe ketosis.
6. List some of the hazards of fasting.
7. List two ways the body spends energy.
8. Describe basal metabolism.
9. List some factors that affect a person's basal metabolic rate.

NUTRITION IN PRACTICE 6

The Exchange System

This Nutrition in Practice introduces the most widely used basis for diet planning, the exchange system. It consists of lists that organize foods by their nutrient and energy contents. Foods on any single list can be used interchangeably. The exchange system is used to plan diets for weight control, diabetes, and other conditions requiring regulation of kcalories and energy nutrients. You may recall that Chapter 1 introduced food group plans, which help the planner to achieve three of the five goals for diets—adequacy, balance, and variety. The exchange system helps with the other two: kcalorie control and moderation. Originally developed for people with diabetes, the exchange system has proved so useful that it is now in use for weight-control diets, too. Appendix C gives details of the major exchange systems used in the United States and Canada.

Why can't we have just one diet-planning tool? Why must we learn to use both food group plans and exchange lists?

The answer lies in the nature of foods themselves. They are biological products, too complex to fit easily into any single system. Food group plans are useful for describing the protein, vitamin, and mineral contents of foods. The exchange system sorts foods by their energy contents and by the *proportions* of carbohydrate, fat, and protein they contain.

In the exchange system, portion sizes are strictly defined, so that the number of kcalories from any food item on a given list is the same as that from any other item on that list. All of the food portions in a given list provide approximately the same amounts of energy nutrients (protein, fat, and carbohydrate). As a result, any food item on a list can be traded, or exchanged, for any other item on that same list without affecting a diet's balance or total kcalories. This gives the plan great flexibility. You can eat a portion of bread, or rice, or macaroni, or any other starchy food without altering the number of kcalories or the energy-nutrient balance in your meal.

That does sound useful. What do I need to know or remember to learn to use the exchange lists?

As Figure 6–6 (on pp. 134-135) shows, the exchange system organizes foods into six lists. A convenient way to remember the portion sizes and energy values is to keep in mind a typical item from each list:

- Starch/breads—1 slice bread (80 kcalories).
- Meats—1 ounce lean beef (55 kcalories).
- Vegetables—½ cup cooked carrots (25 kcalories).
- Fruits—½ banana (60 kcalories).
- Milks—1 cup nonfat milk (90 kcalories).
- Fats—1 teaspoon butter (45 kcalories).

To apply the system successfully, users must become familiar with portion sizes. Figure 6–6 shows the foods on each list with their accurate portion sizes.

Would you please clarify the kcalorie amounts for each list? For example, on the bread list, a slice of bread has 80 kcalories, but many different kinds of bread are available. They don't all provide 80 kcalories per slice, do they?

Not exactly, but the values are close enough to be treated as the same. Table 6–3 shows the carbohydrate, protein, fat, and energy values that pertain to each list.

Take a moment to study the table and the notes below it, and you will see how the number of kcalories agrees with the number of grams of carbohydrate, fat, and protein in each food. (Remember that a gram of carbohydrate offers 4 kcalories; a gram of fat, 9 kcalories; and a gram of protein, 4 kcalories.)

Notice, too, how useful some lists are for planning weight-control diets. In particular, notice how few kcalories are in a portion of vegetables as compared with meats. At 25 kcalories a half cup, you could eat 4 cups of vegetables for less than the kcalorie cost of a single 3-ounce hamburger patty. A 3-ounce hamburger counts as 3 medium-fat meat exchanges, or 225 kcalories.

Why is cheddar cheese on the meat list? Shouldn't it be on the milk list?

Foods are not always listed in the exchange system where you might first expect them to be because they are grouped by their energy-nutrient contents, rather than by their vitamin and mineral contents. Cheeses, like meats, are composed primarily of protein and fat; they provide negligible carbohydrate. (In the food group plans presented earlier, cheeses are classed with milk because they are dairy products with high calcium contents.)

For similar reasons, corn, lima beans, peas, and potatoes are listed with starch/breads in the exchange system, rather than with the vegetables. Similarly, olives are not classed as a "fruit" as a botanist would claim; they are classified as a "fat" because their fat content makes them more similar to butter than to berries. Bacon is also on the fat list to remind users of its high fat content. These groupings permit you to see the characteristics of foods that are especially significant to energy balance.

The exchange lists point out fiber and sodium, too, whenever they are present in significant quantities (see Figure 6–7, p. 136). In Appendix C, foods high in fiber are identified by the wheat symbol (choose them often). The saltshaker symbol identifies foods high in sodium so that people who must avoid them can do so.

Table 6–3
The Six Exchange Lists

LIST	PORTION SIZE	CARBOHYDRATE (g)	PROTEIN (g)	FAT (g)	ENERGY[a] (kcal)
Starch bread[b]	1 slice	15	3	Trace	80
Vegetable[c]	1/2 c	5	2	—	25
Fruit	1 portion	15	—	—	60
Meat[d]	1 oz				
Lean		—	7	3	55
Medium-fat		—	7	5	75
High-fat		—	7	8	100
Milk	1 c				
Nonfat		12	8	Trace	90
Low-fat		12	8	5	120
Whole		12	8	8	150
Fat	1 tsp	—	—	5	45

Note: This is the U.S. exchange system. The complete details, and those of the Canadian system, are shown in Appendix C.

[a] The energy value for each exchange list represents an approximate average for the group and does not reflect the precise number of grams of carbohydrate, protein, and fat. For example, a slice of bread contains 15 grams carbohydrate (that's 60 kcalories). 3 grams protein (that's another 12 kcalories), and a trace of fat—rounded up to 80 kcalories for ease in calculating. A half cup of vegetables (not including starchy vegetables) contains 5 grams carbohydrate (20 kcalories) and 2 grams protein (8 more), which has been rounded down to 25 kcalories.

[b] This list includes starchy vegetables, such as lima beans and corn, as well as cereal, bread, pasta, and other grain products. For portion sizes, see Appendix C.

[c] This list includes low-kcalorie vegetables only.

[d] This list includes cheese and peanut butter as well as meat.

How do food combinations, such as casseroles, fit in the exchange system of planning diets?

Users of the exchange system lists learn to view mixtures of foods, such as casseroles and soups, as combinations of foods from different exchange lists. A piece of cherry pie, for instance, is not simply a fruit exchange. If it contains 12 large cherries, it contains "1 fruit," but it also has a crust made of flour, butter, and sugar. These might count as "2 breads, and 3 fats, with 2 tablespoons added sugar." Some single foods such as legumes also fit on more than one list.

I notice that legumes are on both the starch/bread list and the meat list. Please explain.

Legumes share qualities with both meats and starchy vegetables. Like meats, legumes are rich in protein, but most are lower in fat than meats. Like starchy vegetables, legumes are rich in complex carbohydrates and fiber.

Used as a meat substitute, legumes are counted as follows:

1 c legumes = 1 lean meat + 2 starch.

Used as a bread or starchy vegetable to accompany a meat, they are counted as follows:

1/3 c cooked beans, peas, lentils = 1 starch.
1/4 c cooked baked beans = 1 starch.

Similarly, food group plans allow you to count 1/2 cup cooked legumes as either 1 ounce meat or 1/2 cup vegetables. However you count legumes on paper, use them often in your meals; they are an inexpensive, land-sparing, and health-promoting food.

Figure 6–6 The Exchange System

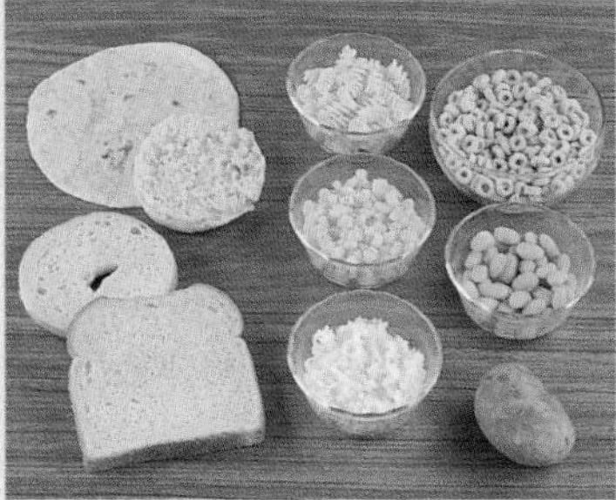

Starch/breads
⅓ slice bread is like:
¾ c ready-to-eat cereal.
½ c cooked pasta.
⅓ c cooked rice.
⅓ c cooked beans.
½ c corn.
1 small (3 oz) potato.
½ bagel or English muffin.
1 tortilla
(1 bread = 15 g carbohydrate, 3 g protein, trace of fat, and 80 kcal.)

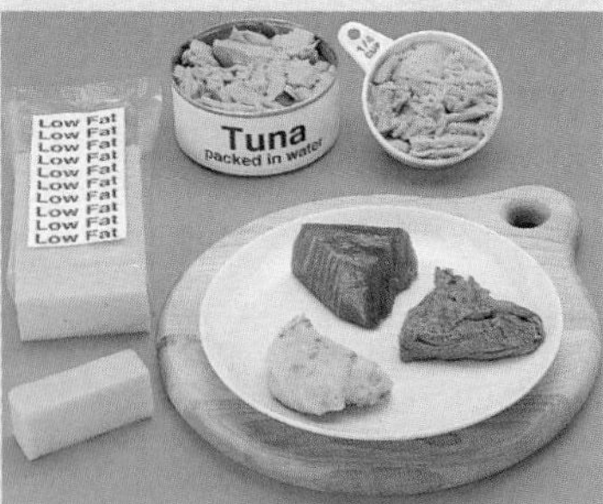

Meats (lean)[a]
1 oz lean meat is like:
1 oz beef or pork tenderloin.
1 oz chicken (without skin)
1 oz fresh fish.
¼ c tuna (canned in water).
1 oz low-fat cheese.
(1 lean meat = 7 g protein, 3 g fat, and 55 kcal.)

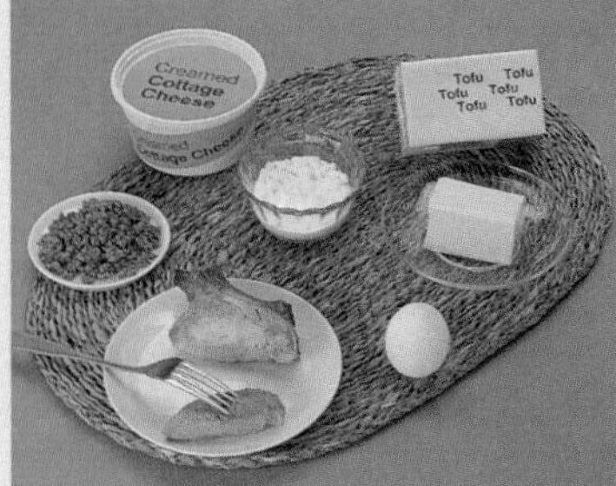

Meats (medium-fat)
1 oz medium-fat meat has the protein content of 1 oz lean meat, but with 5 g fat (2 g more fat than lean meat).
Examples:
1 oz ground beef.
1 oz pork chop.
1 egg.
¼ c creamed cottage cheese or ricotta.
4 oz tofu.
(1 medium-fat meat = 7 g protein, 5 g fat, and about 75 kcal.)

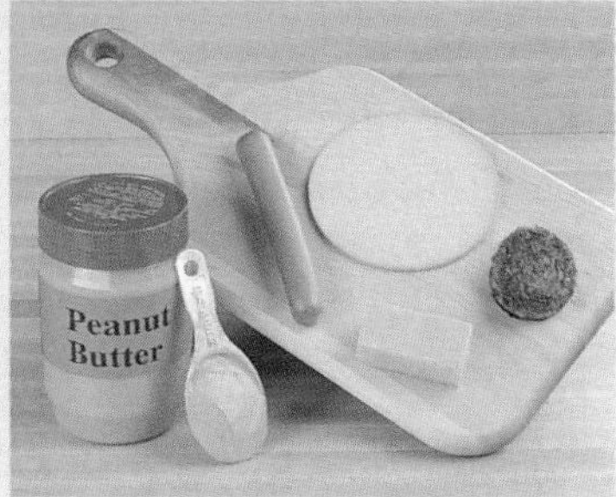

Meats (high-fat)
1 oz high-fat meat has the protein content of 1 oz lean meat, but with an estimated extra "1 fat"—that is, the 3 g fat of a lean meat plus 5 g additional fat.
Examples:
1 oz pork sausage.
1 oz luncheon meat (such as bologna).
1 oz cheddar cheese.
1 small hot dog (frankfurter).[b]
1 tbs peanut butter.
(1 high-fat meat = 7 g protein, 8 g fat, and 100 kcal.)

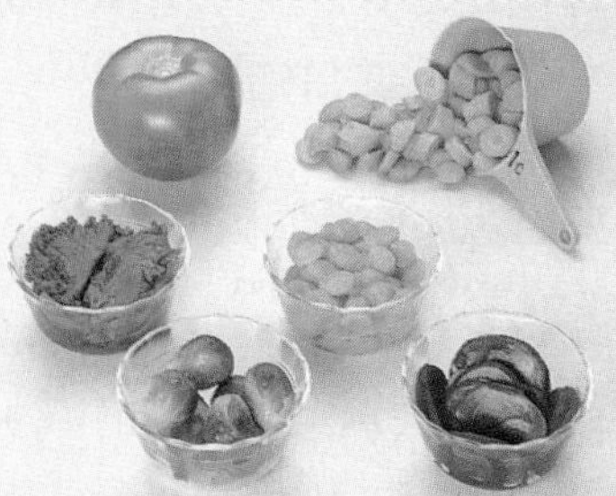

Vegetables[c]
½ c cooked carrots is like:
½ c cooked greens.
½ c cooked brussels sprouts.
½ c cooked beets.
1 c raw carrots.
1 lg tomato.
(1 vegetable = 5 g carbohydrate, 2 g protein, and 25 kcal.)

---

[a]If beans are used as a meat substitute: 1 c cooked beans = 1 lean meat exchange.
[b]The frankfurter counts as 1 high-fat meat exchange plus 1 fat exchange.
[c]Some vegetables such as lettuce, celery, cucumbers, and mushrooms can be eaten freely because their energy value is less than 20 kcalories per serving.

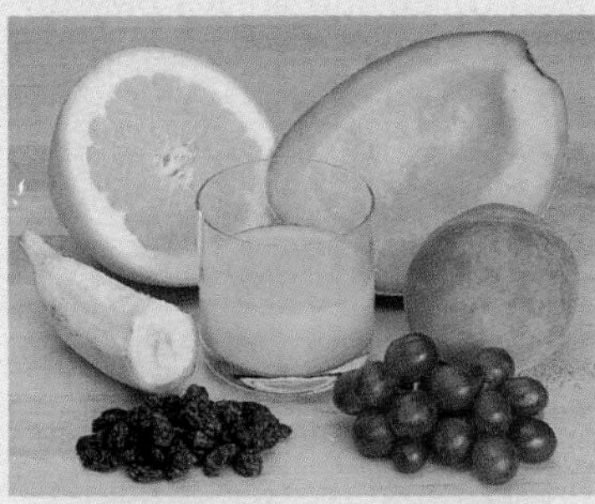

Fruits
½ small banana is like:
1 small apple, peach, orange, or pear.
½ grapefruit.
½ c orange, apple, or grapefruit juice.
15 small grapes.
⅓ cantaloupe.
2 tbs raisins.
(1 fruit = 15 g carbohydrate and 60 kcal.)

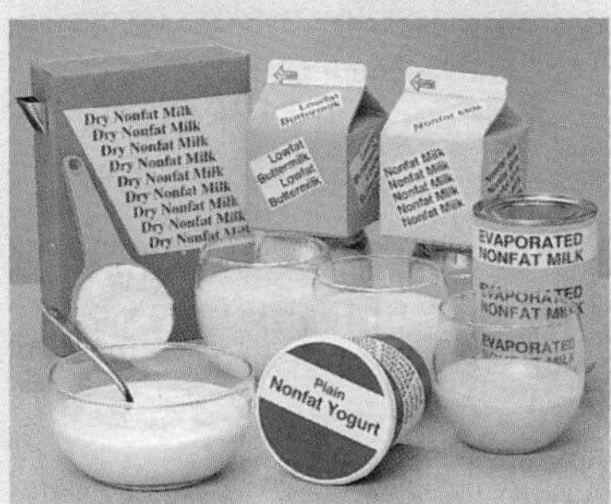

Milks (nonfat and very-low-fat)
1 c nonfat milk is like:
1 c nonfat yogurt, plain.
1 c low-fat buttermilk.
½ c evaporated nonfat milk.
⅓ c dry nonfat milk.
(1 nonfat milk = 12 g carbohydrate, 8 g protein, trace of fat, and 90 kcal.)

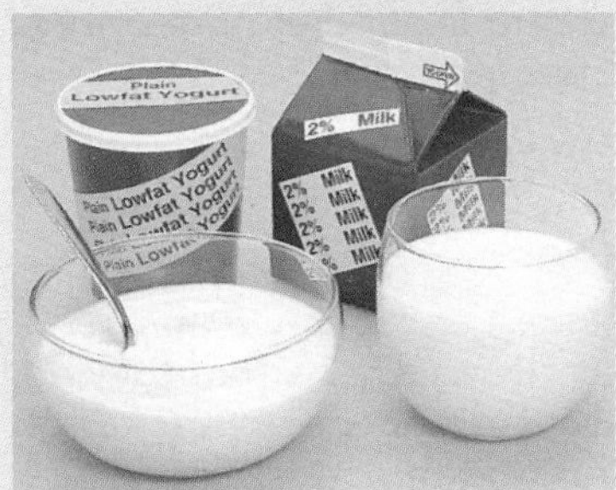

Milks (low-fat)
1 c low-fat milk has the protein and carbohydrate content of 1 c nonfat milk, but with 5 g fat.
Examples:
1 c 2% milk.
1 c low-fat yogurt, plain.
(1 low-fat milk = 12 g carbohydrate, 8 g protein, 5 g fat, and 120 kcal.)

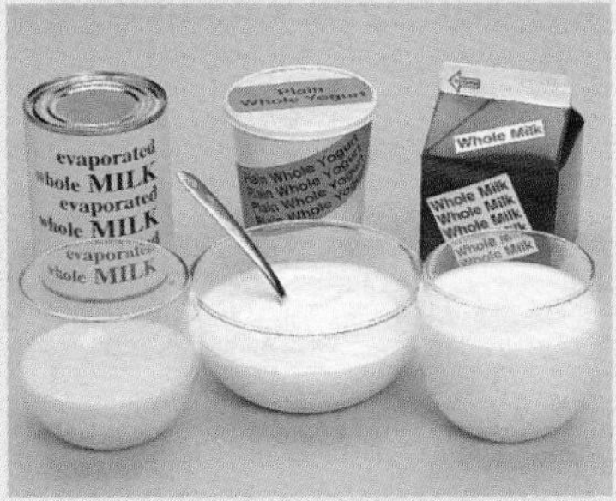

Milks (whole)
1 c whole milk has the protein and carbohydrate content of 1 c nonfat milk, but with 8 g fat.
Examples:
1 c whole milk.
½ c evaporated whole milk.
1 c whole yogurt, plain.
(1 whole milk = 12 g carbohydrate, 8 g protein, 8 g fat, and 150 kcal.)

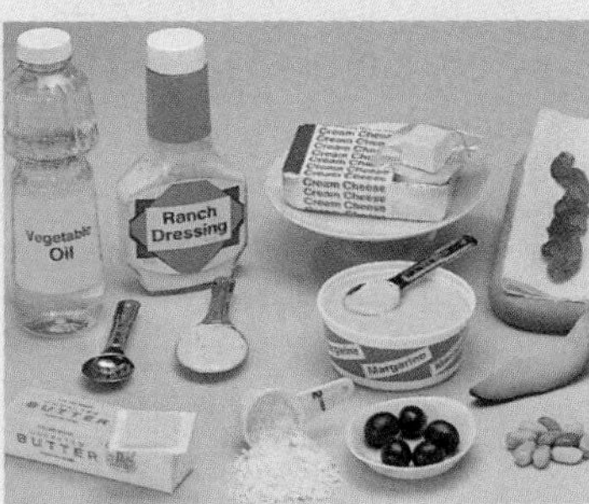

Fats
1 tsp butter is like:
1 tsp margarine.
1 tsp any oil.
1 tbs salad dressing.
5 large olives.
10 large peanuts.
⅛ medium avocado.
1 slice bacon.
2 tbs shredded coconut.
1 tbs cream cheese.
(1 fat = 5 g fat and 45 kcal.)

Figure 6–7
Exchange System Symbols for Fiber and Sodium

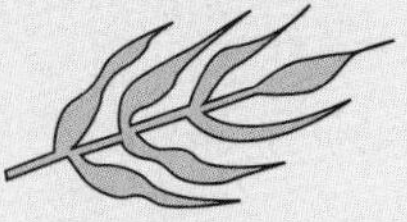

Fiber symbol

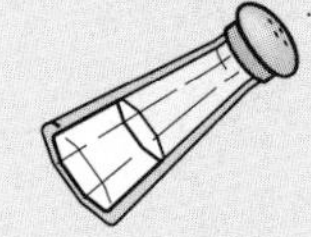

Sodium symbol

The exchange system booklets identify foods high in fiber and sodium with these symbols, so that users can choose foods wisely. In Appendix C these foods are identified using miniature versions of the same symbols. To obtain the original booklet, which is handy to carry around, write to the American Dietetic Association (ADA) at the address given in Appendix D.

You said planners can use the exchange system to control energy intakes and fat intakes. Please explain.

The system's chief usefulness is in the clear definitions it gives to foods. For example, the vegetable list includes only low-kcalorie vegetables, so that 1/2 cup (cooked, or 1 cup raw) of any of them provides about 25 kcalories. The fruit list specifies "without added sugar"—not necessarily to forbid people's eating fruits with sugar, but to help them keep track of sugar consumption (remember, the system was originally intended for people with diabetes). Portion sizes are adjusted so that foods on a given list are equal in their energy value. For example, one-half banana counts as 1 fruit; 15 grapes also count as 1 fruit.

The exchange system also helps users to see the fat in foods. By including items like bacon and avocados, the fat list alerts consumers to foods that are unexpectedly high in fat. Even the starch/bread list specifies which grain products contain added fat (such as biscuits, muffins, and waffles). In addition, the exchange system encourages users to think of nonfat milk as milk and of whole milk as milk with added fat, and to think of lean meats as meats and of medium- and high-fat meats as meats with added fat. To that end, foods on the milk and meat lists are separated into three categories based on their fat contents. The milk group is classed as nonfat, lowfat, and whole; the meat group as lean, medium-fat, and high-fat. Notice, too, that the exchange system lists meats in single ounces. That is, 1 *exchange* of meat is 1 ounce, whereas a *serving* may be 2 or 3 ounces (2 or 3 exchanges). Calculating meat by the ounce encourages the planner to keep close track of meat portion sizes, which eases control of energy and fat intakes.

Thus a person wishing to control food energy intake can be highly successful using the exchange system. Table 6–4 presents a sample balanced 1400-kcalorie diet plan using the exchange system. Table 6–5 provides examples of diet patterns for different energy intakes.

If the exchange system is so useful, why do we need food group plans, too?

A weakness of exchange plans used by themselves is that they do not guarantee adequate intakes of vitamins and minerals. Food group plans work better from that

Table 6–4
A Sample Balanced Weight-Loss Diet Plan

EXCHANGE ITEM	NUMBER OF EXCHANGES	CARBOHYDRATE (g)	PROTEIN (g)	FAT (g)	ENERGY (kcal)
Starch/bread	7	105	21	Trace	560
Meat (lean)	4	0	28	12	220
Vegetables	4	20	8	0	100
Fruit	3	45	0	0	180
Milk (nonfat)	2	24	16	Trace	180
Fat	4	0	0	20	180
Total		194 g	73 g	32 g	1420 kcal

Note: This 1400-kcalorie diet provides approximately 55 percent carbohydrate, 20 percent protein, and 20 percent fat. (Carbohydrate supplies 776 kcalories; protein, 292 kcalories; and fat, 228 kcalories.)

standpoint because the food groupings are based on similarities in vitamin-mineral content. In the exchange system, for example, iron-rich and calcium-poor meats are grouped together with iron-poor and calcium-rich cheeses. To take advantage of the strengths of both food group plans and exchange patterns, and to compensate for their weaknesses, diet planners often combine these two diet-planning tools.

Using the two tools together is not hard to do. Take the plan shown in Table 6–4 as an example. To ensure vitamin and mineral adequacy for this plan, just apply the Daily Food Guide rules:

- For iron, make sure to fill the meat exchanges with iron-rich foods such as meats or legumes (or use legumes as starches).
- For calcium, make sure to fill the milk exchanges with milk products or calcium-rich alternates (or use some cheese in place of meat).
- For vitamins A and C, be sure to include fruits and vegetables rich in these nutrients every day.

As it turns out, when you apply these guidelines, the foods you select will provide ample vitamin B_6, folate, zinc, magnesium, and other vitamins and minerals, too.

As you can see, a diet plan based on the exchange system can deliver an ideal balance of energy nutrients within a controlled number of kcalories and with a moderate fat intake. Use of the Daily Food Guide's rules ensures adequate vitamin and mineral intakes. The two tools used together allow for great flexibility in diet planning. People who understand and apply these principles can design diets that offer a pleasing variety of foods in an array of nutritious and healthful meals.

TABLE 6–5
Diet Patterns for Different Energy Intakes

EXCHANGE	ENERGY LEVEL (kcal)						
	1200	1500	1800	2000	2200	2600	3000
Starch/bread	6	7	8	9	11	13	15
Meat (lean)	4	5	6	6	6	7	8
Vegetable	3	4	5	5	5	6	6
Fruit	2	3	4	4	4	5	6
Milk (nonfat)	2	2	2	3	3	3	3
Fat	3	5	6	7	8	10	12

Note: These patterns follow the Daily Food Guide plan and supply less than 30 percent of kcalories as fat.

■ NOTES ■

1. P. M. Suter, Y. Schutz, and E. Jequier, The effect of ethanol on fat storage in healthy subjects, *New England Journal of Medicine* 326 (1992): 983–987.
2. S. Klein and coauthors, Effect of plasma glucose concentration on the lipolytic response to fasting (abstract), *American Journal of Clinical Nutrition* 45 (1987): 856; J. P. Flatt, The biochemistry of energy expenditure, in P. Bjorntorp and B. N. Brodoff, *Obesity* (Philadelphia: J. B. Lippincott, 1992), pp. 100–116.
3. M. C. Linder, Nutrition and metabolism of proteins, in *Nutritional Biochemistry and Metabolism,* 2nd ed., ed. M. C. Linder (New York: Elsevier, 1991), pp. 87–109.
4. M. E. Sweeney and coauthors, Severe vs. moderate energy restriction with and without exercise in the treatment of obesity: Efficiency of weight loss, *American Journal of Clinical Nutrition* 57 (1993): 127–134.
5. T. J. Horton and C. A. Geissler, Effect of habitual exercise on daily energy expenditure and metabolic rate during standardized activity, *American Journal of Clinical Nutrition* 59 (1994): 13–19.

7

The Vitamins

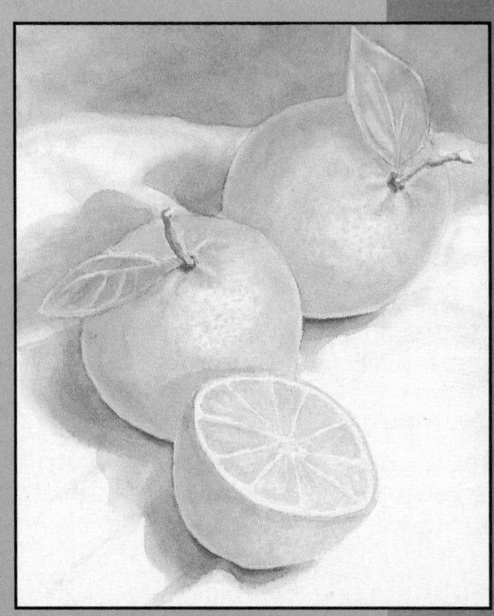

CONTENTS

The last five chapters focused primarily on the energy-yielding nutrients—carbohydrate, fat, and protein. This chapter and the next one discuss the nutrients everyone thinks of when nutrition is mentioned—the vitamins and minerals.

The vitamins occur in foods in much smaller quantities than do the energy-yielding nutrients, and they themselves contribute no energy to the body. Instead, they serve mostly as facilitators of body processes. They are a powerful group of substances, as their absence attests. Vitamin A deficiency can cause blindness; a lack of niacin can cause mental illness; and a lack of vitamin D can retard growth. The consequences of deficiencies are so dire and the effects of restoring the needed nutrients so dramatic that they make wonderful stories for faddists to tell: Are you bald? Impotant? Tired? Do you have pimples? Are you nearsighted? The right vitamin will cure whatever ails you. Vitamins certainly contribute to sound nutritional health, but they do not cure all ills. Actually, a vitamin can cure only the disease caused by a deficiency of that vitamin.

vitamins: essential, noncaloric, organic nutrients needed in tiny amounts in the diet.

The only disease a vitamin can cure is the one caused by a deficiency of that vitamin.

A child once defined vitamins as "what, if you don't eat, you get sick." The description is both insightful and accurate. A more prosaic definition is that vitamins are potent, essential, noncaloric, organic nutrients needed from foods in trace amounts to perform specific functions that promote growth or reproduction or maintain health and life. Two characteristics distinguish vitamins from energy nutrients:

1. Vitamins do not yield energy when broken down, but assist the enzymes that release energy from carbohydrate, fat, and protein.
2. Vitamins are needed in much smaller amounts than the energy nutrients.

As the individual vitamins were discovered, they were named or given letters, numbers, or both. This led to the confusion that still exists today. This chapter uses the names shown in Table 7–1; alternative names are given in Tables 7–2, 7–3, and 7–4, which appear later in the chapter.

Table 7–1
Vitamin Names

FAT-SOLUBLE VITAMINS
Vitamin A
Vitamin D
Vitamin E
Vitamin K
WATER-SOLUBLE VITAMINS
B vitamins
Thiamin
Riboflavin
Niacin
Pantothenic acid
Biotin
Vitamin B_6
Folate
Vitamin B_{12}
Vitamin C

Vitamins fall naturally into two classes—fat soluble and water soluble. The solubility of a vitamin confers on it many characteristic behaviors and determines how it is absorbed and transported, whether it can be stored, and how easily it is lost from the body. This discussion of vitamins begins with the fat-soluble vitamins.

The Fat-Soluble Vitamins

The fat-soluble vitamins—A, D, E, and K—usually occur together in the fats and oils of foods, and the body absorbs them in the same way as it absorbs lipids. Therefore, any condition that interferes with fat absorption can precipitate a deficiency of the fat-soluble vitamins. Once absorbed, fat-soluble vitamins are stored in the liver and fatty tissues until the body needs them. They are not readily excreted, and unlike most of the water-soluble vitamins, they can build up to toxic concentrations.

The capacity to store fat-soluble vitamins affords a person some flexibility as to dietary intakes. When blood concentrations begin to decline, the body can retrieve the vitamins from storage. Thus a person need not eat a day's allowance of each fat-soluble vitamin every day, but need only make sure that over time, average daily intakes approximate the RDA. In contrast, water-soluble vitamins must be consumed more regularly because the body does not store them to any great extent.

Vitamin A and Beta-Carotene

Vitamin A has the distinction of being the first fat-soluble vitamin to be recognized. Today, after more than 75 years of research and revelations, vitamin A and its plant-derived precursor, beta-carotene, are the focus of attention and interest for researchers around the world. Much of this intensive research effort is based on accumulating evidence that both the active vitamin and beta-carotene may protect against some types of cancer.

precursor: a compound that can be converted into another compound.

beta-carotene: a vitamin A precursor made by plants and stored in human fat tissue; an orange pigment.

vitamin A: a fat-soluble vitamin. Its three chemical forms are *retinol* (the alcohol form), *retinal* (the aldehyde form, which is active in the pigments of the eye), and *retinoic acid* (the acid form).

retinol-binding protein (RBP): the specific protein responsible for transporting retinol.

Measurement of the blood concentration of RBP is a sensitive test of vitamin A status.

Metabolic Roles of Vitamin A Vitamin A is a versatile vitamin, playing diverse roles in vision, maintenance of body linings and skin, and immune defenses. Three different forms of vitamin A are active in the body: retinol, retinal, and retinoic acid. Each form of vitamin A performs specific tasks. Retinol is the major transport and storage form of the vitamin; the cells convert retinol to its other active forms as needed. A special transport protein, retinol-binding protein (RBP) picks up retinol from the liver where it is stored and carries it in the blood.

cornea (KOR-nee-uh)**:** the hard, transparent membrane covering the outside of the eye.

retina (RET-in-uh)**:** the layer of light-sensitive nerve cells lining the back of the inside of the eye; consists of rods and cones.

night blindness: slow recovery of vision after exposure to flashes of bright light at night; an early symptom of vitamin A deficiency.

Vitamin A in Vision Vitamin A plays two indispensable roles in the eye. It helps maintain a healthy, crystal-clear outer window, the cornea; and it participates in the events of light detection at the retina. Figure 7–1 shows vitamin A's site of action inside the eye.

When vitamin A is lacking, the eye has difficulty adapting to changing light levels. At night, after the eye has adapted to darkness, a lag occurs before the eye can see again after a flash of bright light. This lag in the recovery of night vision is known as night blindness. Because night blindness is easy to test, it aids in the diagnosis of vitamin A deficiency. Night blindness is only a symptom, however, and may indicate a condition other than vitamin A deficiency.

epithelial (ep-i-THEE-lee-ul) **cells:** cells on the surface of the skin and mucous membranes.

mucous membranes: the membranes composed of mucus-secreting cells that line the surfaces of body tissues. (Reminder: *Mucus* is the smooth, slippery substance secreted by these cells.)

Vitamin A in Epithelial Cells The role that vitamin A plays in vision is undeniably important, but only one-thousandth of the body's vitamin A is in the retina. Much more is in the skin and the linings of organs, where it helps maintain the integrity of the epithelial cells. It is important that each of these surfaces be smooth: the linings of the mouth, stomach, and intestines; the linings of the lungs and the passages leading to them; the lining of the bladder; the linings of the uterus and vagina; and the linings of the eyelids and sinus passageways. The cells lining the surfaces of these and other organs secrete a smooth, slippery substance (mucus) that coats and protects them from invasive microorganisms and other harmful particles. The mucous lining of the stomach also shields its cells from digestion by gastric juices.

Vitamin A, Defense against Infection Based on its role in maintaining these defensive barriers, vitamin A might be expected to play an integral role in fighting infection.[1] Research confirms that this is true in

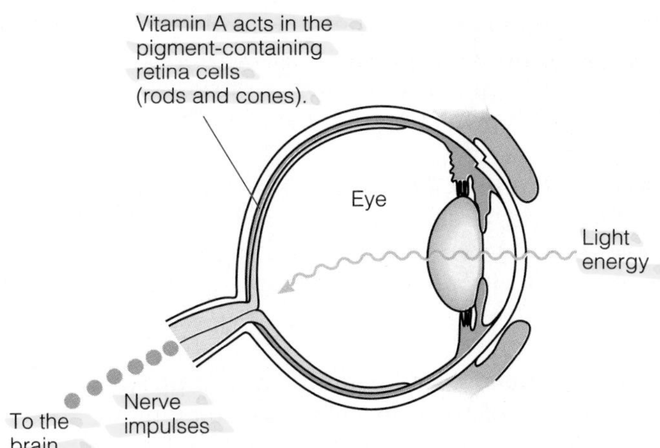

Figure 7–1
Vitamin A's Role in Vision
As light enters the eye, pigments within the cells of the retina absorb the light and generate nerve impulses that travel into the brain. Each pigment contains retinal, the active form of vitamin A.

practice as well as in theory: when children with measles complicated by infections such as pneumonia, diarrhea, or both were given vitamin A supplements, their recovery times and hospital stays were shorter, and their overall survival rates significantly greater, than those of similar children who did not receive vitamin A.[2]

The evidence that Vitamin A reduces the severity of measles and measles-related infections such as pneumonia and diarrhea has prompted the World Health Organization (WHO) and UNICEF (the United Nations International Children's Emergency Fund) to make control of vitamin A deficiency a major goal in their quest to improve child survival throughout the developing world. The American Academy of Pediatrics has issued a formal statement recommending vitamin A supplementation for certain groups of measles-infected infants and children in the United States.[3]

Vitamin A also serves the body in many other ways. It supports normal bone and body growth, reproduction, and cell development.

Metabolic Roles of Beta-Carotene For many years scientists believed beta-carotene to be of interest solely as a vitamin A precursor. Eventually, researchers began to recognize beta-carotene as an extremely effective antioxidant in the body. Antioxidants are compounds that protect other compounds (such as lipids in cell membranes) from attack by oxygen. Oxygen triggers the formation of compounds known as free radicals that can start chain reactions in cell membranes. If left uncontrolled, these chain reactions can damage cell structures and impair cell functions. Oxidative and free radical damage to cells are suspected of instigating some early stages of cancer and heart disease.[4]

antioxidant: a compound that protects other compounds from oxygen by itself reacting with oxygen.

free radical: a highly reactive chemical form that can cause destructive changes in nearby compounds, sometimes setting up a chain reaction.

Beta-Carotene and Cancer Studies of populations suggest that people whose diets are low in beta-carotene have higher incidences of certain types of cancer than those whose diets contain generous amounts of foods rich in beta-carotene.[5] While research has yet to confirm the protective effect of dietary beta-carotene against these diseases, it may turn out that people need both the active form of vitamin A and beta-carotene to stay healthy.

keratin (KERR-uh-tin)**:** a water-insoluble protein; the normal protein of hair and nails. Keratin-producing cells may replace mucus-producing cells in vitamin A deficiency.

keratinization: accumulation of keratin. The progression of this condition to the extreme is **hyperkeratosis.**
hyper = too much

xerophthalmia (zer-off-THAL-mee-uh)**:** progressive blindness caused by vitamin A deficiency.
xero = dry
ophthalm = eye

An early sign is **xerosis** (drying of the cornea); the last and most severe stage is **keratomalacia** (kerr-uh-to-mal-AY-shuh), or total blindness
malacia = softening, weakening

follicle (FOLL-i-cul)**:** a group of cells in the skin from which a hair grows.

The accumulation of the hard material keratin around each hair follicle is **follicular hyperkeratosis.**

preformed vitamin A: vitamin A in its active form.

Vitamin A Deficiency In vitamin A deficiency, the epithelial cells flatten and begin to produce keratin—the hard, inflexible protein of hair and nails. In the eye, this process leads to drying and hardening of the cornea, which may progress to permanent blindness.

Blindness Vitamin A deficiency is the major cause of childhood blindness in the world, causing more than half a million children to lose their sight every year. More than 100 million children worldwide endure less severe forms of vitamin A deficiency, making them vulnerable to infectious diseases.[6]

Infection Proneness In the mouth, a vitamin A deficiency results in drying and hardening of the salivary glands, making them susceptible to infection. Secretions of mucus in the stomach and intestines are reduced, hindering normal digestion and absorption of nutrients. Infections of other mucous membranes also become likely.

All body surfaces, both inside and out, maintain their integrity with the help of vitamin A. When vitamin A is lacking, cells of the skin harden and flatten, making it dry, rough, scaly, and hard. An accumulation of hard material makes a lump around each hair follicle.

Timing of Deficiency Up to a year's supply of vitamin A can be stored in the body, 90 percent of it in the liver. If a healthy adult were to stop eating vitamin A–rich foods, deficiency symptoms would not begin to appear until after stores were depleted, which would take one to two years. Then, however, the consequences would be profound and severe. Table 7–2, later in this chapter, itemizes some of them.

Vitamin A Toxicity When the body stores excess vitamin A, toxicity is possible. Normally, toxicity symptoms are likely only when animal-derived foods or supplements are the source of the excess vitamin, for in these sources the vitamin is already active; it is called *preformed* vitamin A. Plant foods contain the vitamin only in its inactive, precursor form, as beta-carotene. The precursor does not convert to active vitamin A rapidly enough to cause toxicity.

Overdoses of vitamin A damage the same body systems that exhibit symptoms in vitamin A deficiency (see Table 7–2 later in the chapter). Children are most vulnerable to vitamin A toxicity because, being smaller, they need less than adults, and it is easy to give them too much in pill form. The availability of breakfast cereals, instant meals, fortified milk, and chewable candylike vitamins, each containing 100 percent or more of the recommended daily intake of vitamin A, makes it possible for a well-meaning parent to provide several times the daily allowance of the vitamin to a child within a few hours. Serious toxicity is seen in infants and young children when they are given more than ten times the recommended amount every day for weeks at a time. A child who regards vitamin pills as candy may also self-overdose.[7]

Certain vitamin A relatives are available by prescription as acne treatments. When applied directly to the skin surface, these preparations help relieve the symptoms of acne. Taking massive doses of vitamin A internally will *not* cure acne, however, and may cause the miseries itemized in

ized in Table 7–2. Foods are always a better choice than supplements for needed nutrients. The best way to ensure a safe vitamin A intake is to eat generous servings of vitamin A–rich foods. Well-nourished, healthy people need no supplements.

Beta-Carotene Conversion and Toxicity When beta-carotene is converted to retinol in the body, losses occur. This is why, rather than expressing the amounts of beta-carotene in foods, nutrition scientists use the RE (retinol equivalent), which expresses the amount of retinol the body actually derives from a plant food after conversion. The body can make one unit of retinol from about three molecules, or six units, of beta-carotene.

The units in which vitamin A amounts in foods are expressed are **RE (retinol equivalents).** A unit used earlier was the **IU (international unit)**.

Beta-carotene from plant foods is not converted to the active form of vitamin A rapidly enough to be hazardous. It has, however, been known to turn people bright yellow if they eat too much. Beta-carotene builds up in the fat just beneath the skin and imparts a yellow cast.

Vitamin A in Foods In the United States, about half of the vitamin A activity consumed in foods comes from fruits and vegetables. Half of this in turn comes from the plant foods that supply the vitamin as its precursor, beta-carotene. The other half of vitamin A activity consumed in foods comes from preformed vitamin A supplied in milk, cheese, butter, and other dairy products; eggs; and meats. Liver is a rich source of preformed vitamin A. Liver offers many nutrients, so eating it periodically may benefit nutritional health, but once every week or so is enough.

1 RE = 3.33 IU from animal foods or 10 IU from plant foods. (On the average, 1 RE = about 5 IU.)

Because vitamin A is fat soluble, it is lost when milk is skimmed. Nonfat milk is thus often fortified with vitamin A to compensate. Margarine is usually fortified so as to provide the same amount of vitamin A as butter. Snapshot 7–1 shows a sampling of the richest food sources of both preformed vitamin A and beta-carotene.

Fast-food meals often lack vitamin A. When fast-food restaurants offer salads with cheese, carrots, and other vitamin A–rich foods, the nutritional quality of their meals greatly improves.

Beta-Carotene in Foods Many foods from plants contain beta-carotene. Carrots, sweet potatoes, pumpkins, cantaloupe, and apricots are all rich sources, and their bright orange color enhances the eye appeal of the plate. Another colorful group, *dark* green vegetables, such as spinach, other greens, and broccoli, owe their color to both chlorophyll and beta-carotene. The orange and green pigments together give a deep, murky, dark green color to the vegetables. Other colorful vegetables, such as iceberg lettuce, beets, and sweet corn, can fool you into thinking they contain beta-carotene, but these foods derive their color from other pigments and are poor sources of beta-carotene. As for "white" plant foods such as grains and potatoes, they have none. Recommendations to eat *dark* green or *deep* orange vegetables and fruits at least every other day help people to meet their vitamin A needs.

Vitamin D

Vitamin D is different from all the other nutrients in that the body can synthesize it with the help of sunlight. Therefore, in a sense, vitamin D is

Sunlight promotes vitamin D formation in the skin.

Snapshot 7–1 Vitamin A and Beta-Carotene

RDA for men: 1000 μg RE/day
RDA for women: 800 μg RE/day

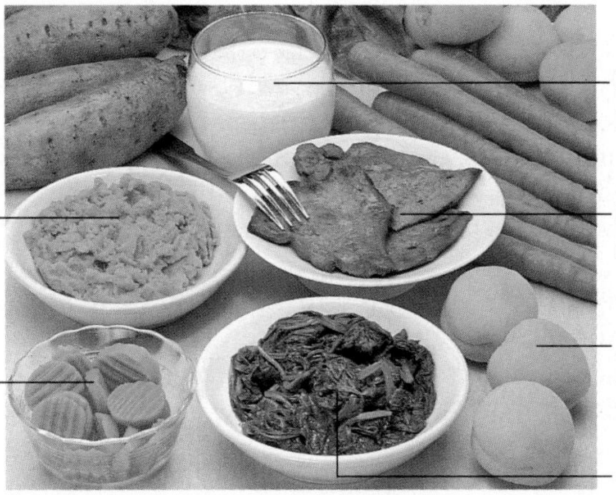

Sweet potato: 1936 RE[b] per ½ c mashed

Carrots: 1915 RE[b] per ½ c cooked

Fortified milk: 150 RE[a] per cup

Beef liver: 9119 RE[a] per 3 oz fried

Apricots: 280 RE[b] per 3 fresh apricots

Spinach: 737 RE[b] per ½ c cooked

[a]Preformed vitamin A.
[b]Beta-carotene.

not an essential nutrient. Given enough sun, you need no vitamin D from foods.

The precursor of vitamin D made in the liver is 7-dehydrocholesterol, which is made from cholesterol. This is one of the body's many "good" uses for cholesterol.

The final, active vitamin is 1.25 dihydroxycholecalciferol, or more simply, dihydroxy vitamin D.

Vitamin D's Metabolic Conversions The liver manufactures a vitamin D precursor, which migrates to the skin and is there converted to a second precursor with the help of the sun's ultraviolet rays. Research suggests that the photosynthesis of vitamin D may be important in enhancing resistance to tuberculosis (TB).[8] This finding helps provide a scientific explanation for the observation that sunshine seems to benefit those with TB.

Next, the liver and then the kidneys alter the second precursor to produce the active vitamin. Vitamin D precursors from plants require the same two conversions by the liver and kidneys to become active. The biologic activity of the active vitamin is 500- to 1000-fold higher than that of its precursor.[9] Diseases that affect either the liver or the kidneys may impair the transformations of precursor vitamin D to active vitamin D and therefore produce symptoms of vitamin D deficiency.

Vitamin D's Actions Vitamin D acts very much like a hormone—a compound manufactured by one organ of the body that has effects on another. The best-known vitamin D target organs are the intestine, the kidneys, and the bones, but recently, scientists have discovered many other vitamin D target tissues, including the brain, the pancreas, the skin, the reproductive organs, and some cancer cells.[10] The abundance of these discoveries suggests that numerous additional functions for vitamin D may surface, including the regulation of the immune system.[11]

Vitamin D's Roles in Bone Vitamin D is a member of a large, cooperative bone-making and maintenance team composed of nutrients and other compounds, including vitamin C; the hormones parathormone and calcitonin; the protein collagen; and the minerals calcium, phosphorus, magnesium, and fluoride. The special function of vitamin D in bone making is to promote normal bone mineralization. Its actions help to make calcium and phosphorus available in the blood that bathes the bones; from there, they are deposited as the bones harden.

Vitamin D acts in three ways to maintain blood concentrations of calcium and phosphorus: it stimulates their absorption from the GI tract; it mobilizes calcium and phosphorus from bones into the blood; and it stimulates their retention by the kidneys.

Vitamin D Deficiency The symptoms of vitamin D deficiency are those of calcium deficiency, shown in Table 7–2. The bones fail to calcify normally and may grow so weak that they become bent when they have to support the body's weight. A child with rickets who is old enough to walk characteristically develops bowed legs, often the most obvious sign of the disease. Worldwide, rickets afflicts a large number of children.

rickets: the vitamin D–deficiency disease in children.

Adult rickets, or osteomalacia, occurs most often in women who have low calcium intakes and little exposure to sun and who go through repeated pregnancies and periods of lactation. The bones of the legs may soften to such an extent that a young woman who is tall and straight at 20 may be condemned by repeated pregnancies to become bent, bowlegged, and stooped before she is 30.

osteomalacia (os-tee-o-mal-AY-shuh)**:** a bone disease characterized by softening of the bones; symptoms include bending of the spine and bowing of the legs. The disease occurs most often in adult women.
osteo = bone
mal = bad (soft)

Vitamin D Toxicity Whereas vitamin D deficiency depresses calcium absorption, blood calcium, and bone mineralization, an excess of vitamin D does the opposite, as shown in Table 7–2. It enhances calcium absorption, produces high blood calcium, and promotes return of bone calcium into the blood. The excess calcium then tends to precipitate in the soft tissues, forming stones, including kidney stones. Calcification may also harden the blood vessels and is especially dangerous in the major arteries of the heart and lungs, where it can cause death.

Vitamin D in excess is the most toxic of all the vitamins. Half the recommended intake is too little, but over a few times the recommended intake may be too much. The amounts of vitamin D found in foods available in the United States and Canada are well within safe limits, but pills containing the vitamin in concentrated form are not. Adults should use caution when taking vitamin D supplements and keep them out of the reach of children.

Vitamin D from the Sun Most of the world's population relies on natural exposure to sunlight to maintain adequate vitamin D nutrition.[12] The sun imposes no risk of toxicity. Prolonged exposure to sunlight degrades the vitamin D precursor in the skin, preventing its conversion to the active vitamin. Even lifeguards on southern beaches are safe from vitamin D toxicity from the sun.

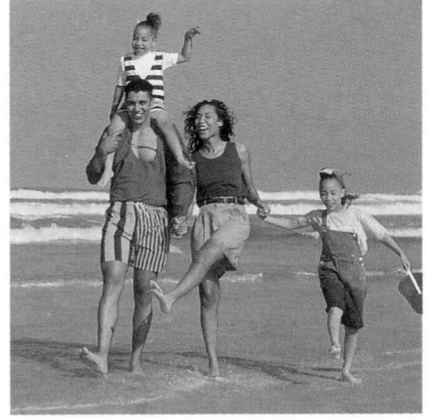

Sunlight promotes vitamin D synthesis in the skin. Exposure to the sun should be moderate, however; excessive exposure may cause skin cancer.

Effects of Sunscreens Prolonged exposure to sunlight has other undesirable consequences such as premature wrinkling of the skin and the increased risk of skin cancer. These risks may be reduced by using sunscreens. Unfortunately, sunscreens with sun protection factors (SPF) of 8 and above also retard vitamin D synthesis.[13] A strategy to avoid this dilemma is to apply sunscreen after enough time has elapsed to provide sufficient vitamin D. For most people, exposing hands, face, and arms on a clear summer day for 10 minutes, a few times a week, should be sufficient to maintain vitamin D nutrition.[14] Dark-skinned people require longer exposure than light-skinned people, but by three hours, vitamin D synthesis in heavily pigmented skin arrives at the same plateau as in fair skin in 30 minutes.

Tanning Lamp Effects The ultraviolet rays from tanning lamps and tanning booths may also stimulate vitamin D synthesis, but the hazards outweigh any possible benefits. The Food and Drug Administration (FDA) warns that if the lamps are not properly filtered, people using tanning booths risk burns, damage to blood vessels, skin cancer, and damage to the eyes.[15]

Smog filters out ultraviolet rays of the sun.

Smog Effects The ultraviolet rays of the sun that promote vitamin D synthesis may be filtered out by heavy clouds, smoke, or smog. Together with skin pigmentation, smog probably accounts for the fact that dark-skinned people in northern, smoggy cities are prone to rickets. For these people, and for those who are unable to go outdoors frequently, dietary vitamin D is important.

Vitamin D activity was previously expressed in international units (IU), but as of 1980, it is expressed in micrograms of cholecalciferol, the active form of vitamin D. To convert, use the following factor:
100 IU = 2.5 μg
400 IU = 10 μg

Vitamin D for Children Rapidly growing children require daily intakes of close to 10 micrograms of vitamin D; mature adults need half as much. Only a few animal foods, notably eggs, liver, and some fish, supply significant amounts of the vitamin. Even in these foods, the vitamin D content varies greatly, depending on the animal's exposure to sun and on its consumption of the vitamin in its foods. Neither cow's milk nor human breast milk supplies enough vitamin D to meet human needs reliably; hence cow's milk is fortified. Infant formulas are fortified with vitamin D in amounts adequate for daily intake. Breast milk is notoriously low in vitamin D, so vitamin D supplements are routinely prescribed for breastfed infants in the United States and Canada. These sources, plus any exposure to the sun, provide babies with more than enough of this vitamin. Well-meaning parents who give their infants extra vitamin drops are risking vitamin D—toxicity symptoms including increased calcium withdrawal from the bones, an effect just the opposite of the desired outcome of strong bones.

Importance of Milk The fortification of milk with vitamin D is the best guarantee that children will meet their vitamin D needs and underscores the importance of milk in children's diets. Strict vegetarians, and especially their children, may have low vitamin D intakes because no fortified plant source except margarine exists. In the United States, breakfast cereals may be fortified with vitamin D, as their labels indicate.[16]

Vitamin D for Adults Most adults, especially in sunny regions, need not make special efforts to obtain vitamin D in food. People who are not outdoors much or who live in northern or predominantly cloudy or smoggy areas, however, are advised to make sure their milk is fortified with vitamin D, to drink at least two cups a day, and to make frequent use of eggs and periodic use of liver in menu planning.

Vitamin E

Like beta-carotene, vitamin E is a fat-soluble antioxidant; it protects other substances from oxidation by being oxidized itself. It is one of the body's primary defenders against oxidation.

Reminder: *Oxidation* is a type of chemical reaction, so named because oxygen is one of the agents that often brings it about.

Cell Membrane Antioxidant If there is plenty of vitamin E in the membranes of cells exposed to an oxidant, chances are this vitamin will take the brunt of any oxidative attack, protecting the lipids and other vulnerable components of the membranes.[17] Vitamin E is especially effective in preventing the oxidation of the polyunsaturated fatty acids (PUFA), but it protects all other lipids (for example, vitamin A) as well. Table 7–2 summarizes important information about vitamin E.

Lung Antioxidant Vitamin E exerts an especially important antioxidant effect in the lungs, where the cells are exposed to high concentrations of oxygen. Vitamin E also protects the lungs from air pollutants that are strong oxidants.

Immune System Protector The role of vitamin E in protecting red blood cell membranes has led researchers to ask whether the vitamin might protect white blood cells as well and perhaps participate in the body's immune defenses. Indeed, vitamin E supplements significantly enhance the immune response of the elderly.[18]

Possible Role in Heart Disease Prevention More research is needed to determine whether vitamin E in amounts greater than the RDA can offer protection against heart disease. Two large population studies lend support to this idea. Researchers found that large doses of vitamin E supplements were associated with a significant reduction in the risk of heart disease.[19]

erythrocyte (en-REETH-ro-cite) **hemolysis** (he-MOLL-uh-sis)**:** rupture of the red blood cells, caused by vitamin E deficiency.
erythro = red
cyte = cell
hemo = blood
lysis = breaking

Vitamin E Deficiency When vitamin E intake is deficient and the blood concentration falls below a certain critical level, the red blood cells tend to break open and spill their contents, probably because the PUFA in their membranes oxidize. This classic vitamin E–deficiency symptom, known as erythrocyte hemolysis, is seen in premature infants, born before the transfer of vitamin E from the mother to the infant that takes place in the last weeks of pregnancy.

Two other conditions appear to respond to vitamin E therapy. One is a nonmalignant breast disease, and the other is an abnormality of blood flow that causes cramping in the legs.

Both diseases have unwieldy names. One is **fibrocystic breast disease,** the other is **intermittent claudication.**
fibr = fibrous lumps
cystic = in sacs
intermittent = at intervals
claudicare = to limp

Caution: Other serious conditions can cause lumps in the breast and pain in the legs. Don't self-diagnose; see a physician.

Causes of Vitamin E Deficiency In human beings, vitamin E deficiency is usually associated with diseases, notably those that cause malabsorption of fat. These include diseases of the liver, gallbladder, and pancreas, as well as various hereditary diseases involving digestion and use of nutrients.

It may be, however, that rare vitamin E deficiencies are seen in people without diseases. They are most likely in people who for years eat diets extremely low in fat; or use fat substitutes, such as diet margarines and salad dressings, as their only sources of fat; or consume diets composed of highly processed or "convenience" foods. Vitamin E is destroyed by extensive heating in the processing of foods.

Vitamin E Myths While research continues to reveal possible roles for vitamin E, it has also clearly discredited claims that vitamin E improves athletic skill, enhances sexual performance, or cures sexual dysfunction in males. Vitamin E also does not prevent or cure hereditary muscular dystrophy, nor does it slow or prevent processes of aging, such as graying of the hair, wrinkling of the skin, or reduced activity of body organs.

muscular dystrophy (DIS-tro-fee): a hereditary disease in which the muscles gradually weaken; its most debilitating effects arise in the lungs. This disease should not be confused with *nutritional* muscular dystrophy, a vitamin E–deficiency disease of animals characterized by gradual paralysis of the muscles.

Vitamin E Toxicity Even though many vitamin E claims have been discredited, people continue to take vitamin E supplements for a variety of reasons. As a result, signs of toxicity are now known or suspected, although vitamin E toxicity is not nearly as common, and its effects are not as serious, as vitamin A or vitamin D toxicity. According to the American Medical Association's Council on Scientific Affairs, the most significant toxic effects of high doses of vitamin E are interference with the blood-clotting action of vitamin K and enhancement of the action of anticoagulant drugs, leading to hemorrhage.[20] For most individuals, however, daily doses below 300 milligrams seem to be harmless.[21]

On vitamin bottles, vitamin E activity is often expressed in IU. One IU is the same as 1 mg of the active form of vitamin E.

The RDA gives values for vitamin E in units known as alpha TE (alpha-tocopherol equivalents). One of these units, 1 alpha TE, equals 1 mg of active vitamin E.

Vitamin E in Foods Vitamin E is widespread in foods. About 20 percent of the vitamin E in the diet comes directly or indirectly from vegetable oils and the products made from them, such as margarine, salad dressings, and shortenings (see Snapshot 7–2). Another 20 percent comes from fruits and vegetables. Fortified cereals and other grain products contribute about 15 percent of the vitamin E in the diet, and smaller percentages come from meats, poultry, fish, eggs, nuts, and seeds.[22] Soybean oil and wheat germ oil have especially high concentrations of vitamin E. Animal fats, such as butter and milk fat, contain little or no vitamin E. Because vitamin E is readily destroyed by heat processing and oxidation, fresh or lightly processed foods are the most desirable sources of this vitamin.

Vitamin K

K stands for the Danish word *koagulation* (coagulation or "clotting").

Vitamin K has long been known for its role in blood clotting, where its presence can make the difference between life and death. The vitamin is now known to act with vitamin D in synthesizing a bone protein.[23]

Blood Clotting At least 13 different proteins and the mineral calcium are involved in making a blood clot. Vitamin K is essential for the synthesis of at least four of these proteins, among them prothrombin, the

Snapshot 7–2 Vlitamin E

RDA for men: 10 mg α-TE/day
RDA for women: 8 mg α-TE/day

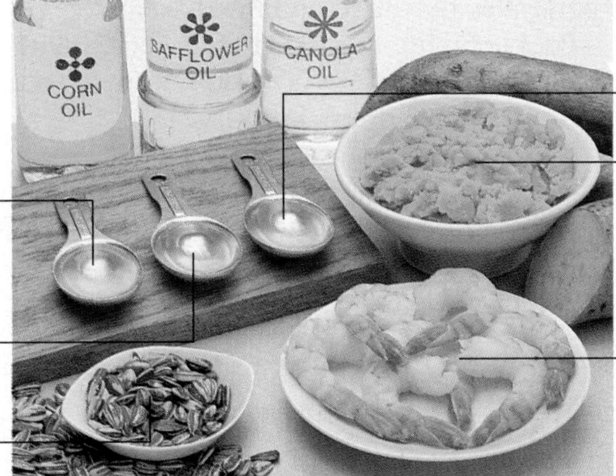

Corn oil: 2.9 mg per tablespoon

Safflower oil: 4.7 mg per tablespoon

Sunflower seeds (shelled): 9 mg per 2 tbs

Canola oil: 2.9 mg per tablespoon

Sweet potato: 4.5 mg per ½ c mashed

Shrimp: 3.2 mg per 3 oz boiled

precursor of the protein thrombin. When any of the blood-clotting factors is lacking, hemorrhagic disease results. If an artery or vein is cut or broken, bleeding goes unchecked. Of course, this is not to say that the cause of hemorrhaging is always a vitamin K deficiency.

hemorrhagic (hem-o-RAJ-ik) **disease:** the vitamin K–deficiency disease in which blood fails to clot.

Reminder: The bacterial inhabitants of the digestive tract are known as the *intestinal flora.*
flora = plant inhabitants

Intestinal Synthesis Like vitamin D, vitamin K can also be obtained from a nonfood source. Bacteria in the intestinal tract synthesize vitamin K that the body can absorb, although people cannot depend on bacterial synthesis alone for their vitamin K.

Vitamin K Deficiency Vitamin K deficiency is seldom seen except when unusual combinations of circumstances conspire to bring it about. When it does occur, however, it can be fatal. The scenario goes like this: a hospital client with marginal vitamin K stores is given antibiotics to prevent or overcome infection and is fed a formula diet that does not include vitamin K. The antibiotics kill the intestinal bacteria, and the vitamin K stores are depleted. During surgery, the blood fails to clot normally, and the client bleeds to death. The combination of antibiotics, inadequate vitamin K intake, and surgery raises a warning flag and requires that clotting time be checked before surgery is performed.[24] People taking sulfa drugs, which destroy intestinal bacteria, may also become deficient in vitamin K.

Vitamin K for Newborns Newborn babies present a unique case of vitamin K nutrition. A baby is born with a sterile digestive tract, and some weeks pass before the vitamin K–producing bacteria become fully established in the baby's intestines. At the same time, plasma prothrombin concentrations are low (this helps prevent blood clotting during the stress of birth, which might otherwise be fatal). A modest dose of vitamin K, usu-

sterile: free of microorganisms, such as bacteria.

The synthetic substitute usually given for vitamin K is **menadione** (men-uh-DYE-own).

ally in a water-soluble form, may therefore be given at birth to prevent hemorrhagic disease in the newborn.

jaundice: yellowing of the skin due to spillover of bile pigments from the liver into the general circulation.

Vitamin K Toxicity A high intake of vitamin K can reduce the effectiveness of anticoagulant drugs used to prevent the blood from clotting. People taking these drugs should eat vitamin K–rich foods in moderation. Vitamin K–toxicity symptoms include red cell hemolysis, jaundice, and brain damage (see Table 7–2).

Vitamin K in Foods Many foods contain ample amounts of vitamin K, notably green leafy vegetables, members of the cabbage family, and liver. Milk, meats, eggs, cereal, fruits, and vegetables provide smaller, but still significant, amounts.

The Water-Soluble Vitamins

The B vitamins and vitamin C are the water-soluble vitamins. These vitamins are found in the watery compartments of foods, and they are distributed into water-filled compartments of the body. They are easily absorbed into the bloodstream and are just as easily excreted if their blood concentration rises too high. Thus the water-soluble vitamins are less likely to reach toxic concentrations in the body than the fat-soluble vitamins. Foods never deliver toxic doses of the water-soluble vitamins, but the large doses concentrated in vitamin supplements can reach toxic levels.

The B Vitamins

Despite advertisements that claim otherwise, the B vitamins do not give you energy. Carbohydrate, fat, and protein—the *energy-yielding* nutrients—are used for fuel. The B vitamins help to burn that fuel, but do not serve as fuel themselves.

coenzyme (co-EN-zime)**:** a small molecule that works with an enzyme to promote the enzyme's activity. Many coenzymes have B vitamins as part of their structure.
co = with

Coenzymes The eight B vitamins are listed in Table 7–3 on page 153. Each is part of an enzyme helper known as a coenzyme. Each B vitamin has other important functions in the body as well, but the roles these vitamins play as parts of coenzymes are the best understood. A coenzyme is a small molecule that combines with an enzyme to make it active. With the coenzyme in place, the substance to be worked on is attracted to the enzyme, and the reaction proceeds instantaneously. Figure 7–2 on page 153 illustrates coenzyme action.

Thiamin, riboflavin, niacin, pantothenic acid, and biotin are each a part of distinct coenzymes necessary for the production of energy from glucose, amino acids, and fats. A coenzyme containing vitamin B_6 assists enzymes that metabolize amino acids. The making of new cells depends on a folate coenzyme, and the making of this coenzyme depends on vitamin B_{12}. Folate and vitamin B_{12} together are, among other things, involved in duplicating genetic material when cells divide. A coenzyme already mentioned in the last chapter was coenzyme A, or CoA, made from the vitamin pantothenic acid.

Table 7–2
The Fat-Soluble Vitamins—A Summary

VITAMIN A

Other Names
Retinol, retinal, retinoic acid; main precursor is beta-carotene

Chief Functions in the Body
Vision: health of cornea, epithelial cells, mucous membranes; skin health; bone and tooth growth; reproduction; hormone synthesis and regulation; immunity; cancer protection

Deficiency Disease Name
Hypovitaminosis A

Significant Sources
Retinol: fortified milk, cheese, cream, butter, fortified margarine, eggs, liver
Beta-carotene: spinach and other dark leafy greens; broccoli; deep orange fruits (apricots, cantaloupe) and vegetables (squash, carrots, sweet potatoes, pumpkin)

	Deficiency Symptoms	Toxicity Symptoms
Blood/Circulatory System	Anemia (small-cell type)[a]	Red blood cell breakage, nosebleeds
Bones/Teeth	Cessation of bone growth, painful joints; impaired enamel formation, cracks in teeth, tendency to decay	Bone pain; growth retardation; increase of pressure inside skull mimicking brain tumor; headaches
Digestive System	Diarrhea, changes in lining	Abdominal cramps and pain, nausea, vomiting, diarrhea, weight loss
Immune System	Depression; frequent respiratory, digestive, bladder, vaginal, and other infections	Overreactivity
Nervous/Muscular Systems	Night blindness (retinal)	Blurred vision, pain in calves, fatigue, irritability, loss of appetite
Skin and Cornea	Keratinization, corneal degeneration leading to blindness,[b] rashes	Dry skin, rashes, loss of hair
Other	Kidney stones, impaired growth	Cessation of menstruation, liver and spleen enlargement

VITAMIN D

Other Names
Calciferol, cholecalciferol, dihydroxy vitamin D; precursor is cholesterol

Chief Functions in the Body
Mineralization of bones (raises blood calcium and phosphorus via absorption from digestive tract, and by withdrawing calcium from bones and stimulating retention by kidneys)

Deficiency Disease Name
Rickets, osteomalacia

Significant Sources
Self-synthesis with sunlight; fortified milk or margarine, eggs, liver, small fish (sardines)

	Deficiency Symptoms	Toxicity Symptoms
Blood/Circulatory System		Raised blood calcium
Bones/Teeth	Abnormal growth, misshapen bones (bowing of legs), soft bones, joint pain, malformed teeth	Increased calcium withdrawal
Nervous System	Muscle spasms	Excessive thirst, headaches, irritability, loss of appetite, weakness, nausea
Other		Kidney stones, stones in arteries, mental and physical retardation

[a]Small-cell anemia is termed *microcytic anemia;* large-cell type is *macrocytic* or *megaloblastic anemia.*
[b]Corneal degeneration progresses from *keratinization* (hardening) to *xerosis* (drying) to *xerophthalomia* (thickening, opacity, and irreversible blindness).

(continued)

Table 7–2 *(continued)*

VITAMIN E		
Other Names Alpha-tocopherol, tocopherol **Chief Functions in the Body** Antioxidant (detoxicification of strong oxidants), stabilization of cell membranes, regulation of oxidation reactions, protection of PUFA and vitamin A **Deficiency Disease Name** (No name) **Significant Sources** Polyunsaturated plant oils (margarine, salad dressings, shortenings), green and leafy vegetables, wheat germ, whole-grain products, nuts, seeds	**Deficiency Symptoms**	**Toxicity Symptoms**
	Blood/Circulatory System	
	Red blood cell damage, anemia	Augments the effects of anticlotting medication
	Digestive System	
		General discomfort
	Nervous/Muscular System	
	Degeneration, weakness, difficulty walking, leg cramps	(No symptoms reported)
	Other	
	Fibrocystic breast disease	(No symptoms reported)

VITAMIN K		
Other Names Phylloquinone, naphthoquinone **Chief Functions in the Body** Synthesis of blood-clotting proteins and a blood protein that regulates blood calcium **Deficiency Disease Name** (No name) **Significant Sources** Bacterial synthesis in the digestive tract; liver, green leafy vegetables, cabbage-type vegetables, milk	**Deficiency Symptoms**	**Toxicity Symptoms**
	Blood/Circulatory System	
	Hemorrhaging	Interference with anticlotting medication; vitamin K analogues may cause jaundice

These eight B vitamins play many specific roles in helping the enzymes to perform thousands of different molecular conversions in your body. They must be present in every cell continuously for the cells to function as they should. As for vitamin C, its primary role, discussed later, is as an antioxidant.

B Vitamin Deficiencies In academic and clinical discussions of the vitamins, different sets of deficiency symptoms are ascribed to each individual vitamin. Such clear-cut symptoms are found only in laboratory animals that have been fed contrived diets that lack just one nutrient. In reality, a deficiency of any single B vitamin seldom shows up in isolation because people do not eat nutrients one by one; they eat foods containing mixtures of nutrients. If a major class of foods is missing from the diet, all of the nutrients delivered by those foods will be lacking to various extents.

Table 7–3
The Water-Soluble Vitamins

Many of the vitamins have both names and numbers, a mixture of terminologies that confuses newcomers to the study of nutrition. A single set of names for the vitamins has been agreed on and published, and those names are used in this book.[a] Still, to read the many worthwhile writings published prior to this nomenclature policy, you have to be aware of the alternative names.

STANDARD VITAMIN NAME	OTHER NAMES COMMONLY USED
B vitamins	
Thiamin	Vitamin B_1
Riboflavin	Vitamin B_2
Niacin	Nicotinic acid, nicotinamide, niacinamide, vitamin B_3
Pantothenic acid	(None)
Biotin	(None)
Vitamin B_6	Pyridoxine, pyridoxal, pyridoxamine
Folate	Folacin, folic acid, pteroylglutamic acid
Vitamin B_{12}	Cobalamin
Vitamin C	Ascorbic acid

[a]The vitamin names used here are those agreed on, and published by, the International Union of Nutritional Sciences Committee on Nomenclature, in Nomenclature policy: Generic descriptors and trivial names for vitamins and related compounds, *Journal of Nutrition* 117 (1987): 7–15.

In only two cases have dietary deficiencies associated with single B vitamins been observed on a large scale in human populations. Diseases have been named for these deficiency states. One of them, beriberi, was first observed in Southeast Asia when the custom of polishing rice became widespread. Rice contributed 80 percent of the energy intake of the people in these areas, and rice hulls were their principal source of thi-

beriberi: the thiamin-deficiency disease; it pointed the way to the first discovery of a B vitamin, thiamin.

Figure 7–2
Coenzyme Action

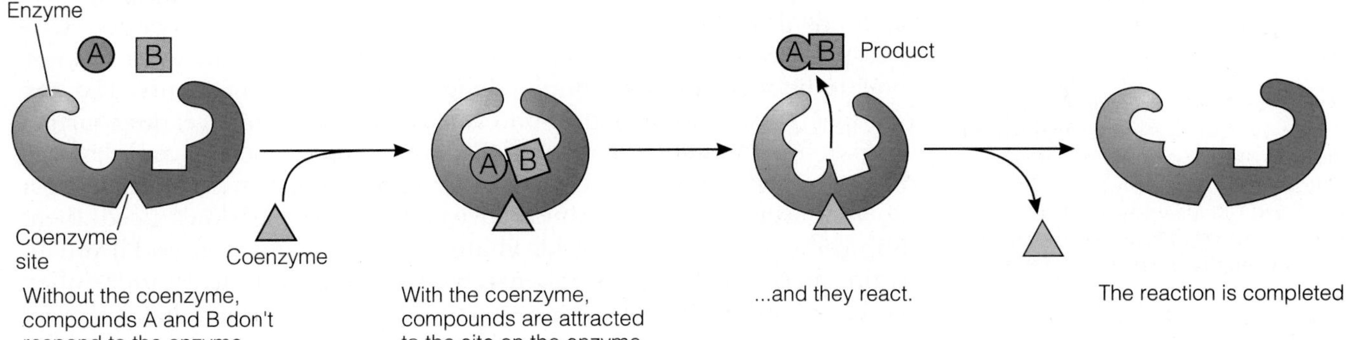
Enzyme
A
B
Coenzyme site
Coenzyme
Without the coenzyme, compounds A and B don't respond to the enzyme.
With the coenzyme, compounds are attracted to the site on the enzyme...
Product
...and they react.
The reaction is completed

amin. When the hulls were removed to make the rice whiter, beriberi spread like wildfire.

pellagra (pell-AY-gra)**:** the niacin-deficiency disease.
pellis = skin
agra = seizure

The niacin-deficiency disease, pellagra, became widespread in the southern United States in the early part of this century among people who subsisted on a low-protein diet with a staple grain of corn. This diet was unusual in that it supplied neither enough niacin nor enough of its amino acid precursor tryptophan to make the niacin intake adequate.

Even in the cases of beriberi and pellagra, the deficiencies were probably not pure. When foods were provided containing the one vitamin known to be needed, other vitamins that may have been in short supply came as part of the package.

Interdependent Systems Table 7–4, at the end of this chapter, sums up a few of the better-established facts about B vitamin deficiencies. A look at the table will make another generalization possible. Different body systems depend to different extents on these vitamins. Processes in nerves and in their responding tissues, the muscles, depend heavily on glucose metabolism and hence on thiamin, so paralysis sets in when this vitamin is lacking, but thiamin is important in all cells, not just in nerves and muscles. Similarly, because the red blood cells and GI tract cells divide the most rapidly, two of the first symptoms of a deficiency of folate are a type of anemia and GI deterioration—but again, all systems depend on folate, not just these. The list of symptoms in Table 7–4 is far from complete.

Subtle Deficiencies Major deficiency diseases such as pellagra and beriberi no longer occur in the United States and Canada, but more subtle deficiencies of nutrients, including the B vitamins, sometimes are observed. When they do occur, it is usually in people whose food choices are poor because of poverty, ignorance, illness, or poor health habits such as alcohol abuse. If the staple grain food is made from refined grain, vitamin B deficiencies are especially likely.

refined grain: a product from which the bran, germ, and husk have been removed, leaving only the endosperm.

fortification: the addition of nutrients to a food to correct or prevent a widespread nutrient deficiency, to balance the total nutrient profile of a food, or to restore nutrients lost in processing. Often, the added nutrients were not originally present and have been added in amounts greater than might be found there naturally.

enrichment: now considered synonymous with fortification; previously, the addition of four specific nutrients—iron, thiamin, riboflavin, and niacin—to refined breads and cereals in amounts approximately equivalent to those originally present in the whole grain.

B Vitamin Enrichment of Foods One way to protect people from deficiencies is to add nutrients to their staple food, a process known as fortification or enrichment. The enrichment of refined breads and cereals has drastically reduced the incidence of iron and B vitamin deficiencies.

The preceding discussion has shown both the great importance of the B vitamins in promoting normal, healthy functioning of all body systems and the severe consequences of deficiency. Now you may want to know how to be sure you are getting enough of these vital nutrients. The next sections present information on each B vitamin. While reading further, keep in mind that *foods* can provide all the needed nutrients and that supplements are a poor second choice. Some supplements are absurdly costly; but even if they are inexpensive, most people don't need them. Supplementing with fat-soluble vitamins can be dangerous, and if you are eating an adequate diet, supplementing with water-soluble vitamins offers no benefit other than to increase the dollar value of your urine. Nutrition in Practice 7 discusses uses and choices of supplements in more detail.

Thiamin

All cells use thiamin, which plays a critical role in their energy metabolism. Thiamin also occupies a special site on nerve cell membranes. Consequently, processes in nerves and in their responding tissues, the muscles, depend heavily on thiamin.

Thiamin Need Provided that you are consuming enough food energy to meet your needs—and obtaining that energy from thiamin-containing foods—your thiamin intake will adjust to your need. However, people who derive a large proportion of their energy from empty-kcalorie items, like sugar or alcohol, risk thiamin deficiency, a condition that seems to be reappearing as the population of malnourished and homeless people rises.[25] A person who is fasting or who has adopted a very-low-kcalorie diet needs as much thiamin as when eating enough to meet energy needs.

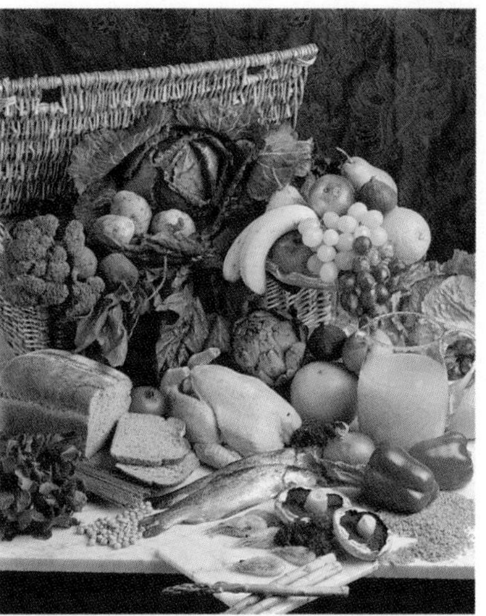

Thiamin: most nutritious foods contribute about 10 percent of daily needs per serving.

Thiamin in Foods Thiamin occurs in small quantities in virtually all nutritious foods, but it is concentrated in only a few foods, of which pork and ham are the most commonly eaten. A useful guideline for meeting thiamin needs is to keep empty-kcalorie foods to a minimum in your diet and to include ten or more different servings of nutritious foods each day, assuming that each serving will contribute, on the average, about 10 percent of your needs. Foods chosen from the bread and cereal group should be either whole grain or enriched. Thiamin is not stored in the body to any great extent, so daily intake is important.

Riboflavin: milk contributes about 50%; meat, about 25%; whole-grain or enriched breads and cereals, additional amounts. The person who does not drink milk should substitute large amounts of dark green vegetables.

Riboflavin

Like thiamin, riboflavin facilitates energy production in the body. Riboflavin recommendations are stated in terms of milligrams per 1000 kcalories. Differences in the riboflavin RDA for different age-sex groups primarily reflect differences in energy intakes. Infants', children's, and pregnant women's needs rise rapidly during periods of active growth.

Riboflavin in Foods Unlike thiamin, riboflavin is not evenly distributed among the food groups. The major contributors of riboflavin to people's diets are milk, milk products, meats, and green vegetables (broccoli, turnip greens, asparagus, and spinach). The riboflavin richness of milk and milk products is a good reason to include these foods in every day's meals. No other commonly eaten food can make such a substantial contribution. People who omit milk and milk products from their diets can substitute generous servings of dark green, leafy vegetables. Among the meats, liver and heart are the richest sources, but all lean meats, as well as eggs, offer some riboflavin.

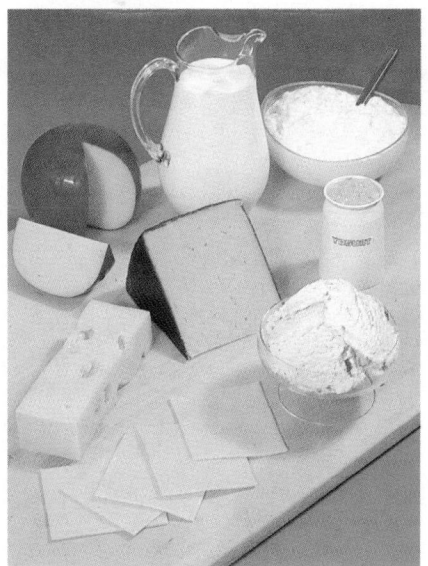

Milk and milk products supply much of the riboflavin in people's diets.

Effects of Light Riboflavin is light sensitive; it can be destroyed by the ultraviolet rays of the sun or of fluorescent lamps. For this reason, milk is seldom sold in transparent glass or translucent plastic containers. Cardboard or opaque plastic containers protect the riboflavin in the milk from light. In contrast, riboflavin is heat stable, so ordinary cooking does not destroy it.

Niacin

Like thiamin and riboflavin, niacin participates in the energy metabolism of every body cell. Niacin is unique among the B vitamins in that the body can make it from protein. The amino acid tryptophan can be converted to niacin in the body: 60 milligrams of tryptophan yield 1 milligram of niacin. Recommended niacin intakes are therefore stated in "equivalents," reflecting the body's ability to convert tryptophan to niacin.

niacin equivalents: the amount of niacin present in food, including the niacin that can theoretically be made from its precursor tryptophan present in the food.

A food containing 1 mg of niacin and 60 mg tryptophan contains the niacin equivalent to 2 mg, or 2 mg NE.

Niacin Used as a Drug Certain forms of niacin supplements in amounts ten times or more the RDA cause "niacin flush," a dilation of the capillaries of the skin with perceptible tingling that, if intense, can be painful. Physicians sometimes use diet and large doses of niacin, along with a drug to lower blood cholesterol, to treat atherosclerosis. When used this way, niacin leaves the realm of nutrition to become a pharmacological agent, a drug. As with any drug, self-dosing with niacin is ill-advised; large doses may injure the liver, cause ulcers, and produce some symptoms of diabetes.[26]

Niacin in Foods Meat, poultry, and fish contribute about half the niacin equivalents most people consume; enriched breads and cereals contribute about a fourth. Among the vegetables, mushrooms, asparagus, and green leafy vegetables are the richest niacin sources. Niacin is less vulnerable to losses during food preparation and storage than other water-soluble vitamins. Being fairly heat-resistant, niacin can withstand reasonable cooking times, but like other water-soluble vitamins, it will leach into cooking water.

Pantothenic Acid and Biotin

Two other B vitamins—pantothenic acid and biotin—are also important in energy metabolism. Pantothenic acid was first recognized as a substance that stimulates growth. It is a component of a key enzyme that makes possible the release of energy from the energy nutrients. Pantothenic acid is involved in more than 100 different steps in the synthesis of lipids, neurotransmitters, steroid hormones, and hemoglobin.[27] Biotin plays an important role in metabolism as a coenzyme that serves as a carrier of carbon dioxide. This role is critical in the TCA cycle.

Pantothenic Acid and Biotin in Foods Both pantothenic acid and biotin are more widespread in foods than the other vitamins discussed so far. There seems to be no danger that people who consume a variety of foods will suffer deficiencies. Claims that pantothenic acid and biotin are needed in pill form to prevent or cure disease conditions are at best unfounded and at worst intentionally misleading.

Biotin Deficiency in the Hospital Biotin deficiencies have been reported in adults fed artificially by vein. Even then, however, deficiencies are unlikely because intestinal bacteria may be able to synthesize enough biotin to meet the host's needs. Biotin deficiency becomes likely only when a person is receiving both intravenous feedings and antibiotics.

Vitamin B_6

Vitamin B_6 has been called the "sleeping giant" of vitamins.[28] A surge of research interest in the last decade has revealed not only new knowledge but new questions about it. For example, unlike other water-soluble vitamins, vitamin B_6 is stored extensively in muscle tissue.[29] Tentative research findings suggest that this vitamin B_6 reservoir becomes available to the rest of the body under conditions of intensified energy use, such as physical activity.

Metabolic Roles of Vitamin B_6 Vitamin B_6 has long been known to play roles in protein and amino acid metabolism. In the cells, vitamin B_6 helps to convert one kind of amino acid, which the cells have in abundance, to another, which they need in larger amounts. It also aids in the conversion of tryptophan to niacin and plays important roles in the synthesis of hemoglobin. Vitamin B_6 also assists in releasing stored glucose from glycogen and thus contributes to the regulation of blood glucose. Research suggests new roles for vitamin B_6 in immune function, hormone response, and possibly in the origins and treatments of some diseases.[30] The association between vitamin B_6 and immune function is related to the critical role the vitamin plays in protein metabolism. Vitamin B_6 deficiency can significantly impair the immune response perhaps by way of impaired antibody production.[31]

Vitamin B_6 Deficiency Besides a weakening immune response, vitamin B_6 deficiency is expressed in general symptoms, such as weakness, irritability, and insomnia. Other symptons include a greasy, flaky dermatitis, anemia, and, in advanced cases, convulsions.

Vitamin B_6 Toxicity For years it was believed that vitamin B_6, like other water-soluble vitamins, could not reach toxic concentrations in the body. Toxic effects of vitamin B_6 became known when a physician reported them in seven different women who had been taking more than 2 grams of vitamin B_6 daily for two months or more. Most of these women had been attempting to cure symptoms of premenstrual syndrome (PMS), the cluster of physical, emotional, and psychological symptoms that some women experience prior to menstruation. The first symptom of toxicity was numb feet; then the women lost sensation in their hands; then they became unable to walk. Since then other researchers have reported neurological symptoms in more than 100 women who took supplements for as long as five years.[32] The women recovered after they discontinued the supplements.

When a normal dose of a nutrient clears up a deficiency condition, the effect is a physiological one. When a megadose (100 times larger) overwhelms some system and acts like a drug, the effect is a pharmacological one.

The specific cause or causes of PMS remain undefined, although researchers agree that the hormonal changes of the menstrual cycle must be responsible. Despite a lack of conclusive evidence that vitamin B_6 is an effective treatment for PMS, the vitamin and many other unproven remedies remain popular among PMS sufferers. Nutrition in Practice 16 offers a discussion of nutrition and PMS.

Vitamin B_6 and Protein Intake Vitamin B_6's many roles in amino acid metabolism are reflected in dietary needs that are roughly proportional to protein intakes. The RDA for vitamin B_6 is more than adequate to handle average protein intakes of 100 grams per day for men and 60 grams per day for women.[33]

Vitamin B_6 in Foods Data on the amounts of vitamin B_6 in foods are not extensive enough to permit the vitamin to be included in the table of food composition in Appendix A. Averaged amounts of vitamin B_6, derived from the available data, reveal that the richest food sources are liver, fish, poultry, potatoes, a few other vegetables, fruits, and whole-grain cereals.

Folate

The B vitamin folate is active in cell division. During periods of rapid growth and cell division, such as pregnancy and adolescence, folate needs increase, and deficiency is especially likely. When a deficiency occurs, the rapidly dividing cells of the blood and the GI tract stop dividing and begin to deteriorate. Not surprisingly, then, two of the first symptoms of a folate deficiency are a type of anemia and GI tract deterioration (see Table 7–4).

Folate, Alcohol, and Drugs As discussed in Nutrition in Practice 8, alcohol-addicted people are at risk of folate deficiency because alcohol impairs folate's absorption and increases its excretion.[34] Furthermore, as people's alcohol intakes rise, their folate intakes decline.[35] Many medications, including aspirin, oral contraceptives, and anticonvulsants, impair folate status. Smoking also exerts a negative effect on folate status. Folate deficiency during pregnancy has been linked to birth defects known as neural tube defects, an association discussed in Nutrition in Practice 7 and Chapter 15.

Folate in Foods The best food sources (see Snapshot 7–3) of folate are liver, legumes, green leafy vegetables (the name of the vitamin is related to the word *foliage*), and beets. Among the fruits, oranges, orange juice, and cantaloupe are the best sources.

Vitamin B_{12}

Vitamin B_{12} and folate share a special relationship: vitamin B_{12} assists folate in its role in cell division. Their roles intertwine, but each performs a specific task that the other cannot perform.

Vitamin B_{12}, Folate, and Cell Division Vitamin B_{12} (in coenzyme form) stands by to accept carbon groups from folate as folate removes them from other compounds. The passing of these carbon groups from folate to vitamin B_{12} regenerates the active form of folate so it can continue its dismantling tasks. In the absence of vitamin B_{12}, folate is trapped in its inactive, metabolically useless form, unable to do its job. When folate is either trapped due to vitamin B_{12} deficiency or unavailable due to a deficiency of folate itself, cells that are growing most rapidly, notably, the blood cells, are the first to be affected. Thus a deficiency of either

Snapshot 7–3 Folate

RDA for men: 200 μg/day
RDA for women: 180 μg/day

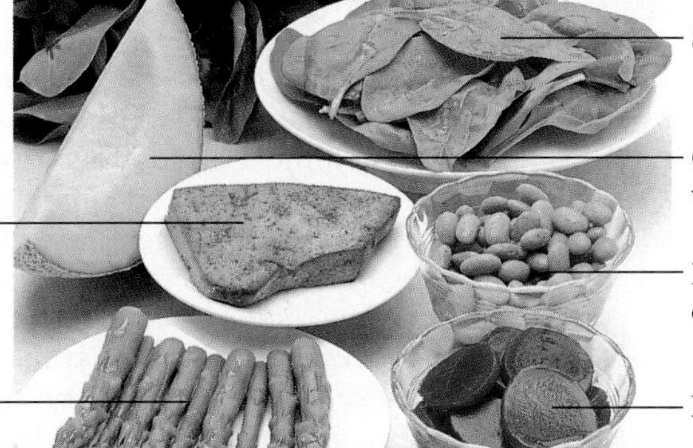
Spinach: 108 μg per 1 c raw
Cantaloupe: 15 μg per small wedge (⅙ melon)
Liver: 187 μg per 3 oz fried
Pinto beans: 147 μg per ½ c cooked
Asparagus: 131 μg per ½ c cooked
Beets: 45 μg per ½ c cooked

nutrient—vitamin B_{12} or folate—impairs maturation of the blood cells and produces anemia. The anemia is identifiable by microscopic examination of the blood, which reveals many large, immature red blood cells. Either vitamin B_{12} or folate will clear up the anemia.

Vitamin B_{12} and the Nervous System Although either vitamin will clear up the anemia caused by vitamin B_{12} deficiency, if folate is given when vitamin B_{12} is needed, the result is disastrous, not to the blood but to the nervous system. The reason: vitamin B_{12} also helps maintain nerve fibers. Devastating neurological symptoms, undetectable by a blood test, can ultimately result from an undetected vitamin B_{12} deficiency. A deceptive folate "cure" of the blood symptoms in vitamin B_{12} deficiency allows the nerve symptoms to progress, leading to paralysis and permanent nerve damage.

The way folate masks vitamin B_{12} deficiency underlines a point already made several times: it takes a skilled diagnostician to make a correct diagnosis. The risk you take when you diagnose yourself on the basis of a single observed symptom is clearly intolerable.

Vitamin B_{12} Absorption Vitamin B_{12} is unique in that it requires an "intrinsic factor"—a compound made inside the body—for absorption from the intestinal tract into the bloodstream. The intrinsic factor is made in the stomach, where it attaches to the vitamin; the complex then passes to the small intestine and is gradually absorbed.

intrinsic: inside the system. The **intrinsic factor** necessary to prevent pernicious anemia is now known to be made in the stomach and to aid in the absorption of vitamin B_{12}. The extrinsic factor necessary to prevent pernicious anemia is vitamin B_{12} itself, which must be obtained outside the system from food.

Loss of Intrinsic Factor In some cases, intrinsic factor production becomes inadequate or ceases altogether—for example, after surgical removal of the stomach. Because vitamin B_{12} deficiency in the body may be caused either by a lack of the vitamin in the diet or by the body's inability to absorb the vitamin, a change in diet alone may not correct it. When an absorption failure is the problem, vitamin B_{12} must be supplied by injection to prevent vitamin B_{12}–deficiency symptoms from developing. The vitamin B_{12} deficiency caused by lack of intrinsic factor is known as pernicious anemia.

Vitamin B_{12} is found exclusively in animal-derived foods.

Vitamin B_{12} in Foods Another unique characteristic of vitamin B_{12} is that it is found almost exclusively in animal-derived foods. People who eat meat are guaranteed an adequate intake, and lacto-ovo vegetarians (who use milk, cheese, and eggs) are also protected from deficiency. It is a myth, however, that fermented soy products, such as miso (a soybean paste), or sea algae, such as spirulina, provide vitamin B_{12} in its active form. Extensive research shows that the amounts of vitamin B_{12} listed on the labels of these plant products are inaccurate and misleading because the vitamin B_{12} in these products occurs in an inactive, unavailable form.[36] Strict vegetarians must take vitamin B_{12} supplements or find other sources of active vitamin B_{12}.

Vitamin B_{12} Deficiency in Vegans Strict vegetarians are at special risk for undetected vitamin B_{12} deficiency for two reasons: first, they receive none in their diets, and second, they consume large amounts of folate in the vegetables they eat. Because the body can store 1000 times the amount of vitamin B_{12} used each day, a deficiency may take years to develop in a new vegetarian. When a deficiency does develop, though, it may progress to a dangerous extreme because the deficiency of vitamin B_{12} may be masked by the high folate intake.

Non-B Vitamins

Other compounds are sometimes inappropriately called B vitamins because like the true B vitamins, they serve as coenzymes in metabolism. Even if they were essential, however, supplements would be unnecessary because these compounds are abundant in foods.

Inositol, Choline, and Lipoic Acid Among the non-B vitamins are a trio of coenzymes known as inositol, choline, and lipoic acid. Researchers are exploring the possibility that these substances may be essential and one day might be considered for an RDA.

Hazards of Supplements Numerous false claims have been made about choline and its relative, lecithin (which contains choline as part of its structure). Consequently, many people rush to buy and consume bottles of them. Physicians have witnessed and reported on the effects of overdoses of these compounds. Overdoses can cause not only short-term discomforts, such as GI distress, sweating, salivation, and anorexia, but also long-term health hazards from the disturbance of the nervous and cardiovascular systems.

Other Non-B Vitamins Other substances have also been mistaken for essential nutrients. They include para-aminobenzoic acid (PABA), bioflavonoids (vitamin P or hesperidin), and ubiquinone. Other names you may hear are "vitamin B_5" (another name for pantothenic acid), "vitamin B_{15}" (a hoax), "vitamin B_{17}" (laetrile, a fake cancer-curing drug and not a vitamin by any stretch of the imagination), "vitamin B_T" (carnitine, an important piece of cell machinery but not a vitamin), and more. There is, however, one other water-soluble vitamin of great interest and importance—vitamin C.

Vitamin C

Two hundred years ago, any man who joined the crew of a seagoing ship knew he had only half a chance of returning alive—not because he might be slain by pirates or die in a storm, but because he might contract the dread disease scurvy. Then a British physician found that citrus fruits could cure the disease, and thereafter, all ships were required to carry lime juice for every sailor. (This is why British sailors are still called "limeys" today.) Nearly 200 years later, the antiscurvy factor in citrus fruits was isolated from lemon juice and named ascorbic acid. Today, hundreds of millions of vitamin C pills are produced in pharmaceutical laboratories.

scurvy: the vitamin C–deficiency disease.

ascorbic acid: one of the two active forms of vitamin C. Many people consistently and incorrectly refer to all vitamin C by this name.
a = without
scorbic = having scurvy

Metabolic Roles of Vitamin C Vitamin C's action defies a simple, tidy description. It plays many important roles in the body, and its modes of action differ in different situations (see Table 7–4).

Collagen Formation The best-understood action of vitamin C is that it helps to form collagen, the single most important protein of connective tissue. Collagen serves as the matrix on which bone is formed, the material of scars, and an important part of the "glue" that attaches one cell to another. This latter function is especially important in the artery walls, which must expand and contract with each beat of the heart, and in the walls of the capillaries, which are thin and fragile.

collagen: the characteristic protein of connective tissue.
kolla = glue
gennan = produce

Antioxidant Vitamin C is also an important antioxidant. Recall that the antioxidants beta-carotene and vitamin E protect fat-soluble substances from oxidizing agents; vitamin C protects water-soluble substances the same way. Vitamin C's antioxidant action is twofold. First, by being oxidized itself, vitamin C regenerates already-oxidized substances such as iron and copper to their original, active form. Second, in the process, the vitamin removes the damaging oxidizing agent.[37] In the intestines, it protects iron from oxidation. In the cells and body fluids, it helps to protect other molecules, including the fat-soluble compounds vitamin A, vitamin E, and the polyunsaturated fatty acids.

Amino Acid Metabolism Vitamin C is also involved in the metabolism of several amino acids. Some of these amino acids may end up being converted to hormones of great importance in body functioning, among them norepinephrine and thyroxine.

Role of Stress During stress, the adrenal glands release large quantities of vitamin C together with the stress hormones epinephrine and norepinephrine. What the vitamin has to do with the stress reaction is unclear, but it is known that stress increases vitamin C needs somewhat.

Possible Antihistamine Newspaper headlines touting vitamin C as a cure for colds and cancer have appeared frequently over the years. Some research suggests that vitamin C (2 grams per day for two weeks) may reduce the severity and duration of cold and allergy symptoms by reducing blood histamine concentrations.[38] In other words, vitamin C acts as an antihistamine. If further research confirms vitamin C's antihistamine effect, its use may permit people to rely less heavily on antihistamine drugs when suffering from cold and allergy symptoms.

Protection of Lungs Researchers continue to explore the relationship between vitamin C and upper respiratory infections. In one study of people with respiratory infections, vitamin C supplements significantly improved their symptoms.[39] In a study of runners in South Africa, vitamin C supplements reduced the incidence of respiratory symptoms after participation in a marathon.[40] Earlier studies have shown that marathon and ultramarathon competitors have a significantly higher incidence of upper respiratory symptoms immediately following a race than do sedentary controls.

Role in Cancer Prevention and Treatment The role of vitamin C in the prevention of, or therapy for, cancer is still being studied. Large-scale studies of populations offer strong support for a protective effect of vitamin C for certain types of cancer, in particular, cancers of the mouth, larynx, and esophagus.[41] In a dozen or so different well-controlled studies, researchers identified individuals with and without cancer and assessed their dietary intakes of vitamin C.[42] They found that people with high vitamin C intakes had lower risks of these cancers than did people with low intakes. The correlation may reflect not just an association with vitamin C, but the broader benefits of a diet rich in fruits and vegetables and low in fat. It does not support the taking of vitamin C supplements to treat or prevent cancer.

latent: the period in the course of a disease when the conditions are present but the symptoms have not begun to appear.
latens = lying hidden

overt: out in the open, full-blown.
ouvrire = to open

Vitamin C Deficiency When intake of vitamin C is inadequate, the body's vitamin C pool dwindles in size, and latent scurvy appears. The blood vessels show the first deficiency signs. The gums around the teeth begin to bleed easily and capillaries under the skin break spontaneously, producing pinpoint hemorrhages. Then the symptoms of overt scurvy appear. Muscles, including the heart muscle, may degenerate. The skin becomes rough, brown, scaly, and dry. Wounds fail to heal because scar tissue will not form. Bone rebuilding falters; the ends of the long bones become softened, malformed, and painful; and fractures appear. The teeth may become loose in the jawbone, and fillings may loosen and fall out. Anemia and infections are common. Sudden death is likely, perhaps because of massive bleeding into the joints and body cavities.

It takes only 10 or so milligrams of vitamin C a day to prevent overt scurvy, and not much more than that to cure it. Once diagnosed, scurvy is readily reversible with moderate doses, in the neighborhood of 100 milligrams per day. The RDA for adults is a generous 60 milligrams a day, and the latest food intake information for the United States shows that nearly all people's intakes either meet or exceed the RDA.[43]

Vitamin C Toxicity The easy availability of vitamin C in pill form and the publication of books recommending vitamin C to prevent colds and cancer have led thousands of people to take megadoses of vitamin C. Not surprisingly, instances of vitamin C causing harm have surfaced.

Some of the suspected toxic effects of vitamin C megadoses have not been confirmed, but others have been seen often enough to warrant concern. Nausea, abdominal cramps, and diarrhea are often reported. Several instances of interference with medical regimens are known. The large amounts of vitamin C excreted in the urine obscure the results of tests used to detect diabetes. People taking anticoagulants may unwittingly abolish the effect of these medicines if they also take massive doses of vitamin C. Vitamin C megadoses can enhance iron absorption too much, resulting in iron overload (see Chapter 8).

Doses of 10 to 30 or more times the recommended intake of a nutrient are termed megadoses. In the case of vitamin C, any amount over 1 g (1000 mg) is considered a megadose.

The anticoagulants with which vitamin C interferes are warfarin and dicumarol.

People with sickle-cell anemia may be especially vulnerable to megadoses of vitamin C. Those who have a tendency toward gout, as well as those who have a genetic abnormality that alters the way they metabolize vitamin C, are more prone to forming stones if they take megadoses of vitamin C.

gout (GOWT)**:** a metabolic disease in which crystals of uric acid precipitate in the joints.

Withdrawal Reaction The body of a person who has taken large doses of vitamin C for a long time adjusts by limiting absorption and destroying and excreting more of the vitamin than usual.[44] If the person then suddenly reduces intake to normal, the accelerated disposal system can't put on its brakes fast enough to avoid destroying too much of the vitamin. Some case histories have shown that adults who discontinue megadosing develop scurvy on intakes that would protect a normal adult. An innocent victim of this kind of error is the newborn baby of a megadoser, because the baby has adjusted to high levels of vitamin C in the mother's womb. Once born into an environment providing much smaller amounts, the baby develops scurvy, a withdrawal reaction.

The temporary condition manifested by withdrawal symptoms and experienced by the person who stops overdosing is vitamin C dependency. The body has adjusted to a high intake and so "needs" a high intake until it can readjust.

withdrawal reaction: a reaction to the withdrawal of a drug, revealing in most cases that the user has become dependent.

Recommended Intakes of Vitamin C As mentioned, the RDA for vitamin C is 60 milligrams for adults, with an extra 10 milligrams recommended for pregnant women and an additional 35 milligrams for lactating women. This amount is midway between two extremes. At one extreme is the requirement, 10 milligrams per day, to prevent overt scurvy; at the other extreme is the amount at which the body's pool of vitamin C would be full to overflowing: about 100 milligrams per day.

Remember the distinction between the requirement and the recommended allowance or standard (see p. 8).

Special Needs for Vitamin C As is true of all nutrients, unusual circumstances may raise vitamin C needs. Among the stresses known to do so are infections; burns; surgery; extremely high or low temperatures; toxic doses of heavy metals, such as lead, mercury, and cadmium; and the chronic use of certain medications, including aspirin, barbiturates, and oral contraceptives. Smoking, too, has adverse effects on vitamin C status.[45] Accordingly, the vitamin C recommendation for people who smoke is 100 milligrams per day.

Safe Limits Few instances warrant the taking of more than 100 to 300 milligrams a day. Adults may not be exposing themselves to severe risks if they choose to dose themselves with 1 to 2 grams a day, but those taking more than 2 grams, and especially those taking above 8 grams per day, should be aware of the distinct possibility of harm.

Vitamin C in Foods The inclusion of intelligently selected fruits and vegetables in the daily diet guarantees a generous intake of vitamin C. Even those who wish to ingest amounts well above the recommended 60 milligrams can easily meet their goals by eating certain foods (see Snapshot 7–4). Citrus fruits are rightly famous for their vitamin C contents. Some other fruits and certain vegetables are also rich sources: cantaloupe, strawberries, broccoli, and brussels sprouts. No animal foods other than organ meats, such as liver and kidneys, contain vitamin C. The humble potato is an important source of vitamin C in Western countries, where potatoes are eaten so frequently that they make substantial vitamin C contributions overall. They provide about 20 percent of all the vitamin C in the diet.

Vitamin C and Iron Absorption Eating foods containing vitamin C at the same meal with foods containing iron can double or triple the absorption of iron from those foods. For women and children, whose energy intakes are not large enough to guarantee that they will get enough iron from the foods they eat, this strategy is highly recommended. Table 7–4 summarizes functions, deficiency and toxicity symptoms, and food sources of vitamin C and the other water-soluble vitamins.

Snapshot 7–4 Vitamin C

RDA for adults: 60 mg/day

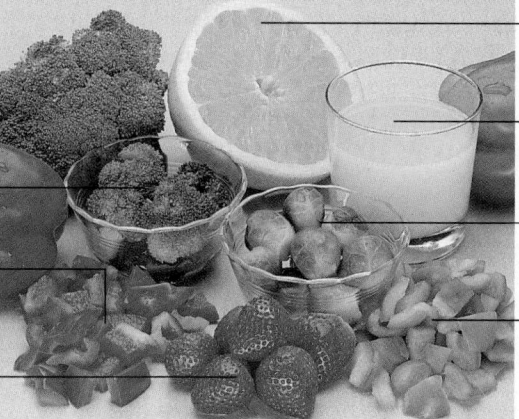

Grapefruit: 47 mg per ½ grapefruit

Orange juice: 93 mg per ¾ c

Broccoli: 58 mg per ½ c cooked

Brussels sprouts: 48 mg per ½ c cooked

Sweet red pepper: 95 mg per ½ c chopped fresh

Green pepper: 45 mg per ½ c chopped fresh

Strawberries: 42 mg per ½ c fresh

Table 7–4
The Water-Soluble Vitamins—A Summary

THIAMIN

	Deficiency Symptoms	Toxicity Symptoms
Other Names Vitamin B_1 **Chief Functions in the Body** Part of a coenzyme used in energy metabolism, supports normal appetite and nervous system function **Deficiency Disease Name** Beriberi **Significant Sources** Occurs in all nutritious foods in moderate amounts; pork, ham, bacon, liver, whole grains, legumes, nuts	*Blood/Circulatory System*	
	Edema, enlarged heart, abnormal heart rhythms, heart failure	(No symptoms reported)
	Nervous/Muscular Systems	
	Degeneration, wasting, weakness, pain, low morale, difficulty walking, loss of reflexes, mental confusion, paralysis	(No symptoms reported)

RIBOFLAVIN

	Deficiency Symptoms	Toxicity Symptoms
Other Names Vitamin B_2 **Chief Functions in the Body** Part of a coenzyme used in energy metabolism, supports normal vision and skin health **Deficiency Disease Name** Ariboflavinosis **Significant Sources** Milk, yogurt, cottage cheese, meat, leafy green vegetables, whole-grain or enriched breads and cereals	*Mouth, Gums, Tongue*	
	Cracks at corners of mouth,[a] magenta tongue	(No symptoms reported)
	Nervous System and Eyes	
	Hypersensitivity to light,[b] reddening of cornea	(No symptoms reported)
	Other	
	Skin rash	(No symptoms reported)

NIACIN

	Deficiency Symptoms	Toxicity Symptoms
Other Names Nicotinic acid, nicotinamide, niacinamide, vitamin B_3; precursor is dietary tryptophan **Chief Function in the Body** Part of a coenzyme used in energy metabolism; supports health of skin, nervous system, and digestive system **Deficiency Disease Name** Pellagra	*Digestive System*	
	Diarrhea	Diarrhea, heartburn, nausea, ulcer irritation, vomiting
	Mouth, Gums, Tongue	
	Black, smooth tongue[c]	(No symptoms reported)
	Nervous System	
	Irritability, loss of appetite, weakness, dizziness, mental confusion progressing to psychosis or delirium	Fainting, dizziness

[a]Cracks at the corners of the mouth are termed *cheilosis* (kee-LOH-sis).
[b]Hypersensitivity to light is *photophobia*.
[c]Smoothness of the tongue is caused by loss of its surface structures and is termed *glossitis* (gloss-EYE-tis).

(continued)

Table 7–4 *(continued)*

NIACIN *(continued)*		
Significant Sources Milk, eggs, meat, poultry, fish, whole-grain and enriched breads and cereals, nuts, and all protein-containing food	*Skin*	
	Flaky skin rash on areas exposed to sun	Painful flush and rash ("niacin flush"), sweating
	Other	
		Abnormal liver function, low blood pressure
PANTOTHENIC ACID		
Other Names (None) **Chief Functions in the Body** Part of a coenzyme used in energy metabolism **Deficiency Disease Name** (No name) **Significant Sources** Widespread in foods	**Deficiency Symptoms**	**Toxicity Symptoms**
	Digestive System	
	Vomiting, intestinal distress	(No symptoms reported)
	Nervous System	
	Insomnia, fatigue	(No symptoms reported)
	Other	
		Water retention (infrequent)
BIOTIN		
Other Names (None) **Chief Functions in the Body** Part of a coenzyme used in energy metabolism, fat synthesis, amino acid metabolism, and glycogen synthesis **Deficiency Disease** (No name) **Significant Sources** Widespread in foods	**Deficiency Symptoms**	**Toxicity Symptoms**
	Blood/Circulatory System	
	Abnormal heart action	(No symptoms reported)
	Digestive System	
	Loss of appetite, nausea	(No symptoms reported)
	Nervous/Muscular Systems	
	Depression, muscle pain, weakness, fatigue	(No symptoms reported)
	Skin	
	Drying, rash, loss of hair	(No symptoms reported)
VITAMIN B_6		
Other Names Pyridoxine, pyridoxal, pyridoxamine **Chief Functions in the Body** Part of a coenzyme used in amino acid and fatty acid metabolism, helps convert tryptophan to niacin, helps make red blood cells	**Deficiency Symptoms**	**Toxicity Symptoms**
	Blood/Circulatory System	
	Anemia (small-cell type)[d]	Bloating
	Mouth, Gums, Tongue	
	Smooth tongue[c]	(No symptoms reported)

[c]Smoothness of the tongue is caused by loss of its surface structures and is termed *glossitis* (gloss-EYE-tis).
[d]Small-cell anemia is termed *microcytic anemia;* large-cell type is *macrocytic* or *megaloblastic anemia.*
[e]The name *pernicious anemia* refers to the vitamin B_{12} deficiency caused by lack of intrinsic factor, but not to that caused by inadequate dietary intake.

Table 7–4 *(continued)*

VITAMIN B_6 *(continued)*		
Deficiency Disease Name (No name) **Significant Sources** Green and leafy vegetables, meats, fish, poultry, shellfish, legumes, fruits, whole grains	*Nervous/Muscular Systems*	
	Abnormal brain wave pattern, irritability, muscle twitching, convulsions	Depression, fatigue, impaired memory, irritability, headaches, numbness, damage to nerves, difficulty walking, loss of reflexes, weakness, restlessness
	Skin	
	Irritation of sweat glands, rashes, greasy dermatitis	(No symptoms reported)
	Other	
	Kidney stones	(No symptoms reported)

FOLATE		
Other Names Folic acid, folacin, pteroylglutamic acid **Chief Functions in the Body** Part of a coenzyme used in new cell synthesis **Deficiency Disease** (No name) **Significant Sources** Leafy green vegetables, legumes, seeds, liver	**Deficiency Symptoms**	**Toxicity Symptoms**
	Blood/Circulatory System	
	Anemia (large-cell type)[d]	(No symptoms reported)
	Digestive System	
	Heartburn, diarrhea, constipation	(No symptoms reported)
	Immune System	
	Suppression, frequent infections	(No symptoms reported)
	Mouth, Gums, Tongue	
	Smooth red tongue[c]	(No symptoms reported)
	Nervous System	
	Depression, mental confusion, fainting	(No symptoms reported)
	Other	
		Masks vitamin B_{12} deficiency

VITAMIN B_{12}		
Other Names Cyanocobalamin **Chief Functions in the Body** Part of a coenzyme used in new cell synthesis, helps maintain nerve cells **Deficiency Disease** (No name[e])	**Deficiency Symptoms**	**Toxicity Symptoms**
	Blood/Circulatory System	
	Anemia (large-cell type)[d]	(No symptoms reported)
	Mouth, Gums, Tongue	
	Smooth tongue[c]	(No symptoms reported)

[c]Smoothness of the tongue is caused by loss of its surface structures and is termed *glossitis* (gloss-EYE-tis).
[d]Small-cell anemia is termed *microcytic anemia;* large-cell type is *macrocytic* or *megaloblastic anemia.*

(continued)

Table 7–4 *(continued)*

VITAMIN B_{12} *(continued)*		
Significant Sources Animal products (meat, fish, poultry, milk, cheese, eggs)	*Nervous System*	
	Fatigue, degeneration progressing to paralysis	(No symptoms reported)
	Skin	
	Hypersensitivity	(No symptoms reported)
VITAMIN C		
Other Names Ascorbic acid **Chief Functions in the Body** Helps in collagen synthesis (strengthens blood vessel walls, forms scar tissue, provides matrix for bone growth), thyroxine synthesis, and amino acid metabolism, serves as an antioxidant; strengthens resistance to infection; helps in absorption of iron **Deficiency Disease Name** Scurvy **Significant Sources** Citrus fruits, cabbage-type vegetables, dark green vegetables, cantaloupe, strawberries, peppers, lettuce, tomatoes, potatoes, papayas, mangoes	**Deficiency Symptoms**	**Toxicity Symptoms**
	Blood/Circulatory System	
	Anemia (small-cell type),[d] atherosclerotic plaques, pinpoint hemorrhages	(No symptoms reported)
	Digestive System	
		Nausea, abdominal cramps, diarrhea, excessive urination
	Immune System	
	Suppression, frequent infections	(No symptoms reported)
	Mouth, Gums, Tongue	
	Bleeding gums, loosened teeth	(No symptoms reported)
	Muscular/Nervous Systems	
	Muscle degeneration and pain, hysteria, depression	Headache, fatigue, insomnia
	Skeletal System	
	Bone fragility, joint pain	(No symptoms reported)
	Skin	
	Rough skin, blotchy bruises	Rashes
	Other	
	Failure of wounds to heal	Interference with medical tests, aggravation of gout symptoms, deficiency symptoms may appear at first on withdrawal of high doses.

[d]Small-cell anemia is termed *microcytic anemia;* large-cell type is *macrocytic* or *megaloblastic anemia.*

In conclusion, a summary of the key points about vitamins—both fat soluble and water soluble—seems in order:

- Vitamins are essential, noncaloric, organic nutrients needed in tiny amounts in the diet.
- Vitamins A, D, E, and K are the fat-soluble vitamins. The B vitamins and vitamin C are the water-soluble vitamins.
- The only disease a vitamin will cure is the one caused by a deficiency of that vitamin.
- Vitamins yield no energy for the body when broken down, but they facilitate the release of energy from carbohydrate, fat, and protein.
- Nutritious foods, not supplements, are the best sources of vitamins.

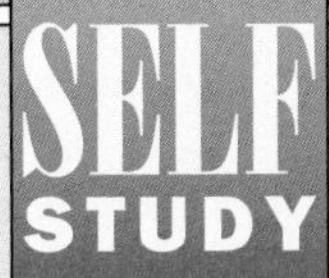

How Are Your Vitamin Intakes?

Compare your average daily intakes of vitamins with the RDA (inside front cover) or the Recommended Nutrient Intakes for Canadians (Appendix B). Express each intake as a percentage of the recommended intake. For example, suppose you ingested 0.9 milligram thiamin, and your RDA is 1.1 milligrams. You ingested (0.9 ÷ 1.1) x 100, or 82 percent of your RDA. If you had ingested 1.4 milligrams of thiamin, you would have ingested (1.4 ÷ 1.1) x 100, or 127 percent of your RDA. Use Form 8 to record your findings.

Comment on your intakes. Look closely at any vitamins for which your intakes fell below 80 percent of the recommendations. What are your best food sources of those vitamins? Could you eat more of these foods to bring your intake up to the recommended level? If not, what food or foods could you eat to improve your intake?

Health care professionals often see clients whose poor nutrition hampers their recovery; those who are alert to this possibility can often provide significant help and advice. Describe the differences between vitamin deficiency diseases and diseases that increase the likelihood of vitamin deficiency. Discuss ways a vitamin deficiency might weaken the body's resistance to disease.

Pull together information from Chapter 1 about the vitamins in different food groups and the significant sources of vitamins shown in the Snapshots throughout this chapter. Consider which vitamins might be lacking in the diet of a client who reports the following:

- Dislikes green leafy vegetables.
- Never uses milk, milk products, or cheese.
- Follows a very-low-fat diet.
- Eats a fruit or vegetable once a day.

What additional information would help you pinpoint a problem with vitamin intake?

Form 8
Vitamin Intakes Compared with Recommended Intakes

	VITAMIN A	VITAMIN C	THIAMIN	RIBOFLAVIN	NIACIN	FOLATE	VITAMIN B6
My intake							
Recommended intake[a]							
My intake as a percentage of the recommended intake							

[a]RDA or RNI (Appendix B)

STUDY QUESTIONS

1. How do the vitamins differ from the energy nutrients?
2. Describe some general differences between fat-soluble vitamins and water-soluble vitamins.
3. List one major function of each of the fat-soluble vitamins A, D, E, and K.
4. Why is vitamin D unique among the vitamins?
5. What is a coenzyme?
6. Name two B vitamin–deficiency diseases.
7. What do vitamin B_{12} and folate have in common?
8. What is a major function of vitamin C?
9. What are the risks associated with vitamin C megadoses?

NUTRITION IN PRACTICE 7

Vitamin Supplements

About 40 percent of U.S. adults collectively spend more than $3 billion a year on vitamin supplements.[46] Promoting this trend, scientists are discovering more and more links between nutrition and disease prevention. Notably, many recent reports indicate that the antioxidant nutrients beta-carotene, vitamin C, and vitamin E may be potent protectors against both cancer and heart disease. Before you race out to buy bottles of antioxidant supplements, it is important to know that the role of antioxidants in preventing disease remains to be confirmed by hundreds of scientific studies that are currently under way. The findings so far are promising, but nevertheless tentative. The main message of this Nutrition in Practice is that most healthy people can get the nutrients they need from food only. Supplements cannot substitute for a healthy diet.

Do foods really contain enough vitamins and minerals to supply all that most people need?

Emphatically, yes, for both healthy adults and children who choose a variety of foods in moderation.[47] The Daily Food Guide and the Food Guide Pyramid described in Chapter 1 are the guides to follow to achieve adequate intakes. People who meet their nutrient needs from foods, rather than supplements, have low risks of toxicity as well as of deficiency.

You said most healthy people do not need supplements. Are there some people who do?

Yes, some people may suffer marginal nutrient deficiencies due to illness, alcohol or drug addiction, or other conditions that limit food intake.[48] People who may benefit from nutrient supplements in amounts consistent with the RDA include:

- People with low energy intakes, such as habitual dieters.
- People with illnesses that take away the appetite.
- People with illnesses that impair nutrient absorption, such as diseases of the liver, gallbladder, pancreas, and digestive system.
- People taking medications that interfere with nutrient metabolism.
- Women who bleed excessively during menstruation (iron supplements).
- Women who are pregnant or lactating (iron and other nutrients under special circumstances as described in Chapter 15).
- Strict vegetarians (calcium, iron, zinc, and vitamin B_{12}).
- Newborn infants (a single dose of vitamin K at birth under the direction of a physician).

A few other special cases exist:

- People who have infections or injuries or who have undergone surgery. The increased metabolic needs associated with these severe stresses are discussed in Chapters 18 and 19.
- Infants, depending on whether they are receiving breast milk or formula, and on whether their water contains fluoride (see Chapter 15).

These people are in the minority. For the majority, supplements are not recommended. Nutrients are potentially toxic when taken in large doses and individual tolerances vary depending on health and age. Whenever a health care professional finds a person's diet inadequate, the right corrective step is to improve the person's food choices and eating patterns, not to begin supplementation.

I recently read that all women of childbearing age, not just those who are pregnant, need more than the RDA for folate. Please clarify.

All women of childbearing age do need to consume more than double the RDA for folate, but *not from supplements.* The U.S. Public Health Service recommends 400 micrograms of folate a day for women, from *foods.*[49]

The reason is this. Folate deficiency is associated with a group of devastating birth defects known as neural tube defects. These defects affect 1 in every 1000 births, making them the second most common form of birth defect after Down's syndrome. Neural tube defects range from slight problems in the spine to mental retardation, severely diminished brain size, and death shortly after birth.[50]

Neural tube defects arise early in pregnancy. By recommending extra folate *before* pregnancy, the Public Health Service hopes to prevent about half of these defects and to see many more of these infants born normal.[51]

To obtain the recommended amount of folate from foods, women need to make conscious efforts to eat folate-rich foods. Just three half-cup servings of these vegetables, for example, can provide 403 micrograms of folate:

- ½ cup cooked asparagus: 131 micrograms.
- ½ cup chickpeas (garbanzo beans): 141 micrograms.
- ½ cup cooked spinach: 131 micrograms.

If people don't like those foods, should they take folate supplements instead?

No, because high folate doses from supplements are a threat. One hazard, of course, is that in folate's presence a dangerous vitamin B_{12} deficiency can advance unnoticed. Also, 800 micrograms, the amount of folate in just two of many types of multivitamin pills, can alter zinc metabolism in men.[52] Prescription folate supplements contain huge therapeutic doses of about 20 times the RDA, doses that are recommended only for women who have already given birth to infants with neural tube defects.[53]

If only a few situations merit the use of supplements, why do so many people take them?

People frequently take supplements for the wrong reasons, such as "They give me energy" or "They make me strong."[54] Other invalid reasons why people may take supplements include:

- Their feeling of insecurity about the nutrient content of the food supply.
- Their belief that extra vitamins and minerals will help them cope with stress.
- Their desire to prevent, treat, or cure symptoms or diseases ranging from the common cold to cancer.

Ironically, at least one study showed that supplement users eat more nutrient-dense diets than nonusers and therefore need supplements less. In addition, little relationship exists between the nutrients people need and the ones they take in supplements.[55] In fact, an argument against supplements is that they may lull people into a false sense of security. A person might eat irresponsibly, thinking, "My supplement will cover my needs."

OK, so people can eat well enough to meet normal needs. But what about taking antioxidant supplements to prevent cancer and heart disease?

Again, it is better advice to eat a very nutritious diet. Evidence from population studies shows a correlation between low intakes of antioxidant nutrients and a high incidence of disease. Many studies show that low intakes of vegetables and fruits, and specifically of those containing beta-carotene and its relatives, are consistently linked with an increased incidence of lung cancer.[56] Researchers note, however, that other constituents of fruits and vegetables have not been ruled out as contributors to the effect.

Similar findings exist regarding vitamin C and vitamin E. Research shows that people with high vitamin C intakes have lower risks of cancer than people with low intakes.[57] Results of a large population study showed that people with low blood concentrations of vitamin E had a greater risk of certain cancers than those with higher blood concentrations of vitamin E.[58]

Almost 200 population studies have examined the effects of fruits and vegetables on cancer risk, and the vast majority show that people who eat more of these foods are less likely to develop cancer.[59] Many experts agree that the antioxidant vitamins in these foods are probably the most important protective factors.

The way to apply this information is to eat nutritious foods. Before supplementation is recommended as a strategy to prevent cancer or other diseases, researchers must find out the optimal doses to reduce risk and the potential adverse effects of long-term supplementation.

When I do need a vitamin-mineral supplement, what kind should I use?

Take your health care professional's advice, if it is offered. If you are selecting a supplement yourself, a single, balanced vitamin-mineral supplement should suffice. Choose the kind that provides all the RDA nutrients in amounts equal to, or very close to, the RDA (remember, you get some nutrients from foods). Avoid preparations that are in excess of the RDA. Avoid preparations that contain items not needed in human nutrition such as choline or inositol.

Can I trust what I read on supplement labels?

Yes. To enable consumers to make more informed choices about nutrient supplements, the Food and Drug Administration (FDA), with the encouragement of the American Dietetic Association (ADA), has published new labeling regulations for supplements.[60]

The new regulations subject supplements to the same general labeling requirements that apply to foods. Specifically:

- **Nutrition labeling for dietary supplements is required, and nutrient content claims ("high," "low") may be made.**
- **The FDA authorizes health claims on supplement labels about the relationship between folate and the risk of neural tube defects.**
- **Supplement labels are not allowed to include health claims on a number of other nutrient-disease relationships (dietary fiber and cancer, dietary fiber and cardiovascular disease, antioxidant vitamins and cancer, omega-3 fatty acids and coronary heart disease, and zinc and immune deficiency in the elderly).**

Health claims made on supplement labels must be based on significant scientific agreement. The $4-billion-a-year supplement industry is expected to continue fighting against the regulations, however, by trying to get overruling legislation.

■ NOTES ■

1. A. C. Ross, Vitamin A and protective immunity, *Nutrition Today,* July/August 1992, pp. 18–26; K. P. West, Jr., G. R. Howard, and A. Sommer, Vitamin A and infection: Public health implications, *Annual Review of Nutrition* 9 (1989): 63–86; P. P. Glasziou and D. E. M. Mackerras, Vitamin A supplementation in infectious diseases: A meta-analysis, *British Medical Journal* 306 (1993): 366–370.
2. Vitamin A administration reduces mortality and morbidity from severe measles in populations nonendemic for hypovitaminosis A, *Nutrition Reviews* 49 (1991): 89–91; W. W. Fawzi and coauthors, Vitamin A supplementation and child mortality: A meta-analysis, *Journal of the American Medical Association* 269 (1993): 898–903; L. J. Machlin and H. E. Sauberlich, New views on the function and health effects of vitamins, *Nutrition Today,* January/February 1994, pp. 25–29.
3. American Academy of Pediatrics, Committee on Infectious Diseases, Vitamin A treatment of measles, *Pediatrics* 91 (1993): 1014–1015.
4. A. T. Diplock, Antioxidant nutrients and disease prevention: An overview, *American Journal of Clinical Nutrition* 53 (1991): 189S–193S; T. V. Ringer and coauthors, Beta-carotene's effects on serum lipoproteins and immunologic indices in humans, *American Journal of Clinical Nutrition* 53 (1991): 688–694.
5. Diplock, 1991.
6. J. H. Humphrey, K. P. West, Jr., and A. Sommer, Vitamin A deficiency and attributable mortality among under-5-year-olds, *Bulletin of the World Health Organization* 70 (1992): 225–232.
7. Keep vitamins out of children's hands, *Tufts University Diet and Nutrition Letter,* August 1991, p. 7.
8. R. Weiss, Study sheds light on TB resistance, *Science News,* 133 (1988): 60.
9. H. Reichel, P. Koeffler, and A. W. Norman, The role of the vitamin D endocrine system in health and disease, *New England Journal of Medicine* 320 (1989): 980–991.
10. A. W. Norman, Intestinal calcium absorption: A vitamin D–hormone—mediated adaptive response, *American Journal of Clinical Nutrition* 51 (1990): 290–300; H. F. DeLuca, Vitamin D: 1993, *Nutrition Today,* November/December 1993, pp. 6–11.
11. Norman, 1990; H. F. DeLuca, New concepts of vitamin D functions, *Annals of the New York Academy of Sciences* 669 (1992): 59–68.
12. A. R. Webb and M. F. Holick, The role of sunlight in the cutaneous production of vitamin D_3, *Annual Review of Nutrition* 8 (1988): 375–399.
13. L. Y. Matsuoka and coauthors, Sunscreens suppress cutaneous vitamin D_3 synthesis, *Journal of Clinical Endocrinology and Metabolism* 64 (1987): 1165–1168, as cited in Webb and Holick, 1988.
14. Webb and Holick, 1988.
15. A Greely, Dodging the rays, *FDA Consumer,* July/August 1993, pp. 30–33.
16. C. Lamberg-Allardt and coauthors, Low serum 25-hydroxy vitamin D concentrations and secondary hyperthyroidism in middle-aged white, strict vegetarians, *American Journal of Clinical Nutrition* 58 (1993): 684–689.
17. L. Packer, Protective role of vitamin E in biological systems, *American Journal of Clinical Nutrition* (Supplement) 53 (1991): 1050–1055.
18. S. N. Meydani and coauthors, Vitamin E supplementation

enhances cell-mediated immunity in healthy elderly subjects, *American Journal of Clinical Nutrition* 52 (1990): 557–563; S. N. Meydani, M. Hayek, and L. Coleman, Influence of vitamins E and B_6 on immune response, *Annals of the New York Academy of Sciences* 669 (1992): 125–139.
19. M. J. Stampfer and coauthors, Vitamin E consumption and the risk of coronary disease in women, *New England Journal of Medicine* 328 (1993): 1444–1449; E. B. Rimm and coauthors, Vitamin E consumption and the risk of coronary disease in men, *New England Journal of Medicine* 328 (1993): 1450–1456.
20. American Medical Association, Council on Scientific Affairs, Vitamin preparations as dietary supplements and therapeutic agents, *Journal of the American Medical Association* 257 (1987): 1929–1936, as cited in C. W. Marshall, Vitamin E supplementation (letter), *American Journal of Clinical Nutrition* 49 (1989): 701–702.
21. D. A. Bender, Vitamin E: Tocopherols and tocotrienols, in *Nutritional Biochemistry of the Vitamins* (New York: Cambridge University Press, 1992), pp. 87–105.
22. S. P. Murphy, A. F. Subar, and G. Block, Vitamin E intakes and sources in the United States, *American Journal of Clinical Nutrition* 52 (1990): 361–367.
23. P. A. Price, Role of vitamin K–dependent proteins in bone metabolism, *Annual Review of Nutrition* 8 (1988): 565–583.
24. Vitamin K deficiency causes coagulopathy (abstract), *Journal of the American Dietetic Association* 88 (1988): 267.
25. Thiamin deficiency, *Nutrition and the M.D.,* May 1990, p. 3.
26. M. L. Schwartz, Severe reversible hyperglycemia as a consequence of niacin therapy, *Archives of Internal Medicine* 153 (1993): 2050–2052.
27. W. O. Song, Pantothenic acid: How much do we know about this B-complex vitamin? *Nutrition Today,* March/April 1990, pp. 19–25.
28. J. E. Leklem, Vitamin B_6: Of reservoirs, receptors, and requirements, *Nutrition Today,* September/ October 1988, pp. 4–10.
29. S. P. Coburn and coauthors, Human vitamin B_6 pools estimated through muscle biopsies, *American Journal of Clinical Nutrition* 48 (1988): 291–294; J. E. Leklem, Vitamin B_6, in *Modern Nutrition in Health and Disease,* 8th ed., eds, M. E. Shils, J. A. Olson, and M. Shike (Philadelphia: Lea & Febiger, 1994), pp. 383–394.
30. S. N. Meydani and coauthors, Vitamin B_6 deficiency impairs interleukin 2 production and lymphocyte proliferation in elderly adults, *American Journal of Clinical Nutrition* 53 (1991): 1275–1280; J. E. Leklem, Vitamin B-6 reservoirs, receptors, and red-cell reactions, *Annals of the New York Academy of Science* 669 (1992): 34–41.
31. L. C. Rall and S. N. Meydani, vitamin B_6 and immune competence, *Nutrition Reviews* 51 (1993): 217–225.
32. K. Dalton and M. J. T. Dalton, Characteristics of pyridoxine overdose neuropathy syndrome, *Acta Neurologica Scandinavica* 76 (1987): 8–11, as cited in National Academy of Sciences, Food and Nutrition Board, *Recommended Dietary Allowances,* 10th ed. (Washington, D.C.: National Academy Press, 1989).
33. National Academy of Sciences, 1989, pp. 142–149.
34. L. B. Bailey, The role of folate in human nutrition, *Nutrition Today,* September/October 1990, pp. 12–19.
35. P. F. Jacques and coauthors, Moderate alcohol intake and nutritional status in nonalcoholic elderly subjects, *American Journal of Clinical Nutrition* 50 (1989): 875–883.
36. V. Herbert, Vitamin B_{12}: Plant sources, requirements, and assay, *American Journal of Clinical Nutrition* 48 (1988): 852–858; P. C. Dagnelie, W. A. van Staveren, and H. van den Berg, Vitamin B_{12} from algae appears not to be bioavailable, *American Journal of Clinical Nutrition* 53 (1991): 695–697.
37. H. Padh, Vitamin C: Newer insights into its biochemical functions, *Nutrition Reviews* 49 (1991): 65–70.
38. Vitamin C suppresses histamine (Newsbreaks), *Nutrition Today,* May/June 1991, p. 4; C. S. Johnston, K. R. Retrum, and J. C. Srilaskshmi, Antihistamine effects and complications of supplemental vitamin C, *Journal of the American Dietetic Association* 92 (1992): 988–989.
39. C. Bucca, G. Rolla, and J. C. Farina, Effect of vitamin C on transient increase of bronchial responsiveness in conditions affecting the airways, *Annals of the New York Academy of Sciences* 669 (1992): 175–186.
40. E. M. Peters and coauthors, Vitamin C supplementation

reduces the incidence of postrace symptoms of upper-respiratory-tract infection in ultramarathon runners, *American Journal of Clinical Nutrition* 57 (1993): 170–174.
41. G. Block, Vitamin C and cancer prevention: The epidemiologic evidence, *American Journal of Clinical Nutrition* (supplement) 53 (1991): 270–282.
42. Block, 1991; G. Block, Vitamin C status and cancer: Epidemio-logic evidence of reduced risk, *Annals of the New York Academy of Sciences* 669 (1992): 280–290.
43. H. S. Wright and coauthors, The 1987–88 Nationwide Food Consumption Survey: An update on the nutrient intake of respondents, *Nutrition Today,* May/June 1991, pp. 21–27.
44. S. T. Omaye, J. H. Skala, and R. A. Jacob, Rebound effect with ascorbic acid in adult males (letter), *American Journal of Clinical Nutrition* 48 (1988): 379–380.
45. G. Schectman, J. C. Byrd, and H. W. Gruchow, The influence of smoking on vitamin C status in adults, *American Journal of Public Health* 79 (1989): 158–162.
46. V. Srinivasan and coauthors, Standards setting for nutritional supplements: A new approach, *Nutrition Today,* November/December 1993, pp. 26–33.
47. Recommendations concerning supplement usage: ADA statement (commentary), *Journal of the American Dietetic Association* 87 (1987): 1342–1343.
48. Recommendations concerning supplement usage, 1987; D. Herber, W. Mertz, and R. E. Shucker, Food versus pills versus fortified foods, *Dairy Council Digest,* March/April 1987; A. E. Harper, "Nutrition insurance"—A skeptical view, *Nutrition Forum,* May 1987, pp. 33–37.
49. Centers for Disease Control and Prevention, Recommendations for use of folic acid to reduce number of spina bifida cases and other neural tube defects, *Journal of the American Medical Association* 269 (1993): 1233, 1236, 1238.
50. J. M. Scott, P. N. Kirke, and D. G. Weir, The role of nutrition in neural tube defects, *Annual Review of Nutrition* 10 (1990): 277–295.
51. J. L. Mills and coauthors, Maternal vitamin levels during pregnancies producing infants with neural tube defects, *Journal of Pediatrics* 120 (1992): 863–871; A. E. Czeil and I. Dudás, Prevention of the first occurrence of neural-tube defects by periconceptional vitamin supplementation, *New England Journal of Medicine* 327 (1992): 1832–1835; Scott, Kirke, and Weir, 1990.
52. USDA human nutrition research and education report, *Nutrition Today,* November/December 1991, p. 5.
53. D. Rush, Folate supplements and neural tube defects, *Nutrition Reviews* 50 (1992): 25–26.
54. P. A. Thomsen, R. D. Terry, and R. J. Amos, Adolescents' beliefs about and reasons for using vitamin/mineral supplements, *Journal of the American Dietetic Association* 87 (1987): 1063–1065.
55. A. Looker and coauthors, Vitamin-mineral supplement use: Association with dietary intake and iron status of adults, *Journal of the American Dietetic Association* 88 (1988): 808–814.
56. R. G. Ziegler, Vegetables, fruits, and carotenoids and the risk of cancer, *American Journal of Clinical Nutrition* (supplement) 53 (1991): 251–259.
57. Block, 1991.
58. P. Knekt and coauthors, Vitamin E and cancer prevention, *American Journal of Clinical Nutrition* (supplement) 53 (1991): 283–286.
59. K. Meister, Fruits, vegetables, and cancer, *Priorities* (a publication of the American Council on Science and Health), Fall/Winter 1993, pp. 27–30.
60. ADA applauds new FDA labeling rules that regulate health claims on dietary supplements, *Journal of the American Dietetic Association* 94 (1994): 146.

8

Water and Minerals

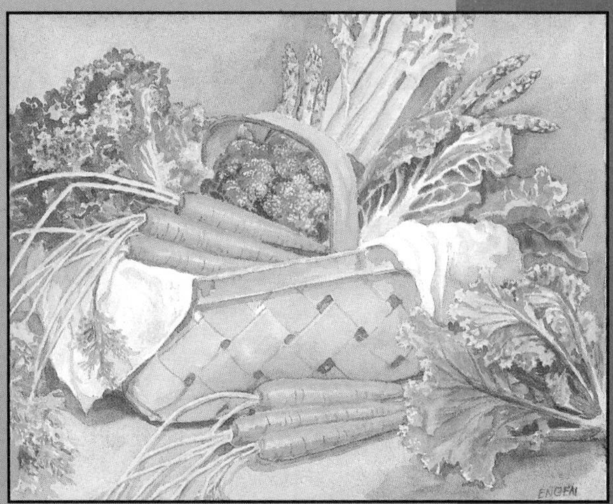

CONTENTS

The body's water cannot be considered separately from the minerals dissolved in it. A person can drink pure water, but in the body it mingles with minerals to become fluids in which all life processes take place. This chapter begins by discussing the body's fluids and their chief minerals. The focus then shifts to other functions of the minerals.

Table 8–1 lists the major and trace minerals in the body, and Figure 8–1 shows the amounts found in the body. As you can see, the most prevalent minerals are calcium and phosphorus, the chief minerals of bone. The distinction between the major and the trace minerals does not mean that one group is more important than the other. A deficiency of the few micrograms of iodine needed daily is just as serious as a deficiency of the several hundred milligrams of calcium. Because of their larger total quantities, however, the major minerals exert a greater influence on the body fluids.

Table 8–1
The Major and Trace Minerals

MAJOR MINERALS	TRACE MINERALS
▸ Calcium	▸ Arsenic
▸ Chloride	▸ Boron
▸ Magnesium	▸ Chromium
▸ Phosphorus	▸ Cobalt
▸ Potassium	▸ Copper
▸ Sodium	▸ Fluoride
▸ Sulfur	▸ Iodine
	▸ Iron
	▸ Manganese
	▸ Molybdenum
	▸ Nickel
	▸ Selenium
	▸ Silicon
	▸ Zinc

Water and Body Fluids

Every cell in the body is bathed in a fluid of the exact composition that is best for that cell. The body fluids bring to each cell the exact ingredients it requires and carry away the end products of the life-sustaining reactions that take place within the cell's boundaries. The cells themselves regulate the composition and amounts of fluids within and surrounding them. The entire system of cells and fluids remains in a delicate but firmly maintained state of dynamic equilibrium. The water in the fluids:

- Actively participates in many chemical reactions.
- Serves as the solvent for minerals, vitamins, amino acids, glucose, and a multitude of other small molecules.
- Acts as a lubricant and cushion around joints.
- Serves as a shock absorber inside the eyes, spinal cord, and amniotic sac surrounding a fetus in the womb.
- Aids in the body's temperature maintenance.

Because water is so vital to these and other functions, the body accurately regulates its influx to match outflow.

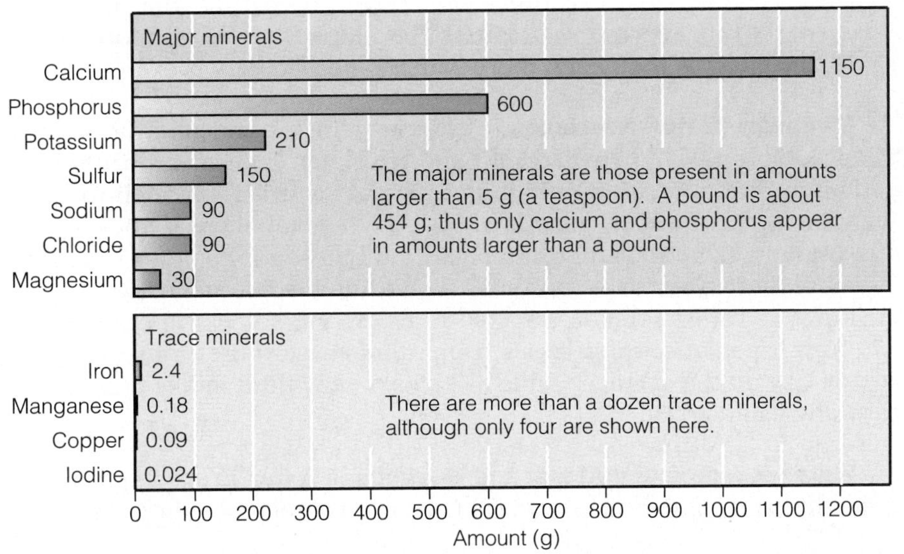

Figure 8–1
The Amounts of Minerals in a 60-kilogram (132-pound) Human Body

Water Balance

Water constitutes about 55 to 60 percent of an adult's body weight and a higher percentage of a child's. The total amount of water in the body is kept constant by delicate balancing mechanisms. Imbalances such as dehydration and water intoxication can occur, but the body quickly restores the balances to normal if it can. The body controls both water intake and water excretion.

dehydration: loss of water from the body that occurs when water output exceeds water input. The symptoms progress rapidly from thirst, to weakness, to exhaustion and delirium and end in death if not corrected.

water intoxication: the rare condition in which body water contents are too high. The symptoms may include confusion, convulsion, coma, and even death in extreme cases.

water balance: the balance between water intake and water excretion, which keeps the body's water content constant.

hypothalamus (high-poh-THALL-uh-mus)**:** a part of the brain that helps regulate many body balances, including fluid balance.

Water Intake Regulation The body can survive for only a few days without water. Thirst and satiety govern water intake. Thirst in healthy people is finely adjusted to ensure a water intake that meets the body's needs. When the blood is too concentrated (having lost water but not salt and other dissolved substances), the mouth becomes dry and the person's response is to drink. The brain center known as the hypothalamus also monitors the blood, and can initiate drinking behavior.

Thirst lags behind water lack. A water deficiency that develops slowly can switch on drinking behavior in time to prevent serious dehydration, but a deficiency that develops quickly may not. Also, thirst itself does not remedy a water deficiency; you have to take the time to get a drink.[1] The long-distance runner, the gardener in hot weather, the busy child at play, and the elderly person whose thirst sensations may be blunted can experience serious dehydration if they fail to drink promptly in response to their needs for water.

pituitary (pit-TOO-ih-tary) **gland:** in the brain, the "king gland" that regulates the operation of many other glands.

ADH (antidiuretic hormone): a hormone released by the pituitary gland in response to high osmotic pressure of the blood. The kidneys respond by reabsorbing water.

This is the enzyme **renin** (REEN-in), released by the kidneys in response to low blood pressure. Renin aids the kidneys in retaining water through the **renin-angiotensin mechanism.**

aldosterone (al-DOS-ter-own): a hormone secreted by the adrenal glands that stimulates the reabsorption of sodium by the kidneys: aldosterone also regulates chloride and potassium concentrations.

500 ml = about ½ qt.

Water Excretion Regulation Water excretion involves the brain and the kidneys. The cells of the brain's hypothalamus, which monitor blood salts, stimulate the pituitary gland to release antidiuretic hormone (ADH) whenever the salts are too concentrated, or the blood volume or blood pressure is too low. ADH stimulates the kidneys to hold back (actually, to reabsorb) water so that the water recirculates rather than being excreted. Thus the more water you need, the less you excrete.

If too much water is lost from the body, blood volume and blood pressure fall. Cells in the kidneys respond to the low blood pressure by releasing an enzyme. By a roundabout route involving the hormone aldosterone, this enzyme also causes the kidneys to retain more water. Again, the effect is that when more water is needed, less is excreted.

Minimum Water Needed These mechanisms can maintain water balance, but only if a person drinks enough water. The body must excrete a minimum of about 500 milliliters each day as urine—enough to carry away the waste products generated by a day's metabolic activities. Above this amount, excretion adjusts to balance intake, and the more you drink the more dilute your urine becomes. In addition, some water is lost from the lungs as vapor, some is excreted in feces, and some evaporates from the skin. A person's water losses from all of these routes total about 2½ liters a day on the average. Table 8–2 shows how fluid intake and output naturally balance out.

Water Recommendations and Sources Water needs vary greatly depending on the foods a person eats, the environmental temperature and humidity, the person's activity level, and other factors. Accordingly, a general water requirement is difficult to establish. The committee on RDA recommends that under normal dietary and environmental conditions adults should consume between 1 and 1½ milliliters of water for each kcalorie spent during the day.[2] For the person who expends about 2000 kcalories a day, this works out to 2 to 3 liters, or about 6 to 8 cups. As a rule of thumb, you can tell from the color of your urine whether you need more water. Pale yellow urine reflects appropriate dilution.

In addition to the plain water people may drink, nearly all foods provide water. Most fruits and vegetables contain up to 95 percent water; many meats and cheeses contain at least 50 percent. The energy nutrients in foods also give up water during metabolism. As Table 8–2 shows, a person's daily water intake from water, foods, and metabolism totals about 2½ liters (about 2½ quarts) on the average.

Table 8–2
Water Balance

WATER SOURCE	AMOUNT (ml)
Liquids	550 to 1500
Foods	700 to 1000
Metabolic water	200 to 300
	1450 to 2800
WATER OUTPUT	
Kidneys	500 to 1400
Skin	450 to 900
Lungs	350
Feces	150
	1450 to 2800

Fluid and Electrolyte Balance

When mineral salts dissolve in water, they separate (dissociate) into charged particles known as ions, which can conduct electricity. For this reason, a salt that partly dissociates in water is known as an electrolyte. The body fluids, which contain water and partly dissociated salts, are electrolyte solutions.

The body's electrolytes are vital to the life of the cells and therefore must be closely regulated to help maintain the appropriate distribution of body fluids. The major minerals form salts that dissolve in the body fluids; the cells direct where these salts go; and the movement of the salts determines where the fluids flow because water follows salts. Cells use this force to move fluids back and forth across their membranes. Thanks to the electrolytes, water can be held in compartments where it is needed.

Proteins in the cell membranes move ions in or out of cells. These protein pumps tend to concentrate sodium and chloride outside cells and potassium and other ions inside. By maintaining certain amounts of sodium outside and potassium inside, cells can regulate exactly the amounts of water inside and outside their boundaries. Physicians apply the same principle when treating kidney failure; they use an electrolyte solution to draw excess fluid out of the blood (see *dialysis* in Chapter 27).

Healthy kidneys regulate the body's sodium, as well as its water, with remarkable precision. The intestinal tract absorbs sodium defenselessly, and it travels freely in the blood, but the kidneys excrete unneeded amounts. The kidneys actually filter all of the sodium out of the blood; then, with great precision, they return to the bloodstream the exact amount the body needs to retain. Thus the body's total electrolytes remain constant, while the urinary electrolytes fluctuate according to what is eaten.

Normally, the body defends itself successfully against fluid and electrolyte imbalances. However, a person may be thrown into situations of imbalance for which the thirst instinct, cell membranes, and kidneys cannot compensate. This is the case when large amounts of fluid and electrolytes are suddenly lost. Vomiting, diarrhea, heavy sweating, fever, burns, wounds, and the like may incur great fluid and electrolyte losses, precipitating an emergency that demands medical management.

salts: compounds composed of charged particles (ions). An example is potassium chloride (K^+Cl^-).

Exceptions: a compound in which the positive ions are hydrogen ions (H^+) is an acid (example: hydrochloric acid, or H^+Cl^-); a compound in which the negative ions are hydroxyl ions (OH^-) is a base (example: potassium hydroxide, or (K^+OH^-).

electrolytes: salts that dissolve in water and dissociate into charged particles called **ions.**

electrolyte solutions: solutions that can conduct electricity.

The simple statement that water follows salt describes the force that chemists call *osmosis.*

Acid-Base Balance

The body uses its ions not only to help maintain water balance but also to help regulate the acidity (pH) of its fluids. Electrolyte mixtures in the body fluids, as well as proteins, protect the body against changes in acidity by acting as buffers—substances that can accommodate excess acids or bases.

Reminder: *Buffers* are compounds that help keep a solution's acidity or alkalinity constant; buffers are capable of neutralizing both acids and bases and thereby maintaining the original concentration of hydrogen ions (pH) in the solution.

The body's buffer systems serve as a first line of defense against changes in the fluids' acid-base balance. The lungs, skin, GI tract, and kidneys provide other defenses. Of these organ systems, the kidneys play the primary role in maintaining acid-base balance.

Disorders of the kidneys, therefore, impair the body's ability to regulate its acid-base balance, as well as its fluid and electrolyte balances. For a person with renal disease, the physician may order, in addition to many medical procedures, adjustment of the electrolyte intake from food. Chapter 27 gives more information about renal disease.

Not only do all of the major minerals help maintain fluid and electrolyte balance in the body, but they have other important functions as well, as the next sections describe. Table 8–6, at the end of this chapter, offers a summary of the minerals and their functions.

The Major Minerals

The major minerals, especially sodium, potassium, and chloride, influence the body's fluid balance. Each major mineral also plays other specific roles in the body. Sodium, potassium, calcium, and magnesium are critical to nerve transmission and muscle contractions. Phosphorus and magnesium are involved in energy metabolism. Calcium, phosphorus, and magnesium contribute to the structure of the bones. Sulfur helps determine the contour of proteins.

Sodium

Sodium is the principal electrolyte in the extracellular fluid and the primary regulator of the extracellular fluid volume. When the blood concentration of sodium rises, as when a person eats salted foods, thirst ensures that the person will drink water until the appropriate sodium-to-water ratio is restored. Sodium also helps maintain acid-base balance and is essential to muscle contraction and nerve transmission.

Estimated minimum requirement for sodium: 500 mg/day. Recommended maximum intake of salt: 6 g/day (2400 mg sodium).

Sodium Recommendations and Food Sources Diets rarely lack sodium. For this reason, no RDA is set; instead an estimated *minimum* sodium requirement was established. The *Diet and Health Recommendations* (Table 1–2 in Chapter 1), which emphasize moderation, not adequacy, set a *maximum* intake of *salt,* primarily to help prevent high blood pressure.

Cultures vary in their use of salt. The most recent food intake survey in the United States estimates that men consume a daily average of 3300 milligrams of sodium (equivalent to about 8 grams of salt).[3] Asian people, whose staple sauces and flavorings are based on soy sauce and monosodium glutamate (MSG or Accent), consume the equivalent of about 30 to 40 grams of salt per day. In China, Japan, and Korea, high blood pressure is as prevalent, or more so, than in the United States.[4]

Figure 8–2
What Processing Does to the Sodium and Potassium Contents of Foods

Note how potassium is lost and sodium is gained as foods become more processed.

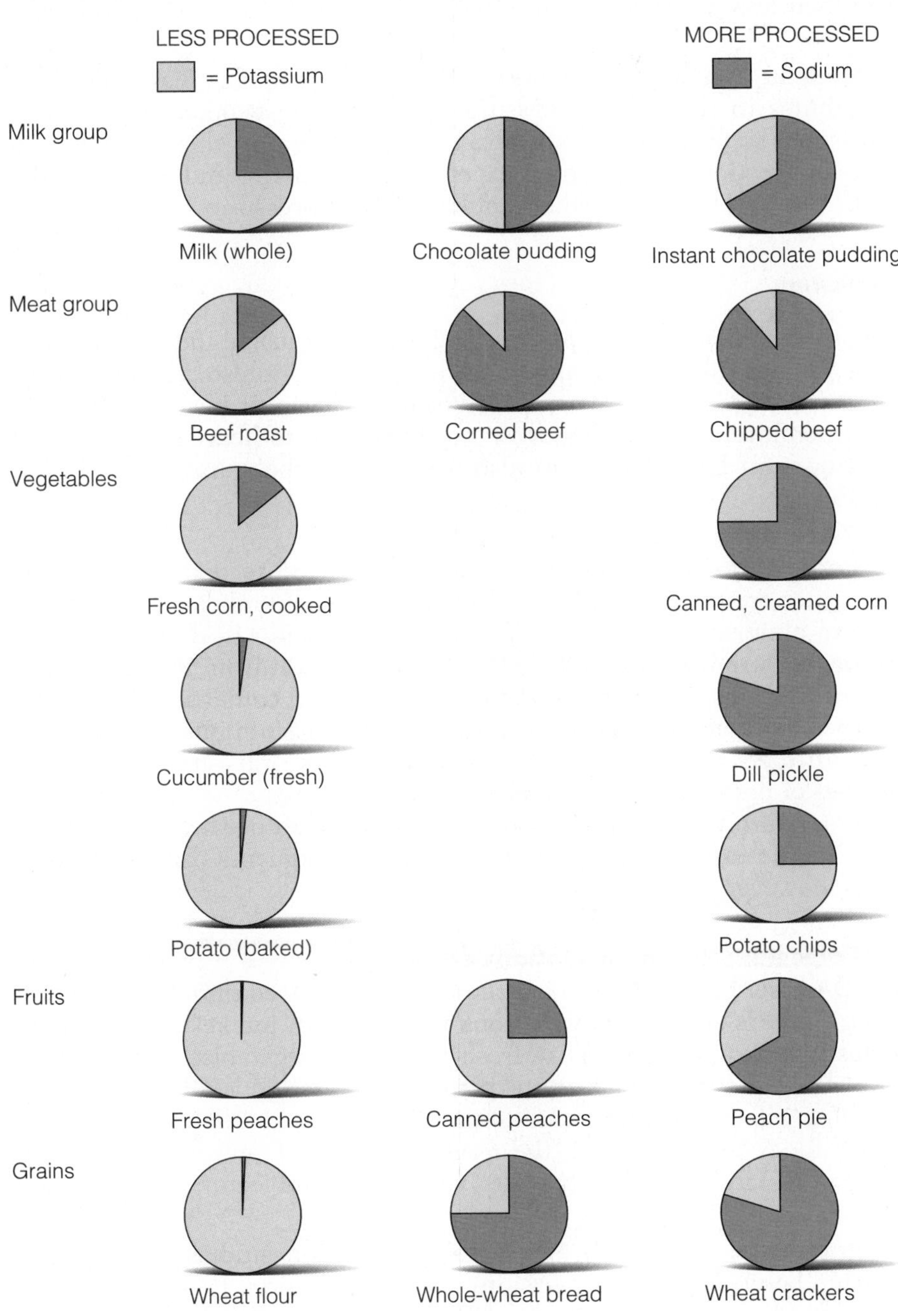

Sodium intakes vary widely, but foods usually supply more sodium than the body needs. In general, people who eat mostly processed foods have the highest sodium intakes, while those who eat mostly whole, unprocessed foods, such as fresh fruits and vegetables, have the lowest intakes.[5] In fact, about three-fourths of the sodium in people's diets comes from salt added to foods by manufacturers.[6] Figure 8–2 shows that

5 g salt is about 2 g sodium.
1 g salt = ⅕ tsp salt.

processed foods contain not only more sodium but also less potassium than their less-processed counterparts.

Sodium and Blood Pressure Sodium, or the salt that delivers it, contributes to high blood pressure in susceptible people. So does low potassium, so processed foods have two strikes against them. Chapter 26 offers suggestions for avoiding excessive salt intakes, and describes the relationship of these and other factors to blood pressure.

Potassium

Potassium is the principal positively charged ion inside the body cells. It plays a major role in maintaining cell integrity and is also critical to keeping the heartbeat steady. The sudden deaths that occur in severe diarrhea and in children with kwashiorkor are likely due to heart failure caused by potassium loss. Potassium also assists in carbohydrate and protein metabolism.

Potassium Deficiency and Toxicity Potassium deficiency results more often from excessive losses than from deficient intakes. Deficiencies arise in abnormal conditions such as diabetic acidosis, dehydration, or prolonged vomiting or diarrhea; they can also result from the regular use of certain drugs, including diuretics, steroids, and cathartics. One of the earliest symptoms is muscle weakness. Low potassium intakes are possible with diets low in fresh fruits and vegetables, but out-and-out deficiencies of potassium are unlikely in healthy people.

Potassium toxicity from foods is not a problem because healthy kidneys excrete excess potassium. Potassium supplements can reach toxic levels, however, and can cause death.

diuretic (dye-yoo-RET-ic)**:** a drug that promotes the excretion of water through the kidneys. Only some diuretics increase the urinary loss of potassium. Others, called potassium-sparing diuretics, are less likely to result in a potassium deficiency.

steroid (STARE-oid)**:** a drug used to reduce tissue inflammation, to suppress the immune response, or to replace certain steroid hormones in people who cannot synthesize them.

cathartic (ca-THART-ic)**:** a strong laxative.
cata = down

Estimated minimum requirement for potassium: 2000 mg/day.

Potassium Recommendations and Food Sources As with sodium, no RDA is set for potassium, but there is an estimated minimum requirement. Surveys show wide variations in potassium intakes in the United States; people who emphasize fresh fruits and vegetables in their diets have intakes as high as 11 grams per day.[7] Potassium is abundant inside all living cells, both plant and animal, and because cells remain intact unless foods are processed, the richest sources of potassium are *fresh* foods of all kinds—especially fruits, vegetables, and legumes.

Potassium and Blood Pressure Population studies show a relationship between dietary potassium and hypertension. Primitive populations worldwide eat diets that are low in sodium and high in potassium; hypertension among such people is virtually nonexistent. Conversely, among populations who eat diets that are low in potassium, the incidence of cardiovascular disease conditions such as hypertension and stroke is abnormally high.[8] Evidence of potassium's influence on blood pressure is continuing to accumulate. One long-term study in California showed that people with a high dietary potassium intake had a risk of stroke as much as 40 percent lower than in other people.[9] A reminder is important here: these findings are based on *food* intakes of potassium, not supplements.

In the United States, where strokes are a leading killer, the potential exists for people to reap substantial health benefits simply by including many potassium-rich fresh fruits, vegetables, and juices in their diets.

Figure 8–3
Cross Section of Bone
The lacy structural elements are **trabeculae** (tra-BECK-you-lee), which can be drawn on to replenish blood calcium.

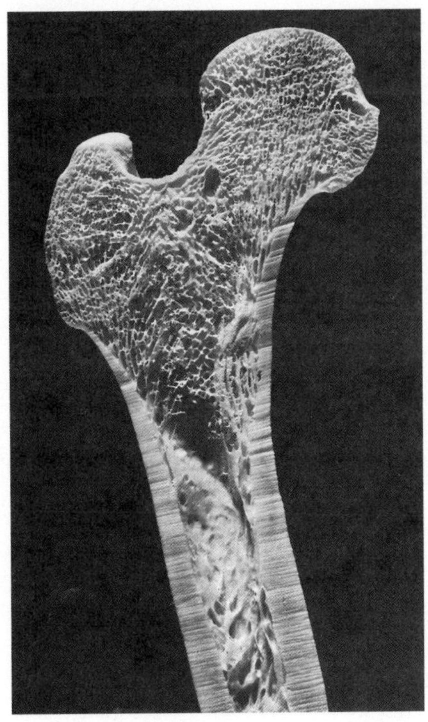

Calcium

Calcium occupies more space in this chapter than does any other major mineral. Other minerals are revisited in Part III of this book, where they play key roles in heart disease and kidney disease. Calcium, though, deserves emphasis here in the normal nutrition part of the book because an adequate intake of calcium early in life helps grow a healthy skeleton and prevent bone disease in later life.

Calcium owns the distinction of being the most abundant mineral in the body. Ninety-nine percent of the body's calcium is stored in the bones, where it plays two important roles. First, it is an integral part of bone structure. Second, it serves as a calcium bank available to the body fluids. Many people have the idea that bones are inert, like rocks. Not so. Bones are in a state of constant flux, with formation and dissolution taking place every minute of the day and night. Figure 8–3 shows the lacy network of calcium-containing crystals in the bone.

Calcium in Body Fluids The 1 percent of the body's calcium that circulates in the fluids as ionized calcium is vital to life. It helps regulate muscle contraction, transmit nerve impulses, clot blood, and secrete hormones, digestive enzymes, and neurotransmitters. Calcium also helps convey signals received at the cell surface to the inside of the cell.[10] Calcium is a cofactor for several enzymes as well.

Because blood calcium is so important, its concentration is tightly controlled. Whenever blood calcium rises too high, a system of hormones and vitamin D promotes its deposit into bone. Whenever blood calcium falls too low, the regulatory system acts in three locations to raise it:

1. The intestine absorbs more calcium.
2. The bones release more calcium.
3. The kidneys excrete less calcium.

Thus blood calcium rises to normal.

cofactor: a mineral element that, like a coenzyme, works with an enzyme to facilitate a chemical reaction.

The regulators are hormones from the thyroid and parathyroid glands, as well as vitamin D. One hormone, parathormone, raises blood calcium. Others, calcitonin and thyrocalcitonin, lower blood calcium by inhibiting release of calcium from bone. The hormonelike vitamin D raises blood calcium by acting at the three sites listed.

Calcium in Bone The calcium stored in bone provides a nearly inexhaustible source of calcium for the blood. Even in a calcium deficiency, blood calcium remains normal. Blood calcium changes only in response to abnormal regulatory control, not to diet. Blood calcium above normal causes calcium rigor: the muscles contract and cannot relax. Blood calcium below normal causes calcium tetany—also characterized by uncontrolled muscle contraction. These conditions are caused by a lack of vitamin D or by abnormal concentrations of the hormones that regulate calcium homeostasis.

Although a chronic *dietary* deficiency of calcium or a chronic deficiency due to poor absorption does not change blood calcium, it does deplete the savings account in the bones. Because this is an important concept, we repeat: it is the bones, not the blood, that are robbed by calcium deficiency.

calcium rigor: hardness or stiffness of the muscles caused by high blood calcium.

calcium tetany: intermittent spasms of the extremities due to nervous and muscular excitability, which is caused by low blood calcium.

osteoporosis (oss-tee-oh-pore-OH-sis): literally, porous bones; reduced density of the bones. Also known as *adult bone loss,* it is a condition in which the bones become porous and fragile. The causes of osteoporosis are multiple.
osteo = bone

Calcium Deficiency Bone mass peaks at the time of skeletal maturity (between the ages of 30 and 35), and a high peak bone mass is the best protection against later age-related bone loss and fracture. Calcium deficiencies impair the acquisition of peak bone mass and density, and they are widespread in human societies.[11] Most research suggests that all adults lose bone as they grow older, although one study of nutrition and bone loss suggests that calcium intakes in the range of the RDA are adequate to prevent bone loss in healthy premenopausal women.[12] Following menopause, women lose about 15 percent of their bone mass, as do middle-aged and older men. When bone loss has reached such an extreme that bones fracture under even common, everyday stresses, the condition is known as osteoporosis. Osteoporosis afflicts as many as 20 million people, mostly women 45 years of age or older.

Both genetic and environmental factors contribute to osteoporosis. Table 8–3 summarizes risk factors for osteoporosis. Osteoporosis is eight times more prevalent in women than men for several reasons. First, women consume only about half as much dietary calcium as men do. Second, at all ages, women's bone mass is lower than men's because women generally have a smaller body size. Finally, bone loss begins earlier in women than in men, and it accelerates after menopause.

Bone Loss Prevention Many minerals and vitamins are required to form and stabilize the structure of bones, including magnesium, fluoride, and vitamin A. Any or all of these elements are needed to prevent bone loss. The first, most obvious lines of defense, however, are to maintain a

Table 8–3
Risk Factors for Osteoporosis

Age
Gender
Race
Family history of osteoporosis
Low calcium intake
Excessive caffeine use
Excessive fiber in the diet
Menopause
Never having given birth
Inactivity or extreme activity with cessation of menstruation
Low body weight
Lean body composition
Short stature, small frame size
Heavy alcohol use
Stomach or intestine surgery (surgery can reduce calcium absorption)
Disease states or long-term medications (consult a physician)

Source: Adapted from B. L. Riggs and L. J. Melton, Involutional osteoporosis, *New England Journal of Medicine* 314 (1986): 1676–1686; L. W. Turner and E. N. Whitney, Nature versus nurture: The calcium controversy, *Nutrition Clinics,* September/October 1989.

lifelong adequate intake of calcium and to "exercise it into place." Moderate weight-bearing exercise, such as walking, running or dancing, prompts the bones to lay down minerals. Nonweight-bearing activity such as swimming or stretching is less effective in terms of bone strength. It has long been known that when people are confined to bed, both their muscles and their bones lose strength. Muscle strength and bone strength go together: when muscles work, they pull on the bones, and both are stimulated to grow stronger.

Rickets The disease rickets was mentioned in Chapter 7 because vitamin D deficiency is its most common cause. Vitamin D deficiency causes rickets by depressing the production of the calcium-binding protein. Dietary calcium is often adequate in a person with rickets, but the calcium passes through the intestinal tract without being absorbed into the body, leaving the bones undersupplied. The symptoms of rickets were listed in Table 7–2.

Reminder: *Rickets* is the calcium-deficiency (or vitamin D–deficiency) disease in children.

Reminder: The vitamin D deficiency-related condition in which the bones become soft is osteomalacia, sometimes called *adult rickets*.

Calcium and Hypertension Emerging evidence suggests that calcium helps prevent hypertension.[13] Studies of populations prone to developing hypertension show that low dietary calcium correlates with a high blood pressure.[14] Reports indicate that calcium supplements can lower blood pressure.[15] Some researchers speculate that calcium's effect on blood pressure is related to its action on the smooth muscle surrounding blood vessels.

Calcium Recommendations and Food Sources The calcium RDA for adults is 800 milligrams, but adult women consume an average of 600 milligrams, and one woman in four consumes less than 300 milligrams of calcium per day.[16] Some authorities advocate calcium recommendations as high as 1500 milligrams per day for women over 50 to guard against bone loss.

Calcium is found almost exclusively in a single class of foods—milk and milk products. As a result, dietary recommendations advise daily consumption of low-fat or nonfat milk products. A cup of nonfat milk offers about 300 milligrams of calcium, so an adult who drinks 2 to 3 cups of milk a day is well on the way to meeting daily calcium needs. Pregnant and lactating teenagers need more (see Table 8–4). The other dairy food that contains comparable amounts of calcium is cheese. One slice of cheese (1 ounce) contains about two-thirds as much calcium as a cup of milk. Cottage cheese, however, is a poor source of calcium. Snapshot 8–1 on page 186 shows foods that are rich in calcium, and the next box suggests ways of adding calcium to meals.

Table 8–4
Recommended Fluid Milk Intakes

AGE	RECOMMENDED INTAKE
Children	2 c
Teenagers and young adults	3 c
Adults	2 c
Pregnant and lactating women	3 c
Pregnant and lactating teens	4 c
Women past menopause	3 c

Some foods offer large amounts of calcium because of fortification. Calcium-fortified orange juice, high-calcium milk (milk with extra calcium added), and calcium-fortified bread are examples.

Among the vegetables, mustard greens, kale, parsley, watercress, and broccoli are good sources of available calcium. Some dark green, leafy vegetables—notably spinach and Swiss chard—appear to be calcium rich but actually provide very little, if any, calcium to the body. These foods contain binders that prevent calcium absorption.

Apparently, all fibers in plant foods—cellulose, hemicellulose, pectin, and others—bind calcium to some extent, as do phytic, oxalic, and uronic acids.

Snapshot 8–1 Calcium

RDA for adults: 800 mg/day

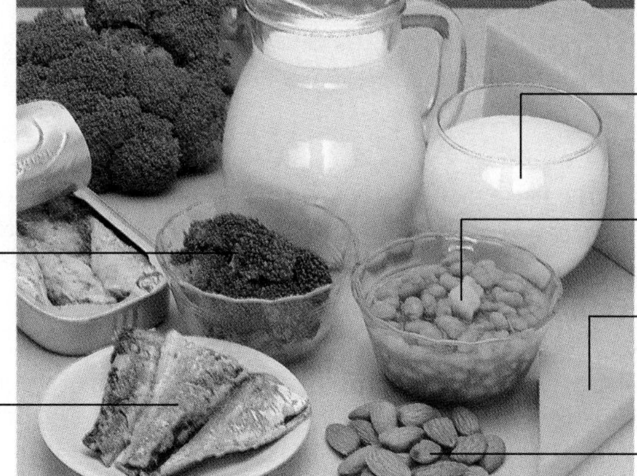
Milk: 316 mg per cup
Pork and beans: 77 mg per ½ c
Broccoli: 36 mg per ½ c cooked
Cheddar cheese: 305 mg per 1½ oz
Sardines: 324 mg per 3 oz
Almonds: 80 mg per 2 tbs

Two cups of milk supply the following percentages of the nutrients an adult man needs:

- Calcium: 75%
- Vitamin D: 50%
- Protein: 25%
- Vitamin A: 30%
- Thiamin: 13%
- Riboflavin: 50%
- Plus 24 g of carbohydrate in the form of lactose.

People may think that taking a calcium supplement is preferable to getting calcium from food, but foods offer important fringe benefits. For example, drinking 2 cups of milk fortified with vitamins A and D will supply substantial percentages of the nutrients listed in the margin. Furthermore, calcium absorption is enhanced by the vitamin D, lactose, fat, and possibly other nutrients in the milk. A calcium supplement supplies only calcium, and in a less absorbable form.

HOW TO Add Calcium to Daily Meals

Many people cannot or will not drink enough milk to meet recommendations. To help deliver calcium, try the following suggestions:

1. Powdered nonfat milk is an excellent and inexpensive source of calcium and can be added to many foods (such as baked products and meatloaf) during preparation.
2. Yogurt and kefir (fermented dairy products) are acceptable substitutes for regular milk.
3. Puddings, custards, and baked goods can be prepared using appreciable amounts of milk.
4. Strict vegetarians and people who are either allergic to milk or lactose intolerant can use calcium-rich milk and cheese substitutes such as calcium-fortified soy milk or tofu (bean curd).
5. Small fish, such as canned sardines, and other canned fish prepared with their bones, such as canned salmon, are also rich in calcium.

milk allergy: the most common food allergy; caused by the protein in raw milk. Milk allergy is sometimes overcome by cooking the milk to denature the protein and is sometimes cured by abstinence from, and gradual reintroduction to, milk.

The body is able to regulate its absorption of calcium by altering its production of the calcium-binding protein aided by vitamin D. More of this protein is made if more calcium is needed. Infants and children absorb up to 75 percent of ingested calcium; and pregnant women, about 50 percent. Other adults, who are not growing, absorb about 30 percent. Also, calcium seems to be better absorbed if accompanied by an approximately equal amount of phosphorus.

Phosphorus

Phosphorus is the second most abundant mineral in the body. About 85 percent of it is found combined with calcium in the crystals of the bones and teeth.

The concentration of phosphorus in the blood is less than half that of calcium. But as part of one of the body's major buffers (phosphoric acid), phosphorus is found in all body cells. Phosphorus is a part of DNA and RNA, the genetic code material present in every cell. Thus phosphorus is necessary for all growth. Phosphorus also plays many key roles in energy transfers occurring during cellular metabolism.

Animal protein is the best source of phosphorus because the mineral is so abundant in the cells of animals. Recommended intakes for phosphorus are the same as those for calcium, except during infancy. Deficiencies are unknown. A summary of facts about phosphorus appears in Table 8–6.

Magnesium

Magnesium barely qualifies as a major mineral. Only about 1¾ ounces of magnesium are present in the body of a 130-pound person, over half of it in the bones. Most of the rest is in the muscles, heart, liver, and other soft tissues, with only 1 percent in the body fluids. Bone magnesium seems to be a reservoir to ensure that some will be on hand for vital reactions regardless of recent dietary intake.

Magnesium is critical to the operation of hundreds of enzymes. Magnesium acts in all the cells of the soft tissues, where it forms part of the protein-making machinery and is necessary for the release of energy. Magnesium helps relax muscles after contraction and promotes resistance to tooth decay by holding calcium in tooth enamel.

Magnesium Deficiency Magnesium deficiency can result from vomiting, diarrhea, alcohol abuse, or protein malnutrition; after surgery in people who have been fed incomplete fluids intravenously for too long; or in people using diuretics. A severe deficiency causes tetany, an extreme and prolonged contraction of the muscles much like the reaction of the muscles when calcium levels fall. Magnesium deficiencies are also thought to cause the hallucinations experienced during withdrawal from alcohol intoxication.

Some research suggests a link between magnesium deficiency and heart problems such as heart rhythm disturbances and heart disease.[17] For example, a five-year follow-up study of men who were part of a large

Snapshot 8–2 Magnesium

RDA for men: 350 mg/day
RDA for women: 280 mg/day

Oysters: 93 mg per 3 oz steamed

Dried figs: 33 mg per ¼ c

Black-eyed peas: 45 mg per ½ c cooked

Spinach: 78 mg per ½ c cooked

Baked potato: 55 mg per whole small potato

Sunflower seeds (shelled): 21 mg per 2 tbs

heart disease study found that those with heart disease had significantly lower daily magnesium intakes than those without heart disease.[18]

Magnesium shows promise in the treatment of heart attacks. In one large study of more than 2000 heart attack victims, treatment with magnesium reduced complications and death as effectively as drugs.[19]

Magnesium Intakes and Food Sources Dietary intakes of magnesium average about three-quarters of the RDA for both men and women in the United States.[20] Dietary intake data do not, however, assess the nutrient contribution of water. In various parts of the country, the water contains both calcium and magnesium and is known as "hard" water. Hard water can contribute significantly to magnesium intakes.

Magnesium-rich food sources (Snapshot 8–2) include dark green, leafy vegetables, nuts, legumes, whole-grain breads and cereals, seafood, chocolate, and cocoa. Magnesium is easily lost from foods during processing, so unprocessed foods are the best choices.

Chloride

The chloride ion is the major negative ion of the fluids outside the cells, where it occurs primarily in association with sodium. Chloride can move freely across cell membranes and so is also found inside the cells in association with potassium. Like sodium, chloride is critical to maintaining fluid, electrolyte, and acid-base balance in the body. In the stomach, the chloride ion is part of hydrochloric acid, which maintains the strong acidity of the stomach.

Estimated minimum requirement for chloride: 750 mg/day.

Salt is a major food source of chloride, and as with sodium, processed foods are a major contributor of this nutrient in people's diets. There is not an established RDA for chloride, but an estimated minimum requirement has been determined for adults.

Sulfur

The body does not use sulfur by itself as a nutrient. Sulfur is included here because it occurs in essential nutrients that the body does use, such as thiamin and certain amino acids. Sulfur is present in all proteins and plays its most important role in helping strands of protein to assume a particular shape and hold it. Thus sulfur helps the proteins to do their specific jobs, such as enzyme work. Skin, hair, and nails contain some of the body's more rigid proteins, and they have a high sulfur content.

Amino acids containing sulfur are methionine and cysteine. Cysteine in one part of a protein chain can bind to cysteine in another part of the chain by way of a sulfur-sulfur bridge, thus helping to stabilize the protein structure.

There is no recommended intake for sulfur, and no deficiencies are known. Only a person who lacks protein to the point of severe deficiency will lack the sulfur-containing amino acids.

The Trace Minerals

Figure 8–1, at the beginning of this chapter, shows how tiny the quantities of trace minerals in the human body are. If you could remove all of them from your body, you would have only a bit of dust, hardly enough to fill a teaspoon. Yet each of the trace minerals performs some vital role for which no substitute will do. A deficiency of any of them can be fatal, and an excess of many can be equally deadly.

The committee on RDA has established recommended dietary intakes for the best-known trace elements—iron, zinc, iodine, and selenium. Tentative ranges for safe and adequate daily intakes of others are also published. Still others are recognized as essential nutrients for some animals, but not proven to be required for human beings (see Table 8–5). Still others are under study to determine whether they, too, perform indispensable roles in the body.

Table 8–5
Trace Minerals

RDA NUTRIENTS
Iron
Zinc
Iodine
Selenium
SAFE AND ADEQUATE DAILY DIETARY INTAKES ESTABLISHED
Copper
Manganese
Fluoride
Chromium
Molybdenum
KNOWN ESSENTIAL FOR ANIMALS; HUMAN REQUIREMENTS UNDER STUDY
Arsenic
Nickel
Silicon
Boron
KNOWN ESSENTIAL FOR SOME ANIMALS; NO EVIDENCE THAT INTAKE BY HUMANS IS EVER LIMITING; NO RDA NECESSARY
Cobalt

Note: The evidence for requirements and essentiality is weak for the trace minerals cadmium, lead, lithium, tin, and vanadium.

Iron

Every living cell—both plant and animal—contains iron. Most of the iron in the body is a component of the proteins hemoglobin in red blood cells and myoglobin in muscle cells. Hemoglobin in the blood carries oxygen from the lungs to tissues throughout the body. Myoglobin holds oxygen for the muscles to use when they contract. Both the hemoglobin and myoglobin molecules contain iron, which helps them carry and hold oxygen and then release it. As part of many enzymes, iron is vital to the processes by which cells generate energy. Iron is also needed to make new cells, amino acids, hormones, and neurotransmitters.

The special provisions the body makes for iron's handling show that it is as precious as gold is to a king. For example, when a red blood cell dies, the liver saves the iron and returns it to the bone marrow, which uses it to build new red blood cells. Thus only tiny amounts of iron are lost, principally in urine, sweat, shed skin, and blood (if bleeding occurs).

Only about 10 to 15 percent of dietary iron is normally absorbed; but if the body's supply is diminished or if the need increases for any reason (such as pregnancy), absorption increases. The body makes several provisions for absorbing iron. A special protein in the intestinal cells captures iron and holds it in reserve for release into the body as needed; another protein transfers the iron to a special iron-carrier in the blood. The blood

hemoglobin: the oxygen-carrying protein of the red blood cells.
hemo = blood
globin = globular protein

myoglobin: the oxygen-carrying protein of the muscle cells.
myo = muscle

transferrin (trans-FERR-in)**:** the body's iron-carrying protein.

The storage proteins are **ferritin** (FERR-i-tin) and **hemosiderin** (heem-oh-SID-er-in).

One common test for iron deficiency measures the **hemoglobin concentration** of blood.
Norms for adults:
Men: 13–16 g/100 ml.
Women: 12–16 g/100 ml.
Norms for children:
Ages 2–5: 11 g/100 ml.
Ages 6–12: 11.5 g/100 ml.
Note that hemoglobin is measured in grams per 100 ml, but often just the number of grams alone is used in speaking of it: "hemoglobin, 14."

Another common test, the **hematocrit,** represents the percentage of red blood cells in a whole blood sample.
Norms for adults:
Men: 40 to 54%.
Women: 37 to 47%.
Norms for children:
Ages 2 to 5: 34%.
Ages 6 to 12: 37%.

Transferrin can be measured directly or estimated by measuring the **total iron-binding capacity (TIBC)** and the **transferrin saturation.**

iron deficiency: having depleted iron stores.

iron-deficiency anemia: a blood iron deficiency that results in small, pale, red blood cells.

In all people including those who are dark skinned, a sign of iron deficiency can be observed by looking in the corner of the eye. The eye lining, normally pink, will be very pale, even white. The skin of a fair person who is anemic may be noticeably pale.

protein (transferrin) carries the iron to tissues throughout the body. When more iron is needed, more of these special proteins are produced so that more than the usual amount of iron can be absorbed and carried. If there is a surplus of iron, special storage proteins in the liver, bone marrow, and other organs store it.

Iron Deficiency If absorption cannot compensate for losses or low dietary intakes, and stores are used up, iron deficiency sets in. Because so much of the body's iron is in the blood, iron losses are greatest whenever blood is lost. Women's menstrual losses make a woman's iron needs twice as great as a man's. Women are also prone to iron deficiency because they are, on average, smaller than men and eat less food. Pregnancy places further iron demands on women. The information about iron in foods that appears later in this section is especially important for women. The iron needs of physically active people are discussed in Chapter 10.

Tests for Iron Deficiency The most common tests for iron deficiency measure the number and size of the red blood cells and the cells' hemoglobin content. Before these levels fall, at the very beginning of an iron deficiency, the transferrin concentration *rises.* A sensitive test that will detect a developing iron deficiency before it is full-blown measures the amount of transferrin in the blood and the amount of iron it is carrying. Other tests measure iron stores.

Iron Deficiency and Anemia The distinction between iron deficiency and anemia is important. They often go hand in hand, but people can be iron deficient without being anemic. The term *iron deficiency* refers to depleted body iron *stores.* The term *anemia* refers to the depletion of iron in the red blood cells, a severe deficiency that results in a lowered *hemoglobin* concentration. In anemia, new red blood cells are smaller and lighter red than normal (Figure 8–4). The depleted cells cannot carry enough oxygen from the lungs to the tissues, so energy release in the cells is hindered. Every cell of the body feels the effect.

The classic symptoms of iron deficiency, long known, are fatigue, weakness, headaches, apathy, and pallor. A more recently recognized symptom is poor tolerance to cold. One way the body accelerates heat production when the environmental temperature falls involves the neurotransmitter norepinephrine and the thyroid hormones, which speed up the metabolic rate. Iron deficiency impairs temperature regulation in both animals and human beings, probably by interfering with the normal production of these compounds.[21]

Iron deficiency less severe than anemia produces symptoms too. Long before the mass of the red blood cells is affected and anemia is diagnosed, a developing iron deficiency affects behavior. Even at slightly lowered iron levels, the complete oxidation of pyruvate is impaired, reducing physical work capacity and productivity. Children deprived of iron become irritable, restless, and unable to pay attention. These symptoms are among the first to appear when the body's iron begins to fall and among the first to disappear when iron intake is increased again.

Several mechanisms by which iron deficiency may affect behavior have been proposed. The one most often discussed and researched pro-

Figure 8–4
Normal and Anemic Blood Cells

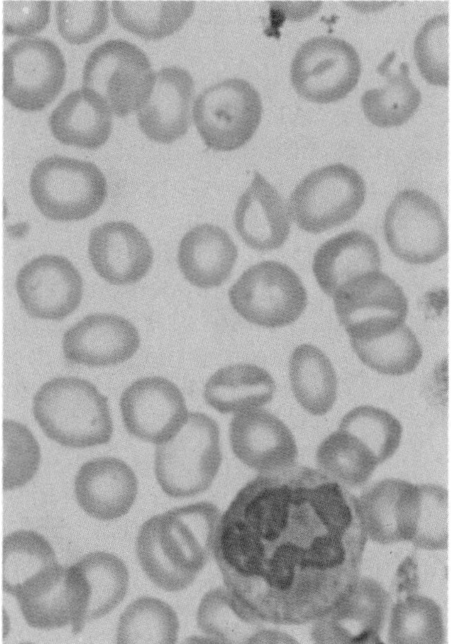

Normal blood cells. Both size and color are normal. The one large, purple cell is a normal white blood cell, stained purple.

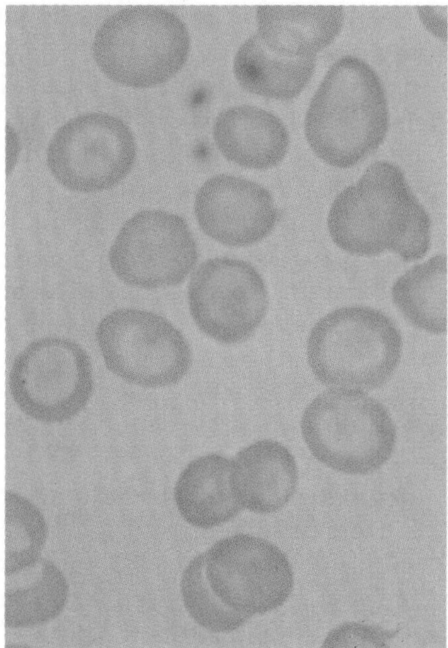

Blood cells in microcytic hypochromic anemia such as that caused by iron deficiency. These cells are small and pale because they contain less hemoglobin.

poses that even in the earliest stages of iron deficiency, a deficit of iron-dependent neurotransmitter receptors in the brain alters behavior.[22]

A curious symptom seen in some iron-deficient individuals is an appetite for ice, clay, paste, and other nonnutritious substances. Such people have been known to eat as many as eight trays of ice in a day, for example. This behavior, which has been named *pica,* has been observed for years, especially in women and children of low-income groups who are deficient in either iron or zinc. Pica clears up dramatically within days after iron is given, long before the red blood cells respond.

microcytic hypochromic anemia: small, pale, red blood cells.
micro = small
cytic = cells
hypo = too little
chrom = color

There is more about the effects of iron deficiency on children's behavior in Chapter 16.

pica (PIE-ka)**:** a craving for nonfood substances; also known as *geophagia* (jee-oh-FAY-jee-uh) when referring to clay-eating behavior.
picus = woodpecker or magpie
geo = earth
phagein = to eat

Caution on Self-Diagnosis Low hemoglobin may reflect an inadequate iron intake, and if it does, the physician may prescribe iron supplements. However, any nutrient deficiency or disease or agent that interferes with hemoglobin synthesis, disrupts hemoglobin function, or causes a loss of red blood cells can precipitate anemia. Nutrient deficiencies other than iron that can cause anemia include, among others, those of protein, vitamin B_6, folate, vitamin B_{12}, vitamin C, vitamin A, vitamin E, and copper. Nonnutritional causes of anemia include excessive blood loss, infections, and some chronic diseases.

Feeling fatigued, weak, and apathetic is thus a sign that something is wrong, but does not indicate that a person should take iron supplements; it means that the person should consult a physician. In fact, taking iron supplements may be the worst possible thing a person can do, because such supplements can mask a serious medical condition, such as hidden bleeding from cancer or an ulcer. Furthermore, a person can waste precious time in not seeking treatment. Remember, don't self-diagnose.

Prevalence of Iron Deficiency Worldwide, iron deficiency is the most common nutrient deficiency.[23] Iron-deficiency anemia affects an estimated 15 percent of the world's population, with the highest prevalence in developing countries.[24] Infants (6 months old or older), young children, and pregnant women are especially vulnerable. In the United States, the overall prevalence of iron-deficiency anemia has declined considerably in the last decade or so. Adult women's improved iron status may be attributed to such factors as improved socioeconomic status, iron fortification, increased use of vitamin C and iron supplements, and reduced menstrual blood loss thanks to birth control pills.[25] The iron status of infants and young children in the United States has also improved in the last decade thanks to more widespread breastfeeding and greater use of iron-fortified infant formula.[26]

Causes of Iron Deficiency The cause of iron deficiency is usually inadequate intake from ignorance of what foods to choose, from sheer lack of food altogether, or from high consumption of iron-poor foods. In the Western world, high sugar and fat intakes are often responsible for low iron intakes. Blood loss is the primary nonnutritional cause, especially in poor regions of the world where parasitic infections of the GI tract may lead to blood loss.

Binding proteins in the intestinal cells (mucosal ferritin and mucosal transferrin) capture and hold unneeded iron to be shed with the cells, thereby forming a **mucosal block** to iron absorption.

iron overload: toxicity from iron overdose. There are two types, hemochromatosis and hemosiderosis.

hemochromatosis (heem-oh-crome-a-TOE-siss)**:** iron overload characterized by deposits of iron-containing pigment in many tissues, with tissue damage. Hemochromatosis is a hereditary defect in iron metabolism.

hemosiderosis (heem-oh-sid-er-OH-sis)**:** iron overload characterized by excessive iron deposits in hemosiderin, the normal iron-storage protein.

Iron Overload Iron toxicity is rare but not unknown. Normally, the body protects itself against absorbing too much iron by setting up a block in the intestinal cells. The system can be overwhelmed, however, and iron overload is the result.

Two kinds of iron overload are known. One (hemochromatosis) is caused by a hereditary defect, the other (hemosiderosis) by the ingestion of too much iron, usually in combination with excessive alcohol consumption. The alcohol abuser is particularly prone to iron overload because alcohol enhances the absorption of iron. In addition, certain wines contain substantial amounts of iron. Regardless of the cause, tissue damage, especially to the liver, results. Infections are likely because bacteria thrive in iron-rich blood.

Iron overload occurs more commonly in men than in women. An argument against the fortification of foods with iron to protect women is that it might put more men at risk of overload. Indeed, some evidence from Sweden, where foods are generously fortified with iron, indicates that food fortification has increased the incidence of iron overload in men.

Iron Poisoning The rapid ingestion of massive amounts of iron can cause sudden death. The most common cause of accidental poisoning in small children is ingestion of iron supplements or vitamins with iron.[27] The American Academy of Pediatrics has urged the Food and Drug Administration (FDA) to improve the labeling of iron-containing drugs and supplements. As few as 6 to 12 tablets have caused death in a child.[28] A child suspected of iron poisoning should be rushed to the hospital to have the stomach pumped. Thirty minutes can make a crucial difference.

Iron Recommendations The usual Western mixed diet provides only about 6 to 7 milligrams of iron in every 1000 kcalories. The recom-

Snapshot 8–3 Iron

RDA for men: 10 mg/day
RDA for women: 15 mg/day

Swiss chard: 2.0 mg per ½ c cooked

Clams: 25.2 mg per 3 oz steamed

Navy beans: 2.2 mg per ½ c cooked

Sirloin steak: 2.8 mg per 3 oz cooked

Dried figs: 1.3 mg per ¼ c

Tofu: 6.7 mg per ½ c

mended daily intake for an adult man is 10 milligrams; most men easily eat more than 2000 kcalories, so a man can meet his iron needs without special effort. The recommendation for women during childbearing years, however, is 15 milligrams.[29] Because women have higher iron needs and typically consume fewer than 2000 kcalories per day, they have trouble achieving appropriate iron intakes. On the average, women receive only 10 to 11 milligrams of iron per day. A woman who wants to meet her iron needs from foods must emphasize the most iron-rich foods in every food group.

About 40 % of the iron in meat, fish, and poultry is bound into molecules of **heme** (HEEM), the iron-holding part of the hemoglobin and myoglobin proteins. This heme iron is much more absorbable than nonheme iron.

Iron in Foods Iron occurs in two forms in foods, one of which is up to ten times more absorbable than the other. The absorbable form is heme iron, which is bound into the iron-carrying proteins hemoglobin and myoglobin in meats, poultry, and fish. The less absorbable form is nonheme iron, found in meats and also in plant foods. Heme iron contributes a smaller portion of the iron consumed by most people, but healthy people absorb it at a fairly constant rate of about 23 percent. People absorb nonheme iron at a lower rate (2 to 20 percent); its absorption depends on dietary factors and iron stores. Most of the iron people consume is nonheme iron from vegetables, grains, eggs, meat, fish, and poultry. Snapshot 8–3 shows the iron found in usual serving sizes of different foods.

To absorb a maximum of iron from the foods you eat, you need to know what enhances iron absorption: MFP factor and vitamin C. Meat, fish, and poultry contain a factor (MFP factor) other than heme that promotes the absorption of iron. MFP factor even enhances the absorption of nonheme iron from other foods eaten at the same time. Vitamin C eaten in the same meal also doubles or triples nonheme iron absorption. Additionally, cooking with iron skillets can contribute iron to the diet. Tea and coffee interfere with iron absorption. The next box offers suggestions on obtaining adequate iron.

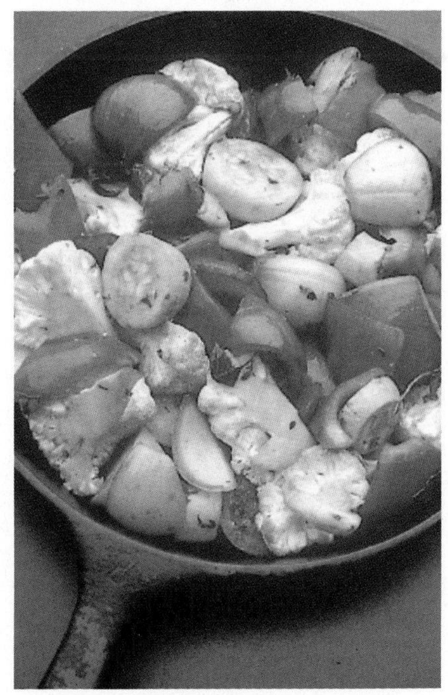

The old-fashioned iron skillet contributes additional iron to foods.

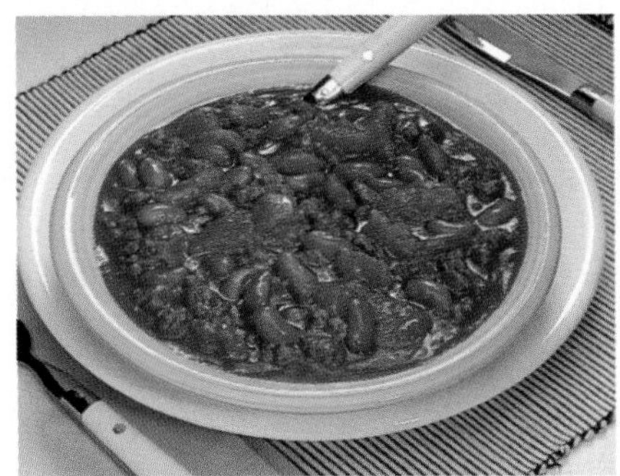

The meat and tomatoes in this chili help the eater to absorb iron from the beans.

Overconsumption of milk can easily lead to iron deficiency in children; the resulting anemia is known as *milk anemia.*

Enrichment and fortification are defined on p. 154.

HOW TO Add Iron to Daily Meals

The following set of guidelines can be used for planning an iron-rich diet:

- *Milk and cheese.* Don't overdo foods from the milk group; they are poor sources of iron. But don't omit them either, because they are rich in calcium. Drink nonfat milk to free kcalories to be invested in iron-rich foods.
- *Meats.* Use liver and other organ meats frequently, perhaps every week or two. Meat, fish, and poultry are excellent iron sources.
- *Meat alternates.* Include legumes frequently. A cup of peas or beans can supply up to 7 milligrams of iron.
- *Breads and cereals.* Use only whole-grain, enriched, and fortified products (iron is one of the enrichment nutrients).
- *Vegetables.* The dark green, leafy vegetables are rich in vitamin C and iron. Eat vitamin C–rich vegetables often to enhance absorption of the iron from foods eaten with them.
- *Fruits.* Dried fruits, such as raisins, apricots, peaches, and prunes, are high in iron. Eat vitamin C–rich fruits often with iron-containing foods.

Zinc

Zinc is a versatile, active trace element. Wherever protein is, zinc is, too, helping with the jobs that proteins do. More than 100 enzymes require zinc as a cofactor. These zinc-requiring enzymes perform tasks in the eyes, liver, kidneys, muscles, skin, bones, and male reproductive organs. Zinc works with the enzymes that make genetic material; manufacture heme; digest food; metabolize carbohydrate, protein, and fat; liberate vitamin A from storage in the liver; and dispose of damaging free radicals. Zinc also interacts with platelets in blood clotting, affects thyroid hormone function, assists in immune function, and affects behavior and learning performance. Zinc is needed to produce the active form of vitamin A in visual pigments and is essential to wound healing, taste perception, the making of sperm, and fetal development. When zinc deficiency occurs, it impairs all these and other functions.

The body's handling of zinc differs from that of iron, but with some interesting similarities. For example, like iron, extra zinc that enters the body is held within the intestinal cells, and only the amount needed is released into the bloodstream. As with iron, a person's zinc status influences the percentage of zinc the person absorbs from the diet; if more is needed, more is absorbed.

Zinc's main transport vehicle in the blood is the protein albumin. Research suggests that circulating albumin is a main determinant of zinc absorption.[30] This may account for observations that zinc absorption declines in conditions that lower plasma albumin concentrations—for example, pregnancy and malnutrition.

Zinc Deficiency Zinc deficiency in human beings was first reported in the 1960s from studies of growing children and male adolescents in Egypt, Iran, and Turkey. Their diets were typically low in zinc and high in fiber and phytates (which impair zinc absorption). The zinc deficiency was marked by dwarfism or severe growth retardation, as well as arrested sexual maturation—symptoms that were responsive to zinc supplementation.

Since that time, zinc deficiency has been recognized elsewhere and is known to affect more than growth. It drastically impairs immune function, causes loss of appetite, and, during pregnancy, may lead to developmental disorders.[31] A detailed list of symptoms of zinc deficiency is presented later in Table 8–6. Conditions other than poor diet that contribute to the development of zinc deficiency include loss of blood due to parasitic infections, climates that increase sweat losses, and clay eating.

Clay eating: see *pica,* p. 191.

Pronounced zinc deficiency is not widespread in developed countries, but deficiencies do occur in the most vulnerable groups of the U.S. population—pregnant women, young children, the elderly, and the poor. Research shows that even mild zinc deficiency can result in metabolic changes such as impaired immune response, abnormal taste, and abnormal dark adaptation (zinc is required to produce the active form of vitamin A, retinal, in visual pigments).[32]

Pregnant teenagers are particularly vulnerable because they need zinc for their own ongoing growth, as well as for the developing fetus. Persons on limited food intakes, such as those on weight-control regimens, may also be at risk. A warning to those following very-low-kcalorie or starvation diets: such diets cause not only a low zinc intake but also a loss of zinc from body tissues being broken down as a source of energy. Older people who eat little food may also have limited zinc intakes. People in the hospital with poor appetites or those receiving inadequate nutrition support are at risk. Certain drug therapies can impair zinc absorption.

Vegetarians, especially pregnant vegetarians, who consume large amounts of fiber, phytate, and dairy foods or low levels of protein need to scrutinize their diets for possible zinc deficiency. Populations dependent on food staples or cultural foods high in phytate and fiber content need to be evaluated as well for zinc status.

Zinc Toxicity Zinc is a relatively nontoxic element; however, it can be toxic if consumed in large enough quantities. A high zinc intake is known to produce copper-deficiency anemia by inducing the intestinal cells to synthesize large amounts of a protein that captures copper in a nonabsorbable form. Accidental consumption of high levels of zinc can cause vomiting, diarrhea, fever, exhaustion, and a host of other symptoms (see Table 8–6, later in the chapter). Large doses can even be fatal.

Zinc Recommendations and Food Sources The zinc RDA for men is 15 milligrams per day; for women, 12 milligrams. Survey data indicate that zinc intakes of adults in the United States fall short of the RDA.[33]

Zinc is most abundant in foods high in protein, such as shellfish (especially oysters), meats, and liver. As a rule of thumb, two ordinary servings a day of animal protein provide most of the zinc a healthy per-

Snapshot 8–4 Zinc

RDA for men: 15 mg/day
RDA for women: 12 mg/day

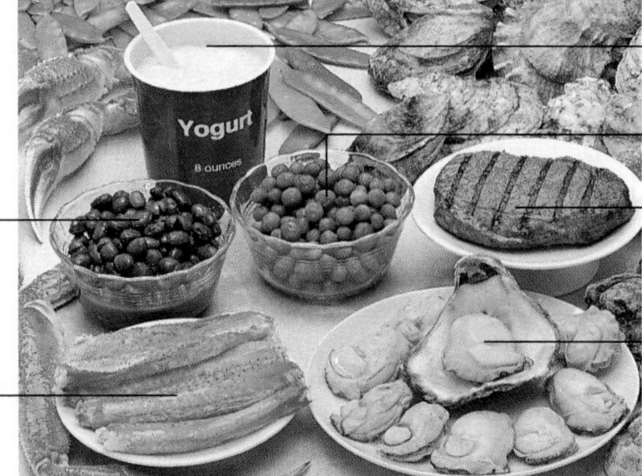
Yogurt
8 ounces
Yogurt: 2.2 mg per cup
Green peas: 1.0 mg per ½ c
Sirloin steak: 5.5 mg per 3 oz cooked
Oysters: 154 mg per 3 oz steamed
Black beans: 1.0 mg per ½ c cooked
Crabmeat: 3.6 mg per 3 oz steamed

son needs. Milk, eggs, and whole-grain products are good sources of zinc if eaten in large quantities. For infants, breast milk is a good source of zinc, which is more efficiently absorbed from human milk than from cow's milk. Commercial infant formulas are fortified with zinc, of course. Snapshot 8–4 shows zinc-rich foods.

Zinc supplements are not recommended except for an accurately diagnosed zinc deficiency or when needed for use as a drug to displace other ions in unusual medical circumstances. Normally, it should be possible to obtain enough zinc from the diet.

Selenium

selenium (se-LEEN-ee-um)**:** a trace element.

The enzyme of which selenium is a part is glutathione peroxidase, which destroys oxidative compounds that could otherwise oxidize other compounds in the cell.

The heart disease associated with selenium deficiency is named *Keshan disease* for one of the provinces of China where it was studied.

Selenium is a trace element that functions as part of an antioxidant enzyme. Selenium has a sparing effect on vitamin E and can substitute for vitamin E in some of that vitamin's antioxidant activities.[34] The question of whether selenium protects against the development of some cancers is currently under investigation. So far, the results are inconclusive. A recent discovery about selenium is that it plays a role in converting thyroid hormone to its active form.[35]

Selenium Deficiency Selenium's function as an antioxidant was, at first, the only evidence of its essentiality for human beings. The discovery that selenium deficiency has been the cause of heart disease in hundreds of thousands of children in China has spurred greater interest in selenium and intensified research efforts to learn more about this mineral.

Selenium Toxicity High doses of selenium are toxic. Selenium toxicity causes vomiting, diarrhea, loss of hair and nails, and lesions of the skin and nervous system. The inappropriate use of selenium supplements as an anticancer agent opens the way to selenium overdose.[36]

Selenium Recommendations and Intakes Anyone who eats a normal diet composed mostly of unprocessed foods need not worry about meeting the selenium RDA. Selenium is widely distributed in foods such as meats and shellfish and in vegetables and grains grown on selenium-rich soil. Some regions in the United States and Canada produce crops on selenium-poor soil, but people are protected from deficiency because they eat selenium-rich meat and supermarket foods transported from other regions.

Selenium RDA:
55 μg/day (women).
70 μg/day (men).

Iodine

Iodine occurs in the body in minuscule amounts, but its principal role in human nutrition is well known, and the amount needed is well established. Iodine is an integral part of the thyroid hormones, which regulate body temperature, metabolic rate, reproduction, growth, the making of blood cells, nerve and muscle function, and more.

Iodine Deficiency When the iodine concentration in the blood is low, the cells of the thyroid gland enlarge in an attempt to trap as many particles of iodine as possible. If the gland enlarges until it is visible, the swelling is called a simple goiter. As many as 800 million people are at the borderline of iodine deficiency, and 200 million people worldwide have goiter.[37] In all but 4 percent of these cases, the cause is iodine deficiency. As for the 4 percent (8 million), those people have goiter because they overconsume plants of the cabbage family and others that contain an antithyroid substance whose effect is not counteracted by dietary iodine.

In addition to causing sluggishness and weight gain, an iodine deficiency may have serious effects on the development of a fetus. Severe thyroid undersecretion during pregnancy causes the extreme and irreversible mental and physical retardation known as cretinism. A cretin has an IQ as low as 20 (100 is normal) and a face and body with many abnormalities. Iodine deficiency is one of the world's most common preventable causes of mental retardation.[38] Much of the mental retardation associated with cretinism can be averted if the pregnant woman's deficiency is detected and treated in time.

goiter (GOY-ter)**:** an enlargement of the thyroid gland due to an iodine deficiency, malfunction of the gland, or overconsumption of a thyroid antagonist. Goiter caused by iodine deficiency is *simple goiter.*

A thyroid antagonist found in food, which causes *toxic goiter,* is called a **goitrogen.**

cretinism (CREE-tin-ism)**:** an iodine-deficiency disease characterized by mental and physical retardation.

Iodine Toxicity Excessive intakes of iodine can enlarge the thyroid gland, just as deficiencies can. In infants, the goiterlike condition can be so severe as to block the airways and cause suffocation.

Iodine Sources and Intakes The ocean is the world's major source of iodine. In coastal areas, seafood, water, and even iodine-containing sea mist are important iodine sources. Further inland, the amount of iodine in the diet is variable and generally reflects the amount present in the soil in which plants are grown or on which animals graze. In areas of the United States with iodine-poor soil (most notably in the Plains states), the use of iodized salt has largely wiped out the iodine deficiency that once was widespread.

People sometimes wonder whether sea salt, made by drying ocean water, is preferable to purified sodium chloride for use in the saltshaker. Sea salt does contain trace minerals, but it loses its iodine during the drying process. Thus, in regions where goiter is a risk, iodized sodium chloride is the salt to choose.

The need for iodine is easy to meet by consuming seafood, vegetables grown in iodine-rich soil, and (in iodine-poor areas) iodized salt. In the United States, you have to read the label to find out whether salt is iodized; in Canada, all table salt is iodized.

Iodine RDA: 150 μg/day.

Iodine intakes in the United States rose dramatically for several decades but are currently declining. The emphasis on salt-restricted diets to control high blood pressure is no doubt a contributing factor to declining intakes. The FDA has found the typical intake to be about 250 micrograms for men and about 170 micrograms for women, excluding intakes from iodized salt; thus deficiency is not a problem.[39]

Copper

The body contains about 100 milligrams of copper.[40] The primary function of copper in the body is to serve as a constituent of enzymes. The copper-containing enzymes have diverse metabolic roles: they catalyze the formation of hemoglobin, help manufacture the protein collagen, assist in the healing of wounds, and help maintain the sheaths around nerve fibers. One of copper's most vital roles is to help cells use iron. Like iron, copper is needed in many reactions related to respiration and energy release.

Copper Deficiency Copper deficiency is rare but not unknown. It has been seen in children with kwashiorkor and with iron-deficiency anemia, and it can severely disturb growth and metabolism. Excess zinc interferes with copper absorption and can cause deficiency.

Copper Toxicity Toxicity from foods is unlikely, but supplements can cause it. Intakes of 10 to 15 milligrams cause toxicity symptoms, notably diarrhea and vomiting.[41] Larger amounts can be fatal.

Estimated safe and adequate dietary intake for copper: 1.5 to 3.0 mg/day.

Copper Recommendations and Food Sources No RDA is set for copper, but an estimated safe and adequate daily dietary intake has been established. The best food sources of copper include organ meats, seafood, nuts, and seeds.

Manganese

The human body contains a tiny 20 milligrams of manganese, mostly in the bones and glands. Animal studies suggest that manganese cooperates with many enzymes, helping to facilitate dozens of different metabolic processes. Deficiencies of manganese have not been noted in people, but toxicity may be severe. Miners who inhale large quantities of manganese dust on the job over prolonged periods show many symptoms of a brain disease, with frightening abnormalities in appearance and behavior. This example of manganese underscores the fact that it is as important not to overdose as it is to have an adequate intake. The committee on RDA emphasizes this point by adding a special warning to its trace mineral table: "not to exceed the upper end of the range of recommended intakes."

Beware of supplements containing trace minerals. It is safer to consume a diet that provides foods from a variety of sources than to try to put together a combination of pills that will meet all your needs without causing toxicity.

Manganese requirements are low, and many plant foods contain significant amounts of this trace mineral. Deficiencies are therefore unlikely.

Estimated safe and adequate dietary intake for manganese: 2.5 to 5.0 mg/day.

Fluoride

Only a trace of fluoride occurs in the human body, but research demonstrates that where diets are high in fluoride during the growing years, crystalline deposits in bones and teeth are larger and more perfectly formed. When bones and teeth become mineralized, first a crystal called hydroxyapatite forms from calcium and phosphorus. Then fluoride replaces the hydroxy portion of hydroxyapatite, forming fluorapatite, which makes the bones and teeth more resistant to decay. Once the teeth have erupted, the topical application of fluoride by way of toothpaste or mouth rinse continues to exert a caries-reducing effect.[42]

fluorapatite (floor-APP-uh-tite)**:** the stabilized form of bone and tooth crystal, in which fluoride has replaced the hydroxy portion of hydroxyapatite.

Fluoride Deficiency Where fluoride is lacking in the water supply, the incidence of dental decay is high. Fluoridation of water to raise its fluoride concentration to 1 part per million is recommended as an important public health measure. Those fortunate enough to have had sufficient fluoride during the tooth-forming years of infancy and childhood are protected throughout life from dental decay.[43] Dental problems are of great concern because they can lead to a multitude of other health problems affecting the whole body. Despite fluoride's value, violent disagreement often surrounds the introduction of fluoride to a community. Figure 8–5 shows the extent of fluoridation nationwide.

Fluoride Sources All normal diets include some fluoride, but drinking water is usually the most significant source. Fish and tea may supply substantial amounts.

In some areas, the natural fluoride concentration in water is high, and children's teeth develop with mottled enamel. Although this condition, called fluorosis, may not be harmful, it violates some people's prejudice that teeth should be white. In fact, such children's teeth may be extraordinarily decay resistant. Fluorosis does not usually occur in communities where fluoride is added to the water supply.

Estimated safe and adequate dietary intake for fluoride: 1.5 to 4.0 mg/day.

fluorosis (floor-OH-sis)**:** mottling of the tooth enamel from ingestion of too much fluoride during tooth development.

Chromium

Chromium is an essential mineral that participates in carbohydrate and lipid metabolism. Experiments on animals have shown that chromium works closely with the hormone insulin, facilitating the uptake of glucose into cells. One form of chromium occurs in association with several different complexes in foods. Best absorbed and most active is a small organic compound named the glucose tolerance factor (GTF). This compound has been purified from brewer's yeast, but its complete structure and function continue to elude researchers.

GTF (glucose tolerance factor)**:** a small organic compound containing chromium, which enhances insulin's action.

Figure 8–5
Fluoridation in the United States

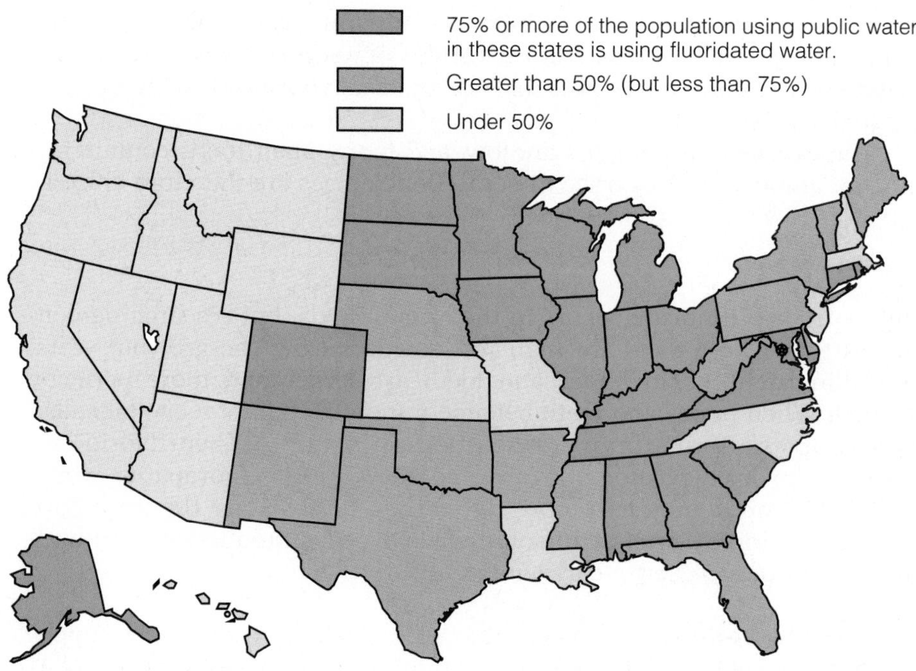

Source: Fluoridation Census 1989 Summary, U.S. Department of Health and Human Services, Public Health Service, Centers for Disease Control and Prevention, National Center for Prevention Services, Division of Oral Health, Atlanta, Ga. April 1993.

Estimated safe and adequate dietary intake for chromium: 50 to 200 µg/day.

Chromium deficiency is unlikely, given the small amount required and its presence in a variety of foods.[44] The more people eat refined foods, however, the less chromium they obtain from their diets. Unrefined foods such as liver, brewer's yeast, whole grains, nuts, and cheeses are the best sources.

Chromium deficiency is difficult to detect, but the effectiveness of insulin is severely impaired when chromium is lacking in the diet. A diabetes-like condition results. Chromium has been shown to remedy impaired carbohydrate metabolism in several groups of older people in the United States. Depleted tissue concentrations have been linked to growth failure in children with protein-energy malnutrition. Chromium toxicity from eating food sources of this element is unknown.

Other Trace Minerals

molybdenum (mo-LIB-duh-num): a trace element.

Estimated safe and adequate dietary intake for molybdenum: 75 to 250 µg/day.

The trace minerals have been known for decades, but their roles as nutrients are a recent surprise. Molybdenum has been recognized as an important mineral in human and animal physiology. It functions as a working part of several metal-containing enzymes, some of which are giant proteins. Deficiencies or toxicities of molybdenum are unknown in human beings.

Nickel is now recognized as important for the health of many body tissues. Nickel deficiencies harm the liver and other organs. Silicon is known to be involved in bone calcification, at least in animals. Tin is necessary for growth in animals, and probably in people also. Cobalt is recognized as the mineral in the large vitamin B_{12} molecule. The future may reveal that other trace minerals also play key roles: silver, mercury, lead, barium, and cadmium, for example. Even arsenic—famous as the death potion in many murder mysteries and known to be a carcinogen—may turn out to be an essential nutrient in tiny quantities.

In summary, the body requires trace minerals in tiny amounts, and they function in similar ways—assisting enzymes all over the body. Eating a diet that consists of a variety of foods is the best way to ensure an adequate intake of these important nutrients. Many dietary factors, including the trace minerals themselves, affect the absorption and availability of these nutrients.

Like the vitamins, the minerals perform a multitude of functions throughout the body. Table 8–6 offers a summary of facts about minerals in the body.

Table 8–6
The Minerals—A Summary

MINERAL NAME	CHIEF FUNCTIONS IN THE BODY	DEFICIENCY SYMPTOMS	TOXICITY SYMPTOMS	SIGNIFICANT SOURCES
Major Minerals				
Sodium	With chloride and potassium (electrolytes), maintains cells' normal fluid balance and acid-base balance in the body. Also critical to nerve impulse transmission.	Muscle cramps, mental apathy, loss of appetite.	Hypertension.	Salt, soy sauce, processed foods.
Potassium	Facilitates reactions, including the making of protein; the maintenance of fluid and electrolyte balance; the support of cell integrity; the transmission of nerve impulses; and the contraction of muscles, including the heart.	Deficiency accompanies dehydration; causes muscular weakness, paralysis, and confusion; can cause death.	Causes muscular weakness; triggers vomiting; if given into a vein, can stop the heart.	All whole foods: meats, milk, fruits, vegetables, grains, legumes.
Calcium	The principal mineral of bones and teeth. Also acts in normal muscle contraction and relaxation, nerve functioning, blood clotting, blood pressure, and immune defenses.	Stunted growth in children; adult bone loss (osteoporosis).	Excess calcium is excreted except in hormonal imbalance states (not caused by nutritional deficiency).	Milk and milk products, oysters, small fish (with bones), tofu (bean curd), greens, legumes.

(continued)

Table 8–6 *(continued)*

MINERAL NAME	CHIEF FUNCTIONS IN THE BODY	DEFICIENCY SYMPTOMS	TOXICITY SYMPTOMS	SIGNIFICANT SOURCES
Major Minerals *(continued)*				
Phosphorus	Important in cells' genetic material, in cell membranes as phospholipids, in energy transfer, and in buffering systems.	Phosphorus deficiency unknown.	Excess phosphorus may cause calcium excretion.	All animal tissues.
Magnesium	Another factor involved in bone mineralization, the building of protein, enzyme action, normal muscular contraction, transmission of nerve impulses, and maintenance of teeth.	Weakness; confusion; depressed pancreatic hormone secretion; if extreme, convulsions, bizarre movements (especially of eyes and face), hallucinations, and difficulty in swallowing. In children, growth failure.[a]	Not known; large doses have been taken in the form of the laxative Epson salts, without ill effects except diarrhea.	Nuts, legumes, whole grains, dark green vegetables, seafoods, chocolate, cocoa.
Chloride	Part of the hydrochloric acid found in the stomach and necessary for proper digestion.	Growth failure in children; muscle cramps, mental apathy, loss of appetite; can cause death (uncommon).	Normally harmless (the gas chlorine is a poison but evaporates from water); can cause vomiting.	Salt, soy sauce; moderate quantities in whole, unprocessed foods, large amounts in processed foods.
Sulfur	A component of certain amino acids; part of the vitamins biotin and thiamin and the hormone insulin; combines with toxic substances to form harmless compounds; stabilizes protein shape by forming sulfur-sulfur bridges.	None known; protein deficiency would occur first.	Would occur only if sulfur amino acids were eaten in excess; this (in animals) depresses growth.	All protein-containing foods.
Trace Minerals				
Iron	Part of the protein hemoglobin, which carries oxygen in the blood; part of the protein myoglobin in muscles, which makes oxygen available for muscle contraction; necessary for the utilization of energy.	Anemia: weakness, pallor, headaches, reduced resistance to infection, inability to concentrate, lowered cold tolerance.	Iron overload: infections, liver injury, possible increased risk of heart attack, acidosis, bloody stools, shock.	Red meats, fish, poultry, shellfish, eggs, legumes, dried fruits.

[a] A still more severe deficiency causes tetany, an extreme, prolonged contraction of the muscles similar to that caused by low blood calcium.

Table 8–6 *(continued)*

MINERAL NAME	CHIEF FUNCTIONS IN THE BODY	DEFICIENCY SYMPTOMS	TOXICITY SYMPTOMS	SIGNIFICANT SOURCES
Trace Minerals *(continued)*				
Zinc	Part of the hormone insulin and many enzymes; involved in making genetic material and proteins, immune reactions, transport of vitamin A, taste perception, wound healing, the making of sperm, and normal fetal development.	Growth failure in children, sexual retardation, loss of taste, poor wound healing.	Fever, nausea, vomiting, diarrhea, muscle incoordination, dizziness, anemia, accelerated atherosclerosis, kidney failure.	Protein-containing foods: meats, fish, shellfish, poultry, grains, vegetables.
Selenium	Part of an enzyme that breaks down reactive chemicals that harm cells; works with vitamin E.	Muscle discomfort, weakness, pancreas damage, heart disease (cardiomyopthy).	Nausea, abdominal pain, nail and hair changes, nerve damage.	Seafoods, organ meats, other meats, grains and vegetables depending on soil conditions.
Iodine	A component of the thyroid hormone thyroxine, which helps to regulate growth, development, and metabolic rate.	Goiter, cretinism.	Depressed thyroid activity; goiterlike thyroid enlargement.	Iodized salt; seafood; bread; plants grown in most parts of the country and animals fed those plants.

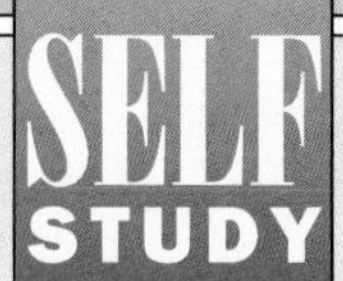

How Are Your Mineral Intakes?

1. Compare your intakes of minerals with the RDA (inside front cover) or RNI (Appendix B). Express each intake as a percentage of the recommended intake. For example, suppose you ingested 640 milligrams of calcium and your RDA is 800 milligrams. You ingested 80 percent (640 ÷ 800 × 100) of your RDA. If you had ingested 1400 milligrams of calcium, you would have ingested 175 percent (1400 ÷ 800 × 100) of your RDA. Use Form 9 to record your findings.

   Comment on your mineral intakes. For any mineral for which your intake fell below 80 percent of the recommendation, what were your best food sources? Could you eat more of them to bring your intake up to the recommended level? If not, what food or foods could you eat to increase your intake?
2. Compute your iron absorption from a meal of your choosing. Three factors go into the calculation. First, how much of the iron in the meal was heme iron and how much was nonheme iron? Second, how much vitamin C was in the meal? Third, how much total meat, fish, and poultry (MFP) was consumed? Here's how it works. Begin by answering these six questions:

(continued)

Self-Study (continued)

a. How much iron was from animal tissues (MFP)? ___ milligrams.
b. Forty percent of this is heme iron. ___ milligrams heme iron.
c. How much iron was from other sources? ___ milligrams.
d. This, plus 60 percent of the iron from animal tissues (MFP), is nonheme iron. ___ milligrams nonheme iron.
e. How much vitamin C was in the meal? Less than 25 milligrams is low; 25 to 75 milligrams is medium; more than 75 milligrams is high.
f. How much MFP was in the meal? Less than 1 ounce lean MFP is low; 1 to 3 ounces is medium; more than 3 ounces is high.

Now you're ready to calculate your iron absorption. You absorbed 23 percent of the heme iron (see step b) or ___ milligrams heme iron. Now, for nonheme iron, take your best response from step e or f. If either vitamin C or MFP was high, the availability of your nonheme iron was high. If neither was high but either was average, the availability of your nonheme iron was medium. If both were low, your nonheme iron had poor availability. You absorbed:

- High availability: 8 percent of the nonheme iron.
- Medium availability: 5 percent of the nonheme iron.
- Poor availability: 3 percent of the nonheme iron.
- Your absorption: ___ milligrams nonheme iron absorbed

Now compute your iron absorption by adding the two together:

___ milligrams heme iron absorbed.
___ milligrams nonheme iron absorbed.
Total = ___ milligrams iron absorbed.

Form 9
Mineral Intakes Compared with Recommended Intakes

	CALCIUM	IRON	ZINC	MAGNESIUM	PHOSPHORUS	POTASSIUM	SODIUM
My intake							
Recommended intake[a]							
My intake as a percentage of the recommended intake							

[a]RDA or RNI (Appendix B).

STUDY QUESTIONS

1. Describe some of the functions of water in the body.
2. List three sources of water intake and four routes for water excretion in the body.
3. What is ADH? Where does it exert its actions? What is aldosterone? How does it work?
4. How does the body use electrolytes to regulate fluid balance?
5. List the major minerals and describe a role of each mineral.
6. Where does most of the sodium in the diet come from?
7. Describe osteoporosis and list some of its risk factors.
8. Describe some of the body's special provisions for iron.
9. Why is the risk of iron deficiency greater for women than for men?
10. What is pica?
11. Why might pregnant vegetarian women be at risk for zinc deficiency?
12. What do selenium and vitamin E have in common?
13. Describe goiter.
14. How is fluoride important to the body?

NUTRITION IN PRACTICE 8

Nutrition and the Alcohol Abuser

Chapter 8 has discussed the last of the nutrients—water and the minerals. Next to the nutrients, probably the most influential substance people normally ingest is alcohol. Its impacts on nutrition are so profound that they deserve attention here.

Like all drugs, alcohol—properly termed ethanol, the active ingredient of alcoholic beverages—offers both benefits and hazards. Wine, beer, and other fermented beverages have been associated with pleasure and relaxation for more than 5000 years. People have always known that these beverages affected their moods, sensations, and behavior. Taken in moderation, alcohol can relax people, reduce their inhibitions, and encourage social interactions. Taken in excess, alcohol can be devastatingly destructive. This discussion focuses on the nutrition implications of alcohol abuse and alcohol addiction.

How many drinks constitute moderate use? And how much is a "drink"?

A drink is any alcoholic beverage that delivers ½ ounce of *pure ethanol:*

- 4 to 5 ounces of wine.
- 10 ounces of wine cooler.
- 12 ounces of beer.
- 1¼ ounce of hard liquor (80 proof whiskey, scotch, brandy, rum, gin, or vodka).

Because people's tolerances to alcohol differ, it is impossible to name an exact amount of alcohol per day that is appropriate for everyone, but authorities have attempted to set limits that are acceptable for most healthy adults. An accepted definition of moderation is not more than two drinks a day for the average-sized man and not more than one drink a day for the average-sized woman. This amount is supposed to be enough to elevate mood without causing any long-term harm to health. Doubtless, some people could consume slightly more; others could not handle nearly so much without significant risk.

Many people drink much more than one or two drinks a day, don't they?

Yes, and they may incur long-term harm to health as a result. Alcohol is the most widely abused drug in the world. Most people who choose to drink alcohol do so with few, if any, adverse consequences. Some people, however, encounter problems related to alcohol consumption. *Alcohol abuse* refers to patterns of drinking that result in health problems, social problems, or both. Alcohol abusers can often change their drinking behavior in response to simple warnings or explanations, thereby alleviating their alcohol-related problems. *Alcohol addiction,* often called alcoholism, refers to a disease that is characterized by abnormal alcohol-seeking behavior that leads to impaired control over drinking.*[45] Alcohol abusers and alcohol-addicted individuals experience many of the same harmful effects of alcohol consumption; the distinguishing characteristics of alcohol addiction are physical dependence on alcohol and an impaired ability to control alcohol intake. Alcohol abuse and addiction exert a heavy toll on the health of the 15.3 million people in the United States who meet the criteria for alcohol abuse, alcohol addiction, or both. The effects of alcohol on nutrition and metabolism—both directly and as a consequence of alcohol-related diseases—are significant. Every alcohol abuser and alcohol-addicted person should be considered at risk for poor nutrition status.

Would you please clarify exactly what alcoholism is?

In the *Eighth Special Report to the U.S. Congress on Alcohol and Health,* the U.S. Department of Health and Human Services defines alcoholism as a disease. The term is essentially synonymous with alcohol addiction. Alcoholism has four main clinical features:

- Tolerance—more and more alcohol is needed to produce the desired effects.
- Physical dependence—when alcohol consumption is interrupted, a characteristic withdrawal syndrome appears that is relieved by more alcohol.
- Impaired ability to regulate alcohol intake—at any time, once drinking has begun.

*Alcohol addiction means the same thing as alcohol dependence. This book uses the term addiction because it is more self-explanatory.

- Discomfort of abstinence—a "craving" for alcohol that can lead to relapse.

The alcohol-addicted person's craving for alcohol becomes marked by several features. The person thinks about alcohol a lot (*obsession*), drinks in spite of resolving not to (*broken promises*), and then suffers *remorse.* Such strong feelings about any substance signify addiction, but note that these feelings do not reflect personal inferiority. The person is simply someone whose internal makeup reacts in a special way to alcohol.

Some misconceptions about alcoholism can be dangerous and demand correction. For example, some people believe that alcoholism is related to the type of alcohol-containing beverage a person drinks. This is not true. People who drink only beer and wine can become alcohol addicts just as readily as people who drink hard liquors. It is not what people drink, but how much, that makes the difference. Another common misconception is that only morally degenerate people become addicted. Alcohol addiction does not single out people of low moral character or people of any particular age, race, education, social class, or income. It is true, however, that people of certain races and cultures tend to be more susceptible to alcohol addiction than others. Environment and heredity can contribute to such differences.

Why do you say that all alcohol abusers and alcohol-addicted people are at risk for poor nutrition status?

Alcohol produces euphoria, which depresses appetite, so heavy drinkers tend to eat poorly. Alcohol is rich in energy (7 kcalories per gram), but like pure fat or sugar kcalories, the kcalories from alcohol are empty kcalories. The more alcohol a person drinks, the less likely that he or she will eat enough food to obtain adequate nutrients. Table 8–7 shows the kcalories in typical alcoholic beverages. Nutrient deficiencies are an almost inevitable result of alcohol abuse, not only because the person who drinks obtains fewer nutrients from food but also because alcohol interferes with the body's ingestion, digestion, absorption, metabolism, and excretion of nutrients.

Alcohol is directly toxic to the liver. Studies of human beings and animals show that even when the diet is adequate, alcohol damages the liver.[46] Since alcohol can

Table 8–7
kCalories in Alcoholic Beverages and Mixers

BEVERAGE	AMOUNT (oz)	ENERGY (kcal)
Beer		
Regular	12	150
Light	12	100
Nonalcoholic	12	32
Distilled liquor (gin, rum, vodka, whiskey)		
80 proof	1½	100
86 proof	1½	105
90 proof	1½	110
Liqueurs		
Coffee liqueur	1½	175
Coffee and cream liqueur	1½	155
Crème de menthe	1½	185
Mixers		
Club soda	12	0
Cola	12	150
Cranberry juice cocktail	8	145
Diet drinks	12	2
Ginger ale	12	125
Grapefruit juice	8	95
Orange juice	8	110
Tomato or vegetable juice	8	45
Tonic	12	124
Wine		
Dessert	3½	160
Nonalcoholic	8	14
Red	3½	75
Rosé	3½	75
White	3½	70
Wine cooler	12	150

affect virtually every organ, other complications frequently develop that also change nutrient requirements. Some of these include anemia (Chapter 8), gastritis and ulcers (Chapter 20), pancreatitis (Chapter 21), and liver disease (Chapter 24).

Just how does alcohol alter nutrient metabolism?

With alcohol in the system, major changes occur in the way the body metabolizes many nutrients, particularly carbohydrate, fat, and protein. Dietary glucose and dietary fat are diverted to making fat, which may accumulate to the liver. In addition, alcohol metabolism in the liver results in structural changes in liver cells that can permanently alter the liver's ability to metabolize fatty acids, causing further fat accumulation.[47] Fatty liver, the first stage of liver deterioration in the heavy drinker (which can be reversed by abstinence from alcohol), can progress to cirrhosis (which is irreversible).

Alcohol also interferes with the body's use of protein in several ways. Large doses of alcohol inhibit protein synthesis in the brain. Alcohol has also been shown to inhibit the release of proteins in the liver, causing them to accumulate in liver cells.[48] Protein deficiency can develop, both from the depression of protein synthesis in the cells and from a poor diet. Alcohol also interferes with amino acid metabolism. The absorption and transport of several amino acids are impaired by high concentrations of alcohol, so that even the amino acids that a person eats are not used efficiently.

Does alcohol affect vitamin and mineral metabolism, too?

Yes. Alcohol interferes with the availability and activation of virtually every vitamin and many minerals. For example, as Figure 8–6 shows, alcohol impairs absorption of thiamin, folate, and other nutrients. Alcohol-induced liver injury impairs the activity of the liver enzyme that activates thiamin to its active form.

Alcohol's effect on folate is dramatic. When alcohol is present, the body behaves as if it were actively trying to expel folate from all its sites of action and storage. The liver, which normally contains enough folate to meet all needs, leaks folate into the blood. As the blood folate concentration rises, the body appears to have an excess of folate, and the kidneys are deceived into excreting it. The intestine normally releases and retrieves folate continuously, but it becomes damaged by folate deficiency and alcohol toxicity, so it fails to retrieve its own folate and misses out on any that may trickle in from food as well. Alcohol abuse causes a folate deficiency that devastates digestive system function.

Alcohol abuse alters metabolism of many other vitamins, including vitamins B_6, B_{12}, and A. One of the products of alcohol metabolism dislodges vitamin B_6 from its protective binding protein so that it is destroyed. Alcohol inhibits vitamin B_{12} absorption, both directly and indirectly, by suppressing the secretion of the factor that facilitates

Figure 8–6
Alcohol's Effect on Vitamin Absorption (Example)
In the presence of alcohol, intestinal cells fail to absorb thiamin, except at very high concentrations.

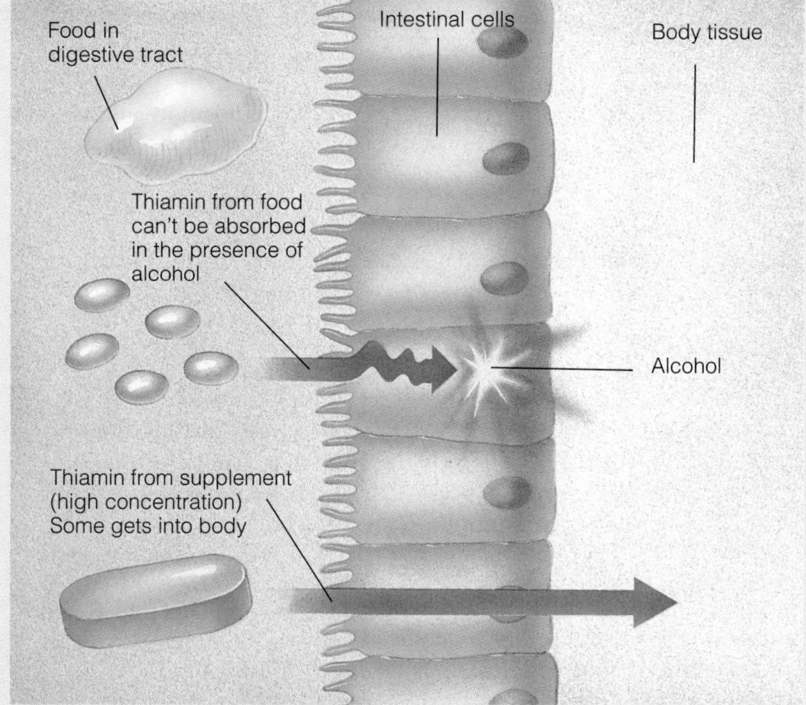

the vitamin's absorption from the intestine to the bloodstream. Alcohol does not impair absorption of vitamin A, but even moderate alcohol use has been shown to deplete liver stores of the vitamin.[49]

Alcohol also promotes water excretion by the kidneys. Important minerals, such as zinc, magnesium, and potassium, are lost with the water. So you see, alcohol profoundly affects nutrition status.

I see. What about alcohol's effect on body weight? I though alcohol had a lot of kcalories, but I had an uncle who abused alcohol and became thinner and thinner.

It is true that the energy contribution of alcohol is relatively high. Alcohol yields about 7 kcalories per gram—more than protein and carbohydrate (4 kcalories per gram) and only slightly less than fat (9 kcalories per gram). In some cases, as mentioned in Chapter 6, excess energy from alcohol can contribute to obesity.[50] That is, when alcohol is consumed as *added* energy, it seems to be a risk factor for obesity. Chronic alcohol ingestion seems to have the opposite effect, however. Some researchers attribute the incomplete energy utilization of large doses of alcohol to an alternate metabolic pathway for alcohol that consumes energy rather than generating it.

What are the long-term nutrition effects of alcohol abuse?

By far, the longest-term effect of alcohol is the damage done to a child whose mother has abused alcohol during pregnancy. The devastating effects of alcohol on the unborn, and the messages pregnant women should hear, are presented in Chapter 15. For nonpregnant adults, long-term alcohol abuse damages different organs in different individuals, but always affects all organs and organ systems to various extents.

The most common damage is to the liver, where the function of affected cells may be lost forever unless abstinence from alcohol and sound nutrition intervene in time to reverse the damage. The injury to the liver results in many side effects; one is high blood pressure, which may lead to heart damage and stroke. The protein deficiencies that develop contribute to increased susceptibility to infection. As the synthesis of fat speeds up, fat is deposited in the heart, arteries, and liver. Although alcohol was at one time believed to reduce heart disease risk, the lipoproteins that are elevated by alcohol use are not the same ones that are protective against heart disease.[51]

Alcohol abuse also increases the risks of cancer of the mouth, throat, esophagus, and lungs.[52] Alcohol interferes with the body's ability to detoxify and excrete cancer-causing compounds.

The central nervous system is particularly sensitive to alcohol. The brain shrinks even in people who drink only moderately, but the extent of damage from alcohol is proportional to the amount consumed. The following are a few of the other effects of alcohol:

- Inflammation of the intestines; ulcers of the stomach and intestines.
- Deterioration of the muscles, including the heart muscle.[53]
- Reduced capacity for exercise; heart discomfort sooner during exercise.
- Kidney damage, bladder damage, prostate gland damage.
- Reduced resistance to disease.
- Loss of function of the testicles and damage to the adrenal glands, leading to feminization and sexual impotence in men.
- Failure of the ovaries and early menopause in women.
- Increased susceptibility to lung infections.

If you make a point of eating well, can you drink alcohol and escape harm to health?

No. Eating well and even taking supplements of protein, vitamins, and minerals do not protect the drinker. There is no set level of safe drinking where no adverse effects take place. Even just a couple of drinks set in motion the destructive processes described, but if the drinking has been moderate, the next day's abstinence can repair the damage. Someplace between total abstinence and the extreme of alcoholism, there may be alcohol intakes moderate enough not to harm health, but the more a person drinks, the closer to a dangerous extreme that person comes.

■ NOTES ■

1. P. H. Baylis, Osmoregulation and control of vasopressin secretion in healthy humans, *American Journal of Psychology* 235 (1987): 671–678.
2. Food and Nutrition Board, *Recommended Dietary Allowances,* 10th ed. (Washington, D.C.: National Academy Press, 1989), pp. 247–261.
3. H. S. Wright and coauthors, The 1987–88 Nationwide Food Consumption Survey: An update on the nutrient intake of respondents, *Nutrition Today,* May/June 1991, pp. 21–27.
4. Committee on Diet and Health, Food and Nutrition Board, *Diet and Health: Implications for Reducing Chronic Disease Risk*

(Washington, D.C.: National Academy Press, 1989), pp. 99–135.
5. Food and Nutrition Board, 1989, pp. 250–255.
6. Food and Nutrition Board, 1989.
7. Food and Nutrition Board, 1989, pp. 255–257.
8. L. Tobian, Potassium and hypertension, *Nutrition Reviews* 8 (1988): 282–283.
9. K. T. Khaw and E. Barrett-Connor, Dietary potassium and stroke-associated mortality: A 12-year prospective population study, *New England Journal of Medicine* 316 (1987): 235–240.
10. H. Rasmussen, The cycling of calcium as an intracellular messenger, *Scientific American*, October 1989, pp. 66–73.
11. V. Matkovic, Calcium metabolism and calcium requirements during skeletal modeling and consolidation of bone mass, *American Journal of Clinical Nutrition* supplement 54 (1991): 245–260.
12. R. P. Heaney, Nutrition factors in osteoporosis, *Annual Review of Nutrition* 13 (1993): 287–316.
13. Joint National Committee on Detection, Evaluation, and Treatment of High Blood Pressure, *Archives of Internal Medicine* 153 (1993): 154–183.
14. D. A. McCarron and coauthors, Dietary calcium and blood pressure: Modifying factors in specific populations, *American Journal of Clinical Nutrition* supplement 54 (1991): 215–219.
15. K. Clark, Calcium and hypertension: Does a relationship exist? *Nutrition Today,* July/August 1989, pp. 21–26; J. T. Repke and J. Villar, Pregnancy-induced hypertension and low birth weight: The role of calcium, *American Journal of Clinical Nutrition* (supplement) 54 (1991): 237–241.
16. Wright and coauthors, 1991; R. P. Heaney, J. A. Creighton, and M. J. Barger-Lux, Calcium nutrition and prevention of disease, *Food and Nutrition News,* March/April 1991, pp. 7–9.
17. Magnesium: Potential benefits for heart, bones and more, *University of Texas Lifetime Health Letter,* May 1993, pp. 1, 6, and 8; P. C. Elwood and coauthors, Dietary magnesium and prediction of heart disease, *Lancet* 340 (1992): 483.
18. Elwood and coauthors, 1992.
19. K. L. Woods and coauthors, Intravenous magnesium sulphate in suspected acute myocardial infarction: Results of the second Leicester Intravenous Magnesium Intervention Trial (LIMIT-2), *Lancet* 339 (1992): 1553–1558.
20. Wright and coauthors, 1991.
21. J. Beard and M. Borrel, Iron deficiency and thermoregulation, *Nutrition Today,* September/October 1988, pp. 41–45; D. E. Danford and coauthors, Report on the Fourth Conference for Federally Supported Human Nutrition Research Units and centers, *American Journal of Clinical Nutrition* 54 (1991): 164–168.
22. E. Pollitt, Iron deficiency and cognitive function, *Annual Review of Nutrition* 13 (1993): 521–537.
23. P. R. Dallman, Iron, in *Present Knowledge in Nutrition,* 6th ed., ed. M. L. Brown (Washington, D.C.: International Life Sciences Institute—Nutrition Foundation, 1990), pp. 241–250.
24. R. D. Baynes and T. H. Bothwell, Iron deficiency, *Annual Review of Nutrition* 10 (1990): 133–148.
25. Baynes and Bothwell, 1990.
26. R. Yip, The Changing characteristics of childhood iron nutritional status in the United States, in *Dietary Iron: Birth to Two Years,* ed. L. J. Filer (New York: Raven Press, 1989), pp. 37–56.
27. Pediatricians seek FDA's help in preventing poisoning deaths, *Journal of the American Dietetic Association* 93 (1993): 529.
28. Keep iron tablets away from children, *FDA Consumer,* May 1993, p. 2.
29. Food and Nutrition Board, 1989.
30. R. J. Cousins and M. J. Hempe, Zinc, in *Present Knowledge in Nutrition,* 6th ed., ed. M. L. Brown (Washington, D.C.: International Life Sciences Institute—Nutrition Foundation, 1990), pp. 251–260.
31. Food and Nutrition Board, 1989, pp. 205–211.
32. A. S. Prasad, Discovery of human zinc deficiency and studies in an experimental human model, *American Journal of Clinical Nutrition* 53 (1991): 403–412.
33. Wright and coauthors, 1991.
34. R. E. Litov and G. F. Combs, Selenium in pediatric nutrition, *Pediatrics* 87 (1991): 339–351; Food and Nutrition Board, 1989, pp. 217–223.
35. J. R. Arthur, F. Nicol, and G. J. Beckett, Selenium deficiency, thyroid hormone metabolism, and thyroid hormone deiodinases, *American Journal of Clinical Nutrition* (supplement) 57 (1993): 236–239.
36. Acute and chronic selenium toxicity (Diet Therapy/Obesity Update), *Nutrition and the M. D.,* January 1991, p. 7.
37. B. S. Hetzel, The iodine deficiency disorders: Their nature and prevention, *Annual Review of Nutrition* 9 (1989): 21–38.
38. G. R. Delong, Effects of nutrition on brain development in humans, *American Journal of Clinical Nutrition* (supplement) 57 (1993): 286–290.
39. J. A. T. Pennington, B. E. Young, and D. B. Wilson, Nutritional elements in U.S. diets: Results from the Total Diet Study,

1982–1986, *Journal of the American Dietetic Association* 89 (1989): 659–664.

40. M. A. Johnson and S. E. Kays, Copper: Its role in human nutrition, *Nutrition Today,* January/February 1990, pp. 6–14.
41. J. R. Turnlund, Copper nutriture, bioavailability, and the influence of dietary factors, *Journal of the American Dietetic Association* 88 (1988): 303–308.
42. The impact of fluoride on dental health, Position Paper of the American Dietetic Association, *Journal of the American Dietetic Association* 89 (1989): 971–974.
43. D. Schultz, Fluoride: Cavity-fighter on tap, *FDA Consumer,* January/February 1992, pp. 34–38.
44. E. G. Offenbacher and F. X. Pi-Sunyer, Chromium in human nutrition, *Annual Review of Nutrition* 8 (1988): 543–563.
45. Secretary of Health and Human Services, *Eighth Special Report to the U.S. Congress on Alcohol and Health* (Rockville, Md.: U.S. Department of Health and Human Services, 1993), pp. 1–15.
46. C. S. Lieber, Herman Award Lecture, 1993: A personal perspective on alcohol, nutrition, and the liver, *American Journal of Clinical Nutrition* 58 (1993): 430–442.
47. Lieber, 1993.
48. M. C. Mitchell, Alcohol, in *Present Knowledge in Nutrition,* 6th ed., ed. M. L. Brown (Washington, D.C.: International Life Sciences Institute—Nutrition Foundation, 1990), pp. 457–462.
49. D. H. Barch and S. Mobarhan, Vitamin deficiencies in the alcoholic patient, *Nutrition and the M. D.,* October 1987, pp. 1–3; Lieber, 1993.
50. P. M. Suter, Y. Schutz, and E. Jequier, The effect of ethanol on fat storage in healthy subjects, *New England Journal of Medicine* 326 (1992): 983–987.
51. National Academy of Sciences, Food and Nutrition Board, Committee on Diet and Health, *Diet and Health: Implications for Reducing Chronic Disease Risk* (Washington, D.C.: National Academy Press, 1989), pp. 443–444.
52. Lieber, 1993.
53. A. Urbano-Marquez and coauthors, The effects of alcoholism on skeletal and cardiac muscle, *New England Journal of Medicine* 320 (1989): 409–415.

9

Overweight, Underweight, and Weight Control

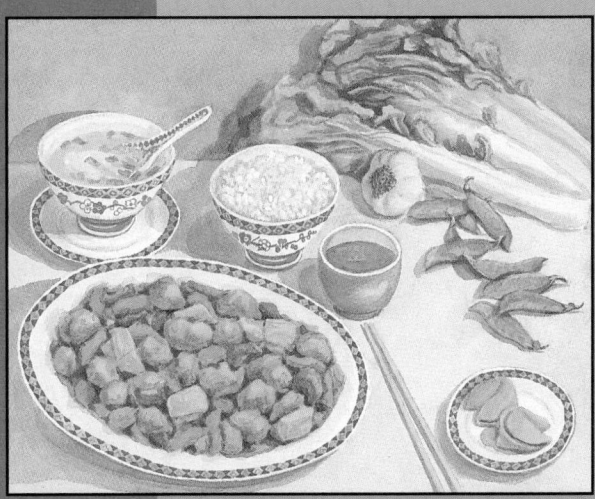

CONTENTS

Are you pleased with your body weight? If you answered yes, you are a rare individual. Nearly all people in our society think they should weigh more or less (mostly less) than they do. Usually, their primary reason is appearance, but they often perceive, correctly, that physical health is also somehow related to weight. At the extremes, both overweight and underweight present definite health risks.

Overweight and underweight both result from unbalanced energy budgets. The simple picture is as follows. Overweight people have consumed more food energy than they have spent and have banked the surplus in their body fat. To reduce fat reserves, overweight people need to spend more energy than they take in from food. In contrast, underweight people have consumed too little food energy to support their activities and so have depleted their bodies' fat stores and possibly their lean tissues as well. To gain weight, they need to take in more food energy than they expend. As you will see, though, the details of the body's weight regulation are quite complex.

This chapter's missions are to examine the problems associated with deficient and excessive body fatness; to present strategies toward solving these problems; and to point out how appropriate body composition, once achieved, can be maintained. This chapter devotes more space to overfatness than to thinness, because it has been more intensively studied and is a more widespread health problem in the developed countries.[1]

The Problems of Underweight and Overweight

Underweight is far less prevalent than overweight, affecting no more than 10 percent of U.S. adults. The health risks of underweight include respiratory disease, tuberculosis, digestive disease, and some cancers.[2] Underweight women may become infertile or may give birth to unhealthy infants. An underweight woman can improve her chances of bearing a healthy infant by gaining weight prior to conception, during pregnancy, or both.

Underweight becomes more hazardous when accompanied by undernutrition. An inadequate supply of nutrients and energy leaves the body underprepared to handle its many metabolic and physical tasks. A person without reserves has a particularly tough battle against medical stresses such as surgery or the wasting diseases of cancer and AIDS. Thus underweight people are urged to gain lean tissue and body fat (as an energy reserve) and to acquire protective amounts of all the nutrients that can be stored.

Overweight is also associated with disease risks, but different ones. For example, it can precipitate hypertension and bring on strokes. Often weight loss alone can normalize the blood pressure of an overfat person; some people with hypertension can tell you exactly at what weight their blood pressure begins to rise. Weight gain can also precipitate diabetes in genetically susceptible people. If hypertension or diabetes runs in your family, you urgently need to attend to weight control.

obesity: a chronic disease characterized by excessively high body fat in relation to lean body tissue. See p. 218 for body fat percentages that define obesity.

Health Risks of Obesity The health risks of overfatness are so many that it has been declared a disease: obesity.[3] Besides diabetes and

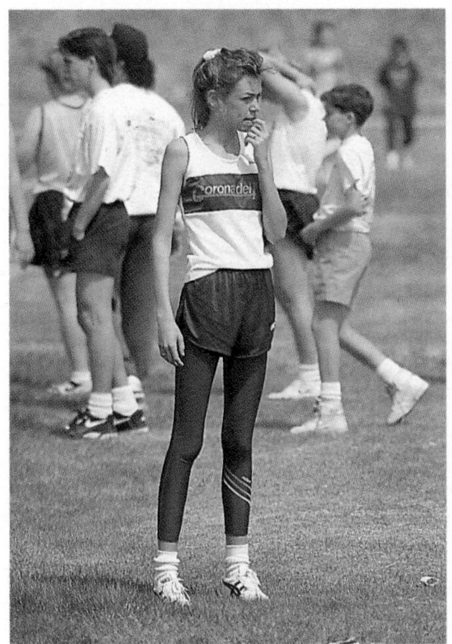

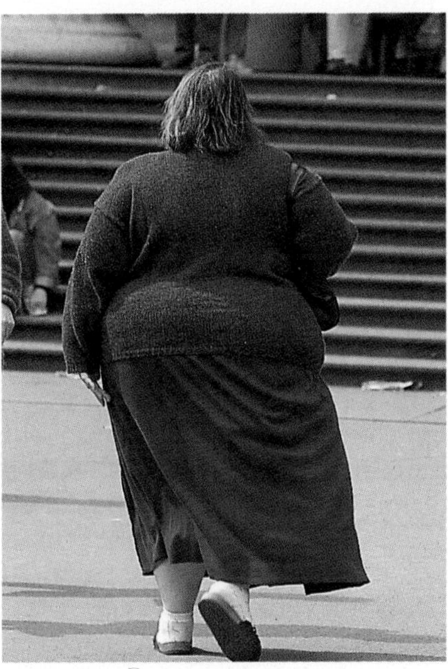

Underweight and overweight both present hazards to health.

hypertension already mentioned, other risks threaten obese adults. Among them are high blood lipids, cardiovascular disease, sleep apnea (abnormal ceasing of breathing during sleep), osteoarthritis, abdominal hernias, some cancers, varicose veins, gout, gallbladder disease, respiratory problems (including Pickwickian syndrome, a breathing blockage linked with sudden death), liver malfunction, complications in pregnancy and surgery, flat feet, and even a high accident rate. Moreover, after the effects of diagnosed diseases are taken into account, the risk of death from other causes remains twice as high for people with lifelong obesity as for others. An estimated 25 percent of U.S. adults are overweight to a degree that incurs such risks.[4]

People want to know exactly how fat is too fat for health, but research results vary on this point. Some evidence indicates that being even mildly or moderately overweight aggravates the risk of heart disease.[5] Even if lean as adults, people who were 20 pounds or more overweight as teenagers may be more likely than others to die of heart disease.[6] On the other hand, some obese people seem to remain healthy and live long despite their body fatness. It may be that genetics determines who among the overweight are susceptible to diseases and who stay well. Still, the majority of obese people do develop associated health problems.

Central Obesity Even more than total fatness, fat that collects in the central abdominal area of the body may be especially likely to lead to diabetes, stroke, hypertension, and coronary artery disease.[7] The risk of death from all causes may be higher for those with central obesity than for those whose fat accumulates elsewhere in the body.[8] In fact, central obesity may raise the risk of heart disease as much as the leading three risk factors (high blood cholesterol, hypertension, and smoking) do.[9] Unlike the fat layers lying just beneath the skin of the abdomen and else-

central obesity: excess fat on the abdomen and around the trunk of the body.

intra-abdominal fat: fat stored within the abdominal cavity in association with the internal abdominal organs, as opposed to the fat stored directly under the abdominal skin (subcutaneous fat).

waist-to-hip ratio: a valuable, commonly used indicator of fat distribution; waist-to-hip ratio = waist circumference ÷ hip circumference. A ratio of 0.8 or greater for a woman or 0.95 or greater for a man suggests a risk to health.

where, the intra-abdominal fat, when mobilized, goes directly to the liver where it is made into cholesterol-carrying low-density lipoprotein (LDL).[10] Fat from elsewhere may arrive in the liver eventually, but it takes a circuitous route that first allows other tissues the chance to pull it from the circulation and metabolize it.

Intra-abdominal fat creates the "apple" profile of central obesity. Fat around the hips and thighs creates more of a "pear" profile. Men of all ages and women past menopause are likely to carry more intra-abdominal fat than are women in their reproductive years.[11] Some women change profile at menopause, and lifelong "pears" may suddenly become "apples" and face increased risks of diseases. Smokers, too, may carry more of their body fat centrally. A smoker may weigh less than the average nonsmoker, but the smoke's waist-to-hip ratio may be greater, leading researchers to think that smoking may directly affect body fat distribution.[12] Two other factors that may affect body fat distribution are intakes of alcohol (associated positively with central obesity) and exercise (associated negatively).

Other Risks of Obesity While some overfat people seem to escape health problems, no one who is fat in our society quite escapes the social and economic handicaps. People who have been overweight as adolescents are still, seven years later, less likely to be married and more likely to have low household incomes than those who were not overweight earlier.[13] This is especially true for women. In contrast, people with other chronic conditions such as asthma, diabetes, and epilepsy do not differ in these characteristics from nonoverweight people.

Our society places enormous value on thinness. Overfat people pay more for insurance and for clothing. Psychologically, too, fat people are made to feel rejected and embarrassed, and this hurts self-esteem.

Traditional medical advice urges all obese people to reduce their weight to reduce associated health risks. Lately, though, experts have been debating whether this advice applies equally to all overweight people. Some people may risk more in the process of losing weight than in remaining obese.

Body Weight and Body Composition

The body's weight reflects its composition—the proportions and composition of its bone, muscles, fat, fluids, and other tissues. All of these body components can vary in quantity and quality—the bones can be dense or porous; the muscles can be well developed or underdeveloped; fat can be abundant or scarce; and so on. By far the most variable tissue, though, is body fat. More than any other component, fat responds to changes in food intake or exercise; and it is fat that is usually the target of efforts at weight control.

Body Weight

At one time, identifying a person's "ideal" body weight was thought to be a simple matter. Now the term *ideal weight* is obsolete, and establishing the point where obesity begins is not a simple matter. One way to choose the cutoff point is to identify the weight at which a correlation to ill health becomes apparent. Epidemiological data show that body weights above a certain line are associated with increased disease risks and excess mortality.

Instead of "ideal weight," researchers now generally speak in terms of "healthy weight" or "reasonable weight." The *Dietary Guidelines for Americans* define healthy weight by three criteria:[14]

- A weight within the suggested range for height and age, as shown in Table 9–1.

Table 9–1
Suggested Weights for Adults

	WEIGHT (lb) [b]			
	19 TO 34 YEARS		35 YEARS AND OLDER	
HEIGHT[a]	MIDPOINT	RANGE	MIDPOINT	RANGE
5'0"	112	97–128	123	108–138
5'1"	116	101–132	127	111–143
5'2"	120	104–137	131	115–148
5'3"	124	107–141	135	119–152
5'4"	128	111–146	140	122–157
5'5"	132	114–150	144	126–162
5'6"	136	118–155	148	130–167
5'7"	140	121–160	153	134–172
5'8"	144	125–164	158	138–178
5'9"	149	129–169	162	142–183
5'10"	153	132–174	167	146–188
5'11"	157	136–179	172	151–194
6'0"	162	140–184	177	155–199
6'1"	166	144–189	182	159–205
6'2"	171	148–195	187	164–210
6'3"	176	152–200	192	168–216
6'4"	180	156–205	197	173–222
6'5"	185	160–211	202	177–228
6'6"	190	164–216	208	182–234

Note: The higher weights in the ranges generally apply to men, who tend to have more muscle and bone, the lower weights more often apply to women, who have less muscle and bone. The higher weights for people aged 35 and older reflect recent research that seems to indicate that people can carry a little more weight as they grow older without added risk to health.

[a] Without shoes.

[b] Without clothes.

Source: U.S. Department of Agriculture and U.S. Department of Health and Human Services, Home and Garden Bulletin No. 232, *Nutrition and Your Health: Dietary Guidelines for Americans,* 3rd ed. (Washington, D.C.: Government Printing Office, 1990).

- A fat distribution pattern that is not associated with a high risk of illness or death.
- The absence of any medical condition for which weight loss would be indicated.

People who meet these three criteria may gain no health advantage from changing their weights. Anyone who does not meet all of these criteria may want to consult with a health care professional, who should carefully consider each criterion in relation to the others.[15] For example, a person with a weight in the suggested range who has high blood cholesterol may need to lose weight. A person who has an "apple" profile, but is within the healthy weight range and in good health, may not need to lose weight.

frame size: the size of a person's bones and musculature. Appendix E describes how to take measures to estimate body frame size and provides tables of standards used in assessment.

overweight: body weight above some standard of acceptable weight that is usually defined in relation to height (such as the weight-for-height tables).

The 1983 Metropolitan Height and Weight tables appear in Appendix E.

Weight for Height Scale weight often fails to reflect body fatness accurately. Still, health care providers typically compare people's weights with weight-for-height tables, which are specific for height, gender, and frame size. Normally, the assessor uses the midpoint of the weight range for a person of a given height and medium build as a standard. If the person's actual weight is 10 to 20 percent above that, then the person is considered overweight; if 20 percent or more above the standard, the person is obese; and if 10 percent below the standard, the person is underweight. Note, however, that weight tables such as Table 9–1 present ranges rather than pinpointing one ideal weight, a good reminder that there is no one perfect weight for anyone. The traditional Metropolitan Height and Weight tables are not reliable for identifying the weights most closely associated with minimal health risks.[16]

body mass index (BMI): an index of a person's weight in relation to height, determined by dividing the weight (in kilograms) by the square of the height (in meters).

To convert pounds to kilograms, divide by 2.2.
To convert inches to meters, divide by 39.37.

Body Mass Index A single standard, derived by manipulating the height and weight measures mathematically, is the body mass index (BMI):

$$\text{BMI} = \frac{\text{weight (kg)}}{\text{height (m)}^2}.$$

A person who takes measurements in pounds and inches can convert them to metric units or can use this modified equation:[17]

$$\text{BMI} = \frac{\text{weight (lb)}}{\text{height (in)}^2} \times 705.$$

Appendix E presents a nomogram that permits people to scan for their BMI rather than calculating it. The inside back covers show weight ranges for various heights using the BMI to define underweight, appropriate weight, overweight, and obesity.

The BMI associated with the lowest overall risk to health is between 22 and 25.[18] Overweight may be defined by a BMI between 25 and 30; obesity may be defined by a BMI above 30.[19] The BMI that indicates the lowest mortality rises with age. Accordingly, the weight ranges in Table 9–1 were based on a BMI of 22 for younger adults, but on a BMI of 24 for older adults. Figure 9–1 presents visual images associated with various BMI values.

BMI values correlate with disease risks as Table 9–2 shows.[20] Most people with a BMI between 20 and 25 have few of the health risks typi-

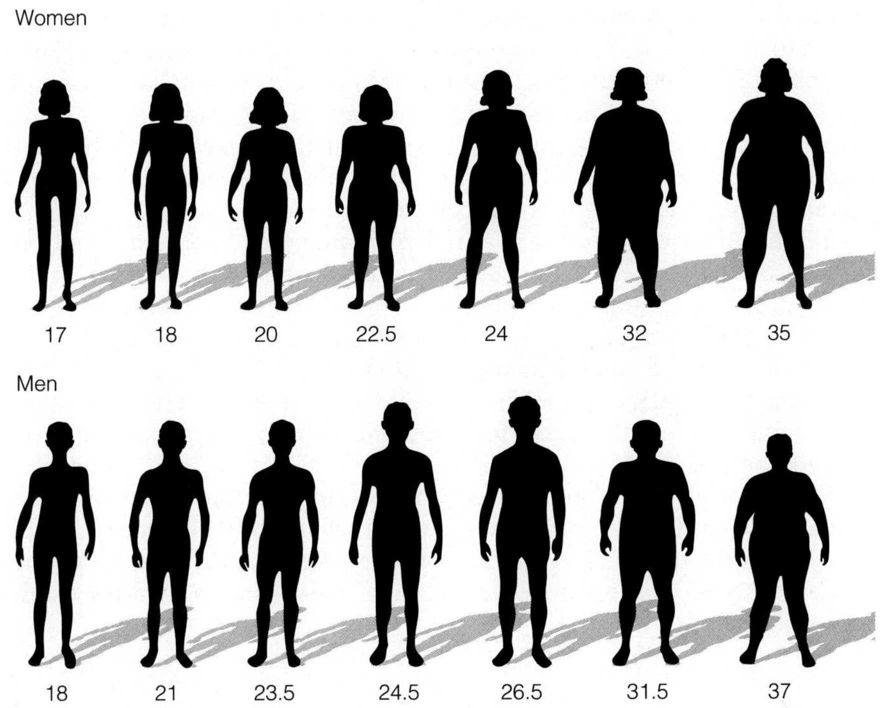

Figure 9–1
Silhouettes and BMI (Actual BMI Shown)

Source: Reprinted from *The Body Test* material of the Canadian Dietetic Association.

cally associated with too-low or too-high body weight. Risks increase as BMI falls below 20 or rises above 25, reflecting the reality that both underweight and overweight impair health status. Factors such as high blood pressure or tobacco use raise risks independently of BMI.

- BMI < 20 = underweight.
- BMI 20 to 25 = normal.
- BMI 25 to 30 = overweight.
- BMI > 30 = obese.

Weight measures are inexpensive, easy to take, and highly accurate, but they fail to reveal two valuable pieces of information in assessing disease risk: how much of the weight is fat and where the fat is located. For this knowledge, measures of body composition are needed.

Body Composition

For many people, being overweight compared with the standard means that they are overfat. This is not the case, though, for athletes with dense bones and well-developed muscles; they may carry little body fat. Conversely, inactive people may seem to have acceptable weights, but may carry too much body fat. In addition, the distribution of fat on the body, as discussed earlier, may be even more critical than overfatness alone. Chapter 13 and Appendix E describe clinical techniques to estimate body fat and its distribution, including fatfold tests, waist-to-hip ratio, bioelectrical impedance, and underwater weighing.

Table 9–2
BMI Values and Disease Risks

BMI	DISEASE RISK
20 to 25	Very low
25 to 30	Low
30 to 35	Moderate
35 to 40	High
40 and over	Very high

How Much Is Too Much Body Fat?

The ideal amount of body fat depends partly on the person. A man with a BMI within the recommended range may have, on average, 15 to 22 per-

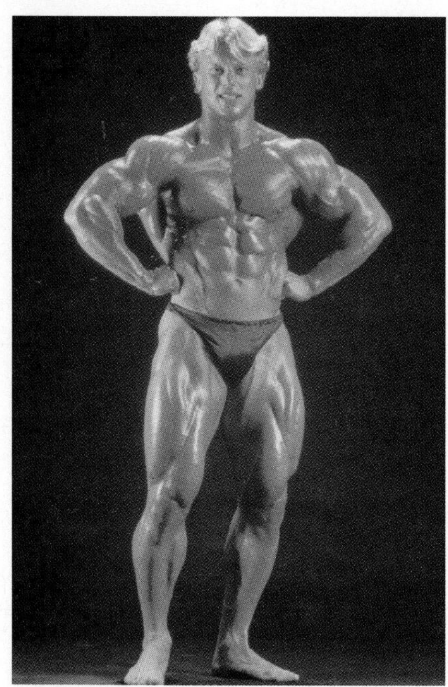

At 5 feet 7½ inches and 200 pounds, Andreas Cahling would be considered overweight by most weight-for-height standards, but he is clearly not overfat. In fact, his body fat is only 10 percent.

cent body fat; a woman, because of her greater quantity of indispensable fat, 18 to 32 percent. For many athletes, a lower-than-average percentage of body fat may be ideal—just enough fat to provide fuel, insulate and protect the body, assist in nerve impulse transmissions, and support normal hormone activity, but not so much as to contribute excess weight for the muscles to carry. Clinicians recommend an absolute *minimum* of 5 to 10 percent for men and 12 to 16 percent for women.[21]

For an Alaskan fisherman, a higher-than-average percentage of body fat is probably beneficial because fat helps prevent heat loss in cold weather. A woman starting a pregnancy needs sufficient body fat to support conception and fetal growth. Below a certain threshold for body fat, individuals may become infertile, develop depression, experience abnormal hunger regulation, or become unable to keep warm. These thresholds differ for each function and for each individual; much remains to be learned about them.

Clearly, the most important criterion of appropriate fatness is health. Researchers find health problems develop when body fat exceeds 22 percent in young men, 25 percent in older men, 32 percent in younger women, and 35 percent in older women; these are the values used to define obesity.[22]

Causes of Obesity

Henceforth, the term *obesity* refers to excess body fat. Excess body fat accumulates when people take in more food energy than they need to provide for the day's metabolic, muscular, and digestive activities. Why do they do this? Is it genetic? Metabolic? Psychological? Behavioral? All of these? Most likely, obesity has many interrelated causes: some experts in the field speak of several different *obesities*.

Genetics and Weight Limited evidence strongly suggests a role for genetic factors in the development of obesity. When both parents are obese, the chances that their children will be obese are quite high (up to 90 percent), whereas when neither parent is obese, the chances are relatively small (less than 10 percent). Adoption studies find a similarity in obesity between biological parents and their natural children, but not between adoptive parents and their adopted children.[23]

To determine the relative contributions of genetic and environmental factors to body weight, one group of researchers studied over 600 pairs of identical and fraternal twins reared together or apart.[24] Like previous studies, this study found that identical twins were twice as likely to have similar weights as fraternal twins—even when reared apart. The researchers concluded that heredity was the most significant determinant of each person's weight.

According to another study of 12 pairs of identical twins, some people have a genetic tendency to store more fat than others, even when energy intakes are comparable.[25] When these twins ate an extra 1000 kcalories a day for 100 days, some of the pairs gained 9 pounds while others gained up to 29 pounds. Within each pair, the amount of fat gained, percentage of body fat, and distribution of fat were similar, suggesting that genetic factors were in control of the process.

Genetics and Energy Expenditure Genetics may also influence how much energy the body spends. For example, the differences in BMR between individuals are greater than can be explained by age, sex, and body composition alone. Similarities within families suggest a genetic influence on BMR. A low metabolic rate is a major risk factor for weight gain.[26]

Lipoprotein Lipase Some of the research investigating the genetic influence on obesity focuses on the enzyme lipoprotein lipase (LPL), which promotes fat storage in fat cells and muscle cells. People with high LPL activity are especially efficient at storing fat. As you might expect, obese people have much more LPL activity than lean people.[27]

lipoprotein lipase (LPL): an enzyme mounted on the surface of fat cells (and other cells). It hydrolyzes triglycerides in the blood into fatty acids and glycerol for absorption into the cells. There they are metabolized or reassembled for storage.

Fat Cell Development Another cause of obesity may be the development of excess fat cells during childhood. The amount of fat on a person's body reflects both fat cell *number* and *size*. The number of fat cells increases during the growing years and then levels off during adulthood. Fat cell number increases more rapidly in obese children than in lean children, and obese children entering their teen years may already have as many fat cells as do adults of normal weight.

Fat cells can expand eight to tenfold in size. When the cells reach their maximum size, they may also divide. Fat cells of obese people contain more LPL, so they are likely to reach a large size quickly.[28] With fat loss, the size of the fat cells shrinks, but not their number and perhaps not their LPL concentrations either.[29] For this reason, people with extra fat cells may tend to regain lost weight rapidly. Prevention of obesity, then, is most critical during the growing years when fat cell number is increasing.

Set-Point Theory One popular theory of why the obese person's body may store too much fat is the set-point theory. Researchers have noted that most people who lose weight on reducing their diets later quickly regain all the lost weight.[30] This seems to suggest that somehow the body chooses a weight that it wants to be and defends that weight by regulating eating behaviors and hormonal actions.[31] This theory is supported by research that shows that some types of obese rats defend their body overweightness as precisely as normal rats defend their normal weight. The set-point theory is unproven and controversial, but many researchers seem to agree that the body somehow (probably by way of genetics) regulates its weight.

set-point theory: the theory that proposes that the body tends to maintain a certain weight by means of its own internal controls.

Environmental Stimuli To a degree, obesity may be environmentally determined. People may overeat because they are pushed to do so by factors such as the availability of many delectable foods. One food constituent is perceived as especially palatable—fat.[32] As Nutrition in Practice 3 pointed out, a high percentage of fat in a person's diet more strongly predicts high body fat than does a high number of total kcalories.

Learned Behavior Psychological stimuli also trigger inappropriate eating behavior in some people. Appropriate eating behavior is a response to hunger. Hunger is a drive programmed into people by their heredity. Appetite, in contrast, is learned and can lead people to ignore hunger or to overrespond to it. Hunger is physiological, whereas appetite is psychological, and the two do not always coincide.

hunger: the physiological need to eat, experienced as a drive for obtaining food; an unpleasant sensation that demands relief.

appetite: the psychological desire to eat, a learned motivation and a pleasant sensation that accompanies the sight, smell, or thought of appealing foods.

Food behavior is also intimately connected to deep emotional needs such as the primitive fear of starvation. Yearnings, cravings, and addictions with profound psychological significance can express themselves in people's eating behavior. An emotionally insecure person might eat rather than call a friend and risk rejection. Another person might use eating to relieve boredom or to ward off depression.

Physical Activity The possible causes of obesity mentioned so far all relate to the input side of the energy equation. What about output? People may be obese, not because they eat too much, but because they spend too little energy. The control of hunger/appetite actually works quite well in active people and only fails when activity falls below a certain minimum. Obese people observed closely are often seen to eat less than lean people, but they are sometimes so extraordinarily inactive (or efficient in their way of moving) that they still manage to accumulate an energy surplus. Chapter 10 discusses the many benefits of regular physical activity.

No two obese people are alike, and many factors may contribute to obesity in one person, so no panacea is likely to be found. The top priority should be prevention, but where prevention has failed, the treatment of obesity must involve a simultaneous attack on many fronts.

Strategies for Weight Loss

1 lb body fat = 3500 kcal.
To lose a pound a week, cut 500 kcal/day.

Whether a person wants to lose 10 pounds or 50, the only realistic and sensible way to maintain a healthy body weight is to cut kcalories (primarily those from fat) increase activity, and maintain this changed lifestyle for life. This is a tall order. Only 5 to 10 percent of people who try achieve long-term success.[33] To succeed, one must modify all the factors that have contributed to the problem in the first place, and sometimes these can't be changed. Still, long-term weight loss can be, and has been, achieved.

The way a person loses weight is a highly individual matter. Two weight-loss plans may both be successful and yet have little or nothing in common. Dietitians often recommend weight-reduction diets based on the exchange list system discussed in Nutrition in Practice 6, but many other weight-reduction plans are also in use. Some are adequate; others are not. The accompanying box provides a way of judging weight-loss programs and diets according to sound nutrition principles. Inappropriate ways of treating obesity are listed in the glossary on page 223.

HOW TO Rate Sound and Unsound Weight-Loss Schemes and Diets

Start by giving each diet or program 160 points. Subtract points as instructed, whenever a diet falls short of ideals.

Scoring: 160 = fine
140–150 = possibly safe with some disadvantage
120–130 = needs improvement
110 or below = dangerous to use

Does the diet or program:

1. Provide a reasonable number of kcalories (not fewer than 1200 kcalories for an average-size person)? If not, give it a minus 10.
2. Provide enough, but not too much, protein (at least the recommended intake or RDA, but not more than twice that much)? If no, minus 10.
3. Provide enough fat for balance but not so much fat as to go against current recommendations (between 20 and 30 percent of kcalories from fat)? If no, minus 10.
4. Provide enough carbohydrate to spare protein and prevent ketosis (100 grams of carbohydrate for the average-size person)? Is it mostly complex carbohydrate (not more than 10 percent of the kcalories as concentrated sugar)? If no to either or both, minus 10.
5. Offer a balanced assortment of vitamins and minerals—that is, foods from all food groups? If it omits a food group (for example, meats), does it provide a suitable substitute? Count five food groups in all: milk/milk products, meat/fish/poultry/eggs/legumes; fruits; vegetables; and starches/grains. For *each* food group omitted and not adequately substituted for, subtract 10 points.
6. Offer variety, in the sense that different foods can be selected each day? If you'd class it as boring or monotonous, give it a minus 10.
7. Consist of ordinary foods that are available locally (for example, in the main grocery stores) at the prices people normally pay? Or does the dieter have to buy special, expensive, or unusual foods to adhere to the diet? If you would class it as "bizarre" or "requiring special foods," minus 10.
8. Promise dramatic, rapid weight loss (substantially more than 1 percent of total body weight per week)? If yes, minus 10.
9. Encourage permanent, realistic lifestyle changes, including regular exercise and the behavioral changes needed for weight maintenance? If not, minus 10.
10. Misrepresent salespeople as "counselors" supposedly qualified to give guidance in nutrition and/or general health without a profit motive, or collect large sums of money at the start, or

(continued)

How To (continued)

require that clients sign contracts for expensive long-term programs? If so, minus 10.

11. Fail to inform clients about the risks associated with weight loss in general or the specific program being promoted? If so, minus 10.
12. Promote unproven or spurious weight-loss aids such as human chorionic gonadotrophin (HCG), starch blockers, diuretics, sauna belts, body wraps, passive exercise, ear stapling, acupuncture, electric muscle stimulating (EMS) devices, spirulina, amino acid supplements (e.g., arginine, ornithine), glucomannan, appetite suppressants, "unique" ingredients, and so forth? If so, minus 10.

To heighten the sense of individuality, the following sections are written in terms of advice to "you." This is not intended to put "you" under pressure to take the advice personally, but to give you the illusion of listening in on a conversation in which an obese person (with, say, 50 pounds to lose) is being competently counseled by someone familiar with the techniques known to be effective. Margin notes at intervals highlight the principles involved.

Diet

Weight-Loss Pointers:
- Be involved in planning.
- Keep in mind that you will want to maintain your lost weight. Practice needed behaviors as you go.

No particular diet is magical, and no particular food must either be included or avoided. You are the one who will have to live with the diet, so you had better be involved in its planning. Don't think of it as a diet you are going "on"—because then you may be tempted to go "off." The diet is successful only if the pounds do not return. Think of it as an eating plan that you will adopt for life. It must consist of foods that you like, that are available to you, and that are within your means.

- Adopt a realistic plan.

A Realistic Energy Level Choose an energy level you can live with. A rule of thumb is that you need at least 10 kcalories per pound of current weight. Nutritional adequacy is difficult for most people to achieve on fewer than 1200 kcalories a day, and most healthy adults should not consume any less than that. You will experience a healthier, more successful weight loss with a small energy deficit that provides an adequate intake than with a large energy deficit that creates feelings of starvation and deprivation, which can lead to an irresistible urge to binge.

- Make the diet adequate by emphasizing nutrient-dense foods.

Nutritional Adequacy Nutritional adequacy should be a high priority. Take a look at the 1200-kcalorie food plan in Table 6–5 (on p. 137). Notice that this pattern offers the minimum number of servings suggested in the Daily Food Guide (introduced in Chapter 1) and allows a teaspoon of fat at each of three meals. Such an intake would allow most people to lose weight at a satisfactory rate and still meet their nutrient needs with careful food selections. (Women might need an iron supplement.) The other plans consist of exchange patterns for higher energy intakes.

Carbohydrates, Not Fats Center meals and snacks on complex-carbohydrate foods of low energy density: fresh fruits, vegetables, and whole grains. They offer abundant vitamins and minerals. They also offer more fiber (which provides bulk and satiety) and far less fat and food energy than smooth, refined foods. They also taste better. Researchers compared a diet in which fat was restricted, but complex carbohydrates were eaten freely, with a more conventional energy-restricted diet, used over six months by obese women.[34] Women in both diet groups lost substantial weight, but those who ate the fat-restricted, complex carbohydrate–rich diet rated it higher in terms of satiety and taste. A person who makes low-fat food selections habitually can lose excess body fat without having to limit portions and meal sizes. Even given the same number of kcalories, less fat in the diet means less fat in the body. Dietary fat correlates positively with body fat, whereas dietary carbohydrate and fiber correlate negatively with body fat.[35]

► Select low-fat foods regularly.

► Make grains, vegetables, and fruits central to your diet plan.

Other studies have also found that when women followed a low-fat diet (20 percent kcalories from fat), they lost weight and body fat.[36] In fact, the only way the women could *maintain* weight was to raise their

Glossary of Poor Treatment Choices for Obesity

diet pills: pills that depress the appetite temporarily; often, physician-prescribed amphetamines (speed). It is generally agreed that these drugs are of little value for weight loss and that their use can cause a dangerous dependency.

diuretic abuse: use of diuretics to promote water excretion by dieters who believe their weight excesses are due to water accumulation.

fad diets: diets based on exaggerated or false theories of weight loss; such diets are usually inadequate in energy and nutrients. Some fad diets are more dangerous to health than obesity itself.

HCG or **human chorionic gonadotropin** (core-ee-ON-ic go-nad-o-TROPE-in)**:** a hormone excreted in the urine of pregnant women, which, given by injection, has been believed to enhance weight loss and reduce hunger. It does neither.

intestinal bypass surgery: surgery that involves removing or disconnecting a portion of the small intestine to reduce absorption of energy nutrients. Such surgery has severe side effects, including deranged fluid and electrolyte balance and liver failure.

low-carbohydrate diets: diets designed to bring about metabolic responses similar to those of fasting (see Chapter 6, pp. 123–126). Without sufficient carbohydrate, the body cannot use its fat in the normal way, and ketosis results. Many physiological hazards accompany low-carbohydrate diets: high blood cholesterol, mineral imbalances, hypoglycemia, and more.

protein-sparing fast: a variant on fasting and low-carbohydrate diets; the technique of eating only protein in the hope that the protein will spare a person's lean tissue while body fat is broken down. Protein-sparing fasts have a low long-term success rate, and worse, they present serious health risks.

very-low-kcalorie diets (VLCD): diets that provide from 400 to 800 kcalories per day to promote weight loss; they may be appropriate for carefully selected, supervised clients, but in general, the long-term outlook for those who use them is bleak: weight regain is almost certain. The diets pose health risks as well.

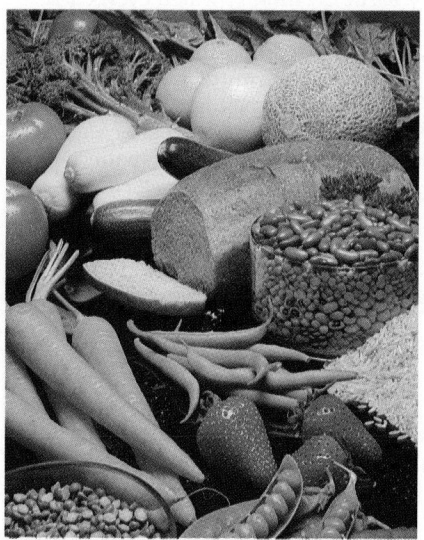

Delicious, low-fat, carbohydrate-rich foods such as fresh fruits, vegetables, whole grains, and legumes offer abundant vitamins, minerals, and fiber.

total energy intakes. A person trying to achieve or maintain a healthy weight needs to pay attention not only to fat, but to sugar and alcohol, too. Using them for pleasure on occasion is compatible with health as long as most daily choices are of nutrient-dense foods.

▸ Limit concentrated sweets and alcoholic beverages.

Adequate Water Learn to satisfy thirst with water. Water fills the stomach between meals and dilutes the metabolic wastes generated from the breakdown of fat, easing their excretion. It meets the water need that was formerly met by eating extra food (remember that food provides water).

▸ Drink plenty of water (8 glasses or more a day).

An Eating Plan, Not a Diet Adopt an "eating plan for good health" rather than a "diet for weight loss." That way, you will be able to keep the lost weight off.

▸ Learn, practice, and follow a healthful eating plan for the rest of your life.

Physical Activity

Either dieting or physical activity alone can produce some weight loss. Clearly, however, the combination is most effective.

weight cycling: repeated cycles of weight loss and subsequent regain that affect body composition and metabolism. With intermittent dieting, a person rebounds to a higher weight (and a higher body fat content) after each round. The weight-cycling pattern is popularly called the *ratchet effect* or *yo-yo effect* of dieting.

Weight Cycling Those who endeavor to lose weight without exercise often become trapped in weight cycling, the endless repeating rounds of weight loss and regain from "yo-yo" dieting. Nearly a third of all women interviewed in one poll reported themselves to be perpetual dieters who dieted at least once a month. At any one time, estimates place 25 percent of adult men and more than 40 percent of adult women on weight-loss diets, with another 25 or so percent struggling to maintain recent losses.[37]

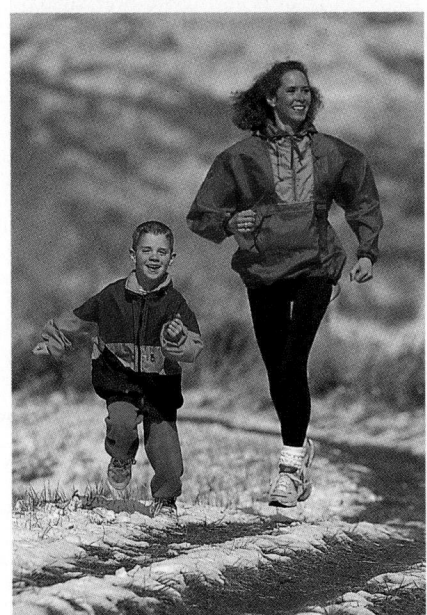

Regular physical activity helps people achieve and maintain healthy weights.

Harm from Weight Cycling Weight cycling may disrupt body composition. In rats repeatedly placed on weight-loss diets, weight losses become slower and slower with less and less weight lost each time, perhaps because weight loss reduces the body's lean tissue and weight regain adds to body fatness. The same effect sometimes shows up in human beings.[38] A recent review found little evidence to support the idea that dieting produces permanent changes in human body composition, however.[39]

Whether or not body composition changes, a serious risk may await those whose weight cycles. A recent study reported a link between repeated fluctuations in body weight and increased risks of death from heart disease and other causes.[40] No conclusions are yet possible, and previous dieters are probably not in danger, so long as they have stopped weight cycling.

Physical Activity and Energy Expenditure Physical activity makes many contributions to weight loss and maintenance. For one thing, it directly increases energy output by the muscles and cardiovascular system. A 150-pound person walking a brisk 4 miles per hour for 30 minutes spends an extra 185 kcalories on that activity. A football player in training may spend several thousand extra kcalories on a day of heavy training.

Benefits of physical activity in a weight-control program:

- Short-term increase in energy expenditure (from exercise and from a slight rise in BMR).
- Long-term increase (slight) in BMR.
- Appetite control.
- Stress reduction and control of stress eating.
- Physical, and therefore psychological, well-being.
- High self-esteem.

Activity and BMR Activity also contributes to energy output in an indirect way—by speeding up basal metabolism. It does this both immediately and over the long term. On any given day, after intense and prolonged exercise, basal metabolism remains elevated for several hours.[41] Over the long term, daily vigorous activity for many weeks gradually shifts body composition towards more lean tissue, which is more active metabolically than fat tissue. Then the ongoing metabolic rate rises accordingly, and this makes a contribution toward continued weight loss or maintenance.

The raised metabolic rate continues for as long as the person keeps exercising regularly. The more energy expended in metabolic activities, the greater the energy requirement. This means that a person can eat more without gaining weight, and this, in turn, brings both pleasure and nutrients.

Activity and Appetite Control Physical activity also helps to control appetite. People think that exercising will make them hungry, but this is not entirely true. Yes, active people do have healthy appetites, but immediately after a good workout, most people do not feel like eating. They want to shower and may be thirsty, but they are not hungry. The reason is that the body has responded to the stress of exercise by mobilizing fuels from storage: glucose and fatty acids are abundant in the blood. At the same time, the body has suppressed its digestive functions. Hard physical work and eating are not compatible.

Physical activity helps especially to curb the inappropriate appetite that prompts a person to eat when bored, anxious, or depressed. Weight-control programs encourage people to go out and exercise when they're tempted to eat but not really hungry.

Activity and Psychological Benefits Activity also helps reduce stress. Since stress itself is a cue to inappropriate eating behavior for many people, activity can help here, too.

Activity offers still more psychological advantages. The fit person looks and feels healthy, and high self-esteem accompanies these benefits. High self-esteem tends to support a person's resolve to persist in a weight-control effort, rounding out a beneficial cycle.

Choosing Activities What kind of physical activity is best? People seeking to lose weight should choose activities that they enjoy and that they are willing to do regularly. In addition to activities such as walking or aerobic dance, there are hundreds of ways to incorporate energy-spending activities into daily routines: take the stairs instead of the elevator, walk to the neighbor's apartment instead of making a phone call, and rake the grass clippings instead of using a bagger. These activities burn only a few kcalories each, but over a year's time they become significant.

Spot Reducing People sometimes ask about "spot reducing." Unfortunately, no one part of the body gives up fat in preference to another. Fat cells all over the body release fat in response to demand, and the fat is then used by whatever muscles are active. No exercise can remove the fat from any one particular area—and, incidentally, neither can a massage machine that claims to break up fat on trouble spots.

Exercise can help with trouble spots in another way, though. Strengthening muscles in a trouble area can help to improve their tone; stretching to gain flexibility can help with associated posture problems. Thus aerobic, strength, and flexibility workouts all have a place in fitness programs (see Chapter 10, which is devoted entirely to physical activity).

Behavior Modification

behavior modification: the changing of behavior by the manipulation of *antecedents* (cues or environmental factors that trigger behavior), the behavior itself, and *consequences* (the penalties or rewards attached to behavior).

Sound nutrition and regular physical activity are not the only prerequisites to achieving and maintaining a healthy body weight and composition. Behavior and attitude are important supporting factors. Behavior modification works to change the behaviors of overeating and underexercising that lead to, and perpetuate, obesity.

Becoming Aware of Behaviors The first step in modifying behavior is to become aware of current behaviors. A person who is aware of all the behaviors that create a problem has a head start toward solving the problem. A person beginning a behavior-modification program should establish a baseline (a record of present eating and exercise behaviors) against which to measure future progress. It is best to keep a diary (see Figure 9–2) that includes the time and place of meals and snacks, the type and amount of foods eaten, the persons present when food is eaten, and a

Figure 9–2
Food Diary
A record of diet and exercise habits reveals problem areas, the first step toward improving behaviors.

Time	Place	Activity or food eaten	People present	Mood
10:30	School vending machine	6 peanut butter crackers and 12 oz. cola	by myself	Starved
12:15	Restaurant	Sub sandwich and 12 oz. cola	friends	relaxed & friendly
3:00	Gym	45 min weight training	work out partner	tired
4:00	Snack bar	Small frozen yogurt	by myself	OK

description of the individual's feelings when eating. The diary should also record physical activities: the kind, the intensity level, the duration, and the person's feelings about them. These entries will help the individual identify possible behaviors to change.

Making Small Changes Next, behavior-modification strategies can be applied to make changes in many small, individual daily behaviors. Behavior-modification experts see each behavior as the second part of a three-part sequence. Its antecedents precede it, and its consequences follow it:

A (antecedents) → B (behavior) ↔ C (consequences).

A behavior occurs in response to antecedents (cues or stimuli); the more intense the antecedents are, the more likely the behavior will occur. The behavior in turn leads to consequences. The more intense these consequences are, postively or negatively, the more or less likely the behavior is to occur again.

Applying Behavior-Modification Principles To encourage the repeated occurrence of desired eating and exercise behaviors and to eliminate the occurrence of unwanted behaviors, use behavior-modification principles as follows:

1. Eliminate inappropriate eating cues.
2. Suppress the cues you cannot eliminate.
3. Strengthen cues to appropriate eating and exercise.
4. Engage in the desired eating and exercise behaviors.
5. Arrange or emphasize negative consequences of inappropriate eating.
6. Arrange or emphasize positive consequences of appropriate eating and exercise behaviors.

The box on pp. 228–229 shows how a person might apply each of these strategies to a weight-control program. A particularly attractive feature of these strategies is that they do not involve blaming oneself or putting oneself down—an important element in fostering self-esteem.

Maintaining Weight Finally, be aware that it can be hard to maintain weight loss. On arriving at the goal weight after months of self-discipline and new habit formation, the victorious weight loser must not "celebrate" by resuming old eating habits. Membership in an ongoing weight-control organization and regular, continued physical activity can provide indispensable support for the formerly overweight person who wants to remain trim.

Personal Attitude

When behavior therapists view overeating and underexercising as maladaptive behaviors that people can change, they ignore the positive contribution that overeating plays in a person's life. They also miss that being overweight may have become part of a person's identity. For many people, overeating and being overweight have become integral aspects of their

HOW TO Modify Behaviors

Start simply and don't try to master all the behavior changes all at once. Attempting too many changes at one time is never successful; a person must set priorities. A person may begin by limiting meals to three a day. When between-meal snacking is no longer a problem, the person may want to change another behavior.

1. To eliminate inappropriate eating cues:

- Don't buy problem foods (such as ready-to-eat foods).
- Don't shop when you are hungry.
- Don't serve rich sauces and toppings.
- Let other family members buy, store, and serve their own sweets.
- Change channels or look away when the television shows food commercials.
- Shop only from a list and stay away from convenience stores.
- Carry appropriate snacks from home and avoid vending machines.

2. To suppress the cues you cannot eliminate:

- Eat only in one place and in one room.
- Clear plates directly into the garbage.
- Create obstacles to the eating of problem foods (for example, make it necessary to unwrap, cook, and serve each one separately).
- Minimize contact with excessive food (serve individual plates, don't put serving dishes on the table, and leave the table when you have finished eating).
- Make small portions of food look large (spread food out, serve on small plates).
- Control states of deprivation (eat regular meals, don't skip meals, avoid getting tired, avoid boredom by keeping cues to fun activities in sight).

3. To strengthen the cues to appropriate eating and exercise:

- Eat only at planned times; plan not to eat after a specified time (say, 7:00 or 8:00 P.M.).
- Encourage others to eat appropriate foods with you.
- Keep your favorite appropriate foods in the front of the refrigerator.
- Learn appropriate portion sizes and prepare one portion at a time.
- Save permitted foods from meals for snacks (and make these your only snacks).
- Prepare permitted foods attractively.
- Keep your hiking boots (ski poles, tennis racket) by the door.

How To (continued)

4. To engage in desired eating or exercise behaviors:
   - Slow down (pause several times during a meal, put down utensils between mouthfuls, chew thoroughly before swallowing, swallow before reloading the fork, always use utensils).
   - Leave some food on the plate.
   - Engage in no other activities while eating (such as reading or watching television).
   - Move more (shake a leg, pace, fidget, flex your muscles).
   - Join in and exercise with a group of active people.
5. To arrange or emphasize negative consequences of inappropriate eating:
   - Eat your meals with other people.
   - Ask that others respond neutrally when you deviate from your plan (make no comment). This is a negative consequence because it withholds attention.
6. To arrange or emphasize positive consequences of appropriate behaviors:
   - Update records of food intake, physical activity, and weight change regularly.
   - Arrange for rewards for each unit of behavior change or weight loss.
   - Ask family and friends for reinforcement (praise and encouragement).

activities, work, health, self-concept, and emotional states. Changing diet and exercise behaviors without attention to a person's self-concept invites failure.

Many people overeat to cope with the stresses of life. To break out of that pattern, they must first identify the particular stressors that trigger their urges to overeat. Then, when faced with these situations, they must learn to practice problem-solving skills. When the problems that trigger the urge to overeat are dealt with in alternative ways, people may find that they eat less and that their eating during stressful times has become appropriate. The message is that sound emotional health supports your ability to take care of your health in all ways—including nutrition, weight control, and fitness.

Strategies for Weight Gain

Weight gain, like weight loss, is an individual matter. People who are healthy at their present weights may stay there; those who are at risk for illness should try to gain.

Some people are unalterably thin by reasons of heredity or early physical influences. Those who wish to gain weight for appearance's sake or to

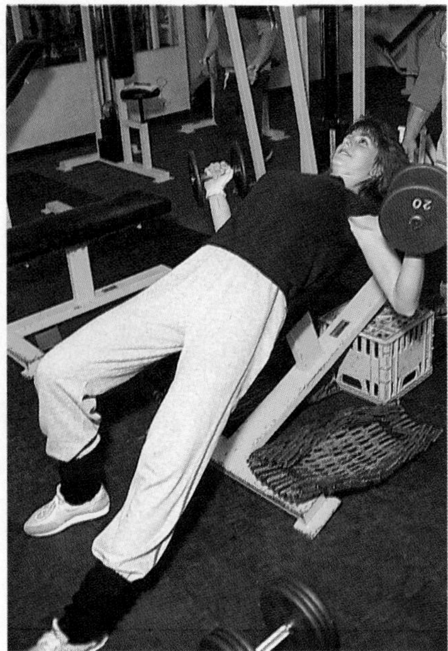

Strength training is essential to a sound plan for gaining weight.

improve athletic performance should be aware that a healthful weight can be achieved only through physical activity, particularly strength training, combined with a high energy intake. Eating many high-kcalorie foods can bring about weight gain, but it will be mostly fat, and this can be as detrimental to health as being slightly underweight. In an athlete, such a weight gain can impair performance. Therefore, in weight gain, as in weight loss, physical activity is an essential component of a sound plan.

Weight-Gain Pointers:

- Exercise and eat to build muscles.

Exercising to Build Muscles The person who wants to gain weight should use strength training primarily. As exercise is added, energy intake must be increased to support that exercise—otherwise, weight (body fat) will be lost. A person who eats just enough to support the exercise will build muscle, but at the expense of body fat; that is, fat will be used to support the muscle building. If more food is eaten, the person will gain both muscle and fat.

In theory, it takes an excess of about 2000 to 2500 kcalories to support the gain of a pound of pure lean tissue.[42] The rate at which a person can build muscle tissue also depends on the person. Men and women have mixtures of both male and female hormones; those with more male hormones build muscle more easily than others, but it is not known what the limits are. About 700 to 1000 kcalories a day above normal energy needs is enough to support both the exercise and the building of muscle.

- Eat energy-dense foods regularly.

Energy-Dense Foods Energy-dense foods (the very ones eliminated from a successful weight-loss diet) hold the key to weight gain. Pick the highest-kcalorie items from each food group—that is, milkshakes instead of nonfat milk, peanut butter instead of lean meat, avocados instead of cucumbers, and whole-wheat muffins instead of whole-wheat bread. Because fat contains more than twice as many kcalories per teaspoon as sugar does, fat adds kcalories without adding much bulk.

Be aware that a low-fat diet plan is recommended for the general U.S. population because the general population is overweight and at risk for heart disease. Consumption of high-fat foods is not healthy for most people, of course, but may be essential for an underweight individual who needs to gain weight. An underweight person who is physically active and eating a nutritionally adequate diet can afford a few extra kcalories from fat.

- Eat at least three hearty meals a day.

Three Meals Daily People wanting to gain weight should eat at least three hearty meals a day. Most people who are underweight have simply been too busy (sometimes for months) to eat enough to gain or maintain weight. Therefore, they need to make meals a priority and plan them in advance. Taking time to prepare and eat each meal can help, as can learning to eat more food within the first 20 minutes of a meal. Another suggestion is to eat meaty appetizers or the main course first and leave the soup or salad until later.

Large Portions It is also important to learn to eat more food at each meal. Have two sandwiches for lunch instead of one, drink milk from a larger glass, and eat cereal from a larger bowl.

The person should expect to feel full. Most underweight individuals are accustomed to small quantities of food. When they begin eating significantly more, they feel uncomfortable. This is normal and passes over time.

▸ Eat large portions of foods and expect to feel full.

Extra Snacks Since a substantially higher energy intake is needed each day, in addition to eating more food at each meal, it is necessary to eat more frequently. Between-meal snacking offers a solution. For example, a student might make three sandwiches in the morning and eat them between classes in addition to the day's three regular meals.

▸ Eat snacks between meals.

Juice and Milk Beverages provide an easy way to increase energy intake. Consider that 6 cups of cranberry juice add almost 1000 kcalories to the day's intake. kCalories can be added to milk by mixing in powdered milk or packets of instant breakfast.

▸ Drink plenty of juice and milk.

For people who are underweight due to illness, concentrated liquid formulas are often recommended because a weak person can swallow them easily. A physician or registered dietitian can recommend high-protein, high-kcalorie formulas to help the underweight person maintain or gain. Used in addition to regular meals, these can help considerably.

An extreme underweight condition known as anorexia nervosa is sometimes seen in young people who exercise heroic self-denial in order to control their weight. They go to such extremes that they become severely undernourished, achieving final body weights of 70 pounds or even less. The distinguishing feature of a person with anorexia nervosa, as opposed to other thin people, is that the starvation is intentional.

Anorexia nervosa is one of two eating disorders seen in our society today. The other is bulimia—compulsive overeating, sometimes with purging. These two disorders are the subject of the Nutrition in Practice that follows this chapter.

SELF STUDY

Choose a Goal Weight and Develop a Weight-Control Plan

What weight is appropriate for you? When physical health alone is considered, a wide range of weights is acceptable for a person of a given height. Within the safe range, the choice of a weight is up to the individual.

Choose a Goal Weight

1. Determine whether your current weight is appropriate for your height.

▸ Record your height: ___ in (or ___ cm).

▸ Record your weight: ___ lb (or ___ kg).

Look up the weight range for a person your age in Table 9–1 on p. 215.

▸ Record the entire range: ___ to ___ lb.

Does your weight fall within the suggested range? Now calculate your BMI using the equations on p. 216.

▸ Record your BMI: ___ kg/m^2.

Look up the disease risk for a person with your BMI value in Table 9–2 on p. 217.

(continued)

Self-Study (continued)

▸ Record your risk of disease based on your BMI: ______________________.

If this level of risk is unacceptable, calculate the weight needed for a desired BMI value (divide the desired BMI by the appropriate height factor in the accompanying table). For example, a 165 pound person who is 5 feet 5 inches tall has a BMI of 27.5. To obtain a BMI of 22, the person would need to weigh about 133 pounds (22 ÷ 0.166).

▸ Record your desired weight based on your height and desired BMI: ______________.

If your weight is below the range in Table 9–1 and your BMI is below 20, you may need to gain weight for your health's sake. If your weight is over the suggested weight range and your BMI value is associated with an unacceptable risk of disease, you may want to examine your body's fat distribution.

2. Determine whether your fat distribution is associated with health risks.

▸ Record your waist measurement: ___.
▸ Record your hip measurement: ___.

Calculate the waist-to-hip ratio by dividing the number of inches (or centimeters) around your waistline by the number of inches (or centimeters) around your hips.

▸ Record your waist-to-hip ratio: ___.

Women with a ratio of 0.8 or greater and men with a ratio of 0.95 or greater are at high risk of obesity-related health problems.

3. Check your health history. A family or personal medical history of diabetes (non-insulin-dependent type), hypertension, or high blood cholesterol signals the need to pay attention to diet and exercise habits.

Based on these three considerations, how does your current weight compare with standards that are compatible with health? If your current weight compares favorably, you probably want to maintain your weight. If you want to gain weight or lose weight, indicate a sensible goal weight here: ___ lb goal weight.

Choose weight loss or weight gain as a goal for yourself. (If you are at the perfect weight, pretend that you are not, for purposes of this exercise, and develop a plan to change your weight by ten pounds.)

Develop a Weight-Control Plan

To *lose* weight, you would need to adjust your energy balance by reducing your energy intake, increasing your energy output, or both. To *gain* weight, you would need to increase your energy intake. (It is hardly ever desirable to reduce energy expenditure.)

HEIGHT	HEIGHT FACTOR	HEIGHT	HEIGHT FACTOR	HEIGHT	HEIGHT FACTOR
4'7"	0.232	5'3"	0.177	5'11"	0.139
4'8"	0.224	5'4"	0.172	6'0"	0.136
4'9"	0.216	5'5"	0.166	6'1"	0.132
4'10"	0.209	5'6"	0.161	6'2"	0.128
4'11"	0.202	5'7"	0.157	6'3"	0.125
5'0"	0.195	5'8"	0.152	6'4"	0.122
5'1"	0.189	5'9"	0.148	6'5"	0.119
5'2"	0.183	5'10"	0.143	6'6"	0.116

To obtain the weight needed for a certain BMI, divide the desired BMI by the height factor appropriate for your height.

Source: R. P. Abernathy, Body mass index: Determination and use. Copyright the American Dietetic Association. Reprinted by permission from *Journal of the American Dietetic Association* 91 (1991): 843.

Self-Study (continued)

1. Review your energy intake. Return to Self-Study 1, Form 2, and record from it your average daily energy intake:

▸ My energy intake is ___ kcal/day.

2. Review your energy output. The Self-Study in Chapter 6 helped you estimate your energy expenditure for a day. Record it here:

▸ My energy output is ___ kcal/day.

3. Estimate your rate of weight gain or loss. Compare your energy intake with your output. Recall that a difference of 3500 kcalories between energy intake and output will make a difference of one pound, and estimate the rate at which you must be gaining or losing weight.

   Example: If your intake is 2000 kcalories per day and your output is 1500 kcalories per day, then you are acquiring an excess of 500 kcalories per day beyond your need, or 3500 kcalories each week. That means you should be gaining 1 pound per week:

▸ With an intake of ___ kcal/day and an output of ___ kcal/day, I must be gaining/losing (circle one) 1 pound every ___ days.

4. Now choose a goal and a balance that will achieve it. Do not plan to gain or lose weight at a rate greater than 2 pounds per week, and do not plan to eat less than 10 kcalories per pound of your current weight each day.

▸ I wish to gain/lose (circle one) 1 pound every ___ days. That means my energy intake should be ___ kcal per day and my energy output should be (or remain at) ___ kcal per day.

This exercise assumes you will adjust your energy output appropriately and focuses on the input side, the diet.

5. Choose an appropriate diet. Table 6–5 on page 137 offers diet patterns for different energy intakes, starting with a 1200-kcalorie plan using the minimum number of servings suggested in the Daily Food Guide. This pattern would allow most people to lose weight at a satisfactory rate and still meet all nutrient needs. The other plans offer patterns for higher energy intakes. All of the patterns in the table supply less than 30 percent of kcalories from fat:

▸ I choose the ___-kcalorie diet.

6. Now plan a day's menus, following the pattern. What will you have for breakfast, lunch, dinner, and snacks (if any)?

■ STUDY QUESTIONS ■

1. What are the risks associated with underweight?
2. What are the risks associated with excess body fat?
3. What is central obesity and how is it related to disease?
4. Distinguish between body weight and body composition.
5. What factors are thought to cause obesity?
6. Discuss dietary strategies suitable for losing weight and maintaining a healthy body weight.
7. Why is physical activity so important in a weight-loss program?
8. Describe the behavior-modification techniques recommended for changing a person's dietary habits.
9. Describe strategies for successful weight gain.

NUTRITION IN PRACTICE 9

Eating Disorders

When and how does dieting to lose weight progress to the point that it is dangerous and obsessive? The specific causes of eating disorders baffle clinicians. Some speculate that society's excessive pressure to be thin is to blame; others point to neurological links with depression and impulsive behaviors or other biological malfunctions; and still others believe the cause is an inability to cope. They agree that the disorders, like obesity itself, are most likely multifactorial—sociocultural, neurochemical, and psychological. They also agree that the treatment requires a multidisciplinary approach.

What are eating disorders?

The two major types of eating disorders of concern today are anorexia nervosa and bulimia. An estimated 2 million people in the United States, primarily girls and women, meet the criteria that define these disorders. Many more do not meet the strict criteria, but still endanger their health. Psychologists refer to this category of eating disorders as unspecified eating disorders.[43] Furthermore, some evidence indicates that certain characteristics of disorderd eating such as restrained eating, binge eating, purging, fear of fatness, and distortion of body image may be extraordinarily common among young middle-class girls.[44] The alarming incidence of these disorders challenges health care professionals to prevent and treat them.

People with anorexia nervosa suffer from an extreme preoccupation with weight loss that seriously endangers their health and even their lives. People with bulimia engage in episodes of binge eating alternating with periods of severe dieting or self-starvation. Some bulimics also follow binge eating with self-induced vomiting, laxative abuse, or diuretic abuse to "undo the damage." The accompanying glossary defines the relevant terms.

You said girls and women are most vulnerable to anorexia nervosa and bulimia nervosa. Are there other vulnerable groups?

Yes. Athletes seem to be vulnerable, too.[45] To succeed in competition, athletes must often meet stringent weight requirements. Many athletes report that they

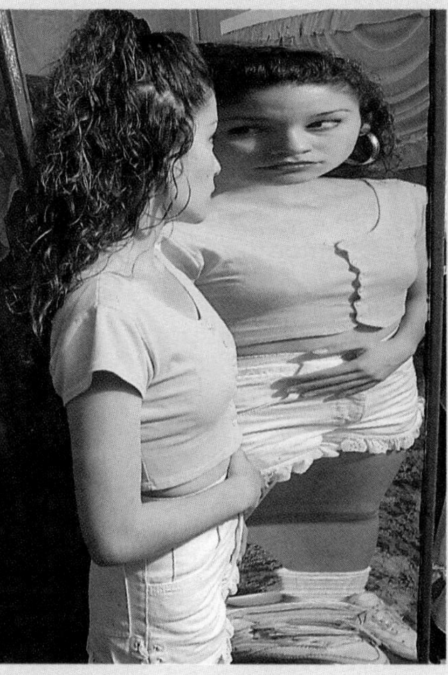

Women with anorexia nervosa see themselves as fat, even when they are dangerously underweight.

engage in behaviors that are typical of people with eating disorders. Female competitors often report being terrified of becoming fat, being obsessed with food, and using laxatives in attempting to control weight. They judge them-

Glossary of Eating Disorders

anorexia nervosa: a disorder involving a marked fear of fatness, self-starvation to the extreme, and a disturbed perception of body image, seen (usually) in teenaged girls and young women.

anorexia = without appetite

nervos = of nervous origin

bulimia (byoo-LEEM-ee-uh) **nervosa:** recurring binge eating combined with a morbid fear of becoming fat, sometimes followed by self-induced vomiting or purging.

compulsive overeating: an eating disorder characterized by uncontrolled chronic episodes of overeating without other symptoms of eating disorders.

eating disorder: a disturbance in eating behavior that jeopardizes a person's physical or psychological health.

unspecified eating disorders: eating disorders that do not meet the criteria for specific eating disorders previously defined.

selves to have suffered anorexia at some time.[46] Ballet dancers, jockeys, wrestlers, distance runners, gymnasts, and others whose body weight and appearance are frequently judged in comparison with an "ideal" are especially prone to develop problems. Also, people with eating disorders often pursue athletics as a means of ridding the body of energy from food.

Men account for about 1 in 20 cases in the general population, but among male athletes and dancers, eating disorders are much more common, possibly equaling the incidence among their female peers.[47] Male teenagers normally average about 15 percent of body weight as fat, but some high school athletes strive to carry only 5 percent or so of their body weight as fat.

I remember a high school friend who had anorexia nervosa. She was a very bright girl and seemed to have it all. Is that uncommon for a girl with anorexia nervosa?

Not at all. The person with anorexia almost always comes from an educated, middle- or upper-class family. A typical psychological profile includes depression, early developmental failure, and a characteristic cluster of family circumstances. The family values achievement and outward appearances more than an inner sense of self-worth and self-actualization.

The person with anorexia nervosa is often a perfectionist who works hard to please her parents. She may identify so strongly with her parents' ideals and goals for her that she sometimes feels she has no identity of her own. She earnestly desires to control her own destiny, but she feels controlled by others. When she does not eat, she gains control.

Many people go on diets. How do you know when a diet is going too far?

Many young women diet to lose weight. However, when a person loses weight to well below the average for her height and is no longer slim, but too slim, and still doesn't stop, she has gone too far. Regardless of how thin she is, she looks in the mirror and sees herself as fat. Central to the diagnosis of anorexia nervosa is a distorted body image that overestimates body fatness. Table 9–3 shows the criteria that professionals use to diagnose anorexia nervosa. Anorexia nervosa resembles an addiction. The characteristic behavior is obsessive and compulsive. Before drawing conclusions about someone who is extremely thin or who eats very little, remember that diagnosis of anorexia nervosa requires professional assessment.

What is the harm in being very thin?

Anorexia nervosa damages the body much as starvation does. In young people growth ceases and normal development falters. They lose so much lean tissue that

Table 9–3
Criteria for Diagnosis of Anorexia Nervosa

A person with anorexia nervosa demonstrates the following:

A. Refusal to maintain body weight at or above a minimal normal weight for age and height, e.g., weight loss leading to maintenance of body weight less than 85% of that expected; or failure to make expected weight gain during period of growth, leading to body weight less than 85% of that expected.
B. Intense fear of gaining weight or becoming fat, even though underweight.
C. Disturbance in the way in which one's body weight or shape is experienced; undue influence of body weight or shape on self-evaluation, or denial of the seriousness of the current low body weight.
D. In females past puberty, amenorrhea, i.e., the absence of at least three consecutive menstrual cycles. (A woman is considered to have amenorrhea if her periods occur only following hormone, e.g., estrogen, administration.)

Two types:

- *Restricting type:* During the episode of anorexia nervosa, the person does not regularly engage in binge eating or purging behavior (i.e., self-induced vomiting or the misuse of laxatives or diuretics).
- *Binge eating/purging type:* During the episode of anorexia nervosa, the person regularly engages in binge eating or purging behavior (i.e., self-induced vomiting or the misuse of laxatives or diuretics).

Source: Reprinted with permission from the American Psychiatric Association: *DSM-IV Draft Criteria* (3/1/93), Washington, D.C., American Psychiatric Association, 1993.

basal metabolic rate slows, an effect that may remain even after treatment and regain of weight.[48] In athletes, the loss of lean tissue affects physical performance unfavorably. Hormonal changes and nutrient deprivation compromise bone density and lead to stress fractures.[49] Losses of bone density are especially pronounced in female athletes who cease menstruating because of overtraining. In fact, eating disorders, premature bone loss, and irregular menstruation are a triple threat to overtrained female athletes.[50] Additionally, the heart pumps inefficiently and irregularly, the heart muscle becomes weak and thin, the chambers diminish in size, and the blood pressure falls. Electrolytes that help to regulate heartbeat become unbalanced. Many deaths from heart failure occur in people with anorexia.

Starvation brings other physical consequences as well: impaired immune response, anemia, and a loss of digestive function that worsens malnutrition. Digestive functioning becomes sluggish, the stomach empties slowly, and the lining of the intestinal tract shrinks. The ailing digestive tract fails to provide sufficient digestion of any food the victim may eat. The pancreas slows its production of digestive enzymes. The person may suffer from diarrhea, further worsening malnutrition.

Starvation also brings altered blood lipids, high concentrations of vitamin A and vitamin E in the blood, low blood proteins, dry skin, abnormal nerve functioning, low body temperature, and the development of fine body hair (the body's attempt to keep warm). The electrical activity of the brain becomes abnormal, and insomnia is common. Both women and men lose their sex drives.

What kind of treatment helps people with anorexia nervosa?

Treatment artfully combines medical, psychosocial, and dietary facets to initiate and sustain weight gain with psychological techniques to resolve personal and family problems. Teams of physicians, nurses, psychiatrists, family therapists, and dietitians work together to treat people with anorexia nervosa. Appropriate diet is crucial and must be tailored individually to each client's needs. Seldom are clients willing to eat for themselves, but if they are, chances are they can recover without other interventions.

High-risk clients may require hospitalization and may need to be force-fed by tube at first to forestall death. This step causes psychological trauma.[51] Drugs are commonly prescribed, but to date, they play a limited role in treatment.[52]

Denial runs high among those with anorexia nervosa. Few seek treatment on their own. Almost half of the women who are treated can maintain their body weight within 15 percent of healthy weight; at that weight, many of them begin menstruating again. The other half have poor or fair treatment outcomes and two-thirds of those treated fight an ongoing mental battle with recurring morbid thoughts about food and body weight.[53] Many relapse into abnormal eating behaviors to some extent. About 5 percent die during treatment, 1 percent by suicide.

How does bulimia nervosa differ from anorexia nervosa?

Bulimia nervosa is distinct from anorexia nervosa and is more prevalent. More men suffer from bulimia nervosa than from anorexia, but bulimia is still more common in women. The secretive nature of bulimic behaviors makes recognition of the problem difficult, but once it is recognized, diagnosis is based on the criteria listed in Table 9–4.

The typical person with bulimia is well educated, in her early twenties, and close to ideal body weight. She is a high achiever, with a strong feeling of dependence on her parents. She experiences considerable social anxiety and has difficulty establishing personal relationships. She is sometimes depressed and often exhibits impulsive behavior.

Like the person with anorexia nervosa, the person with bulimia spends much time thinking about her body weight and food. Her preoccupation with food manifests itself in secretive binge-eating episodes followed by self-induced vomiting, fasting, or the use of laxatives or diuretics. Such behaviors typically begin in late adolescence after a long series of various unsuccessful weight-reduction diets. People with bulimia commonly follow a pattern of restrictive dieting interspersed with bulimic behaviors and experience weight fluctuations of more than 10 pounds up and down over short periods of time.

Unlike the person with anorexia nervosa, the person with bulimia is aware of the consequences of her behavior, feels that it is abnormal, and is deeply ashamed of it. She feels inadequate and unable to control her eating, so she tends to be passive and to look to men for confirmation of her sense of self-worth. When she is rejected, either in reality or in her imagination, her bulimia becomes worse.

Table 9–4
Criteria for Diagnosis of Bulimia Nervosa

A person with bulimia nervosa demonstrates the following:

A. Recurrent episodes of binge eating. An episode of binge eating is characterized by both of the following:

1. eating, in a discrete period of time (e.g., within any two-hour period), an amount of food that is definitely larger than most people would eat during a similar period of time and under similar circumstances, and,
2. a sense of lack of control over eating during the episode (e.g., a feeling that one cannot stop eating or control what or how much one is eating).

B. Recurrent inappropriate compensatory behavior in order to prevent weight gain, such as self-induced vomiting; misuse of laxatives, diuretics, or other medications; fasting; or excessive exercise.
C. Binge eating and inappropriate compensatory behaviors that both occur, on average, at least twice a week for three months.
D. Self-evaluation unduly influenced by body shape and weight.
E. The disturbance does not occur exclusively during episodes of anorexia nervosa.

Two types:

- *Purging type:* The person regularly engages in self-induced vomiting or the misuse of laxatives or diuretics.
- *Nonpurging type:* The person uses other inappropriate compensatory behaviors, such as fasting or excessive exercise, but does not regularly engage in self-induced vomiting or the misuse of laxatives or diuretics.

Source: Reprinted with permission from the American Psychiatric Association: *DSM-IV Draft Criteria* (3/1/93), Washington, D.C., American Psychiatric Association, 1993.

If she gets carried away by bulimia, she may not only experience a deepening of her depression, but may move on to drug or alcohol abuse.

What exactly is binge eating?

Binge eating is not like normal eating. It is not primarily a response to hunger, and the food is not consumed for its nutritional value. It is a compulsion to eat. A typical binge occurs periodically, is done in secret, usually at night, and lasts an hour or more. A binge frequently follows a period of rigid dieting, so that binge eating is accelerated by hunger. During a binge the person with bulimia may consume between one thousand and many thousands of kcalories of food. The food typically contains little fiber or water, has a smooth texture, and is high in sugar and fat, so that it is easy to consume vast amounts rapidly with little chewing.

What are the consequences of this behavior?

After a binge, the person develops swollen hands and feet, bloating, fatigue, headache, nausea, and pain. Repeated binges result in more serious consequences. A fluid and electrolyte imbalance caused by vomiting can lead to abnormal heart rhythms and injury to the kidneys, which have to cope with the altered balance. Infections of the bladder and kidneys can lead to kidney failure. Vomiting causes irritation and infection of the pharynx, esophagus, and salivary glands; erosion of the teeth; and dental caries. The esophagus may rupture or tear, as may the stomach. Sometimes the eyes become red from pressure during vomiting. The hands may be bruised and lacerated from scraping on the teeth while inducing vomiting.

Some people use cathartics—violent laxatives that can injure the lower intestinal tract. Others use emetics, drugs that induce vomiting. Repeated use can lead to heart failure due to poisoning. It was emetic abuse that caused the death of popular singer Karen Carpenter in 1983.

What is the treatment for bulimia?

As for people with anorexia nervosa, a team approach provides the most effective treatment for

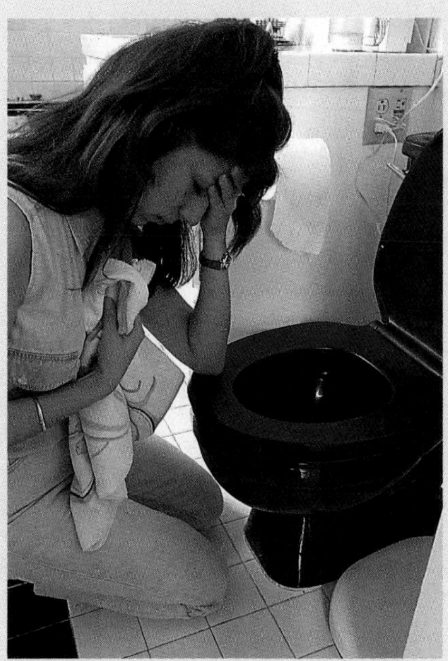

For many people with bulimia, guilt, depression, and self-condemnation follow a binge-eating episode.

people with bulimia. Bulimia is easier to treat than anorexia nervosa in many respects because it seems to be more of a chosen behavior. People with bulimia know that their behavior is abnormal, and many are willing to try to cooperate.

The goal of the dietary plan to treat bulimia is to help clients gain control, establish regular eating patterns, and restore nutritional health.[54] Energy intake should not be severely restricted. The person needs to learn to eat a quantity of nutritious food sufficient to nourish her body and to satisfy hunger (at least 1600 kcalories a day). The accompnying box offers some ways to begin correcting bulimia nervosa.

A mental health professional should be on the treatment team. Almost 90 percent of people with bulimia are clinically depressed, and the rates of alcohol, marijuana, and cigarette abuse are high.

Anorexia nervosa and bulimia nervosa are distinct eating disorders, each having a specific set of diagnostic criteria and medical complications. Yet they also sometimes overlap. Anorexia victims may purge, and victims of both conditions share an overconcern with body weight and the tendency to drastically undereat. The two disorders can also appear in the same person, or one can lead to the other.

At so tender an age as 12 years, beautifully growing, normal-weight female youngsters are already worried that they are too fat. Most are "on diets." Maga-zines, newspapers, and television all present the message that to be thin is to be beautiful and happy. Anorexia nervosa and bulimia are not a form of rebellion against these unreasonable expectations, but rather the exaggerated acceptance of them. Perhaps a person's best defense against these disorders is to learn to appreciate her own uniqueness. The author Eda LeShan beautifully described her recovery from overeating: "Deep inside there had always been a small child begging for my attention. . . . All I gave her was food. Now I give her love."[55] To respect and value oneself may be lifesaving.

HOW TO Combat Bulimia Nervosa

The following advice has proven useful for people fighting bulimia nervosa:

- Avoid finger foods; eat foods that require the use of utensils.
- Enhance satiety by eating warm foods.
- Include vegetables, salad, and/or fruit at meals to prolong eating time.
- Choose whole-grain and high-fiber breads and cereals to maximize bulk.
- Eat a well-balanced diet and meals consisting of a variety of foods.
- Use foods that are naturally divided into portions, such as potatoes (rather than rice or pasta); 4- and 8-ounce containers of yogurt, ice cream, or cottage cheese; precut steak or chicken parts; and frozen entrees.
- Include foods containing ample complex carbohydrates (for satiety) and some fat (to slow gastric emptying).
- Eat meals and snacks sitting down.
- Plan meals and snacks, and record plans in a food diary prior to eating.

Source: Reproduced with permission from Nutrition & Eating Disorders. Copyright © 1989, Quest Publishing Company, division of Raven Press, 1351 Titan Way, Brea, CA 92621, (714) 738-6400.

NOTES

1. Parts of this discussion have been adapted with permission from E. N. Whitney and S. R. Rolfes, *Understanding Nutrition,* 6th ed. (St. Paul, Minn.: West Publishing Co., 1993), pp. 242–283; F. S. Sizer and E. N. Whitney, *Nutrition: Concepts and Controversies,* 6th ed. (St. Paul, Minn.: West Publishing Co., 1994), pp. 310–348.
2. G. A. Bray, Obesity: Classification of subtypes, an address presented at the North American Association for the Study of Obesity and Emory University School of Medicine Conference on Obesity Update: Pathophysiology, Clinical Consequences, and Therapeutic Options, Atlanta, Georgia, August 31–September 2, 1992.
3. F. X. Pi-Sunyer, Health implications of obesity, *American*

Journal of Clinical Nutrition 53 (1991): 1595S–1603S.

4. R. J. Kuezmarski, Prevalence of overweight and weight gain in the United States, *American Journal of Clinical Nutrition* 55 (1992): 4955–5025.
5. J. E. Manson and coauthors, A prospective study of obesity and risk of coronary heart disease in women, *New England Journal of Medicine* 322 (1990): 882–889.
6. A. Must and coauthors, Long-term morbidity and mortality of overweight adolescents, *New England Journal of Medicine* 327 (1992): 1350–1355; G. A. Bray, Adolescent overweight may be tempting fate, *New England Journal of Medicine* 327 (1992): 1378–1380.
7. Pi-Sunyer, 1991; E. M. Emery and coauthors, A review of the association between abdominal fat distribution, health outcome measures, and modifiable risk factors, *American Journal of Health Promotion,* May/June 1993, pp. 342–353.
8. Committee on Diet and Health, Food and Nutrition Board, *Diet and Health: Implications for Reducing Chronic Disease Risk* (Washington, D.C.: National Academy Press, 1989), p. 117; Emery and coauthors, 1993; A. R. Folsom and coauthors, Body fat distribution and 5-year risk of death in older women, *Journal of the American Medical Association* 269 (1993): 483–487.
9. C. Bouchard, G. A. Bray, and V. S. Hubbard, Basic and clinical aspects of regional fat distribution, *American Journal of Clinical Nutrition* 52 (1990): 946–950.
10. P. Björntorp, Regional obesity, in P. Björntorp and B. N. Brodoff, eds., *Obesity* (Philadelphia: J. B. Lippincott, 1992), pp. 579–586.
11. C. Ley, B. Lees, and J. C. Stevenson, Sex- and menopause-associated changes in body fat distribution, *American Journal of Clinical Nutrition* 55 (1992): 950–954.
12. R. J. Troisi, Cigarette smoking, dietary intake, and physical activity: Effects on body fat distribution—The Normative Aging study, *American Journal of Clinical Nutrition* 53 (1991): 1104–1111; Emery and coauthors, 1993.
13. S. L. Gortmaker and coauthors, Social and economic consequences of overweight in adolescence and young adulthood, *New England Journal of Medicine* 329 (1993): 1008–1012.
14. U.S. Department of Agriculture and U.S. Department of Health and Human Services, Home and Garden Bulletin No. 232, *Nutrition and Your Health: Dietary Guidelines for Americans,* 3rd ed. (Washington, D.C.: Government Printing Office, 1990).
15. C. W. Callaway, New weight guidelines for Americans, *American Journal of Clinical Nutrition* 54 (1991): 171–172.
16. Addresses presented at the North American Association for the Study of Obesity and Emory University School of Medicine Conference on Obesity Update: Pathophysiology, Clinical Consequences, and Therapeutic Options, Atlanta, Georgia, August 31–September 2, 1992.
17. S. H. Stensland and S. Margolis, Simplifying the calculation of body mass index for quick reference, *Journal of the American Dietetic Association* 90 (1990): 856.
18. Committee on Diet and Health, 1989, pp. 563–592.
19. Committee on Diet and Health, 1989, pp. 99–135.
20. G. A. Bray, Pathophysiology of obesity, *American Journal of Clinical Nutrition* 55 (1992): 488S–494S.
21. T. G. Lohman, Body composition assessment in sports medicine, *Sports Medicine Digest,* September 1990, pp. 1–2.
22. G. A. Bray, Definition and characterization of obesity, an address presented at the North American Association for the Study of Obesity and Emory University School of Medicine Conference on Obesity Update: Pathophysiology, Clinical Consequences, and Therapeutic Options, Atlanta, Georgia, August 31–September 2, 1992.
23. C. Bouchard and L. Perusse, Genetics of obesity, *Annual Review of Nutrition* 13 (1993): 337–354.
24. A. J. Stunkard and coauthors, The body-mass index of twins who have been reared apart, *New England Journal of Medicine* 322 (1990): 1483–1487.
25. C. Bouchard, The response to long-term overfeeding in identical twins, *New England Journal of Medicine* 322 (1990): 1477–1482.
26. E. Ravussin and C. Bogardus, A brief overview of human energy metabolism and its relationship to essential obesity, *American Journal of Clinical Nutrition* 55 (1992): 242S–245S.
27. R. H. Eckel, Lipoprotein lipase regulation in obesity and after weight loss, an address presented at the North American Association for the Study of Obesity and Emory University School of Medicine Conference on Obesity Update:

Pathophysiology, Clinical Consequences, and Therapeutic Options, Atlanta, Georgia, August 31–September 2, 1992.
28. Eckel, 1992.
29. P. Lönnroth and U. Smith, Intermediary metabolism with an emphasis on lipid metabolism, adipose tissue, and fat cell metabolism, in *Obesity,* eds. P. Björntorp and B. N. Brodoff (Philadelphia: Lippincott, 1992), pp. 3–14.
30. Failure to maintain weight loss: Permissive role of lipoprotein lipase, *Nutrition Reviews,* October 1989, pp. 328–331.
31. A. J. Stunkard, Body weight regulation, an address presented at the North American Association for the study of Obesity and Emory University School of Medicine Conference on Obesity Update: Pathophysiology, Clinical Consequences, and Therapeutic Options, Atlanta, Georgia, August 31–September 2, 1992.
32. D. J. Mela and D. A. Sacchetti, Sensory preferences for fats: Relationships with diet and body composition, *American Journal of Clinical Nutrition* 53 (1991): 908–915.
33. G. K. Goodrick and J. P. Foreyt, Why treatments for obesity don't last, *Journal of the American Dietetic Association* 91 (1991): 1243–1247.
34. M. Shah and coauthors, Comparison of a low-fat, ad libitum complex-carbohydrate diet with a low-energy diet in moderately obese women, *American Journal of Clinical Nutrition* 59 (1994): 980–984.
35. D. M. Dreon and coauthors, Dietary fat: Carbohydrate ratio and obesity in middle-aged men, *American Journal of Clinical Nutrition* 47 (1988) 995–1000.
36. L. Sheppard, A. R. Kristal, and L. H. Kushi, Weight loss in women participating in a randomized trial of low-fat diets, *American Journal of Clinical Nutrition* 54 (1991): 821–828; T. E. Prewitt and coauthors, Changes in body weight, body composition, and energy intake in women fed high- and low-fat diets, *American Journal of Clinical Nutrition* 54 (1991): 304–310.
37. NIH Technology Assessment Conference Panel, Methods for voluntary weight loss and control, *Annals of Internal Medicine* 116 (1992): 942–949.
38. G. L. Blackburn and coauthors, Weight cycling: The experience of human dieters, *American Journal of Clinical Nutrition* 49 (1989): 1105–1109.
39. A. M. Prentice and coauthors, Effects of weight cycling on body composition, *American Journal of Clinical Nutrition* 56 (1992): 209S–216S.
40. L. Lissner and coauthors, Variability of body weight and health outcomes in the Framingham population, *New England Journal of Medicine* 324 (1991): 1839–1844: L. Lissner and K. D. Brownell, Weight cycling, mortality, and cardiovascular disease: A review of epidemiologic findings, in P. Björntorp and B. N. Brodoff, eds., *Obesity* (Philadelphia: J. B. Lippincott, 1992), pp. 653–661.
41. E. T. Poehlman and E. S. Horton, The impact of food intake and exercise on energy expenditure, *Nutrition Reviews* 47 (1989): 129–137.
42. W. D. McArdle, F. I. Katch, and V. L. Katch, *Exercise Physiology: Energy, Nutrition, and Human Performance,* 2nd ed. (Philadelphia: Lea & Febiger, 1991), pp. 634–655.
43. Task force on DSM-IV, 307–50, Eating Disorder Not Otherwise Specified, DSM-VI *Draft Criteria* (Washington, D.C.: American Psychiatric Association, 1993), p. P:2.
44. L. M. Mellin, C. E. Irwin, and S. Scully, Prevalence of disordered eating in girls: A survey of middle-class children, *Journal of the American Dietetic Association,* 92 (1992): 851–853.
45. K. K. Yeager and coauthors, The female athlete triad: Disordered eating, amenorrhea, osteoporosis, *Medicine and Science in Sports and Exercise* 25 (1993): 775–777.
46. J. L. Walbery and C. S. Johnston, Menstrual function and eating behavior in female recreational weight lifters and competitive body builders, *Medicine and Science in Sports and Exercise* 23 (1991): 30–36.
47. "Anorexia athletica," Special report on nutrition and the athlete, *Sports Medicine Digest,* 1989, p. 10; S. N. Steen and K. D. Brownell, Patterns of weight loss and regain in wrestlers: Has the tradition changed? *Medicine and Science in Sports and Exercise* 22 (1990): 762–768.
48. R. C. Casper and coauthors, Total daily energy expenditure and activity level in anorexia nervosa, *American Journal of Clinical Nutrition* 53 (1991): 1143–1150; L. Scalfi and coauthors, Bioimpedance analysis and resting energy expenditure in undernourished and refed anorectic patients, *European Journal of Clinical Nutrition* 47 (1993): 61–67.
49. R. B. Mazess, H. S. Barden, and E. S. Ohlrich, Skeletal and body-composition effect of anorexia nervosa, *American*

Journal of Clinical Nutrition 52 (1990): 438–441: L. K. Bachrach and coauthors, Decreased bone density in adolescent girls with anorexia nervosa, *Pediatrics* 86 (1990): 440–447.

50. R. C. Henderson, Bone health in adolescence: Anorexia and athletic amenorrhea, *Nutrition Today,* March/April 1991, pp. 25–29; F. Munning, Tackling women's health issues, *Physician and Sportsmedicine,* September 1992, p. 33.
51. B. R. Carruth, Adolescence, in *Present Knowledge in Nutrition,* ed. M. L. Brown (Washington, D.C.: International Life Sciences Institute—Nutrition Foundation, 1990), pp. 325–332.
52. L. G. Tolstoi, The role of pharmacotherapy in anorexia nervosa and bulimia, *Journal of the American Dietetic Association* 89 (1989): 1640–1646.
53. American Psychiatric Association Workgroup on Eating Disorders, Practice guidelines for eating disorders, I. Disease definition, epidemiology, and natural history, *American Journal of Psychiatry* 150 (1993): 212–228.
54. S. H. Krey, Eating disorders: The clinical dietitian's changing role, *Journal of the American Dietetic Association* 89 (1989: 41–43.
55. E. LeShan, *Winning the Losing Battle: Why I Will Never Be Fat Again* (New York: Crowell, 1979).

10

Fitness and Nutrition

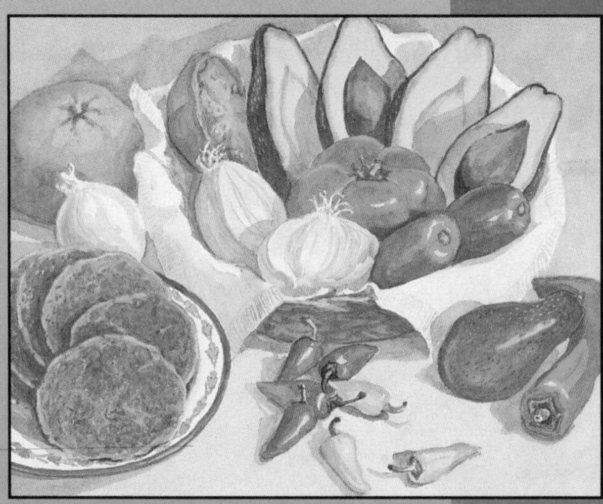

CONTENTS

Extensive evidence confirms that regular physical activity promotes health and prevents disease.[1] Still, despite an increasing awareness of the health benefits that physical activity confers, as many as 60 percent of adults in the United States are either irregularly active or completely inactive.[2]

Physical inactivity is linked to the major degenerative diseases—heart disease, cancer, stroke, and hypertension—that are the primary killers of adults in developed countries.[3] Therefore, one of the most important challenges health care professionals face is to motivate more people to become physically active. To motivate others, health care professionals must first become more physically active themselves, thereby enhancing their own health. Second, they can include regular physical activity as a component of therapy for their clients.

People don't have to run marathons to reap the health rewards of physical activity. In fact, anyone who is extremely inactive stands to gain the greatest health benefits by engaging in a regular program of moderate-intensity, endurance-type activity.[4] Researchers who conducted an extensive study on physical fitness and mortality concluded that "moderate levels of physical fitness that are attainable by most adults appear to be protective against early mortality."[5] It makes sense, then, to promote activities that can readily be performed by the least active people, since they can benefit most. Table 10–1 shows that regular physical activity protects against many diseases and conditions.[6]

Table 10–1
Regular Physical Activity Helps to Protect against These Physical Conditions

- Backaches
- Cancer (colon cancer, breast cancer, and others)
- Diabetes
- Digestive disorders (ulcers, constipation, diarrhea, and others)
- Headaches
- Heart and blood vessel disease (heart attacks and strokes)
- High blood cholesterol, high blood pressure
- Infections (colds, flu, and many others)
- Kidney disease
- Menstrual irregularities
- Obesity
- Osteoporosis (adult bone loss)

In 1990, the American College of Sports Medicine (ACSM) updated an earlier (1978) position statement on the quantity and quality of exercise recommended for developing and maintaining fitness in healthy adults (see Table 10–4 on p. 250).[7] The main objective of these guidelines was to outline the types and amounts of physical activity needed for improving *physical fitness*. These familiar guidelines have helped adults develop programs to improve their cardiorespiratory endurance and body composition. However, the types and amounts of physical activity needed to promote *fitness* may differ from those needed to obtain *health* benefits. For health's sake, the ACSM specifies that people should spend an accumulated minimum of 30 minutes in some sort of physical activity on most days of each week.[8] The activity need not be sports. A few minutes spent climbing up stairs, another few spent pulling weeds, and several more spent walking the dog all contribute to the day's total. The guidelines for developing fitness (listed in Table 10–4) are still optimal, though, because they produce superb results in terms of health and improve the heart's capacity to do its work.

This chapter begins by defining fitness and presenting its benefits. Then it goes on to show how nutrition supports fitness.

Fitness

Perhaps you are already physically fit. If so, the following description applies to you. You are graceful and move with ease. You are strong and meet physical challenges without strain. You have endurance, and your energy lasts for hours. You can meet normal physical challenges with ease and have plenty of energy in reserve to handle emergencies. What is more, you are likely to be well able to meet mental and emotional challenges, too—for physical fitness undergirds mental and emotional, as well as physical, energy and resilience.

If these statements do not describe you as you are today, then you can gain fitness through practice. Activities that promote fitness are themselves enjoyable, and they quickly lead to rewards in terms of physical improvements. Feeling fit can build your confidence in other areas of life, too: social, academic, professional—you name it.

Three Definitions of Fitness

Narrowly defined, the term fitness describes *the characteristics of the body that enable it to perform physical activity.* These characteristics include flexibility of the joints; strength and endurance of the muscles, including the heart muscle; and a healthy body composition. A broader definition of fitness is *the ability to meet routine physical demands with enough reserve energy to rise to a sudden challenge.* This definition shows how fitness relates to everyday life: ordinary tasks such as carrying heavy suitcases, opening a stuck window, or climbing four flights of stairs, which might strain an unfit person, can be well within the capacity of the fit person. Still another definition is *the body's ability to withstand stress,* meaning stress of all kinds, including psychological stress. There is no contradiction among these three definitions; they are three different descriptions of the same wonderful condition of the body.

fitness: the characteristics of the body that enable it to perform physical activity; more broadly, the ability to meet routine physical demands with enough reserve energy to rise to a sudden challenge; or the body's ability to withstand stress of all kinds.

The Lack of Fitness Fitness is the reward of a person who leads a physically active life. The opposite of such a life is a sedentary life, which means, literally, "sitting down a lot." Today's world permits many people to lead inactive lives and even rewards them for it. It provides elevators, escalators, cars, and golf carts so that people can exert a minimum of physical effort. Unfortunately, people are attracted to labor-saving devices, but the more they use the devices, the more weak and unfit they become, and the less well they feel. The body responds to inactivity by losing muscle and skill, just as it responds to activity by gaining them.

sedentary: physically inactive (literally, "sitting down a lot").

Fitness and Physical Activity A person who practices a physical activity *adapts* by becoming better able to perform it after each session—more flexible, stronger, more enduring. Moreover, a person who gains physical fitness also gains in abilities to take exams in school and to take on major responsibilities in society or on the job. Activity promotes fitness; fitness promotes stress resistance in general; and stress resistance benefits health in many ways.[9]

Physical activity and fitness are so closely connected that the rest of this chapter makes no distinction between them. The benefits of fitness are the benefits of physical activity, and vice versa. Table 10–2 summarizes these benefits.

A person seeking fitness does not have to be an elite athlete. Rather, a person needs to develop enough flexibility, muscular strength, and endurance to meet the everyday demands of life with some to spare and to achieve a reasonable body weight and body composition.

Table 10–2
Benefits of Fitness (Summary)

- Sound, beneficial rest and sleep.
- Improved nutritional health.
- Reduced fatness and increased lean body tissue.
- Improved resistance to colds, other infectious diseases, and cancer.
- Reduced risk of heart and blood vessel disease, diabetes, and other diseases.
- Reduced probability of accidents; fewer and less severe injuries.
- Reduced incidence and severity of anxiety and depression.
- Freedom from drug (including alcohol) abuse.
- Improved self-image and self-confidence.
- Better learning ability.
- Greater interpersonal, social, and spiritual strengths.
- Improved quality of life in the later years.
- Longer life.

Components of Fitness

Physical fitness expresses itself in body characteristics. Some are health related, some are skill related. The health-related components of fitness include flexibility, muscle endurance and strength, cardiorespiratory endurance, and body composition. Flexibility allows the joints to move without injury. Muscle endurance and strength enable muscles to work without fatigue. Cardiorespiratory endurance supports the ongoing action of the heart and lungs. Fitness also expresses itself in body composition—the proportions of muscle, fat, bone, and other tissue that make up a person's total body weight. Physical activity augments desirable lean body tissue and eliminates excess body fat. Thus, as a person becomes physically fit, the health of the entire body improves.

The person who wants to go beyond general health and enhance athletic performance in specific sports will also value skill-related components of fitness such as agility, balance, coordination, power, reaction time, and speed. The importance of each characteristic varies widely with individual sports, and athletes practice endless hours to develop them. The glossary on page 246 describes these characteristics.

Principles of Conditioning

Training, or practice, sessions develop fitness and skills. The way to achieve conditioning is by training, primarily by applying overload—that is, by asking a little more of the body in each practice session. During conditioning, the body adapts microscopically to perform the work asked of it. Whatever component of fitness a person seeks to develop, whether flexibility, strength, or endurance, the principles of conditioning apply.

The Overload Principle You can apply the progressive overload principle in several different ways. You can perform the activity more often, that is, increase its frequency; you can perform the activity more strenuously, that is, increase its intensity; or you can do it for longer times, that is, increase its duration. All three strategies work well, and you

flexibility: the capacity of the joints to move through a full range of motion; the ability to bend and recover without injury.

muscle endurance: the ability of a muscle to contract repeatedly within a given time without becoming exhausted.

muscle strength: the ability of muscles to work against resistance.

cardiorespiratory endurance: the ability to perform large-muscle, dynamic exercise of moderate to high intensity for prolonged periods.

body composition: the proportions of muscle, bone, fat, and other tissue that make up a person's total body weight.

conditioning: the physical effect of *training;* improved flexibility, strength, and endurance.

training: practicing an activity, which leads to conditioning. Training is what you do; conditioning is what you get.

overload: an extra physical demand placed on the body; an increase in the *frequency, duration,* or *intensity* of exercise.

progressive overload principle: the training principle that a body system, in order to improve, must be worked at frequencies, durations, or intensities that gradually increase physical demand.

frequency: the number of occurrences per unit of time (for example, the number of exercise sessions per week).

intensity: the degree of exertion while exercising (for example, the amount of weight lifted or the speed of running).

duration: length of time (for example, the length of time spent in each exercise session).

Glossary of Skill-Related Fitness Components

agility: the ability to move the entire body quickly.

balance: the ability to maintain equilibrium in a fixed position or in motion.

coordination: the harmonious functioning of the senses and the muscles to accurately perform complex movements, such as hitting a baseball or juggling two or more objects.

power: the combination of strength and speed that allows a person to move quickly and forcefully, such as in jumping, shot-putting, or spiking a ball.

reaction time: the amount of time between a stimulus and a response to the stimulus, such as when starting a race.

speed: the ability to move fast, as in running or swimming.

can pick one or a combination, depending on your preferences. For example, if you really love your workout, do it more often. If you do not have much time, increase intensity. If you hate hard work, take it easy and go longer. If you desire continuous improvements, remember to overload progressively as you gain higher levels of fitness.

Applying Overload When you are increasing the frequency, intensity, or duration of your workout, exercise to a point that only *slightly* exceeds your comfortable capacity to work. It is better to progress too slowly than to risk serious injury by overexertion. Here are other pointers about applying overload:

- Be active all week. Don't be a weekend athlete.
- Train hard only once or twice a week, not every time you work out. Between times, do light workouts.
- Pay attention to body signals. Symptoms such as the following demand immediate medical attention: abnormal heartbeats; pain or pressure in the middle of the chest, teeth, jaw, neck, or arm; dizziness; lightheadedness; cold sweat; or confusion.
- Use proper equipment and attire.
- Perform approved exercises using proper form.

Cautions on Starting Before you begin any fitness program, make sure it is safe for you to do so. The ACSM classifies individuals into three groups based on coronary risk factors (see Table 10–3). The classification "apparently healthy" applies to those individuals who have no more than one of the major coronary risk factors listed in Table 10–3. The second category, "individuals at higher risk," pertains to those who have two or more of the risk factors in Table 10–3 and/or symptoms suggestive of disease. The third category, "individuals with disease," applies to those individuals with known cardiac, pulmonary, or metabolic disease.

Most "apparently healthy" people can begin moderate exercise programs such as walking or increasing daily activities without the need for medical examination, but people in either of the other two classifications

Table 10–3
Major Coronary Risk Factors

1. Diagnosed hypertension or systolic blood pressure ≥160 or diastolic blood pressure ≥90 mmHg on at least two separate occasions, or on antihypertensive medication.
2. Serum cholesterol ≥6.20 mmol/L (≥240 mg/dl).
3. Cigarette smoking.
4. Diabetes mellitus.[a]
5. Family history of coronary or other atherosclerotic disease in parents or siblings prior to age 55.

[a]Persons with insulin-dependent diabetes mellitus (IDDM) who are over 30 years of age, or have had IDDM for more than 15 years, and persons with non-insulin-dependent diabetes mellitus who are over 35 years of age should be classified as patients with disease and treated according to the guidelines specific for those individuals. Chapter 25 describes coordination of diet and exercise for people with diabetes.

Source: American College of Sports Medicine, *Guidelines for Exercise Testing and Prescription,* 4th ed. (Philadelphia: Lea & Febiger, 1991), pp. 1–10.

need medical advice.[10] The ACSM describes *moderate exercise* as activity that can be sustained comfortably for 60 minutes or so. It does not make sense to start with activities so demanding that pain stops you within two days. Learn to enjoy small steps toward improvement. Fitness builds slowly.

moderate exercise: exercise that can be sustained comfortably for 60 minutes or so.

Warm-Up and Cool-Down Within training sessions, gradualness is a key to success. Sudden intense activity can cause injury, and abrupt discontinuance can hamper recovery, so it is best to ease into and out of activity sessions. All strenuous workouts should therefore be fitted inside a frame composed of warm-up and cool-down activities.

A warm-up facilitates gradual warming of the body and helps prepare muscles, ligaments, and tendons for activity to come. Most important, the onset of activity stimulates the release of the hormone epinephrine, which mobilizes fuels to support strength and endurance activities.

Cool-down activity eases the transition from exercising to normal functioning. A few minutes of light activity facilitate the relaxation of tight muscles and enhance the circulation of blood through them. The circulation in turn brings accumulated heat from the body's core to the surface, where it can radiate away. As you approach the end of your workout, gradually ease up on the intensity of the activity (for example, if you are running, begin to slow to a light jog), reaching a minimum intensity over 5 to 10 minutes. Stretching exercises to promote flexibility are particularly well suited to the end of the cool-down.

Cool-down activities can also help to prevent symptoms—dizziness, for example—that you may experience if you abruptly stop exercising. A cool-down facilitates a gradual drop in blood pressure; an abrupt drop would stress the heart. A cool-down can also help to prevent muscle cramps that might otherwise occur.

warm-up: five to ten minutes of light exercise, such as easy jogging or cycling, to warm up the body in preparation for vigorous exercise.

cool-down: five to ten minutes of light exercise following a vigorous workout to gradually cool the body's core to near-normal temperature.

epinephrine (ep-ih-NEFF-rin)**:** one of the stress hormones. It is secreted whenever emergency action is called for; it readies body systems for fast action and mobilizes fuel to support that action.

Unlike a poorly maintained car, which will break down when consistently overloaded, the body responds to overload in a positive way—it gets itself into better shape to meet the demand next time. As the next section shows, the overload principle applies to the heart muscle in the same way that it does to the other muscles of the body: the heart becomes stronger.

Cardiorespiratory Endurance

As you know, the heart beats faster during exercise than during rest. The length of time a person can keep exercising with an elevated heart rate—that is, the ability of the heart, lungs, and blood to sustain a given demand—defines the person's cardiorespiratory endurance. Training can improve ability to sustain a vigorous activity such as running, brisk walking, or swimming. Cardiorespiratory endurance training enhances the ability of the heart, lungs, and blood to deliver oxygen to, and remove waste from, the body's cells during such activity. The benefits of this training are not only physical, though, because all of the body's cells, not just the muscle cells, require oxygen to function. When the cells receive more oxygen more readily, both the body and mind benefit.

Working muscles need especially large amounts of oxygen to produce energy. Cardiorespiratory endurance training requires the heart and lungs to work extra hard for a sustained period to deliver oxygen to the muscle cells. Cardiorespiratory endurance training, therefore, is *aerobic* (oxygen-requiring). As the cardiorespiratory system gradually adapts to the demands of aerobic exercise, the body delivers oxygen more efficiently.

aerobic (air-ROE-bic)**:** refers to energy-producing processes involving the immediate use of oxygen.
aero = air

Benefits of Aerobic Conditioning The changes brought about by aerobic workouts are called cardiorespiratory conditioning. Among its benefits, the total blood volume increases, so that the blood can carry more oxygen. The heart becomes larger and stronger, and each beat pumps more blood. As the heart pumps more blood with each beat, fewer beats are necessary, and the pulse rate slows down. The average resting pulse rate for adults is around 70 beats per minute, but people who have cultivated cardiorespiratory conditioning may have resting pulse rates of 50 or even lower. The muscles that work the lungs become stronger, too, so breathing becomes more efficient. Circulation through the arteries and veins improves. Blood moves easily, and blood pressure falls.

cardiorespiratory conditioning: improvements in the heart and lung function and increased blood volume, brought about by aerobic training.

Training for cardiorespiratory conditioning:

- Increases blood volume and oxygen delivery.
- Increases heart strength and stroke volume.
- Slows resting pulse.
- Increases breathing efficiency.
- Improves circulation.
- Reduces blood pressure.

stroke volume: the amount of oxygenated blood the heart ejects toward the tissues at each beat.

Cardiorespiratory endurance is the physical achievement that many people appropriately prize the most highly, because it reflects the health of the heart and circulatory system, on which all other body systems depend. Figure 10–1 shows the major relationships among the heart, circulatory system, and lungs.

To improve your cardiorespiratory endurance, you must train at an intensity that elevates your heart rate a certain amount above its resting rate. Although formulas based on maximal oxygen uptake (VO_2 max) or maximal heart rate are available, a person's own perceived effort is usually a reliable indicator of activity intensity. In general, when you're working out, do so at an intensity that raises your breathing and heart rate, but still leaves you able to talk comfortably with a friend. If you are more competitive and want to work to your limit on some days, a treadmill test can reveal your maximal heart rate. You can work out safely at up to 90

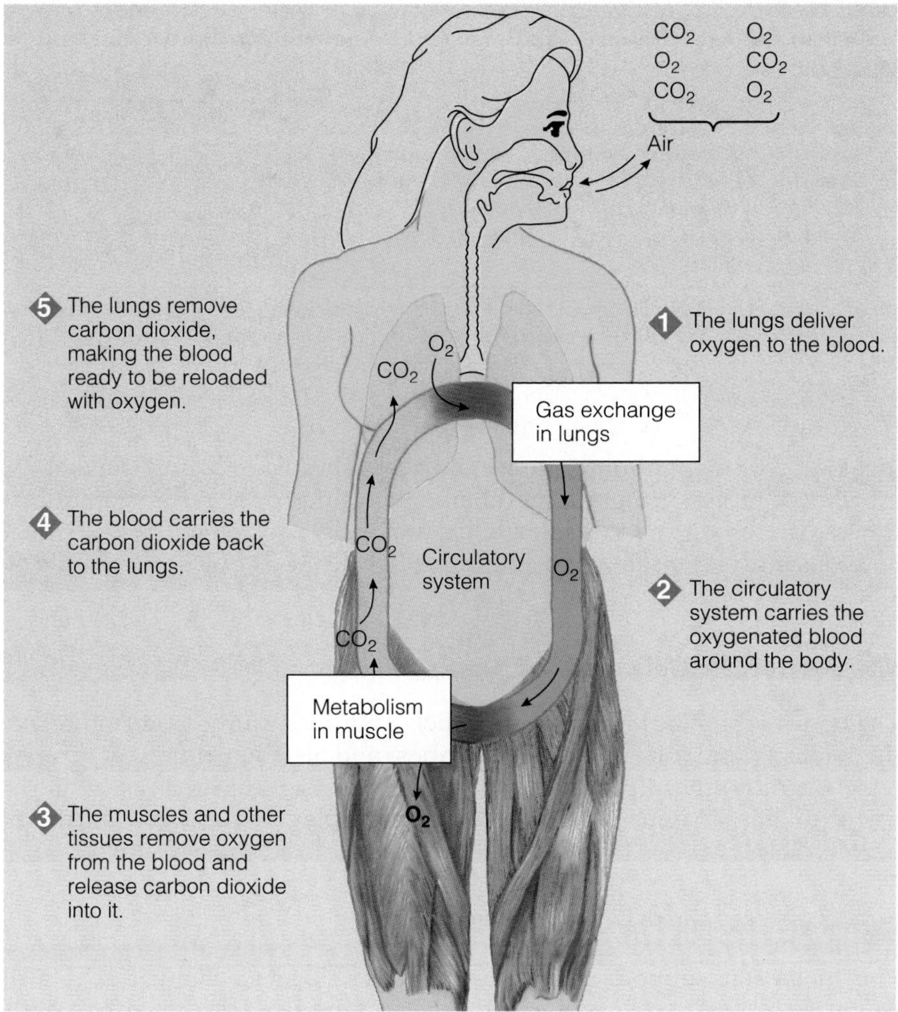
CO2 O2
O2 CO2
CO2 O2
Air
5 The lungs remove carbon dioxide, making the blood ready to be reloaded with oxygen.
O2
CO2
1 The lungs deliver oxygen to the blood.
Gas exchange in lungs
4 The blood carries the carbon dioxide back to the lungs.
CO2
Circulatory system
O2
2 The circulatory system carries the oxygenated blood around the body.
CO2
Metabolism in muscle
O2
3 The muscles and other tissues remove oxygen from the blood and release carbon dioxide into it.

Figure 10–1
Delivery of Oxygen by the Heart and Lungs to the Muscles
The more fit a muscle is, the more oxygen it draws from the blood. That oxygen is drawn from the lungs, so the person with more fit muscles extracts more oxygen from the inhaled air than a person with less fit muscles. The cardiorespiratory system responds to the demand for oxygen by building up its capacity to deliver oxygen.

percent of that rate. The ACSM guidelines for developing and maintaining cardiorespiratory fitness are listed in Table 10–4 on page 250.[11]

Cardiorespiratory Training Benefits Muscles A fringe benefit of aerobic training is its effect on muscles. The more fit a muscle is, the more oxygen it draws from the blood. That oxygen is drawn from the lungs, so the person with more fit muscles extracts more oxygen from the inhaled air than a person with less fit muscles. This improves the efficiency of the cardiorespiratory system still further, reducing the heart's workload. An added bonus is that muscles that can use more oxygen can burn fat longer—a plus for body composition and weight control.

Anaerobic Training In contrast to aerobic activity, anaerobic activity generally does not bring about cardiorespiratory conditioning, but develops strength and bulk of muscles. Anaerobic activity involves sudden, all-out exertions of muscles that last less than 90 seconds. Examples

Table 10–4
American College of Sports Medicine Guidelines for Cardiovascular and Muscular Fitness

- **Frequency of training:** three to five days per week.
- **Intensity of training:** 60 to 90% of maximum heart rate.
- **Duration of activity:** 20 to 60 minutes of continuous activity.
- **Mode of activity:** any activity that uses large muscle groups.
- **Resistance training:** strength training of moderate intensity at a minimum of two times per week.

Note: The ACSM notes that duration and intensity are interrelated, so that 40 to 50 minutes of brisk walking may be needed to gain the same result as 20 to 30 minutes of jogging.

Table 10–5
A Sample Balanced Fitness Program (45 Minutes a Day)

Monday, Wednesday, Friday:
- 10 minutes of warm-up activity and stretching.
- 25 minutes of aerobic exercise.
- 10 minutes of cool-down activity.

Tuesday, Thursday:
- 10 minutes of warm-up activity and stretching.
- 25 minutes of weight training.
- 10 minutes of cool-down activity.

Saturday or Sunday:
- Softball, walking, hiking, biking, or swimming.

include sprinting, jumping a fence, doing push-ups, or lifting weights. In a balanced fitness program, aerobic activity improves cardiorespiratory fitness, stretching enhances flexibility, and weight training or calisthenics develops muscle strength and endurance. Table 10–5 shows an example of a balanced fitness program.

The Active Body's Use of Fuels

The body uses different mixtures of fuels at different times, depending on the intensity and duration of its activities, and also depending on its own prior conditioning. For athletes who seek the highest levels of achievement in sports, some knowledge of the interplay of fuels and nutrients permits selection of a diet that will best support the chosen activity.

Carbohydrate and Physical Activity

The fuels that support activity are glucose (from carbohydrate), fatty acids (from fat), and, to a small extent, amino acids (from protein). Glucose and its stored form, glycogen, are particularly crucial to athletes who compete in endurance events.

During rest, the body derives a little more than half of its energy from fatty acids and most of the rest from glucose, along with a small percentage from amino acids. During exertion, the liver releases its glucose into the bloodstream. The muscles pick up this glucose and use it in addition to glucose from their own glycogen stores. Although glycogen supplies are ample to support everyday activity, they are less abundant than body fat stores; in other words, glycogen is limited.

Glycogen Storage Depends on Diet The body constantly uses and replenishes its glycogen. How much glycogen a body stores depends partially on the amount of carbohydrate in the diet. How much carbohydrate a person eats affects how much glycogen is stored, which in turn influences how much will be used during activity.[12] Thus diet bears on performance because the more glycogen you store, the longer the stores will last as you work.

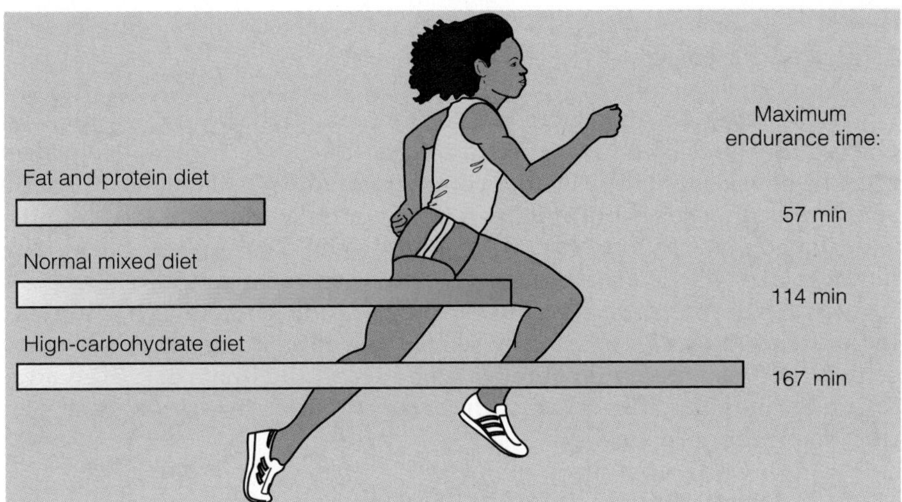
Maximum
endurance time:
Fat and protein diet
57 min
Normal mixed diet
114 min
High-carbohydrate diet
167 min

Figure 10–2
The Effect of Diet on Physical Endurance
A high-carbohydrate diet can triple an athlete's endurance.

A classic study compared fuel use during exercise among three groups of runners, each on a different diet. For several days before testing, one of the groups consumed a normal mixed diet (55 percent of kcalories from carbohydrate), the second group consumed a high-carbohydrate diet (83 percent of kcalories from carbohydrate), and the third group consumed a high-fat diet (94 percent of kcalories from fat). Figure 10–2 shows that the high-carbohydrate diet allowed the athletes to keep going longer before they became exhausted. This study and many others that followed suggest that a high-carbohydrate diet enhances endurance by promoting the storage of ample glycogen. A later section of this chapter describes how to choose a performance diet, paying special attention to carbohydrate.

Intensity of Activity Affects Glycogen Use How long an exercising person's glycogen lasts depends not only on diet, but also partly on the intensity of the exercise. The most intense activities—the kind that make it difficult to "catch your breath" such as a quarter-mile race—use glycogen quickly. Other, less-intense activities, such as jogging, during which breathing is steady and easy, use glycogen more slowly. But joggers still use it, and if they run long enough, eventually they run out of it. Glycogen depletion usually occurs within about two hours from the onset of moderately intense exercise.

The more intense the exercise, the more glycogen is used, because glucose from glycogen can serve as a fuel even when oxygen is in short supply, as when a person is "out of breath." Glucose can "burn" without oxygen; it can serve as an anaerobic fuel.

During *moderate* activity, the lungs and circulatory system have no trouble keeping up with the muscles' need for oxygen—the activity is aerobic. During aerobic activity, energy derives from both glucose and fatty acids.

During *intense* activity, the demand for oxygen becomes too high to permit much use of fat as fuel. When a person exercises faster than the heart and lungs can supply oxygen to the muscles, aerobic metabolism cannot meet energy needs. The muscles must instead draw more heavily on glucose for energy.

lactic acid: a compound produced in muscles when they break down glucose anaerobically; it can cause burning pain if not promptly drained away.

Lactic Acid: An Anaerobic Waste Product When muscles are using glucose as a fuel without sufficient oxygen to "burn" it completely, they break it down only partway, to a compound known as lactic acid. Lactic acid builds up, causes burning pain in the muscles, and can lead to muscle exhaustion within seconds if it is not cleared away. The blood can, however, carry lactic acid to the liver, which can reconvert it to glucose. A strategy for dealing with the pain caused by lactic acid buildup is to relax the muscles at every opportunity so that the circulating blood can carry acid away. Tired mountain climbers can ascend the final peak, even after severe burning pain has set in, if they relax their leg muscles at each step (the "mountain rest step").

These factors affect glycogen use in exercise:

- Dietary and stored carbohydrate.
- Intensity of the activity.
- Duration of the activity.
- Degree of training.

Duration of Activity Affects Glycogen Use Glycogen use during exercise depends not only on the *intensity* of the activity, but also on its *duration*—how long it continues. Within the first 20 minutes or so of moderate exercise, a person uses mostly glycogen for fuel. A person who continues exercising moderately for longer than 20 minutes begins to use less and less glycogen and more and more fat. Still, glycogen use continues, and if the activity is long and hard enough, glycogen stores run out almost completely. Exercise can continue for a short time thereafter only because the liver scrambles to produce from the available lactic acid and amino acids a small amount of glucose that can briefly forestall total depletion. When glycogen and glucose depletion hits, it brings nervous system function almost to a halt, making continued exertion almost impossible.

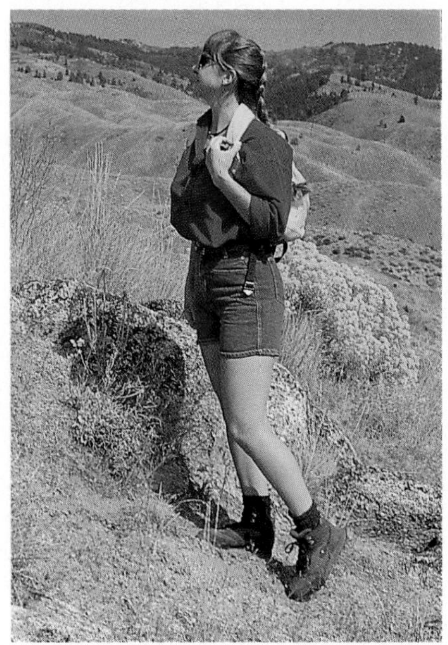

The mountain rest step permits muscles to relax and recover even during strenuous hikes.

Degree of Training Affects Glycogen Use Training also affects how much glycogen muscles store—muscles that deplete their glycogen through work adapt to store greater amounts of glycogen to support that work. The more glycogen the muscles store, the longer the stores last during physical activity. Muscles make still another adaptation to training that affects glycogen use during activity—conditioned muscles rely less on glycogen and more on fat for energy, so the rate of glycogen breakdown in trained individuals is lower than in untrained individuals at the same intensity of work.

Glycogen stores can be depleted within just a few days of exercise if an exerciser eats a diet that is high in protein and low in carbohydrates. Then the exerciser may feel burned out and sluggish. The exerciser may attribute these symptoms to vitamin deficiencies, but they indicate a need for glycogen, which comes from a carbohydrate-rich diet. To prevent the fatigue caused by glucose depletion, endurance athletes try to maintain their blood glucose concentrations for as long as they can. Three dietary strategies and one exercise strategy may help maintain glucose concentrations.

- Eat a high-carbohydrate diet (60 to 70 percent of energy intake) regularly.
- Take glucose (usually in fruit juice or other sweet beverage) periodically during exercise that lasts for 90 minutes or more.

- Eat carbohydrate-rich foods following exercise.
- Train the muscles, so they will store as much glycogen as possible.

Before concluding that sugar might be good for your own performance, though, consider whether you engage in *endurance* activity. Do you run, swim, bike, or ski nonstop at a steady pace for more than an hour and a half at a time? If not, the sugar picture changes. For an everyday jog, swim, or game match, sugar probably will not help performance because such activity is not limited by carbohydrate availability. The body's glycogen stores are usually sufficient.

Fat and Physical Activity

An active person who eats a fat-rich diet with little carbohydrate will burn more fat during activity, but will sacrifice performance, as Figure 10–2 showed. Since even physically active people are not immune to heart attacks and strokes, it is no wonder that every reliable source speaks out against high-fat diets for active people. The active person's body can supply fat and will make more when it needs to as long as food energy is adequate.

Duration of Activity Affects Fat Use Unlike glycogen stores, which are limited, body fat stores can fuel hours of activity without running out, as long as the exercise is not too intense. Fat is a virtually unlimited source of energy. Early in an activity, the muscles draw on and use the fatty acids already available to them from the blood. If the activity continues for more than a few minutes, the fat cells get the message that more fat is needed for energy, and they begin rapidly breaking down their stored fat to keep the supply going. After about 20 minutes of sustained, moderate exercise, the fat cells are significantly shrinking in size as they empty out their lipid stores.

Intensity of Activity Affects Fat Use In addition to duration, intensity also affects fat use. As intensity increases, fat makes less and less of a contribution to the total fuel used. Fat can be broken down for energy in one way only—aerobically. Thus, for fat to fuel exercise, oxygen is indispensable. (Remember, if you are breathing easily during exercise, your muscles are getting all the oxygen they need and are able to burn fat.)

Degree of Training Affects Fat Use The body adapts in response to aerobic activity. For one thing, the trained person's heart and lungs become stronger and better able to deliver oxygen at high exercise intensities. For another, as already mentioned, the muscle cells develop greater capacity to use fat as fuel. For still another, the trained person's hormones slow glucose release from the liver and encourage fat use instead. The person who wishes to burn fat by exercising can conclude that patient, persistent training is worthwhile and that steady, long-duration activity works best.

The key to burning fat is steady, long-duration exercise.

Table 10–6 summarizes fuel use during physical activity as discussed so far. You may wonder why the third energy-yielding nutrient, protein, is not listed in the table. The reason is that protein donates only a little ener-

Table 10–6
Carbohydrate and Fat Use during Activity

FUEL USED	PERFORMANCE TIME	OXYGEN NEEDED?	EXERCISE INTENSITY	ACTIVITY EXAMPLES
Carbohydrate	30 seconds to 3 minutes	No	Very high	1/4-mile sprint, a football play
Mostly carbohydrate (and some fat)	3 to 20 minutes	Yes	High	Distance swimming or running
Mostly fat (and some carbohydrate)	More than 20 minutes	Yes	Moderate	Distance running or jogging, cross-country skiing

Sources: Adapted in part from M. H. Williams, Human energy, in *Nutritional Aspects of Human Physical Performance,* 2nd ed. (Springfield, Ill.: Charles C. Thomas, 1985), pp. 21–57; E. L. Fox, Sports activities and the energy continuum, in *Sports Physiology,* 2nd ed. (New York: Saunders, 1984), pp. 26–39.

gy to physical activity. However, it does provide the structural material of muscle tissue, so it is important to active people.

Protein and Physical Activity

The body handles protein differently during activity than at rest. Synthesis of body proteins is suppressed during activity and for several hours afterward. In the hours following this period, though, protein synthesis rebounds beyond normal resting levels.[13] The body must adapt and build the tissues it needs for the next period of activity. Whenever the body remodels a part of itself, it must tear down old structures to make way for new ones. Repeated activity, with just a slight overload, triggers the equipment of each muscle cell to do so—that is, the muscle cells adapt.

Activity Triggers Protein Synthesis The physical work of each muscle cell acts as a signal to its protein-building systems to begin producing the kinds of proteins that best support that work.[14] Take jogging, for example. In the first difficult sessions, the body is not yet well prepared to perform. The muscle fibers have not adapted to producing the energy needed for aerobic work. But with each session, the cells get the message that an overhaul is needed. In the hours that follow the session, muscle cells busily break down any unneeded protein structures and begin producing the needed new structures. Just one or two exercise sessions do not appreciably affect the muscles, but within a few weeks, remodeling occurs, and jogging becomes easier.

Protein Recommendations for Active People All athletes, as well as those who work like athletes, probably need a little more protein than do sedentary people. A joint position paper from the American Dietetic Association (ADA) and the Canadian Dietetic Association (CDA) recommends 1.0 to 1.5 grams of protein per kilogram of body weight each day, an amount somewhat higher than the 0.8 grams per kilogram of body weight a day recommended for sedentary people.[15] Because most U.S. and Canadian adults eat diets containing plenty of protein, though, no one needs protein supplements, or even large servings of meat, to obtain the protein they need. A later section translates protein recommendations into diet.

Vitamins, Minerals, and Water

Popular belief has it that vitamin supplements can lead to both health benefits and improved performance for those who are physically active. It goes without saying that active people need adequate vitamins and minerals to do what they do, as Table 10–7 shows. But research confirms that nutrient supplements do not enhance the performance of well-nourished people.[16] In a well-controlled study of 30 runners, substantial nutrient supplementation for three months did not improve performance.[17] Active people do not need supplements—they can get the nutrients they need from food.

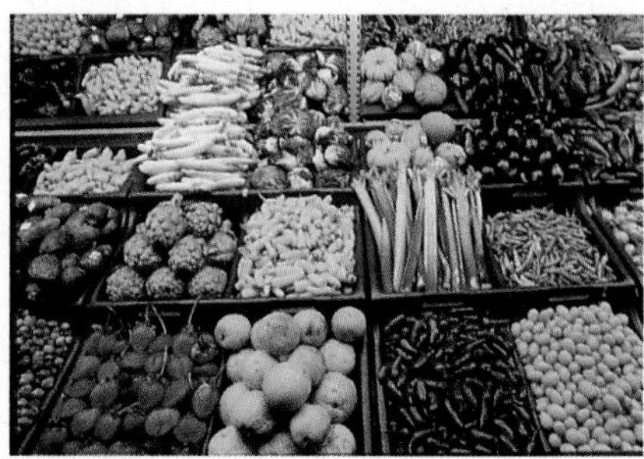

Vitamins and minerals in abundance are best obtained from foods, not supplements.

Like the vitamins, all of the nutrient minerals are essential to physical activity. Three are of special current interest: chromium, zinc, and copper, which people excrete in their urine in larger amounts when they exercise than when they are sedentary.[18] So far, though, it is too early to say whether these added losses increase people's nutrient needs. In general, the minerals are probably like the vitamins in that active people do not need them in supplement form. For the most part, active people who choose foods with care can be sure of meeting their vitamin and mineral needs without supplements.

Iron Deficiency in Women Athletes Iron is an exception to the rule just stated. Physically active young women, especially those who engage in endurance activities such as distance running, are prone to iron deficiency. Iron status may be affected by exercise in any of several ways. One possibility is that iron lost in sweat creates the deficiency, although the sweat of trained athletes contains less iron than the sweat of others (an

Table 10–7
Roles of Vitamins and Minerals in Exercise

VITAMIN OR MINERAL	FUNCTION
Thiamin, riboflavin, niacin, magnesium	Energy-releasing reactions
Vitamin B_6, zinc	Building of muscle protein
Folate, vitamin B_{12}	Building of red blood cells to carry oxygen
Vitamin C	Collagen formation for joint and other tissue integrity; hormone synthesis
Vitamin E	Protection of cell membranes against oxidative damage
Iron	Transport of oxygen in blood and in muscle tissue; energy transformation reactions
Calcium	Building of bone structure; muscle contractions; nerve transmissions
Phosphorus	Energy-releasing reactions
Sodium, potassium, chloride	Maintenance of fluid balance; transmission of nerve impulses for muscle contraction
Chromium	Assistance in insulin's energy-storage function
Magnesium	Cardiac and other muscle contraction

Note: This is just a sampling. Other vitamins and minerals play equally indispensable roles in exercise.

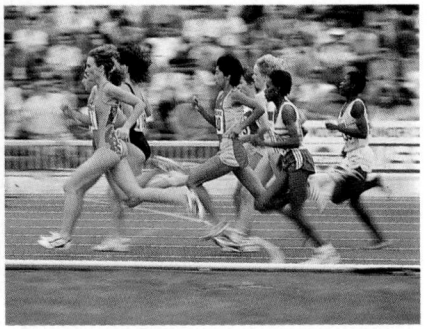

Women athletes may be at special risk of iron deficiency.

adaptation to conditioning). Still, athletes sweat more copiously than sedentary people. Another possible route to iron loss is red blood cell destruction: blood cells are squashed when body tissues (such as the soles of the feet) make high-impact contact with an unyielding surface such as the ground. In addition, physical activity may cause small blood losses through the digestive tract, at least in some athletes. Research studies show that as many as 45 percent of female runners of high school age have low iron stores.[19] Habitually low intakes of iron-rich foods, combined with iron losses aggravated by physical activity, may cause iron deficiency in physically active young women.

Iron deficiency impairs physical performance because iron is crucial to the body's handling of oxygen. One consequence of iron-deficiency anemia is impaired oxygen transport. This reduces aerobic work capacity, so the person tires easily. Whether marginal deficiency without anemia impairs physical performance is a point of debate among researchers.[20]

Sports Anemia Early in training, athletes may develop low blood hemoglobin for a while. This condition, sometimes called "sports anemia," probably reflects a normal adaptation to physical training. Aerobic training enlarges the blood volume, and with the added fluid, the red blood cell count per unit of blood drops. True iron deficiency requires treatment with prescribed iron supplements, but the temporary reduced red blood cell count seen early in training goes away by itself after a while.

Iron Supplements May Be Needed Because true iron deficiency is a real possibility for all people, and especially for active people and athletes, it is important to keep track of your own iron status. (All routine physical examinations that include blood work check you for the extreme deficiency state, anemia, but you should also be aware that such tests will not tell you if your iron stores are low.) Consider your individual needs. Many young menstruating women probably border on iron deficiency even without the additional iron losses incurred through exercise. Active teens of both genders, because they are growing, have high iron needs, too. Especially for women and teens, then, supplements may be needed to maintain iron stores or to correct a deficiency of iron.

Iron supplements are available over the counter, but because the absorption of iron from them is poor, it may take a dose as high as twice the RDA or more for several weeks to deliver sufficient iron to replenish depleted stores. Taking a self-prescribed supplement may mask symptoms of a dangerous condition such as gastrointestinal bleeding from ulcers or cancer, though, so anyone considering this course of action should consult a health care professional before adopting it.

Electrolyte Losses in Sweat Electrolytes—the charged minerals sodium, potassium, chloride, and magnesium—are lost from the body in sweat. Beginners lose electrolytes to a much greater extent than do trained athletes; as the body adapts to physical activity, it becomes better at conserving most electrolytes. People normally need to make no special effort to replenish lost electrolytes. A regular diet that meets their energy and nutrient needs also supplies all the electrolytes they need.

Moderate Electrolyte Replacement During physical activity, electrolyte replacement is also not necessary unless a person works up a drenching sweat amounting to the loss of 5 to 10 pounds or more each day (3 percent of body weight) for several consecutive days. In that case, drinking plain water and relying on food to replace lost electrolytes may not suffice, and a commercial "sweat replacer" beverage, diluted by half with water, may be drunk for fluid and electrolyte replacement. A homemade mixture of ⅓ teaspoon of table salt and 1 cup of fruit juice added to each quart of water will also serve the purpose. Avoid electrolyte or salt tablets; they can irritate the stomach and cause vomiting, and they always cause water to flow into the digestive tract from the tissues at first, thereby temporarily worsening dehydration and impairing performance. As for potassium, avoid potassium supplements unless prescribed by a physician; although they better some conditions, they worsen others.

Water Is Key to Performance Water is a crucial nutrient for everyone, especially those engaged in physical activity. Exercise blunts the thirst mechanism, especially in cold weather. During physical activity, thirst signals too late, after fluid stores are depleted, so don't wait to feel thirsty before drinking. To find out how much water you need to replenish exercise losses, weigh yourself before and after the activity—the difference is all water. One pound equals roughly 2 cups of fluid. You will feel better and your workout will seem easier if you consistently tend to your body's fluid needs. Plain, cool water is the best fluid for the exercising body for two reasons: it rapidly leaves the digestive tract to enter the tissues, and it cools the body. Table 10–8 offers a schedule of hydration for exercise.

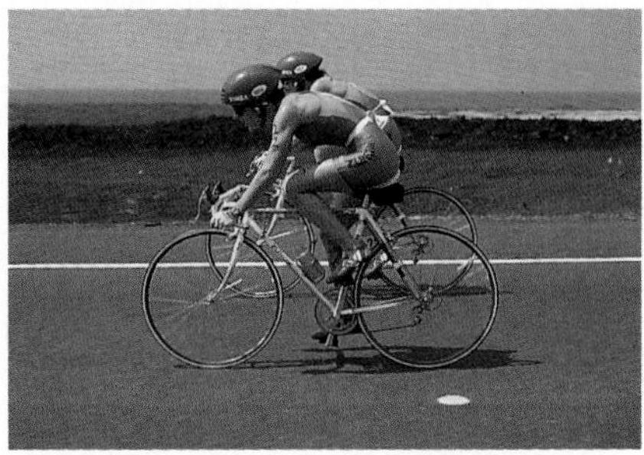

Those who compete in endurance activities require fluid and carbohydrate fuel.

Food for Fitness

No one diet best supports physical performance. Many different diets can be excellent for active people. However, food choices must be made within the framework of rules for diet planning presented in Chapter 1. The active person needs a diet composed mostly of nutrient-dense foods, the kind that supply a maximum of vitamins and minerals for the energy they provide. When active people eat mostly refined, processed foods that have suffered nutrient losses and that contain added sugar and fat, nutrient status suffers.[21]

Table 10–8
Schedule of Hydration before, during, and after Exercise

WHEN TO DRINK	TOTAL AMOUNT OF FLUID
2 hours before exercise	About 3 c
10 to 15 minutes before exercise	About 2 c
Every 15 minutes during exercise	About 1 c
After exercise	Replace each pound of body weight lost with 2 c fluid

Source: Clark, N. Fluid facts. *The Physician and Sportsmedicine,* 1992 (11), pp. 33–36.

Active people need to eat both for adequacy and for energy. Active people are not immune to heart disease and cancer and so must limit fats. A diet that is high in carbohydrate (60 percent of total kcalories or more), low in fat (25 percent or less), and adequate in protein (12 to 15 percent) ensures full glycogen and other nutrient stores. Such a diet helps to control weight (thus reducing risks of diabetes and other diseases) and provides adequate fiber while supplying abundant nutrients. Table 10–9 shows some sample diet plans for people who wish to increase their energy and carbohydrate intakes to allow for a physically active lifestyle, and Figure 10–3 displays the foods a person at the 3000-kcalorie level might eat in a day to fit the recommended pattern. Notice how abundant carbohydrate is in the athlete's meals.

On certain occasions the active person's high-carbohydrate, fiber-rich diet may require temporary adjustment. Both of these exceptions involve training for competition rather than fitness. During intensive training, energy needs may outstrip the person's capacity to eat enough to meet them. At that point, added sugar and fat may be needed. The other special occasion is the pregame meal, when fiber-rich, bulky foods are best avoided. Carbohydrate-rich foods such as pasta and fruit juices—low in fat, protein, and fiber—are the basis of the pregame meal. The recommended pregame meal includes plenty of fluids and is light and easy to digest. The meal or snack should provide between 300 and 800 kcalories, primarily from carbohydrate-rich foods that are familiar and well-tolerated. The meal should end three to five hours before competition to allow the stomach enough time to empty before exertion.

The person who chooses to live a physically active life can expect to enjoy the rewards of fitness and good overall health as well as the pleasures of the chosen activities themselves. Another benefit accompanies these: when you spend more kcalories, you can eat more food, which can bring

Table 10–9
High-Carbohydrate Food Patterns for Various Energy Levels

	1500 kcal	2000 kcal	2500 kcal	3000 kcal	3500 kcal	4000[a] kcal
Food Group	**Number of Exchanges**					
Milk	3	3	4	4	4	4
Fruit	5	6	7	9	10	12
Vegetable	3	3	3	5	6	7
Grain	7	11	16	18	20	24
Fat	2	3	5	6	8	10
Meat	5	5	5	5	6	6
Percent carbohydrate:	58%	58%	63%	64%	60%	62%

[a]A way to add more energy to the diet without adding much bulk is to include snacks of milkshakes or "complete meal" liquid supplements.

Figure 10–3
An Example of What an Athlete Might Eat in a Day
These meals deliver over 3000 kcalories, 61% of them from carbohydrate, 24% from fat, and 15% from protein.

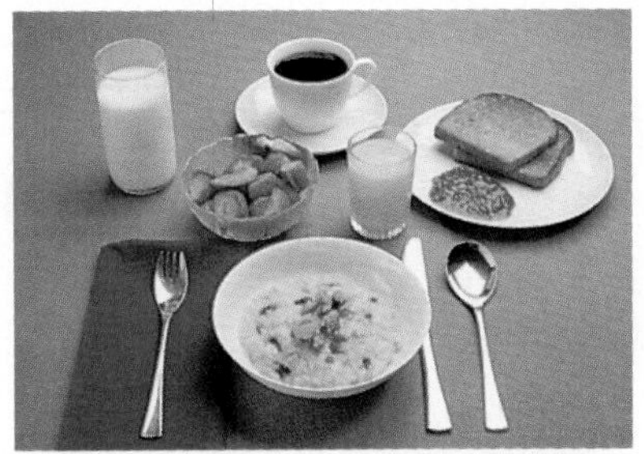

Breakfast:

8 oz	low-fat milk.
½ c	strawberries.
½ c	orange juice.
1 c	oatmeal with raisins and 2 tsp brown sugar.
2 slices	whole-wheat toast with 4 tsp jelly.
1 c	coffee.

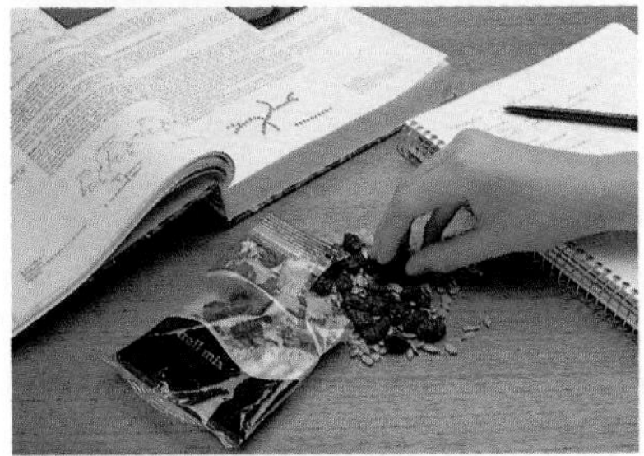

Snack:

4 tbs	trail mix.

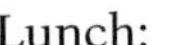

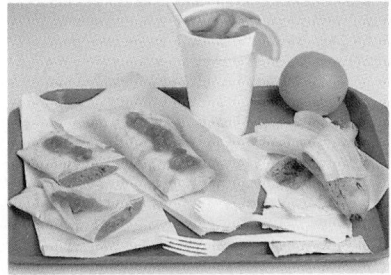

Lunch:

3	beef and bean burritos.
1	orange.
1	banana.
12 oz	iced tea with sugar.

Snack:

1 c	low-fat milk.
1 piece	angel-food cake.

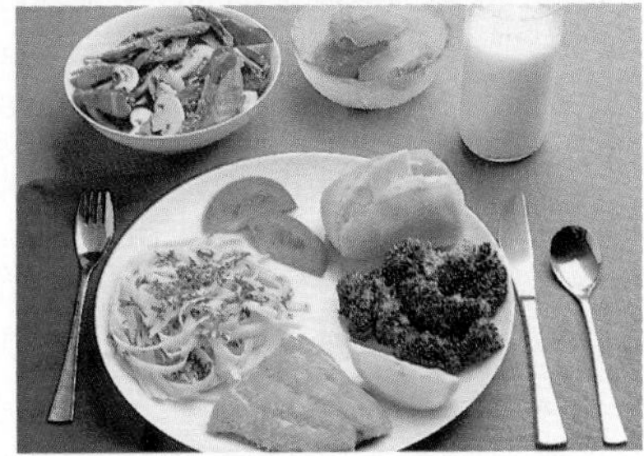

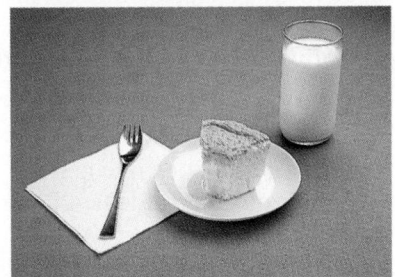

Dinner:

1 c	spinach salad with 1 tbs salad dressing.
8 oz	low-fat milk.
1	dinner roll with 2 tsp margarine.
1 c	broccoli.
4 oz	salmon.
¾ c	noodles with parsley and 2 tsp margarine.
¼	tomato.
1 c	sherbet.

you added pleasure and improved nutrition status. The next chapter focuses on foods themselves, and specifically on the food choices that best support health.

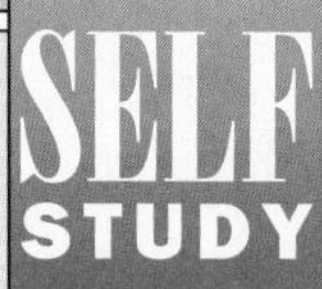

How Physically Active Are You?

"The road to fitness is physical activity." To find out how physically active you are, answer the following questions and record your answers on Form 10 on p. 261. For each question answered yes, give yourself the number of points indicated. Then total your points to determine your score. Don't take this quiz too seriously; it is intended only to help you become aware of opportunities for improving your fitness.

A. Formal, Vigorous Exercise Routines

1. I participate in active recreational sports such as tennis or handball for an hour or more.
   a. About once a week. (*2 points*)
   b. About twice a week. (*4 points*)
   c. Three times a week. (*6 points*)
   d. Four times a week. (*8 points*)

(Adjust your point score if your answer is less or more than these. For example, if you play sports six days a week, give yourself more points—say, 12 points. If you play once a week for only 30 minutes, give yourself 1 point. Note: Any session of less than 20 minutes counts as zero.)

2. At least once a week, I participate in vigorous fitness activities like aerobic dancing, jogging, or swimming (at least 20 continuous minutes each session):
   a. About once a week. (*3 points*)
   b. About twice a week. (*6 points*)
   c. Three times a week. (*9 points*)
   d. Four times a week. (*12 points*)

(Adjust your point score upward or downward if your answer is slightly different from these. For example, if you work out *six* days a week, give yourself more points—say, 18 points.)

B. Other Formal Exercise Routines

3. At least two times a week, I perform floor workouts (sit-ups, push-ups) for at least ten minutes:
   a. Two sessions a week. (*2 points*)
   b. Three sessions a week. (*3 points*)
   c. Four or more sessions a week. (*4 points*)

(No points for a session of less than ten minutes; no points for only one session a week; maximum is 4 points.)

4. At least two times a week, I participate in yoga or perform stretching exercises for at least ten minutes:
   a. Two sessions a week. (*2 points*)
   b. Three sessions a week. (*3 points*)
   c. Four or more sessions a week. (*4 points*)

(No points for a session of less than ten minutes; no points for only one session a week; maximum is 4 points.)

5. At least two times a week, I work out with weights for at least ten minutes:
   a. Two sessions a week. (*2 points*)
   b. Three sessions a week. (*3 points*)
   c. Four or more sessions a week. (*4 points*)

(No points for a session of less than ten minutes; no points for only one session a week; maximum is 4 points.)

C. Occupation and Daily Activities

6. I walk to and from school, work, and shopping (½ mile or more each way), two or three times a week or more. (*1 point*)
7. I climb stairs rather than using elevators or escalators, every other day or more. (*1 point*)
8. My school, job, or household routine involves physical activity that fits the following description:

Self-Study (continued)

Form 10
Physical Activity Scorecard

Record your point scores here for the Self-Study:

Category	Score
A. Formal, Vigorous Exercise Routines	___ (A high score would be 20.)
B. Other Formal Exercise Routines	___ (A high score would be 12.)
C. Occupational and Daily Activities	___ (A high score would be 12.)
D. Leisure Activities	___ (A high score would be 11.)
Total:	___ (A high score would be 50.)

Evaluation of total score (circle one):

- Inactive (0 to 5 points).
- Moderately active (6 to 11 points).
- Active (12 to 20 points).
- Very active (21 points or over).

If your score categorized you as inactive or only moderately active, return to Parts A through D, reread the questions, and choose some activities that you would like and could realistically undertake to raise your score to "active" (12 points or more). List these activities below. You are not committing yourself to doing these things, just acknowledging that you could.

A. Formal, Vigorous Exercise Routines

I could: ______________________________

____

____

State for how long and how many times a week: ______________________________

____

B. Other Formal Exercise Routines

I could: ______________________________

____

____

State for how long and how many times a week: ______________________________

C. Occupation and Daily Activities

I could: ______________________________

____

____

State for how long and how many times a week: ______________________________

____

D. Leisure Activities

I could: ______________________________

____

____

State for how long and how many times a week: ______________________________

____

(continued)

Self-Study (continued)

a. It is mostly desk work or light physical activity. (*0 points*)
b. It is mostly farm activities, moderate physical activity, brisk walking, or the like. (*4 points*)
c. Many of my typical days include several hours of heavy physical activity such as shoveling or lifting. (Don't include sports practice here. See Part A.) (*2 points per day*)

(Part C maximum: 12 points.)

D. Leisure Activities

9. I do several hours of gardening, lawn work, or equally active hobby work each week. (*1 point*)
10. I fish or hunt once a week or more on the average. (This must involve active work such as rowing a boat or tracking game. Dock and truck sitting don't count.) (*1 point*)
11. At least once a week I dance vigorously (folk or square dance) for an hour or more. (*1 point*)
12. In season, I play 9 to 18 holes of golf at least once a week, and I do not use a power cart. (*2 points*)
13. I walk for exercise or recreation.
    a. One to two hours a week. (*1 point per hour*)
    b. Three to four hours a week. (*2 points*)
    c. Five hours or more a week. (*3 points*)
14. In *addition* to the above, I choose to engage in other forms of physical activity:
    a. One to two hours a week. (*1 point*)
    b. Three to four hours a week. (*2 points*)
    c. Five hours or more a week. (*3 points*)

(For Part D, don't count sports practice. See Part A.)

(Part D maximum: 11 points.)

STUDY QUESTIONS

1. Define fitness in three ways.
2. Explain how fitness benefits physical health.
3. Describe the health-related components of fitness.
4. Discuss the differences between conditioning and training.
5. Describe the progressive overload principle.
6. Why are warm-up and cool-down activities important to fitness?
7. Describe some of the conditioning effects of cardiorespiratory endurance training.
8. Explain how glycogen use during exercise is related to the intensity of the exercise.
9. What is sports anemia?
10. Why is plain, cool water the best fluid for the exercising body?
11. What kinds of foods should active people emphasize in their diets?

NUTRITION IN PRACTICE 10

Athletic Hocus-Pocus: Ergogenic Aids Athletes Use

In a world where body condition and skill are hard won, athletes gravitate to promises that they can easily improve their performance by taking pills or potions. Athletes too often hear well-intended, but unsubstantiated, advice from their coaches and peers recommending that they use special nutrients, drugs, or procedures to enhance performance. The wish to win is strong but no amount of wishing can change the fact that an overwhelming majority of supplements sold for athletes are frauds. If the products that are tried have no effect and are harmless, they are only a waste of money; but some products are harmful or actually impair performance, and these are a waste of athletic potential as well. This Nutrition in Practice looks at some of the so-called magical potions that promise to improve physical performance.

What does ergogenic mean?

Ergogenic means work enhancing or work producing. In connection with athletic performance, ergogenic aids are substances or treatments that purportedly improve athletic performance above and beyond what is possible through training alone. Research findings do not, for the most part, support the claims made for ergogenic aids. When you hear a claim that a product is ergogenic, remember to consider the source of the claim and ask who may gain from the sale.[22]

My coach told me to take protein supplements. Should I take them?

Protein and amino acid supplements are advocated to improve both strength and endurance, but as discussed in Chapter 10, well-nourished active people and athletes do not need them. Extra protein cannot be forced into the muscles to make them grow. Muscle cells accept nutrients only when they are needed. The cells "decide" what they need, based on the messages they receive from the hormones that regulate them and from demands put upon them. The way to make muscle cells grow, therefore, is to make them work. The only role for diet in this process is to make protein available, and good diets always do. Although the protein needs of some endurance and strength athletes may be slightly higher than those of sedentary people, the additional protein is already present in a well-chosen diet as Chapter 10 described.

What about vitamin-mineral supplements for athletes? I have a friend who is a bodybuilder. She takes several vitamin pills right before each competition.

Tell your friend that this practice is pointless, though probably harmless. For one thing, vitamins taken right before competition have no effect; during the event, they are still waiting in the blood and have not yet been assembled into working molecules.

Besides, research shows that most bodybuilders' diets provide adequate amounts of vitamins and minerals, and when a nutrient is lacking, the supplements chosen are seldom the ones needed to remedy the deficiencies. In one study, researchers noted that the diets of the women bodybuilders were so deficient in calcium that supplementation by itself could probably not compensate fully. The women had omitted all dairy products from their diets for as many as four months before competition.[23] All of the women and 90 percent of the men in this study used supplements, but these supplements did not supply calcium, and many of the supplements did not even carry standard nutrient label information.

If a diet lacks nutrients, it should be modified to provide the needed nutrients. Only if a health professional identifies a clinical nutrient deficiency should nutrient supplements be prescribed—and then only if dietary modification alone cannot remedy the deficiency.

An ordinary multivitamin and mineral supplement may be prudent if an athlete's need for energy consistently outstrips the ability to eat the quantity of food required to supply it. In this case, many athletes must turn to concentrated energy sources, such as candies and fats—foods that lack vitamins and minerals. The energy that foods supply requires processing by vitamin- and mineral-containing enzymes, so the greater the energy spent, the greater the need for these nutrients. Thus, for a short time during the heaviest training, a supplement might be appropriate. Chapter 10 described the other instance when supplementation is justified: iron deficiency in endurance athletes, especially women and teen athletes, for whom iron supplements may help to provide a remedy.

I have heard of a technique for improving endurance called glycogen loading. What is glycogen loading?

The fuel for intense muscular activity is carbohydrate, stored in the muscle as glycogen. Athletes who compete in long-distance endurance events naturally want to have as much energy stored in their muscles as they can. Various techniques called glycogen loading were used in the past to trick muscles into storing more glycogen than normal. These techniques involved sudden, drastic changes in diet that caused nausea or cramping in some athletes. Other athletes experienced more dangerous effects such as abnormal heart and kidney function.

Exercise physiologists now recommend a modified plan of glycogen loading that confers benefits without such side effects. First, about two or three weeks before competition, the athlete increases exercise intensity while eating a normal, high-carbohydrate diet. Then, during the last week before competition, the athlete modifies both exercise and diet. With respect to exercise, the athlete gradually cuts back, resting completely on the day before the event. Meanwhile, with respect to foods, the athlete eats carbohydrate as usual until three days before the competition and then eats a very-high-carbohydrate diet.[24] Endurance athletes who follow this plan can keep going longer than their competitors without ill effects. In a hot climate, extra glycogen confers an additional advantage: as glycogen breaks down, it releases water, which helps to meet the athlete's fluid needs.

Extra glycogen benefits only those who exercise long (90 minutes or more) and hard enough to deplete their stores; the regular, everyday exerciser will not benefit from having larger stores. What that person does need, though, is *adequate* glycogen from eating a diet high in complex carbohydrates.

I have heard that steroids are dangerous, but I have a friend who takes them. His mother is a doctor, and she constantly monitors his blood pressure when he is taking steroids. Are they safe in his case?

Steroids are not safe in your friend's case or in any case; they have dangerous side effects and are illegal. Technically called androgenic-anabolic steroid drugs, they are derivatives of the male sex hormone testosterone. Testosterone promotes the development of male characteristics (androgenic) and lean body mass (anabolic). Athletes take steroids to stimulate muscle bulking. The American College of Sports Medicine and the American Academy of Pediatrics condemn the use of steroids by athletes, and the International Olympic Committee has banned their use.[25] In support of its position, the committee cites the known toxic side effects and maintains that steroid use is a form of cheating. Competitors who use the drugs put other athletes in the difficult position of either conceding an unfair advantage to abusing competitors or taking steroids and accepting the risk of untoward side effects.

The list of hazards and adverse reactions from steroids continues to grow amid only a slight decline in use of the drugs. Among the side effects and adverse reactions that steroids produce are cancerous liver tumors that impair liver function, causing it to rupture and hemorrhage; testicular shrinkage in men and masculinization of women; cardiovascular problems; and sterility.

The blood lipid profile of a steroid user also changes abruptly to a profile associated with a high risk of heart disease. In one study, at the peak of steroid use, all users had blood lipid profiles indicative of a very high risk of heart disease. Even six months after cessation of steroid use, the users demonstrated an increased risk.[26] Your friend is sure to develop side effects no matter how closely a trainer or doctor monitors him. Table 10–10 lists side effects and adverse reactions to anabolic steroids.

The dangers of steroid use cannot be overemphasized. Health care professionals are obligated to warn athletes of these dangers. Speak simply and emphatically: the price for the potential competitive edge that steroids confer is damaged health and sometimes life itself. The safest effective way to build muscle has always been through hard training, and always will be.

What about caffeine? I've heard that it can improve endurance performance.

Although some research findings support this notion, other findings suggest that caffeine has no effect on endurance.[27] If caffeine does enhance endurance, the effect probably occurs because caffeine stimulates fatty acid release, thereby slowing glycogen use. Caffeine is a drug that stimulates the nervous system. The possible benefits must be weighed against caffeine's adverse effects—stomach upset, nervousness, irritability, headache, and diarrhea. Caffeine induces fluid losses that can be potentially hazardous if

Table 10–10 Anabolic Steroids: Side Effects and Adverse Reactions

ESTABLISHED SIDE EFFECTS AND ADVERSE REACTIONS	
Acne	Liver disease
Cancer	Liver tumors
Cholesterol increase	Male pattern baldness (in women—irreversible)
Clitoris enlargement	Oily skin (females only)
Death	Peliosis hepatitis (a liver disease)
Edema (water retention in tissue)	Penis enlargement (young boys)
Fetal damage	Priapism (painful, prolonged erections)
Frequent or continuing erections	Prostate enlargement
HDL (which helps reduce cholesterol) decrease	Sterility (reversible)
Heart disease	Stunted growth
Hirsutism (hairiness in women—irreversible)	Swelling of feet or lower legs
Increased risk of coronary artery disease (heart attack, stroke)	Testicular atrophy
Jaundice	Yellowing of the eyes or skin
OTHER POSSIBLE SIDE EFFECTS AND ADVERSE REACTIONS	
Abdominal or stomach pains	Insomnia
Aggressive, combative behavior ("roid rage")	Kidney disease
Anaphylactic shock (from injections)	Kidney stones (from hypercalcemia)
Black, tarry, or light-colored stool	Listlessness
Bone pain	Menstrual irregularities
Breast development (sore or swelling—male)	Muscle cramps
Chills	Nausea or vomiting
Dark-colored urine	Purple- or red-colored spots on body, inside of mouth or nose
Depression	Rash
Diarrhea	Septic shock (blood poisoning from injections)
Fatigue	Sexual problems
Feeling of abdominal or stomach fullness	Sore tongue
Feeling of discomfort	Unexplained darkening of skin
Fever	Unexplained weight loss
Frequent urge to urinate (mature males)	Unnatural hair growth
Gallstones	Unpleasant breath odor
Headache	Unusual bleeding
High blood pressure	Unusual weight gain
Hives	Urination problems
Hypercalcemia (too much calcium)	Vomiting blood
Impotence	
Increased chance of injury to muscles, tendons, and ligaments, plus longer recovery period from injuries	

Source: K. L. Ropp, No-win situation for athletes, *FDA Consumer,* December 1992, pp. 8–12; National Academy of Sports Medicine policy statement and position paper: Anabolic androgenic steroids, growth hormones, stimulants, ergogenics, and drug use in sports, in B. Goldman and R. Klats, *Death in the Locker Room II: Drugs and Sports* (Chicago: Elite Sports Medicine Publications, 1992) , pp. 328–373.

caffeine-containing fluids are used in place of other fluids by athletes competing in hot environments. The use of caffeine is banned by the International Olympic Committee when it exceeds a dosage equivalent to 5 or 6 cups of coffee in a 2-hour period prior to competition.[28]

I've heard that among endurance athletes, blood doping is gaining popularity as a way to enhance performance. What is it and how does it work?

Blood doping involves removing about one liter of blood from an athlete approximately two or three months before competition, freeze-storing the blood, and then returning it to the body a few days before the event. By the time the blood is reintroduced, the athlete's body has compensated for its loss by making many new red blood cells, so that the added blood becomes "extra." This creates a 5 to 10 percent excess in hemoglobin concentration, which temporarily enhances the oxygen-carrying capacity of the blood and improves cardiorespiratory endurance.[29] Blood doping does seem to improve aerobic performance temporarily, but is not without risks. For endurance athletes competing in hot weather, dehydration increases the relative volume of red blood cells, and blood doping augments the volume further, enhancing the possibility that blood clots may develop. Besides the health hazard, blood doping is considered unethical; it is also illegal, and the International Olympic Committee forbids it.

OK, protein supplements and vitamin supplements are ineffective performance enhancers except when used to treat a true deficiency. Glycogen loading works, but is unnecessary unless a person works out hard for longer than 90 minutes at a time. Caffeine may or may not be effective, but can have adverse side effects and is illegal. Steroids pose serious health risks and are illegal. Blood doping is risky and illegal. Do any of the substances athletes use to boost performance work?

You guessed it: no. Many of these substances have been studied and found to be worthless. The accompanying glossary lists and describes ineffective ergogenic aids.

Health professionals can positively influence athletes and others interested in boosting athletic performance by stressing the measures that do help to enhance performance. They are, of course, regular training and sound nutrition.

■ NOTES ■

1. R. S. Paffenbarger and coauthors, The association of changes in physical-activity level and other lifestyle characteristics with mortality among men, *New England Journal of Medicine* 328 (1993): 538–545; L. Sandvik and coauthors, Physical fitness as a predictor of mortality among healthy, middle-aged Norwegian men, *New England Journal of Medicine* 328 (1993): 533–537.
2. Public Health Service, U.S. Department of Health and Human Services, *Year 2000 Health Objectives for the Nation* (Washington, D.C.: Government Printing Office, 1990).
3. K. E. Powell and coauthors, Physical activity and chronic diseases, *American Journal of Clinical Nutrition* 49 (1989): 999–1006; S. N. Blair and coauthors, Physical fitness and all-cause mortality: A prospective study of healthy men and women, *Journal of the American Medical Association* 262 (1989): 2395–2401; American Heart Association Position Statement on Exercise: Benefits and recommendations for physical activity programs for all Americans, *Circulation* 86 (1992): 340–344; A. M. Bovens and coauthors, Physical activity, fitness, and selected risk factors for CHD in active men and women, *Medicine and Science in Sports and Exercise* 25 (1993): 572–576.
4. W. L. Haskell, Health consequences of physical activity: Understanding and challenges regarding dose-response, *Medicine and Science in Sports and Exercise* 26 (1994): 649–660.
5. Blair and coauthors, 1989.
6. Source notes for table: For can cer, R. E. Frisch and coauthors, Lower lifetime occurrence of breast cancer and cancers of the reproductive system among former college athletes, *American Journal of Clinical Nutrition,* 45 (1987: 328–355; E. R. Eichner, Exercise and cancer prevention, *Sports Medicine Digest,* January 1991, p. 5; J. A. Woods and J. M. Davis, Exercise, monocyte/macrophage function, and cancer, *Medicine and Science in Sports and Exercise* 26 (1994): 147–157; Blair and coauthors, 1989. For diabetes, S. P. Helmrich and coauthors, Physical activity and reduced occurrence of non-insulin-dependent diabetes mellitus, *New England Journal of Medicine* 325 (1991): 147–152; J. E. Manson and coauthors, A prospective study of exercise and incidence of diabetes

Glossary of Ineffective Ergogenic Aids

bee pollen: a product consisting of bee saliva, plant nectar, and pollen that confers no benefit on athletes and may cause an allergic reaction in individuals sensitive to it.

blood doping: the process of injecting red blood cells to enhance the blood's oxygen-carrying ability. Risks include dangerous blood clotting, especially in athletes who become dehydrated, infections from nonsterile equipment, transfusion reactions, and dangers of improperly transferred blood. Blood doping is banned in Olympic competitions.

branched-chain amino acids: the amino acids leucine, isoleucine, and valine, which are present in large amounts in skeletal muscle tissue.

caffeine: a stimulant that in small amounts may produce alertness and reduced reaction time in some people, but that also creates fluid losses. Overdoses cause headaches, trembling, an abnormally fast heart rate, and other undesirable effects.

calcium pangamate: a compound once thought to enhance aerobic metabolism, now known to have no such effect.

carnitine: an organic compound found in most body cells that serves as a carrier of unoxidized fatty acids. It is advertised as a "fat burner" to bodybuilders and as a means of sparing glycogen to endurance athletes, but studies show it does neither. Low-fat dairy products and lean meats are good sources of carnitine for athletes and active people.

cell salts: a mineral preparation supposedly prepared from living cells.

coenzyme Q10: a lipid found in cells (mitochondria) shown to improve exercise performance in heart disease patients, but not effective in improving performance of healthy athletes.

DNA and RNA (deoxyribonucleic acid and ribonucleic acid): the genetic materials of cells necessary in protein synthesis, falsely promoted as ergogenic aids.

glycine: a nonessential amino acid, promoted as an ergogenic aid because it is a precursor of the high-energy compound phosphocreatine. Other amino acids commonly packaged for athletes and that are equally useless include ornithine, arginine, lysine, and the branched-chain amino acids.

growth hormone releasers: herbs or pills falsely promoted for enhancing athletic performance.

inosine: an organic chemical that is falsely said to "activate cells, produce energy, and facilitate exercise," but has been shown actually to reduce the endurance of runners.

octacosanol: an alcohol extracted from wheat germ, often falsely promoted to enhance athletic performance.

phosphate salt: a salt that has been demonstrated to raise the concentration of a metabolically important compound (diphosphoglycerate) in red blood cells and enhance the cells' potential to deliver oxygen to muscle cells; the salts may cause calcium losses from the bones if taken in excess.

plant sterol: lipid extracts of plants, called *ferulic-acid, oryzanol, phytosterols,* or *adaptogens,* marketed with false claims that they contain hormones or balance hormonal activity.

royal jelly: a substance produced by worker bees and fed to the queen bees, often falsely promoted as enhancing athletic performance.

sodium bicarbonate: baking soda; an alkaline salt believed to neutralize blood lactic acid and thereby reduce pain and enhance possible workload. Some studies show that sodium bicarbonate in recommended doses can enhance performance of high-intensity exercise (in 1- to 5-minute exercise sessions) but its effects on endurance exercise are unknown; "soda loading" may cause intestinal bloating and diarrhea.

among U.S. male physicians, *Journal of the American Medical Association* 268 (1992): 63–67. For heart disease, Paffenbarger and coauthors, 1993. For infections, D. C. Nieman, Exercise, upper respiratory tract infection, and the immune system, *Medicine and Science in Sports and Exercise* 26 (1994): 128–139; D. C. Nieman and coauthors, Physical activity and immune function in elderly women, *Medicine and Science in Sports and Exercise* 25 (1993): 823–831. For osteoporosis, R. R. Recker and coauthors, Bone gain in young adult women, *Journal of the American Medical Association* 268 (1992): 2403–2408; A. M. Fehily and coauthors, Factors affecting bone density in young adults, *American Journal of Clinical Nutrition* 56 (1992): 579–586; B. P. Conroy and coauthors, Bone mineral density in elite junior Olympic weightlifters, *Medicine and Science in Sports and Exercise* 25 (1993): 1103–1109.

7. American College of Sports Medicine, The recommended quality and quantity of exercise for developing and maintaining fitness in healthy adults, *Medicine and Science in Sports and Exercise* 22 (1990): 265–274.
8. U.S. Centers for Disease Control and Prevention and American College of Sports Medicine, Summary statement: Workshop on physical activity and public health, *Sports Medicine Bulletin* 28 (1993): 7.
9. Parts of this discussion are based on L. K. DeBruyne, F. S. Sizer, and E. N. Whitney, *The Fitness Triad: Motivation, Training, and Nutrition* (St. Paul, Minn.: West Publishing Co., 1991).
10. American College of Sports Medicine, *Guidelines for Exercise Testing and Prescription,* 4th ed. (Philadelphia: Lea & Febiger, 1991).
11. American College of Sports Medicine, 1990.
12. W. M. Sherman, Carbohydrate, muscle glycogen, and improved performance, *Physician and Sportsmedicine* 15 (1987): 157–164.
13. M. J. Zackin, Protein requirements for athletes, *Sports Medicine Digest,* March 1990, pp. 1–2.
14. P. Babij and F. W. Booth, Biochemistry of exercise: Advances in molecular biology relevant to adaptation of muscle to exercise, *Sports Medicine* 5 (1988): 137–143.
15. Position of the American Dietetic Association and the Canadian Dietetic Association: Nutrition for physical fitness and athletic performance in adults, *Journal of the American Dietetic Association* 93 (1993): 691–695.
16. A. Singh, F. M. Moses, and P. A. Deuster, Chronic multivitamin-mineral supplementation does not enhance physical performance, *Medicine and Science in Sports and Exercise* 24 (1992): 726–732.
17. L. M. Weight, K. H. Myburgh, and T. D. Noakes, Vitamin and mineral supplementation: Effect on the running performance of trained athletes, *American Journal of Clinical Nutrition* 47 (1988): 192–195.
18. W. W. Campbell and R. A. Anderson, Effects of aerobic exercise and training on the trace minerals chromium, zinc, and copper, *Sports Medicine* 4 (1987): 9–18.
19. T. W. Rowland, S. A. Black, and J. F. Kelleher, Iron deficiency in adolescent endurance athletes, *Journal of Adolescent Health Care* 8 (1987): 322–326; H. J. Nickerson, M. C. Holubets, and B. R. Weiler, Causes of iron deficiency in adolescent athletes, *Journal of Pediatrics* 114 (1989): 657–663.
20. W. B. Strong and coauthors, The effect of iron therapy on the exercise capacity of nonanemic iron-deficient adolescent runners, *American Journal of Diseases of Children* 142 (1988): 165–169.
21. S. A. Tilgner and M. R. Schiller, Dietary intakes of female college athletes: The need for nutrition education, *Journal of the American Dietetic Association* 89 (1989): 967–969.
22. Adapted in part from E. N. Whitney and S. R. Rolfes, *Understanding Nutrition,* 6th ed. (St. Paul, Minn.: West Publishing Co., 1993), pp. 471–475 and F. S. Sizer and E. N. Whitney, *Nutrition: Concepts and Controversies,* 6th ed. (St. Paul, Minn.: West Publishing Co., 1994), pp. 375–379.
23. S. M. Kleiner, T. L. Bazarre, and M. D. Litchford, Metabolic profiles, diet, and health practices of championship male and female bodybuilders, *Journal of the American Dietetic Association* 90 (1990): 962–967.
24. W. M. Sherman, Carbohydrate, muscle glycogen, and improved performance, *Physician and Sports-medicine* 15 (1987): 157–161, 164.
25. P. G. Dyment and B. Goldberg, Anabolic steroids and the adolescent, *Nutrition* 49 (1989): 1066–1069.
26. S. M. Kleiner and coauthors, Dietary influences on cardiovascular disease risk in anabolic steroid using and nonusing bodybuilders, *Journal of the American College of Nutrition* 8 (1989): 109–119.
27. G. I. Wadler and B. Hainline, *Drugs and the Athlete* (Philadelphia: F. A. Davis, 1989), pp. 107–113, as cited in J. A. Work, Are java junkies poor sports? *Physician and Sportsmedicine* 19 (1991): 83–88.
28. M. H. Williams, Nutritional ergogenic aids and athletic performance, *Nutrition Today,* January/February 1989, pp. 7–14.
29. D. C. Nieman, *Fitness and Sports Medicine: An Introduction* (Palo Alto, Calif.: Bull Publishing, 1990), pp. 221–268.

11

Consumer Concerns about Foods

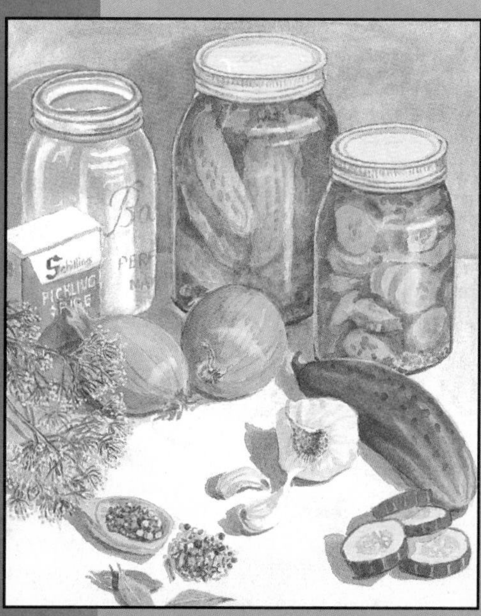

CONTENTS

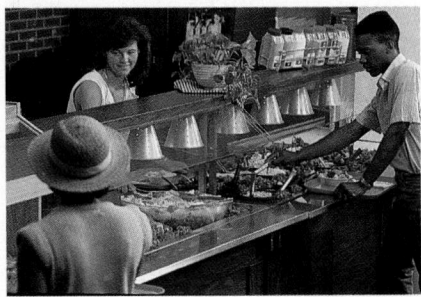

Which foods are best?

The preceding chapters have presented a basic course in nutrition. This chapter wraps up the course by tying nutrition to the world of foods. Nutrition is, after all, delivered in the form of foods, and to use foods correctly, consumers need to know how best to select and prepare them. The first half of this chapter is devoted to the nutritional value of grocery-store foods. The second half is devoted to food safety.

Nutritional Value of Grocery-Store Foods

People want to know how to choose the best foods—those that are most nutritious. Which are the best foods, anyway? Are canned foods OK? Frozen foods? Are fresh foods better? What about fast foods?

Processed Foods

Most of the foods consumed today, whether eaten in restaurants or at home, have been prepared in some way by industry. People often ask what processing does to foods and which kinds of foods are most and least nutritious.

Goals of Food Processing Many forms of processing aim to extend the usable life of a food—that is, they preserve the food. To preserve food, a process must prevent three detrimental changes. It must:

- Prevent microbial growth.
- Prevent oxidative changes.
- Prevent enzymatic destruction of food molecules.

Canning, freezing, drying, salting, and adding preservatives are all ways of achieving these objectives.

Costs of Processing In general, food processing involves a trade-off. It makes foods safer, it gives them a longer usable lifetime than fresh foods, or it cuts preparation time—but at the cost of some vitamin and mineral losses. A process such as pasteurization is clearly worth the cost because the safety gains are great and the nutrient losses small. Some processed foods gain a nutritional edge over their unprocessed counterparts; the removal of fat from milk or other foods by processing is an example. This section describes the most common processing techniques and explains their effects on nutrients.

pasteurization: the treatment of milk with heat sufficient to kill certain pathogens (disease-causing microbes) commonly transmitted through milk. It is not a sterilization process; pasteurized milk retains bacteria that cause milk spoilage. Raw milk, even if labeled "certified," transmits many food-borne diseases to people each year and should be avoided.

Canned Foods Canning is one of the better methods for protecting food against the growth of microbes (bacteria, fungi, and yeasts) that might otherwise spoil it, but canning, unfortunately, does incur nutrient losses.

Like other heat treatments, the canning process is based on time and temperature. Each small increase in temperature has a major killing effect on microbes with only a minor effect on nutrients, so industry chooses canning treatments that employ high temperatures for short times.

To determine how much of a food's nutritional value is lost in canning, food scientists have performed many experiments. They have paid particular attention to three vulnerable water-soluble vitamins—thiamin, riboflavin, and vitamin C.

Acid stabilizes thiamin, but heat rapidly destroys it, so low-acid canned foods such as lima beans, corn, and meat lose up to half, or even more, of their thiamin. Unlike thiamin, riboflavin is stable to heat but sensitive to light; so glass-packed, not canned, foods are most likely to lose riboflavin. Vitamin C's special enemy is an enzyme present in fruits and vegetables and in microorganisms. By destroying this enzyme, canning actually helps preserve some vitamin C, although some is destroyed by the heat of the process. As for the fat-soluble vitamins, they are relatively stable and are not affected much by canning.

To see the effect of canning on thiamin in foods, look at Appendix A, items 890 and 891—½ c canned green peas versus ½ c frozen green peas. While you are looking, what other effects of canning on thiamin do you see?

Minerals are unaffected by heat processing because they cannot be destroyed, as vitamins can be. Some minerals are added when foods are canned. Important in this regard is sodium chloride, table salt, added for flavoring. Because salt tends to raise some people's blood pressure, many food companies have begun making low-salt versions of their products. Unfortunately, though, these may cost more than the higher-salt versions.

Frozen Foods Frozen foods' nutrient contents are similar to those of fresh foods; losses are minimal. The freezing process itself does not destroy any nutrients, but some losses may occur during the steps taken in preparation for freezing, such as the quick dunking into boiling water (blanching), washing, trimming, or grinding. Vitamin C losses are especially likely because they occur whenever tissues are broken and exposed to air (oxygen destroys vitamin C). Uncut fruits, especially if they are acidic, do not lose their vitamin C. Strawberries, for example, may be kept frozen for over a year without losing any vitamin C. Mineral contents of frozen foods are much the same as those of fresh foods.[1]

Fresh foods are often shipped long distances, and to ensure that they make the trip without bruising or spoiling, they are often harvested unripe. Frozen foods are shipped frozen, so that produce is allowed to ripen in the field where nutrients develop to their fullest potential. If foods are frozen and stored under proper conditions, they will often contain more nutrients when served at the table than fresh fruits and vegetables that have stayed in the produce department of the grocery store for even a day.

Frozen foods have to be kept frozen to retain their nutrients. To be solidly frozen, a food has to be colder than 32°F or 0°C. Conversion of vitamin C to its inactive forms occurs rapidly at warmer temperatures. Food may seem frozen at 36°F or 2°C, but enzymes can work at these temperatures. Under these conditions the vitamin C in a frozen food can be completely lost in as short a time as two months. If you want to maximize the nutritive value of the foods you store at home, invest in a freezer thermometer, monitor the temperature of your frozen-food storage place, and keep it at or below 32°F.

Dried Foods Dried or dehydrated foods have their own special characteristics. Drying offers several advantages. It eliminates microbial spoilage (because microbes need water to grow), and it greatly reduces the weight and volume of foods (because foods are mostly water).

Commercial drying does not destroy many nutrients, but foods dried in heated ovens at home may sustain dramatic nutrient losses. Vacuum puff drying and freeze drying, which take place in cold temperatures, conserve nutrients especially well.

Sulfite additives are added during the drying of fruits such as peaches, grapes (raisins), and plums (prunes) to prevent browning. (Some people suffer allergic reactions when they consume sulfites.) Sulfur dioxide, a commonly used sulfite, helps to preserve vitamin C as well, but it is highly destructive of thiamin. This is of small concern, however, because most dehydrated products with added sulfur dioxide are not major sources of thiamin anyway.

Some dried foods are heated, ground, and pushed through various kinds of screens to yield different shapes, such as pieces of breakfast cereal or the "bits" you sprinkle on salad—so-called food novelties. Considerable nutrient losses occur during these processes, and nutrients are usually added to compensate. But foods this far removed from the original fresh state are still lacking significant nutrients (notably, vitamin E), and consumers should not rely on them as staple foods. Enjoy them, but only as occasional snacks and as additions to enhance the appearance, taste, and variety of meals.

Making Wise Choices

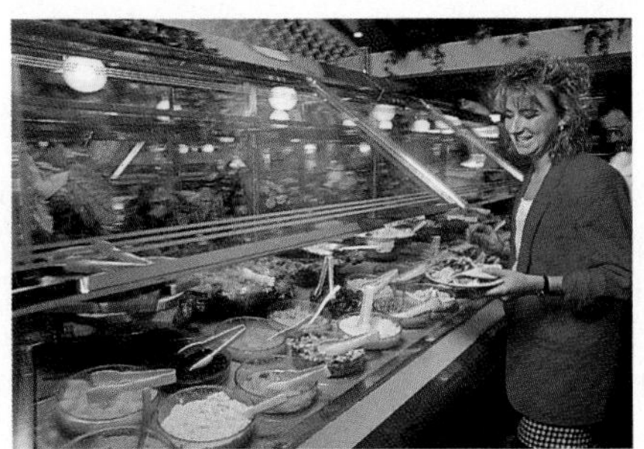

With the privilege of abundance comes the responsibility to choose wisely.

In general, the more heavily processed foods are, the less nutritious they become. Does that mean, then, that everyone should avoid all processed foods? It depends on the food and on the process.

Some Processed Foods Are Fine Consider the case of orange juice and vitamin C. Orange juice is available in several forms, each processed a different way. Fresh juice is simply squeezed from the orange, a process that extracts the fluid juice from the fibrous structures that contain it. The fresh-squeezed juice contains 124 milligrams of vitamin C per cup. When this juice is condensed by heat, frozen, and then reconstituted by adding water, a cup of juice contains just 97 milligrams of vitamin C, because the condensing process destroys the vitamin. Canning is even harder on vitamin C: a cup of canned orange juice has only 86 milligrams.

These figures may seem to indicate that fresh juice is the superior food, and so it may be. But consider this: most people's RDA of vitamin C (60 milligrams) is easily met by a cup of any of the above choices. In this case, at least for vitamin C, the losses due to processing are not a problem.

On the other hand, refusing to process orange juice would be a big mistake. Fresh orange juice spoils. Shipping fresh juice to distant places in refrigerated trucks would cost much more than shipping frozen juice (which takes up less space) or canned juice (which requires no refrigeration). Fresh juice still contains active enzymes that continue to destroy its nutrients (including vitamin C), but frozen and canned juices remain virtually unchanged for long periods. Without canned or frozen juice, people with limited incomes or those with no access to fresh juice would be deprived of this excellent food.

Some Processed Foods Are Inferior Some processing stories are not so rosy. In Chapter 8, for instance, you saw how processed foods are often loaded with sodium as their potassium is leached away. A related mischief of processing is the addition of sugar and fat—palatable, high-kcalorie additives that reduce nutrient density. Nuts and raisins covered with "natural yogurt" are an example. This may sound like one healthy food being added to another, but a look at the ingredient panel warns that generous amounts of fat and sugar accompany the yogurt. About 75 percent of the weight of the product is fat and sugar; only about 8 percent is yogurt.

To pick just one nutrient for an example, here is what happens to the iron density of raisins as they become yogurt-coated raisins: 100 kcalories of raisins contains 0.71 milligrams of iron; 100 kcalories of "yogurt" raisins contain 0.26 milligrams of iron. These foods taste so good that wishful thinking can easily take hold, but the reality is that fat-coated, sugar-coated food is candy. The word *yogurt* on the label means only that one of the ingredients of the candy coating is some small amount of yogurt. Names, even whole-food names, written on labels do not prove that the foods so named provide any nutritional benefit to consumers unless the foods themselves are nutritious.

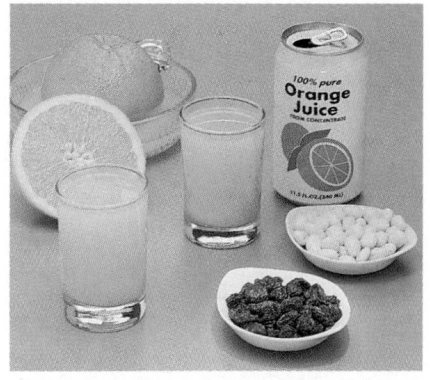

In terms of nutrient density, canned juice is almost as nutritious as fresh, but yogurt-covered raisins are not *as nutritious as plain raisins.*

Virtues of Whole Foods A good general rule for making food choices is to choose whole foods to the greatest extent possible and, among processed foods, to choose only those that processing has improved nutritionally. The nutrient contents of processed foods exist on a continuum:

Whole-grain bread > refined white bread > sugared doughnuts.
Milk > fruit-flavored yogurt > canned chocolate pudding.
Corn on the cob > canned creamed corn > caramel popcorn.
Oranges > orange juice > orange-flavored drink.
Baked ham > deviled ham > fried bacon.

Another continuum parallels it—the nutrition status of the consumer.

Chosen by these guidelines, even fast foods can contribute to a nutritious diet. Just choose the tomatoes rather than the catsup, the low-fat milk rather than the milkshake, and the chicken salad rather than the fried chicken sandwich.

At home, be realistic. Few people have the time to bake all their own bread from scratch, to shop every few days for fresh meats, or to wash, peel, chop, and cook fresh fruits and vegetables at every meal. This is where food processing comes in. Commercially prepared whole-grain breads, frozen cuts of meats, bags of frozen vegetables, and canned or frozen fruit juices do little disservice to nutrition and enable the consumer to eat a variety of foods at great savings in time and human energy. It is true that the closer to the farm the foods you eat, the better nourished you are, but that doesn't mean you have to live in the fields.

In modern commercial processing, losses of vitamins seldom exceed 25 percent. In contrast, losses in food preparation at home can be close to 100 percent, and losses in the 60 to 75 percent range are not unusual. These facts put the matter of food processing into perspective and reveal

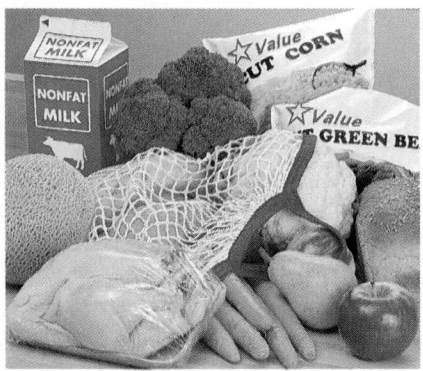

1. *Purchase mostly fresh foods or those that processing has benefited nutritionally.*

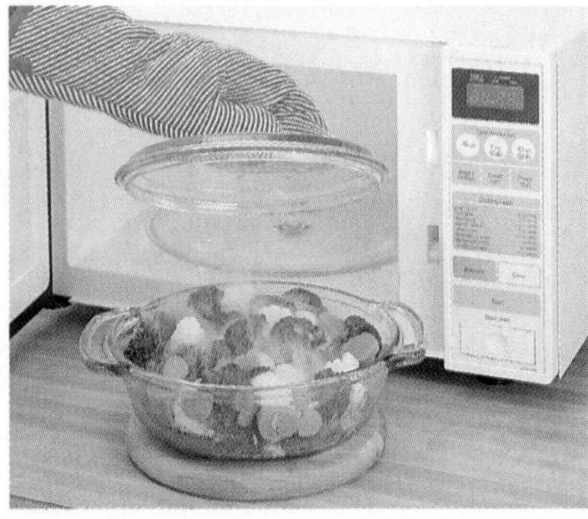

2. *Steam vegetables or cook them in a microwave oven.*

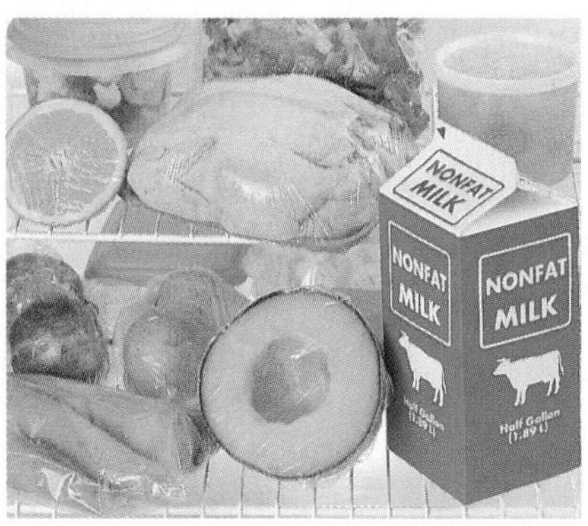

3. *Wrap foods tightly and refrigerate them. Space foods to allow chilled air to circulate around them.*

that while the kinds of foods you buy certainly make a difference, what you do with them in your kitchen can make an even greater difference.

Cooking to Preserve Nutrients

Once you have selected nutritious foods at the market and brought them home, you have the task of storing and preparing them so that they deliver their nutritional benefits to you. This requires some understanding of how cooking and storing foods affect nutrients.

Keep Fresh Produce Cold Vitamins are organic compounds synthesized and broken down by enzymes found in the foods that contain them. The enzymes that break down nutrients in fruits and vegetables work best at the temperatures at which the plants grow, which are near room temperature. Chilling fresh produce slows down enzymatic destruction of nutrients. To protect the vitamin content, most fruits and vegetables should be vine ripened (if possible), chilled immediately after picking, and kept cold until used.

Keep Meats Cold For meats purchased in bulk, divide the package into portions and immediately refrigerate meats to be used within two days. Wrap the portions of meat to be used later in coverings that exclude air, and freeze them.

Keep Milk Products in the Dark Riboflavin is light sensitive; it can be destroyed by the ultraviolet rays of the sun or by fluorescent light. For this reason milk is not sold (and should not be stored) in transparent glass containers. Cardboard or opaque plastic containers screen out light, protecting the riboflavin.

Do Not Cut before Use Some vitamins are acids or antioxidants and so are most stable in an acid solution, away from air. Citrus fruits, tomatoes, and many juices are acid. As long as the skin is uncut or the can is unopened, their vitamins are protected from air. If you store a cut vegetable or fruit or an opened carton of juice, cover it with an airtight wrapper or close it tightly and store it in the refrigerator.

Save Nutrient-Rich Water Water-soluble vitamins and minerals in cut vegetables readily dissolve into the water in which they are canned, washed, or boiled. If the water is discarded, as much as half of the vitamins and minerals in foods go down the drain with the water. A bit of southern folk wisdom is to serve the liquid with the vegetable rather than throwing it away; this liquid is known as the "pot liquor." The liquid may also be used to moisten cornbread or to make gravies, soups, or stews.

Conserve Water-Soluble Nutrients Other ways to minimize cooking losses are to steam vegetables over water rather than in it, stir-fry them in small amounts of oil, or microwave them. Wash intact foods vigorously and briefly; don't soak them. Cut vegetables after washing, except for those such as broccoli that you have to cut to wash adequately. For peeled vegetables such as potatoes, add them to water that is vigorously boiling, not to cold water. Microwave ovens are excellent for conserving nutrients. They cook fast without requiring the addition of fats or excess liquid.

Other Tactics During other types of cooking, minimize the destruction of vitamins by avoiding high temperatures and long cooking times. Iron destroys vitamin C by catalyzing its oxidation, but the increased iron content of foods achieved by cooking in iron utensils may outweigh this disadvantage. Each of these tactics is small by itself, but saving a small percentage of the vitamins in foods daily can mean saving significant amounts in a year's time.

Meanwhile, however, a law of diminishing returns operates. Most vitamin losses under reasonable conditions are not catastrophic. You need not fret over small vitamin losses that occur in your kitchen; doing so may waste energy or time that is valuable to you in other ways. Be assured that if you start with fresh, whole foods containing ample amounts of vitamins and are reasonably careful in preparing those foods, you will receive a bounty of the nutrients that they contain.

Food Safety

A vitally important aspect of food preparation is safety. Episodes of food poisoning cause illness in at least one-third of the U.S. population each year. Some 20 to 80 million cases of diarrhea, and possibly even more, are caused yearly by food poisoning. Many cases of "the flu" may actually be cases of food poisoning.

food poisoning: illness transmitted to human beings through food, caused by infectious agents or by toxins that they produce.

Other aspects of food safety include avoiding the toxins that grow naturally in some foods as part of their normal composition and avoiding the contaminants (including pesticides) that can get into foods before they are harvested. Consumers also want to know whether food additives are safe or should be avoided. The next sections take up these issues in the order just mentioned, which is roughly the order of concern. Food poisoning is far and away the most important issue; food additives are the matter of least concern.

Preventing Food Poisoning

The term *food poisoning* refers to either food-borne infection or food intoxication. A food-borne infection is an illness caused by microorganisms, such as *Salmonella* varieties, that infect people, whereas food intoxication is caused by toxins produced by microorganisms in food or within the digestive tract. In most food-borne illnesses, the symptoms are mild, but for people who are otherwise ill or malnourished or for the very old or young, even these relatively mild disturbances can be fatal. If abdominal cramps, headache, vomiting, and diarrhea are the major or only symptoms of your next bout of "flu," chances are excellent that what you really have is food poisoning.

The symptoms of one toxin stand alone as severe and commonly fatal—those of botulism, caused by the toxin of a microbe that grows

toxins: poisons. Toxins produced by bacteria come in two varieties: *enterotoxins,* which act in the GI tract, and *neurotoxins,* which act on the nervous system.

botulism: an often-fatal food poisoning caused by botulin toxin, a toxin produced by bacteria that grow without oxygen in nonacidic canned foods.

Warning signs of botulism:

- Double vision.
- Weakening muscles.
- Difficulty swallowing.
- Difficulty breathing.

inside improperly canned, home-canned, or vacuum-packed foods. Botulism danger signs constitute a true medical emergency (see margin). Even with medical assistance, survivors can suffer the effects for months, years, or a lifetime. So potent is the botulin toxin that an amount as tiny as a single grain of salt can kill several people within an hour. The botulin toxin is destroyed by heat, so canned foods that have been boiled for ten minutes are generally safe from this threat. Home-canned foods are safe if prepared by following proper canning techniques to the letter.*

Food Safety in the Marketplace Commercially prepared food is usually safe, but when rare accidents happen, the effect can be dramatic. Milk producers, for example, rely on pasteurization to kill off many disease-causing organisms and make the milk safe to drink. When the pasteurization system at a major dairy developed a flaw, over 16,000 confirmed, and as many as 200,000 suspected, cases of food-borne illness resulted. In another episode 100 people died of infection. On another occasion a fast-food restaurant served undercooked burgers tainted with an infectious organism that cost one child's life and made many other patrons ill. This incident attracted the national spotlight to two standard food-safety concerns. First, live, disease-causing organisms are routinely found in raw meats. Second, only thorough cooking can ensure the safety of animal-derived foods.

Consumers have little protection against such large-scale calamities; they must trust government inspectors to enforce strict standards to prevent all but truly unavoidable accidents. Luckily, large-scale incidents, though dramatic, make up only a fraction of the total food-poisoning cases each year. Most arise from one person's error in a small setting and affect just a few victims. Some people have come to accept a yearly bout or two of intestinal illness as inevitable, but in truth, most of these illnesses can be prevented. To protect themselves, consumers need to learn how to select, prepare, and store food safely.

Canned and packaged foods as sold in grocery stores are almost invariably safe. When accidental contamination does occur, batch numbering makes it possible to recall all the foods of a contaminated batch through public announcements in newspapers, on television, and on the radio. You can avoid buying foods that are contaminated, too. Reject packages with defective seals and wrappers. Reject leaking or bulging cans. Many jars have safety "buttons," areas of the lid designed to pop up once opened; reject those that have popped up. Frozen foods should be solidly frozen and those in a chest-type freezer case should be stored below the frost line. Notice how the majority of the packages on the shelf appear. If the one you have chosen looks ragged, soiled, or punctured, do not buy it—turn it in to the store manager.

Raw foods, especially meats and poultry, always contain microbes. You can keep these microbes from multiplying and causing illness by handling these foods correctly when you get them home.

---

*Complete, up-to-date, safe home canning instructions are included in the USDA's 172-page *Complete Guide to Home Canning* available for $11.00 from the Superintendent of Documents, Government Printing Office, Washington, DC 20402.

Food Safety in the Kitchen Foods can provide ideal conditions for bacteria to thrive and produce their toxins. Disease-causing bacteria require:

- Warmth (40 to 140°F).
- Moisture.
- Nutrients.

To defeat the bacteria, people who prepare foods can do these things: cook foods thoroughly, keep hot foods hot, keep cold foods cold, keep dry foods dry, and keep the kitchen clean.

Keep Hot Foods Hot Cook foods for long enough to reach an internal temperature that will kill microbes. When holding cooked food, keep it at 140°F or higher until it is served to prevent bacterial growth. When serving food cold, let it stay at cool room temperature (about 68°F) for no more than two hours. If the room is warm (about 80°F), refrigerate the food after just one hour.

Keep Cold Foods Cold Keeping cold foods cold starts when you leave the grocery store. If you are running errands, shop last, so that the groceries will not stay in the car too long. (If the ice cream has begun to melt, it has been too long.) Upon arrival at home, load foods into the refrigerator or freezer immediately. Table 11–1 lists some safe keeping times for foods stored in the refrigerator at 40°F.

Keeping foods cold applies to defrosting foods before use, too. Bacterial growth begins on thawed portions of food even while the inner core is solidly frozen, so thaw meats or poultry in the refrigerator, not at room temperature. If you must hasten thawing, use cool running water or a microwave oven set to defrost.

Keep Dry Foods Dry Cereals, breads, powdered mixes, and the like will keep for a long time if you don't let moisture get to them. Store them in cool, dry places, and keep them well sealed against humid air.

Keep the Kitchen Clean Keeping the kitchen clean includes using freshly washed utensils and laundered towels and washing your hands frequently. If you are ill or have open sores, stay away from food so as not to contaminate it.

To eliminate microbes, you have three choices, each with benefits and drawbacks. One is to poison the microbes where they reside by washing countertops, cutting boards, sponges, and such items with toxic chemicals such as bleach (one capful per gallon of water). The benefit here is that chlorine can kill even the hardiest organism. The obvious drawback is that chlorine that washes down household drains into the water supply forms chemicals that can harm waterways and fish.

A second option is to use heat. Soapy water heated to 140°F kills most harmful organisms and washes most others away. This takes effort, though, for you have to use truly scalding water heated well beyond the temperature of the tap. (Most tap water called "hot" is not hotter than 130°F.)

Table 11–1
Safe Refrigerator Storage Times (40°F)

1 TO 2 DAYS
Raw ground meats, breakfast or other raw sausages, raw fish or poultry; gravies
3 TO 5 DAYS
Raw steaks, roasts, or chops; cooked meats, vegetables, and mixed dishes; ham slices; mayonnaise salads (chicken, egg, pasta, tuna)
1 WEEK
Hard cooked eggs, bacon or hot dogs (opened packages); smoked sausages
2 TO 4 WEEKS
Raw eggs (in shells); bacon or hot dogs (packages unopened); dry sausages (pepperoni, hard salami); most aged and processed cheeses (swiss, brick)
2 MONTHS
Mayonnaise (opened jar); most dry cheeses (parmesan, romano)

Sources: A. Hecht, Preventing food-borne illnesses, *FDA Consumer,* January/February 1991, p. 21; Refrigerator storage times for selected foods, *Consumer Reports on Health,* December 1991, p. 93.

The third option is to use clean nonporous boards for cutting and washable dishcloths that can be laundered often for wiping. (Save sponges for car washing and other heavy cleaning chores, and keep them away from surfaces that come in contact with raw foods.) For a small initial investment, you can create a truly safe environment in which to prepare your food.

Troublesome Foods Some foods are more hospitable to microbial growth than are others. Especially vulnerable are moist foods, nutrient-rich foods, and foods that are chopped or ground.

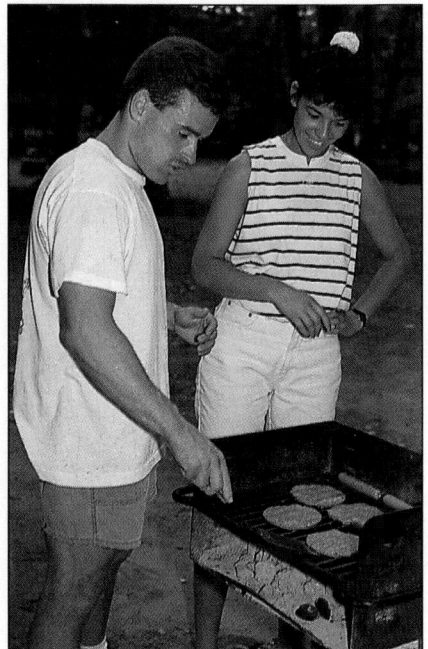

Use a clean plate to hold grilled meats.

Meats Because raw meats require special handling, they now bear labels to instruct consumers on meat safety. Meats may contain all sorts of bacteria, and they provide a moist, nutritious environment that is ideal for microbial growth. Do not leave raw meat at room temperature for more than a very short time. Chill it thoroughly or cook it promptly, preferably the latter. Remember that every surface and utensil that raw meat has touched is contaminated with microbes; wash all such surfaces and utensils with hot, soapy water right away. Never put cooked meat back on a countertop or plate on which the raw meat has stood. The microbes will resume growing in it immediately.*

Ground meat is handled more than other kinds of meat and has much more surface exposed to the air for bacteria to land on, so it poses special risks. It is best to cook hamburger to at least medium–well done. For a meatloaf, use a thermometer to test the internal temperature (see Figure 11–1).

Do not use or even taste a food with an "off" appearance or odor. However, don't trust your senses of smell or sight alone to tell you that foods are safe. Most contamination is not detectable by odor, taste, or appearance. Even hot cooked food, if handled improperly prior to cooking, can cause illness.

The cardinal rule to protect yourself is to remember, always, that food poisoning is a possibility. For example, the meatballs in a warming tray at a lovely buffet may be warm but not hot. Despite the beautiful setting, their low temperature is a warning flag. Food at 140°F feels hot, not just warm. The likelihood of illness is strong when food is not hot enough, and the pleasure of eating meatballs isn't worth the risk, even if you must go hungry for a while.

In Florida, containers of raw oysters must bear this warning: "There is a risk associated with consuming raw oyster or any raw animal protein. If you have chronic illness of the liver, stomach or blood or have immune disorders, you are at greater risk of serious illness from raw oysters and should eat oysters fully cooked. If unsure of your risk, consult a physician."

Seafood For adults and children alike, eating raw or lightly steamed seafood is a risky proposition even when the food is prepared by a master Japanese chef. The microorganisms that lurk there are undetectable even to an expert.

People who like Japanese *sushi* know that not all varieties are made from raw fish. Many types are made with cooked crabmeat and vegetables, avocado, or other delicacies and are perfectly safe to enjoy. Also, rumor has it that freezing fish will make it safe to eat raw, but this is only partly true.

*The USDA's meat and poultry hotline answers questions about meat and poultry safety: 1-800-535-4555.

Freezing fish will kill mature parasitic worms, but only cooking can kill all worm eggs and other microorganisms that can cause illness.

As population density increases along the shores of seafood-harvesting waters, pollution of those waters inevitably invades the seafood living there.* Watchdog agencies monitor commercial fishing waters and try to keep harvesters out of the worst areas, and they eventually do catch cheaters. Still, unwholesome foods can reach the market. In one season alone, black-market dealers may sell millions of dollars worth of clams and oysters taken illegally from polluted harvesting areas.[2] Experts are unanimous in saying that the risk of eating raw or lightly cooked seafood have become unacceptably high due to environmental contamination.[3]

Picnics Picnics are fun and can be safe, too. Choose foods that last without refrigeration, such as fresh fruits and vegetables, breads and crackers, and canned spreads and cheeses that you can open and use on the spot. Aged cheeses, such as cheddar and swiss, do well for an hour or two, but for longer periods, carry them in an ice chest. Mayonnaise resists spoilage because of its acid content, but when mixed with chopped ingredients, such as pasta, meat, or vegetable salads, it spoils quickly. The chopped ingredients offer an extensive surface area for bacteria to invade, and the foods have been in contact with cutting boards, hands, and kitchen utensils that have transmitted bacteria to them. Chill chopped salads well before, during, and after the picnic. Keep mayonnaise itself cold.

Honey Another danger lurks in honey. Honey has been found to contain dormant bacterial spores that can awaken in the human body to produce the deadly botulin toxin mentioned earlier. Adults are big and strong enough to withstand the doses usually encountered, but infants under one year of age should never be fed honey. (It can also be contaminated with environmental pollutants picked up by the bees.) Honey has been implicated in several cases of sudden infant death.

Travel Special food safety concerns arise when people travel. In many parts of the world, food-borne illness is likely to strike tourists even while the local people, eating exactly the same foods prepared the same way, remain healthy. That is because the locals have developed immunity to local disease-causing organisms, while tourists have no such protection. The box on p. 280 offers tips to travelers on avoiding food-borne infection.

Natural Toxins in Foods

Consumers concerned about food contamination may naively think that they can eliminate all poisons from their diets by eating only "natural" foods. On the contrary, nature has provided natural foods with the natural poisons they need to fend off diseases, insects, and other predators. However, while the potential for harm exists, actual harm rarely occurs.

Figure 11–1
Safe Internal Temperatures for Meats and Poultry (Fahrenheit)

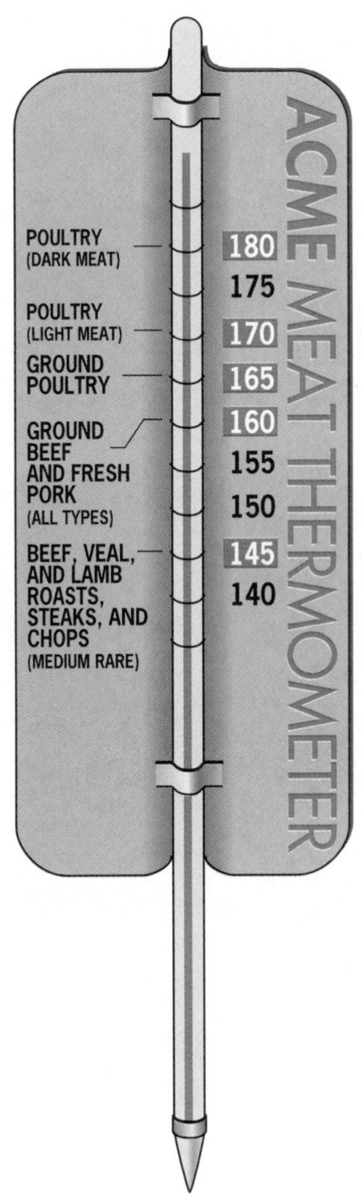

*To speak with an expert about seafood safety, call the FDA seafood hotline: 1–800–FDA–4010.

HOW TO Achieve Food Safety while Traveling

Food-borne illnesses contracted while traveling are colloquially known as traveler's diarrhea. A bout of this ailment can ruin the most enthusiastic tourist's trip. To avoid food-borne illness while traveling:

- Wash your hands often with soap and water, especially before handling food or eating.
- Eat only cooked food and canned foods. Eat raw fruits or vegetables only if you have washed them in boiled water and peeled them yourself. Skip salads, raw fish, and shellfish.
- Be aware that water, and ice made from it, may be unsafe, too. Take along disinfecting tablets or an element that boils water in a cup.
- Drink no beverages made with tap water. Drink only treated, boiled, canned, or bottled beverages, and drink them without ice, even if they are not chilled to your liking. Refuse dairy products unless they have been properly pasteurized and refrigerated.
- Do not use the local water supply, even to brush your teeth, unless you boil or disinfect it first.
- Before you leave on the trip, ask your physician to recommend medicines to take with you in case your efforts to avoid illness fail.

One journalist succinctly sums up these recommendation, "Boil it, cook it, peel it, or forget it."[a] Chances are excellent that if you follow these rules, you will remain well.

[a] R. D. Williams, Boil it, cook it, peel it or forget it, *FDA Consumer,* September 1991, p. 17.

Most people would recognize the names *belladonna* and *hemlock*—both classic deadly poisons in the form of natural herbs. Few people know, however, that the herb *sassafras* contains a cancer-causing agent and is banned from addition to commercially produced foods and beverages. Equally surprising is that cabbage, turnips, mustard greens, and radishes all contain small quantities of harmful goitrogens—compounds that can enlarge the thyroid gland and aggravate thyroid problems.

Cabbages and their relatives are celebrated for containing nonnutrients associated with low cancer incidence. An unexpected twist to the cabbage-family story is that some of the nonnutrients celebrated as protective against cancer are themselves carcinogenic. The protection they confer on the body seems to result because these mild toxins prompt the body to build up defenses, in somewhat the same way as it builds immunity.[4] Then, when a potent carcinogen arrives, the prepared body deals with it swiftly, detoxifies it, and excretes its remnants before cancer can begin.

The cyanogens are another natural poison. These precursors to the deadly poison cyanide are found in lima beans and fruit seeds such as apricot pits. Many countries allow commercial growers to grow only those varieties of lima beans with the lowest cyanogen contents. As for fruit seeds, they are seldom deliberately eaten. An occasional swallowed seed or two presents no danger, but a couple of dozen seeds could be fatal to a small child.

Potatoes contain many natural poisons. One is solanine, a bitter, powerful, narcotic-like substance. The small amounts of solanine normally found in potatoes are harmless, but if potatoes are stored in the light, the solanine in them can build up to toxic levels. Cooking does not destroy solanine, but because most of a potato's solanine is in the green layer that develops just beneath the skin, it can be peeled off, making the potato safe to eat. If the potato tastes bitter, however, throw it out.

At some times of the year, seafood may become contaminated with the so-called red tide toxin that occurs during algae blooms. Consumption of seafood contaminated with red tide causes a paralyzing form of food poisoning. The Food and Drug Administration (FDA) monitors fishing waters for red tide algae and closes waters to fishing whenever it appears.

Environmental Contaminants in Foods

A justifiably high-ranking concern about our food supply is contamination of foods by environmental pollutants. As populations increase worldwide and nations become more industrialized, this problem looms even larger.

The potential harmfulness of a contaminant depends in part on the extent to which it lingers in the environment or in the human body—how persistent it is. Some contaminants are short-lived, because microorganisms or agents such as sunlight or oxygen can break them down. Some contaminants linger in the body only for a short time, because the body can rapidly excrete them or metabolize them to harmless compounds. These contaminants present little cause for concern. Some contaminants, however, resist breakdown and interact with the body's systems without being metabolized or excreted. These can pass unchanged from food to the eater, and if the same food is eaten every day, larger and larger quantities of the contaminant may accumulate in the eater's body. Figure 11-2 on p. 282 shows how toxins accumulate at higher concentrations at each level of the food chain (bioaccumulation).

persistent: of a stubborn or enduring nature; with respect to food contaminants, the quality of persisting, rather than breaking down, in the bodies of animals and human beings.

bioaccumulation: The accumulation of toxins in living tissues at concentrations that increase at higher levels of the food chain.

Lead A contaminant of great concern in foods today is lead, a heavy metal that appears everywhere in the environment due to human industrial processes and easily finds its way into foods and water. One out of every six children from six months to five years old and one out of every nine fetuses are exposed to harmful doses of lead.[5] Lead toxicity is most prevalent among children under six—as many as 3 to 4 million children may have blood lead concentrations high enough to cause mental, behavioral, and other health problems (see Table 11-2).[6]

Lead poisoning in infants is most likely to derive from infant formula made with contaminated water.[7] The water, in turn, receives its lead burden from lead-soldered plumbing. The first water drawn from the tap

Table 11–2
Symptoms of Lead Toxicity

- Learning disabilities
- Low IQ
- Behavior problems
- Slow growth
- Iron-deficiency anemia
- Nervous system disorders
- Impaired concentration
- Reduced short-term memory
- Slow reaction time
- Seizures
- Impaired hearing
- Poor coordination

Figure 11–2
Bioaccumulation of Toxins in the Food Chain

A person whose principal animal protein source is fish may consume about 100 pounds of fish in a year. These fish will, in turn, have consumed a few tons of plant-eating fish in the course of their lifetimes. The plant eaters, in their lifetimes, will have consumed several tons of photosynthetic producer organisms. If the producer organisms have become contaminated with toxic chemicals, these chemicals become more concentrated in the bodies of the fish that consume them. If none of the chemicals are lost along the way, *one person,* ultimately eats the same amount of contaminant as was present in the original *several tons* of producer organisms.

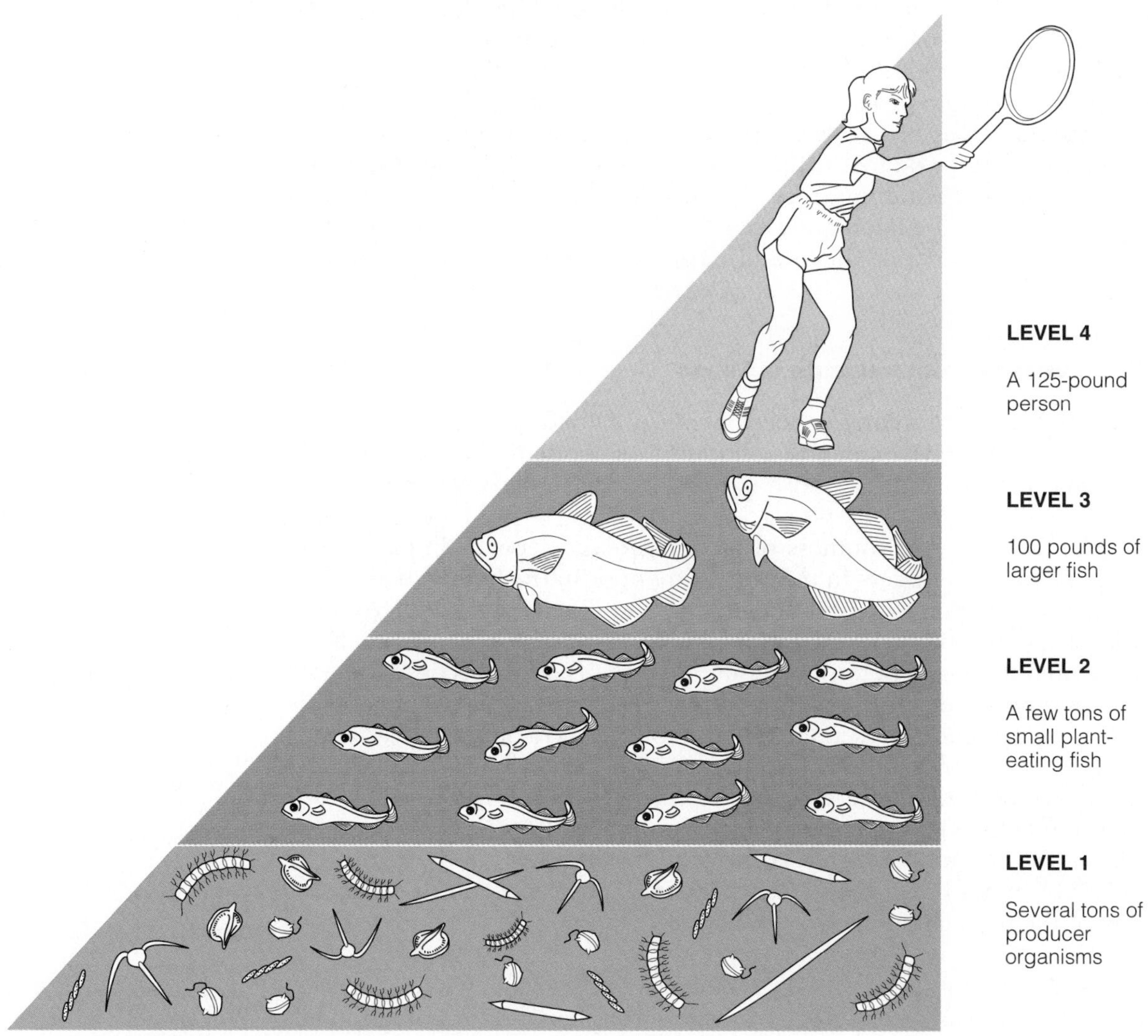

each day is highest in lead—therefore, a person should let the water run a few minutes before drinking or using it to prepare formula or food.

Lead intoxication in young children results from their behaviors and activities—putting their hands in their mouths, playing in dirt, and eating nonfood items (see Figure 11–3). Consequently, the toddler years see a marked rise in blood lead.[8] Tragically, a child's neuromuscular system is maturing at precisely the same time. As a result, children with high blood

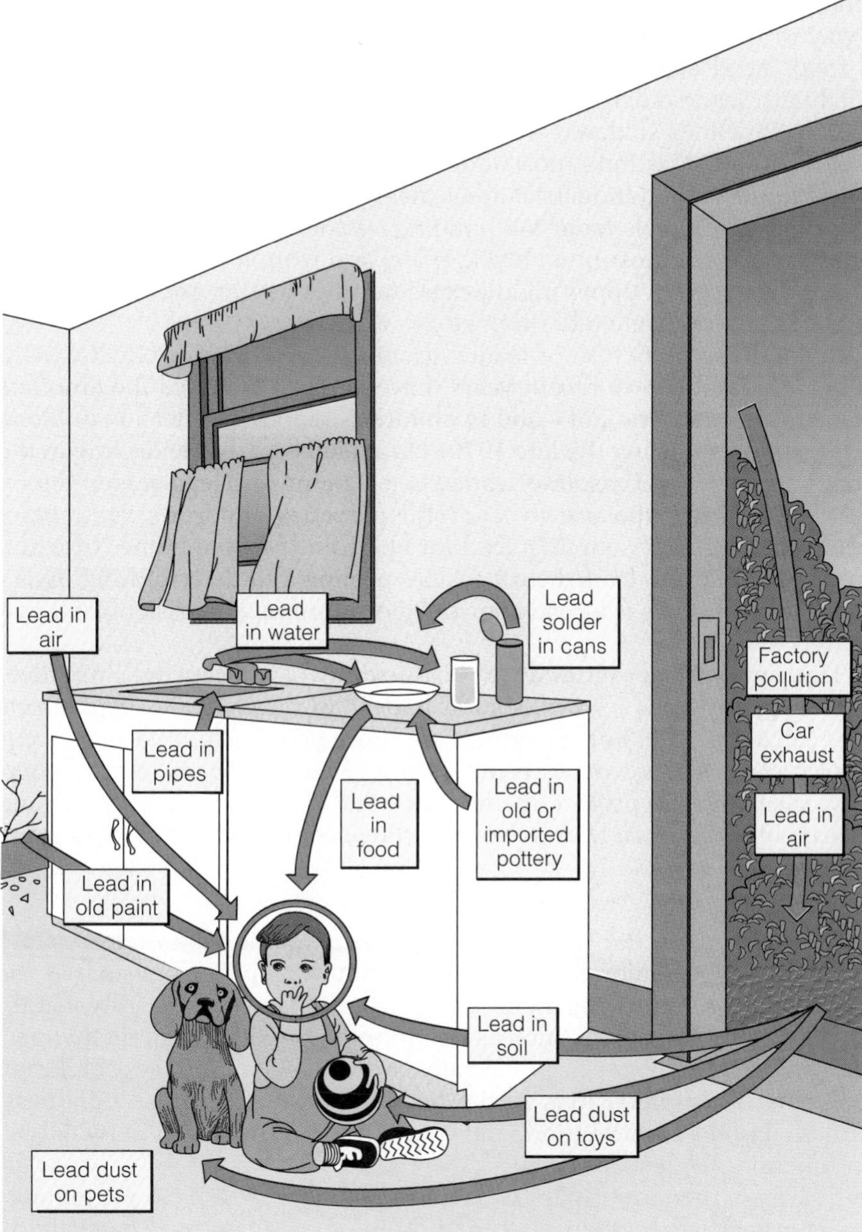
Lead in air
Lead in water
Lead solder in cans
Factory pollution
Car exhaust
Lead in air
Lead in pipes
Lead in food
Lead in old or imported pottery
Lead in old paint
Lead in soil
Lead dust on toys
Lead dust on pets

Figure 11–3
Sources of Lead Exposure

lead experience impairment of balance, motor development, and the relaying of nerve messages to and from the brain. Children with the highest blood lead when they are two and three years old suffer the greatest developmental delays at age four.[9] Researchers studying young children's development must now consider the possibility that lead poisoning may affect their results.[10]

All foods contain some lead. Much, perhaps all, of it is from industrial pollution. People are exposed to lead in some types of gasoline, paint, newspaper ink, batteries, shotgun ammunition, and pesticides as well as in the air and water that carry lead from industrial processes. Lead works its way through rainfall and soil into plants and animals that people use for food. Lead also enters food from food containers such as tin cans sealed with lead solder and old or imported pottery decorated with lead glazes.[11] Pipelines soldered with lead also release it into drinking water, in which it is the nation's most significant contaminant.[12] Exposures are highest in urban and industrial areas, near highways, and in slums where old leaded paint peels from the buildings. People suffering the effects of lead exposure are most often black, male, and from low-income families, but it is also seen in upper-middle-class families as they move into inner-city areas and renovate older homes.

Reductions in the use of leaded gasolines and other products, mandated by federal law in recent years, have helped to reduce the amounts of lead in the environment—and in children's blood. The decline in blood lead in children during the late 1970s paralleled exactly the decline in the nation's use of leaded gasoline, leaded house paint, and lead-soldered food cans.[13] Even so, exposure to lead still pervades children's lives. Paint remains the primary source of lead for children.[14] In the homes of 3 million young children, leaded surfaces are peeling and deteriorating. Every child in these homes is already poisoned or at immediate risk of lead poisoning.

Three major discoveries about lead toxicity have occurred simultaneously. Not only does lead poisoning appear to have more *subtle* effects than realized before, but the effects are more *permanent,* and they occur at *lower levels of exposure.* Consumers would be wise to take ultraconservative measures to protect themselves, and especially their small and unborn children, from lead poisoning; the accompanying box offers suggestions.

Mercury Mercury is another heavy metal that industry releases into the environment. Major contributors are industrial processes such as the burning of coal and the incineration of wastes. Mercury is readily metabolized by living organisms such as fish into the organic form, methylmercury, which is highly toxic, especially to growing infants and children. Displacing other metal ions in the body, mercury can cause blindness, deafness, loss of coordination, and other forms of impaired nervous system function. Higher doses kill.

Like lead, mercury is persistent and so bioaccumulates to the greatest extents in the tissues of animals high on the food chain, and particularly in the large fish that eat smaller fish in freshwater lakes and rivers and in the ocean. Also like lead, mercury finds its most vulnerable victims among the young. To protect yourself and your family against mercury poisoning, obey public health advisories about the fish caught in your local area, and do not eat any one kind of fish from one source too often.

Lead and mercury have been used here to show the potential seriousness of food and water contamination by persistent contaminants and the best defenses against them. Thousands of other contaminants exist, but in all cases two principles apply. First, remain alert to the possibility of contamination of foods, and keep an ear open for public health announce-

HOW TO Avoid Lead Poisoning

To protect yourself and your family against lead poisoning, take these steps:

- Test children for lead poisoning.
- In contaminated environments, keep small children from putting dirty or old painted objects in their mouths, and make sure children wash their hands before eating.
- Do not make baby formula from lead-soldered canned milk or with lead-contaminated water.
- Once you have opened canned food, immediately move it to a lead-free storage container to prevent lead migration into the food.
- Do not store acidic foods or beverages (such as orange juice) in ceramic dishware.
- Do not heat coffee in ceramic cups.
- Do not store alcoholic beverages in pewter or crystal decanters.
- Confirm with the publisher that your newspaper uses no lead in its ink before using the paper to wrap food, mulch garden plants, or add to your compost.
- Have the water in your home tested by a competent laboratory.
- Use only cold water for drinking, cooking, and making formula (cold water absorbs less lead).
- When water has been standing in lead-soldered pipes, flush the cold-water pipes until it is as cold as it can get (this may take as long as two minutes). If possible, replumb your home with plastic (PVC) piping, at least for drinking-water lines.
- If lead contamination of your water supply seems probable, obtain additional information and advice from the Environmental Protection Agency and your local public health agency.[a]

By taking these steps, parents can protect themselves and their children from this preventable danger.

[a]A cure that's worse than the ailment, *Science News* 135 (1989): 135.

ments and advice. Second, do not eat any one food too often; vary your diet. Switching from food to food is an effective defensive strategy against the accumulation of toxins in your body. This is the principle of dilution: each food eaten dilutes contaminants that may be present in other components of the diet.

Pesticide Residues in Foods

Pesticides are a special category of contaminants, different from those just discussed in that they are applied to foods on purpose and in a manner that is regulated and controlled. Their use is controversial. Pesticides do help to ensure the survival of some crops, but the damage they do to

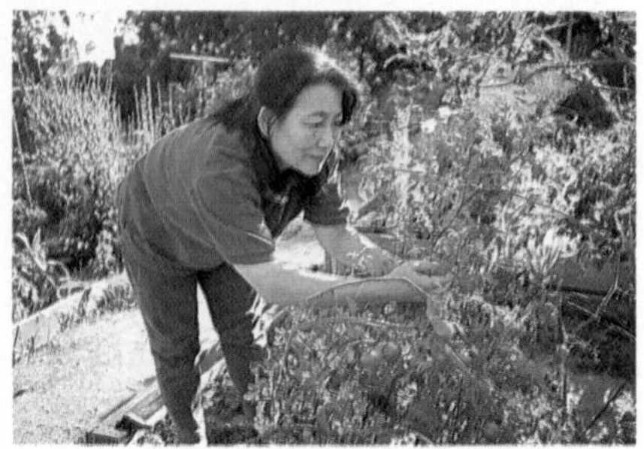

In some small gardens, handwork can take the place of pesticides.

the environment is considerable and increasing. Moreover, there is some question about whether the widespread use of pesticides has really improved the overall yield of food. Even with extensive pesticide use, U.S. agriculture loses about one-fifth of its crops to pests every year. Worldwide, pests destroy about one-third of the food crops every year.

Hazards of Pesticides Many pesticides are broad-spectrum poisons that damage all living cells, not just those of pests. Their use, therefore, is hazardous to those who work with them: manufacturers, field workers, truck drivers, and anyone else who is exposed to them. The danger of misuses or spills is ever present, and serious accidents are not always successfully prevented despite safety regulations and precautions applying to pesticide use.

Consumers of produce in the marketplace have reason to be concerned about pesticides, too, because they may still linger in the foods to which they were applied in the field.[15] Risks to health from pesticide exposure are probably small for healthy adults, but children may be vulnerable to some types of pesticide poisoning.[16]

Regulation of Pesticides The FDA sets legal limits on the types and amounts of pesticides permitted in foods. Over 10,000 separate regulations in the law regulate some 300 separate pesticide chemicals used in the United States. If a pesticide is misused, growers risk fines, lawsuits, and destruction of their crops. In 25 years of testing, the FDA has seldom found residues above tolerance levels, so it appears that pesticides are generally used according to regulations. This makes sense because growers are not eager to spend extra money on unneeded chemicals. Pesticides, along with fertilizers and fuels, make up one of the conventional farmer's major capital expenses each year.[17]

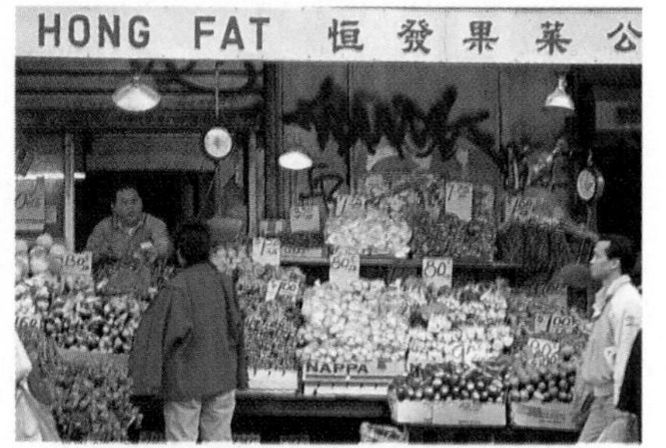

Foods imported from other countries may contain residues of pesticides that are banned from use here.

Pesticides from Other Countries What about foods imported from other countries, though, consumers may wonder. Indeed, a loophole in federal law does allow U.S. companies to produce pesticides that are banned here and sell them in other countries. Those countries then use the banned pesticides on their foods and ship the foods back to U.S. consumers, the so-called circle of poison. Federal inspectors do monitor incoming foods, however, and refuse to let them enter the country if they are found to contain illegal residues.

Testing Procedures The FDA analyzes foods using methods that can detect residues well below tolerances. If the FDA finds violative levels, it can seize the products or order them destroyed. Four times a year, FDA surveyors buy over 200 foods in U.S. grocery stores in several cities, prepare the foods table ready, and then analyze them, not only for pesticides but for essential minerals, industrial chemicals, heavy metals, and radioactive materials. Food preparation often reduces levels of contaminants in foods, so the FDA looks for levels at least five times lower than permitted limits. Findings confirm that the bulk of the U.S. food supply is safe from excessive pesticide residues.[18] In 1990, FDA tests found that more than 97 percent of the foods produced in the United States or imported from 92

HOW TO Rid Foods of Pesticide Residues

No matter where your food comes from, it is wise to remove parts that might contain pesticide residues:

- Trim the fat from meat and remove the skin from poultry and fish; discard fats and oils in broths and pan drippings. Avoid fish oil capsules. (Pesticide residues concentrate in the animal's fat.)
- Wash fresh produce in water. Use a scrub brush, and rinse thoroughly.
- Use a knife to peel an orange or grapefruit; do not bite into the peel.
- Discard the outer leaves of leafy vegetables such as cabbage and lettuce.
- Peel waxed fruit and vegetables; waxes don't wash off and can seal in pesticide residues.
- Peel vegetables such as carrots and fruits such as apples when appropriate. (Peeling removes pesticides that remain in or on the peel, but also removes fibers, vitamins, and minerals.)

other countries had either no residues or residues within federally permitted limits.[19]

A problem, though, is that budget restraints limit the FDA's testing capacity. The FDA does not sample *all* food shipments or test for *all* pesticides. Fewer than 700 inspectors and scientists test food samples from the multitude of farms, groves, docks, airports, warehouses, and processing plants the agency oversees. The FDA cannot (nor can it be expected to) guarantee 100 percent safety in the food supply. Instead, it sets conditions so that substances do not become a hazard and acts promptly when problems or suspicions arise.

Avoiding Pesticides Consumers, therefore, have some responsibility for their own health and safety with respect to pesticides. They can learn about the potential benefits and dangers of pesticide use, discuss regulations and alternatives with others, advise their government representatives about their findings, and apply pressure wherever it will help change inappropriate procedures.* Meanwhile, people can minimize their risks by following the guidelines offered in the accompanying box.

In addition to the suggestions in the box, consumers can buy fresh foods grown locally, especially when they can confirm that the produce has been grown using responsible methods. Consumers who want pesticide-free produce shouldn't look for "perfect" fruits and vegetables; pesticide-free produce may have a few blemishes, but minor blemishes are not a hazard.

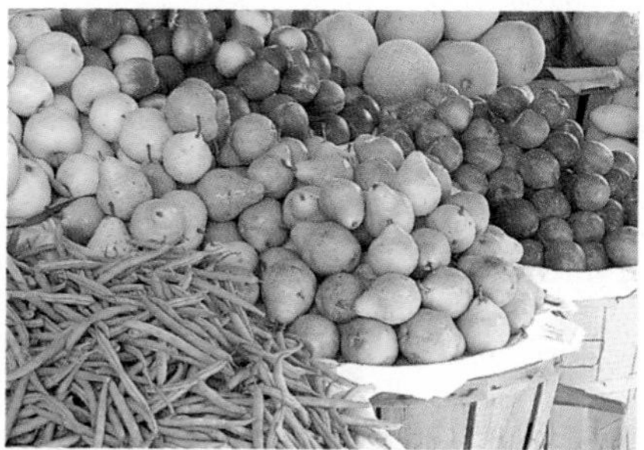

Pesticide-free produce may not be perfectly free of blemishes, but may be a healthy choice.

*For answers to any questions about any sort of pesticides, call the EPA's 24-hour National Pesticide Hotline: 1–800–858–PEST.

Incidental Food Additives

incidental food additives: substances that can get into food not through intentional introduction but as a result of contact with the food during growing, processing, packaging, storing, or some other stage before the food is consumed. The terms *accidental additives* and *indirect additives* mean the same thing.

Here's a way to tell if glass or other containers are made of microwave-safe materials. Microwave the empty container for one minute and carefully touch it.

- Warm = unsafe for microwave.
- Lukewarm = safe for short reheating use.
- Cool = safe for long microwave cooking times.

dioxins: toxic organic compounds containing chlorine, arising in industry as (among other things) by-products of the bleaching process.

Indirect or incidental additives are really contaminants that find their way into food as a result of some phase of production, processing, storage, or packaging. Examples of incidental additives include tiny bits of plastic, glass, paper, tin, and other substances from packages, as well as chemicals from processing, such as the solvent used to decaffeinate some types of coffee.

Some microwave products are sold in "active packaging" that participates in cooking the food. Pizza, for example, may rest on a cardboard pan coated with a thin film of metal that absorbs microwave energy and may heat up to 500°F. Exposed to the intense heat, some particles of the packaging components migrate into the food.[20] Regular microwave packages heat up less, but particles still migrate, and the materials from both kinds of packaging are under study to determine their safety for consumption. Until more is known, a wise choice is to use only glass or ceramic containers designed for microwaving and to avoid reusing disposable containers, such as margarine tubs, for heating foods.

Coffee filters, milk cartons, paper plates, and frozen food packages can all be made of bleached paper and so can contaminate foods with trace amounts of compounds known as dioxins. Dioxins form during the chlorination step in making bleached paper. Dioxins can migrate into foods that come in contact with bleached paper, but the amounts entering food are infinitesimally small—one part per trillion, or the equivalent of one second in 32,000 years. Such amounts do not appear to present a health risk to people, and drinking milk from bleached cartons appears to be safe.[21] Dioxins are persistent, however, and they leach into the environment by way of both paper-mill effluent and discarded paper products in landfills. They therefore bioaccumulate as do other contaminants described earlier (Figure 11–2), becoming more and more concentrated in land, water, and animals until they build up to hazardous levels.

Incidental additives sometimes find their way into foods, but adverse effects are rare. These additives are well regulated. All food packagers are required to perform specific tests to discover whether materials from packages are migrating into foods; if they are, their safety must be confirmed by strict procedures similar to those governing intentional additives, discussed next.

Food Additives

additives: substances that are not normally consumed as foods by themselves, but are added to foods.

Of all consumer concerns about food safety, preventing food poisoning is the most important. Next are natural toxins, environmental contaminants, and pesticides. Last is additives. Manufacturers use food additives to give foods desirable characteristics: color, flavor, texture, stability, higher nutrient content, or resistance to spoilage. Consumers see additives mentioned on labels, and wonder or worry about them, but additives are of very little concern compared to the other aspects of foods already covered. Nevertheless, for the sake of completeness, here they are.

Regulations Governing Additives Manufacturers have to go through special procedures that can take many years to get permission to use new additives in food products. The manufacturer must test each new additive to satisfy the FDA of the following:

- It is effective (it does what it is supposed to do).
- It can be detected and measured in the final food product.

Then the manufacturer must study the effects of feeding the additive in large doses to animals under strictly controlled conditions to prove that:

- It is safe (it does not cause cancer, birth defects, or other injury).

Finally, the manufacturer must submit all test results to the FDA. Public hearings follow, where consumers are invited to participate and experts present testimony for and against granting permission to use the additive. Thus consumers' rights and responsibilities are written into the provisions for deeming additives safe.

When the FDA approves an additive, it writes a regulation stating in what amounts, for what purposes, and in what foods the additive may be used. No additives are permanently approved; all are periodically reviewed.

GRAS List Additives Many substances were exempted from complying with this procedure at the time it was first instituted because they had been used a long time and their use entailed no known hazards. Some 700 substances in all were put on the generally recognized as safe (GRAS) list. However, when substantial scientific evidence or public outcry has questioned the safety of a substance on the GRAS list, its safety has been reevaluated. All substances about which any legitimate question was raised have been removed or reclassified.

GRAS (generally recognized as safe) list: a list of food additives, established by the FDA in 1958, that had long been in use and were believed safe.

Toxicity versus Hazard An important distinction governs decisions about an additive's safety—the distinction between toxicity as a property of substances and hazard associated with substances. Toxicity is a general property of all substances; hazard is the capacity of a chemical to produce injury *under conditions of its use.* All substances can be toxic at some level of consumption, but they are called hazardous only if they are actually consumed in sufficiently large quantities to cause harm. An additive is not considered to be a hazard if some immense amount that people never consume is toxic. The additive is a hazard only if it is toxic under the conditions of its actual use. A food additive is supposed to have a wide margin of safety.

toxicity: the ability of a substance to harm living organisms. All substances are toxic if used in high enough concentrations.

hazard: the ability of a substance to produce injury under the conditions of its use.

margin of safety: as used when speaking of food additives, a zone between the concentration normally used and that at which a hazard exists. For common table salt, for example, the margin of safety is ⅕ (five times the concentration normally used would be hazardous).

Testing Procedures Most additives that involve risk are allowed in foods only at levels 100 times below those at which the risk is still known to be zero. Experiments to determine the extent of risk involve feeding test animals the substance at different concentrations throughout their lifetimes. The additive is then permitted in foods at 1/100 the level that causes no harmful effect whatever in the animals. In many foods, *naturally* occurring toxins appear at levels that bring their margins of safety closer to 1/10. Even nutrients, as you have seen, involve risks at high dosage levels. The margin of safety for vitamins A and D is 1/25 to 1/40; it may be less than 1/10 in infants. For some trace elements, it is about 1/5. People consume common table salt daily in amounts only three to five times less than those that cause serious toxicity.

The margin-of-safety concept also applies to nutrients when they are used as additives. Iodine has been added to salt to prevent iodine deficiency, but it has to be added with care because it is a deadly poison in excess. Similarly, iron has been added to refined bread and other grains (enrichment) and has doubtless helped prevent many cases of iron-deficiency anemia in women and children who are prone to that disease. But the addition of too much iron could put men (who usually have enough iron in their bodies) at risk for iron overload. The upper limit has to be remembered.

Benefits versus Risks Most additives used in foods are there because they offer benefits that outweigh their risks or that make the risks worth taking. In the case of color additives that only enhance the appearance of foods and do not improve their health value or safety, no amount of risk may be deemed worth taking. Only 10 of an original 80 synthetic color additives are still approved by the FDA for use in foods, and screening of these continues.[22]

It is also the manufacturers' responsibility to use only the amounts of additives necessary to get the needed effects, not more. Additives must also *not* be used:

- To disguise faulty or inferior products.
- To deceive the consumer.
- Where they significantly destroy nutrients.
- Where their effects can be achieved by economical, sound manufacturing processes.

The regulations in force governing the management of intentional additives are well conceived and have been effective, on the whole. Funding shortages limit the capabilities of watchdog agencies such as the FDA, however, and some mistakes and cases of false reporting are found to slip by.

The next few paragraphs focus on a few individual food additives—notably, those that have received the most negative publicity because people ask questions about them most often. The order is alphabetical; it does not imply an order of importance.

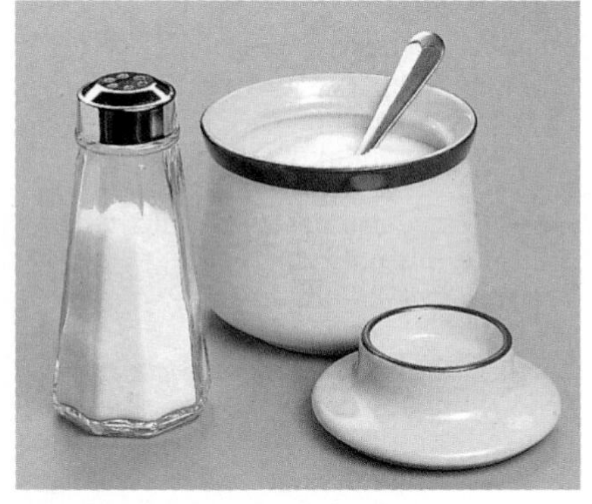

Two long-used preservatives.

preservatives: antimicrobial agents, antioxidants, chelating agents, radiation and other additives that retard spoilage or preserve desired qualities, such as softness in baked goods.

antimicrobial agents: substances used as food additives that prevent growth of illness-causing microorganisms in foods.

nitrites: salts added to food to prevent botulism.

Antimicrobial Agents Foods can go bad in two ways: one dangerous, one not. The dangerous way is by becoming hazardous to health; the other way is by losing their flavor and attractiveness. An example of the dangerous way: bacteria, yeasts, and molds and other fungi growing in foods can cause food poisoning. Preservatives known as antimicrobial agents protect foods from these microbes.

The best-known, most widely used antimicrobial agents are the two common substances salt and sugar. Salt preserves meat and fish; sugar preserves canned and frozen fruits, jams, and jellies. Both salt and sugar work by withdrawing water from the food; microbes cannot grow without water. Today, other additives such as potassium sorbate and sodium propionate are also used to extend the shelf life of baked goods, cheese, beverages, mayonnaise, margarine, and many other products.

Another group of antimicrobial agents, the nitrites, is added to foods for three main purposes: to preserve their color (especially the pink color of hot dogs and other cured meats); to enhance their flavor by inhibiting rancidity (especially in cured meats); and to protect against bacterial growth. In particular, nitrites prevent the growth of the botulinum bacterium that produces the deadly toxin described earlier.

Nitrites clearly perform important jobs, but they have been the object of controversy because in the human body they can be converted to nitrosamines, which cause cancer in animals. Some cured meats are available without nitrites, but reducing nitrites consumed in meats would hardly make a difference in a person's overall exposure to nitrosamine-related compounds. For example, an average cigarette smoker inhales 100 times the nitrosamines that the average bacon eater ingests. Likewise, a beer drinker imbibes up to roughly five times the amount that the bacon eater receives. Cosmetics deliver via absorption through the skin about twice the amount delivered from bacon. Even the air inside automobiles delivers measurable amounts of nitrosamines.[23]

nitrosamines (nigh-TROHS-uh-meens)**:** derivatives of nitrites that may form when nitrites combine with amines.

Antioxidants The other way foods can go bad is by undergoing changes in color and flavor caused by exposure to oxygen in the air (oxidation). Often these changes involve little hazard to health, but they damage the food's appearance, taste, and nutritional quality. Familiar examples of these changes are the ways sliced apples or potatoes turn brown or oils go rancid. Antioxidant preservatives protect foods from this kind of spoilage. A total of 27 antioxidants are approved for use in foods. Vitamin C (ascorbate) and vitamin E (tocopherol) are among them.

The sulfites are another group of antioxidants. They are used to prevent oxidation in many processed foods, in alcoholic beverages (especially wine), and in drugs. They used to be popular with restaurant owners for use on salad bars because they keep raw fruits and vegetables looking fresh, but some people experience allergic reactions to the sulfites—reactions that are sometimes dangerous and, for a few, deadly. The FDA now prohibits sulfite use on foods intended to be consumed raw, with the exception of grapes, and it requires sulfite-containing foods and drugs to include a warning on their labels. For most people, sulfites do not pose a hazard in the amounts used in products.

antioxidants: defined in Chapter 7 as compounds that protect other compounds from oxygen by themselves reacting with oxygen. Antioxidants are used to prevent rancidity of fats in foods and other damage to foods caused by oxygen. Examples are vitamins E and C, BHA, BHT, propyl gallate, and sulfites.

sulfites: salts containing sulfur that are added to fresh and frozen fruits and vegetables to prevent changes in color and texture due to oxidation.

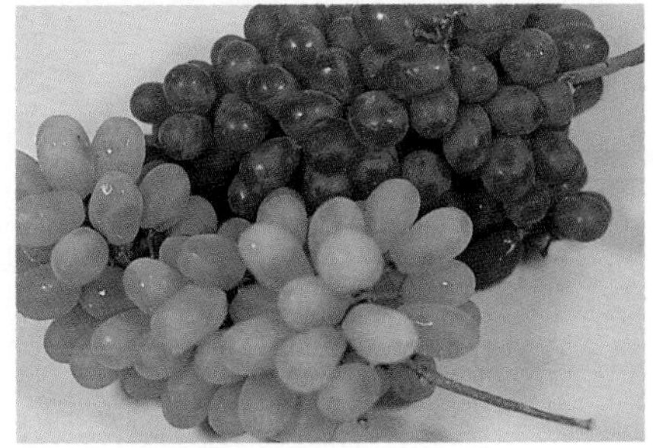

Raw grapes may legally be treated with sulfites. Wash them thoroughly before eating.

Artificial Colors As mentioned, only about ten synthetic artificial colors are still on the GRAS list, a highly select group that has survived considerable screening. They are among the most intensively investigated of all additives. In fact, they are much better known than the *natural* pigments of plants, and the limits on the safety of their use can be stated with greater certainty.

Still, the food colors have been more heavily criticized than almost any other group of additives. This is because, simply stated, they only make foods pretty, whereas other additives, such as preservatives, make foods safe. Hence, with food colors, we can afford to require that their use entail no risk, whereas with other additives we may have to compromise between the risks of using them and the risks of *not* using them.

An infamous food-coloring agent of an earlier time was red dye number 2, which came under suspicion as a carcinogen in 1970 on the basis of two studies conducted in Russia. It was never shown to cause cancer,

artificial colors: certified food colors, added to enhance appearance (*certified* means approved by the FDA).

but it proved impossible to demonstrate that the dye did *not* cause cancer either, and so it was banned in the United States in 1976. On the same evidence, Canada concluded that the dye was not likely to cause cancer and continued to permit its use. (Red candies in this country do not contain red dye number 2.)

Foods containing tartrazine:
- Orange drinks (Tang, Daybreak, Awake).
- Gatorade (lime flavored).
- Gelatin desserts (Jell-O, Royal).
- Golden Blend Italian dressing (Kraft).
- Some cake mixes and icings (Duncan Hines, Pillsbury, Cake Mate).
- Imitation banana or pineapple extract (McCormick).
- Seasoning salt (French's).
- Macaroni and cheese dinner (Kraft).
- "Cheez" curls and balls (Planter's).
- Fruit chews (Skittles).
- Butterscotch squares and candy corn (Brach's).

The food color tartrazine (yellow dye number 5) causes an allergic reaction in susceptible people. Symptoms include hives, itching, and nasal congestion, sometimes severe enough to require medical treatment. It is not a common problem; only one or two in 10,000 individuals may have the reaction. Still, that is more than 20,000 individuals in the nation as a whole. These people rightly demand to know what foods contain the dye so they can avoid it. It is not enough to avoid yellow-colored foods because tartrazine is used to confer turquoise, green, and maroon colors in foods and drugs as well. Legislation is now in force requiring that tartrazine be listed on all labels of foods that contain it.

artificial flavors, flavor enhancers: chemicals that mimic natural flavors and those that enhance flavor.

Artificial Flavors and Flavor Enhancers While only a few artificial colors are currently permitted in foods, close to 2000 artificial flavors and flavor enhancers are approved, making them the largest single group of food additives. One of the best-known members of this group is monosodium glutamate, or MSG (trade name, Accent)—the monosodium salt of the amino acid glutamic acid. MSG is used widely in restaurants, especially Asian restaurants, as a flavor enhancer. Research indicates that in addition to enhancing other flavors, MSG may itself possess a basic taste independent of the well-known sweet, salty, bitter and sour tastes.*[24]

MSG has received publicity because it may produce an adverse reaction called the Chinese restaurant syndrome in some individuals. Symptoms include burning sensations, chest and facial flushing or pain, and throbbing headaches. MSG has been investigated extensively enough to be deemed safe for adults to use (except people who react adversely to it, of course), but it is kept out of foods for infants because very large doses have been shown to destroy brain cells in developing mice. Infants have not yet developed the capacity to fully exclude such substances from their brains and so are more sensitive to them.

Nutrient Additives Another class of additives includes nutrients added to improve or to maintain the nutritional value of foods. Included among nutrient additives are the nutrients added to refined grains to enrich them; the iodine added to salt; vitamins A and D added to dairy products; and the nutrients added to fortified breakfast cereals. When nutrients are added to a nutrient-poor food, it may appear from its label to be nutrient rich. It is, but only in those nutrients chosen for addition. Nutrients are sometimes also added for other purposes. The use of vitamins C and E as antioxidants has already been mentioned. Beta-carotene may be added as a selling point because consumers, who have heard media reports of studies linking beta-carotene to reduced risks of diseases, are buying more products that contain it.

---

*The taste produced by MSG is termed *umami*.

As this section has shown, no two additives are alike, and therefore generalizations about them are meaningless. Whenever questions about the safety of "additives" are being raised, you might as well leave the room, because no valid statement can be made that applies to the 3,000-odd different substances commonly added to foods. Questions about which additives are safe, under what conditions of use, have to be asked and answered on an item-by-item basis.

One thing is clear, though. The U.S. food supply is well monitored and well protected against hazards that might threaten people's health. Provided that consumers apply common sense in selecting and preparing their foods, they can enjoy the great blessing of an abundant and safe food supply.

■ STUDY QUESTIONS ■

1. Are canned and frozen foods nutritionally inferior to fresh foods? Explain.
2. In what ways may processed foods be superior or inferior to fresh foods?
3. What guidelines can help people to preserve nutrients when cooking foods at home?
4. To what extent does food poisoning present a real hazard to U.S. consumers eating U.S. foods? How often does it occur?
5. Identify the guidelines that people can follow to prevent food-borne infections from arising in their own kitchens.
6. What special food-poisoning prevention precautions apply to meats? To seafood? To uncooked fruits and vegetables?
7. What is meant by a "persistent" contaminant of foods? Why are persistent contaminants a hazard to meat-eating animals and humans?
8. In what ways can people protect themselves and their children against lead poisoning?
9. In what ways can people reduce the concentrations of pesticides in and on the foods that they prepare?
10. Name five classes of additives and give an example of each.

NUTRITION IN PRACTICE 11

Environmentally Conscious Foodways

The chapter preceding this discussion viewed foods from many angles and suggested ways of achieving many dietary goals: nutritional adequacy, protection from food poisoning, avoidance of contaminants, and other elements of safety. People who follow the advice given can be satisfied that they have good answers to the questions "How can I get the best health from my foods?" and "How can I keep my foods safe?"

Some people want to achieve another goal when they shop for foods and cook them. They recognize that they will spend thousands of dollars on foods and cook thousands of meals in a lifetime, and they perceive that their money and actions exert effects in the world outside their own personal lives. Increasingly, people today are asking, "What are the environmental impacts of my food choices? How do my actions in the kitchen affect the environment?" They want to make environmentally responsible choices.

What sort of environmental impacts do people's food choices have?

Among the global resources involved in producing food are irrigation water, fertilizers, pesticides, fuel, and land and fisheries. And in the U.S. market, tons of packaging materials and a massive transportation network burning immense quantities of fossil fuel are used to convey foods to consumers. Each truckload of food produced in this country travels, on the average, 1300 miles to reach the market.[25] It costs 800 kcalories in fuel to make a can of diet soda that contains 1 kcalorie of food energy, and more water is used to make the can than to make the soda.[26] An appetizer of shrimp cocktail may contain 4 ounces of shrimp, but to net those shrimp, the shrimpers had to kill 2½ pounds of young fish that otherwise could have grown up to provide food.[27]

More environmentally benign choices are available. In place of vegetables shipped in from far away, people might choose to eat vegetables grown in their own home states, at least during the growing seasons. In place of several sodas in aluminum cans, a soda drinker might use one large recyclable bottle. In place of shrimp cocktail, the diner might choose a crab salad or a few oysters harvested without killing other sea creatures. Environmentally responsible food choices can also be made in the realms of food shopping, cooking, and cleanup.

Give me some examples of environmentally responsible food shopping.

Food shopping involves going to the store, selecting foods once there, choosing among the packages in which those foods are sold, and choosing bags in which to carry the foods home. All of these actions exert impacts on the environment, and consumers can choose to minimize those impacts. Consider the shopping trips first. The environmentally conscious shopper knows that motor vehicles are the world's single largest source of air pollution and so tries to minimize car mileage spent on trips to and from the store. Strategies are to shop nearby and to shop only once a week. To make it possible to shop for a week's meals at a time, a shopper can plan to buy foods with various shelf lives and to eat the most perishable ones first. For example, buy lettuce, cabbage, squash, and carrots. Use up the lettuce first, then the squash. The carrots and cabbage keep longer, so eat these later. Buy fruits of differing ripeness—for example, six bananas: two ripe, two nearly ripe, and two green. Use the ripe ones right away and the others as they become ripe. On first arriving home, cook the meats for the early meals; portion out the rest, and freeze the bread and meat

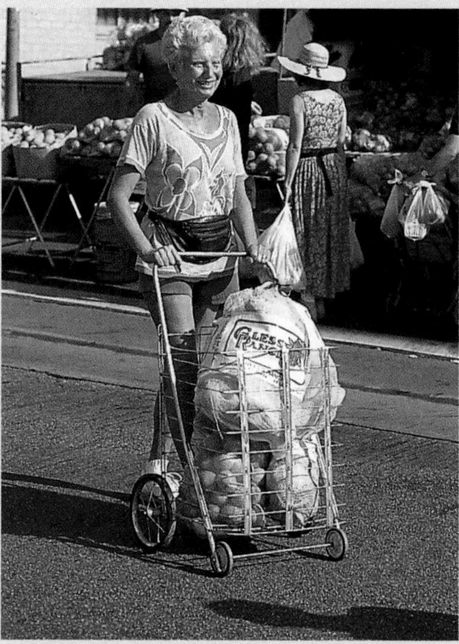

Shopping without a car can be a pleasure, if you can afford the time.

that won't be needed until midweek. These strategies save time and money as well as fossil fuels.

Give some examples of environmentally responsible food choices.

Perhaps the advice most frequently given to save fuel and resources is to "eat low on the food chain." It takes much less land and fuel, and costs much less in pollution, to produce most plant foods than to produce most meats (see Figure 11–4). Following this advice benefits nutritional health, too: recall from Chapter 1 that the Daily Food Guide recommends that adults eat 11 or more servings of plant foods (grains, vegetables, and fruits) daily and only 4 or 5 servings of milk products and meats combined. This is also a good strategy for avoiding food contaminants.

Another guideline is to eat foods that are processed as little as possible. Figure 11–5 on page 296 shows how much more energy it takes to produce canned or frozen corn than fresh corn. Energy costs mean fuel costs, and fuel costs mean pollution.

Other environmentally aware food-shopping practices include buying products whose production benefits the land, or at least harms it minimally, and boycotting products whose production damages the land. Buying food produced locally by farmers known to use a minimum of fertilizers and pesticides and not to waste water is often a positive choice. Refusing to buy tuna fish caught by fishers who slaughter dolphins and avoiding beef grown at the expense of virgin rainforest land are examples of boycotts inspired by environmental awareness.

What about the packages foods come in? Do they exert impacts on the environment?

Figure 11–4
Eating Low on the Food Chain Saves Resources

It takes ten times as much land and fuel to feed people meat as to feed them plants. (Reminder: The *food chain* is the sequence in which living things depend on other living things for food as shown in Figure 11–2.)

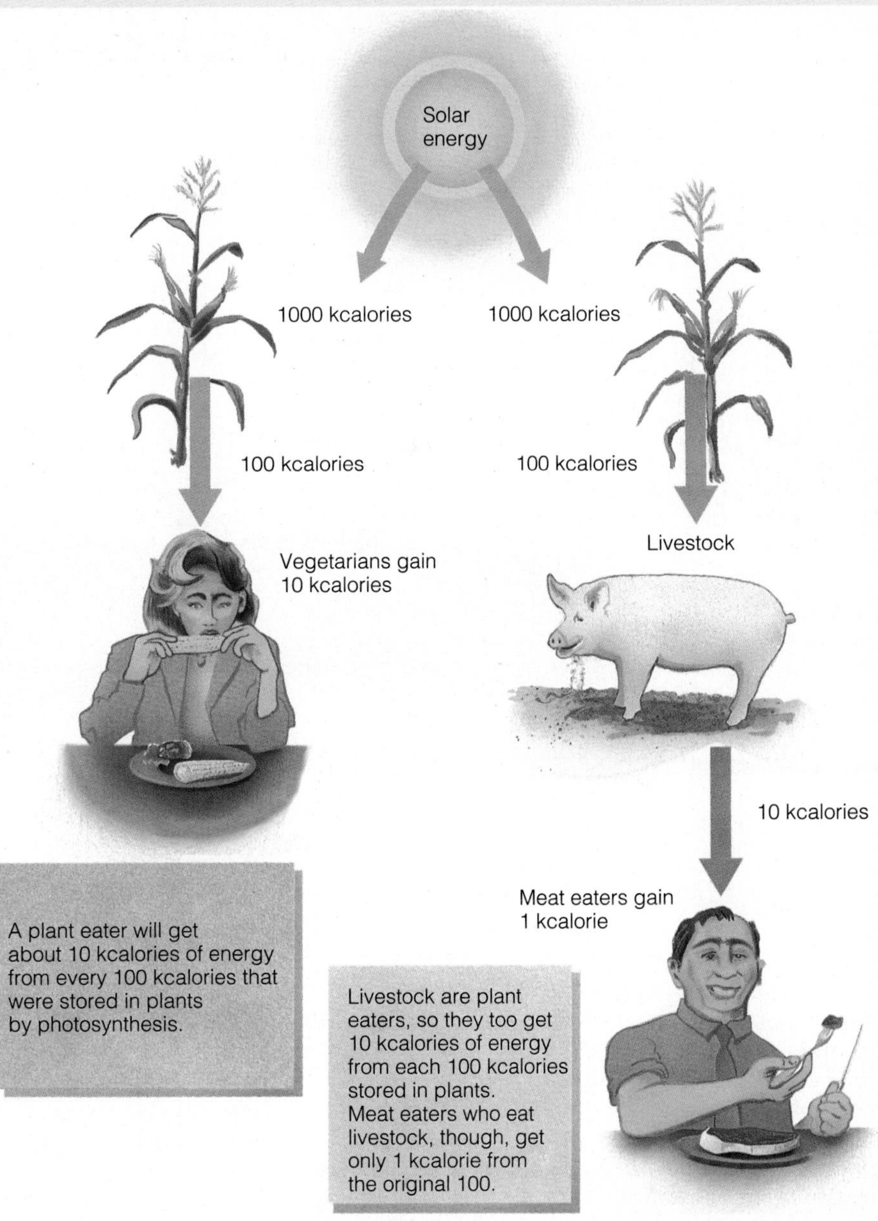

Solar energy
1000 kcalories
1000 kcalories
100 kcalories
100 kcalories
Vegetarians gain 10 kcalories
Livestock
10 kcalories
Meat eaters gain 1 kcalorie
A plant eater will get about 10 kcalories of energy from every 100 kcalories that were stored in plants by photosynthesis.
Livestock are plant eaters, so they too get 10 kcalories of energy from each 100 kcalories stored in plants. Meat eaters who eat livestock, though, get only 1 kcalorie from the original 100.

Figure 11–5
Energy Costs of Canned and Frozen Corn

The corn contains only 825 kcalories per kilogram, but look how much energy goes to produce it.

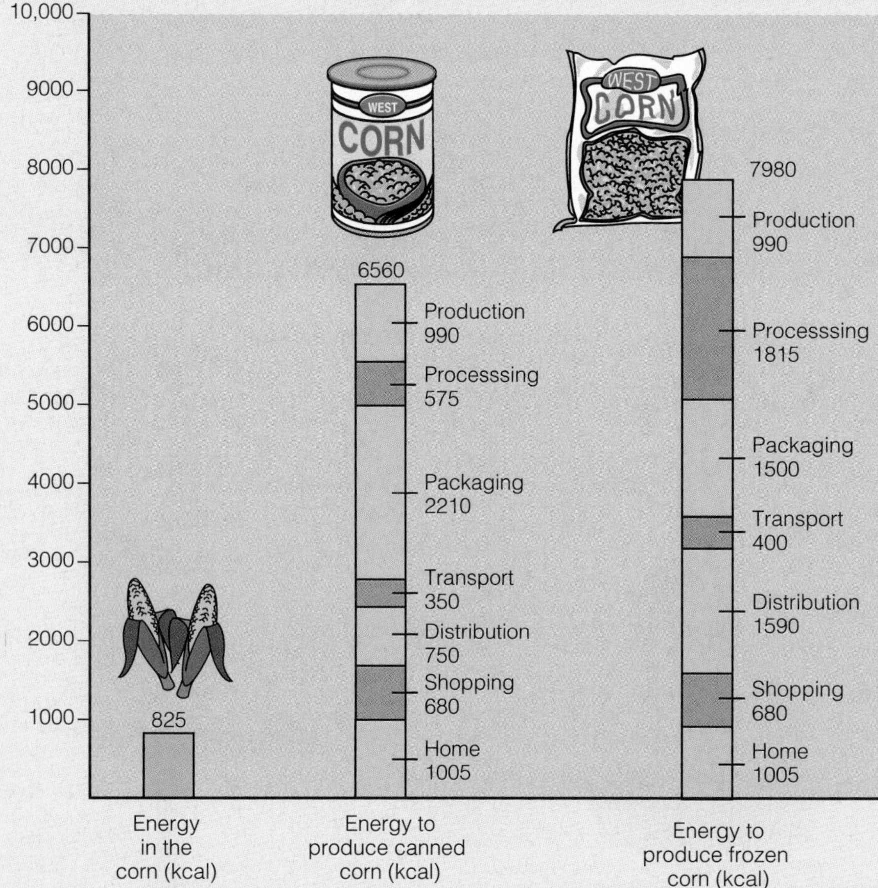

Source: D. Pimentel, *Food, Energy and the Future of Society* (Boulder, Colo.: Associated University Press, 1980).

Yes. It costs energy and resources to make these packages, and it may cost land or pollution to dispose of them. In general, what is best for the environment is no packages; next best are minimal, reusable, or recyclable ones. Even grocery bags represent a huge drain on energy and resources, and many consumers are demanding alternatives to throwaway bags. Many shoppers prefer to carry reusable shopping bags to the store and refuse all others. Failing in this, they ask for plastic bags if they are recyclable—and then take care to recycle them. The third choice would be paper bags, and last would be nonrecyclable plastic.

What are the best ways to cook food from the environmental standpoint?

Fast cooking saves fuel and so pollutes less. Asian meals exemplify this principle: they are made of precut, bite-sized pieces of food, stir-fried fast in small amounts of oil. This cooking style both saves energy and preserves nutrients.

The pressure cooker or the microwave can also cook food fast. The pressure cooker can do the occasional big piece of meat the cook wants to serve whole; the microwave can cook vegetables, casseroles, or leftovers. Both may save using several burners on the stove, and both preserve nutrients better than most stove-top methods.

The oven, in contrast, can be a fuel waster. Efficient oven use is possible if the cook bakes or roasts a lot of food at one time. To use the stove top efficiently, a cook can use flat-bottomed pots with close-fitting lids that completely cover the burners. That way, each burner will donate all its heat to cooking something, not just heating the kitchen (and the

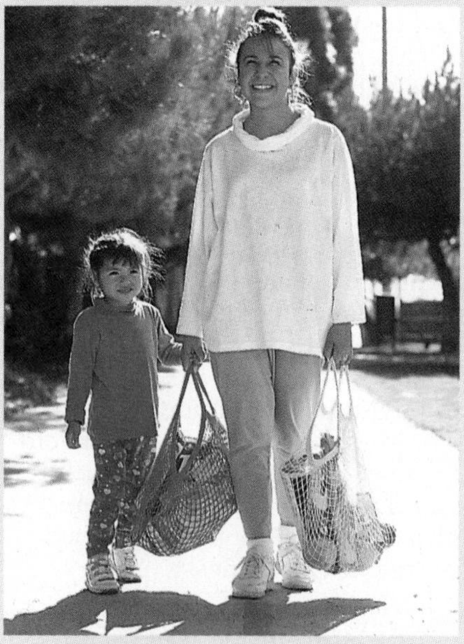

Reusable bags require the fewest resources.

planet). One can also turn electric burners and ovens off before the food is fully cooked and let the cooking finish as the stove cools.

What about cleanup after a meal?

A big energy user associated with food preparation and cleanup is the water heater. The less hot water used, the less fuel must be burned to heat the water. People can save water-heating energy in many ways. They can set the water heater at 130°F, not hotter. They can put it on a timer, so that each day it heats just enough water to meet that day's needs. They can wrap it in insulation to keep it from losing heat to the surroundings. They can wrap the hot-water pipes all the way to the points of use. They can install water-saving faucets and shower heads.

When replacing a water heater or installing a new one, a consumer can opt for a small, instantaneous-type water heater that heats the water only at the point of use, and only when needed. A consumer can choose a gas water heater, rather than an electric one. Natural gas is a cleaner fossil fuel than the coal or oil usually burned to make electricity. Solar water heaters work well in sunny regions.

Someone who washes many dishes at a time should consider using a dishwasher, if it is affordable. People may think that the cost of the water, heat, and soap would be higher than the cost of washing by hand, but this is not the case. One school found that a normal washing machine cycle used on full loads consumed less than two-thirds the water used in hand washing.[28] Using less hot water also means using less electricity to heat it. The savings are greatest if the dishes are not prerinsed and are allowed to air dry.[29]

Are there "right" and "wrong" ways to throw garbage away, too?

An average American household of four people produces about 100 pounds of trash a week, much of it from the kitchen.[30] National concern has focused on this issue because the nation is running out of landfill space in which to dispose of all the trash. Landfill space is only one of many problems associated with trash, however. Every item thrown away is a resource lost: an aluminum can could be used to make a new aluminum can; a cereal box, but for its clay coating, could become recycled paper; a plastic bottle could become part of a beautiful carpet. Trash need not become an undesirable mess; recycled trash could be viewed as a usable resource. Yet as it is now, about 70 percent of all the metal mined in the United States is used only once and then discarded. The aluminum thrown away every three months could rebuild the entire U.S. air fleet.[31]

Garbage is a special case of a resource generated in the kitchen. Vegetable scraps, fruit peelings, and leftover plant foods are organic and biodegradable, like the leaves and grass cuttings people rake up in their yards. All of these materials can be piled up together with some soil and allowed to decompose naturally, forming compost, a rich, crumbly material that can be used as in nature to fertilize growing things. Some communities, recognizing this, conduct composting programs to recycle people's organic debris; some homeowners maintain their own composting piles. College campuses can use composted kitchen waste, mixed with grass cuttings and weeds, to mulch, fertilize, and enrich the soil they use in landscaping. Composting can even be done indoors in small odor-free bins and the resulting material used to pot plants.[32]

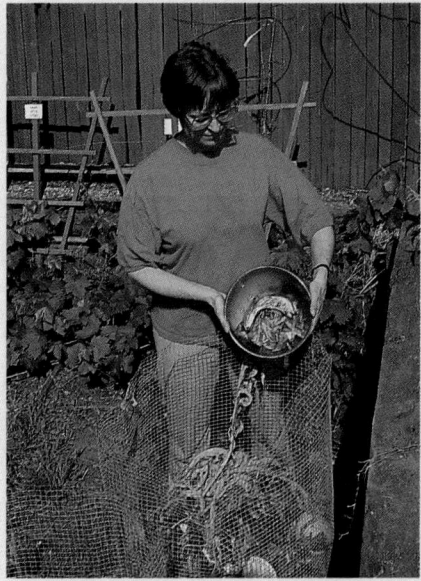

Compost nourishes plants as food nourishes people.

As you can see, environmental awareness can permeate every aspect of food management from start to finish. And each choice made to save resources, cut energy use, or refrain from polluting helps to preserve and protect the environment.

■ NOTES ■

1. M. V. Polo, M. J. Lagarda, and R. Farré, The effect of freezing on mineral element content of vegetables, *Journal of Food Composition and Analysis* 5 (1992): 77–78.
2. V. Modeland, Fishing for facts on fish safety, *FDA Consumer,* February 1989, pp. 16–24.
3. Seafood safety: Highlights of the Executive Summary of the 1991 Report by the Committee on Evaluation of the Safety of

Fishery Products of the Food and Nutrition Board, Institute of Medicine, National Academy of Sciences, *Nutrition Reviews* 49 (1991): 357–363.

4. K. E. Anderson and A. Kappas, Dietary regulation of cytochrome P450, *Annual Review of Nutrition* 11 (1991): 141–167.
5. R. W. Miller, The metal in our mettle, *FDA Consumer,* December 1988/January 1989, pp. 24–27.
6. J. Murphy, Federal agencies gearing up for new efforts against lead, *Nation's Health,* May/June 1991, pp. 1, 23.
7. M. E. Shannon and J. W. Graef, Lead intoxication in infancy, *Pediatrics* 89 (1992): 87–90.
8. J. Raloff, Lead effects show in child's balance, *Science News* 135 (1989): 54.
9. A. J. McMichael and coauthors, Port Pirie Cohort study: Environmental exposure to lead and children's abilities at the age of four years, *New England Journal of Medicine* 319 (1988): 468–475.
10. Environmental exposure to lead and cognitive deficits in children, *New England Journal of Medicine* 320 (1989): 595–596.
11. Miller, 1988/1989.
12. Getting the lead out, *Science News* 132 (1987): 269.
13. E. Yetley, Nutritional applications of the Health and Nutrition Examination Surveys (HANES), *Annual Review of Nutrition* 7 (1987): 441–463.
14. Childhood lead poisoning: A disease for the history texts (editorial), *American Journal of Public Health* 81 (1991): 685.
15. C. F. Chaisson, B. Petersen, and J. S. Douglass, *Pesticides in Foods: A Guide for Professionals* (Chicago: American Dietetic Association, 1991), pp. 2 –3.
16. National Academy of Sciences Committee, as quoted by J. Raloff and D. Pendick, Pesticides in produce may threaten kids, *Science News* 144 (1993): 4–5.
17. P. Weber, A place for pesticides? *World Watch,* May/June 1992, pp. 18–25.
18. Food and Drug Administra-tion Pesticide Program, *Residues in Foods—1990* (Washington, D.C.: Food and Drug Administration, 1991).
19. Food and Drug Administration Pesticide Program, 1991.
20. D. Farley, Keeping up with the microwave revolution, *FDA Consumer,* March 1990, pp. 17–21.
21. D. Blumenthal, Deciding about dioxins, *FDA Consumer,* February 1990, pp. 11–13.
22. I. D. Wolf, Critical issues in food safety, 1991–2000, *Food Technology,* January 1992, pp. 64–70.
23. J. Hotchkiss and R. Cassens, Nitrate, nitrite, and nitroso compounds in foods (a scientific status summary by the Institute of Food Technologists' Expert Panel on Food Safety and Nutrition), April 1987, available from Institute of Food Science, Department of Food Science, Cornell University, Ithaca, NY 14853.
24. M. Naim and coauthors, Interaction of MSG taste with nutrition: Perspectives in consummatory behavior and digestion, *Physiology and Behavior* 49 (1991): 1019–1024.
25. A. D. Basiago, The house where the future lives, *Calypso Log,* September 1986, p. 11.
26. J. E. Young, Aluminum's real tab, *World Watch,* March/April 1992, pp. 26–33; Earth Works Group, *50 Simple Things That You Can Do to Save the Earth* (Berkeley, Calif.: Earthworks Press, 1989), pp. 64–65.
27. Regional perspectives: Gulf of Mexico shrimp fishery, *Marine Conservation News,* Winter 1990, p. 11.
28. At home, *Executive Fitness,* April 1989, p. 8.
29. Ask Garbage, *Garbage,* Spring 1994, p. 63.
30. Earth Works Group, 1989, p. 9.
31. Earth Works Group, 1989, p. 9.
32. R. Kourik, As the worm turns, *Garbage,* January/February 1992, pp. 48–51.

12

Nutrition Assessment: History, Drug History, and Physical Examination

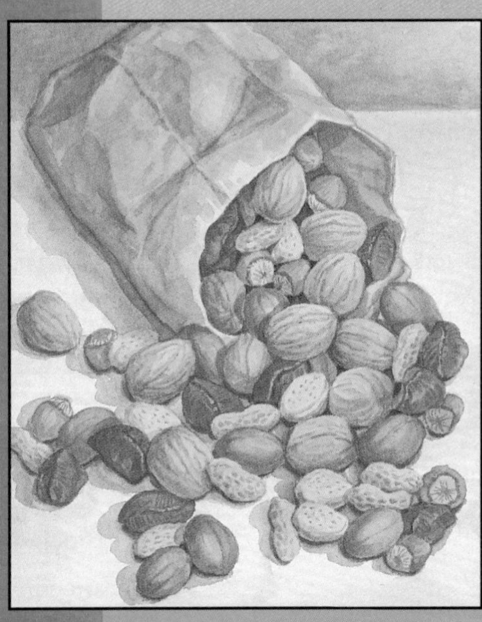

CONTENTS

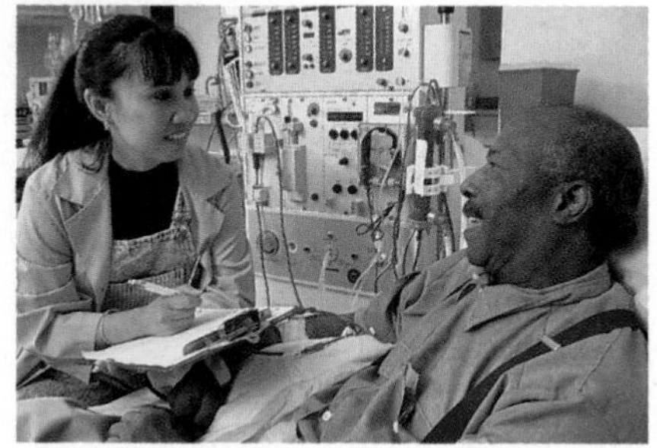

Health care professionals develop nutrition care plans based on information gathered from nutrition assessments.

nutrition assessment: the evaluation of many factors that influence or reflect nutritional health; the tools used for nutrition assessment include historical information, physical examinations, anthopometric measures, and biochemical analyses.

Nurses and registered dietetic technicians are the professionals who most often assist dietitians in completing nutrition assessments.

The first eleven chapters of this book have shown how a physically fit body and an alert mind depend on good nutrition. Turning now to clinical nutrition, the remaining chapters show how to prevent, detect, and correct nutrient imbalances.

Health care professionals who recognize nutrition's indispensable roles in supporting health make a conscientious effort to think "nutrition." They employ the tools of nutrition assessment, described in this chapter and the next, to aid their efforts. They are alert to the signs of malnutrition and act promptly to prevent, retard, or reverse its progress. They look at a child's pale complexion and lack of appetite and investigate to see if the child's diet is adequate; they see an elderly person's poor posture and lethargy and look for possible nutrient imbalances.

Defining Nutrition Status

Nutrition assessment procedures provide the health care team with the information they need to determine how well a client's nutrient needs are being met. From this information, the assessor can develop a plan of action to correct any deficits or imbalances. The assessor, usually a registered dietitian assisted by other qualified health care professionals, uses all of the following as sources of data:

- Historical information.
- Physical examinations.
- Anthropometric measurements.
- Biochemical analyses (laboratory tests).

By accurately gathering this information and carefully interpreting each finding in relation to the others, the assessor obtains the basis for a meaningful evaluation. Assessors frequently use computer programs to perform many of the mathematical calculations required and to check the results against standards.

This chapter describes the uses of histories and physical examinations in nutrition assessments. Chapter 13 shows how anthropometric measurements and biochemical tests complete the assessment process.

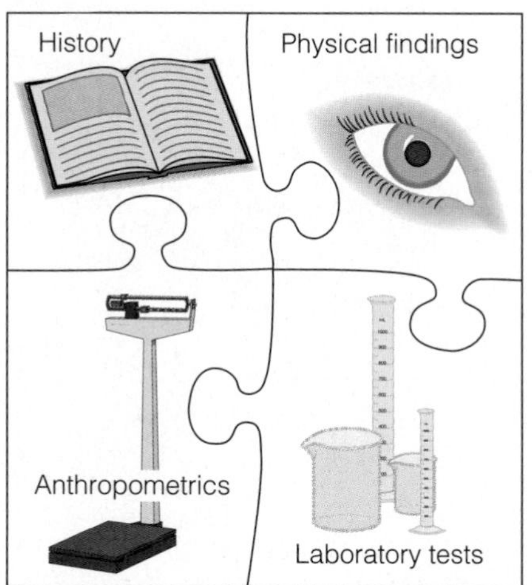

Taken as a whole, the information gathered during a nutrition assessment helps define a person's nutrition status.

Historical Information

Table 12–1 sums up the types of historical data that may yield clues to nutrition status. Form 12–1 (on pp. 305–306) shows the data typically collected in recording a client's history. A thorough history alerts the assessor to potential problems that can be further investigated using other assessment techniques.

An adept history taker uses the interview not only to gather facts, but also to establish rapport with the client and to assess education and ability level. Histories also provide the basis for making realistic nutrition care plans.

Health History

An assessor is wise to review the client's health, or medical, history before visiting the client. During the interview, the assessor can then keep in

Table 12–1
Historical Data Used in Nutrition Assessments

TYPE OF HISTORY	WHAT IT IDENTIFIES
Health history	Health factors that affect nutrition status
Socioeconomic history	Personal, financial, and environmental influences on food intake, nutrient needs, and diet therapy options
Drug history	Medications and nutrient supplements that affect nutrition status
Diet history	Nutrient intake excesses or deficiencies and the reasons for imbalances

mind the factors that may affect the person's nutrition status. Conversations with the client can also uncover valuable health-related information that might otherwise be overlooked because no one thought to ask.

Physical and mental health both affect and reflect nutrition status; the history taker should be alert to conditions that place a client at risk for malnutrition (see Table 12–2). Figure 12–1 on the next page illustrates some of the relationships between illness and nutrition.

health history: the medical record. Traditionally, the health history has been called the *medical history.* The term *health history* now seems more appropriate, however, because the contents describe the client's health status. Current trends in the medical profession are now emphasizing health promotion and disease prevention.

Appetite and Food Intake Loss of appetite commonly accompanies illness. A child with a fever frequently is unable to eat; so is an adult with cancer. Nausea, mouth dryness, problems with chewing or swallowing, and obstructions in the digestive tract can all lead to poor food intake and result in malnutrition.

Table 12–2
Health Factors That Can Affect or Reflect Nutrition Status

- Acquired immune deficiency syndrome (AIDS)
- Alcoholism
- Anorexia (lack of appetite)
- Anorexia nervosa
- Bulimia
- Cancer
- Chewing or swallowing difficulties (including poorly fitted dentures, dental caries, and missing teeth)
- Chronic obstructive pulmonary disease
- Circulatory problems
- Constipation
- Crohn's disease
- Decubitus ulcers
- Dementia
- Depleted blood proteins
- Diabetes mellitus
- Diarrhea
- Diseases of the GI tract
- Drug addiction
- Dysphagia
- Fever
- Heart disease
- Hormonal imbalance
- Hyperlipidemia
- Hypertension
- Infection
- Kidney disease
- Liver disease
- Lung disease
- Malabsorption
- Mental illness
- Mental retardation or deterioration
- Multiple pregnancies
- Nausea
- Neurologic disorders
- Organ failure
- Overweight
- Pancreatic insufficiency
- Paralysis
- Physical disability
- Pneumonia
- Pregnancy
- Radiation therapy
- Recent major illness
- Recent major surgery
- Recent weight loss or gain
- Smoking
- Surgery of the GI tract
- Trauma
- Ulcerative colitis
- Ulcers
- Underweight
- Vomiting

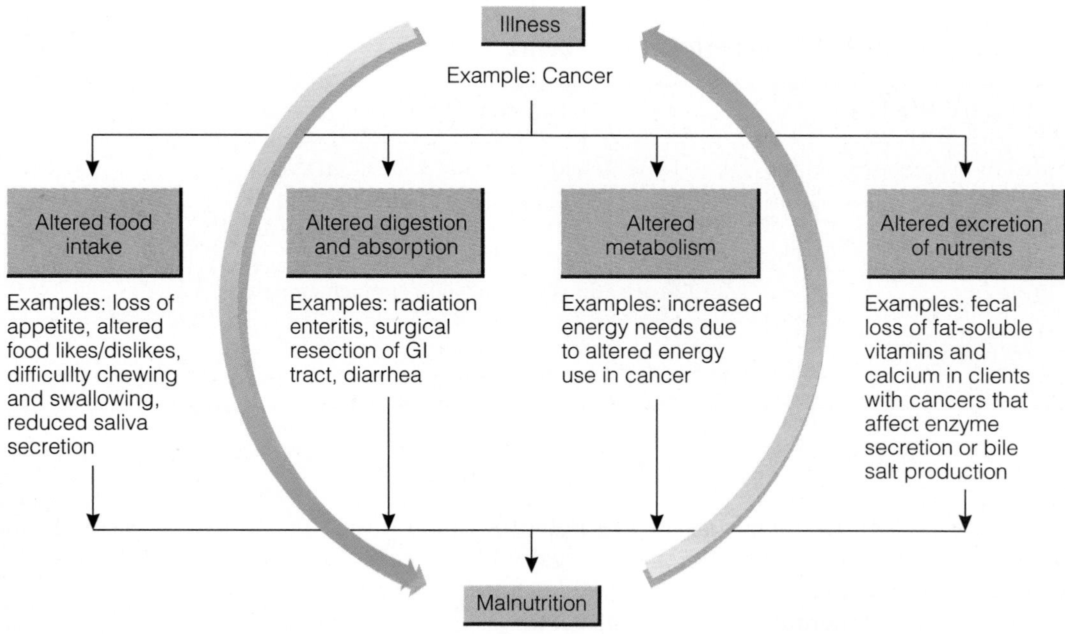

Figure 12–1 Relationships between Illness and Nutrition (Nutrition for people with cancer is discussed in Chapter 28.)

The secondary effects of illness can also affect nutrient intake. Pain and anxiety associated with illness can make it difficult or impossible to eat; pain in the mouth or throat is especially problematic. Anxiety stimulates stress hormone activity and suppresses digestive activity, making clients lose their appetites. Medical treatments and procedures may require that a person not eat at the very time when nutrient needs are especially high due to illness.

Digestion and Absorption Illnesses that interfere with digestion or absorption usually affect several nutrients and can cause nutrition status to deteriorate rapidly. Examples include cystic fibrosis, pancreatitis, and inflammatory bowel diseases. (Chapter 21 describes these disorders in more detail.)

Metabolism Illnesses can directly alter metabolism (Chapters 18 and 19) and change nutrient needs. They can also alter organ function and thereby alter metabolism indirectly; examples are liver disease (Chapter 24), renal failure (Chapter 27), cancer (Chapter 28), and AIDS (Chapter 29).

Excretion Illnesses can also interfere with the excretion of nutrients. The result can be either excessive retention of nutrients, as in renal failure, or excessive loss of nutrients, as in diarrhea or nephrotic syndrome (Chapter 27).

Nutrition in Practice 8 describes nutrition concerns associated with alcohol abuse (one type of substance abuse), and Nutrition in Practice 9 explores eating disorders and their nutrition consequences.

Mental Health The effects of mental illnesses on nutrition status may be less readily apparent than the effects of physiological illnesses, but are no less important. Nutrition in Practice 12 describes some major interactions between emotional health and nutrition status.

Drug History

Medical drugs are often involved in the treatment of illness, and nearly every drug affects nutrition status to some degree. Therefore, obtaining a drug history is an important part of the assessment process. Of interest are all drugs: prescription drugs, nonprescription over-the-counter (OTC) drugs, illicit drugs, and even nutrient supplements. If a person is taking any drug routinely, the assessor records the name of the drug or supplement with the dose, frequency, and duration of intake; the reason for taking it; and signs of any adverse or positive effects (see Form 12–1).

Hundreds of drugs interact with nutrients, making imbalances or deficiencies likely. This discussion focuses on medical drugs. Adverse drug-nutrient interactions are most likely if drugs are taken over long periods, if several drugs are taken, or if nutrition status is poor or deteriorating. Understandably, then, elderly people and people with serious illnesses that raise nutrient needs are most at risk. A recent study of institutionalized elderly people found that multiple drug use (an average of more than six medications daily) significantly affects nutrition status.[1]

Nutrients and drugs may interact in many ways:

- Drugs can alter food intake and the absorption, metabolism, and excretion of nutrients.
- Foods and nutrients can alter the absorption, metabolism, and excretion of drugs.

Table 12–3 lists the general categories of drugs notable for their interactions with nutrients. The following sections describe these interactions, and Table 12–4 on the next page summarizes this information and provides specific examples. Table E–1B in Appendix E provides details on specific interactions, drug by drug.

Drugs and Food Intake Many drugs can lead to malnutrition by interfering with food intake. Amphetamines used to treat hyperactivity in children provide an example: they may effectively improve behavior, but they also suppress appetite, alter taste perceptions, dry the mouth, and cause nausea. Conversely, some drugs stimulate the appetite and lead to undesirable weight gain. An example is astemizole (Hismanal), an antihistamine used by some people to relieve allergy symptoms.

Absorption and Drugs A classic example of how drugs can interfere with nutrient absorption involves laxatives. A person who uses laxatives daily for a long time may find that the intestines can no longer function without them. This dependence can lead to malnutrition. Laxatives cause foods to move rapidly through the intestine, so that many vitamins have too little time to be absorbed. The use of mineral oil as a laxative robs the person of the fat-soluble vitamins, including vitamin D. The vitamins dissolve in the indigestible oil and are excreted; calcium, too, is excreted.

A classic example of how foods can interfere with drug absorption is that between the antibiotic tetracycline and the minerals calcium and iron. When calcium and tetracycline, or iron and tetracycline, are taken at the same time, they bind to each other, thus reducing the absorption of both. Clients are therefore instructed not to take tetracycline with milk,

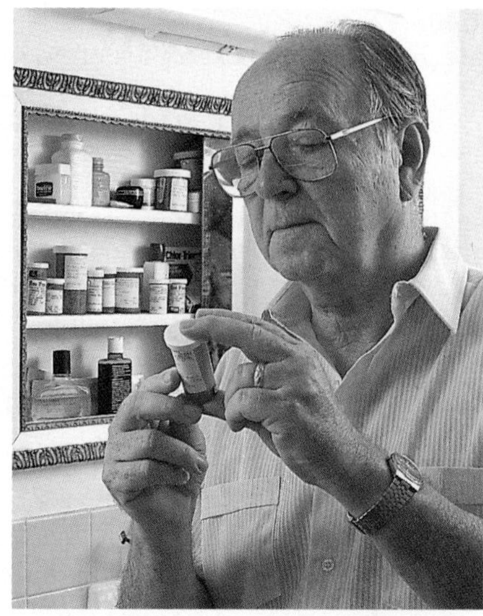

Taking several drugs over long periods intensifies the risk of drug-nutrient interactions.

drug history: a record of all the drugs, over-the-counter and prescribed, that a person takes routinely.

Table 12–3
Classes of Drugs That Can Affect Nutrition Status

- Amphetamines and other stimulants
- Analgesics
- Antacids
- Antibiotics
- Anticancer agents
- Anticonvulsant agents
- Antidepressant agents
- Antidiarrheal agents
- Antihyperlipemic agents
- Antihypertensive agents
- Antiulcer agents
- Catabolic steroids
- Diuretics
- Hormonal agents
- Immunosuppressive agents
- Laxatives
- Oral contraceptives
- Sulfonylurea agents
- Vitamin and other nutrient preparations

Note: Specific examples, drug by drug, appear in Appendix E, Table E-1B.

Table 12–4
Mechanisms and Examples of Food-Drug Interactions

DRUGS CAN ALTER FOOD INTAKE BY:	
▸ Altering the appetite (amphetamines suppress the appetite). ▸ Interfering with taste or smell (methotrexate changes taste sensations). ▸ Inducing nausea or vomiting (digitalis can do both). ▸ Changing the oral environment (phenobarbital can cause dry mouth). ▸ Irritating the GI tract (cyclophosphamide induces mucosal ulcers). ▸ Causing sores or inflammation of the mouth (methotrexate can cause painful mouth ulcers to form).	
DRUGS CAN ALTER NUTRIENT ABSORPTION BY:	**FOODS CAN ALTER DRUG ABSORPTION BY:**
▸ Changing the acidity of the digestive tract (antacids can interfere with iron absorption). ▸ Altering digestive juices (cimetidine can improve fat absorption). ▸ Altering motility of the digestive tract (laxatives speed motility, causing the malabsorption of many nutrients). ▸ Inactivating enzyme systems (neomycin may reduce lipase activity). ▸ Damaging mucosal cells (chemotherapy can damage mucosal cells). ▸ Binding to nutrients (antacids bind phosphorus).	▸ Changing the acidity of the digestive tract (candy can change the acidity, thereby causing slow-acting asthma medication to dissolve too quickly). ▸ Stimulating secretion of digestive juices (griseofulvin is absorbed better when taken with foods that stimulate the release of digestive enzymes). ▸ Altering digestive processes (aspirin is absorbed more slowly when taken with food). ▸ Binding to drugs (tetracycline binds to calcium in dairy foods, limiting drug absorption). ▸ Competing for absorption sites in the intestines (dietary amino acids interfere with levodopa absorption this way).
DRUGS AND NUTRIENTS CAN INTERACT AND ALTER METABOLISM BY:	
▸ Acting as structural analogs (as anticoagulants and vitamin K do). ▸ Competing with each other for metabolic enzyme systems (as phenobarbitol and folate do). ▸ Contributing pharmacologically active substances (tyramine from cheese and monoamine oxidase inhibitors).	
DRUGS CAN ALTER NUTRIENT EXCRETION BY:	**FOODS CAN ALTER DRUG EXCRETION BY:**
▸ Altering reabsorption in the kidneys (some diuretics increase the excretion of sodium and potassium). ▸ Displacing nutrients from their plasma protein carriers (aspirin displaces folate).	▸ Changing the acidity of the urine (vitamin C can alter urinary pH and limit the excretion of aspirin).

milk products, or calcium-containing antacids (such as Tums). Similarly, clients must take their iron supplements two hours apart from their tetracycline doses.

Another example of how food can interfere with the absorption of a drug is that of nicotine gum and acidic foods. Physicians sometimes prescribe nicotine gum to help people quit smoking cigarettes. Certain acid-containing foods and beverages interfere with the action of this gum: they prevent the absorption of the nicotine through the lining of the mouth into the blood.[2] Unfortunately, three of the interfering beverages are beer, coffee, and colas—favorites chosen by many people who use nicotine gum. When a food or beverage blocks nicotine's absorption from the mouth, the person swallows the nicotine, and this may cause nausea and hiccups.

Foods and beverages that may interfere with the effectiveness of nicotine gum:

- Apple juice.
- Beer.
- Catsup.
- Coffee.
- Colas.
- Grape juice.
- Lemon-lime soda.
- Mustard.
- Orange juice.
- Pineapple juice.
- Soy sauce.
- Tomato juice.

Form 12–1
Historical Data

Name________________________ Date________________________
Address________________________ Date of last medical checkup ________________________
________________________ Age__________ Sex __________
________________________ Height__________ Weight__________
Phone________________________ Usual weight________________________
Reason for admission________________________ Ideal weight range ________________________
____

Health History

1. Have you been told that you have (check any that apply):
   ____Diabetes ____Heart disease ____Ulcers
   ____GI disorders ____Lung disease ____Cancer
   ____High blood pressure ____Kidney disease ____Other
   ____Hardening of arteries ____Liver disease ____________
2. Do you have complaints about any of the following:
   ____Lack of appetite ____Diarrhea ____Nausea
   ____Difficulty chewing or swallowing ____Indigestion ____Vomiting
   ____Constipation ____Fever ____Other
3. Do you use tobacco in any way?____ How much?____
4. For females:
   Are you pregnant?__________ How many months?__________
   How many pregnancies have you carried to term? __________
   When was your last child born? __________
   Are your menstrual periods normal? _____If not, please explain: __________

Drug History

1. Do you take medication, either prescribed by a doctor or over-the-counter?

Name of drug	Reason for taking	Dose	Frequency	Duration of intake
________	________	________	________	________
________	________	________	________	________
________	________	________	________	________

2. Have you noticed any side effects from taking these medications?_____ If so, please explain: __________
3. Do you take vitamins or any kind of supplements?_____ Which ones? __________
   How often?__________ For what reason? ____

Socioeconomic History

1. Last grade of school completed __________Still in school?__________
2. Are you employed? _____ Occupation __________
3. Does someone else live with you?_____ Who? __________
4. Do you regularly eat alone or with others?__________
5. Do you have a refrigerator?__________Stove?__________
6. How often do you shop for food?__________
   Where? __________

(continued)

Form 12–1 *(continued)*

Diet History

1. Have you recently lost or gained more than 10 lbs? ________ If yes, explain the surrounding circumstances (including associated illness, dietary changes, and time frame)`: ________
2. Do you eat at regular times each day? ________ How many times per day? ________
3. Where do you eat most of your meals? ________
4. Do you usually eat snacks? ________When? ________
5. What foods do you particularly like? ________
6. Are there foods you don't eat for other reasons? ________
7. Do you have difficulty eating? ________
8. How would you describe your feelings about food? ________
9. How do your eating habits change when you are emotionally upset? ________
10. Are you, or any member of your family, on a special diet? ____ If yes, who and what kind?________
11. Do you drink alcohol? ________ How much? ________ How often? ________
12. How would you describe your exercise habits?________ Type of exercise ________
    Intensity________ Duration ________ Frequency ________
13. Are there any other facts about your lifestyle that you think might be related to your nutritional health? ________
    Explain ________

Note: Use the appropriate form to record food intake data (Form 12–2 and 12–3).

These interactions may explain why nicotine gum helps only about one fourth of the people who use it to quit smoking. For maximum effectiveness, people should refrain from ingesting foods and beverages during and immediately after chewing the gum.

Some drugs are absorbed better with foods than without them. For this reason, the antifungal drug griseofulvin is always given with meals. In many cases, though, foods delay the rate at which drugs are absorbed, although in some instances this too can be helpful. An aspirin taken on an empty stomach works faster than when it is given with food, but because aspirin can irritate the GI tract, taking it with food can reduce nausea.

Metabolism and Drugs To appreciate how drug-nutrient interactions can affect metabolism, consider the example of vitamin K and the anticlotting medication warfarin (Coumadin). Warfarin opposes clotting by interfering with vitamin K, so the warfarin dose has to be large enough to counteract whatever vitamin K is in the person's diet. If a person's vitamin K intake increases, as it may do in summer when lettuces and greens are in season, then the physician has to increase the drug dose.

The effects of tyramine provide another example. Tyramine is a substance found in some foods, and it interacts with monoamine oxidase inhibitors (MAO inhibitors), which are prescribed to treat certain forms of severe depression. An enzyme in the brain normally inactivates tyramine, and MAO inhibitors block the action of that enzyme. When people take the drug, the enzyme fails to act, and tyramine remains active and stimulates the release of norepinephrine. This can cause severe hypertension and headaches, and if blood pressure rises high enough, it can be

Table 12–5
Foods Restricted in a Tyramine-Controlled Diet

Beverages	Red wines including chianti, sherry[a]
Cheeses	Aged cheeses, American, camembert, cheddar, gouda, gruyère, mozzarella, parmesan, provolone, romano, roquefort, stilton[b]
Meats	Liver; dried, salted, smoked, or pickled fish; sausage; pepperoni; salami; dried meats
Vegetables	Fava beans; Italian broad beans; sauerkraut; snow peas; fermented pickles and olives
Other	Brewer's yeast;[c] all aged and fermented products; soy sauce in large amounts, cheese-filled breads, crackers, and desserts, salad dressings containing cheese

Note: The tyramine contents of foods vary from product to product depending on the methods used to prepare, process, and store the food. In some cases, as little as 1 ounce of cheese can cause a severe hypertensive reaction in people taking monoamine oxidase inhibitors. In general, the following foods contain small enough amounts of tyramine that they can be consumed in small quantities: ripe avocado, banana, yogurt, sour cream, acidophilus milk, buttermilk, raspberries, and peanuts.

[a]Most wine and domestic beer can be consumed in small quantities.

[b]Unfermented cheeses, such as ricotta, cottage cheese, and cream cheese, are allowed.

[c]Products made with baker's yeast are allowed.

fatal. For this reason, people taking MAO inhibitors should restrict their intakes of foods rich in tyramine (see Table 12–5).

Drugs that resemble vitamins in structure can interfere with normal metabolism. Methotrexate, used to treat cancer and psoriasis, and pyrimethamine, used to prevent malaria, are examples (see Figure 12–2). Both are structurally similar to folate and can cause severe folate deficiencies. Aspirin can also alter folate metabolism. Aspirin competes with

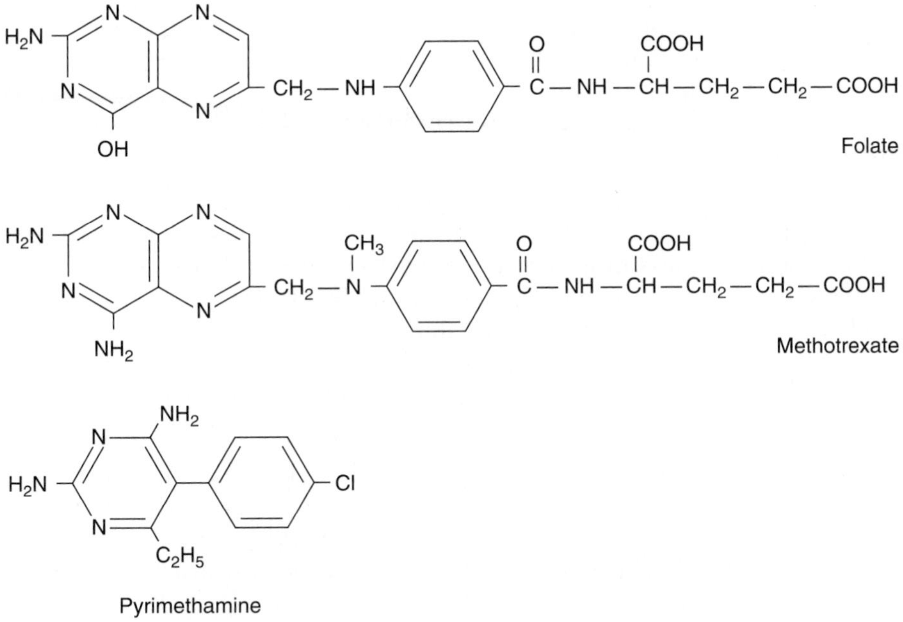

Folate

Methotrexate

Pyrimethamine

Figure 12–2
Folate and Two Antivitamins Used in Cancer Chemotherapy

folate for its protein carrier, thus hindering the body's use of the vitamin. When these drugs are used, health care professionals should ensure that either the diet or supplements are supplying sufficient folate to meet the added demands.

Excretion and Drugs Urinary acidity affects drug reabsorption from the kidneys back into the blood. For example, acidic urine limits the excretion of acidic drugs like aspirin. When large doses of vitamin C are given with aspirin, this increases the urine's acidity and aspirin remains in the blood longer.

Drugs can also alter urinary excretion of nutrients. For example, some diuretics accelerate the excretion of calcium, potassium, magnesium, and zinc.

Nutrients in Drugs The contribution that drugs make to nutrient intakes often goes unnoticed. Many liquid preparations contain sizable doses of sugar to make them taste better. Antibiotics and antacids often contain sodium. A person who takes Alka-Seltzer may not realize it, but a single 2-tablet dose exceeds some people's safe sodium intakes for a whole day. Another antacid (Tums) claims to supplement calcium to the diet, but its action as a drug makes it unsuitable for this purpose. It neutralizes stomach acid, on which the absorption of many nutrients (possibly including calcium itself) depends. Taking Tums or any other antacid regularly will cause the body to excrete many nutrients as wastes, rather than absorb them.

Medications given by vein provide water and frequently provide sodium, potassium, and other electrolytes, or dextrose (a form of sugar). Assessors must consider these contributions when clients' diets must be modified in any of these nutrients. Administering drugs through a feeding tube requires additional precautions (see Chapter 22).

A Note to Assessors The number of drug-nutrient interactions that have been identified is mind-boggling, and it continues to grow. It would be difficult, if not impossible, to memorize all the potential effects of drug-nutrient interactions on nutrition status. Instead, assessors serve their clients best if they:

- Keep in mind that drug-nutrient interactions can and do occur.
- Record the complete drug and diet histories of clients.
- Develop awareness of groups of people who are likely to develop drug-related nutrient deficiencies and be prepared to look up the nutrition effects of drugs these clients are taking.
- Reassess nutrition status frequently for high-risk clients.
- Become familiar with the nutrient interactions of the drugs commonly used to treat the disorders of their clients.

For example, nurses working with people who have heart disease should become familiar with the nutrition effects of drugs used to treat that condition. Better yet, they might keep a reference handy, such as Table E–1B in Appendix E, and check it frequently whenever drugs are prescribed.

Socioeconomic History

Socioeconomic factors profoundly affect nutrition status (see Table 12–6 and Form 12–1). Age affects both nutrient requirements and food choices (see Chapters 15–17). Infants and children depend on caretakers to provide nutritious and acceptable foods; so do adults who are unable to care for themselves. Assessors must therefore evaluate caretakers sometimes, as well as clients.

A person's occupation provides clues to the person's education and income. It can also reveal certain eating habits and physical activity levels. One job, for example, may entail desk work and eating out; another may require vigorous physical activity and permit only a short lunch break.

A client's ethnic identity, religious affiliation, and education may dictate certain food choices. These factors also suggest how the interviewer should word questions and interpret answers. The community environment may also influence nutrition status. The interviewer should be familiar with the foods typically eaten by the neighborhood's major ethnic and religious groups, the regional food preferences, local crops, and the nutrition resources and programs available in the community. Health departments and social agencies often can provide such information.

People's incomes also affect their diet. In general, diet quality declines as income falls, and an inadequate income puts an adequate diet out of reach. Agencies use poverty indexes to identify people at risk for poor nutrition and to qualify people for government food assistant programs. Nutrition in Practice 13 addresses additional issues regarding poverty and hunger.

A low income affects not only the power to purchase foods but also the ability to shop for, store, and cook them. A skilled assessor will note whether a person has transportation to a grocery store that sells a sufficient variety of low-cost foods and whether the person has access to a refrigerator and stove.

Table 12–6
Socioeconomic Factors That Can Affect Nutrition Status

Access to grocery stores
Activities
Age
Education
Ethnic identity
Income
Kitchen facilities
Number of people in household
Occupation
Religious affiliation

socioeconomic history: a record of a person's social and economic background, including such factors as education, income, and ethnic identity.

Diet History

A diet history provides a record of eating habits and food intake and can help identify possible nutrient imbalances (see Table 12–7 on the next page). Information about the person's eating habits provides the basis for developing realistic and attainable nutrition goals.

Constructing an accurate diet history requires skill. Eating habits are an important part of lifestyle and often reflect a person's philosophy. The assessor who asks nonjudgmental, open-ended questions about eating habits and food intake encourages trust and enhances the likelihood of obtaining accurate information.

Form 12–1 (on pp. 305–306) shows questions about eating habits and lifestyle that can clue assessors to possible nutrient imbalances and factors that affect food intake. In addition to determining food habits, assessors evaluate food intake using various tools such as the 24-hour recall, the usual intake record, the food frequency checklist, the food record, and direct observation of food intake. Food models or photos and measuring

diet history: a record of eating behaviors and the foods a person eats.

Judgmental versus nonjudgmental responses:

- *Helper:* Do you take any type of vitamin or mineral supplements?
- *Client:* I take a vitamin E capsule and 2 grams of vitamin C every day.
- *Judgmental helper response:* You know, of course, that there is no reason for taking these vitamin supplements?
- *Nonjudgmental helper response:* For what reasons do you take these vitamin supplements?

Closed- versus open-ended questions:

- *Closed-ended:* You feel fine about your new diet, don't you?
- *Open-ended:* How do you feel about your new diet?
- *Closed-ended:* Do you drink orange or tomato juice with breakfast?
- *Open-ended:* Do you drink anything with breakfast?

Table 12–7
Dietary Factors That Can Affect Nutrition Status

Deficient or excessive food intake
Frequently eating out
Intravenous fluids (other than total parenteral nutrition) for 7 or more days
No intake for 7 or more days
Omission from diet of any food group (for example, vegetables)
Poor appetite
Restrictive or fad diets
Monotonous diet (lack of variety)

24-hour recall: a record of foods eaten by a person for one 24-hour period.

devices can help clients identify the types of foods and quantities consumed. The assessor also needs to know how the foods are prepared and when they are eaten. In addition to asking about foods, assessors ask about beverage consumption, including beverages containing alcohol or caffeine.

24-Hour Recall The 24-hour recall provides data for one day only and is commonly used in nutrition surveys to obtain estimates of the typical food intakes for a population. The assessor asks the client to recount everything eaten or drunk in the past 24 hours or for the previous day. Form 12–2 shows a typical 24-hour recall form.

An advantage of the 24-hour recall is that it is easy to obtain. It is also more likely to provide accurate data, at least about the past 24 hours, than a person's estimates of average intakes over long periods. It does not, however, provide enough information to allow accurate generalizations about an individual's usual food intake. Only when 24-hour recalls are collected on several nonconsecutive days, including both weekdays and weekend days, is this limitation overcome.

Form 12–2
Food Intake Form for a 24-Hour Recall or Usual Intake Pattern

Name and address ______________________________ Date __________

____

____

Did [or Do] you take a vitamin-mineral supplement? ______________________________

If yes, what kind? ______________________________ Dose __________

Please record the amount and type of foods and beverages consumed today. [Or: Please record the amounts and types of foods and beverages you typically consume each day.]

Time of Day	Food	Amount (c, tbs, or piece)	Description (how cooked, how served)

Usual Intake To obtain data about a person's usual intake, an inquiry might begin with "What is the first thing you usually eat or drink during the day?" Similar questions follow until a typical daily intake pattern emerges. This method uses the same form as the 24-hour recall (Form 12–2), and can be useful, especially in verifying food intake when the past 24 hours have been atypical. It also helps the assessor verify food habits. For example, one person may always eat an afternoon snack; another may never eat breakfast. A person whose intake varies widely from day to day, however, may find it difficult to answer such general questions, and in such a case, another food intake tool should be used.

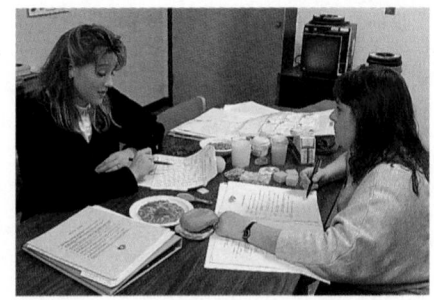

Clients provide food intake data most accurately when guided by a dietitian who is equipped with plastic models of foods to illustrate portion sizes.

Food Frequency Checklist Another approach is to use a food frequency checklist. The purpose of this record is to ascertain how often an individual eats a specific type of food per day, week, or month, using a long list of foods or types of foods. This information helps pinpoint food groups, and therefore nutrients, that may be excessive or deficient in the diet. That a person ate no vegetables yesterday may not seem particularly significant, but never eating vegetables is a warning sign of possible nutrient deficiencies. When used with the usual intake or 24-hour recall approach, the food frequency record enables the assessor to double-check the accuracy of the information obtained. Form 12–3 (on pp. 312–313) is a food frequency checklist.

food frequency checklist: a checklist of foods on which a person can record the frequency with which he or she eats each food.

Food Records A food record maintained over several days or more can be a valuable tool for gathering food intake data. The assessor instructs the person keeping the record to write down the times foods are eaten, all foods and beverages consumed, the amounts consumed, and methods of preparation. Often the person must record other information as well, depending on the purpose of the food record. When the purpose of the record is to help a person change eating behaviors and lose weight, the record might also include information about the person's mood, the occasion (party, holiday, family meal), behaviors associated with eating food (ate while watching TV, ate in the car on the way to work, ate at the table while reading), and physical activity. Figure 9–2 in Chapter 9 provided an example of this type of record. When the purpose of the food record is to establish blood glucose control (see Chapter 25), records include details of drug administration, physical activity, and the results of blood glucose monitoring. When the purpose of the record is to establish food tolerances (such as the amount of lactose a person can handle), food records also include symptoms associated with eating (for example, cramps, diarrhea, nausea, or hives).

food record: an extensive, accurate log of all food eaten over a period of several days or weeks. A food record that includes associated information such as when, where, and with whom each food is eaten is sometimes called a **food diary**.

Food records help the assessor and the record keeper to analyze food behaviors with negative consequences and find solutions. The record keeper plays an active role and learns to take responsibility for personal food choices and eating habits.

Observing Food Intake Direct observation of clients' food intakes is possible in health care facilities such as hospitals or nursing homes. Dietitians, dietary technicians, and nurses frequently work together to

Form 12–3
Food Frequency Checklist

	NUMBER OF SERVINGS	FREQUENCY (PER DAY, WEEK, OR MONTH)
1. How often do you eat the following foods?[a]		
Bread, toast, rolls, muffins	______	______
Cereal (which kind?) ____________	______	______
Rice or other cooked grains	______	______
Noodles (macaroni, spaghetti)	______	______
Pancakes or waffles	______	______
Crackers or pretzels	______	______
Fruits or fruit juices	______	______
Vegetables other than potatoes	______	______
Vegetable juice	______	______
Potatoes	______	______
Dried beans and peas	______	______
Beef	______	______
Pork or ham	______	______
Veal	______	______
Poultry	______	______
Fish	______	______
Organ meats (such as liver)	______	______
Bacon	______	______
Sausage	______	______
Lunch meat	______	______
Hot dogs	______	______
Other meats (which?) ____________	______	______
Eggs	______	______
Peanut butter or nuts	______	______
Milk (including on cereal)	______	______
Cheese or cheese dishes	______	______
Yogurt or tofu	______	______
Other milk products (type?)____________	______	______
Butter	______	______
Margarine (type?) ____________	______	______
Salt pork	______	______
Mayonnaise or salad dressing (type?)______	______	
Oil (type?) __________	______	______
Cream	______	______
Sugar, jam, jelly, syrup, honey	______	______
Sweet rolls or doughnuts	______	______
Bakery goods (cake, cookies)	______	______

[a]The assessor helps the client estimate portion sizes and frequency of use.

Form 12–3 *(continued)*

Candy . . . . ______ ______
Soft drinks (types?) __________ . . . . ______ ______
Potato or snack chips (type?)__________ . . . . ______ ______
Coffee or tea (type?) __________. . . . . ______ ______
Wine . . . . ______ ______
Beer . . . . ______ ______
Whiskey, vodka, rum, etc. ______ ______
Fast foods eaten out . . . . ______ ______
TV dinners, pot pies, other prepared meals . . . . . ______ ______
Instant meals such as breakfast bars or diet meal beverages (which)__________ . . . . ______ ______

2. What specific kinds of the following foods do you eat? Include the name of the food; whether it is fresh, canned, or frozen; and how it is prepared.
   Fruits and fruit juices ______________________________
   Vegetables ______________________________
   Milk and milk products ______________________________
   Meats and meat alternates ______________________________
   Breads and cereals ______________________________
   Desserts ______________________________
   Snack foods ______________________________
3. Please list the names of any liquid, powder, or pill forms of vitamin or mineral products you take, and state how often you take them. Please also list any diet supplement you use (such as protein milkshakes or brewer's yeast), how much you use, and how often you use it. ______________________________
   ____
4. Is there anything else we should know about your food/nutrient intake?
   ____

keep records of the kinds and quantities of foods a client receives and leaves on the plate. From these records, the dietitian deduces what has been eaten and estimates nutrient intakes as described in the next section. Often, direct observations are used to generate estimates of a client's energy and protein intake, and the procedure is simply called a *kcalorie count.*

Analysis of Food Intake Data After collecting food intake data, the assessor estimates nutrient intakes, either informally by using food guides or formally by using food composition tables. Food intakes are then compared to standards, either nutrient recommendations or food guides, to determine how well a diet measures up. Are the types and amounts of proteins, carbohydrates (including fiber), and fats (including cholesterol) appropriate? Are all food groups included in appropriate amounts? Is caffeine or alcohol consumption excessive? Are intakes of any vitamins or minerals (such as sodium and iron) excessive or deficient?

Formal calculations can be performed either manually (by looking up each food in a table of food composition, recording its nutrients, and adding them up) or by using a computer diet analysis program. The assessor then compares the intakes with standards such as the RDA.

Limitations of Food Intake Analysis Food intake data can be informative, but the skillful assessor also keeps their limitations in mind. A computer diet analysis tends to imply greater accuracy than is possible to obtain from data as uncertain as the starting information. Nutrient contents of foods listed in tables of food composition or stored in computer databases are averages, and for some nutrients, incomplete. In addition, the available data on nutrient contents of foods do not reflect the amounts of nutrients a person actually absorbs. Iron is a case in point: its availability from a given meal may vary from as high as 50 percent to below 2 percent. (Chapter 8 explains how to calculate iron absorption from a meal.)

Help clients estimate food sizes by using food models and measuring utensils. When these items are not available, provide comparisons. For example, a small chicken leg is about 2 ounces; a slice of luncheon meat is about 1 ounce.

Reported portion sizes may also not be correct. The person who reports eating "a serving" of greens may not distinguish between ¼ cup and 2 whole cups. Children tend to remember the serving sizes of foods they like as being larger than serving sizes of foods they dislike.

Interpretation of Food Intake Data The assessor must remember that adequate nutrient *intakes* do not guarantee adequate nutrient *status* for an individual. Likewise, insufficient intakes do not always indicate deficiencies, but instead alert the assessor to possible problems. Each person digests, absorbs, metabolizes, and excretes nutrients in a unique way; individual needs vary. Intakes of nutrients identified by diet histories are only pieces of a puzzle that must be put together with other indicators of nutrition status in order to extract meaning.

Histories alert health care professionals to potential nutrition problems. To substantiate findings, other assessment tools including physical examinations (described next) and anthropometric and biochemical measurements (described in the next chapter) are useful.

Physical Examinations

An assessor can use a physical examination to search for signs of nutrient deficiency or toxicity. Like the other assessment methods, such an examination requires knowledge and skill. Many physical signs are nonspecific; they can reflect any of several nutrient deficiencies, as well as conditions not related to nutrition (see Table 12–8). For example, cracked lips may be caused by sunburn, windburn, dehydration, or any of several B vitamin deficiencies, to name just a few possible causes. For this reason, physical findings are especially unreliable for diagnosis of nutrition problems. Instead, like the data from histories, they are puzzle pieces. Their value often lies in suggesting problems that indicate a need for investigation using other assessment techniques.

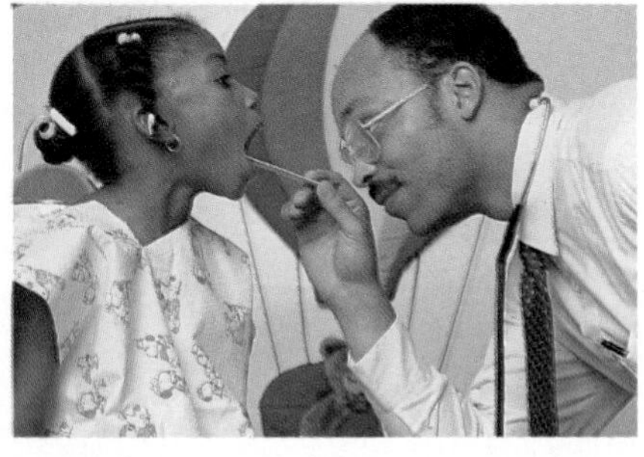

A physical examination provides valuable clues about a person's nutrition status.

Many tissues and organs can reflect signs of malnutrition. The signs appear most rapidly in parts of the body where cell replacement occurs at a high rate, such as the hair, skin, and digestive tract (including the mouth and tongue). The summary tables in Chapters 7 and 8 list additional physical signs of vitamin and mineral malnutrition.

Table 12–8
Physical Findings Used in Nutrition Assessments

BODY SYSTEM	ACCEPTABLE FINDINGS	MALNUTRITION FINDINGS	WHAT THE FINDINGS REFLECT
Hair	Shiny, firm in the scalp	Dull, brittle, dry, loose; falls out	PEM
Eyes	Bright, clear pink membranes; adjust easily to light	Pale membranes; spots; redness; adjust slowly to darkness	Vitamin A, the B vitamins, zinc and iron status
Teeth and gums	No pain or caries, gums firm, teeth bright	Missing, discolored, decayed teeth; gums bleed easily and are swollen and spongy	Mineral and vitamin C status
Face	Clear complexion without dryness or scaliness	Off-color, scaly, flaky, cracked skin	PEM, vitamin A, and iron status
Glands	No lumps	Swollen at front of neck, cheeks	PEM and iodine status
Tongue	Red, bumpy, rough	Sore, smooth, purplish, swollen	B vitamin status
Skin	Smooth, firm, good color	Dry, rough, spotty; "sandpaper" feel or sores; lack of fat under skin	PEM, essential fatty acid deficiency, vitamin A, the B vitamins, and vitamin C status
Nails	Firm, pink	Spoon-shaped, brittle, ridged	Iron status
Internal systems	Regular heart rhythm, heart rate, and blood pressure; no impairment of digestive function, reflexes, or mental status	Abnormal heart rate, heart rhythm, or blood pressure; enlarged liver, spleen; abnormal digestion; burning, tingling of hands, feet; loss of balance, coordination; mental confusion, irritability, fatigue	PEM and mineral status
Muscles and bones	Muscle tone; posture, long bone development appropriate for age	"Wasted" appearance of muscles; swollen bumps on skull or ends of bones; small bumps on ribs; bowed legs or knock-knees	PEM and vitamin D status

Histories and physical examinations provide a general picture of a person's nutrition status. The next chapter describes anthropometric and biochemical measurements that further define nutrition status.

■ STUDY QUESTIONS ■

1. Identify the four components of nutrition assessment.
2. How can a client's health history affect nutrition status?
3. What factors in a client's drug history suggest a likelihood of drug-nutrient interactions? Describe the mechanisms by which drugs and nutrients can interact.
4. List two important uses for diet histories.
5. Describe ways of gathering food intake data and suggest uses for each method.
6. For two methods of analyzing food intake data, itemize the major limitations.

■ CLINICAL APPLICATION ■ QUESTIONS

1. Describe the possible nutrition implications of these findings from a client's history and physical examination: age 73, lives alone, recently lost spouse, uses a walker, has no teeth, pale skin, lack of energy, history of hypertension and diabetes, several prescribed medications.
2. Nurses and nurses' aides often shoulder much of the responsibility for collecting food intake data for kcalorie counts because they often deliver food trays and snacks and later retrieve them. Why would it be important for a nurse or aide to verify and record what the client receives (both the foods and the amounts) and to look at the foods that remain uneaten? When might clients be enlisted to aid in the collection of food intake data and when might such a course be unwise?
3. A busy nurse is working with three people who are taking drugs that may be affecting their nutrition status. The drugs are: Probucol, Cyclophosphamide, and Prednisone. How much time might it take the nurse to check the nutrition side effects of each drug and record them in each person's chart? (Look up each drug in Appendix E, Table E–1A to find its class. Then turn to that class of drugs in Table E–1B and discover the drug's side effects. Jot down a note on each drug and record the time this took.)

NUTRITION IN PRACTICE 12

Nutrition and Emotional Health

Emotional health and nutritional health go together. Emotionally healthy people feed themselves well. Well-nourished people bear none of the burdens of malnutrition that might impair their emotional health.

By the same token, when either type of health is impaired, both are affected. People with emotional illness often have poor diets; and people who are malnourished are often emotionally handicapped. It is important to understand these connections, for they affect everyone from the man or woman on the street to the hospitalized person with a severe psychiatric illness. The health professional who recognizes the nutrition implications of emotional disorders can sometimes offer effective help.

I'm interested to hear more about the man or woman on the street. Are you saying that all people's emotional states affect their nutritional health?

Certainly they do. Consider what ordinary anxiety does to your own eating habits. You may be unable to eat at all, you may eat the wrong things, or you may vastly overeat, depending on your personality type. If your anxiety becomes prolonged or chronic, the resulting changes in your eating habits can make you underweight, or cause nutrient deficiencies, imbalances, or obesity.

The same is true of ordinary depression. People who are depressed often eat poorly—as with anxiety, they may eat too little, too much, the wrong things, or not at all. Thus prolonged depression, too, can affect nutrition status.

What nutrition advice do you give to people whose anxiety or depression is making them unable to eat?

Help them to understand how their bodies may be reacting to stress and how this may affect their health. A later chapter describes the physical effects of severe stresses, but even in mild emotional stress, nutrition status may decline.

The person who is well nourished to begin with can best withstand such times, but nutrition is only one part of the problem. Seeking counseling or therapy can help resolve underlying conflicts and can improve stress management skills. Learning to relax can bolster the appetite and ease digestion. Exercise can reduce stress and improve appetite. Attending to vitamin and mineral needs can help maintain stores that may become depleted during stressful times. Drinking enough fluid helps the body function optimally. When the stressful time is over, eating appropriately restores nutrient balances. Meanwhile, learning attitudes to prevent the next stressful event from being so overwhelming can help.

A lot of people, especially elderly people, seem to be lonely and eat very little. How would you advise them?

You have identified one of the most profound connections between nutrition and emotional health: loneliness. For human beings, eating is as much a social and psychological event as a biological one. Without companionship, appetite falters.

Many authorities believe that malnutrition among the elderly is most often due to loneliness. Some six million adults over age 65 live alone. Their most pressing need seems to be for companionship; food takes second place. Social interaction is important to emotional health, and elderly people of all classes in our society, both the financially secure and the poverty-stricken, tend to become isolated.

Jack Weinberg, professor of psychiatry at the University of Illinois, wrote perceptively of this problem:

> In our efforts to provide the aged with a proper diet, we often fail to perceive it is not

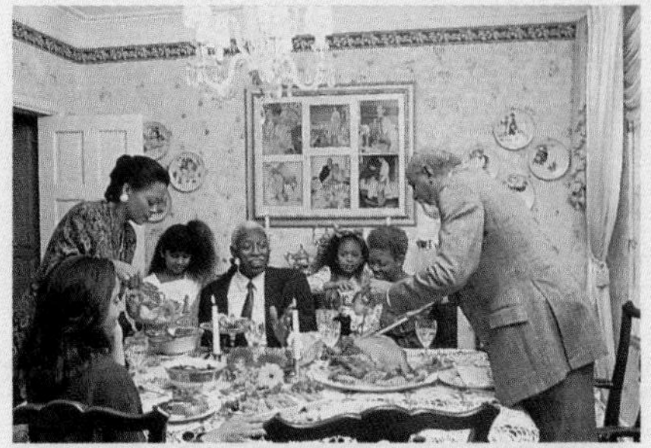

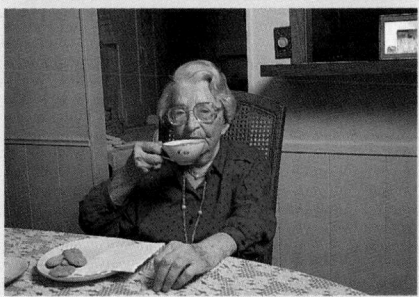

It is not just what people eat, but with whom, that makes the difference to emotional and physical health.

what the older person eats but with whom that will be the deciding factor in proper care for him. The oft-repeated complaint of the older patient that he has little incentive to prepare food for only himself is not merely a statement of fact but also a rebuke to the questioner for failing to perceive his isolation and aloneness and to realize that food . . . for one's self lacks the condiment of another's presence which can transform the simplest fare to the ceremonial act with all its shared meaning.[3]

A sad spiral can set in when a lonely person begins to neglect to eat well. Malnutrition worsens the apathy felt due to loneliness. Then the person has even less energy with which to secure nourishment. Watch for this spiral in all people, and especially in elderly people who live alone and in those who have recently lost a spouse or other loved one and are grieving.

When an old person seems senile, is it possible that malnutrition is responsible?

Sometimes yes, sometimes no. Sometimes the confusion caused by a vitamin or mineral deficiency is incorrectly diagnosed as senility.[4] An elderly person may even be wrongly confined to a nursing home. The story is told of a women who exhibited the classic signs of senility—mental confusion, inability to make decisions, and forgetting to perform important tasks, such as turning off a stove burner. The woman's family decided to move her into a nursing home. While she was waiting for a place there, her family took her into their own home. After several weeks of eating good meals and enjoying social stimulation, the woman became her old self again and was able to return to her home. This story has been repeated with many variations and serves to remind us to think about loneliness and nutrition before concluding that a person is senile and needs institutional care. What harm could there be in first trying good, balanced meals served with tender, loving care?

Suppose a person is truly mentally ill. Then what nutrition considerations apply?

Nutrition in psychiatric care is a specialty all its own because there are so many connections. Mental illnesses characterized by depression, illogical thinking, dementia, paranoia, delusions, and inappropriate eating habits can alter food intake and thus interfere with nutrition status. Such disorders include schizophrenia, Alzheimer's disease, mood disorders, substance abuse, and eating disorders. The accompanying glossary defines terms related to mental illness.

Individuals suffering from depression, illogical thinking, or dementia may have little interest in food. Those who are paranoid may believe that foods are being used to poison them. People suffering from delusions may attribute magical powers to certain foods and insist on eating only those foods. Drugs used in the treatment of mental illness can also interact with nutrients in significant ways.

Abnormal nutrient intakes can also affect mental health. For example, some psychiatric conditions are caused by nutrient deficiencies and can be corrected by repleting the nutrients. Although rare, classical nutrient-deficiency diseases such as pellagra, beriberi, and others include "mental" symptoms ranging from insomnia and fatigue to schizophrenia-like behavior.

What are the mental effects of malnutrition on children?

Protein-energy malnutrition in pregnant women can cause mental retardation in their children. Children malnourished early in life show behavioral and social deficits as well as physical retardation. Also, children who are neglected early in life show a greater tendency to suffer from severe malnutrition than children who receive love

Glossary of Mental Illness Terms

Alzheimer's (ALTZ-high-mers) **disease:** a degenerative disease of the brain involving memory loss and major structural changes in the brain's nerve cells.

delusions: inappropriate beliefs not consistent with the individual's own knowledge and experience.

dementia (dee-MEN-she-ah)**:** irreversible loss of mental function.

mood disorders: mental illnesses characterized by episodes of severe depression or excessive excitement (mania) or both.

paranoia (PARA-NOY-ah)**:** mental illness characterized by delusions of persecution.

schizophrenia (SKITS-oh-FREN-ee-ah)**:** mental illness characterized by an altered concept of reality and, in some cases, delusions and hallucinations.

and attention. Wherever you see abnormal nutrition status in a child, ask yourself if the child requires emotional as well as physical support. And wherever you see emotional illness, look to the child's nutrition, too.

What mental disorders affecting nutrition are especially common?

Alcoholism is one, and it is treated elsewhere in this book (see Nutrition in Practice 8). You almost always see abnormal energy balance and vitamin and mineral deficiencies in cases of severe alcoholism. Anorexia nervosa and bulimia nervosa are other examples (see Nutrition in Practice 9).

Nutrition affects the brain and the mind, and the brain and the mind affect the way people eat. It all goes together, and the wise health care professional will keep the whole picture in mind.

■ NOTES ■

1. R. N. Varma, Risk for drug-induced malnutrition is unchecked in elderly patients in nursing homes, *Journal of the American Dietetic Association* 94 (1994): 192–194.
2. J. E. Henningfield and coauthors, Drinking coffee and carbonated beverages blocks absorption of nicotine from nicotine polacrilex gum, *Journal of the American Medical Association* 264 (1990): 1560–1564.
3. J. Weinberg, Psychological implications of the nutritional needs of the elderly, *Journal of the American Dietetic Association* 60 (1972): 293–296.
4. V. R. Newburn, Is it really Alzheimer's? *American Journal of Nursing* 91 (1991): 51–54.

13

Nutrition Assessment: Anthropometric and Biochemical Data

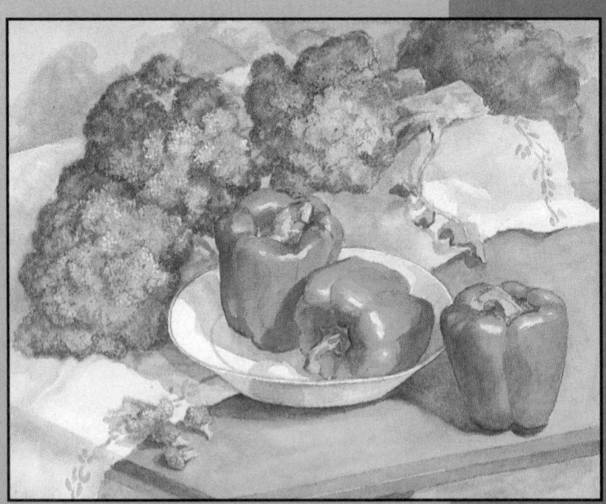

CONTENTS

Chapter 12 introduced nutrition assessments and showed how the assessor can use historical information and physical examinations to look for signs of nutrient imbalances. This chapter shows how measurements of the body, both physical and biochemical, further aid in the assessment process.

Anthropometric Measurements

Anthropometrics are physical measurements that reflect body composition and development (see Table 13–1). They serve three main purposes: first, to evaluate the progress of growth in pregnant women, infants, children, and adolescents; second, to detect undernutrition and overnutrition in all age groups; and third, to measure changes in body composition over time.

anthropometric: relating to measurement of the physical characteristics of the body, such as height and weight.
anthropos = human
metric = measuring

Assessors compare anthropometric measurements taken on an individual with population standards specific for gender and age to see how body composition compares to norms. Assessors may also take measurements periodically and compare them with previous measurements to detect changes in an individual's status.

Height and weight are well-recognized anthropometrics; others include fatfold measurements and various measures of lean tissue. Still other measures are useful in specific situations. A head circumference measurement may help to assess brain development in an infant, and an abdominal girth measurement supplies information about abdominal fluid retention in individuals with liver disease.

Mastering the techniques for taking anthropometric measurements requires proper instruction and practice. Once the correct techniques are learned, however, taking the measurements is easy and generally requires minimal equipment.

Measures of Growth and Development

Height and weight are among the most common and useful anthropometric measurements. Length measurements for infants and children up

Table 13–1
Anthropometric Measurements Used in Nutrition Assessments

TYPE OF MEASUREMENT	WHAT IT REFLECTS
Abdominal girth measurement	Abdominal fluid retention
Height-weight	Overnutrition and undernutrition; growth in children
%IBW, %UBW,[a] recent weight change	Overnutrition and undernutrition
Head circumference	Brain growth and development in infants and children under two
Fatfold	Subcutaneous and total body fat
Midarm muscle circumference	Muscle mass (i.e., protein status)

[a]%IBW = percent ideal body weight; %UBW = percent usual body weight.

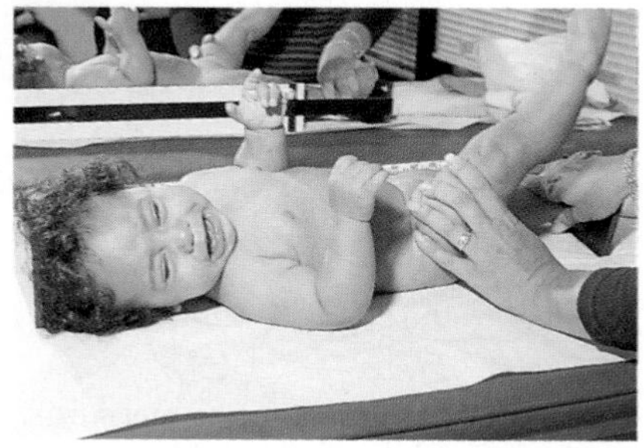

Lying still with legs straight for a length measurement can be a trying experience.

to age three and height measurements for children over three are particularly valuable in assessing growth, which depends on adequate nutrition. Poor growth in children is an important indicator of malnutrition. For adults, height measurements alone do not reflect current nutrition status but are necessary for estimation of desirable weight, for interpretation of other assessment data, and for estimation of energy needs. Once adult height has been reached, changes in body weight may reveal either overnutrition or undernutrition.

Height For infants and children younger than three, health care professionals may use special equipment to measure length. The assessor lays the barefoot infant on a measuring board that has a fixed headboard and movable footboard attached at right angles to the surface. Often two people are needed to obtain an accurate measurement: one to hold the infant's head against the headboard and keep the legs straight, and the other to do the measuring. This method provides the most accurate measure possible, but many health care professionals use a less exacting method. They may simply hold the infant straight with its head against the headboard or other vertical support, mark the blanket with a chalk or pen at the infant's heel, and then measure the distance from the headboard to the mark. Even more informally and less accurately, they may lay the infant on a flat surface and extend a nonstretchable measuring tape along the side of the infant from the top of the head to the heel of the foot.

To measure the height of a child who can stand erect and cooperate, the procedure is the same as for an adult. The best way to measure standing height is with the person's back against a flat wall to which a nonstretchable measuring tape or stick has been fixed. The person stands erect, without shoes, with heels together. The person's line of sight should be horizontal, with the heels, buttocks, shoulders, and head touching the wall. The assessor places a ruler, book, or other stiff object on top of the head at a right angle to the wall; carefully checks the height measurement; and records it immediately in either inches or centimeters. Immediate recording prevents the assessor from forgetting the correct measurement.

The measuring rod of a scale is commonly used to measure height but is less accurate because it bends easily. The assessor follows the same general procedure, asking the person to face away from the scale and to take extra care to stand erect.

Unfortunately, many health care professionals merely ask clients how tall they are rather than measuring their height. Self-reported height is often inaccurate and should be used only as a last resort when measurement is impractical (in the case of an uncooperative client, an emergency admission, or the like).

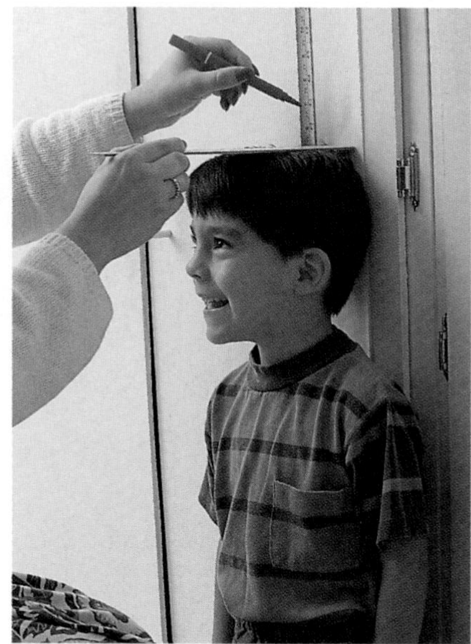

Standing "at attention" allows for an accurate height measurement.

Weight Valid weight measurements require functional scales that have been carefully maintained, calibrated, and checked for accuracy at regular intervals.[1] Beam balance and electronic scales are the most accurate types of scales. To measure an infant's weight, assessors use special scales that allow the infant to lie or sit. Weighing infants naked, without diapers, is standard procedure. Children who can stand are weighed in the same way as adults. Standardized conditions are necessary if repeated measures are to be useful. Each weighing should take place at the same time of day (preferably before breakfast), in the same amount of clothing (without shoes), after the person has voided, and on the same scale.

Special scales are available for weighing people who are bedridden. State-of-the-art hospital beds equipped with built-in scales are also available. Bathroom scales are inaccurate and inappropriate for use in professional settings. As with all measurements, the assessor records observed weight immediately in either pounds or kilograms.

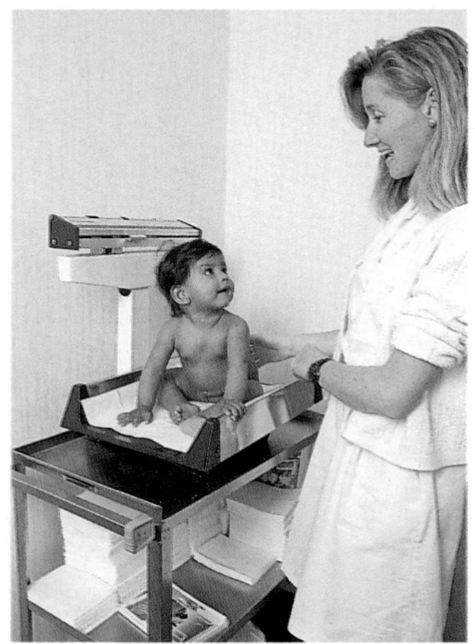

Special scales allow infants to sit and watch while they are being weighed.

Head Circumference Assessors may also measure head circumference in infants and young children to confirm that growth is proceeding normally or to help detect protein-energy malnutrition (PEM) and evaluate the extent of its impact on brain size. Head circumference is measured by encircling the largest part of the infant's or child's head with a nonstretchable tape: the tape goes just above the eyebrow ridges, just above the point where the ears attach, and around the occipital prominence at the back of the head. To ensure accurate recording, the assessor immediately notes the measure in either inches or centimeters.

Analysis of Measures in Infants and Children Health professionals generally evaluate physical development by monitoring the growth of a child over time and plotting the data on standard charts (see Appendix E for more information). Standard charts compare weight to age, height to age, and weight to height; ideally, height and weight are at roughly the same percentile. Although individual growth patterns may vary, a child's growth curve will generally stay at about the same percentile throughout childhood. Measurements below this percentile for height, weight, or head circumference in infants and young children indicate growth retardation, which is an important sign of poor nutrition status. In children whose growth has been retarded, nutrition rehabilitation will ideally induce height and weight to increase to higher percentiles. In overweight children, the goal is for weight to remain stable as height increases, until weight becomes appropriate for height.

Head circumference is a useful indicator of brain growth in children under two years of age. Since the brain grows rapidly before birth and during early infancy, malnourished children may have fewer brain cells and smaller head circumferences than normal. The assessor plots head circumference measurements on a percentile growth chart; head circumference percentile should be similar to the child's weight and height percentiles. Nonnutritional factors, such as certain disorders and genetic variation, can also influence head circumference.[2]

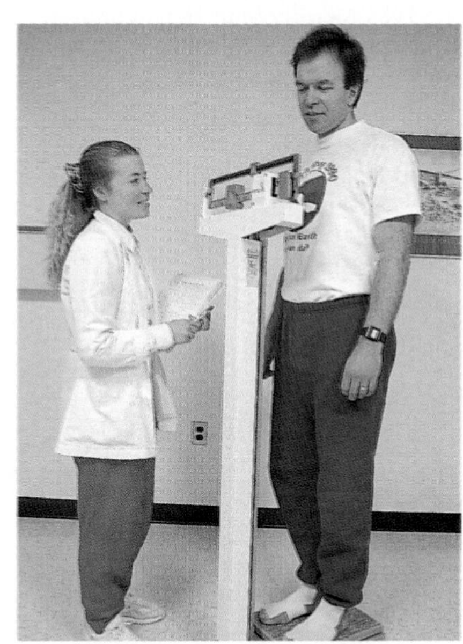

Beam balance scales provide accurate weight measurements for adults.

Analysis of Weight Measures for Adults For adults, health care professionals typically compare weights with weight-for-height standards. Today, however, the standards are changing. To identify the weight most consistent with an individual's health requires good clinical judgment. One standard is the body mass index (BMI), described in Chapter 9 (pp. 216–217), which is useful for estimating the risk to health associated with overnutrition. The weight ranges presented in Chapter 9 (Table 9–1, p. 215) are based on the BMI most consistent with health. This table pre-

Reminder: Height and weight tables suggest a weight range rather than pinpointing one ideal weight—a helpful reminder that there is no single perfect weight for anyone.

Table 13–2
Quick Estimation of Ideal Body Weight

MEN
For 5 feet, consider 106 pounds a reasonable weight.
For each inch over 5 feet, add 6 pounds.
Subtract six pounds for each inch under 5 feet.
Add 10% for a large-framed individual; subtract 10% for a small-framed individual.
Example: A man 5 feet 8 inches tall (medium frame) would start at 106 pounds, add 48, and arrive at a reasonable weight of 154 pounds.
WOMEN
For 5 feet, consider 100 pounds a reasonable weight.
For each inch over 5 feet, add 5 pounds.
Subtract 5 pounds for each inch under 5 feet.
Add 10% for a large-framed individual; subtract 10% for a small-framed individual.
Example: A woman 5 feet 6 inches tall (medium frame) would start at 100 pounds, add 30, and arrive at a reasonable weight of 130 pounds.

The 1983 Metropolitan Height and Weight tables appear in Appendix E.

Reminder: The *body mass index (BMI)* is an index of a person's weight in relation to height, determined by dividing the weight in kilograms by the square of the height in meters:

$$BMI = \frac{\text{weight (kg)}}{\text{height}^2\ (m^2)}$$

sents wide ranges of weights appropriate for heights without regard to gender and allows higher weights for older people. Other weight-for-height tables, used earlier, are specific for gender and frame size and make no allowance for age. The classic example of these, the Metropolitan height-weight table, is shown in Appendix E (Table E–2), together with two methods of estimating frame size.

In the health care setting, the professional may bypass these tables and simply use a rule of thumb to calculate ideal weight based on height and gender (see Table 13–2). While easy to use, this rule is of limited usefulness. The weights it deems ideal are low compared to the BMI standard, especially for taller and older people. Still, it offers a rough estimate of weights near the low end of the range consistent with health.

The standard chosen can be used to generate a figure known as the percent ideal body weight (%IBW), calculated and evaluated as shown in the next box. However, a more valuable parameter for assessing weight changes in the person who has weighed considerably more or less than

Table 13–3
Weight as an Indicator of Nutrition Status

%IBW	%UBW	NUTRITION STATUS
>120	—	Obese
110–120	—	Overweight
90–109	—	Adequate
80–89	85–95	Mildly undernourished
70–79	75–84	Moderately undernourished
<70	<75	Severely undernourished

the average throughout life is the percent usual body weight (%UBW), which considers what is normal for a particular individual. The client, family, friends, and older medical records can provide the usual body weight. The %UBW, used in conjunction with Table 13–3, is a useful indicator of the risk of malnutrition, especially for a person whose usual weight is higher than the average.

Besides %IBW and %UBW, the assessor looks closely at the rate of any recent weight change. A 5 percent weight loss within a month might be significant, yet the same loss over five months might not be. The accompanying box shows how all three of these parameters are used.

HOW TO Estimate %IBW and %UBW

To estimate %IBW, compare the individual's current weight with the ideal body weight from standard height-for-weight tables; to estimate %UBW, compare the current weight with the individual's typical weight. For example, to calculate %IBW and %UBW in a 45-year-old man of medium frame who is 5 feet 8 inches tall, weighs 115 pounds, and has lost 15 pounds in the last month, follow these steps:

1. $\%IBW = \frac{\text{actual weight}}{\text{ideal weight}} \times 100.$

For ideal weight, the assessor chooses to use the midpoint of the weight range in Table E–2 in Appendix E, in this case 151 pounds.

2. $\%IBW = \frac{115 \text{ lb}}{151 \text{ lb}} \times 100 = 76\%.$

The man in this example is at 76 percent of his ideal body weight. Look to Table 13–3 to find that 76% IBW indicates that the person is moderately undernourished.

To calculate %UBW for this man, follow these steps:

1. $\%UBW = \frac{\text{actual weight}}{\text{usual weight}} \times 100.$

Calculate the usual weight (130 pounds) by adding the weight loss (15 pounds) to the current body weight (115 pounds).

2. $\%UBW = \frac{115 \text{ lb}}{130 \text{ lb}} \times 100 = 89\%.$

The man is at 89 percent of his usual body weight. A look at Table 13–3 reveals that a person at 89% UBW is mildly undernourished.

The recent weight change is highly significant. The man has lost weight at a rate of almost 4 pounds per week for four weeks. From all three standpoints, attention to this man's nutrition needs will be important to his recovery.

Weight measurements in hospitalized clients are sometimes difficult to evaluate. Diseases or therapies can cause fluid retention and mask significant weight loss. In fact, starvation itself is accompanied by an expanded extracellular fluid volume.

Weight Gain during Pregnancy One of the most important anthropometric measures predictive of an infant's birthweight is the mother's amount and pattern of weight gain during pregnancy. Chapter 15 describes normal weight gains related to pregnancy, and Appendix E provides an example of a chart used to monitor weight gain during pregnancy. Patterns of weight gain that deviate from these require further investigation.

Measures of Body Fat and Lean Tissue

Significant weight changes in both children and adults can reflect overnutrition and undernutrition with respect to energy and protein. To estimate the degree to which various body compartments (fat stores or lean tissues) are affected by overnutrition or undernutrition, several anthropometric measurements are useful (as listed earlier in Table 13–1).

Fatfold Measures Approximately half the fat in the body is located directly beneath the skin, and its thickness reflects total body fat. In some parts of the body, this fat is loosely attached; a person can pull it up between the thumb and forefinger and obtain a measure of fatfold thickness. Although fatfold measures can be taken from a variety of body sites, these sites are not always practical in clinical settings, so most often, the triceps fatfold measurement is used. The fatfold test is a valuable and practical diagnostic procedure when performed with skilled hands and with proper equipment. The proper techniques for measuring triceps fatfold, as well as standards for comparison, are given in Appendix E.

Midarm Circumferences To determine whether a person has depleted lean body mass, an indirect measure of muscle size is useful: the midarm *muscle* circumference. This measure is estimated by subtracting the area of fat on the arm from the total area (derived from its circumference). Appendix E shows how this is done and presents standards for comparison.

Reminder: Fat around the abdomen is associated with a greater risk of chronic disorders such as diabetes and cardiovascular diseases than fat found elsewhere on the body.

Waist-to-Hip Ratio Chapter 9 described how fat distribution correlates with health risks and mentioned that the waist-to-hip ratio is a valuable indicator of fat distribution. To calculate the waist-to-hip ratio, divide the number of inches (or centimeters) around the waistline by the number of inches (or centimeters) around the hips. For example, a person with a 28-inch waist and 38-inch hips would have a ratio of 28/38 or 0.74. Women with a ratio of 0.8 or greater and men with a ratio of 0.95 or greater are considered likely to develop obesity-related health problems.

Analysis of Measures The accuracy and value of anthropometric measurements are limited by several factors: the skills of the measurer, the accuracy of the equipment used for measurement, and the interpretation of the measurements. Changes in body composition, such as fluid retention or dehydration, affect anthropometric measures. Furthermore, exercise influences muscle size independently of nutrition factors, and lack of exercise may alter muscle mass.[3] Fatfold and circumference measurements can be difficult to determine for people who are obese or for elderly individuals with loose skin hanging on the upper arm. Furthermore, significant changes in measurements occur slowly in adults. When changes do occur, they represent prolonged alterations in nutrient intake. Therefore, anthropometrics cannot be used to describe small changes in body composition that occur over short periods of time.

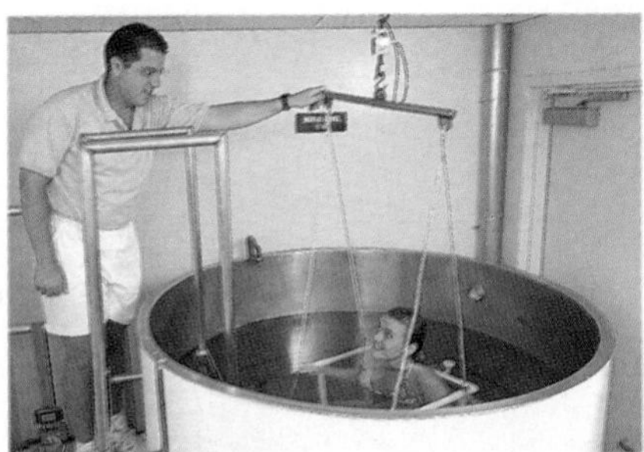

Researchers may use underwater weighing to estimate percent body fat.

Hydrodensitometry (underwater weighing) and bioelectrical impedance techniques are two additional methods for assessing body composition. Both of these techniques are useful in research and are popular among athletes. They are used most frequently in research centers, health clubs, weight training centers, and exercise physiology clinics.

hydrodensitometry: measurement of body density by submerging the person underwater.

bioelectrical impedance: a method for estimating body fat using low-intensity electrical current.

Hydrodensitometry Underwater weighing, or hydrodensitometry, measures body density—an indirect measure of body compostition. Body fat is estimated from body weight and the volume of water that the body displaces when submerged in water. Underwater weighing generates a good estimate of body fat and is useful in research, but requires bulky, expensive, nonportable equipment. Furthermore, submerging some people (especially those who are ill or fearful) under water is not always practical.

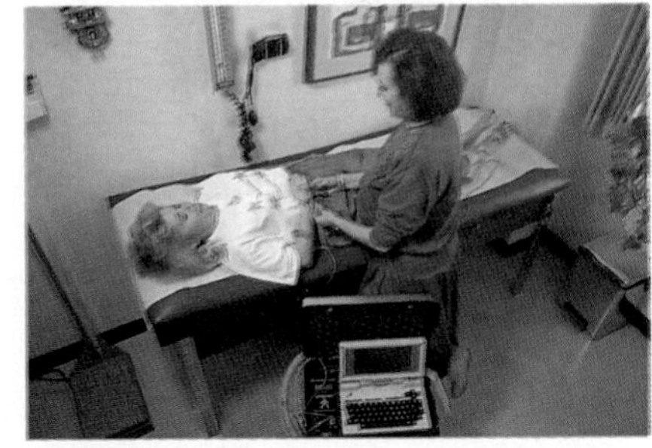

Bioelectrical impedance provides a simple and painless way to estimate body fat.

Bioelectrical Impedance Using bioelectrical impedance techniques to determine body composition is less expensive than underwater weighing, the equipment is portable, and the procedure is painless. To measure body fat using the bioelectrical impedance technique, an electrical current of very low intensity is briefly sent through the body by way of electrodes placed on the wrist and ankle. The leaner the person, the less resistance to the electrical current.

Hand Grip Strength The measurement of hand grip strength is a practical and inexpensive method of assessing nutrition status by measuring muscle function. The assessor asks the person to grip an instrument (called a dynamometer) as tightly as possible. Low grip strength (weak muscle function) suggests poor nutrition status, which must be confirmed by other tests. People with severe arthritis or muscular disorders may have low grip strengths unrelated to nutrition status.

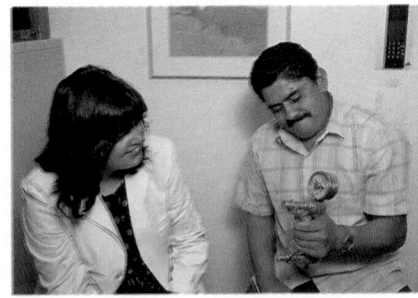

An instrument called a dynamometer measures hand grip strength.

Biochemical Analysis

All of the approaches to nutrition assessment discussed so far are external approaches. Biochemical analyses or laboratory tests help to determine what is happening to the body internally. Most tests are based on analysis of blood and urine samples, which contain nutrients, enzymes,

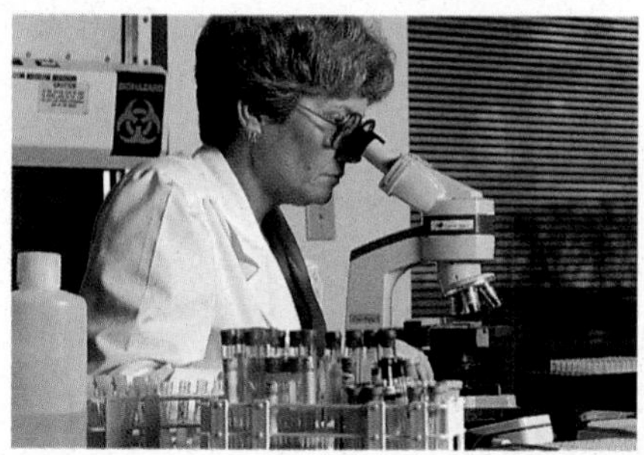

Blood and urine samples offer valuable clues for assessing nutrition status.

The taking of several measurements during a single blood test is referred to as **SMA (simultaneous multiple analysis).** SMA is followed by a number (for example, SMA–12) that indicates how many tests will be run.

The **serum** is the watery portion of the blood that remains after removal of the cells and clot-forming material; **plasma** is the fluid that remains when unclotted blood is centrifuged. In most cases, serum and plasma concentrations are similar. Lab technicians usually prefer serum samples because plasma samples occasionally clog mechanical blood analyzers.

and metabolites that reflect protein, vitamin, and mineral status. Other tests, such as serum glucose, help pinpoint disease-related problems with nutrition implications. Tests that define fluid and electrolyte balance, acid-base balance, and organ function also have nutrition implications. Table 13–4 identifies some lab tests commonly encountered in health care settings and shows what these tests reflect. Some tests are important in specific situations and will be discussed in the appropriate chapters.

The interpretation of biochemical data requires skill. The person's state of hydration greatly influences laboratory values. With dehydration, lab results may be deceptively high; with overhydration, lab results may be deceptively low. No single test by itself is sufficient to diagnose the cause of poor nutrition status because many factors influence test results. The low blood concentration of a nutrient may reflect a primary deficiency of that nutrient, but it may also be secondary to a deficiency of one or several other nutrients or to a nonnutrition-related factor. Nutrient concentrations present in the blood and urine sometimes reflect recent intakes rather than long-term intakes. Thus blood concentrations of a nutrient may be normal, even when tissue levels are deficient. Assessors who keep these limitations in mind and use lab tests along with other assessment data, however, can create a total picture that becomes clear with careful interpretation.

It is beyond the scope of this text to describe all lab tests used to assess nutrition status. Instead, the emphasis is on common lab tests used to detect protein-energy malnutrition and nutrition-related anemias.

Protein-Energy Malnutrition (PEM)

Protein-energy malnutrition (PEM) is pervasive in illness and can dramatically worsen outcome. Recall from Chapter 4 that body proteins conduct all metabolic activities including the management of fluid balances, digestion of nutrients, physical work, synthesis of hormones, maintenance of immune defenses, and much more. Many of the upcoming chapters repeatedly make note of the prevalence of PEM in illness, so this special section focuses on its assessment and classification.

Assessment of Protein-Energy Malnutrition

Tests available to determine protein status include serum albumin, serum transferrin, other serum proteins, the total lymphocyte count, and other tests of immune function. Of these, serum albumin and total lymphocyte count are the most commonly used. Physicians may also order additional tests, such as urinary creatinine.

Serum Albumin Albumin accounts for over 50 percent of the total serum proteins and its concentrations reflect the protein status of the blood and internal organs. Serum albumin tends to decline slowly, so albumin is slow to reflect changes in nutrition status.* Therefore, when low serum albumin is seen in association with malnutrition, it reflects pro-

*The half-life of albumin is about 20 days, reflecting the protein's slow degradation rate.

Table 13–4
Routine Hospital Laboratory Tests

TEST	USES
Hematology	
Hemoglobin (Hg)	To detect anemia and determine state of hydration.
Hematocrit (Hct)	To detect anemia and determine state of hydration.
White blood cells (WBC)	To detect infection and determine total lymphocyte count.
Mean corpuscular volume (MCV)	To detect anemia and determine its causes.
Mean corpuscular hemoglobin (MCH)	To detect anemia and determine its causes.
Mean corpuscular hemoglobin concentration (MCHC)	To detect anemia and determine its causes.
Blood Chemistry	
Proteins	
Total protein[a]	To detect PEM and various nutrient imbalances.
Albumin	To detect PEM and determine state of hydration.
Transferrin	To detect PEM and monitor responses to refeedings.
Electrolytes	
Sodium	To check state of hydration.
Potassium	To monitor acid-base balance and renal function and detect deficiencies.
Chloride	To monitor acid-base balance and detect GI losses of chloride (from vomiting or nasogastric suctioning).
Carbon dioxide	To monitor acid-base balance.
Other	
Glucose	To detect diabetes mellitus, glucose intolerance, stress, and pancreatic tumors.
Blood urea nitrogen	To monitor renal function and determine state of hydration.
Calcium	To detect hormonal imbalances, certain malignancies, and steatorrhea (malabsorption).
Phosphorus	To detect hormonal imbalances, PEM, and cirrhosis and monitor response to refeeding.
Magnesium	To monitor renal function and response to refeeding and detect PEM.
Cholesterol	To assess risk of heart disease and possibility of obstructive jaundice.
Uric acid	To detect gout and determine state of hydration.
Serum creatinine	To monitor renal function and determine state of hydration.
Serum enzymes	
Creatinine phosphokinase (CPK)	To monitor heart function.
Lactic dehydrogenase (LDH)	To monitor heart and renal function.
Alanine transaminase (ALT, formerly SGPT)	To monitor heart and liver function.
Aspartate transaminase (AST, formerly SGOT)	To monitor heart and liver function.
Alkaline phosphatase	To monitor liver function.
Serum amylase	To monitor pancreatic function.
Serum lipase	To monitor pancreatic function.

Note: This table presents a partial listing of the major uses of certain commonly performed lab tests that have implications for nutrition.
[a]More than half of the total protein is albumin.

Table 13–5
Relationship between Degree of Undernutrition and Serum Proteins

INDICATOR	DEGREE OF DEPLETION			
	Normal	Mild	Moderate	Severe
Albumin (g/100 ml)	≥3.5	2.8–3.4	2.1–2.7	<2.1
Transferrin (mg/100 ml)	>200	150–200	100–149	<100
Prealbumin (mg/100 ml)	16–30	10–15	5–9	<5
Retinol-binding protein[a] (mg/100 ml)	2.6–7.6	—	—	—

Note: To convert albumin (g/100 ml) to international standard units (g/L), multiply by 100. To convert transferrin (mg/100 ml) to standard international units (g/L), multiply by 0.01.
[a]Levels less than normal suggest compromised protein status. The actual degree of depletion (mild, moderate, and severe) has not been defined.

longed protein depletion. Likewise, albumin concentrations increase slowly with appropriate nutrition support, so measuring albumin as an indicator of response to nutrition therapy is of limited value.[4] Serum albumin levels appear to correlate well with survival among people in the hospital.[5] Table 13–5 provides standards for determining the severity of low serum albumin concentrations.

Many other conditions besides malnutrition can depress albumin concentrations, including liver disease, advanced kidney disease (nephrotic syndrome), infection, cancer, AIDS, burns, and eclampsia. Therefore, as is true for all other nutrition assessment measurements, albumin alone cannot determine protein status, but rather serves as one indicator among many.

Serum Transferrin Serum transferrin reflects both protein and iron status. Clinicians consider transferrin a more sensitive indicator of protein malnutrition than albumin because it responds more promptly to changes in protein intake and has a smaller body pool.* Standards for defining the severity of transferrin depletion are given in Table 13–5.

Interpreting transferrin levels as an indicator of protein status may be difficult when an *iron* deficiency is present, however. Transferrin rises as iron deficiency grows worse and falls as iron status improves. In addition, liver disease, nephrotic syndrome, and burns lower blood transferrin, whereas pregnancy and blood loss raise it. Thus all of these factors may complicate the interpretation of transferrin levels.

Other Serum Proteins Two other proteins, prealbumin and retinol-binding protein, quickly reflect PEM and rapidly respond to appropriate refeeding.† These sensitive tests are ordered in the hospital setting for clients who are malnourished or those with disorders that markedly

*Transferrin has a half-life of 4 to 8 days, an indication that it is sensitive to changes in protein intake.
†The half-lives of prealbumin and retinol-binding protein are 2 days and 12 hours, respectively.

change metabolic rates and can rapidly and profoundly affect nutrition status (see Chapter 18). Other serum proteins may be useful in nutrition assessment but are more expensive to measure than albumin and transferrin and therefore are not in common use.

Tests of Immune Function PEM depresses the immune system, a dangerous effect for people with infections, and therefore important to detect. A depressed immune system produces a reduced number of lymphocytes. White blood cell volume and red and white blood cell counts are routinely measured in hospital tests, and the total lymphocyte count can easily be derived (see Appendix E). Another test of immune function is antigen skin testing, in which the person is exposed to organisms that should produce an immune reaction in most people.* In general, a healthy immune response will occur in the well-nourished person, but will not appear in the malnourished person. Many factors other than nutrition can, however, interfere with the immune response, including infections, trauma, surgery, burns, liver diseases, renal diseases, and many drugs.[6]

Classification of Protein-Energy Malnutrition

Health care professionals classify PEM as either acute (kwashiorkor), chronic (marasmus), or a mixture of the two. Such distinctions can be useful, but they are not absolute. These clinical syndromes may overlap, or one may transist into another. This serves as another reminder of the need to assess nutrition status at regular intervals.

To evaluate PEM, assessors use data from all four assessment techniques. Historical information and physical findings alert health care professionals to the possibility of malnutrition. Anthropometric measures and biochemical analyses permit classification into acute or chronic PEM (see Table 13–6 on p. 332).

Chapter 4 used the terms *kwashiorkor* and *marasmus* to classify PEM as seen in developing countries. Because PEM found in industrialized countries often develops for different reasons (as a result of illness, for example), these terms, though frequently used in clinical settings, do not denote exactly the same conditions. We use the term **acute malnutrition** to describe kwashiorkor-type malnutrition and **chronic malnutrition** to describe marasmus-type malnutrition.

Acute Malnutrition The person with acute malnutrition typically has normal or above-standard anthropometric measurements with below-normal indices of blood and organ proteins. Because the individual may be overweight, health care workers can easily overlook malnutrition. Overweight by itself would suggest overnutrition; which again illustrates why no single parameter can be used to define nutrition status.

Chronic Malnutrition Chronic malnutrition manifests itself in an opposite manner from acute malnutrition. The individual has blood and organ protein levels that appear to be adequate, while skeletal muscle and subcutaneous fat are depleted. The emaciated appearance of the person with chronic malnutrition makes this form of malnutrition easier to notice than acute malnutrition.

Mixed PEM Mixed PEM presents signs of depleted blood, organ, and skeletal muscle proteins as well as depleted subcutaneous fat. The

*Typical antigens include *Candida*, mumps, purified protein derivative (PPD), streptokinase-streptodornase (SK-SD), and *Monilla*.

Table 13–6
Different Types of PEM

	FAT STORES AND MUSCLES	BLOOD PROTEIN, INTERNAL ORGANS, AND IMMUNE FUNCTION
CHRONIC MALNUTRITION (MARASMUS)	Depleted	Normal
ACUTE MALNUTRITION (KWASHIORKOR)	Normal	Depleted/compromised
TRANSITION (MIX)	Depleted	Depleted/compromised

person with this type of malnutrition has virtually no energy reserves, has compromised organ function, and is in grave danger, especially if experiencing severe stress as well.

Energy Overnutrition Malnutrition includes both undernutrition and overnutrition. Above-normal anthropometric measures combined with normal blood protein concentrations identify a person consuming energy in excess of needs. Such a person risks obesity and the many chronic diseases associated with it (see Chapter 9).

The assessment of PEM is commonly performed because many people, including the elderly and those who are hospitalized, have this type of malnutrition and it can lead to severe consequences. Vitamin and mineral imbalances can also be assessed using histories and physical examinations (as Chapter 12 discussed), and biochemical tests help confirm suspected deficiencies. Table 13–7 reviews the biochemical tests helpful in assessing vitamin and mineral status. The next section illustrates how biochemical tests can be used to assess nutrition-related anemias caused by iron, folate, or vitamin B_{12} deficiencies.

Nutritional Anemias

Anemia, a symptom of a wide variety of nutrition- and nonnutrition-related disorders, is characterized by a reduced number of red blood cells. Iron, folate, and vitamin B_{12} deficiencies caused by inadequate intake, poor absorption, or abnormal metabolism of these nutrients are the most common nutritional anemias. Some nonnutrition-related causes of anemia include massive blood loss, infections, hereditary blood disorders such as sickle-cell anemia, and chronic liver or kidney disease. Recall from Chapter 8 that anemia in turn slows down all body processes by interfering with normal energy metabolism.

Table 13–7
Biochemical Tests Useful for Assessing Nutrition Status

NUTRIENT	ASSESSMENT TESTS
Vitamins	
Vitamin A	Retinol-binding protein, serum carotene
Thiamin	Erythrocyte (red blood cell) transketolase activity, urinary thiamin
Riboflavin	Erythrocyte glutathione reductase activity, urinary riboflavin
Vitamin B_6	Urinary xanthurenic acid excretion after tryptophan load test, urinary vitamin B_6, erythrocyte transaminase activity
Niacin	Urinary metabolites NMN (N-methyl nicotinamide) or 2-pyridone, or preferably both expressed as a ratio
Folate	Free folate in the blood, erythrocyte folate (reflects liver stores), urinary formiminoglutamic acid (FIGLU), vitamin B_{12} status (folate assessment tests alone do not distinguish between the two deficiencies)
Vitamin B_{12}	Serum vitamin B_{12}, erythrocyte vitamin B_{12}, urinary methylmalonic acid synthesis or DUMP test (from the abbreviation for the chemical name of DNA's raw material, deoxyuridine monophosphate), Schilling test
Biotin	Serum biotin, urinary biotin
Vitamin C	Serum or plasma vitamin C,[a] leukocyte vitamin C, urinary vitamin C
Vitamin D	Serum alkaline phosphatase
Vitamin E	Serum tocopherol, erythrocyte hemolysis
Vitamin K	Blood clotting time (prothrombin time)
Minerals	
Potassium	Serum potassium
Magnesium	Serum magnesium
Iron	Hemoglobin, hematocrit, serum ferritin, total iron-binding capacity (TIBC), transferrin saturation, erythrocyte protoporphyrin, mean corpuscular volume (MCV), serum iron
Iodine	Serum protein-bound iodine, radioiodine uptake
Zinc	Plasma zinc, hair zinc

[a]Vitamin C shifts unpredictably between the plasma and the white blood cells known as leukocytes; thus a plasma or serum determination may not accurately reflect the body's pool. The appropriate clinical test may be a measurement of leukocyte vitamin C. A combination of both tests may be more reliable than either one alone.

Source: Adapted from A. Grant and S. DeHoog, *Nutritional Assessment and Support,* 3rd ed., 1985 (available from Anne Grant and Susan DeHoog, Box 25057, Northgate Station, Seattle, WA 98125).

General Tests for Anemia

A low hemoglobin or hematocrit most frequently alerts the health care professional to the presence of anemia. To help distinguish among the various types of anemias, laboratory tests determine the size and color of the red blood cells. Table 13–8 shows laboratory tests that are helpful in

Table 13–8
Laboratory Tests Useful in Evaluating Nutrition-Related Anemias

TEST OR TEST RESULT	WHAT IT REFLECTS
General Tests for Anemia	
Hemoglobin (Hg)	Total amount of hemoglobin in the red blood cells (RBC)
Hematocrit (Hct)	Percentage of RBC in the blood volume
Red blood cell (RBC) count	Number of RBC
Mean corpuscular volume (MCV)	RBC size; helps to determine if anemia is microcytic or macrocytic
Mean corpuscular hemoglobin concentration (MCHC)	Hemoglobin concentration within the average RBC helps to determine if anemia is hypochromic or normochromic
Bone marrow aspiration	The manufacture of blood cells in different developmental states
Early Stages of Iron Deficiency	
↓ Serum ferritin	Early deficiency state with depleted iron stores
↓ Transferrin saturation	Progressing deficiency state with diminished transport iron
↑ Erythrocyte protoporphyrin	Later deficiency state with limited hemoglobin production
Folate-Deficiency Anemia	
↓ Serum folate	Progressing deficiency state
↓ RBC folate	Later deficiency state
Vitamin B_{12}–Deficiency Anemia	
↓ Serum vitamin B_{12}	Progressing deficiency state
Schilling test	Absorption of vitamin B_{12}

distinguishing among the three most common nutrition-related anemias. Whenever anemia is diagnosed, further tests should be ordered to pinpoint the cause.

Hemoglobin The hemoglobin molecule, carried within the red blood cells, transports oxygen to the cells to help oxidize the energy nutrients. Hemoglobin is measured in grams per 100 milliliters of blood, and low hemoglobin values signal anemia. Table 13–9 provides hemoglobin values used in nutrition assessment.

Hematocrit To measure the hematocrit, a clinician spins a volume of blood in a centrifuge to separate the red blood cells from the plasma. The packed red blood cell volume is the hematocrit, which is expressed as a percentage of the total blood volume. Table 13–10 provides values used in nutrition assessment. Low values indicate a reduced number of red blood cells, and thus anemia.

Mean Corpuscular Volume (MCV) A direct or calculated measure of the mean corpuscular volume (MCV) determines the average size of a red blood cell. Such a measure helps to classify the type of anemia. In iron deficiency, the red blood cells are smaller than average (microcytic). In

Table 13–9
Standards for Hemoglobin Test Results

AGE (YR)	SEX	DEFICIENT (g/100 ML)	ACCEPTABLE (g/100 ML)
<2	M–F	<9.0	10.0 or >
2–5	M–F	<10.0	11.0 or >
6–12	M–F	<10.0	11.5 or >
13–16	M	<12.0	13.0 or >
	F	<10.0	11.5 or >
>16	M	<12.0	14.0 or >
	F	<10.0	12.0 or >
Pregnancy Trimester 2	F	<9.5	11.0 or >
Pregnancy Trimester 3	F	<9.0	10.5 or >

Note: To convert hemoglobin values (g/100 ml) to international standard units (g/L), multiply by 10.

folate and vitamin B_{12} deficiencies, the red blood cells are larger than average (macrocytic).

Assessment of Iron Status

Iron deficiency, a common mineral deficiency, is described in Chapter 8. The deficiency develops in stages, and different laboratory tests can uncover these stages as Table 13–8 shows.[7] Note that the blood symptom, anemia, does not develop until an iron deficiency has progressed quite far, when brain and muscular activity may already be impaired. Unfortunately, though, low hemoglobin and hematocrit test results are often the first indicators of iron deficiency seen in the clinical setting. Other tests that

Stages of iron deficiency:

1. Iron stores diminish.
2. Transport iron decreases.
3. Hemoglobin production falls.

Table 13–10
Standards for Hematocrit Test Results

AGE (YR)	SEX	DEFICIENT (%)	ACCEPTABLE (%)
<2	M–F	<28	31 or >
2–5	M–F	<30	34 or >
6–12	M–F	<30	36 or >
13–16	M	<37	40 or >
	F	<31	36 or >
>16	M	<37	44 or >
	F	<31	38 or >
Pregnancy Trimester 2	F	<30	35 or >
Pregnancy Trimester 3	F	<30	33 or >

Note: To convert hemotocrit values (%) to standard units (decimals), multiply by 0.01.

could pinpoint iron deficiency in its earlier stages are measures of serum ferritin, total iron-binding capacity (a measure of serum transferrin), and serum iron.

Assessment of Other Anemias

Folate deficiency and vitamin B_{12} deficiency present similar clinical pictures, but distinguishing between them is important because their treatments differ. Giving folate to a person with vitamin B_{12} deficiency improves some symptoms, but is a dangerous error because a vitamin B_{12} deficiency causes nerve damage that folate cannot correct. Thus inappropriate folate administration masks vitamin B_{12}–deficiency anemia, and nerve damage worsens. Tests that measure serum folate and serum vitamin B_{12} help to make the distinction.

Vitamin B_{12} deficiency usually arises from malabsorption. To determine whether malabsorption is the cause, a small oral dose of vitamin B_{12} is given, and urinary excretion is measured. This procedure measures vitamin B_{12} absorption and is called the Schilling test.

Nutrition Screening

A complete nutrition assessment as described in this chapter and the last is a tool for uncovering malnutrition or the risk of malnutrition. Rather than performing complete assessments on all clients, however, health care professionals often use short-cut methods to identify high-risk clients and then proceed with complete assessments just on those individuals. Nutrition screening is important in health care settings where nutrition assessments are not routinely performed on each client.

nutrition screening: the use of preliminary nutrition assessment techniques to identify people who are malnourished or are at risk for malnutrition.

Many institutions have nutrition screening policies, although the exact procedures vary from facility to facility.[8] A basic nutrition screening typically includes the following:

- Assessment of the individual's health history. Does the person's history reveal risk factors for poor nutrition status (review Table 12–2 on p. 301)?
- Assessment of height and weight data. Is the person's weight for height adequate, but not excessive? Has the person lost or gained weight? How much? How fast?
- Assessment of available lab reports. Do serum albumin, total lymphocyte count, hemoglobin, and hematocrit suggest malnutrition?

In addition to these screening procedures, health care professionals can use other informal techniques to screen clients:

- Check the client's tray to see if food is being eaten.
- If the client is to receive no food or is unable to eat, note how long it has been since the client has eaten. Ask if the client is expected to be able to eat soon.
- Determine whether adequate nutrients are being delivered by tube or by vein. (A box in Chapter 23 shows how to calculate the nutrient contents of intravenous solutions.)

- Visually observe the person to see if any obvious signs of malnutrition are present (review Table 12–8 on p. 315). Is the client emaciated? Obese? Extremely pale?

Regardless of the health care setting in which the client is seen, communicate any problems that you discover and follow up to make sure the problem is being addressed. Always record problems in the medical record (see Chapter 14) to ensure that whoever cares for a particular client will be alert to the problem. A dietitian will perform a more in-depth nutrition assessment if a problem is detected. Be persistent if you suspect that a problem is being ignored. Use the accompanying case study as a guide to completing the assessment process.

Nutrition assessments can uncover the extremes of both PEM and energy overnutrition. They can help pinpoint vitamin and mineral deficiencies and toxicities, poor food choices, possible drug-nutrient interactions, and a host of other risk factors that alert the assessor that nutrition and health status may be poor or deteriorating. Assessments also highlight conditions that significantly alter nutrient requirements, such as pregnancy or disease. (Later chapters will help clarify how nutrient needs change throughout the life cycle and as a result of medical disorders.) Nutrition status can change at any time. One person, previously healthy, may develop a disorder that leads to malnutrition; another person may correct poor eating habits and improve nutrition status; still another may lose a loved one and develop poor eating habits. Therefore, nutrition assessment repeated at regular intervals is an important tool in helping people to maintain or recover their health.

Armed with information from the assessment, a dietitian can develop a plan of action to either maintain or improve the individual's nutrition status. Chapter 14 provides details of how nutrition assessment information is translated into nutrition care plans.

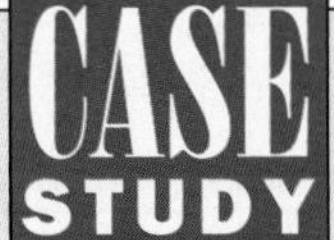

Computer Scientist with Car Accident Injuries

Ms. Green, a 38-year-old computer scientist, was admitted to the hospital for testing following a car accident. Her injuries included several broken bones and a collapsed left lung. Her lab report revealed a mildly depleted serum albumin and a moderately depleted total lymphocyte count. After screening her health record, the health care team decided that a complete nutrition assessment was necessary. The following significant information resulted.

- *Health history:*
  Increased nutrient requirements due to injuries sustained in the car accident.
- *Socioeconomic history:*
  Lives alone; her busy schedule seldom leaves time for her to prepare meals so she often eats out, usually at fast-food restaurants.
  Money for food and facilities for food preparation are adequate.
- *Drug history:*
  One standard multivitamin-mineral supplement daily.
  No other drugs.

(continued)

Case Study (continued)

- *Diet history:*
  Very-low-kcalorie, low-carbohydrate diet over past six weeks.
- *Physical examination:*
  Pale skin, slightly overweight.
- *Anthropometric measurements:*
  Height: 5 feet 7 inches.
  Weight: 150 pounds.
  Usual weight: 175 pounds
  Recent weight loss intentional.
- *Biochemical analyses:*
  Serum albumin: 3 g/100 ml (mildly depleted).
  Total lymphocyte count: 1000 mm^3 (moderately depleted).

1. Reviewing the elements of typical nutrition screening procedures described on pp. 336–337, what factors would alert the health care team to the need for a complete nutrition assessment?
2. What factors in Ms. Green's health, drug, socioeconomic, and diet histories or physical findings suggest malnutrition?
3. Determine Ms. Green's ideal body weight and calculate her percent ideal body weight and usual body weight.
4. Consider Ms. Green's recent weight change. What is a safe rate of weight loss (see p. 221)?
5. How does Ms. Green's weight loss compare with the safe rate?
7. Does her recent weight change and health history suggest a risk of poor nutrition status?
8. What do Ms. Green's lab values indicate with respect to her protein status?
9. Think ahead to Ms. Green's nutrient needs once she goes home from the hospital. What factors in Ms. Green's history will be important in devising a realistic nutrition care plan for her?

■ STUDY QUESTIONS ■

1. How do anthropometric measurements help define nutrition status? What anthropometric measurements are frequently used in nutrition assessments? Describe the limitations of anthropometric measurements.
2. How do lab tests define nutrition status? What factors influence lab test results?
3. Describe the lab tests used to uncover PEM. How is PEM classified?
4. Which lab tests can be used to distinguish between the major types of nutritional anemias?
5. What is the purpose of nutrition screening? List various screening techniques.

■ CLINICAL APPLICATION QUESTIONS ■

1. Calculate percent ideal body weight and percent usual body weight for a man who is 5 feet 11 inches tall with a current weight of 160 pounds and a usual body weight of 180 pounds. What additional information will be important for you to find out about this man's weight loss?
2. Describe the possible implications of these findings from a nutrition assessment: 15-pound weight loss over the last four months (unintentional), normal serum albumin, low hemoglobin and hematocrit.

NUTRITION IN PRACTICE 13

U.S. and World Hunger

Chapters 12 and 13 showed how to detect malnutrition and identified the many factors that can influence a person's nutrition status. This Nutrition in Practice focuses on global and societal problems that can affect the availability of food and thus cause widespread malnutrition.

Today, hundreds of millions of people are suffering from hunger and malnutrition. Tens of thousands die each day of undernutrition. Many are children afflicted by the diseases of poverty: parasitic and infectious diseases such as dysentery, measles, tuberculosis, cholera, and malaria. These diseases interact with poor nutrition to form the vicious cycle that leads to deaths—at the rate of one every two seconds.[9] Because of poverty, infection, and malnutrition, the average life expectancy in some African countries averages 50 years; in Sierra Leone it is only 34.

Even in the United States, hunger is a problem. Some 20 million people, again more than half of them children, are chronically undernourished. Malnutrition and other health problems associated with chronic hunger—stunted growth, failure to thrive, low birthweight, infant mortality, and anemia—are improving more slowly than in earlier decades; some are growing worse. The causes of hunger and malnutrition are many; this Nutrition in Practice looks at three major causes—poverty, environmental degradation, and overpopulation.

I can understand how poverty affects food availability, but I find it hard to believe that 20 million people in the United States suffer from poverty and hunger. Who exactly is affected?

In the United States, poverty and hunger reach into all segments of society—not only the chronic poor (migrant workers, the unskilled and unemployed, the homeless, and some elderly) but also the so-called new poor. Some are displaced farm families. Some are former blue-collar and white-collar workers forced out of their trades and professions into minimum-wage jobs. These new poor, who outnumber the chronic poor, are not on welfare; they have jobs, but the pay is low. Families with incomes below a certain level are simply unable to buy sufficient amounts of nourishing foods, even if they are skilled in food shopping.

Is anything being done to remedy the problem?

At present, many programs aimed at preventing or remediating malnutrition and hunger are in effect in the United States. Among them are food assistance programs for children such as the school lunch, breakfast, and child care food programs; programs to supply nourishing food to low-income pregnant women and mothers; and food assistance programs for older adults such as congregate meals and Meals on Wheels. Another program aimed directly at the poor is the Food Stamp program, administered by the U.S. Department of Agriculture (USDA). The number of stamps a household receives depends on its size and income. Recipients may use the coupons like cash to purchase food and seeds, but not tobacco, cleaning items, alcohol, or other nonfood items.

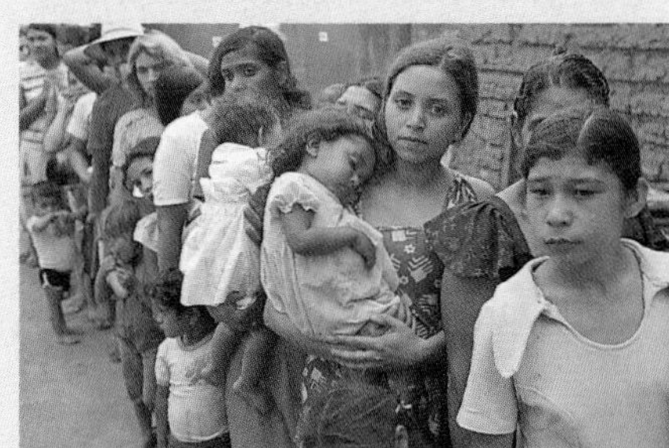

Feeding the hungry—in Nicaragua.

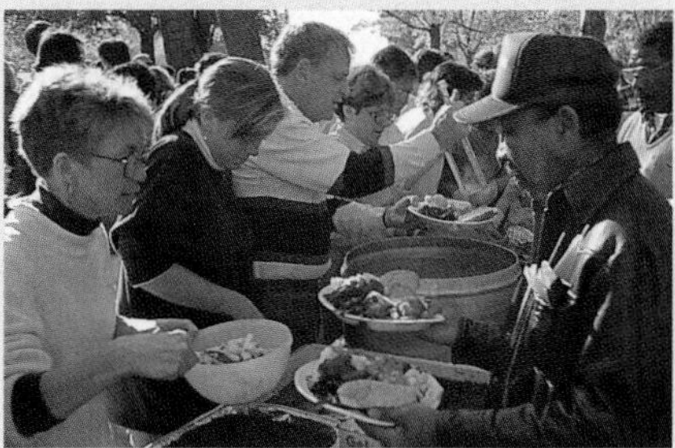

Feeding the hungry—in the United States.

Participation in the Food Stamp program reached a record high in 1992. Still, the program is not fully successful. For example, of the estimated 2 million homeless people in the United States who are eligible for food assistance, only 15 percent of single adults and 50 percent of families receive food stamps.

To supplement federal programs and reach those who are still hungry, private efforts have sprung up in many communities, where concerned citizens work through local agencies and

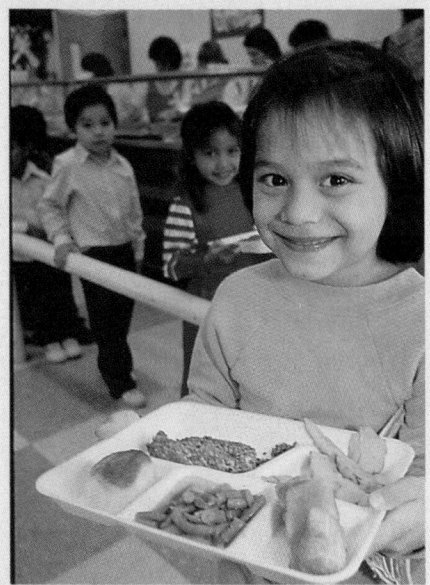

School lunches provide children with nourishment for little or no cost.

churches to help the hungry. Community-based soup kitchens and shelters generally provide good-quality meals, but most homeless people receive fewer than one and a half meals a day. Consequently, few homeless people have adequate nutrient intakes.[10]

How do hunger problems in developing countries compare to those in the United States?

Developing countries face more extreme hunger problems than the United States, and the causes are more diverse. The primary cause of hunger is still poverty, but the poverty is more extreme. Most people find it hard to comprehend the severity of poverty in the developing world. One-fifth of the world's 5 billion people have no land and no possessions *at all.* They survive on less than a dollar a day each, they lack water that is safe to drink, and they cannot read or write.[11] The average U.S. house cat eats twice as much protein every day as one of these people, and the cost of keeping the cat for a year is greater than these people's annual income.[12] Another important aspect of the hunger-poverty problem is its relationships to the environment.

How does the hunger problem relate to the environment?

Today's environmental problems are reducing the world's ability to feed its people. These environmental problems include soil erosion, deforestation, air pollution, and climate changes.

Soil erosion is reducing agricultural productivity in every nation on earth. The resulting crop losses are estimated at 6 percent per year.[13] Soil chemistry is also changing; rising concentrations of salt from irrigation are lowering yields on close to a quarter of the world's irrigated cropland.

Another environmental problem, deforestation, leads to soil erosion and also to both droughts and floods. Deforestation causes droughts because the loss of forests reduces the land's ability to hold water and to produce rain. (Trees transpire groundwater to the air and thus recycle rainfall.) Deforestation increases flooding because water runs off deforested land instead of soaking into the ground. (Trees slow the fall of rain and produce a bed of litter that holds moisture and soil on the ground.) Deforestation also deprives people of the firewood that millions in the past used as fuel; now they burn cow dung and crop residues, which they would otherwise use to build up the soil. Scenes of people starving in drought- and flood-stricken areas are a familiar sight on television. Some of the causes (such as war) are obvious, but the environmental factors that often underlie these situations are less apparent.

Air pollution also reduces crop yields. Damage to crops from air pollution is now measurable in the car-centered societies of Western Europe and the United States and in societies that burn coal to generate electricity—notably, Eastern Europe and China.[14] According to a seven-year study by two government agencies, ground-level ozone, sulfur dioxide, and nitrous oxide, which come from the burning of fossil fuels, are the most damaging air pollutants in the United States.[15] Crops are especially sensitive to ground-level ozone concentrations, which increasingly are being detected in rural as well as urban areas in ranges that reduce crop yields. An estimate puts the increase in annual crop losses ascribable to ozone pollution at 1 percent per year.[16]

Not only is ground-level ozone *pollution* reducing agricultural outputs, but outer-atmosphere ozone *depletion* is doing so, too—especially to radiation-sensitive crops such as soybeans. For each 1 percent loss of outer-atmosphere ozone, the amount of damaging ultraviolet radiation reaching the earth increases by 2 percent. Based on studies of experimental plots, soybean yields fall by the same extent—1 percent for each 1 percent rise in radiation. Soybeans are the world's leading protein crop, and at last report, no one was monitoring radiation-induced yield losses.

Climate change may also affect crop yields. At whatever rate it is occurring, it is potentially extremely disruptive. If hot summers become hotter and more frequent, droughts during the growing season will become more common. A combined hot-dry summer in 1988 pushed the U.S. grain harvest below consumption for the first time in history.[17] The calculations presented in the previous two paragraphs made no assumptions about the effects of climate change because it is too early to know what those effects may be. However, it is clear that much damage may occur. A rise of only a degree or so in average global temperature may reduce soil moisture, impair pollination of major staple food crops such as rice and corn, slow growth rates, weaken disease resistance, worsen forest fires, and disrupt many other factors affecting crop yields. Worse yet, environmental problems are disrupting crop yields at the same time that the world's population is increasing.

How is the increasing world population affecting food availability?

The impact of population growth is extremely serious. The world's population is rising at the rate of 2 percent per year.[18] Many authorities in many fields—more every year—are calling for a reduction in the rate of increase as the only way to enable the world's food output to keep pace with the growing numbers of people.

This conclusion seems inescapable. The rising population threatens the world's capacity to produce adequate food without degrading the environment and threatening future food production. Population stabilization has become one of the most pressing needs of this time in history. Until the nations of the world resolve the population problem, they can neither succeed in supporting the lives of people already born nor remedy global trends toward environmental deterioration. And of the 92 million people being added to the population each year, 88 million are being added in the most poverty-stricken areas of the world.[19]

What role can the United States play in solving these problems?

The challenges are many. For one, we are being asked to reduce our consumption of fossil fuel and thereby reduce our disproportionate contribution to global environmental degradation. For another, we can help directly by supporting family planning programs where people want them.

Also, the developing countries need relief from the gigantic interest payments they have been making to U.S. and international banks. Ten years ago those countries received $50 billion more a year from the developed world than they paid out, and they were able to make some progress toward solving their internal poverty and environmental problems. Today, however, they pay out $50 billion more than they take in, so they are becoming poorer every year.[20] They sell a bounty of cash crops to the developed world, such as cotton, tobacco, coffee, sugar, and palm oil, but they cannot put the proceeds back into their economies. Instead, all the money goes to pay the interest on their loans, and they even have to borrow more. Furthermore, they must use the land for cash crops to pay back debts, rather than for food crops to feed their own people.

Debt relief must reach those who need it, and not just the wealthy. In some poor countries, astronomically wealthy upper classes control all the good cropland and use it to produce luxury cash crops for export while the landless poor starve and multiply. Relieving hunger requires land reform—returning sufficient land to the dispossessed so that they can live and grow food on it and become able to support themselves permanently.

The idea behind these measures is that relieving poverty will help relieve environmental degradation and hunger. To rephrase a well-known adage, if you give a man a fish, he will eat for a day. If you teach him to fish, he will eat for a lifetime and may even help to feed you. Unlike food giveaways and money doles, which are only stopgap measures, social programs that permanently better the lot of the poor can permanently solve the hunger problem.[21]

What can individuals do to help?

All individuals can help by understanding the problems and helping others to understand. They can "talk it up," urging their friends and relatives in powerful positions to assist in the global effort to bring about a sustainable economy. They can support organizations that lobby for the needed changes in economic policy toward developing countries. According to one nutrition educator, "This [lobbying] is probably the most effective single thing that Joe or Jane Average Citizen can do [to help solve the world's hunger and environment problems]."[22]

Another way people can assist the global community in solving its poverty and hunger problems is to join and work for international hunger relief organizations. In addition, all individuals can take many small steps to help in their own homes, schools, and workplaces. All aspects of our lifestyles relate to global problems. Nutrition in Practice 11 recommended personal actions: reduce, reuse, recycle, and cut energy use for cars and homes. Admittedly, these approaches to

solving today's global problems seem simplistic, but because we number 5 billion plus, such actions taken by many people can exert an immense impact. If each of the world's 5 billion people takes one-five-billionth share of the responsibility, the job can get done. Just to be sure, though, those who can do more are encouraged to do so to compensate for those who are too poor, ignorant, powerless, or inflexible to join in.

Finally, it makes sense for everyone in this world, rich or poor, in the United States or in any other country, to plan on bearing no more than one or two children. For those who want large families, there are plenty of children to adopt. And for those who love children and want to help them in other ways, there are numerous opportunities to play with, teach, and nurture the world's children, from the community center downtown to the remotest primitive village on the globe.

■ NOTES ■

1. K. Schlegal-Pratt and W. D. Heizer, The accuracy of scales used to weigh patients, *Nutrition in Clinical Practice* 5 (1990): 254–257.
2. R. S. Gibson, *Principles of Nutrition Assessment* (New York: Oxford University Press, 1990), p. 172.
3. K. N. Jeejeebhoy, A. S. Detsky, and J. P. Baker, Assessment of nutrition status, *Journal of Parenteral and Enteral Nutrition* (supplement) 14 (1990): 193–196.
4. J. P. Doweiko and D. J. Nompleggi, The role of albumin in human physiology and pathophysiology, Part III: Albumin and disease states, *Journal of Parenteral and Enteral Nutrition* 15 (1991): 476–483.
5. J. A. Tayek, Albumin synthesis and nutritional assessment, *Nutrition in Clinical Practice* 3 (1988): 219–221.
6. Jeejeebhoy, Detsky, and Baker, 1990.
7. V. Herbert, Everyone should be tested for iron disorders, *Journal of the American Dietetic Association* 92 (1992): 1502–1509.
8. M. B. Foltz, R. Schiller, and A. S. Ryan, Nutrition screening and assessment: Current practices and dietitians' leadership roles, *Journal of the American Dietetic Association* 93 (1993): 1388–1395.
9. D. R. Gwatkin, How many die? A set of demographic estimates of the annual number of infant and child deaths in the world, *American Journal of Public health* 70 (1980): 1286–1289.
10. J. C. Wolgemuth and coauthors, Wasting malnutrition and inadequate nutrient intakes identified in a multiethnic homeless population, *Journal of the American Dietetic Association* 92 (1992): 834–839; M. A. Drake, The nutritional status and dietary adequacy of single homeless women and their children in shelters, *Public Health Reports* 107 (1992): 312–319; B. E. Cohen, N. Chapman, and M. R. Burt, Food sources and intake of homeless persons, *Journal of Nutrition Education* (1 supplement) 24 (January/February 1992): 45S–51S.
11. World Bank, *World Development Report 1991* (New York: Oxford University Press, 1991); S. Postel, Denial in the decisive decade, in L. R. Brown and coauthors, *State of the World 1992: A Worldwatch Sustainable Society* (New York: Norton, 1992), pp. 3–8.
12. L. Timberlake, *Only One Earth,* cited in Food for thought, *Seeds,* Sprouts edition, 1988.
13. L. R. Brown and J. E. Young, Feeding the world in the nineties, Chapter 4 in L. R. Brown, *State of the World 1990: A Worldwatch Institute Report on Progress toward a Sustainable Society* (New York: Norton, 1990), p. 60.
14. Brown and Young, 1990, p. 62.
15. U.S. Environmental Protection Agency (EPA) and U.S. Department of Agriculture (USDA),as cited in Brown and Young, 1990, p. 62.
16. Brown and Young, 1990, pp. 62–63.
17. Brown and Young, 1990, p. 63.
18. Brown and Young, 1990, pp. 64–65.
19. Postel, 1992.
20. S. Lewis, Food security, environment, poverty, and the world's children, *Journal of Nutrition Education* (1 supplement) 24 (January/February 1992): 3S–5S.
21. K. L. Clancy and J. Bowering, The need for emergency foods: Poverty problems and policy responses, *Journal of Nutrition Education* (1 supplement) 24 (January/February 1992): 12S–17S; J. M. Dodds, S. L. Parker, and P. S. Haines, Hunger in the 80s and 90s: A challenge for nutrition educators, *Journal of Nutrition Education* (1 supplement) 24 (January/February 1992): 2S.
22. S. Smith, professor of nutrition, University of New Hampshire, Durham, personal communication, Summer 1993.

14

Nutrition Intervention

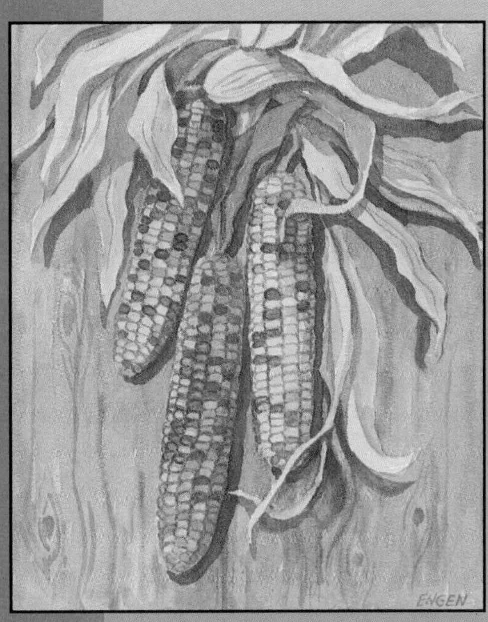

CONTENTS

This chapter describes the process used to correct the nutrition problems identified through nutrition assessment. Because assuring that a person's nutrient needs are met is part of this process, this chapter also describes diet therapy, helping people eat, and communicating clients' needs to the health care team.

The Nutrition Care Process

To correct or prevent nutrition problems, health care professionals use a systematic and logical process that meets both the person's nutrient needs *and* the person's need to understand. Appropriate diet therapy and skillful communication are the two complementary parts of effective nutrition care.

The nutrition care process consists of these five steps:

- Assess nutrition status. (Chapters 12 and 13 described how a nutrition assessment is conducted.)
- Analyze assessment data to determine nutrient requirements.
- Develop a plan of action (a nutrition care plan) for meeting nutrition needs, including client education.
- Implement the nutrition care plan.
- Evaluate the effectiveness of the nutrition care plan through ongoing assessment, and make appropriate changes.

nutrition care process: an organized approach to nutrition intervention that consists of five steps (assessing, analyzing, planning, implementing, and evaluating). The nutrition care process parallels the *nursing care process* except that it focuses on nutrition concerns.

nutrition care plan: a plan that translates nutrition assessment data into a strategy for meeting a client's nutrient and nutrition education needs.

To ensure the success of the nutrition care process, the health care professional or team should make sure that, whenever possible, the client is an active participant in the process. In cases where active participation is not possible, such as for infants and young children, people who are very ill or unconscious, people with mental disabilities, or people who are uncooperative, health care professionals should enlist the involvement of family members or other support people.

The dietitian has the primary responsibility for developing and implementing nutrition care plans. The physician, nurse, dietetic technician, social worker, pharmacist, physical therapist, and occupational therapist also make valuable contributions (see the Nutrition in Practice that follows this chapter). To the extent that all of these people apply their nutrition knowledge, technical skills, and interpersonal skills, the care plan will be realistic and attainable.

Analyzing Assessment Data

The first step following nutrition assessment is to study the nutrition assessment data. What are the potential nutrition problems? Is body weight appropriate? Are lab values normal? Are there physical signs of malnutrition? Are nutrient needs altered due to growth or illness? This information generates a nutrition problem list and forms the basis of the care plan. The problems listed may be past, current, or future conditions that may impair nutrition status or alter nutrient needs. From this information, the dietitian estimates nutrient needs. Always keep in mind that these estimates are just that—estimates. A person's response to the nutrition care plan reveals the person's needs better than estimates can.

The word **illness** as used in this book refers to any medical condition that alters nutrient needs. Not all such conditions are diseases. For example, major surgery can have a significant impact on nutrition status. It is not a disease, but it is a stress that alters nutrient needs.

The nutrition problem list gives rise to the nutrition care plan just as the nursing diagnosis gives rise to the nursing care plan.

Energy Needs If an adult has maintained a desirable weight over a period of time, then that person's energy needs can be estimated from habitual food intake. The person is already consuming the amount of energy needed. For otherwise healthy adults who are not at a desirable weight, energy needs can be calculated as detailed in Chapter 6 (p. 128). As for infants, pregnant women, children, and others, the chapters that follow describe their changing energy needs. Later chapters describe energy needs imposed by different states of health.

Protein Needs The RDA provide an estimate of protein needs for healthy people throughout life. Later chapters describe the protein needs of people who are ill.

Vitamin and Mineral Needs Vitamin and mineral needs are highly variable and are often difficult to estimate. Not only do exact requirements vary from one person to the next, but the same person's needs for certain nutrients can vary dramatically at different stages of the life cycle and in different states of health. For healthy individuals, health care professionals generally use the RDA to estimate nutrient needs. Although the RDA are not intended for this purpose, they are really the only available guidelines. Vitamin and mineral needs in different stages of the life cycle and in medical disorders are discussed in more detail in later chapters.

Once nutrient needs have been assessed and analyzed, a dietitian develops a plan of action that meets the client's nutrition needs. Such a plan will benefit the client only if it also includes attention to the client's eating habits and lifestyle.

Developing a Nutrition Care Plan

A dietitian uses a nutrition care plan for two purposes: first, to provide a clear statement of a client's needs for nutrition care and nutrition information; and second, to set forth a strategy for meeting those needs. Form 14–1 on the next page provides a sample nutrition assessment and care plan summary.

Objectives of a nutrition care plan:
- To meet the client's nutrition needs.
- To meet the client's needs for nutrition information.

With a problem list in hand, a dietitian can develop a plan that specifies the objectives of dietary recommendations, the content of counseling sessions, and a tentative time frame for accomplishing each objective. If, for example, a client needs to lose weight (the objective), the dietitian might set a goal of one pound a week for three months (the time frame). That specific goal helps the dietitian to design the weight-loss program. It determines that the diet will provide 500 kcalories less than the client's energy expenditure each day; that the diet will be low in fat and high in carbohydrate; and that each day will include a certain amount of aerobic activity (the areas of content). The dietitian may plan one counseling session to discuss the nutrition care plan with the client, several sessions to instruct the client about the diet, and another to evaluate the client's understanding.

The nutrition care plan specifies:
- The objectives.
- The areas of content.
- The tentative time frame.

For each nutrition problem, the dietitian must first identify the cause, if known, and then may specify one or several strategies to tackle it. The more detailed the strategies, the better. Consider, for example, a problem

Form 14–1
Sample Nutrition Assessment and Care Plan Summary

After analyzing the assessment data as described in Chapters 12 and 13, the health care professional summarizes significant findings and key points of the care plan using a form such as this one.

Client: ______________________ Diet Order: ______________________

Assessment Summary

Anthropometric Data: ______________________

____

Biochemical Data: ______________________

____

Health History Data: ______________________

____

Socioeconomic History Data: ______________________

____

Drug-Nutrient Interactions: ______________________

____

Dietary Intake Data: ______________________

____

Recommend Additional Screening: Yes/No ______________________

Problem List:

1. ______________________
2. ______________________
3. ______________________
4. ______________________
5. ______________________

Nutrition Care Plan Summary

Plan of Nutrition Care: ______________________

____

Other Therapy: ______________________

____

Education: ______________________

____

Compliance/Understanding: ______________________

____

Follow-Up: ______________________

Date: ______________________ Dietitian: ______________________

of diarrhea. If a drug is causing the diarrhea, an appropriate strategy might be to prevent dehydration by giving ample fluids and electrolytes while the physician tries substituting other drugs. The client should be informed of this plan. If the diarrhea is caused by a milk allergy, then the problem-solving strategy is to eliminate milk and milk products from the diet. The client should receive instructions on how to make the diet adequate despite these omissions.

Implementation of Nutrition Care Plans Once care plans are developed, the next step is to implement them by providing both the appropriate diet and education. In the hospital or in a long-term health care facility (such as a nursing home or inpatient mental health facility), the diet part is simple: meals are simply delivered to clients. Before discharge, though, dietitians should counsel clients so that they will understand and continue their diets at home, if necessary.

Nurses, thanks to their frequent daily contact with clients, can offer important support in this aspect of client care. Clients often think of questions hours after the dietitian has left, and they ask the next person who walks into the room—most often, the nurse. The nurse who is confident of the answers should provide them. If not sure of the answers, the nurse should express honest uncertainty and inform the dietitian that the client needs a follow-up visit to clarify a few points. Nutrition in Practice 14 shows more ways that health care team members work together to improve nutrition care, and the case study on p. 357 affords an opportunity to apply some of the planning principles introduced here.

Ongoing Evaluation While the planned strategies are being implemented, the dietitian must keep track of how they are working. If, for example, a client on a weight-reduction diet fails to lose weight, a change may be needed. Is the client eating too much? Is the client too inactive? Perhaps the client should keep a food diary and increase the intensity, duration, or frequency of physical activity.

If a client's situation changes, so may nutrition status and nutrient needs. For example, when a pregnant woman delivers her baby, she will need instructions on how to feed her infant. She will also need to learn how to revise her diet to support lactation (if she is breastfeeding) or to return to a healthy weight (if she is feeding formula). Dietitians must keep adjusting care plans to meet changing needs.

A care plan may be ideal, but may still fall short if a client is unable or unwilling to comply with it. If the client is unable to comply, communication may help. If the client is unwilling, despite the best efforts of health care professionals, little can be done except to try again later when the client may be more receptive.

Diet Therapy

An essential component of every nutrition care plan is diet therapy. Diet therapy strives to provide the appropriate amounts of energy, protein, carbohydrate, fat, vitamins, major minerals, trace elements, and water in whatever form best meets the client's special needs. For example, a person who cannot chew needs soft foods; a person who is in a coma may need to have a formula delivered by tube into the GI tract; a person with diabetes needs a special diet.

Often, a diet must complement other therapies. A diet plan for an individual with insulin-dependent diabetes mellitus must coordinate meals with the physical activity routine and the insulin-delivery schedule.

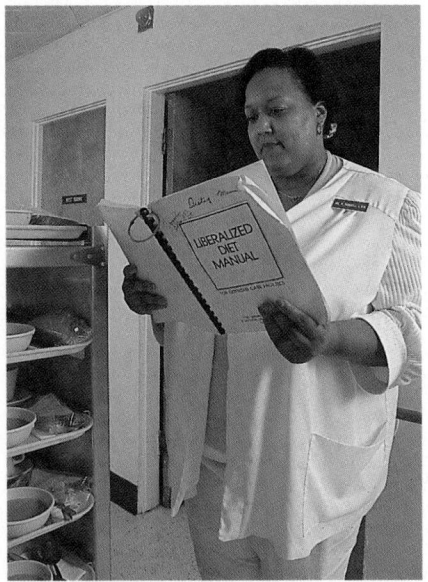

The diet manual specifies which foods to exclude or include on various modified diets.

Diet Manuals and Diet Orders

In health care facilities, the physician and dietitian usually select the therapeutic diet appropriate for each case, and the foodservice department delivers it. The exact foods excluded or included on a specific modified diet differ among health care facilities, generally in minor ways. These variations reflect different schools of thought regarding diet. You can familiarize yourself with a particular institution's diets by reading its diet manual.

diet manual: a book that describes the foods allowed and restricted on different diets, the rationale and indications for use of the diets, and sample menus.

diet order: a physician's written statement in the medical record of what diet a client should receive.

Diet Manuals In large hospitals, the staff of dietitians compiles a diet manual, subject to approval by the hospital administrator, several physicians, and representatives of the nursing service. A small hospital or clinic may adopt the diet manual of another hospital or an organization such as the state dietetic association. The diet manual describes the foods allowed and not allowed on each diet, outlines the rationale and indications for use of each diet, provides information on the nutritional adequacy of the diets, and offers sample menus. In hospitals, the dietary staff uses the manual to design menus for clients.

Diet Orders The physician prescribes the client's diet and writes the diet order into the medical record. The physician often relies on the dietitian or health care team to suggest a diet prescription or make recommendations when changes in the diet orders appear warranted or when clarity seems to be lacking. To avoid confusion, physicians should order diets by the names given in the diet manual and describe exact modifications when appropriate. For example, a low-sodium diet order should specify the amount of sodium; otherwise, "low sodium" could be interpreted to mean any amount from 500 to 4000 milligrams of sodium. In facilities serving meals, the dietary department may send a preselected diet if it receives an unclear order for an uncomplicated diet from the nursing station. For more complicated diets, such as a renal diet, meals will not be sent until the order is clarified.

An order to give a client nothing orally (including food, beverages, and medications) reads "NPO"; **NPO** stands for *nil per os,* which means "nothing by mouth." **PO** stands for *per os,* which means "by mouth" or "orally."

Occasionally, diet orders, even though written in the chart, may be inappropriate. For example, the physician may describe an obese individual as "well-nourished" and order a regular diet. If this occurs, the dietitian will not see the client, and the client will receive an inappropriate diet and no nutrition advice. As another example, a physician may order that a client receive no food or fluids after midnight because a lab test is to be run in the morning. The doctor assumes that the order will be discontinued after the test, but it is not. The client misses several meals before someone notices the error. These examples illustrate opportunities where communication between health care professionals can make a difference in client care. Whenever you notice inappropriate diet orders, contact the dietitian or alert the physician.

Standard and Modified Diets

standard diet: a regular diet—that is, one that includes all foods and meets the nutrient needs of a normal, healthy person.

Standard or regular diets include all foods and provide all the nutrients in amounts appropriate for healthy people. Modified diets are used when standard diets fail to meet the specific needs of clients. Modifying the standard diet is much like tailoring a suit. A tailored suit is the same suit after alterations—only it fits better. In the case of a modified diet, the tailoring may involve changing the consistency; adjusting the amounts of individual nutrients, energy, or fluid; altering the number of meals; or eliminating certain foods. Appendix F shows an example of how a hospital menu can be modified for different diets. Table 14–1 on pp. 350–351 gives examples of modified diets used to treat diseases involving different organ systems. These diets are described further in later chapters.

modified or **therapeutic diet:** a regular diet that is adjusted to meet special nutrition needs. Such diets can be adjusted by changing the consistency, amounts of energy and nutrients, amount of fluid, or number of meals, or by adding or eliminating certain foods.

It is helpful to think about modified diets in terms of the symptoms or conditions they relieve rather than in terms of disorders. Two people with the same disorder may need two different diets. Conversely, people with two different disorders may benefit from the same diet. Consider two people with cancer: one may need a diet that will help control nausea; the other may need a high-kcalorie diet. Now consider a pregnant woman with nausea. She may benefit from the same recommendations as those for the first person with cancer.

Putting the principles of diet therapy into practice does not end with offering foods to clients. It is equally important that the client eat the foods. This is especially important in the hospital environment when attention to nutrition can hasten or slow a client's recovery.

Food in the Hospital

Food in the hospital can be viewed from the perspectives of both those who provide it and those who consume it. The next two sections describe hospital food from these two points of view.

Foodservice in Health Care Facilities

Providing standard and modified diets to clients in health care facilities presents unique problems. Consider that such institutions must provide dozens of diets to hundreds, or thousands, of individuals. In order to prevent errors and facilitate client care, health care professionals need an understanding of the general procedures underlying foodservice in health care facilities. This discussion uses the hospital as an example of a health care facility.

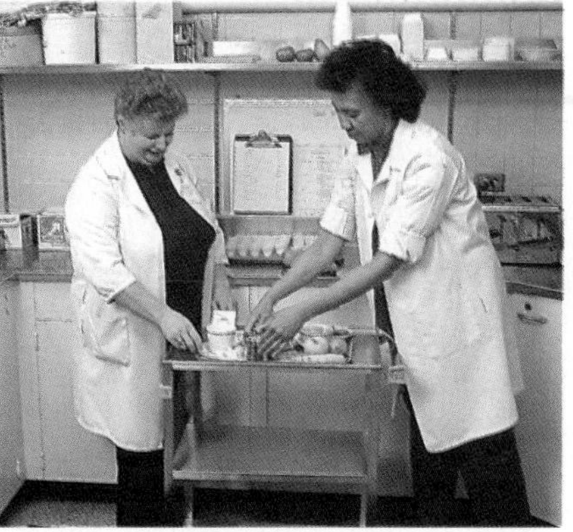

People appreciate receiving the right meal served attractively.

The Personnel The responsibility for preparing and serving food in a health care setting rests with either a chief administrative dietitian or a foodservice manager. (The glossary on p. 352 defines these and related terms.) These professionals direct all aspects of foodservice—from purchasing foods to delivering meals to clients.

The clinical dietitian works directly with clients to assess their nutrition status, plan appropriate diets, and provide nutrition education. In some facilities, dietetic technicians assist dietitians in both administrative and clinical tasks. Other dietary employees include clerks, aides, cooks, porters, and other assistants. Only dietitians should interpret diet orders, develop nutrition care plans, and provide nutrition education. Other dietary employees do not have extensive formal training in nutrition, and their ability to provide accurate information may be limited.

Table 14–1
Summary of Modified Diets by Organ System

DISORDERS	POSSIBLE DIET MODIFICATIONS
Conditions Affecting or Involving the GI Tract, Liver, and Exocrine Pancreas[a]	
Blind loop syndrome	Fat-restricted, fluid and electrolyte replacement
Broken jaw	Mechanical soft
Celiac disease	Gluten-restricted
Cirrhosis	Protein-restricted, sodium-restricted, fluid-restricted
Constipation	High-fiber, increased fluids
Cystic fibrosis	High-kcalorie, high-protein, fat-modified
Dental caries	Mechanical soft
Diarrhea	Liquid, low-fiber, regular, fluid and electrolyte replacement
Difficulty swallowing (dysphagia)	Mechanical soft, tube feeding, total parenteral nutrition (TPN)
Diverticulitis	Low-fiber
Diverticulosis	High-fiber
Dry mouth	Mechanical soft
Dumping syndrome	Carbohydrate-restricted, no concentrated sugars, frequent small feedings, fluid and electrolyte replacement
Gastritis	Low-fiber, bland
Hepatic coma	Protein-restricted, sodium-restricted, fluid-restricted
Hepatitis	Regular, high-kcalorie, high-protein
Hiatal hernia	Frequent small feedings, fat-restricted, bland, kcalorie-restricted
Ill-fitting dentures	Mechanical soft
Indigestion (dyspepsia)	Low-fiber, bland, frequent small feedings
Inflammatory bowel disease	Low-fiber, fat-restricted, high-kcalorie, high-protein, fluid and eletrolyte replacement, lactose-restricted, tube feeding, TPN
Irritable bowel syndrome	High-fiber, fat-restricted
Lactose intolerance	Lactose-restricted
Malabsorption	Fat-restricted, high-kcalorie, high-protein, fluid and electrolyte replacement
Missing teeth	Mechanical soft
Nausea	Low-fiber, bland, frequent small feedings, no liquids with meals
Oral surgery	Mechanical soft
Pancreatitis[a]	Fat-restricted, regular, frequent small feedings, tube feeding, TPN
Peptic ulcer	Bland
Periodontal disease	Mechanical soft
Plastic surgery of head or neck	Mechanical soft, tube feeding, TPN
Reflux esophagitis	Frequent small feedings, fat-restricted, bland, kcalorie-restricted
Short bowel syndrome	Fat-restricted, high-kcalorie, high-protein, fluid and electrolyte replacement
Ulcers of mouth or gums	Mechanical soft, avoid spicy foods and foods with seeds
Vomiting	Fluid and electrolyte replacement
Conditions Affecting the Endocrine Pancreas[a]	
Diabetes mellitus	Carbohydrate-controlled, kcalorie-controlled, fat-restricted, high-fiber, sodium restricted
Hypoglycemia	No concentrated sweets, frequent small feedings
Conditions Affecting the Blood Vessels, Heart and Lungs	
Atherosclerosis	Fat-restricted, low-cholesterol, kcalorie-restricted, sodium-restricted, high-fiber
Congestive heart failure	Sodium-restricted, kcalorie-restricted, low-fiber, bland, frequent small feedings, fluid-restricted
Coronary heart disease	Fat-restricted, low-cholesterol, kcalorie-restricted, sodium-restricted, high-fiber
Hypertension	Sodium-restricted, kcalorie-restricted, high-potassium, fat-restricted
Myocardial infarction	Sodium-restricted, kcalorie-restricted, low-fiber, bland, frequent small feedings, moderate-temperature foods, fat-restricted
Pulmonary disease	High-kcalorie, high-protein

Table 14–1 *(continued)*

Conditions Affecting the Kidneys	
Acute renal disease	Protein-restricted, high-kcalorie, fluid-controlled, sodium-controlled, potassium-controlled, fat-restricted, carbohydrate-controlled
Chronic renal disease	Protein-restricted, low-sodium, fluid-restricted, potassium-restricted, phosphorus-restricted, fat-restricted
Kidney stones	Increased fluid intake, calcium-controlled, low-oxalate
Nephrotic syndrome	Sodium-restricted, high-kcalorie, potassium-restricted
Conditions Affecting Many Organ Systems	
Acquired immune deficiency syndrome (AIDS)	High-kcalorie, high-protein, fat-restricted, low-residue, low-fiber, fluid and electrolyte replacement, lactose-restricted, mechanical soft, tube feeding, TPN (see also specific related conditions such as ulcers of the mouth)
Burns	High-kcalorie, high-protein, increased fluid intake
Cancer	High-kcalorie, high-protein (see also specific related conditions such as nausea)
Food sensitivities	Elimination of offending substance
Galactosemia	Galactose-restricted
Obesity, overweight	kCalorie-restricted, fat-restricted, high-fiber
Phenylketonuria (PKU)	Phenylalanine-restricted
Stroke	Mechanical soft, regular, tube feeding, fat-restricted, low-sodium, high-potassium
Surgery	Regular, high-kcalorie, high-protein, increased fluids
Underweight	High-kcalorie, high-protein

[a]The pancreas produces both external (exocrine) and internal (endocrine) secretions. The external secretions (enzymes) play an important role in the digestion of food; the internal secretions (insulin and other hormones) play a primary role in the regulation of glucose metabolism.

The Menus Many hospitals provide menus from which clients can select their meals. This system helps to ensure that clients will receive foods they enjoy and will eat. It also gives clients the feeling of having some control in an otherwise impersonal hospital environment. Clients who must follow special diets receive menus that list only appropriate food selections. By marking those menus, clients can learn about their diets.

selective menu: a menu from which clients can select the foods they will receive while hospitalized.

Some facilities offer no selective menus. Their dietary departments serve a standard house diet, adjusting it according to dietary orders as necessary. Generally, even these menus provide some flexibility, though. For example, a client can request simple changes, such as the substitution of one vegetable for another.

The Procedures Nurses can help clients greatly, and also save themselves needless aggravation and time, by learning about the foodservice system in the health care facilities where they work. Some of the things to learn include:

- The number to call and procedure to follow to request a physician-ordered diet, make changes in the diet order, or report problems with a client's tray.
- The number to reach the clinical dietitian in case a client needs special nutrition advice.
- The times when meals are plated, so requests can be called in before these times.

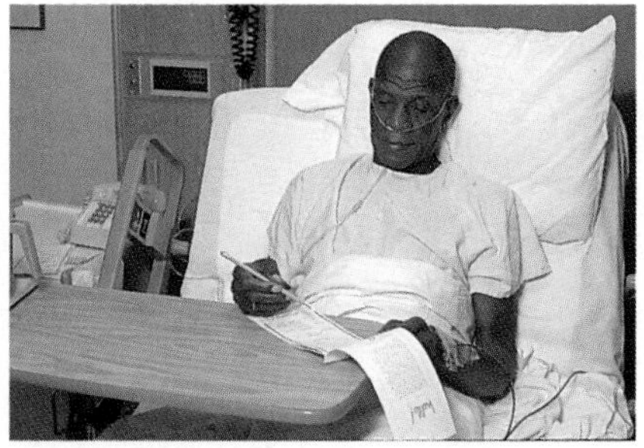

By selecting foods from a menu, clients receive meals they enjoy and gain some control over their hospital stay.

Glossary of Terms Defining Dietetics Professionals

Reminder: A *registered dietitian (R.D.)* is a trained professional with at least a bachelor's degree in nutrition and food science; a year's internship at a facility approved by the American Dietetic Association (ADA) or an equivalent facility; and a passing score on the national registration exam (a four-hour qualifying exam administered over six competency areas by the ADA).

administrative dietitian: a dietitian who is primarily concerned with the management of a foodservice system that provides optimal nutrition and quality food. Administrative dietitians may assume some clinical duties as well.

clinical dietitian: a dietitian responsible for direct client care—assessing nutrition needs, developing and implementing nutrition care plans, and evaluating and reporting the results.

dietetic technician registered (D.T.R.): a technically skilled person with an associate's degree who meets the ADA's educational standards and works under the guidance of an R.D. (registered dietitian). In some states, D.T.R.s are also licensed.

- The location of the diet manual—usually available at each nursing station—and its contents.

You may want to carry a card with this information on your person. Understanding how the dietary department operates, you will know where to turn for help when your clients have problems with meals or nutrition.

Clients' Perspectives on Hospital Food

What do you think of when you see or hear the words "hospital food"? What are your own experiences with hospital food? Viewing hospital food from a client's perspective will add to your skill in offering nutrition care.

The Pleasures of Eating Most people generally look forward to eating, and in the hospital, eating may be especially enjoyable. It offers clients something familiar in an otherwise strange environment. It is also one of the few experiences in the hospital in which clients have a choice. They cannot choose when they will receive tests, how much blood will be drawn, what nurse will care for them, or what time they will have surgery, but they can select their own meals and either eat them or refuse them!

Complaints about Food Of course, clients may complain about hospital food. Food is so important to most people that a bad experience with it can make them, and those who work with them, agitated and angry. Complaining may have little to do with the food itself, but may serve as a way of venting fear, frustration, anger, and physical pain. Clients need opportunities to express their feelings, and often you may find that problems can be eased simply by listening without the need to make any diet changes. The next two boxes offer pointers on how to help a client eat and on how to help a child. Problems with the food itself need to be corrected by the dietary department.

HOW TO Help a Client Eat

If someone has a poor appetite or constantly complains about the food, try to get to the root of the problem and solve it. Here are some things you can do:

1. Care. If the person is frightened, angry, or confused, show that you care.
2. Motivate. Be sure the person understands how important nutrition may be to recovery.
3. Teach. If on a modified diet, does the client know which foods are allowed and which are restricted? Does the client understand how to mark the menu correctly? If a client needs help in any of these areas, provide it. (Call a dietitian, if in your judgment the client needs help in finding acceptable foods.)
4. Coordinate client care. Work with other health care professionals to avoid painful procedures before mealtimes. The stress of pain or fear shuts down digestion and turns off interest in food. Physicians can often prescribe medications to relieve pain prior to mealtimes.
5. Permit foods from home. When it is permissible and possible, let a friend or family member bring favorite foods from outside the hospital if these foods will improve food intake. This may be especially helpful for clients with strong ethnic, religious, or personal food preferences.
6. Encourage. Take a positive attitude toward the hospital's food. Never say something like, "I couldn't eat this stuff either." Instead, say, "The dietary department really tries to make foods the way you like them. Let me call the dietitian. I'm sure we can find a solution." (When a dietitian or foodservice manager is unavailable, look for the dietary department's list of alternative foods at the nursing station.)
7. Help with menu selection. Make sure that clients mark menus, so that they will receive foods they enjoy eating.
8. Help clients prepare for meals. Encourage them to wash their hands and faces and to brush their teeth or rinse their mouths before eating. Help them get comfortable, either in bed or sitting in a chair. Adjust the extension table to a comfortable height and distance, and make sure it is clean. A clean, odor-free room also helps. Take these steps before the tray arrives, so that the meal can be served promptly and at the right temperature.
9. Check for accuracy. When the food cart arrives on the floor, check each tray. Verify that the name on the tray is the client's name. Check to see that the client is receiving the right diet. Compare the tray with the client's marked menu to be sure that

(continued)

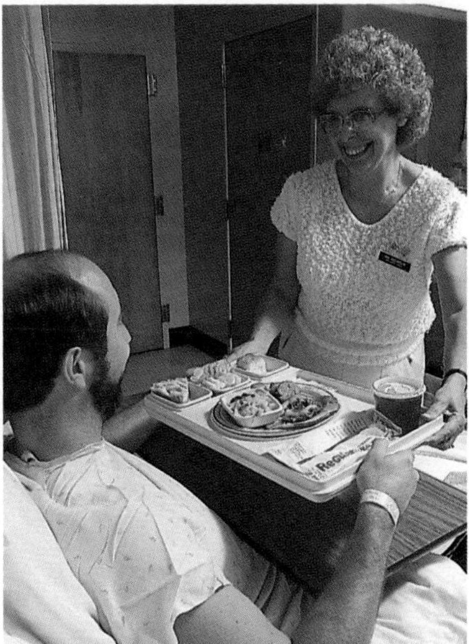

People enjoy eating when they feel comfortable and cared for.

How To (continued)

the foods are those that were ordered. Order a new tray if foods are not appropriate.

10. Make the meal appetizing. Scan the tray and improve its appearance if you can. The client will eat best if the food looks appetizing. Then serve the meal immediately—while hot foods are still hot and cold foods are still cold.
11. Help with eating. Help clients who need assistance in opening containers such as milk cartons or those who are unable to feed themselves. Your efforts can mean a lot to clients whose illnesses, fears, and frustrations significantly interfere with the desire to eat.
12. If needed, help more. In the special case of a client just emerging from a stressful episode, offer further assistance. Imagine feeling almost too sick to move or too tired to sit up. Anorexia and pain associated with severe stresses interfere with eating. Show that you understand how difficult it is to eat. In successive encounters, work closely with clients to find the foods they enjoy most. Encourage clients to eat the most nutritious foods first before they become too full to finish the meal. Encourage clients to select foods that require little effort to eat. For example, eating a roast beef sandwich requires less effort than cutting and eating a steak. Drinking a soup is easier than eating it with a spoon. Finally, encourage clients to get out of bed and begin minimal physical activity (such as walking) as soon as medically safe.

As you can see, helping clients eat requires active communication with each client. Professional communications play a vital role in client care as well.

Professional Communications

Maintaining strong professional communication networks benefits both health care professionals and their clients. Conversely, miscommunication between professionals can result in inappropriate therapy with serious consequences for clients' health. Many opportunities exist for professionals to discuss clients' concerns and progress. One way professionals communicate is through the medical record and other records.

Written Records

Written records, including the medical record and care plans, document a client's problems and what is being done to treat them. Such records allow health care professionals to share information and check the progress of client care.

HOW TO Help a Child Eat

Nutrition care contributes importantly to a child's recovery, even though its effects may not be immediately obvious. A sick child often requires special care around mealtimes. The suggestions for clients in general are valuable for working with ill children. So are many of the hints given in Chapter 16 for helping healthy children to eat. Additional pointers from people experienced in working with children include the following.

1. Notice the child's posture. Body language will tell you if a child feels fear, pain, or discomfort.
2. Touch the child often and lovingly. Your touch communicates more than your words.
3. Smile and be playful. Laughing releases stress and promotes relaxation and good appetite.
4. Notice whether the child eats the food. Putting a tray of food in front of a child is not enough.
5. Stay with the child during the meal, or make sure a loved person is there. The child will eat and assimilate food better if a caring person smoothes away anxiety and loneliness.
6. Let children eat with other children if possible. They'll enjoy mealtimes more, accept more food, and eat for longer periods.

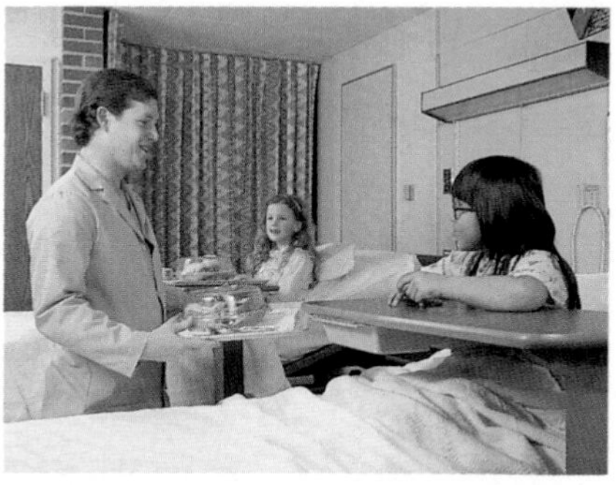

Foods taste better when you're not alone and scared.

The Medical Record The medical record is a legal document that compiles the history, diagnosis, therapy, and prognosis for each client. By reading the medical record at regular intervals, the health care professional obtains a continuous assessment of the client's condition and responses to therapy. By writing in the medical record, the professional documents each action taken in client care. This information helps determine if medical orders are being followed and directs future care.

medical record: a continuous written account of a client's health status, diagnosis, therapy, and prognosis.

Medical records can be organized in many ways. Health care professionals today commonly use the problem-oriented medical record (POMR) approach. In this approach, health care team members list all of the client's problems to generate a problem list. Subsequent entries describe the actions being taken to deal with each problem in the record. As new problems arise, they are added to the list.

The Medical Record and Nutrition Care Learn how to effectively use the record in the facility where you work. Regardless of the approach used, be sure the client's medical record includes important nutrition-related information. Examples of important information include:

- Evaluation of the client's current diet.
- Nutrition assessment data.
- Recommended nutrition therapy.

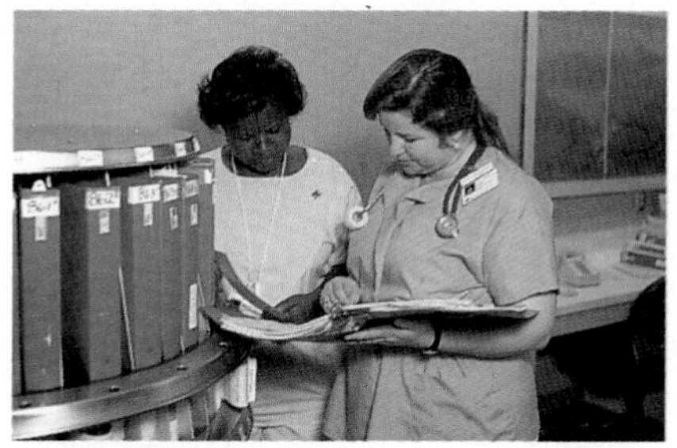

Take time to record important nutrition information in the client's medical record.

- The client's acceptance and tolerance of the diet.
- Problems with the client's food intake.
- Documentation of diet counseling.
- Any planned follow-up or referral to another person or agency.
- The client's response to nutrition care.
- The client's response to diet counseling.

Other Records In addition to the formal medical record, various health care professionals generally keep records of their own. For example, nurses keep nursing care plans, and dietitians keep nutrition care plans (as described earlier). These records contain some of the same information as the formal medical record, but they also include more detailed plans and notes specifically pertinent to the individual health care team member. For example, a nutrition care plan may have details about a client's reaction to a diet, which the dietitian will later use in preparation for diet counseling. Nursing care plans may also include information about a client's nutrition needs. The direct and frequent interactions nurses have with clients generate valuable additions to the care plan.

Other Communication Channels

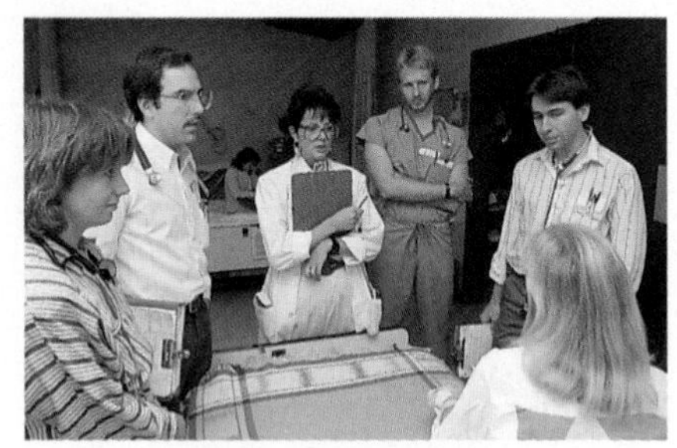

Bedside rounds provide an excellent opportunity to discuss concerns regarding a person's nutrition status.

Health care team members have other opportunities for communication besides written records. Team members in a hospital often phone or page each other when they identify problems or when questions arise. Outside the hospital, health care team members may be reached in their offices or through their answering services.

Bedside rounds provide an ideal opportunity for professional communication as do other times when nurses report to one another at the end of each shift (see the Nutrition in Practice that follows this chapter). Use these times to talk over nutrition problems and to pass along information regarding clients' special nutrition and diet needs and requests.

Nutrition care encompasses much more than diet therapy. Effective nutrition care addresses the unique needs of the individual, framing nutrition needs in the context of the person's educational, socioeconomic, and medical needs. This chapter has described techniques for building effective nutrition care plans. The remaining chapters describe how nutrient needs change due to illness and how therapeutic diets can meet them.

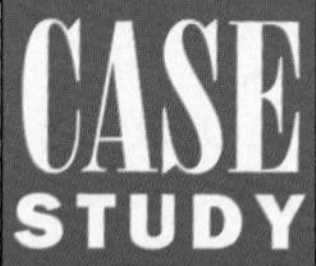

Boy with Diabetes

Sam is a nine-year-old boy who was admitted to the hospital after he passed out while playing with friends. Tests confirmed a diagnosis of insulin-dependent diabetes mellitus. Sam will be in the hospital for several days until his blood glucose is under control. During this time, he and his family will be learning about the special diet he will have to follow, how to use insulin, and how to coordinate diet, insulin, and physical activity.

1. The details of diabetes mellitus are reserved for Chapter 25, but for now, describe the steps that will be necessary to develop a nutrition care plan.
2. From the limited description above, what problems will need to be addressed in the nutrition care plan?
3. Different health care professionals will be working with Sam to help him deal with diabetes. For example, nurses will be teaching him how to give insulin injections, and dietitians will be helping him understand his diet. Describe information these professionals might need to communicate with each other.

■ STUDY QUESTIONS ■

1. What are the steps in the nutrition care process that can be used to identify nutrition problems and take corrective measures?
2. What two services should the nutrition care plan deliver to a client?
3. Discuss the problems that some people encounter with food in the hospital. Describe some ways health care professionals can help both adults and children alleviate these problems.
4. How can you use the medical record to communicate a client's nutrition needs to other health care professionals? What kinds of information about nutrition should you record? Where else can you find written information about a client's nutrient or nutrition education needs?
5. Discuss some ways other than written records that health care professionals can share concerns about a client's nutrition needs.

■ CLINICAL APPLICATION QUESTIONS ■

1. Think for a moment about the foodservice system in a typical hospital, where clients mark menus listing foods appropriate to their respective diets. First, these menus must be marked by the client (who may not be in the room when the menus are delivered, or may be too ill, too apathetic, or simply unable to make food selections); then, the menus must be collected from the client; next, the menus must find their way to the dietary offices; and finally, the foods selected must be correctly assembled on trays, taken to the correct hospital floor, and delivered to the proper client. Do you see how easily errors can occur in the food delivery process? For each step in the delivery process described above, list at least one way an error can occur. Suggest ways for preventing some of these errors. Consider what impacts your suggestions might have on the budget and staff.
2. You are a nurse visiting a client who recently suffered a heart attack and is now on a special diet. The client tells you that the dietitian has talked to him about his diet and he is totally confused. He confides that diet is the last thing on his mind right now. What actions should you take?
3. You are a nurse working with an elderly client who is recovering from surgery and who has been unable to eat food for two days. What steps could help you uncover problems the client might be having with food? What steps might you take to correct the problems you identify?

NUTRITION IN PRACTICE 14

The Health Care Team and Nutrition Support

Teamwork in health care can accomplish many things more efficiently than can individual professionals working solo. Fortunately for many clients, the value of health care teams is increasingly recognized.

Each professional on a health care team possesses specialized knowledge. By working together, the members can integrate their knowledge and provide the client with the benefits of their combined expertise. Team members also benefit—by learning how the others contribute to the care process, each discovers which person can do each job efficiently.

Who serves on a health care team?

A health care team consists of a group of professionals specializing in a particular medical disorder. Core members of many health care teams include physicians, nurses, dietitians, and pharmacists. Other members vary according to the disorder. A respiratory therapist would be a primary member of a pulmonary rehabilitation team, for example. Physical therapists and occupational therapists frequently participate on rehabilitation or burn teams. Social workers work with health care teams to provide solutions to financial problems and to coordinate home care programs.

Whenever nutrition is important to client care, a dietitian serves as a member of the health care team. Additionally, in cases where nutrition is the central concern of therapy, as in the case of people being fed by vein or by tube, a special nutrition support team may oversee client care.

What do team members do?

Team members maintain records and meet frequently to review the progress of each client in their care. They often serve as consultants to the rest of the hospital staff, providing information, answering questions, and solving problems that arise in client care. Team members also carry responsibility for keeping abreast of new developments in their respective fields. They analyze new products, review current research, and communicate their findings to other team members.

The physician assumes primary responsibility for client care: diagnosing the client's medical problems, performing medical procedures, and coordinating and prescribing appropriate therapy. The physician frequently supervises the activities of other team members and makes the final decisions on what steps to take to correct problems.

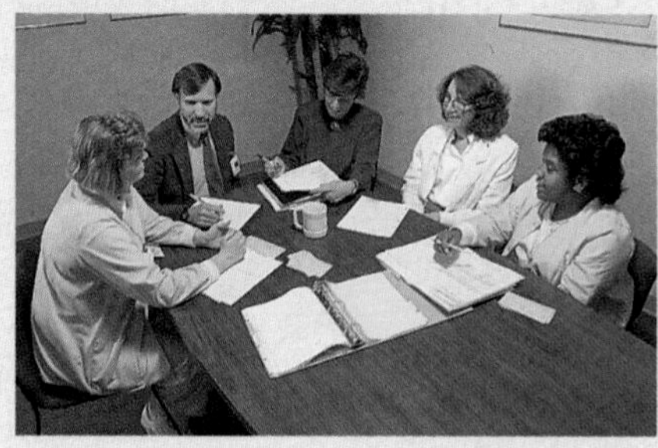

The team approach helps to ensure safe and effective nutrition support.

The nurse plays a central role in client care management and communications with the client, family, and nursing staff. The nurse often explains medical procedures and treatment plans to clients and their caregivers. In addition, the team supervises other nurses who care for each client to assure that they are delivering appropriate and optimal care. The team nurse teaches the staff nurses, as a group and individually, the rationales for various procedures and the appropriate administration techniques. The nurse also assists in training physicians and other health care professionals.

The team nurse often coordinates discharge from the hospital. Discharge responsibilities include discussing with clients any steps they will need to follow at home, making sure clients have written instructions, providing them with appropriate supplies and equipment, and arranging for return visits and follow-up care.

What about the dietitian and the pharmacist?

The dietitian, as the team's nutrition expert, determines the client's nutrition requirements, recommends appropriate diet therapy, and translates diet orders into foods or feedings. The dietitian visits clients regularly to monitor nutrient intakes and nutrition status and to help them understand and cope with their unique feeding situations. The dietitian also instructs clients about their diets and prepares them to follow special diets at home.

Dietitians provide in-service training for other dietitians and nurses on nutrition-related topics in their specialty area. If particular nutrition problems arise, dietitians actively devise solutions and see that they are carried out. The team dietitian also acts as a liaison between the team and the dietary department.

The pharmacist assists the physician in managing the client's drug therapy, alerts team members to interactions of drugs with other drugs and with nutrients, and identifies complications that may be drug related. The pharmacist may recommend an optimal drug administration schedule and educates clients about the proper use of their medications. The pharmacist also serves as a liaison between the pharmacy and the health care team.

Figure 14–1
The Nutrition Support Team

The physician
- Diagnoses medical problems
- Performs medical procedures
- Coordinates and prescribes therapy
- Directs and supervises team
- Approves guidelines and protocols
- Consults with other physicians

The nurse
- Assesses nursing needs
- Performs direct client care
- Explains medical procedures and treatment plans
- Instructs clients regarding medical care
- Acts as a liaison between team and nursing staff
- Coordinates discharge plans

All team members
- Review current research
- Analyze new products
- Develop guidelines
- Provide in-service training
- Monitor clients
- Correct problems
- Educate clients
- Evaluate the outcome of the care provided

The dietitian
- Assesses nutrition status
- Determines clients' nutrient needs
- Recommends appropriate diet therapy
- Reevaluates clients regularly
- Instructs clients about their diets
- Acts as a liaison between the team and the dietary department

The pharmacist
- Recommends appropriate drug therapy
- Identifies drug-drug and drug-nutrient interactions
- Identifies drug-related complications
- Educates clients about their medications
- Acts as a liaison between the team and the pharmacy

Describe how a health care team solves nutrition problems.

Figure 14–1 shows an example of the special version of a health care team that provides nutrition support and shows how the team members interact. Members of the nutrition support team share many of the responsibilities for client care, but each one also provides unique services.

Team members communicate with each other both informally and formally. They may share office space and see each other throughout the day, but their primary time for managing team responsibilities is during rounds, when the entire team visits each client as a group and discusses the client's care.

During rounds, the physician oversees the discussions and takes recommendations for changes. For example, the dietitian may express concern for a client who is unable to eat dinners because painful treatments have been scheduled each day just prior to the meal. The pharmacist recommends pain medication that will be effective through dinner to help alleviate this problem. The physician and pharmacist see no problem with adding this drug to the client's therapy, and the physician writes the medication order. The nurse makes sure that staff nurses working with the client understand the rationale for the new drug therapy and the importance of its timing. Working together, the team has efficiently identified and solved a problem that might have cost great effort otherwise.

Do such teams always work with one client at a time?

No, team rounds often serve as avenues of communication for problems that affect more than one client's care. For example, while discussing a client who has undergone a nitrogen balance study, the dietitian may mention that problems have occurred repeatedly with this procedure in the last month. The nurse then recalls that many of the new nurses are having difficulty with the procedure and suggests an in-service training session on the proper techniques for nitrogen balance studies. The nurse agrees to conduct the in-service training and the dietitian joins in to explain how nitrogen balance studies help determine protein needs.

During rounds, team members may bring up current research that may affect the care they give clients, or they may share information about new products they may wish to consider for their clients. The team then decides if further action is warranted.

Health care teams not only contribute to optimal client care, but they can also effectively reduce hospital costs by providing the most efficient use of personnel and supplies.[1] Nutrition in Practice 19 itemizes other ways nutrition support teams help contain health care costs.

To appreciate the team approach, remember the adage, "Two heads are better than one." In this case, several heads are better still. Clients benefit when they have many eyes noting problems and many brains searching for solutions. In short, teamwork works.

■ NOTES ■

1. M. F. Roberts and G. M. Levine, Nutrition support team recommendations can reduce hospital costs, *Nutrition in Clinical Practice* 7 (1992): 227–230.

15

Nutrition during Pregnancy and Infancy

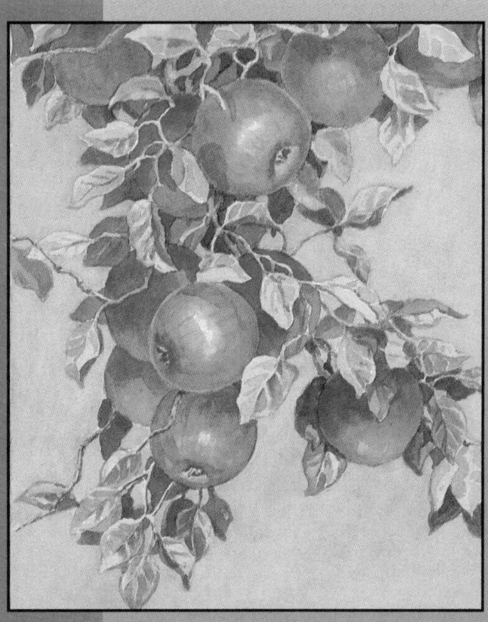

CONTENTS

The effects of nutrition extend over years. A woman's nutrition prior to and throughout pregnancy and lactation affects not only her own health but also the growth, development, and health of her child, even long after it has been born. Similarly, sound nutrition is vital to healthy infant development.

Pregnancy: The Impact of Nutrition on the Future

The woman who enters pregnancy with full nutrient stores, sound eating habits, and a healthy body weight has done a lot already to ensure an optimal pregnancy outcome. Then, during the pregnancy itself, if she eats a variety of nutrient-dense foods, her own and her infant's health will benefit further.

low birthweight (LBW): a birthweight less than 5½ lb (2500 g); indicates probable poor health in the newborn and poor nutrition status of the mother during pregnancy. Normal birthweight for a full-term baby is 6½ to 8¾ lb (about 3000 to 4000 g).

Low-birthweight infants are of two different types. Some are **premature;** they are born early and are of a weight **appropriate for gestational age (AGA).** Others have suffered growth failure in the uterus; they may or may not be born early, but they are **small for gestational age (SGA).**

fetus: (FEET-us): the developing infant from eight weeks after conception until its birth.

placenta (pla-SEN-tuh)**:** an organ that develops inside the uterus early in pregnancy in which maternal and fetal blood circulate in close proximity and exchange materials. The fetus receives nutrients and oxygen across the placenta; the mother's blood picks up carbon dioxide and other waste materials to be excreted via her lungs and kidneys.

amniotic (am-nee-OTT-ic) **sac**: the "bag of waters" in the uterus, in which the fetus floats.

umbilical (um-BIL-ih-cul) **cord**: the ropelike structure through which the fetus's veins and arteries reach the placenta; the route of nourishment and oxygen into the fetus and the route of waste disposal from the fetus.

uterus (YOO-ter-us): the womb, the muscular organ within which the infant develops before birth.

Preparing for Pregnancy

Full nutrient stores *before* pregnancy are essential both to conception and to healthy infant development during pregnancy. In the early weeks, before many women are even aware that they are pregnant, significant developmental changes occur that depend on a woman's nutrient stores.

Prepregnancy Weight Appropriate weight for height prior to pregnancy also benefits pregnancy outcome. Weights outside the normal range (10 percent below, or 20 percent above, standard weight for height and age) present some medical risks.[1] Underweight women are therefore advised to gain weight before becoming pregnant; and overweight women to lose excess weight. Guidelines for weight gain and loss were offered in Chapter 9.

Infant Birthweight Infant birthweight strongly correlates with prepregnancy weight and is the most potent single predictor of the infant's future health and survival. A low-birthweight baby is statistically more likely than a normal-weight baby to contract diseases, and low-birthweight babies are nearly 40 times more likely to die in the first month of life than normal-weight babies are.[2] Low socioeconomic status also impairs fetal development by limiting access to medical care and nutritious foods.[3]

Healthy Support Tissues A major reason why the mother's prepregnancy nutrition is so crucial to a healthy pregnancy is that it determines whether she will be able to grow healthy support tissues: the placenta, the amniotic sac, and the umbilical cord, as well as the uterus (see Figure 15–1). Malnutrition prior to and around conception keeps these tissues from developing fully.[4]

Nutrient Needs during Pregnancy

Between the moment of conception and the moment of birth, innumerable events determine the course and outcome of fetal development and, ultimately, the health of the newborn infant. Each organ needs nutrients most during its own intensive growth period. A nutrient deficiency during

Figure 15–1
The Placenta
The placenta is composed of spongy tissue in which fetal blood and maternal blood flow side by side, each in its own vessels. The maternal blood transfers oxygen and nutrients to the fetus's blood and picks up fetal wastes to be excreted by the mother. Thus the placenta facilitates the nutritive, respiratory, and excretory functions that the fetus's digestive system, lungs, and kidneys will provide after birth.

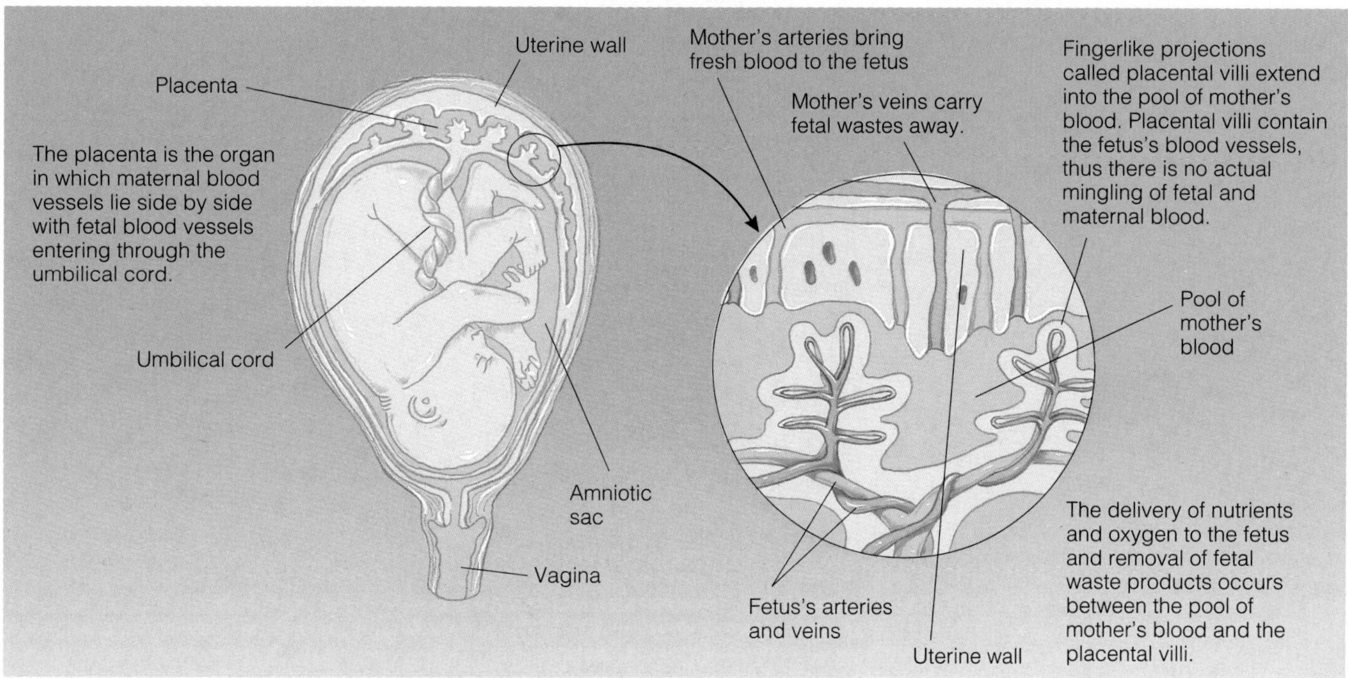

one stage of development might affect the heart and, during another stage, the developing limbs.

A woman's nutrient needs during pregnancy and lactation are higher than at any other time in her adult life and are greater for certain nutrients than for others. Figure 15–2 (see p. 364) compares the nutrient needs of nonpregnant, pregnant, and lactating women. A study of the figure reveals some of the key needs.

Energy During pregnancy, one of the smallest increases is in the need for food energy. An intake of only 15 percent more than the allowance for nonpregnant women is recommended; this amounts to only about 300 kcalories per day and only during the second and third trimesters. Pregnant teenagers, underweight women, or physically active women may need more.

Energy RDA during pregnancy (2nd and 3rd trimesters): +300 kcal/day.

Pregnancy is often divided into thirds called *trimesters*.

Protein The RDA suggests an added 10 grams of protein per day throughout pregnancy. Food consumption surveys indicate that many women in the United States exceed the recommended protein intake each day, and so they already receive the 10 grams of additional daily protein

Protein RDA during pregnancy: +10 g/day.

Figure 15–2
Comparison of Nutrient RDA of Nonpregnant, Pregnant, and Lactating Women

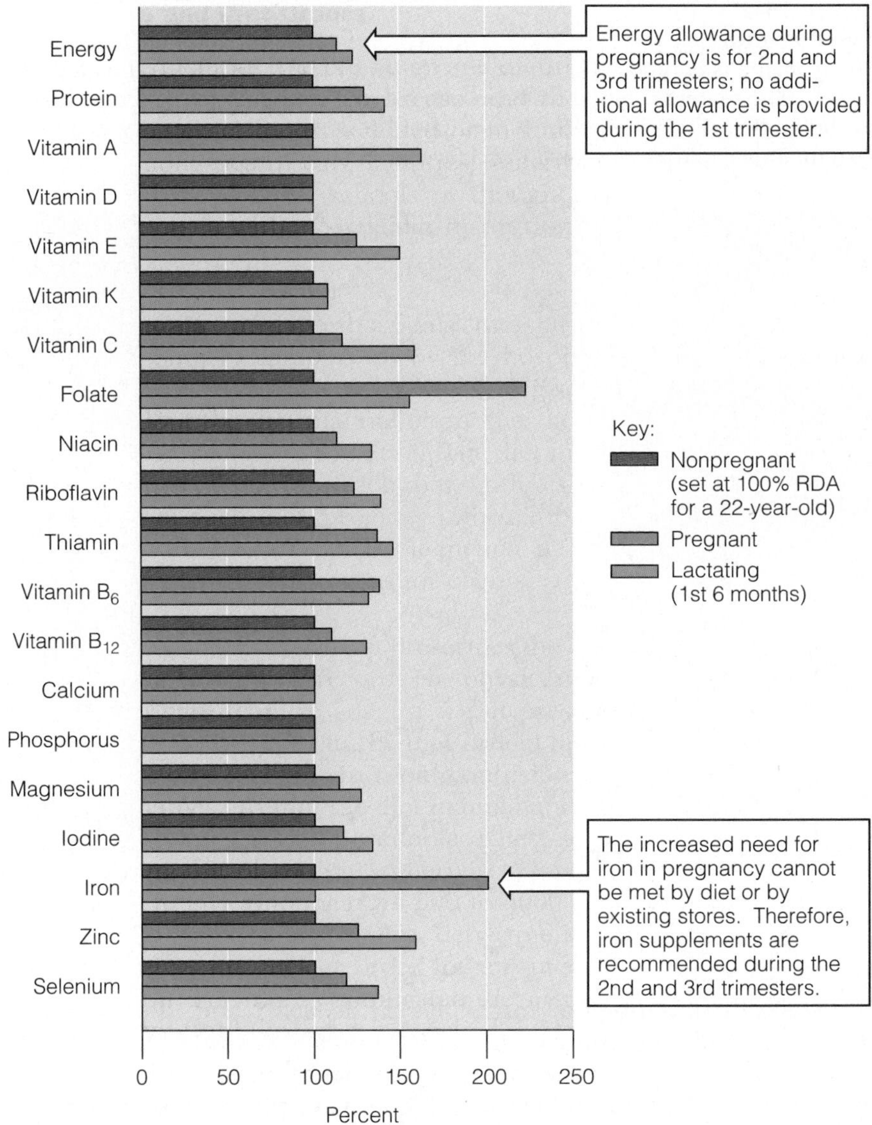

recommended for pregnancy.[5] Adequate protein during pregnancy is important, but excessive protein may have adverse effects, as Chapter 4 described.

For people who eat no meat or other foods of animal origin, available choices of protein-rich foods are limited, and the need for abundant high-quality protein during pregnancy demands careful attention. Consuming adequate food energy each day including several generous servings of plant protein foods such as legumes, whole grains, nuts, and seeds is imperative.

Recommended carbohydrate intake: about 50% of energy intake. In a 2000-kcal/day intake, this represents 1000 kcal of carbohydrate, or about 250 g. Four cups of milk will contribute about 50 g carbohydrate. An apple provides 15 g carbohydrate, and a slice of bread provides 15 g, so generous intakes of fruit and bread are clearly beneficial.

Carbohydrate Pregnant women need generous amounts of carbohydrate to spare the protein they eat. If added energy is needed, it is best obtained from carbohydrate.

Table 15–1
Women at Nutritional Risk during Pregnancy

- Women who ordinarily consume an inadequate diet (for example, those who avoid consumption of all animal-derived foods)
- Women who are lactose intolerant
- Women who are carrying multiple fetuses
- Women who smoke cigarettes or use alcohol or illicit drugs
- Women who are underweight or overweight at conception
- Women who gain insufficient or excessive weight during pregnancy
- Women who lack nutrition knowledge or who have insufficient financial resources to purchase adequate food
- Adolescents

Source: Compiled from information in National Academy of Sciences, Food and Nutrition Board. *Nutrition During Pregnancy* (Washington, D.C.: National Academy Press, 1990).

Vitamins The vitamins required for rapid cell proliferation—folate and vitamin B_{12}—are needed in large amounts during pregnancy. New cells are laid down at a tremendous pace as the fetus grows and develops. At the same time, the mother's red blood cell number rises, so the RDA for folate more than doubles during pregnancy—to 400 micrograms a day.

As described in Nutrition in Practice 7, folate deficiency is associated with a group of birth defects known as neural tube defects. Because neural tube defects arise early in pregnancy, the U.S. Public Health Service recommends ensuring that women derive 400 micrograms of folate (from foods) each day throughout their childbearing years.[6] Routine folate supplementation is not recommended, but if a pregnant woman seems not to be eating well enough to obtain the recommended amount from foods, then folate supplementation of 300 micrograms per day is recommended.[7] For women who eat all-plant diets, a daily vitamin B_{12} supplement is also recommended.[8]

Dietary improvements are always preferred as the means of correcting nutrient inadequacies, but sometimes nutrient supplementation is necessary. The National Academy of Sciences subcommittee for the publication *Nutrition During Pregnancy* identifies certain women as being nutritionally at risk during pregnancy (see Table 15–1).[9] Unfortunately, the categories of "at risk" women undoubtedly include most pregnant women in the United States.[10] The subcommittee recommends a multivitamin-mineral supplement containing the nutrient amounts shown in Table 15–2 for these women.

Folate RDA during pregnancy: 400 μg/day.

Foods containing folate:
- Green leafy vegetables.
- Legumes.
- Liver.
- Orange juice and cantaloupe.
- Other vegetables.
- Whole-wheat products.

Table 15–2
Nutrient Supplements during Pregnancy[a]

NUTRIENT	AMOUNT
Folate	300 μg
Vitamin B_6	2 mg
Vitamin C	50 mg
Vitamin D	5 μg
Calcium	250 mg
Copper	2 mg
Iron	30 mg
Zinc	15 mg

[a]For pregnant women at nutritional risk (see Table 15–1).

Source: Reprinted with permission. *Nutrition During Pregnancy*. Copyright 1990 by the National Academy of Sciences. Courtesy of the National Academy Press, Washington, D.C.

Minerals for Bones: Calcium, Phosphorus, and Magnesium The minerals involved in building the skeleton—calcium, phosphorus, and magnesium—are in great demand during pregnancy. Intestinal absorption of calcium doubles early in pregnancy, when the mother's bones store the mineral. Later, as the fetal bones begin to calcify, there is a dramatic shift of calcium across the placenta. Indirect evidence suggests that the calcium added to the mother's bones early in pregnancy is what is withdrawn to build the fetus's bones later.[11]

Calcium RDA during pregnancy: 1200 mg/day.

Four cups of milk a day will supply 1200 mg calcium. For other food sources, see Chapter 8.

Phosphorus RDA during pregnancy: 1200 mg/day.

Magnesium RDA during pregnancy: 320 mg/day.

For women whose prepregnancy calcium intakes are below recommendations, as most are, increased calcium intakes may be especially important. Milk products offer many advantages over supplements, as emphasized in earlier chapters. Women under 25 who consume less than 600 milligrams of calcium a day, however, are advised to take supplements.[12]

Fluoride Mineralization of the baby's teeth begins in the fifth month after conception. For this and for the bones, fluoride may be needed. Fluoride does cross the placenta, but whether the placenta can defend against excess intakes is questionable. Therefore, fluoride supplements are not recommended for pregnant women who drink fluoridated water. For women who live in communities without fluoridated water, a fluoride supplement may protect fetal teeth.

Iron RDA during pregnancy: 30 mg/day.

Iron The body conserves iron especially well during pregnancy: menstruation ceases, and absorption of iron increases up to threefold due to a rise in the blood's iron-absorbing and iron-carrying protein, transferrin. Still, iron needs are so high that stores dwindle during pregnancy.

The developing fetus draws on the mother's iron stores to create stores of its own to last through the first four to six months of life. Research shows that women who enter pregnancy with iron-deficiency anemia have two to three times the normal risk of delivering low-birthweight or preterm infants.[13] Iron losses also occur with the bleeding that is inevitable at birth.

In pregnancy, hemoglobin values of 12 g are not unusual, and 11 g is where the line defining "too low" is often drawn. It is usually desirable to use more sensitive measures than hemoglobin tests if questions about the woman's iron status arise (see Chapter 13).

Few women enter pregnancy with adequate iron stores. For all women not taking supplements containing iron, a daily iron supplement containing 30 milligrams is recommended during the second and third trimesters of pregnancy.[14]

Food sources of iron:

- Liver, oysters.
- Red meat, fish, other meat.
- Dried fruits.
- Legumes (dried beans, peas, lima beans).
- Dark green vegetables.

Zinc RDA during pregnancy: 15 mg/day.

Zinc Zinc is another nutrient of vital importance in pregnancy; it is required for DNA and RNA synthesis and thus for protein synthesis and low blood zinc predicts low birthweight.[15] Zinc is most abundant in foods of high protein content, such as shellfish, meat, and nuts, but the presence of other trace elements and fiber in foods may adversely affect zinc absorption. Iron interferes with the body's absorption and use of zinc, so women taking iron supplements (more than 30 milligrams per day) may also need zinc supplements.

Food Choices Because food energy needs increase less than nutrient needs, the pregnant woman must select foods of high nutrient density. For most women, appropriate choices include foods like nonfat milk, nonfat plain yogurt, lean meats, eggs, liver, dark green vegetables, vitamin C-rich fruits, legumes, and whole-grain breads and cereals. Table 15–3 provides a suggested food pattern.

WIC A woman of limited financial means may need help in obtaining needed food and information. At the federal level, the WIC program provides nutrition education and nutritious foods to low-income pregnant women and their children. WIC provides eggs, milk, cereal, juice, cheese,

Table 15–3
Daily Food Choices for Pregnant and Lactating Women

FOOD GROUP	NUMBER OF SERVINGS Adult (Select anywhere within the range.)	NUMBER OF SERVINGS Pregnant or Lactating Women (Select higher end of the range.)
Breads/cereals	6 to 11	7 to 11
Vegetables	3 to 5	4 to 5
Fruits	2 to 4	3 to 4
Meat/meat alternates	2 to 3	3
Milk/milk products	2	3 to 4

Note: Figure 1–3 in Chapter 1 provides a detailed summary of foods in each group with serving sizes.

legumes, and peanut butter to infants, children up to age five, and pregnant and breastfeeding women who qualify financially and are at medical or nutritional risk. For infants given formula, WIC also provides iron-fortified formulas. Studies of the nutrition and health effects of WIC have found that participation in the program benefits both the iron status and the growth and development of infants and children. WIC participation during pregnancy has been shown to reduce the risks of delivering preterm or low-birthweight babies.[16]

WIC, pronounced *WICK*, is the acronym for the federal Special Supplemental Food Program for Women, Infants, and Children. The U.S. Department of Agriculture (USDA) funds WIC, and state health departments administer the program.

Food Cravings and Aversions Some women develop cravings for, or aversions to, certain foods and beverages during pregnancy. Individual food cravings during pregnancy do not seem to reflect real physiological needs.[17] In other words, a woman who craves pickles does not necessarily need salt, nor does a chocolate craving indicate a need for caffeine or fat. The craving for ice cream is the most common craving in pregnancy, but does not signify a calcium deficiency. Food aversions and cravings that arise during pregnancy are probably due to hormone-induced changes in taste and sensitivities to smells.

food craving: a deep longing for a particular food.

food aversion: a strong desire to avoid a particular food.

Cravings for nonfood items such as clay, ice, and cornstarch are known as *pica.*

Weight Gain

All pregnant women must gain weight: fetal growth and maternal health depend on it. A pregnancy weight gain of 25 to 35 pounds is recommended for women who begin pregnancy at a normal weight for height and are carrying a single fetus; for others, see the margin.[18] Some women should strive for gains at the upper ends of the target ranges, notably adolescents, who are still growing themselves. Short women (5 feet 2 inches and under) should strive for lower gains. Table 15–4 (see p. 368) shows the components of a weight gain of 30 pounds.

The ideal pattern of weight gain during pregnancy is thought to be about 2 to 4 pounds during the first three months and a pound per week thereafter. Women lose some of the weight gained during pregnancy at

Weight-gain recommendations:
- Underweight women: 28 to 40 lb (12.5 to 18 kg).
- Normal-weight women: 25 to 35 lb (11.5 to 16 kg).
- Overweight women: 15 to 25 lb (7 to 11.5 kg).
- Obese women: 13 lb minimum (6 kg minimum).
- Twin birth: 35 to 45 lb (16 to 20.5 kg).

Table 15–4
Components of Weight Gain during Pregnancy

DEVELOPMENT	WEIGHT GAIN (lb)
Infant at birth	7 ½
Placenta	1 ½
Increase in mother's blood volume to supply placenta	4
Increase in mother's fluid volume	4
Increase in size of uterus and supporting muscles	2
Increase in size of mother's breasts	2
Fluid to surround infant in amniotic sac	2
Mother's fat stores	7
Total	30

Source: The American College of Obstetricians and Gynecologists: *ACOG Guide to Planning for Pregnancy, Birth and Beyond.* ACOG, Washington, D.C.: ©1990.

Weight-for-height categories for prepregnant women are based on body mass index (BMI) measures (see Appendix E):

- Underweight BMI: <19.8.
- Normal BMI: 19.8 to 26.0.
- Overweight BMI: 26.1 to 29.0.
- Obese BMI: >29.

A prenatal weight gain grid (see Appendix E) plots the rate of weight gain during pregnancy.

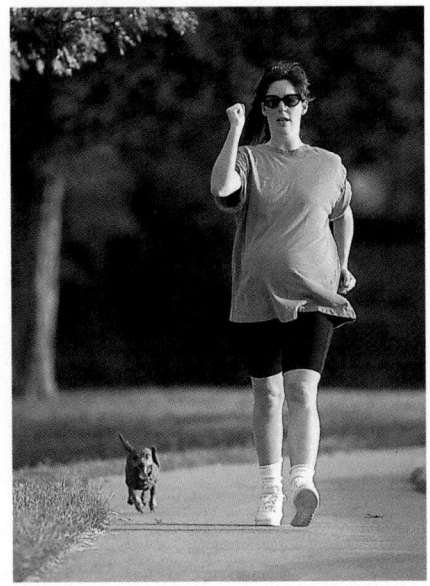

Pregnant women can enjoy the benefits of physical activity.

delivery and most of the remainder within the following few weeks or months, as blood volume returns to normal and accumulated fluids are lost.

If a woman has gained more than the expected amount of weight early in pregnancy, she should not try to diet in the last weeks. A sudden large weight gain, however, is a danger signal that may indicate the onset of pregnancy-induced hypertension (see next page).

Weight gain during pregnancy, like prepregnancy weight, directly relates to infant birthweight.[19] If the mother does not gain all of the weight recommended, she may give birth to an underweight baby.

Physical Activity

Chapter 10 described another lifestyle component that promotes health and well-being: physical activity. The active, physically fit woman experiencing a normal pregnancy can continue her regular activities throughout pregnancy, adjusting the duration and intensity as needed. Her rewards may include reduced stress, better weight control, an easier labor, better posture, less back pain, prevention of gestational diabetes (see next page), an improved mood and body image, and a faster recovery from childbirth.[20] Potential risks of physical activity during pregnancy include acute conditions such as altered fetal heart rate and hyperthermia and other possible hazards such as premature labor or reduced birthweight, but these seldom outweigh the benefits.

As is true for everyone, the frequency, duration, and intensity of the activity affect the likelihood of the benefits or risks. Physically fit, low-risk pregnant women can probably tolerate longer activity sessions and more exertion than is currently recommended.[21] Table 15–5 provides some guidelines for physical activity during pregnancy, but every pregnant women should consult with her own health care provider regarding safe activity limits.

Table 15–5
Exercise Guidelines for Pregnancy

- Limit strenuous activity to 15 minutes or less.
- Stop exercising if you feel overheated.
- Drink plenty of fluids before and after exercise.
- Avoid exercising in hot, humid weather; avoid overheating.
- Protect your abdomen from injury, especially in games like baseball or basketball in which accidents are likely.
- Discontinue any exercise that causes discomfort.
- Do not exercise while lying on your back after the fourth month.
- Do not allow your heart rate to exceed 140 beats per minute.
- Eat enough to support the energy needs of pregnancy and of exercise.

Problems in Pregnancy

Just as adequate nutrition and normal weight gain support the health of the mother and growth of the fetus, maternal diseases detract from health and growth. If discovered early, many diseases can be controlled—another reason why early prenatal care is recommended. Some nutrition measures can help alleviate the most common problems encountered during pregnancy.

Gestational Diabetes Pregnancy precipitates the onset of diabetes in some women because placental hormones alter the way insulin works. This condition is known as gestational diabetes. Blood glucose becomes abnormal during pregnancy but usually returns to normal after the infant is born. In about one-third of such cases, however, diabetes becomes permanent. To ensure that the problems of diabetes are dealt with promptly, women with one or more of the risk factors listed in Table 25-6 (p. 602) receive glucose tolerance tests during the sixth month of pregnancy.[22]

gestational diabetes: the appearance of abnormal glucose tolerance during pregnancy, with subsequent return to normal postpartum.

Risk factors for gestational diabetes:
- Age 30 or older.
- Obesity or excessive weight gain.
- Complications in previous pregnancies.
- Symptoms of diabetes.
- Family history of diabetes.

Without proper management, gestational diabetes can lead to infant sickness and death. Women with gestational diabetes need to select foods rich in complex carbohydrates, such as legumes, vegetables, and whole-grain products, and should limit their intakes of concentrated sweets. Optimal protein intakes are also important. Insulin therapy may be required if blood glucose fails to normalize.

Hypertension Hypertension in pregnancy can cause maternal death, infant death, retarded growth, lung problems, and other birth defects. Prenatal care includes keeping track of maternal blood pressure throughout pregnancy and, if hypertension occurs, initiating treatment promptly. Medical attention is required; salt restriction is not a part of treatment until and unless the kidneys prove unable to handle a normal sodium load. A normal salt intake is necessary for health.

Pregnancy-Induced Hypertension and Preeclampsia Some women develop a type of hypertension during the second half of pregnancy that normalizes afterward, a condition known as pregnancy-induced hypertension (PIH). PIH is a common medical complication seen in pregnancy

pregnancy-induced hypertension (PIH): high blood pressure that develops in the second half of pregnancy.

and may signal the onset of preeclampsia, which involves not only high blood pressure but protein in the urine and fluid retention (edema). The edema of PIH is a whole-body edema, distinct from the localized fluid retention women normally experience late in pregnancy.

Preeclampsia affects almost all of the mother's organs—the circulatory system, liver, kidneys, and brain. If it progresses, she may experience convulsions; when this occurs, the condition is called eclampsia.

preeclampsia: a condition characterized by hypertension, fluid retention, and protein in the urine.

The normal edema of pregnancy responds to gravity: blood pools in the ankles. The edema of PIH is a generalized edema. The distinction helps with diagnosis.

eclampsia: a severe stage of preeclampsia characterized by convulsions.

Morning Sickness Unlike the conditions just discussed, the nausea of "morning" (actually, anytime) sickness is benign, although distressing to some women. It arises from the hormonal changes taking place early in pregnancy, ranges from mild queasiness to debilitating nausea, and afflicts more than half of all pregnant women. One expert who has worked with women hospitalized with the condition notes that a trigger for morning sickness is what she calls the "radar nose of pregnancy."[23] Many women complain that smells, especially cooking smells, make them sick. Thus, minimizing odors is a key to alleviating morning sickness.

After much frustration and failure in treating morning sickness with the traditional saltine crackers and ginger ale, this innovative specialist began to ask her clients the question, "If you could have anything you wanted to eat right now, what would it be?" Much to her surprise, her clients often named foods such as spaghetti and meat sauce, potato chips, and lemonade. When she could serve these foods quickly, the results were positive: the women felt better. While foods such as potato chips are no replacement for more nutritious foods, they can, in some cases, serve a temporary role to keep women out of the hospital. Women like to eat ice chips when feeling nauseated, but plain water often makes them throw up. It seems the tartness or sweetness of lemonade prevents this from happening. In short, morning sickness seems to be alleviated best by the foods and beverages most desired at a given time. The margin note offers further suggestions for alleviating nausea.

Hints for controlling nausea and vomiting:

- Eat frequent small meals. Keep something in your stomach.
- Avoid foods with strong odors if the odors make you feel nauseated.
- Everybody is different. Keep track of what you eat and when you feel nauseated, and do what's best for you.
- Take prenatal vitamin and iron supplements on a full stomach or at a time of day when you feel well.

Heartburn Heartburn, a burning sensation in the lower esophagus near the heart, is common during pregnancy and is also benign. As the growing fetus puts increasing pressure on a woman's stomach, acid may back up and create a burning sensation in her throat. Tips to relieve heartburn are listed in the margin.

To prevent or relieve heartburn:

- Eat frequent small meals.
- Drink liquids between meals.
- Avoid spicy or greasy foods.
- Sit up while eating.
- Wait an hour after eating before lying down.
- Wait 2 hours after eating before exercising.

Constipation As the hormones of pregnancy alter muscle tone and the thriving infant crowds intestinal organs, an expectant mother may complain of constipation, another harmless but annoying condition. A high-fiber diet, exercise, and a plentiful fluid intake will help relieve this condition. Also, responding promptly to the urge to defecate can help. Laxatives should be used only as prescribed by the physician. Mineral oil should not be used, because it robs the body of fat-soluble vitamins.

Practices to Avoid

A general guideline for the pregnant woman is to eat a normal, healthy diet and practice moderation. A woman's daily choices during pregnancy take on enormous importance. Forewarned, pregnant women can choose to abstain from or avoid potentially harmful practices.

Cigarette Smoking Smoking adversely affects the pregnant woman's nutrition status, which in turn impairs fetal nutrition. Cigarette smoking increases iron needs and reduces the availability of vitamin B_{12}, vitamin C, folate, and zinc.[24] Smoking also restricts the blood supply to the growing fetus, and so limits the delivery of oxygen and nutrients and the removal of wastes. Smoking also causes these adverse effects: premature births, spontaneous abortions (fetal deaths), and increased risks of infants' dying early in life.[25] In addition, sudden infant death syndrome (SIDS), the sudden, unexplained death of an infant, has been positively linked to the mother's cigarette smoking during pregnancy and even to postnatal exposure to smoke in the household.[26] Research also shows that children born to women who smoke during pregnancy may be intellectually impaired.[27] Cigarette smoking is by far the single most important modifiable risk factor responsible for fetal growth retardation in developed countries.[28] In short, the scientific and medical literature confirms over and over again that smoking during pregnancy is dangerous.

sudden infant death syndrome (SIDS): the unexpected and unexplained death of an apparently well infant; the most common cause of death of infants between the second week and the end of the first year of life; also called *crib death.*

Caffeine Caffeine crosses the placenta, and the fetus has a limited ability to metabolize it. So far, no convincing evidence indicates that caffeine causes birth defects in human beings (as it does in animals), but limited evidence suggests that moderate-to-heavy use may lower infant birthweight.[29] One well-designed, carefully controlled study of caffeine's effects on pregnancy outcome showed that moderate caffeine consumption (3 cups of coffee daily) is not a risk factor for spontaneous abortion or growth retardation.[30] All things considered, it seems most sensible to limit caffeine consumption to the equivalent of one cup of coffee or two 12-ounce cola beverages a day.

A table of the caffeine amounts in beverages and medications is provided in Nutrition in Practice 20.

Medicines Drugs taken during pregnancy can cause serious birth defects. Even aspirin can do harm, as revealed by research on more than 3000 pregnant women.[31] Aspirin taken late in pregnancy adversely affects fetal circulation and uterine contractions.[32] Chronic use of aspirin may also cause iron deficiency. For reasons such as these, women are advised to take medicines only if their physicians deem it necessary to protect their life and health.

Illicit Drugs Marijuana or cocaine use during pregnancy adversely affects fetal growth and development.[33] Such drugs of abuse pass easily through the placenta and impair fetal development.[34] Moreover, newborns born to drug users face low birthweight, cardiovascular problems, and increased risk of death. If they survive, their behavior at birth is abnormal.[35] Unfortunately, use of illicit drugs is common among pregnant women. One study of about 30,000 women in California found that 11 percent tested positive for alcohol and illicit drugs.[36]

Dieting Dieting, even for short periods, is hazardous during pregnancy. Low-carbohydrate diets or fasts that cause ketosis deprive the growing brain of needed glucose and may impair its development. Energy restriction during pregnancy is dangerous for all women, regardless of their prepregnancy weights.

fetal alcohol syndrome (FAS): the cluster of symptoms seen in a person whose mother consumed excess alcohol during her pregnancy; includes mental and physical retardation with facial and other body deformities.

Alcohol Alcohol can cause irreversible brain damage and mental and physical retardation in the fetus—the abnormalities that define fetal alcohol syndrome (FAS). The potential for fetal damage arises when the mother's liver receives more alcohol than it can detoxify. Alcohol-laden blood then circulates to all parts of the mother's body and freely crosses the placenta to impair fetal development. Alcohol also interferes with placental transport of nutrients to the fetus.[37]

Of the leading causes of mental retardation, FAS is the only one that is totally preventable.[38] The surgeon general has issued a statement that pregnant women should drink absolutely no alcohol. All containers of beer, wine, and liquor now must carry a warning to this effect.

Adolescent Pregnancy

Each year in the United States, about one million adolescent girls between the ages of 15 and 19 become pregnant. Of these, about half choose to continue their pregnancies.[39] Many teenage women, especially the youngest ones, have not had time to store the nutrients needed to support their own rapid growth and development, much less nutrients needed to support pregnancy and the developing fetus. Nutrient shortages place both mother and infant at risk. Pregnant teenagers have more miscarriages, premature births, stillbirths, and low-birthweight infants than do pregnant adult women. Their greatest risk, though, is death of the infant: mothers under 15 bear more babies who die within the first year than do women in any other age group. Clearly, teenage pregnancy is a major public health problem.

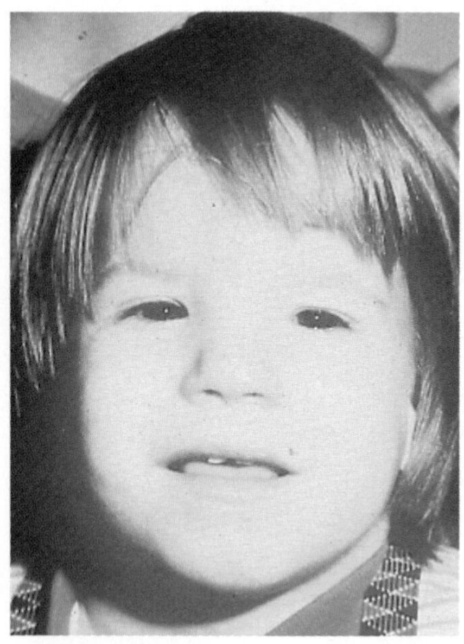

These facial traits are typical of fetal alcohol syndrome, caused by drinking during pregnancy—low nasal bridge, short eyelid opening, underdeveloped groove in center of the upper lip, small midface, short nose, and small head circumference.

Pregnant teenagers suffer many illnesses. The rates of PIH are 50 percent higher in teens than in older women. Other common problems of teen pregnancies are iron-deficiency anemia and prolonged labor.[40]

To support their own and fetal needs, young teenagers (13 to 16 years old) are encouraged to strive for pregnancy weight gains at the upper ends of the ranges recommended for pregnant women.[41] Those who gain between 30 and 35 pounds during pregnancy have lower risks of delivering low-birthweight infants.[42] Adequate nutrition can substantially improve the health of the mother and infant; it is an indispensable component of prenatal care.[43] Pregnant and lactating teenagers can use the Daily Food Guide presented in Table 15–3 (on p. 367), making sure to select at least 4 servings of milk or milk products daily.

Breastfeeding

The American Academy of Pediatrics recommends that infants receive breast milk for the first 6 to 12 months of life.[44] The American Dietetic Association advocates breastfeeding for the nutritional health it confers on the infant as well as for the physiological, social, economic, and other benefits it gives to the mother.[45] Breast milk's unique nutrient composition and protective factors promote optimal infant health and development. The only acceptable alternative to breast milk is iron-fortified formula.[46] Adequate nutrition of the mother supports successful lactation, and without it, lactation is likely to falter or fail.

The Mother's Nutrient Needs

By continuing to eat nutrient-dense foods, not restricting weight gain unduly, and enjoying ample food and fluid at frequent intervals throughout lactation, the mother who chooses to breastfeed her infant will be nutritionally prepared to do so. An inadequate diet does not support the stamina, patience, and self-confidence that nursing an infant demands. Figure 15–2 (p. 364) shows the differences between a lactating woman's nutrient needs and those of a nonpregnant woman, and Table 15–3 (p. 367) shows a food pattern that meets those needs.

Food Energy A nursing mother produces about 25 ounces of milk a day, more or less, depending primarily on the infant's demand for milk.[47] This milk output amounts to about 525 kcalories per day, and the mother's body requires extra energy to produce it. The energy allowance for a woman during the first six months of lactation is a generous 640 kcalories a day above her ordinary need. The Committee on Dietary Allowances suggests that 500 kcalories come from added food, and the rest from the body stores of fat accumulated during pregnancy for that purpose. Some research suggests that many women may need less energy for milk production than current recommendations.[48] Severe energy restriction (less than 1500 kcalories per day), however, hinders milk production and can compromise the mother's health.[49]

Maternal Weight Loss The period of lactation is the natural time for a woman to lose the extra body fat that was accumulated during pregnancy. If she chooses nutrient-dense foods, she will gradually lose weight, even though her energy intake may be greater than normal.[50] One study found that breastfeeding or a combination of breastfeeding and formula feeding led to faster loss of body weight during the first month after women delivered their babies than formula feeding only.[51] After the first month, however, no significant effect of breastfeeding on weight loss was observed. Results of other studies examining the relationship between feeding method and loss of body weight and body fat are inconsistent.[52] Most women lose 1 to 2 pounds a month during the first four to six months of lactation; some may lose more; and others may maintain or even gain weight.

Supplements Most lactating women can obtain all the nutrients they need from a well-balanced diet without taking vitamin-mineral supplements. If a woman's diet is found to be inadequate in one or more nutrients, consumption of foods rich in those nutrients or appropriate nutrient supplementation can be recommended. Women can produce milk that contains adequate protein, carbohydrate, fat, folate, and most

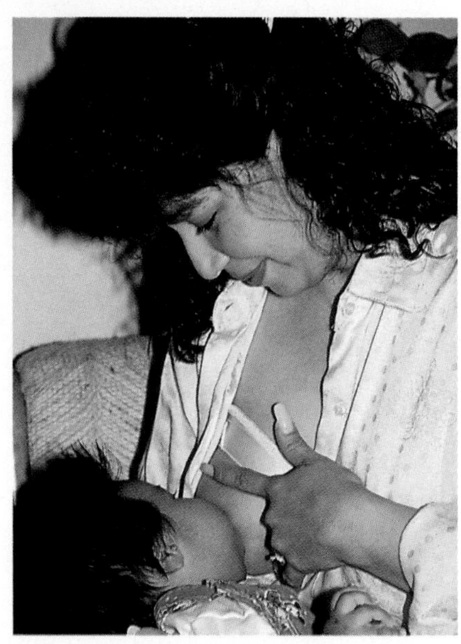

Breastfeeding is a natural extension of pregnancy—the mother's body continues to nourish the infant.

minerals, even when their own supplies are limited.[53] The milk's quality is maintained at the expense of maternal stores. The nutrients in breast milk that are most likely to decline in response to prolonged inadequate maternal intakes are vitamins B_6, B_{12}, A, and D.[54]

Water Despite previous misconceptions, drinking more fluid does not enable a mother to produce more breast milk.[55] Nevertheless, a lactating woman needs to drink at least 2 quarts of liquids each day to protect herself from dehydration. A convenient way to ensure adequate fluid consumption is to drink a glass of milk, juice, or water each time the baby nurses, as well as at each meal.

Particular Foods Foods with strong or spicy flavors (such as garlic or onion) may alter the taste of breast milk. A sudden change in the taste of the milk may annoy some infants. Infants who are sensitive to particular foods such as cow's milk protein may become uncomfortable when the mother's diet includes these foods. Most nursing mothers should drink cow's milk, however; the nutrients it provides contribute significantly to both the infant's and the mother's health.

Contraindications to Breastfeeding

Some substances impair maternal milk production or enter the breast milk and interfere with infant development. Some medical conditions prohibit breastfeeding.

Alcohol Alcohol easily enters breast milk. One study showed that the alcohol concentration of breast milk peaks within one hour after ingestion of even small amounts of alcohol (½ ounce).[56] In this study, alcohol consumption by lactating women significantly reduced the breast milk intakes of their infants. In the past, alcohol has been recommended to lactating mothers to ease milk production, despite a lack of scientific support for such recommendations. The research described here suggests that in general, alcohol consumption by lactating women should be discouraged.

Caffeine Excessive caffeine consumption during lactation may cause irritability and wakefulness in the breastfed infant. As during pregnancy, caffeine consumption should be moderate.

Smoking Health care professionals should actively discourage smoking by lactating women. Research shows that lactating women who smoke produce less milk, and milk with a lower fat content, than mothers who don't smoke.[57] Smoking also exerts numerous harmful effects on both mother and child.[58]

Maternal Illness If a woman has an ordinary cold, she can go on nursing without worry. If susceptible, the infant will catch it from her anyway, and thanks to immunological protection, a breastfed baby may be less susceptible than a formula-fed baby would be. If a woman has a communicable disease such as tuberculosis or hepatitis, which could threaten the infant's health, then mother and baby must be separated. Breastfeeding would be possible only by pumping the mother's breasts several times a day. The Centers for Disease Control recommend that where safe alternatives are available, women who test positive for human immunodeficiency virus (HIV), the virus that causes acquired immune deficiency syndrome (AIDS), should not breastfeed their infants.[59]

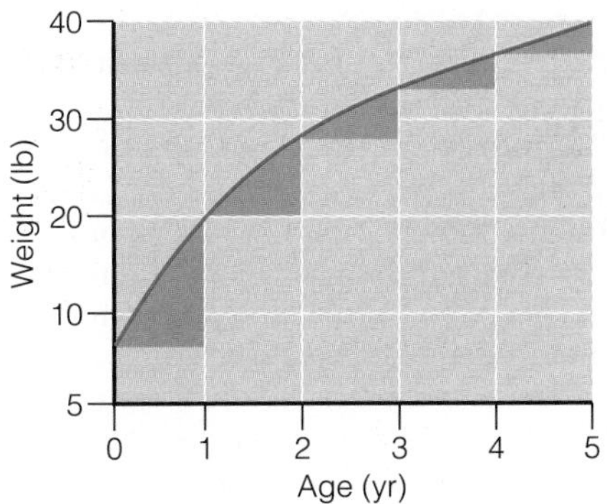

Figure 15–3
Weight Gain of Human Infants in Their First Five Years of Life
In the first year, an infant's birthweight may triple, but over the following several years, the rate of weight gain gradually diminishes.

Maternal Medicine and Drug Use Similarly, if a nursing mother must take medication that is secreted in breast milk and that is known to affect the infant, then breastfeeding is contraindicated.[60] Many prescription drugs do not reach nursing infants in sufficient quantities to affect them adversely. Some, however, do. As a precaution, a nursing mother should consult with the prescribing physician prior to ingesting any drug. Drug addicts, including alcohol abusers, are capable of taking such high doses that their infants can become addicts by way of breast milk; in these cases, too, breastfeeding is contraindicated.

A lactating woman is wise to avoid oral contraceptives until after she has weaned her infant and to use another method of contraception in the meantime. Standard oral contraceptives contain estrogen, which reduces both the volume and the protein content of breast milk.[61]

Nutrition of the Infant

Early nutrition affects later development, and early feeding sets the stage for eating habits that will influence nutrition status for a lifetime. Trends change, and experts argue about the fine points, but properly nourishing a baby is relatively simple, overall. Common sense in the selection of infant foods and a nurturing, relaxed environment go far to promote an infant's health and well-being.

Nutrient Needs

An infant grows faster during the first year than ever again, as Figure 15–3 shows. The growth of infants and children directly reflects their nutritional well-being and is an important parameter in assessing their nutrition status. Health care professionals use growth charts to evaluate the growth and development of children from birth to 18 years of age (see Appendix E).

Nutrients to Support Growth An infant's birthweight doubles by about four to five months of age, and it triples by the age of one year. (Consider that if an adult, starting at 150 pounds, were to do this, the person's weight would increase to 450 pounds in a single year.) By the end of the first year, the growth rate slows considerably. Between the first and second birthdays, the weight gained amounts to less than 10 pounds.

A newborn baby requires only about 650 kcalories per day, whereas most adults require about 2000 kcalories per day. In comparison to body weight, however, the difference is remarkable. Infants require about 100 kcalories per kilogram of body weight per day; most adults require fewer

Figure 15–4
Nutrient RDA of a Five-Month-Old Infant and an Adult Male Compared on the Basis of Body Weight
Infants may be relatively small and inactive, but they use large amounts of energy and nutrients to keep all their metabolic processes going.

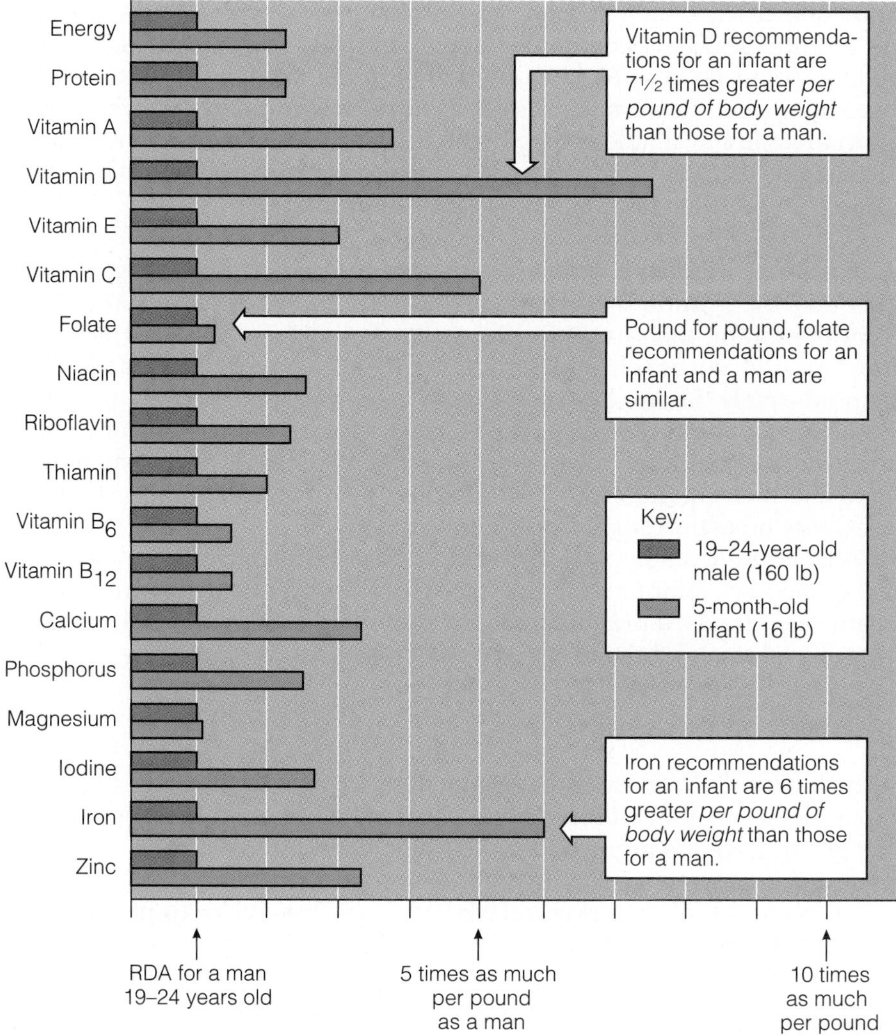

than 40. A 170-pound adult who tried to eat like an infant would have to ingest over 7000 kcalories a day! Figure 15–4 compares a five-month-old infant's needs per kilogram of body weight with those of an adult male; as you can see, some of the differences are extraordinary. After six months, energy needs increase less rapidly as the growth rate begins to slow, but some of the energy saved by slower growth is spent in increased activity.

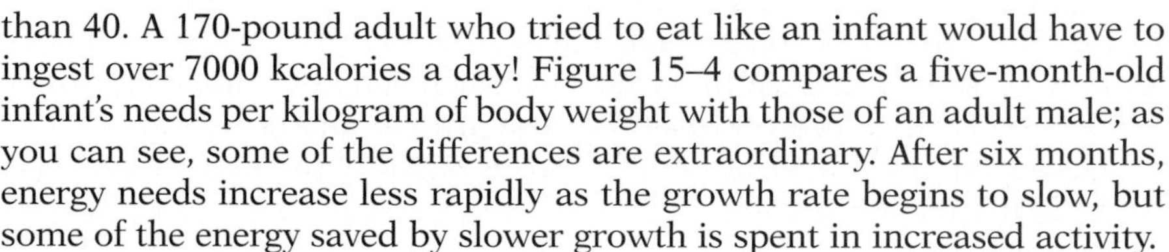

Water The most important nutrient of all, for infants as for everyone, is the one easiest to forget: water. Conditions that cause fluid loss, such as vomiting, diarrhea, sweating, or obligatory urinary loss without replacement, can rapidly propel an infant into life-threatening dehydration. In early infancy, breast milk or formula normally provides enough water for a healthy infant to replace water losses from the skin, lungs, feces, and urine.[62] An infant who is exposed to hot weather, has diarrhea, or vomits repeatedly, however, needs supplemental water to prevent dehydration. Infants cannot tell you what they are crying for; remember that they may need water, and let them drink it until they quench their thirst.

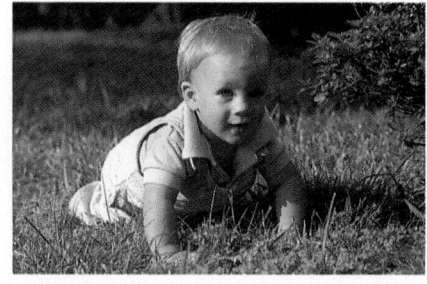

At six months, the energy saved by slower growth is spent on increased activity.

In developed countries with well-nourished populations, such as the United States and Canada, the dietary practices that influence infants' nutrition status the most center upon which type of milk the infant receives and the age at which solid foods are introduced. The remainder of this discussion is devoted to feeding the infant and identifying the nutrients most often deficient in infant diets.

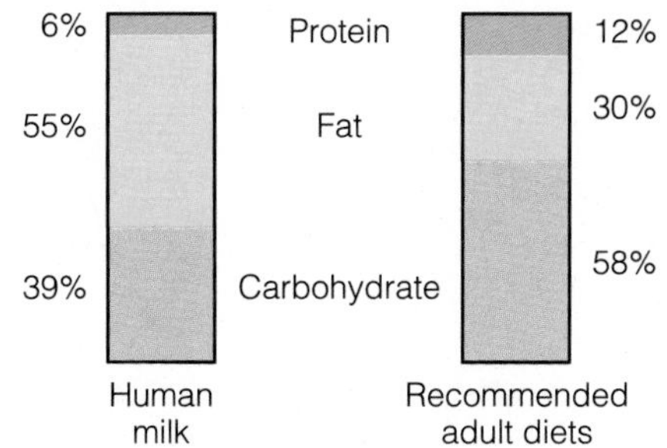

Figure 15–5
Percentages of Energy-Yielding Nutrients in Human Milk and in Recommended Adult Diets
The balance of energy-yielding nutrients in human breast milk is ideal for infants and does not resemble the balance recommended for adults.

Breast Milk

Breast milk excels as a source of nutrients for the young infant. With the possible exceptions of vitamin D and fluoride, breast milk provides all the nutrients a healthy infant needs for the first four to six months of life, and disease-preventive benefits as well.

Energy Nutrients The energy nutrient balance of breast milk differs dramatically from the balance recommended for adults (see Figure 15–5). Yet for infants, breast milk is the most nearly perfect food, proving that people at different stages of life really do have different nutrient needs.

Tailor-made to meet the nutrient needs of the human infant, breast milk offers its carbohydrate as lactose and its fat as a mixture with a generous proportion of the essential fatty acid linoleic acid. The unique composition of the fat in breast milk, in combination with the fat-digesting enzymes present, contributes to highly efficient fat absorption by the breastfed infant. The protein in breast milk is largely alpha-lactalbumin, a protein the human infant can easily digest.

alpha-lactalbumin (lack-AL-byoo-min): the chief protein in human breast milk, as **casein** (CAY-seen) is the chief protein in cow's milk.

Vitamins and Minerals The vitamin content of breast milk is ample. Even vitamin C, for which cow's milk is a poor source, is supplied generously by the breast milk of a well-nourished mother. The concentration of vitamin D in breast milk, however, is low, and vitamin D deficiency causes impaired bone mineralization in children. Manufacturers fortify cow's milk and infant formulas with vitamin D, but physicians routinely prescribe vitamin D supplements for breastfed infants in the United States and Canada.

Calcium, phosphorus, and magnesium are present in breast milk in amounts appropriate for the rate of growth expected in a human infant. Breast milk is healthfully low in sodium, and its iron is highly absorbable. Its zinc, too, is absorbed better than zinc from cow's milk, thanks to the presence of a zinc-binding protein.

Supplements for Infants Normally, given the nutrient composition of breast milk, infants require no nutrient supplements, with the possible exceptions of vitamin D and fluoride. After age four to six months, depending on food intake, infants may also require iron supplements, as Table 15–6 on the next page shows.

Immunological Protection Breast milk offers the infant unsurpassed protection against infection. Protective factors include antiviral agents, antibacterial agents, and other infection inhibitors.

During the first two or three days of lactation, the breasts produce colostrum, a premilk substance containing antibodies and white cells

colostrum (co-LAHS-trum): a milklike secretion from the breast that is rich in protective factors; it is present during the first day or so after delivery, before milk appears.

Table 15–6
Supplements for Full-Term Infants

	VITAMIN D[a]	IRON[b]	FLUORIDE[c]
Breastfed infants:			
Birth to six months of age	√		√
Six months to one year	√	√	√
Formula-fed infants:			
Birth to six months of age			√
Six months to one year		√	√

[a]Vitamin D supplements are recommended only for as long as breast milk is the infant's major milk.
[b]Infants four to six months of age need additional iron, preferably in the form of iron-fortified cereal for both breastfed and formula-fed infants and iron-fortified infant formula for formula-fed infants.
[c]The Committee on Nutrition of the American Academy of Pediatrics recommends initiating fluoride supplements for breastfed infants, formula-fed infants who receive ready-to-use formulas (these are prepared with water low in fluoride), or those who receive formula mixed with water that contains little or no fluoride (less than 0.3 ppm). The committee is evaluating recommendations to delay initiation of fluoride supplementation until six months of age or older.

Source: Adapted from Committee on Nutrition, American Academy of Pediatrics, Vitamin and mineral supplement needs of normal children in the United States, in *Pediatric Nutrition Handbook,* 3rd ed. L. A. Barness (Elk Grove Village, Ill., American Academy of Pediatrics, 1993), pp. 34–42.

from the mother's blood. Colostrum is relatively sterile as it leaves the breast, and the baby cannot contract a bacterial infection from it even if the mother has one. Colostrum contains maternal immune factors that inactivate harmful bacteria within the digestive tract. Later, breast milk also delivers immune factors, although not as many as colostrum. Among them are bifidus factors and lactoferrin.[63]

Breast milk also contains several enzymes, several hormones (including thyroid hormone and prostaglandins), and lipids, all of which protect the infant against infection. Research suggests that breastfeeding offers better protection against wheezing during the first few months of life than formula feeding does.[64] It seems, too, that breastfed babies are less prone to develop stomach and intestinal disorders during the first few months of life, and so experience less vomiting and diarrhea than formula-fed infants do.[65] Research shows that exclusive breastfeeding for at least four months protects babies against middle ear infection, one of the most common illnesses of infancy.[66] Researchers speculate that the upright position in which breastfed babies nurse keeps fluid from entering the tubes that drain the middle ear. Furthermore, the antibodies in breast milk keep bacteria from clinging to the tubes. Much remains to be learned about the composition and characteristics of human milk, but clearly it is a very special substance. Nutrition in Practice 15 offers suggestions for successful breastfeeding.

bifidus (BIFF-id-us, by-FEED-us) **factors:** factors in colostrum and breast milk that favor the growth of the "friendly" bacteria *Lactobacillus* (lack-toh-ba-SILL-us) *bifidus* in the infant's intestinal tract; these bacteria prevent other, less desirable intestinal inhabitants from flourishing.

lactoferrin (lak-toe-FERR-in): a factor in breast milk that binds iron and keeps it from supporting the growth of the infant's intestinal bacteria.

Infant Formula

Because breastfeeding offers so many advantages for both mother and infant, it should be encouraged whenever possible. However, the mother who has decided to use formula should be supported in her choice just as the breastfeeding mother should be. She can offer the same closeness, warmth, and stimulation during feedings as the breastfeeding mother can, and other family members can help with feedings, thus allowing her additional time to rest.

Many mothers choose to breastfeed at first but wean their children within the first 1 to 12 months. Before infants reach a year of age, mothers must wean them onto *infant formula,* not onto plain cow's milk of any kind—whole, low-fat, or nonfat.

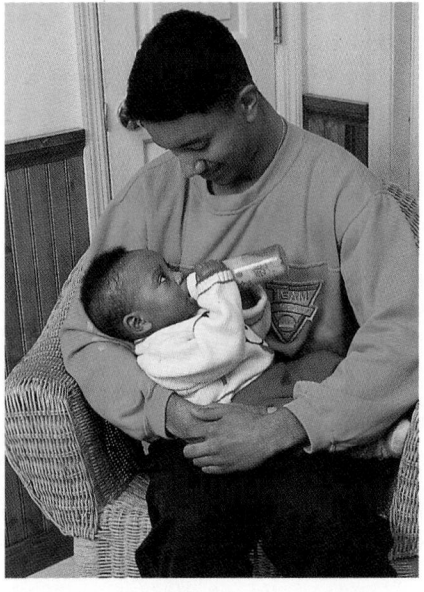

The infant thrives on infant formula offered with affection.

Formula preparation:

- Liquid concentrate (moderately expensive, relatively easy)—mix with equal part water.
- Powdered formula (least expensive, lightest for travel)—read label directions.
- Ready-to-feed (easiest, most expensive)—poor directly into clean bottles.

Infant Formula Composition Formulas can be prepared from cow's milk in such a way that they do not differ significantly from human milk in nutrient content. Figure 15–6 illustrates the energy-nutrient balance of both. Formulas contain no protective antibodies for human babies, but preventive medical care (vaccinations) and reliable public health measures help minimize this disadvantage. The educated mother whose water supply is reliable can prepare safe, sanitary formulas. Lead-contaminated water, however, is a major source of lead poisoning in infants.[67]

Infant Formula Standards National and international standards have been set for the nutrient contents of infant formulas. U.S. standards are based on American Academy of Pediatrics (AAP) recommendations, and the Food and Drug Administration (FDA) mandates quality control procedures to ensure that the standards are met. All standard formulas are therefore nutritionally similar. Small differences in nutrient content are sometimes confusing but usually not important.

Special Formulas Standard formulas are inappropriate for some infants (see Figure 15–7 on p. 380). For example, premature babies require special formulas. Infants allergic to milk protein can drink special formulas based on soy protein. Infants with lactose intolerance need formulas with the lactose replaced. For infants with other special needs, many other variations have been formulated.

Risks of Formula Feeding In developing countries and in poor areas of our country, formula may be unavailable, prepared with contaminated water, or overdiluted in an attempt to save money. Contaminated formula often causes infections leading to diarrhea, dehydration, and failure to absorb nutrients. Wherever sanitation is poor, breastfeeding should take priority over feeding formula. Breast milk is sterile, and its antibodies enhance an infant's resistance to disease.

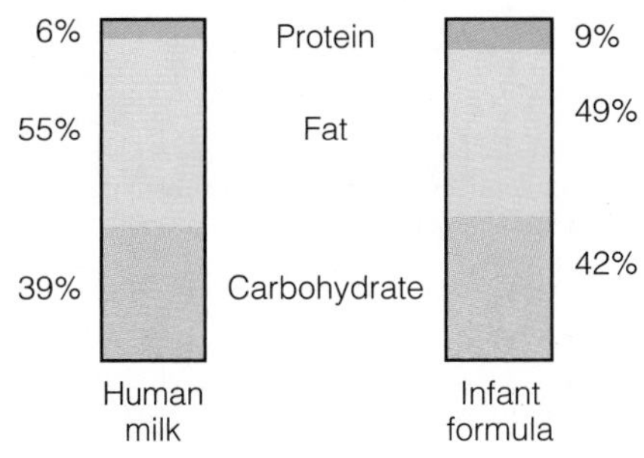

Figure 15–6
Percentages of Energy-Yielding Nutrients in Human Milk and in Infant Formula
The proportions of energy-yielding nutrients in human breast milk and formula differ slightly.

Iron in Formula The AAP recommends iron-fortified formula for all formula-fed infants.[68] Low-iron infant formulas have no role in infant feeding. Use of iron-fortified formulas has risen in recent decades and is credited with the decline of iron-deficiency anemia in U.S. infants.[69] Only iron-fortified formula can support normal development in an infant's first year.

Nursing Bottle Tooth Decay Dentists advise against putting a baby to bed with a bottle. Salivary flow, which normally cleanses the mouth, diminishes as the baby falls asleep. Sucking for long times pushes the jaw-

Figure 15–7
Choosing a Formula

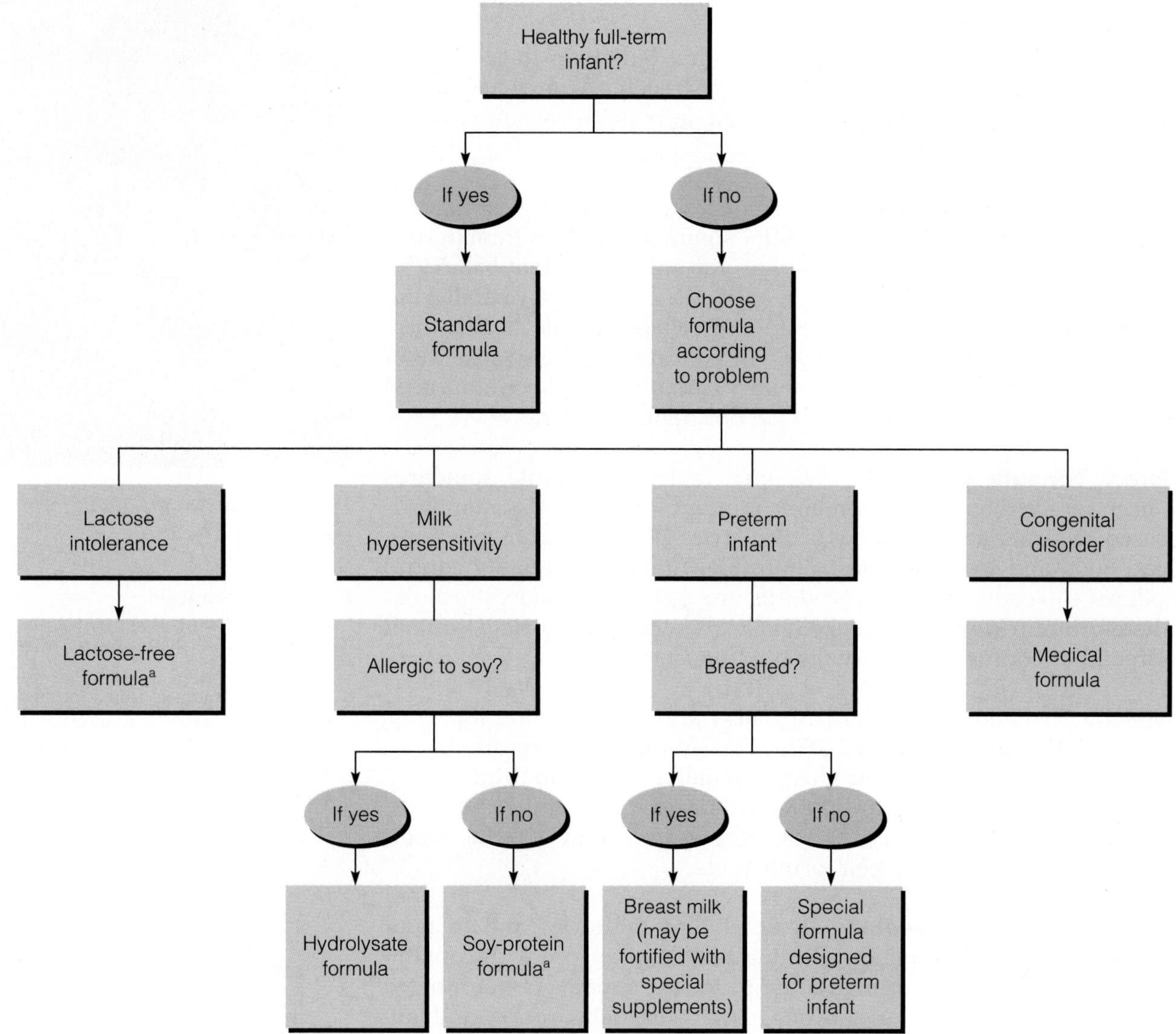

[a]Manufacturers design soy-based formulas for infants with milk sensitivities—whether lactose intolerance or milk allergy. These formulas use corn syrup or sucrose in place of lactose.

line out of shape and causes a bucktoothed profile (protruding upper and receding lower teeth). Furthermore, prolonged sucking on a bottle of formula, milk, or juice bathes the upper teeth in a carbohydrate-rich fluid that nourishes decay-producing bacteria. (The tongue covers and protects most of the lower teeth, but they, too, may be affected.) The result is extensive and rapid tooth decay. To prevent nursing bottle tooth decay, no child should be put to bed with a bottle as a pacifier. If a bottle is given, it should contain water. In fact, a caregiver would do well to offer an infant water after each feeding to rinse the mouth.

nursing bottle tooth decay: extensive tooth decay due to prolonged tooth contact with formula, milk, fruit juice, or other carbohydrate-rich liquid offered to an infant in a bottle.

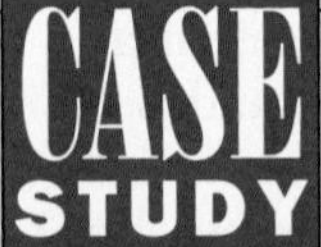

Pregnant Woman with Weight Problem

Ellen is a 24-year-old housewife who is four months pregnant. This is her first pregnancy, and she is eager to learn how to feed herself during pregnancy as well as her infant after birth. She is 5 feet 3 inches tall and currently weighs 150 pounds. Her prepregnancy weight was 148 pounds. Ellen is very concerned about her 2-pound weight gain.

1. Assess Ellen's weight and determine what her desirable weight would be if she were not pregnant.
2. Should Ellen be concerned about her 2-pound weight gain? Why?
3. What advice should you give Ellen about her weight gain during pregnancy?
4. What other dietary advice would you give her?
5. Discuss methods of infant feeding with Ellen and describe some of the advantages breastfeeding would offer her.
6. What are the advantages of formula feeding?
7. What advice will you give Ellen if she decides to breastfeed?
8. What information should Ellen have about formula feeding?

The accompanying case study presents a woman who is four months pregnant. Answering the questions offers practice in thinking through some of the issues related to pregnancy and breastfeeding.

The Transition to Cow's Milk

During an infant's first six months, formula must supply the nutrients of human milk in similar forms and proportions. Ordinary milk is an inappropriate replacement—primarily because cow's milk provides too little vitamin C and iron and too much sodium and protein. After the first year, the exact formulation of the milk selected is less critical, but milk or a suitable substitute still occupies a place in the diet that no other type of food can fill. Children one to two years of age should not drink low-fat or nonfat milk routinely; they need the fat of whole milk. If powdered milk is used, the fat-containing varieties should be chosen.

Introducing First Foods

Changes in the body organs during the first year affect the baby's readiness to accept solid foods. The immature stomach and intestines can digest milk sugar (lactose), but not starch until they are several months old. This is one of the many reasons why breast milk and formula are such good foods for babies; they provide simple, easily digested carbohydrate, supplying energy for the baby's growth and activity.

The Need for Water The infant's kidneys are unable to concentrate waste efficiently, so an infant must excrete relatively more water than an adult to carry off a comparable amount of waste. The risk of dehydration is ever present, and it becomes greater once solid foods are introduced. Foods with a high protein or electrolyte content such as meat and eggs can cause dehydration if offered without water. Water should be offered to infants regularly once they are eating solid food.[70] Water also provides fluid without additional food energy. Many adults would no doubt be healthier had they learned early to quench their thirst with water.

When to Introduce Solid Food For an infant receiving formula or breast milk from a healthy, well-nourished mother, additions to the diet are not needed until the infant is four to six months old. Foods may be started gradually beginning sometime between four and six months, depending on the infant's readiness. Any one of the following indicates readiness:

- The infant's birthweight has doubled.
- The infant can sit with support and can control head movements.
- The infant is six months old.

Infants vary; and the program of additions depends on the individual baby's developmental readiness, not on any rigid schedule. Table 15–7 presents a suggested sequence for introducing new foods.

The addition of foods to an infant's diet should be governed by three considerations: the infant's nutrient needs, the infant's physical readiness

Table 15–7
First Foods for the Infant

Breast milk or iron-fortified formula is the only source of nourishment for the first 4 to 6 months. Throughout the first year, the infant's intake of breast milk or iron-fortified formula will gradually decline as solid food intake increases.

AGE (MO)	ADDITION
4 to 6	Iron-fortified rice cereal, followed by other single-grain cereals, mixed with breast milk, formula, or water
	Pureed vegetables and fruits, one by one (perhaps vegetables before fruits, so the baby will learn to like their less sweet flavors)
6 to 8	Infant breads and crackers
	Mashed vegetables and fruits, and their juices[a]
8 to 10	Breads and cereals from the table
	Soft, cooked vegetables and fruit from the table
	Finely cut meats, fish, chicken, casseroles, cheeses, yogurts, tofu, eggs, and legumes
10 to 12	Continue to introduce a variety of nutritious foods

[a]All baby juices are fortified with vitamin C. Orange juice may cause allergies; apple juice may be a better choice at first. Dilute juices with water and offer in a cup to prevent nursing bottle tooth decay.

Source: Adapted in part from Committee on Nutrition, American Academy of Pediatrics, *Pediatric Nutrition Handbook,* 3rd ed., ed. L. A. Barness (Elk Grove Village, Ill.: American Academy of Pediatrics, 1993), pp. 23–33.

to handle different forms of foods, and the need to detect and control allergic reactions. With respect to nutrient needs, the nutrient needed earliest is iron, then vitamin C.

Foods to Provide Iron and Vitamin C Iron deficiency is common in young children throughout the world, especially between six months and three years when they are growing fast and milk, which is a poor source of iron, has a large place in their diets. The iron an infant has stored from before birth typically runs out after the birthweight doubles, long before the end of the first year. This is why cow's milk should not be offered during the first year: it not only displaces iron-fortified formula but also causes GI blood loss in many infants.[71] Infants can derive adequate iron first from breast milk or formula with iron, then from iron-fortified cereals, and later from meat or meat alternates such as legumes. Once infants are consuming iron-fortified cereals, parents or caretakers should begin selecting vitamin C–rich foods to go with meals to enhance iron absorption. The best sources of vitamin C are fruits and vegetables (see p. 164).

Physical Readiness for Solid Foods The ability to swallow solid food develops at around four to six months, and food offered by spoon helps to develop swallowing ability. Six months is also a good time to introduce the cup. At nine months to a year, a baby can sit up, can handle finger foods, and begins to teethe. At that time, hard crackers and other hard finger foods may be introduced to promote the development of manual dexterity and control of the jaw muscles. These feedings must occur under the watchful eye of an adult because the infant can also choke on such foods.

Some parents want to feed solids at an earlier age, on the theory that "stuffing the baby" at bedtime promotes sleeping through the night. There is no proof for this theory. On the average, babies start to sleep through the night at about the same age (three to four months) regardless of when solid foods are introduced.

Some authorities suggest that the early introduction of sweet fruits to infants' diets might favor the development of a preference for sweets and lessen the liking for vegetables introduced later. To prevent this, the order can be reversed: vegetables first, fruits later. As for fruit juices, they should be diluted and served in a cup, not a bottle.

Allergy-Causing Foods New foods should be introduced singly and at intervals spaced to permit detection of allergies. For example, when cereals are introduced, rice cereal is offered first for several days; it causes allergy least often. Wheat cereal is offered last; it is the most common offender. If a cereal causes an allergic reaction (irritability due to skin rash, digestive upset, or respiratory discomfort), its use should be discontinued before going on to the next food.

Choice of Infant Foods Baby foods commercially prepared in the United States and Canada are safe, and except for mixed dinners and heavily sweetened desserts, they generally have high nutrient density. An alternative for the parent who wants the baby to have family foods is to "blenderize" a small portion of the table food (cooked without salt) at each meal.

Foods to Omit Sweets of any kind (including baby food "desserts") have no place in a baby's diet. The added food energy they contribute can promote obesity, and they convey few or no nutrients to support growth. Canned vegetables are inappropriate for infants; they often contain too much sodium. Honey should never be fed to infants because of the risk of botulism. Babies and even young children have difficulty swallowing foods such as popcorn, whole grapes, whole beans, hot dog slices, and nuts, and they can easily choke on these foods. Also, an infant's caretaker must be on guard against food poisoning and take the precautions against it described in Chapter 11.

Reminder: milk anemia develops when an excessive milk intake displaces iron-rich foods from the diet.

Foods at One Year At a year of age, whole milk is still the best food to supply most of the nutrients the infant needs; 2 to 3½ cups a day meets those needs sufficiently. More milk than this displaces food necessary to provide iron and can cause the iron-deficiency anemia known as milk anemia. Other foods—meat, iron-fortified cereal, enriched or whole-grain bread, fruits, and vegetables—should be supplied in variety and in amounts sufficient to round out total energy needs. Ideally, a one-year-old will sit on the table, eat many of the same foods everyone else eats, and drink liquids from a cup—not a bottle. Table 15–8 shows a meal plan that meets a one-year-old's requirements.

Looking Ahead

Probably the most important single measure to undertake during the first year is to encourage eating habits that will support continued normal weight as the child grows. This means introducing a variety of nutritious

Table 15–8
Meal Plan for a One-Year-Old

Breakfast	**Afternoon snack**
1 c whole milk	½ c whole milk
3 tbs cereal	Teething crackers
2 to 3 tbs fruit[a]	1 tbs peanut butter
Teething crackers	**Dinner**
Lunch	1 c whole milk
1 c whole milk	1 egg
2 to 3 tbs vegetables[b]	2 tbs cereal or potato
2 tbs chopped meat or well-cooked, mashed legumes	2 to 3 tbs vegetables[b]
	2 to 3 tbs fruit[a]

[a]Include citrus fruits, melons, and berries.
[b]Include dark green, leafy and deep yellow vegetables.

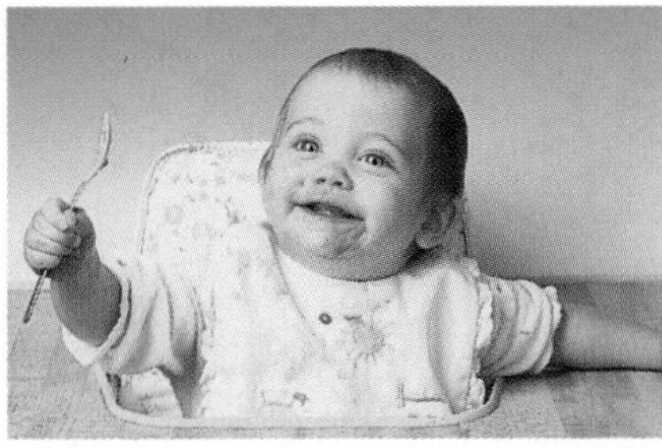

Ideally, a one-year-old eats many of the same foods as the rest of the family.

foods in an inviting way; not forcing the baby to finish the bottle or the baby food jar; avoiding concentrated sweets and empty-kcalorie foods; and encouraging physical activity. Parents should avoid teaching infants to seek food as a reward, to expect food as comfort for unhappiness, or to associate food deprivation with punishment. If infants cry for thirst, give them water, not milk or juice. Infants seem to have no internal "kcalorie counter," and they stop eating when their stomachs feel full. Nutrient-dense, low-kcalorie foods will satisfy as long as they provide bulk.

Normal dental development is also promoted by supplying nutritious foods, avoiding sweets, and discouraging the association of food with reward or comfort. Dental health is the subject of Nutrition in Practice 2.

A "prudent diet," like that recommended for heart clients (restrict fat, increase the ratio of polyunsaturated to saturated fat, and reduce cholesterol intake), is inappropriate for infants. The AAP recommends against a fat-modified diet during infancy, stating that the available evidence does not warrant dietary manipulation to lower serum cholesterol.

Mealtimes

The wise parent of a one-year-old offers nutrition and love together. Both promote growth. Children "fed with love" grow more in both weight and height than children fed the same food in an emotionally negative climate.

The person feeding a one-year-old should be aware that exploring and experimenting are normal and desirable behaviors at this time in a child's life. The child is developing a sense of autonomy that, if allowed to develop, will lay the foundation for later confidence and effectiveness as an individual. The child's impulses, if consistently denied, can turn to shame and self-doubt. In light of the developmental and nutrient needs of one-year-olds, and in the face of their often contrary and willful behavior, a few feeding guidelines may be helpful:

- *Discourage unacceptable behavior (such as standing at the table or throwing food) by removing the child from the table to wait until later to eat.* Be consistent and firm, not punitive. The child will soon learn to sit and eat.
- *Let the child explore and enjoy food.* This may mean the child eats with fingers for a while. Use of the spoon will come in time.
- *Don't force food on children.* Provide children with nutritious foods, and let them choose which ones and how much they will eat. Gradually, they will acquire a taste for different foods. If children refuse milk, provide cheese, cream soups, and yogurt.
- *Limit sweets strictly.* Infants have no room in their 1000-kcalorie daily energy allowance for empty-kcalorie sweets, except occasionally.

These recommendations reflect a spirit of tolerance that serves the best interest of the child emotionally as well as physically.

Nutrition Assessment

Assessing the nutrition status of pregnant women and of infants offers an opportunity to detect and correct potential problems in their future lives.

Accurate histories and measurements of growth and development are especially useful.

- The diet history should uncover normal eating habits in all settings. Have the woman's food choices changed since she became pregnant? How did she eat before? Does the same person always feed the infant? Establish baseline eating habits so that realistic improvements can be recommended. Watch for the use of monotonous or bizarre diets.
- For the pregnant woman, does she eat sufficient folate-rich foods daily to meet the U.S. Public Health Service recommendation of 500 micrograms a day from foods? Are her calcium and iron intakes ample? Does she use alcohol or drugs (prescription or other)? Are her exercise habits appropriate and sustainable for the future?
- The history should pick up on low socioeconomic status in pregnant women and new mothers. Referral to food assistance programs such as WIC may be appropriate. Also be alert for the risk factors for gestational diabetes.
- Accurate measurement of weight of the pregnant woman and plotting against previous measures is useful for keeping tabs on development over time.
- In the lactating mother, a careful history can determine not only eating and exercise habits but also alcohol and caffeine use, smoking, and medicine and drug use as well as maternal illness that might preclude breastfeeding. Is the breastfeeding mother receiving appropriate supplementation?
- In assessing the infant, a careful history should determine whether the infant is or has been breastfed; what formula is in use; and what solid foods are being fed. Are iron and vitamin C needs covered? Is the timing and style of feeding safe for infant tooth development? Are all foods nutrient dense? Are they prepared safely?
- In the infant, accurate measurement of weight, length, and head circumference and plotting against previous measures will reveal any deviations from normal growth.

Other parameters become important when pregnant women or infants have diseases or disorders that require medical intervention. Later chapters cover these conditions.

■ STUDY QUESTIONS ■

1. What is the significance of infant birthweight to a child's future health?
2. Why does a woman's nutrition before pregnancy profoundly influence the course and outcome of her pregnancy?
3. Which nutrients are needed in the greatest amounts during pregnancy? Why are they so important? What foods best supply these nutrients?
4. What is the recommended pattern of weight gain during pregnancy?
5. What practices should be avoided during pregnancy?
6. How do a woman's nutrient needs during lactation differ from her nutrient needs during pregnancy?
7. Describe some of the nutritional and immunological attributes of breast milk.
8. What are the advantages of formula feeding?
9. What three considerations govern the addition of solid foods to an infant's diet?
10. Name some foods that are inappropriate for infants and explain why they are inappropriate.

NUTRITION IN PRACTICE 15

Encouraging Successful Breastfeeding

Breastfeeding offers benefits to both mother and infant. The AAP, the ADA, the WIC program, and the U.S. Department of Health and Human Services advocate breastfeeding as the preferred means of infant feeding for the first six months of life.[72] Nevertheless, breastfeeding has been on the decline since the early 1980s when it reached a high of about 60 percent.[73]

Why has breastfeeding been declining?

Many experts cite two major deterrents: public advertising of infant formula, and the medical community's failure to encourage breastfeeding. As an example of the medical lack of encouragement, some hospitals routinely separate mother and child soon after birth. The child's first feeding then comes from the bottle rather than the breast. Furthermore, many hospitals send new mothers home with free samples of infant formula. The World Health Organization opposes this practice because it sends a misleading message that medical authorities favor infant formula over breast milk for infants.

Even in hospitals where women are encouraged to breastfeed and supported in doing so, little if any assistance is available after hospital discharge, and many breastfeeding women still need assistance. Of mothers who initially breastfeed their infants, up to half stop within a month—seemingly due to lack of knowledge.[74] Research shows that when women receive early and repeated breastfeeding information and support, they breastfeed their infants longer than other women do.[75] Information and instruction are especially important during the prenatal period when most women decide whether to breastfeed or to feed formula. Health professionals can play a vital role in encouraging successful breastfeeding by offering women adequate, accurate information about breastfeeding that permits them to make informed choices.

I thought that breastfeeding was a natural process that didn't require any learning.

Although *lactation* is an automatic physiological process, *breastfeeding* requires some learning. This learning is most successful in a supportive environment. It begins with preparatory steps taken before the baby is born.

What are these preparatory steps?

Toward the end of pregnancy and throughout lactation, a woman who intends to breastfeed should stop using soap and lotions on her breasts. The natural secretions of the breasts themselves lubricate the nipple area best. A few weeks before the baby is due, the woman should allow her breasts to rub against her outer clothing for a little while each day to toughen the nipples somewhat in preparation for the baby's suckling. Also, she should occasionally go without clothing at home to expose her breasts to air and light.

A woman who plans to breastfeed should acquire at least two nursing bras before her baby is born. The bras should provide good support and have drop-flaps so that either breast can be freed for nursing.

How soon after birth should breastfeeding start?

As soon as possible. Immediately after the delivery, for a short period, the baby is intensely alert and intent on suckling. This is the ideal time for the first breastfeeding and facilitates successful lactation.[76]

What does the new mother need to know in order to breastfeed her infant successfully?

She needs to learn how to relax and position herself so that she and the infant will be comfortable and so that the infant can breathe freely while nursing. She also needs to understand that infants have a rooting reflex that makes them turn toward any touch on the face. (The glossary on p. 388 defines this and other relevant terms.) Consequently, she should touch the infant's cheek to her nipple so that the infant will turn the right way and start to nurse. The mother can then squeeze her areola, the colored ring around the nipple, between two fingers and slip enough of it into the infant's mouth to permit a good hold and strong pumping action (see Figure 15–8 on p. 388). The nipple must rest well back on the infant's tongue so that the infant's gums will squeeze on the glands that release the milk and swallowing will be effortless. To break the suction, if necessary, the mother can slip a finger between the infant's mouth and her breast.

Glossary of Breastfeeding Terms

engorgement: overfilling of the breasts with milk.

letdown reflex: the reflex that forces milk to the front of the breast when the infant begins to nurse.

mastitis: infection of a breast.

rooting reflex: a reflex that causes an infant to turn toward whichever cheek is touched, in search of a nipple.

Doesn't it hurt to have the infant sucking so hard on the breast?

No, because the mother has a letdown reflex that forces milk to the front of her breast when the infant begins to nurse, virtually propelling the milk into the infant's mouth. Letdown is necessary for the infant to obtain milk easily, and the mother needs to relax for letdown to occur. The mother who assumes a comfortable position in an environment without interruptions will find it easiest to relax.

How long should the baby be allowed to nurse at each feeding?

Although the infant sucks half the milk from the breast within the first 2 minutes, and 80 to 90 percent of it within 4 minutes, sucking on each breast for 10 to 15 minutes is encouraged. The sucking itself, as well as the complete removal of milk from the breast, stimulates the mammary glands to produce milk for the next nursing session. Successive sessions should start on alternate breasts to ensure that each breast is emptied regularly. This pattern maintains the same supply and demand for each breast and thus prevents either breast from overfilling.

Figure 15–8
Infant's Grasp on Mother's Breast
The mother squeezes the areola, slipping enough of it into the infant's mouth to promote good pumping action. The infant's lips and gums pump the areola, releasing milk from the mammary glands into the milk ducts that lie beneath the areola.

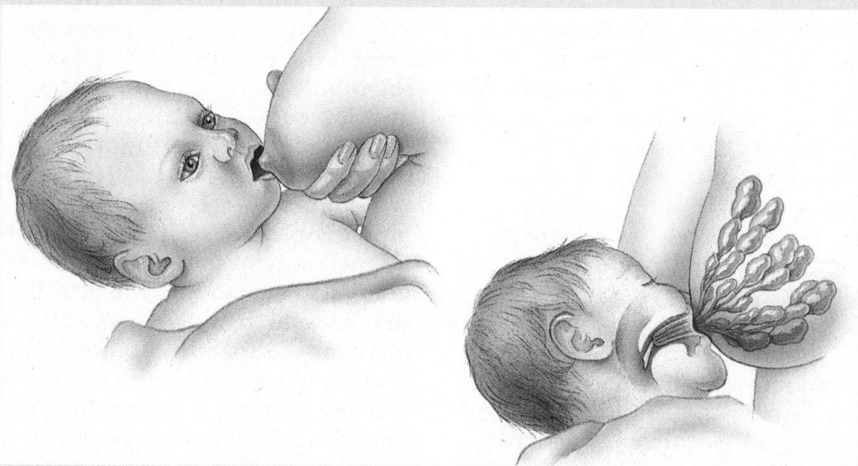

Infants should be fed "on demand" and not held to a rigid schedule. The breastfed baby may average 8 to 12 feedings per 24-hour period during the first month or so. Once the mother's milk supply is well established and the infant's capacity has increased, the intervals between feedings will become longer.

What if a mother wants to skip one or two feedings daily—for example, because she works outside the home?

A mother can substitute formula for those feedings and continue to breastfeed at other feedings. Or, the mother can express breast milk into a bottle ahead of time, freeze the breast milk, and when needed, substitute the expressed breast milk for a nursing session. Breast milk can be kept refrigerated for 48 hours or frozen (at a freezer temperature below 0°F) for several months.

The mother can hand express her breast milk or use one of several different breast pumps available. The bicycle-horn type of manual breast pump is not recommended, however. These pumps are difficult to keep clean. Cylinder-type manual pumps or electric breast pumps are safer and are also more efficient.

What about problems associated with breastfeeding such as sore nipples or infection of the breast?

Most problems associated with breastfeeding can be resolved. Many mothers experience sore nipples during the initial days of breastfeeding. Sore nipples need to be treated kindly, but nursing can continue. Improper feeding position is a frequent cause of sore nipples: the mother should make sure the infant is taking the entire nipple and part of the areola onto the tongue. She should nurse on the less-sore breast first to get letdown going while the infant is sucking hardest; then she can switch to the sore breast. Between times, she should expose her nipples to light and air to heal them.

Before lactation is well established, when the schedule changes, or when a feeding is missed, the breasts may become full and hard—an uncomfortable condition known as engorgement. The infant cannot grasp an engorged nipple and so cannot provide relief by nursing. A gentle massage or warming the breasts with a heating pad or in a shower helps to initiate letdown and to release some of the accumulated milk; then the mother can pump out some of her milk and allow the infant to nurse.

Infection of the breast, known as mastitis, is best managed by *continuing to breastfeed.* By drawing off the milk, the infant helps to relieve pressure in the infected area. The infant is safe because the infection is between the milk-producing glands, not inside them.

Even if everything is going smoothly, the nursing mother should ideally have enough help and support so that she can rest in bed a few hours each day for the first week or so. Successful breastfeeding requires the support of all those who care. This, plus adequate nutrition, ample fluids, fresh air, and exercise, will do much to enhance the well-being of mother and infant.

■ NOTES ■

1. M. C. Mitchell and E. Lerner, Weight gain and pregnancy outcome in underweight and normal weight women, *Journal of the American Dietetic Association* 89 (1989): 634–638, 641.
2. National Academy of Sciences, Food and Nutrition Board, *Nutrition During Pregnancy* (Washington, D.C.: National Academy Press, 1990), pp. 176–211.
3. J. B. Gould and S. LeRoy, Socioeconomic status and low birthweight: A racial comparison, *Pediatrics* 82 (1988): 896–904; C. M. Olson, Promoting positive nutritional practices during pregnancy and lactation, *American Journal of Clinical Nutrition* (supplement) 59 (1994): 525–531.
4. Transplacental nutrient transfer and intrauterine growth retardation, *Nutrition Reviews* 50 (1992): 56–57.
5. H. S. Wright and coauthors, The 1987–1988 Nationwide Food Consumption Survey: An update on the nutrient intake of respondents, *Nutrition Today,* May/June 1991, pp. 21–27.
6. Centers for Disease Control and Prevention, Recommendations for use of folic acid to reduce number of spina bifida cases and other neural tube defects, *Journal of the American Medical Association* 269 (1993): 1233, 1236, 1238.
7. National Academy of Sciences, Food and Nutrition Board, 1990, pp. 1–23.
8. National Academy of Sciences, Food and Nutrition Board, 1990.
9. National Academy of Sciences, Food and Nutrition Board, 1990.
10. J. E. Brown and M. Story, "Let them eat cake" or a prescription for improving the outcome of pregnancy? *Nutrition Today,* November/December 1990, pp. 18–23.
11. National Academy of Sciences, Food and Nutrition Board, 1990, pp. 318–335.
12. National Academy of Sciences, Food and Nutrition Board, 1990, p. 322.
13. T. O. Scholl and M. L. Hediger, Anemia and iron-deficiency anemia: Compilation of data on pregnancy outcome, *American Journal of Clinical Nutrition* (supplement) 59 (1994): 492–501.
14. National Academy of Sciences, Food and Nutrition Board, 1990.
15. Y. H. Neggers and coauthors, A positive association between maternal serum zinc concentration and birth weight, *American Journal of Clinical Nutrition* 51 (1990): 678–684.
16. P. L. Splett, Federal food assistance programs; A step to food security for many, *Nutrition Today,* March/April 1994, pp. 6–13.
17. B. Worthington-Roberts and coauthors, Dietary cravings and aversions in the postpartum period, *Journal of the American Dietetic Association* 89 (1989): 647–651.
18. National Academy of Sciences, Food and Nutrition Board, 1990, pp. 63–96.
19. National Academy of Sciences, Food and Nutrition Board, 1990, pp. 176–211.
20. K. G. Dewey and M. A. McCrory, Effects of dieting and physical activity on pregnancy and lactation, *American Journal of Clinical Nutrition* (supplement) 59 (1994): 446–453.
21. M. C. Hatch and coauthors, Maternal exercise during pregnancy, physical fitness, and fetal growth, *American Journal of Epidemiology* 137 (1993): 1105–1114.
22. *ACOG Guide to Planning for Pregnancy, Birth, and Beyond* (Washington, D.C.: The American College of Obstet-

ricians and Gynecologists, 1990), pp. 128–140.

23. N. I. Hahn and M. Erick, Battling morning (noon and night) sickness: New approaches for treating an age-old problem, *Journal of the American Dietetic Association* 94 (1994): 147–148.
24. National Academy of Sciences, Food and Nutrition Board, 1990.
25. U.S. Department of Health and Human Services, Public Health Service, *The Health Benefits of Smoking Cessation: A Report of the Surgeon General, 1990* (Washington, D.C.: Government Printing Office, 1990).
26. K. C. Schoendorf, Relationship of sudden infant death syndrome to maternal smoking during and after pregnancy, *Pediatrics* 90 (1992): 905–908; B. Haglund and S. Cnattingus, Cigarette smoking as a risk factor for sudden infant death syndrome, *American Journal of Public Health* 80 (1990): 29–32; E. A. Mitchell and coauthors, Smoking and sudden infant death syndrome, *Pediatrics* 91 (1993): 893–896.
27. D. L. Olds, C. R. Henderson, and R. Tatelbaum, Intellectual impairment in children of women who smoke cigarettes during pregnancy, *Pediatrics* 93 (1994): 221–227.
28. National Academy of Sciences, Food and Nutrition Board, 1990, pp. 390–411.
29. National Academy of Sciences, Food and Nutrition Board, 1990.
30. J. L. Mills and coauthors, Moderate caffeine use and the risk of spontaneous abortion and intrauterine growth retardation, *Journal of the American Medical Association* 269 (1993): 593–597.
31. B. M. Sibai and coauthors, Prevention of preeclampsia with low-dose aspirin in healthy, nulliparous, pregnant women, *New England Journal of Medicine* 329 (1993): 1213–1218.
32. New pregnancy warning on aspirin, *FDA Consumer,* September 1990, p. 2.
33. B. Zuckerman and coauthors, Effects of maternal marijuana and cocaine use on fetal growth, *New England Journal of Medicine* 320 (1989): 762–768; I. J. Chasnoff and coauthors, Cocaine/polydrug use in pregnancy: Two-year follow-up, *Pediatrics* 89 (1992): 284–289.
34. D. B. Petitti and C. Coleman, Cocaine and the risk of low birth weight, *American Journal of Public Health* 80 (1990): 25–28. J. J. Volpe, Effect of cocaine use on the fetus, *New England Journal of Medicine* 327 (1992): 399–407.
35. L. C. Mayes and coauthors, Neurobehavioral profiles of neonates exposed to cocaine prenatally, *Pediatrics* 91 (1993): 778–783; M. J. Corwin and coauthors, Effects of in utero cocaine exposure on newborn acoustical cry characteristics, *Pediatrics* 89 (1992): 1199–1203.
36. W. A. Vega and coauthors, Prevalence and magnitude of perinatal substance exposures in California, *New England Journal of Medicine* 329 (1993): 850–854.
37. S. Fisher and P. Karl, Maternal ethanol use and selective fetal malnutrition, *Alcoholism* (New York: Plenum Press, 1988), pp. 277–289.
38. K. R. Warren and R. J. Bast, Alcohol-related birth defects: An update, *Public Health Reports* 103 (1988): 638–642.
39. Position of the American Dietetic Association: Nutrition care for pregnant adolescents, *Journal of the American Dietetic Association* 94 (1994): 449–450.
40. Position of the American Dietetic Association, 1994; J. L. Beard, Iron deficiency: Assessment during pregnancy and its importance in pregnant adolescents, *American Journal of Clinical Nutrition* (supplement) 59 (1994): 502–510.
41. National Academy of Sciences, Food and Nutrition Board, 1990, pp. 1–23.
42. M. L. Hediger and coauthors, Rate and amount of weight gain during adolescent pregnancy: Associations with maternal weight-for-height and birth weight, *American Journal of Clinical Nutrition* 52 (1990): 793–799.
43. Position of the American Dietetic Association, 1994.
44. Committee on Nutrition, American Academy of Pediatrics, The use of whole cow's milk in infancy, *Pediatrics* 89 (1992): 1105–1109.
45. Position of the American Dietetic Association: Promotion and support of breast-feeding, *Journal of the American Dietetic Association* 93 (1993): 467–469.
46. Committee on Nutrition, 1992.
47. K. G. Dewey and coauthors, Maternal versus infant factors related to breast milk and residual milk volume: The DARLING Study, *Pediatrics* 87 (1991): 829–837; National Academy of Sciences, Food and Nutrition Board, *Nutrition during Lactation* (Washington, D.C.: National Academy Press, 1991), pp. 1–19.

48. J. M. A. van Raaij and coauthors, Energy cost of lactation, and energy balances of well-nourished Dutch lactating women: Reappraisal of the extra energy requirements of lactation, *American Journal of Clinical Nutrition* 53 (1991): 612–619; A. Sadurskis and coauthors, Energy metabolism, body composition, and milk production in healthy Swedish women during lactation, *American Journal of Clinical Nutrition* 48 (1988): 44–49.
49. Position of the American Dietetic Association, 1993.
50. M. Brewer, M. R. Bates, and L. P. Vannoy, Postpartum changes in maternal weight and body fat depots in lactating vs. nonlactating women, *American Journal of Clinical Nutrition* 49 (1989): 259–265.
51. F. M. Kramer and coauthors, Breast-feeding reduces maternal lower-body fat, *Journal of the American Dietetic Association* 93 (1993): 429–433.
52. National Academy of Sciences, Food and Nutrition Board, 1991, pp. 197–212.
53. National Academy of Sciences, Food and Nutrition Board, 1991, p. 140.
54. National Academy of Sciences, Food and Nutrition Board, 1991, p. 140.
55. L. B. Dusdieker and coauthors, Prolonged maternal fluid supplementation in breast-feeding, *Pediatrics* 86 (1990): 737–740.
56. J. A. Mennella, and G. K. Beauchamp, The transfer of alcohol to human milk: Effects on flavor and the infant's behavior, *New England Journal of Medicine* 325 (1991): 981–985.
57. Highlights from U.S.D.A. research, *Nutrition Today,* January/February 1993, pp. 4–5.
58. Nutrition during lactation, *Nutrition Today,* May/June 1991, pp. 28–31; American Academy of Pediatrics, Committee on Drugs, The transfer of drugs and other chemicals into human milk, *Pediatrics* 93 (1994): 137–150.
59. B. Lonnerdal and M. F. Picciano, Mechanisms regulating lactation and infant nutrient utilization, *Nutrition Today,* May/June 1991, pp. 32–35; Breast feeding by HIV-positive mothers, *Nutrition Today,* September/October 1992, p. 5.
60. American Academy of Pediatrics, Committee on Drugs, 1994.
61. American Academy of Pediatrics, Committee on Drugs, 1994.
62. Committee on Nutrition, American Academy of Pediatrics, *Pediatric Nutrition Handbook,* 3rd ed., ed. L. A. Barness (Elk Grove Village, Ill.: American Academy of Pediatrics, 1993), pp. 23–33.
63. P. F. Hennart and coauthors, Lysozyme, lactoferrin, and secretory immunoglobulin A content in breast milk: Influence of duration of lactation, nutrition status, prolactin status, and parity of mother, *American Journal of Clinical Nutrition* 53 (1991): 32–39.
64. When deciding between feeding by breast or by bottle, *Tufts University Diet and Nutrition Letter,* December 1990, pp. 3–4.
65. *Tufts University Diet and Nutrition Letter,* 1990.
66. B. Duncan and coauthors, Exclusive breast-feeding for at least 4 months protects against otitis media, *Pediatrics* 91 (1993): 867–872.
67. M. W. Shannon and J. W. Graef, Lead intoxication in infancy, *Pediatrics* 89 (1992): 87–90.
68. Committee on Nutrition, American Academy of Pediatrics, Iron-fortified infant formulas, *Pediatrics* 84 (1989): 1114; Committee on Nutrition, 1992.
69. Committee on Nutrition, 1989.
70. Committee on Nutrition, 1993. pp. 23–33.
71. Committee on Nutrition, 1992.
72. Committee on Nutrition, 1993, pp. 1–10; Position of the American Dietetic Association, 1993; Position of National Association of WIC Directors on breastfeeding promotion in the WIC program, *Journal of the American Dietetic Association* 89 (1989): 1091; *Healthy People 2000: National Health Promotion/Disease Prevention Objectives: Conference Edition* (Washington, D.C.: Government Printing Office, 1990), p. 377.
73. Position of the American Dietetic Association, 1993.
74. S. E. Saunders and J. Carroll, Post-partum breast feeding support: Impact on duration, *Journal of the American Dietetic Association* 88 (1988): 213–215.
75. S. P. Barron and coauthors, Factors influencing duration of breast feeding among low-income women, *Journal of the American Dietetic Association* 88 (1988): 1557–1561; C. I. Dungy and coauthors, Effect of discharge samples on duration of breast-feeding, *Pediatrics* 90 (1992): 233–237.
76. M. Teitel, S. Delaney, and L. Fink, *Breastfeeding: The Art of Mothering* (Port Washington, N.Y.: Alive Productions, 1987).

16

Nutrition for Children, Teenagers, and Young Adults

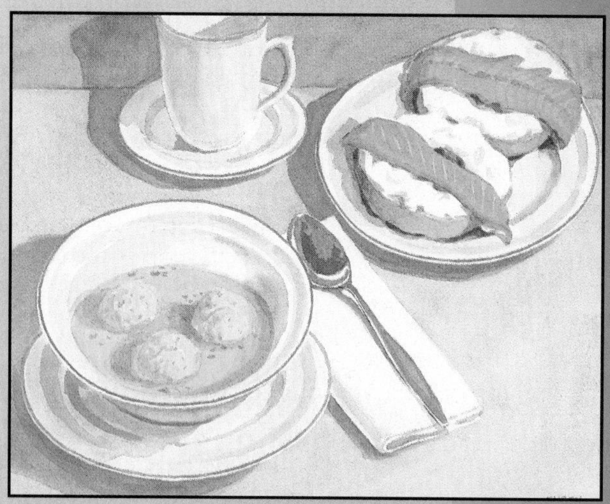

CONTENTS

Nutrient needs change steadily throughout life, depending on people's rates of growth, gender, activity level, and many other factors. Nutrient needs also vary from individual to individual, but generalizations are possible and useful. Sound nutrition throughout childhood promotes normal growth and development; facilitates academic and physical performance; and helps prevent obesity, heart disease, cancer, and other degenerative diseases in adulthood. As children enter the teen years, a foundation built by years of eating nutritious foods best prepares them to meet the upcoming demands of rapid growth.

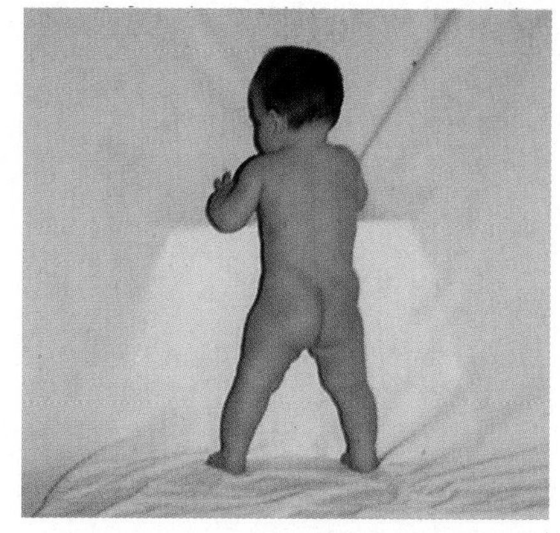

The body shape of a one-year-old (above) changes dramatically by age two (below). The two-year-old has lost much of the baby fat; the muscles (especially in the back, buttocks, and legs) have firmed and strengthened; and the leg bones have lengthened.

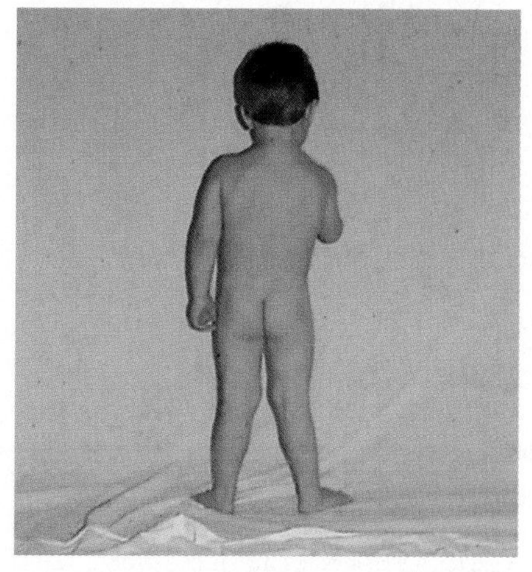

Early and Middle Childhood

After the age of one, a child's growth rate slows, but the body continues to change dramatically. At one, infants have just learned to stand and toddle; by two, they walk confidently and are learning to run, jump, and climb. Nutrition and physical activity have helped them prepare for these new accomplishments by adding to the mass and density of their bone and muscle tissue. Thereafter, their bones continue to grow longer and their muscles to gain size and strength, though unevenly and more slowly, until adolescence.

Energy and Nutrient Needs

An infant's appetite declines markedly around the first birthday, consistent with the slowed growth rate. Thereafter, the appetite fluctuates. At times children seem to be insatiable, and at other times they seem to live on air and water. Parents need not worry about this—a child will need and demand much more food during periods of rapid growth than during slow periods. The perfect regulation of appetite in children of normal weight guarantees that their food energy intakes will be right for each stage of growth.[1]

Children's Appetites Many people mistakenly believe that they must "make" their children eat the right amounts of food, and children's erratic appetites often reinforce this belief. However, research proves otherwise. Researchers studied preschool children's food intakes for six days. Each child's food energy intake was highly variable from meal to meal, but the total daily energy intake was remarkably constant.[2] The children adjusted their energy intakes at successive meals: if they ate less at one meal, they ate more at the next, and vice versa.

Parents do, however, need to help children to choose the right foods, and with overweight children they may need to help more, as described later. Overweight children may not adjust their energy intakes appropriately, but may eat in response to external cues, disregarding appetite-regulation signals.

Energy A one-year-old child needs perhaps 1000 kcalories a day; a three-year-old needs only 300 kcalories more. By age ten, a child needs about 2000 kcalories a day. Total energy needs increase slightly with age, but energy needs per kilogram of body weight actually decline gradually.

Nutrients Steady growth during childhood is reflected in gradually increasing needs for all nutrients. The RDA table (inside front cover) lists average nutrient intakes recommended for each span of three years.

Before adolescence, children accumulate stores of nutrients. Then, when they take off on the adolescent growth spurt and their nutrient intakes cannot keep pace with the demands of rapid growth, they can draw on the nutrient stores accumulated earlier. This is especially true of calcium; the denser the bones are in childhood, the better prepared they will be to support teen growth and still withstand the inevitable bone losses of later life. The way preteen children eat therefore influences their nutritional health during childhood, during their teen years, and for the rest of their lives.

Food Patterns for Children To provide all the needed nutrients, a variety of foods from each food group is recommended. Table 16–1 offers a guide. The portion sizes increase with the children's ages. A rule of thumb appropriate from age two to the teen years is that a portion of meat, fruits, and vegetables for children is loosely defined as 1 tablespoon per year. Thus, at four years of age, a serving of meat, fruit, or vegetable is about 4 tablespoons (¼ cup).

Children's Food Choices A parent or caretaker can do much to foster the development of healthy eating habits in a child. The challenge is to deliver nutrients in the form of meals and snacks that are nutritious and delicious to children, so that they will learn to enjoy a variety of nutritious foods.

Table 16–1
Children's Daily Food Patterns for Good Nutrition

FOOD GROUP	SERVINGS PER DAY	AVERAGE SIZE OF SERVING		
		1 to 3 years	4 to 6 years	7 to 12 years
Bread and cereals (whole grain or enriched)[a]	6 or more	½ slice	1 slice	1 to 2 slices
Vegetables[b]	3 or more	2–4 tbs or ½ c juice	¼–½ c or ½ c juice	½–¾ c or ½ c juice
Fruits[b]	2 or more	2–4 tbs or ½ c juice	¼–½ c or ½ c juice	½–¾ c or ½ c juice
Meat and meat alternates[c]	2 or more	1–2 oz	1–2 oz	2–3 oz
Milk and milk products[d]	3 to 4	½–¾ c	¾ c	¾–1 c

[a]1 slice bread = ¾ c dry cereal, ½ c cooked cereal, ½ c potato, rice, or noodles.
[b]Vitamin C source (citrus fruits, berries, tomatoes, broccoli, cabbage, cantaloupe) daily: vitamin A source (spinach, carrots, squash, tomato, cantaloupe) 3 to 4 times weekly.
[c]1 oz meat, fish, poultry = 1 egg, 1 frankfurter, 2 tbs peanut butter, ½ c legumes.
[d]½ c milk = ½ c cottage cheese, pudding, yogurt; ¾ oz cheese; 2 tbs dried milk.

Source: Adapted from P. M. Queen and R. R. Henry, Growth and nutrient requirements of children, in *Pediatric Nutrition,* eds. R. J. Grand, J. L. Sutphen, and W. H. Dietz, Jr. (Boston: Butterworths, 1987), p. 347.

Candy, cola, and other concentrated sweets must be limited in children's diets. If such foods are permitted in large quantities, the only possible outcomes are nutrient deficiencies, obesity, or both. Children can't be trusted to choose nutritious foods on the basis of taste alone; the preference for sweets is innate, and children naturally gravitate to them. In one study, when children were allowed to create meals freely from a variety of foods, they selected foods that provided 25 percent of the kcalories from sugar.[3] When their parents were watching, or even when they were told that their parents would be watching, the children improved their selections. Overweight children, especially, need help in sticking to nutrient-dense foods that will meet their nutrient needs within their energy intake allowances. Underweight children or active, normal weight children can enjoy higher-kcalorie foods, but these should still be nutritious. Examples are ice cream or pudding in the milk group and whole-grain or enriched pancakes or crackers in the bread group.

Malnutrition in Children

Most U.S. children are well nourished. Their average energy intakes are sufficient to support normal growth, and their average nutrient intakes, except for iron and zinc, meet or exceed recommendations. Survey findings suggest that hunger is prevalent among some groups, however.[4] As of the early 1990s, more than 11 million children under 12 years of age in the United States are hungry or are at risk of hunger.[5]

A root cause of this hunger is poverty. Many more homeless people are hungry than people who are housed, and children are the fastest growing segment of the homeless population. Homeless children from large families and from families with single mothers are especially vulnerable to hunger and its adverse consequences.

Effects of Hunger Both short-term and long-term hunger exert negative effects on behavior and health. Short-term hunger, such as when a child misses a meal, impairs the child's ability to pay attention and to be productive. Hungry children are irritable, apathetic, and uninterested in their environment. Long-term hunger impairs growth and immune defenses. Food assistance programs such as the WIC program and the National School Breakfast and Lunch programs are designed to improve the health of children.

Hunger and School Performance A study of more than 1000 elementary schoolchildren offers evidence that children who eat a nutritious breakfast function better than their peers who do not.[6] Young children who participated in the School Breakfast Program improved their scores on achievement tests and were tardy or absent significantly less often than children who did not participate in the breakfast program. Common sense dictates that it is unreasonable to expect anyone to learn and perform work when no fuel has been provided. By the late morning, discomfort from hunger may become distracting even if a child has eaten breakfast.

The problem that arises for children who attempt morning schoolwork on an empty stomach appears to be at least partly due to low blood

Table 16–2
Iron-Rich Foods Children Like[a]

Breads, cereals, and grains
Canned macaroni (½ c)
Canned spaghetti (½ c)
Cream of wheat (¼ c)
Fortified dry cereals (1 oz)[b]
Noodles, rice, or barley (½ c)
Tortillas (1 flour, 2 corn)
Whole-wheat, enriched, or fortified bread (1 slice)
Vegetables
Baked flavored potato skins (½ skin)
Cooked mushrooms (½ c)
Cooked mung bean sprouts or snow peas (½ c)
Green peas (½ c)
Mixed vegetable juice (1 c)
Fruits
Apple juice (1 c)
Canned plums (3 plums)
Cooked dried apricots (½ c)
Dried peaches (4 halves)
Raisins (1 tbs)
Meats and legumes
Bean dip (¼ c)
Canned pork and beans (⅓ c)
Mild chili or other bean/meat dishes (¼ c)
Liverwurst (½ oz)
Meat casseroles (½ c)
Peanut butter and jelly sandwich (½ sandwich)
Lean roast beef or cooked ground beef (1 oz)
Sloppy joes (½ sandwich)

[a]Each serving provides at least 1 milligram iron, or one-tenth of a child's RDA for iron. Vitamin C–rich foods included with these snacks increase iron absorption.
[b]Some fortified breakfast cereals contain more than 10 milligrams iron per half-cup serving (read the labels).

Source: Many of these ideas reflect data in A. A. Hertzler, Children's food patterns—A review: I. Food preferences and feeding problems, *Journal of the American Dietetic Association* 83 (1983): 551-554.

glucose. The average child up to the age of ten or so needs to eat every four to six hours to maintain a blood glucose concentration high enough to support the activity of the brain and nervous system. A child's brain is as big as an adult's, and the brain is the body's chief glucose consumer. A child's liver is considerably smaller—and the liver is the organ responsible for storing glucose (as glycogen) and releasing it into the blood as needed. A child's liver can't store more than about four hours' worth of glycogen; hence the need to eat fairly often. Teachers aware of the late-morning slump in their classrooms wisely request that a midmorning snack be provided; it improves classroom performance all the way to lunchtime.

Iron Deficiency and Behavior In U.S. children and adolescents, as in infants after six months, iron-deficiency anemia is the most prevalent nutrient deficiency. Iron deficiency is especially common among children and teens from low-income families. Iron deficiency presents the best-known and most widespread effects on behavior. Most people are familiar with the role of iron in carrying oxygen in the blood. Another important function of iron is transporting oxygen within cells, where it is used to help produce energy. A lack of iron not only causes an energy crisis but also directly affects behavior, mood, attention span, and learning ability. Iron is involved in the function of many molecules in the brain and nervous system. Much of the research on iron and behavior has focused on the proposal that even in the early stages of iron deficiency an iron-dependent neurotransmitter is altered. This, in turn, impairs learning ability and behavior.[7]

Iron deficiency is usually diagnosed from a deficit of iron in the *blood*, after the deficiency has progressed all the way to anemia. A child's *brain*, however, is sensitive to slightly lowered iron concentrations long before the blood effects appear. The effects are hard to distinguish from the effects of other factors in children's lives, but it is likely that iron deficiency manifests itself in a lowering of "motivation to persist in intellectually challenging tasks," a shortening of the attention span, and a reduction of overall intellectual performance. Anemic children perform less well on tests and have more conduct disturbances than their nonanemic classmates.[8]

Preventing Iron Deficiency To avert iron-deficiency anemia, children's foods must deliver 10 milligrams of iron or more per day. To achieve this goal, milk intakes must be limited after infancy, because milk is a poor source of iron. Children should receive enough milk products to ensure adequate calcium and riboflavin intakes, but no more. That means 2 to 3 cups of milk per day up to age three, grading on up to 3 to 4 cups per day from ages six to twelve (see Table 16–1). After age two, if low-fat milk is used instead of whole milk, saved kcalories can be invested in iron-rich foods such as lean meats, fish, poultry, eggs, and legumes. Whole-grain or enriched breads and cereals also contribute iron. Table 16–2 lists iron-rich foods children like.

The iron status of children in the United States may be changing for the better. Infant feeding practices such as breastfeeding and use of iron-fortified formulas may be improving iron status in later childhood.[9] Among children from low-income families, the WIC program, which provides supplemental iron-rich foods during infancy and early childhood, appears to be playing a role in improving iron status.

World Focus on Iron Deficiency The prevalence of iron deficiency among children throughout the world has become the focus of major public health efforts. The U.S. Public Health Service lists the reduction of iron deficiency among young children as one of the nation's foremost health priorities.[10] The World Health Organization is collaborating with a United Nations subcommittee on nutrition to develop a ten-year plan to eliminate iron deficiency.[11]

Other Nutrient Deficiencies Iron is only one of several dozen nutrients that can be displaced in a diet high in nutrient-poor foods. Any of the other nutrients may be lacking as well, and the deficiencies of those nutrients may also cause not only physical symptoms but behavioral symptoms, too (see Table 16-3 on p. 398). A child with behavioral symptoms of nutrient deficiencies may be irritable, aggressive, disagreeable, or sad and withdrawn. One might label such a child "hyperactive," "depressed," or "unlikable," but in fact these traits might arise from simple, albeit marginal, malnutrition. Should suspicion of dietary inadequacies be raised, *no matter what other causes may be implicated,* the people responsible for feeding the child should take steps to correct those inadequacies promptly.

Lead Poisoning in Children

The health impairment caused by malnutrition may be compounded by environmental factors such as lead poisoning. A two-way interaction is typical: lead poisoning can cause an iron deficiency, and an iron deficiency can impair the body's defenses against lead absorption. In fact, the interactions between lead poisoning and iron deficiency are so strong that some researchers suggest it may be appropriate to consider lead poisoning an adverse consequence of iron deficiency.[12] Like iron deficiency, mild lead toxicity has nonspecific effects, including diarrhea, irritability, reduced ability of the blood to carry oxygen, and fatigue. The symptoms may be reversible if exposure stops soon enough. With higher levels of lead, the signs become more pronounced, yet pinpointing a cause may still be difficult. Children lose their general cognitive, verbal, and perceptual abilities and develop learning disabilities and behavior problems. Still more severe lead toxicity can cause irreversible nerve damage, paralysis, mental retardation, and death.

Research shows that the ill effects of lead poisoning occur with lower doses than was thought in the past.[13] In response, the Centers for Disease Control have reduced their guideline for the amount of lead in the blood officially considered to cause lead poisoning. The new threshold is 10 micrograms per 100 milliliters of blood, a considerable drop from the previous 25 micrograms per 100 milliliters.[14] The U.S. Department of Health and Human Services has labeled lead poisoning "the most common and societally devastating environmental disease of young children."[15]

You may recall from Chapter 11 that three to four million children may have blood lead concentrations high enough to cause mental and behavioral problems and other health problems. Children's behaviors and

Table 16–3
Signs of Health and Malnutrition in Children

	HEALTHY	MALNOURISHED
Hair:	Shiny, firm in the scalp	Dull, brittle, dry, loose; falls out
Eyes:	Bright, clear pink membranes; adjust easily to darkness	Pale membranes; spots; redness; adjust slowly to darkness
Teeth and gums:	No pain or cavities, gums firm, teeth bright	Missing, discolored, decayed teeth; gums bleed easily and are swollen and spongy
Face:	Good complexion	Off-color, scaly, flaky, skin
Glands:	No lumps	Swollen at front of neck and cheeks
Tongue:	Red, bumpy, rough	Sore, smooth, purplish, swollen
Skin:	Smooth, firm, good color	Dry, rough, spotty; "sandpaper" feel or sores; lack of fat under skin
Nails:	Firm, pink	Spoon-shaped, brittle, ridged
Behavior:	Alert, attentive, cheerful	Irritable, apathetic, inattentive, hyperactive
Internal systems:	Heart rate, heart rhythm, and blood pressure normal; normal digestive function; reflexes and psychological development normal	Heart rate, heart rhythm, or blood pressure abnormal; liver and spleen enlarged; abnormal digestion; mental irritability, confusion; burning, tingling of hands and feet; poor balance and coordination
Muscles and bones:	Good muscle tone and posture; long bones straight	"Wasted" appearance of muscles; swollen bumps on skull or ends of bones; small bumps on ribs; bowed legs or knock-knees

Note: The signs here are consistent with malnutrition but not diagnostic of it.

activities—putting their hands in their mouths, playing in dirt, and eating nonfood items—favor their chances of exposure to lead. Of all the sources of lead for children, paint remains the most important.[16] In the homes of 3 million young children, leaded surfaces are peeling and deteriorating. Each child in these homes is already poisoned or at immediate risk of lead poisoning.

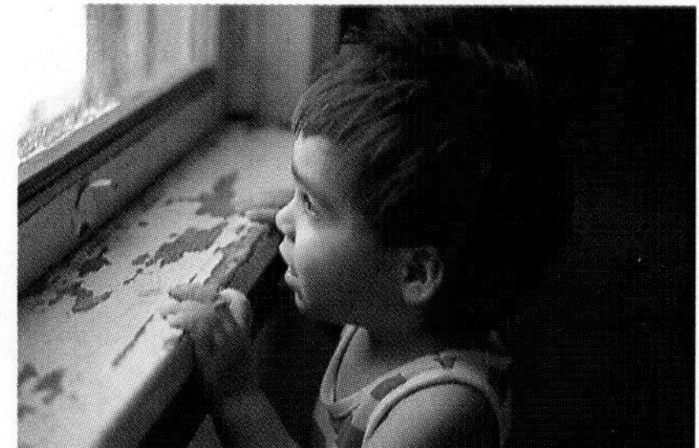

Paint is the number-one source of the lead that poisons children.

Lead toxicity symptoms are widespread among children under six. Lead aggressively attacks fetuses, infants, and children because the body absorbs lead most efficiently during times of rapid growth. Blood concentrations of lead generally reach a peak in two-year-old children; age two is the typical time of exploring surroundings "hand to mouth" and ingesting lead-tainted dirt and debris.[17] Reductions in the use of leaded products (such as leaded gasoline, lead-soldered food cans, and leaded house paint) mandated by federal law in recent years have helped to limit the amount of lead in the environment, but the problem of exposure to lead still pervades children's lives. Chapter 11 offered a How-to box on preventing lead exposure.

Food Allergies

Food allergies are frequently blamed for physical and behavioral abnormalities in children. Food allergies are most common in the first several years of life and tend to decline with age.[18] A true food allergy occurs when a whole food protein or other large molecule enters the system. (Recall that large molecules of food are normally dismantled in the digestive tract to smaller ones before absorption.) The body's immune system reacts to a food protein or other large molecule as it does to an antigen—by producing antibodies or other defensive agents. A problem that does not involve the immune system, but does result from exposure to food substances, is known as a food intolerance.

food allergies: adverse reactions to foods that involve an immune response; also called *food-hypersensitivity reactions.*

Reminder: *Antigens* are substances foreign to the body that elicit the formation of antibodies or an inflammation reaction from immune system cells. Food antigens are usually glycoproteins (large proteins with glucose molecules attached).

Reminder: *Antibodies* are large proteins that are produced in response to antigens and then inactivate the antigens.

food intolerance: an adverse response to a food or food additive that does not involve the immune system.

Asymptomatic and Symptomatic Allergies Allergies may have one or two components. They always involve antibodies; they may or may not involve symptoms. A person may produce antibodies without having any symptoms (known as asymptomatic allergy) or may produce antibodies and have symptoms (known as symptomatic allergy). A person who experiences symptoms without producing antibodies, however, does not have an allergy. This means that allergies have to be diagnosed by testing for antibodies.

Allergy Symptoms A symptomatic allergy will exhibit different symptoms depending on the location of the reaction. In the digestive tract, the allergy may cause nausea or vomiting; in the skin, it may cause rashes; and in the nasal passages and lungs, it may cause inflammation or asthma. A generalized, all-systems shock reaction can also occur.

Parents often mistakenly ascribe children's symptoms to food allergies, especially if the symptoms arise after eating. However, stomach aches, headaches, pain, a rapid pulse rate, nausea, wheezing, hives, bronchial irritation, coughs, and the like usually have other causes. Only proper testing can distinguish the many possibilities, and such testing is seldom done.

Immediate and Delayed Reactions Allergic reactions to food can occur with different timings, simply classified as immediate and delayed. In both, the antigen interacts immediately with the immune system, but symptoms may appear within minutes or not until after several (up to 24) hours. Identifying the food that causes an immediate allergic reaction is easy because symptoms correlate closely with the time of eating the food. Identifying the food that may cause a delayed reaction is more difficult because the symptoms may not appear until a day after the offending food is eaten. By this time, many other foods will have been eaten, too, complicating the picture.

The foods that most often cause immediate allergic reactions are listed in Table 16–4. Almost 75 percent of reactions are caused by three major foods—eggs, peanuts, or milk.[19] Allergic reactions to single foods are common. Reactions to multiple foods are the exception, not the rule.

Table 16–4
Foods That Most Often Cause Allergies

Eggs
Fish
Milk
Peanuts
Shellfish
Soybeans
Wheat

Source: Adapted from R. U. Sorensen, M. C. Porch, and L. C. Tu, Food allergy in children, *Textbook of Pediatric Nutrition,* 2nd ed., eds. R. M. Suskind and L. Lewinter-Suskind (New York: Raven Press, 1993), pp. 457–469.

Other Adverse Reactions to Foods Adverse reactions to foods that are not true food allergies include:

- Allergic reactions to molds, antibiotics, and other contaminants of foods.
- Chinese restaurant syndrome, a reaction specific to the flavor enhancer monosodium glutamate, or MSG (trade name, Accent).
- Reactions to bacterial toxins, such as botulinal toxin, and other food poisoning.
- Reactions to chemicals in foods, such as the natural laxative in prunes.
- Symptoms of digestive diseases such as hernias and ulcers, aggravated by eating any food.
- Enzyme deficiencies, such as lactose intolerance, that cause symptoms superficially indistinguishable from those of food allergy.
- Psychological reactions based on the belief that certain foods cause certain symptoms.

The simple dislike of a food may be a clue to allergy or to any of these reactions.

Food Dislikes Parents are advised to watch for signs of food dislikes and take them seriously. Children's food aversions may be the result of nature's efforts to protect them from allergic or other adverse reactions. Test, and then apply nutrition knowledge conscientiously in deciding how to alter the diet. Don't risk feeding the child an unbalanced diet, which could lead to nutrient deficiencies. Whenever a food is excluded from the diet, care must be taken to include other foods that offer the same nutrients as the omitted food contains. Remember that children who must avoid certain foods need all their nutrients, just as other children do.

Hyperactivity and Diet

Hyperactivity is a behavioral disorder that occurs in 2 to 5 percent of young school-aged children. Left untreated, it can interfere with a child's social development and ability to learn. Parents and teachers need to deal effectively with it wherever it appears to avert the grief it causes.

hyperactivity: a diagnosable syndrome in which the essential features are signs of developmentally inappropriate inattention, impulsivity, and excess motor activity. Other important features are onset before age seven, duration of six months or more, and proven absence of mental illness or mental retardation. Also called *attention deficit disorder.*

Physicians often diagnose hyperactivity by conducting a trial with stimulant drugs. Stimulants normally speed up people's activity, but they have a paradoxical effect with hyperactivity; they normalize it. (Perhaps they stimulate control centers in the brain.) If a child responds to stimulant drugs by calming down, it indicates that the drugs may be correcting a biochemical imbalance in the nervous system, and they can be used to help control the behavior. *In children who are responsive,* prescription medication should at least be considered as the treatment of choice.

Many parents fail to appreciate the utility of drug treatment for hyperactivity and resist its use, especially when they believe that manipulating the diet may help. Diet is one aspect of a child's life that parents may feel they can control. If problems can be solved by adding carrots or eliminating cookies, then parents are eager to give diet advice a try. While nutrition should be considered whenever a person's physical or mental health is less than optimal, it is unwise to jump at appealing solutions that

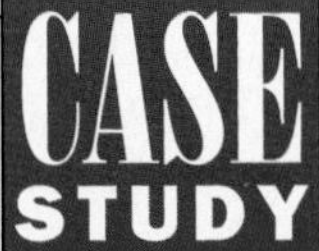

Boy with Disruptive Behavior

Freddie is a six-year-old boy who seldom sits still, often misbehaves, and is frequently sick. Freddie's eating habits are erratic and poor, as is his appetite. He often misses breakfast because he is too tired to get up in time to eat before school. By midmorning, Freddie is irritable and disruptive in the classroom. At lunchtime he trades the fruit his mother packed in his lunchbox for a piece of cake. After school he hurries home to watch television while he eats his favorite snack—root beer and potato chips. At dinnertime Freddie picks at his food because he isn't very hungry. Later on, when it's time for bed, Freddie complains that he's hungry. His parents let him stay up to have a bowl of cereal (the kind with marshmallows) before he finally falls asleep.

1. What factors in Freddie's daily routine might be contributing to his restless behavior?
2. Discuss some changes in diet that may improve Freddie's health and disposition.

are unfounded. The accompanying case study offers an opportunity to think about these issues in relation to a specific child.

Caffeine and Other Stimulants

One dietary excess that can irritate many children is that of caffeine, a matter of some concern to pediatricians. A 12-ounce soft drink may contain as much as 50 milligrams of caffeine. Two or more such beverages in the body of a 60-pound child are equivalent to the caffeine in 8 cups of coffee for a 175-pound man. Chocolate bars also contribute caffeine. Children can be troubled by sleeplessness, restlessness, and irregular heartbeats due to excess caffeine consumption. A survey of over 1000 children between ages 1 and 17 found that 77 percent of them were caffeine consumers.[20] Nutrition in Practice 20 discusses caffeine further and presents a table that lists the caffeine contents of beverages, foods, and medications. As long as such undeniably attractive temptations as cola beverages and candy bars surround children, barriers against their abuse have to be provided by concerned adults until the children learn to control consumption themselves.

Common sense says that all children at times get wild and "hyper." Such behavior has many normal, everyday causes: the desire for attention, lack of sleep, overstimulation, too much TV, or the lack of physical activity. Together, these produce the tension-fatigue syndrome, which can be relieved by giving more consistent care to the child's welfare. In particular, insisting on regular hours of sleep, regular mealtimes, and regular outdoor activity can be helpful.

tension-fatigue syndrome: apparent hyperactivity produced in a child by the combination of lack of sleep, overstimulation, and anxiety.

gatekeeper: with respect to nutrition, a key person who controls other people's access to foods and thereby exerts a profound impact on their nutrition. Examples are the spouse who buys and cooks the food, the parent who feeds the children, and the caretaker in a day-care center.

Food Choices and Eating Habits of Children

The childhood years are a parent's last chance to influence food choices. Parents are gatekeepers, controlling the availability of foods in their children's environments. Gatekeepers who want to promote nutritious choices and healthful habits provide access to healthful foods and opportunities for active play at home. Food choices and regular physical activity not only can promote healthy growth but, as mentioned earlier, also can help prevent the degenerative diseases of later life. Many experts agree that early childhood is the time to put into effect practices that, until recently, were recommended only for adults.[21]

Nutrition at Home

Reminder: *cardiovascular disease (CVD)* is a general term for all diseases of the heart and blood vessels. Atherosclerosis is the main form of CVD (see Chapter 26).

atherosclerosis (ath-er-oh-scler-OH-sis): a type of artery disease characterized by accumulations of lipid-containing material on the inner walls of the arteries.

Disease of the heart and blood vessels, known as cardiovascular disease, or CVD, is the leading cause of death in the United States and Canada each year. Most CVD involves atherosclerosis. Compelling evidence shows that atherosclerosis has its beginnings in childhood and that its development is related to dietary fats and blood lipids.[22] The disease is not inevitable, however; people can reach advanced age with very little atherosclerosis. Strategies begun early in life offer the most promise of prevention.

Preventing Obesity Strong correlations exist between obesity and high blood cholesterol.[23] To prevent obesity, encourage children to eat slowly, to pause and enjoy their table companions, and to stop eating when they are full. Show them how to serve themselves small portions and to take second helpings only after finishing the first, if they wish. Never force children to clean their plates. Encourage physical activity on a daily basis to promote strong skeletal, muscular, and cardiorespiratory development and to instill in children a desire to be physically active that will persist throughout life.

Dealing with Obesity The child who is already obese needs careful management. Weight loss is ordinarily not recommended because it may easily impair growth in children. Instead, aim to maintain a constant weight while the obese child grows taller. The object is to support normal lean body development, while letting children "grow out" of their obesity.

Preventing Cardiovascular Disease To reduce the risk of developing CVD, first and foremost, prevent or treat obesity. This alone may be sufficient to normalize blood cholesterol and benefit cardiac health. Direct evidence that reducing blood cholesterol in children will reduce heart disease risk in adulthood does not exist; such research would necessarily involve following large numbers of people from childhood through several decades. However, many studies show that correcting high blood cholesterol by diet or drug treatment in adults slows the progression of atherosclerosis.[24] Such studies support the belief that control of blood cholesterol in children will reduce the risk of heart disease in adulthood.

Screening for Those at Risk Information from the Bogalusa Heart Study (a long-term study of CVD risks in children and young adults) and other population studies of U.S. children show much obesity and high blood cholesterol.[25] Based on such prevalence data and on evidence that the risks associated with these factors persist into adulthood, some experts recommend routine screening to identify all children with high cholesterol.[26] Other experts argue that universal screening could lead to overuse of cholesterol-lowering drugs during childhood and adolescence.[27] Currently, selective screening for children and adolescents whose parents or grandparents have CVD is recommended. Given these criteria, many children with high cholesterol will not be identified.

Food Choices to Prevent Heart Disease An expert panel on blood cholesterol in children and adolescents recommends that, regardless of family history, beginning at age two, healthy children and adolescents consume a diet containing, on average, no more than 30 percent of total kcalories from fat, less than 10 percent of total kcalories from saturated fat, and less than 300 milligrams of cholesterol per day. The American Academy of Pediatrics recommends a similar diet, but cautions against fat intakes of less than 30 percent of total kcalories for growing children. Translated into foods, this means healthy children over age two need balanced meals that provide lean meat, poultry, fish, and legumes; fruits and vegetables; whole grains; and low-fat dairy products. Such meals provide enough food energy and nutrients to support growth and maintain blood cholesterol within a healthy range.[28]

Avoiding Power Struggles It is not surprising that problems over food often arise during the second or third year, when children are asserting their independence. Many of these problems stem from the conflict between children's developmental stages and capabilities and parents who, in attempting to do what they think is best for their children, try to control every aspect of eating. Such conflicts can disrupt children's abilities to regulate their own food intakes or to determine their own likes and dislikes. For example, many people share the misconception that children must be persuaded or coerced to try new foods. Research with children indicates the opposite. When children are forced to try new foods, even by way of rewards, they are less likely to try those foods again than are children who are left to decide for themselves.[29] The parent is responsible for *what* the child is offered to eat, but the child is responsible for *how much* and even *whether* to eat.[30]

When introducing new foods at the table, parents are advised to offer them one at a time and only in small amounts at first. The more often a food is presented to a young child, the more likely the child will like that food. Whenever possible, the new food should be presented at the beginning of the meal, when the child is hungry, but the child should make the decision to accept or reject it. Parents have their own inclinations and dislikes; so do children. It is best never to make an issue of food acceptance. A power struggle almost invariably sets a firm pattern of resistance and permanently closes the child's mind.

Honoring Children's Preferences Researchers attempting to explain children's food preferences encounter many contradictions. Children say they like colorful foods, yet most often reject green and yellow vegetables while favoring brown peanut butter, white potatoes, apple wedges, and bread. They do like raw vegetables better than cooked ones,

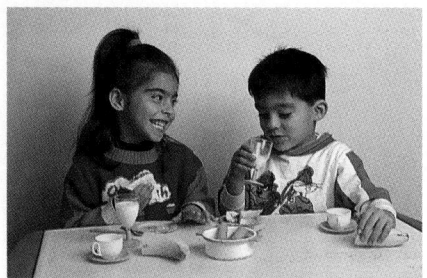

Little children like little tables and little portions.

though, so it is wise to offer vegetables that are raw or slightly undercooked and crunchy and bright in color. They should be warm, not hot, because a child's mouth is much more sensitive than an adult's. The flavor should be mild (a child has more taste buds), and smooth foods such as mashed potatoes or pea soup should have no lumps (a child wonders, with some disgust, what the lumps might be). Vegetables should be served separately and be easy to eat.

Small children like to eat at little tables and to be served little portions of food. They also love to eat with other children and have been observed to stay at the table longer and eat much more when in the company of their peers. Parents who serve food in a relaxed and casual manner, without anxiety, provide the emotional climate in which a child's negative emotions will be minimized.

Preventing Choking When feeding children, parents must always be alert to the dangers of choking. A choking child is a silent child—an adult should be present whenever a child is eating. Make sure the child sits when eating; choking is too likely when a child is running or falling. Round foods such as grapes, nuts, hard candies, and hot dog pieces are hard to control in a mouth with few teeth, and they can easily become lodged in a small opening of a child's trachea. Other potentially dangerous foods include tough meat, popcorn, and chips.

Play First Ideally, each meal is preceded, not followed, by the activity the child looks forward to the most. A number of schools have discovered that children eat a much better lunch if it is served after, rather than before, recess—otherwise, children "hurry up and eat" so that they can go and play.

Child Participation Allowing children to help plan and prepare the family's meals provides enjoyable learning experiences and encourages children to eat the foods they have prepared. Vegetables are pretty, especially when fresh, and provide opportunities for children to learn about color, growing things and their seeds, and shapes and textures—all of which are fascinating to young children. Measuring, stirring, decorating, and arranging foods are skills that even a very small child can practice with enjoyment and pride.

Snacks Parents may find that their children often snack so much that they aren't hungry at mealtimes. Instead of teaching children *not* to snack, teach them *how* to snack. Provide snacks that are as nutritious as the foods served at mealtime. Snacks can even be mealtime foods that are served individually over time, instead of all at once on one plate. When providing snacks to children, think of the food groups and offer such snacks as pieces of cheese, tangerine slices, carrot sticks, and peanut butter on whole-wheat crackers. Snacks that are easy to prepare should be readily available to children, especially if they arrive home after school before their parents.

Sick Children Children sometimes lose their appetites when they are sick with colds or flu and sometimes for no apparent reason at all. On a short-term basis, this is usually nothing to worry about. As children who are ill recover, so will their appetites. The child who is sick should be encouraged to drink plenty of fluids. Chapter 14 gives suggestions to improve the appetite of the hospitalized child.

Television's Influence U.S. children spend more time watching television than doing anything else except sleeping. By some estimates, the average high school senior has spent 15,000 hours watching TV. Survey data show a direct relationship between time spent watching television and the incidence and prevalence of obesity among children and adolescents.[31] This may be because TV watchers eat more energy-rich foods while watching or as a result of the food commercials they see on TV; or it may be because TV time displaces physical activity time. Some research shows that while people are watching TV, their metabolic rates are slower than when they are simply resting.[32] (Another study, however, found that television viewing did not alter metabolic rate.[33]) Regardless of the exact mechanism by which TV watching may promote obesity, common sense dictates that the more time children spend watching TV, the less time they will spend on other activities—including outdoor and active play.

The average child sees about 10,000 commercials a year, and almost all of them urge viewers to purchase sugar-coated breakfast cereals, candy bars, chips, fast foods, and carbonated beverages. Those foods add sugar, fat, and salt to the diet and displace foods that provide needed nutrients. Many parents and pediatricians believe that food ads aimed at children should be banned because they support corporate profits rather than children's health. Alternatively, parents can teach their children how to evaluate food ads and make healthful choices.

Nutrition at School

While parents are attempting to establish good eating habits in their children at home, preschools or grade schools introduce foods prepared and served by outsiders. The U.S. government funds several programs to provide nutritious, high-quality meals for children at school. Both the School Breakfast Program and the National School Lunch Program provide meals at a reasonable cost to children from families with the financial means to pay. Meals are available free or at reduced cost to children from low-income families.

School Breakfast The School Breakfast Program is available in slightly more than half of the nation's schools, and about 5 million children participate in it. The school breakfast must contain at a minimum the food servings listed in the margin. Surveys show that the majority of children who eat school breakfasts are from low-income families. As research results continue to emphasize the positive impact breakfast has on school performance and health, campaigns to expand school breakfast programs are under way.

A school breakfast must offer at least:

- One serving of fluid milk.
- One serving of fruit or vegetable or full-strength juice.
- Two servings of bread or bread alternates, or two servings of meat or meat alternates, or one of each.

School Lunch Nearly 25 million children receive lunches through the National School Lunch Program—half of them at a free or reduced

Table 16–5
School Lunch Patterns for Different Ages

	PRESCHOOL (AGE)		GRADE SCHOOL THROUGH HIGH SCHOOL (GRADE)		
FOOD GROUP	**1 to 2**	**3 to 4**	**K to 3**	**4 to 6**	**7 to 12**
Meat or meat alternate					
1 serving:					
Lean meat, poultry, or fish	1 oz	1 ½ oz	1 ½ oz	2 oz	3 oz
Cheese	1 oz	1 ½ oz	1 ½ oz	2 oz	3 oz
Large egg(s)	½	¾	¾	1	1 ½
Cooked dry beans or peas	¼ c	⅜ c	⅜ c	½ c	¾ c
Peanut butter	2 tbs	3 tbs	3 tbs	4 tbs	6 tbs
Vegetable and/or fruit					
2 or more servings, both to total	½ c	½ c	½ c	¾ c	¾ c
Bread or bread alternate					
Servings[a]	5 per week	8 per week	8 per week	8 per week	10 per week
Milk					
1 serving of fluid milk	¾ c	¾ c	1 c	1 c	1 c

[a]A serving is 1 slice bread; 1 biscuit, roll, or muffin; ½ c cooked rice, pasta, or cereal grain.

Source: U.S. Department of Agriculture, *Food Program Facts—National School Lunch Program,* 1992.

price. School lunches are designed to provide at least a third of the RDA for each nutrient and must include specified numbers of servings of milk, protein-rich food (meat, poultry, fish, cheese, eggs, legumes, or peanut butter), vegetables, fruits, and breads or other grain foods. Table 16–5 shows school lunch patterns for children of different ages.

The Teen Years

The teen years bring many changes, physically, emotionally, intellectually, and socially. Nutrient needs are greatly enhanced during adolescence; only the needs for pregnancy and lactation are greater. Making sure that nutrient needs are met presents a challenge.

A significant transition is that teens make many more choices for themselves than they did as children. Teenagers are not fed; they eat. And they are not sent out to play; they choose whether to invest their energy in physical activity. Social pressures thrust choices at them: whether to drink alcohol or not, or whether to develop their bodies to meet sometimes extreme ideals of slimness or athletic prowess. The person concerned with the nutrition and health of teenagers cannot simply supply food, but must instead deliver motivation. Few teenagers become interested in nutrition for its contribution to health. Lessons (and misinformation) in nutrition come to them by way of personal experiences—eating to improve athletic performance or dieting to lose unwanted pounds. That means that would-be teachers must learn what subjects teenagers are interested in and show how nutrition relates to those subjects. The next few sections examine the nutrient needs of teenagers and the influences that affect their food choices.

Growth

The rate of growth, which has been fairly steady throughout childhood, speeds up abruptly and dramatically with the onset of adolescence. Up to now, girls' and boys' growth patterns have differed little, but with the onset of puberty, they become distinct. A girl's adolescent growth spurt begins at age 10 or 11 and reaches its peak at 12. A boy's growth spurt begins at 12 or 13 and peaks at 14. In girls, fat becomes a larger percentage of the total body weight, and in boys, muscle and bone become much greater. The growth spurt brings not only a dramatic increase in height and weight, but also hormonal changes that profoundly affect every organ of the body, including the brain, and culminate in the emergence of physically mature adults within two or three years.

The growth spurt lasts about two years, but individual experiences vary widely.[34] Growth charts used for children must be abandoned when the signs of puberty begin to appear. Age in years indicates little about development. The only way to be sure a teenager is growing normally is to compare his or her height and weight with previous measures taken at intervals. Rating scales based on stages of adolescent development are available and widely used to record developmental changes during puberty.[35]

Energy and Nutrient Needs

The energy needs of teenagers vary to a great extent, depending on their current rates of growth, body size, and physical activity. The energy needs of teenage boys may be especially high. Boys experience a more intense growth spurt and develop more lean body mass than girls do. An active teenage boy of 15 may need 4000 kcalories or more a day just to maintain his weight. In general, because girls enter their growth spurts earlier and then grow less than boys, their energy needs peak sooner and decline more quickly.[36] Thus teenage girls need to pay special attention to being physically active and selecting foods of high nutrient density in order to meet their nutrient needs without exceeding their energy needs.

Obesity The insidious problem of obesity becomes more apparent in adolescence than before and often continues into adulthood. Those who are obese during childhood or adolescence face a 70 percent risk of becoming obese adults. Overfatness and obesity during adolescence predict later health risks and earlier deaths.[37] Obesity occurs mostly in girls, and especially in black girls.[38] Young women who become interested in nutrition may make choices that benefit their health and fitness, or they may become dangerously obsessed with weight control (see Nutrition in Practice 9).

Iron Iron remains a nutrient of special concern. Iron needs increase in teen girls as they start to menstruate and in boys as their lean body mass develops. Food intake surveys show that adolescent iron intakes often fail to keep pace with increasing needs, especially for girls, who typically consume less meat and fewer total kcalories than boys do.[39]

Calcium Another nutrient of concern during adolescence is calcium. Low calcium intakes, especially during the adolescent growth spurt and especially if paired with physical inactivity, may compromise the development of peak bone mass. The attainment of maximal bone mass is considered the best protection against age-related bone loss and fractures.[40] Once again, teenage girls are at greatest risk, for their milk intakes tend to decline as they begin choosing soft drinks instead of milk at the time when their calcium needs are greatest.[41]

Other Nutrients Other nutrients are also required in greater quantities during adolescence than in childhood. These nutrient requirements either level off or diminish slightly as the adolescent passes into adulthood.

Food Choices and Health Habits

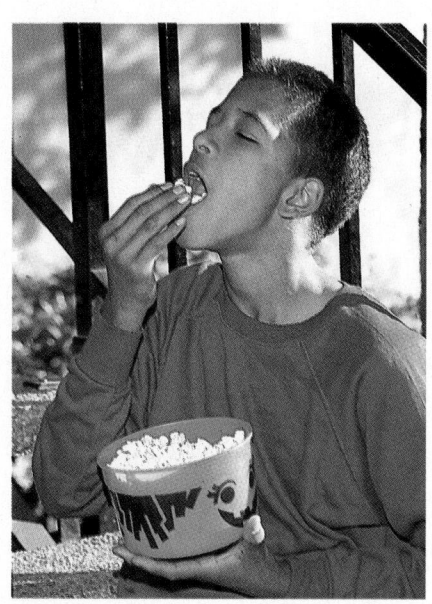

Nutritious snacks play an important role in an active teen's diet.

Teenagers come and go as they choose and eat what they want when they have time. With a multitude of after-school, social, and job activities, they almost inevitably fall into irregular eating habits. The teenage snacker who finds only nutritious foods around the house is well provided for.

Snacks Snacks provide about a fourth of the average teenager's total daily food energy intake. Teens receive substantial amounts of protein, thiamin, riboflavin, vitamin B_6, magnesium, and zinc from snacks. The nutrients they most often fail to obtain are calcium, iron, vitamin A, and folate. Protein usually need not be stressed, but many teenagers need to be encouraged to seek out more dairy products for calcium. Iron-rich snacks include bean burritos, bran muffins, and peanut butter and crackers. Green vegetables are the best sources of vitamin A and folate; the two go together in these vegetables.

Eating Away from Home Inevitably, teenagers do a lot of eating away from home. There, as well as at home, their nutritional welfare is favored or hindered by the choices they make. A lunch of a hamburger, a chocolate shake, and french fries can supply nutrients in the amounts shown in Table 16–6 at a kcalorie cost of 820, a cost some teenagers can afford. With the exception of vitamin A, vitamin C, folate, and zinc, these are substantial percentages of the recommended intakes. Depending on how they adjust their breakfast and dinner choices, lean, active teenagers may easily meet their nutrient needs with this kind of lunch. They need only select fruits and vegetables for vitamins A, C, and folate, good fiber sources, and more good iron and zinc sources at their other meals.

Adult Influence Teenagers are intensely engaged in day-to-day life with their peers and preparing for their future lives as adults. Adults need to remember that teenagers have the right to make their own decisions—even if those decisions are not in line with the adults' own views. Gatekeepers can set up the environment so that nutritious foods are available and can stand by with reliable nutrition information and advice, but the rest is up to the teenagers. Ultimately, they make the choices.

Drugs, Alcohol, Tobacco, and Nutrition

The teen years are a critical time in the development of problem behaviors such as drug, alcohol, and tobacco use. Three of every five high school seniors report that they have at least tried an illicit drug, most commonly marijuana.[42] One in 20 high school seniors reports having used cocaine at least once.[43] Illicit drug use by adolescents rose significantly between 1992 and 1993, reversing the downward trend observed previously.[44]

Marijuana Smoking a marijuana cigarette affects the body in several ways. In some people, it leads to taste changes that temporarily enhance the enjoyment of eating, especially of sweets, commonly known as "the munchies." Why or how this effect occurs is not known; it may be a social effect caused by suggestibility, or it may be that the drug stimulates appetite. Prolonged use of the drug does not seem to bring about a weight gain. Marijuana abusers often consume fewer nutrients than do non-abusers, probably because the extra foods they choose are usually low-nutrient snack foods.

Marijuana users may think that because they usually smoke fewer marijuana cigarettes in a day than they would tobacco cigarettes, they will incur fewer harmful, long-term effects on their lungs. This is a myth. Research shows that one marijuana cigarette is bad for the body as four or five tobacco cigarettes. People who smoke marijuana inhale more smoke and hold it in their lungs longer, so regular smokers of several marijuana cigarettes a day face the same risk of lung cancer as people who smoke a pack of tobacco cigarettes a day.[45]

Cocaine Cocaine elicits effects such as intense euphoria, restlessness, heightened self-confidence, irritability, insomnia, and loss of appetite. The stronger the craving for cocaine, the less a drug abuser wants food. Weight loss is a common side effect, and cocaine abusers often develop eating disorders.[46] Rats given unlimited cocaine will choose the drug over food until they die of starvation.[47] Thus, unlike marijuana use, cocaine use brings major nutritional consequences.

Repeated cocaine use can cause rapid heart rate, irregular heartbeats, heart attacks, and even death. Cocaine use continues to escalate as cheaper and more dangerous forms of the drug become available. Cocaine in its smokable form, crack, is more addicting than any other drug.[48] The addictive power of cocaine is overwhelming. One former crack addict tells of holding a gun to his brother's head to steal money for his next crack purchase.

The effects of other addictive drugs vary in degree, but are similar in kind to those of cocaine. Drug abusers face multiple nutrition problems. They spend money for drugs that could be spent on food; they lose interest in food during "high" times; and some drugs depress the appetite.

Table 16–6
Selected Nutrients in a Hamburger, Low-Fat Chocolate Shake, and Small Serving of French Fries

NUTRIENT	MALE[a] % RDA	FEMALE[a] % RDA
Energy	28	36
Protein	48	60
Fat[b]	25	32
Calcium	38	38
Iron	36	24
Zinc	16	20
Vitamin A	9	11
Thiamin	38	49
Riboflavin	39	50
Niacin	33	42
Folate	18	20
Vitamin C	7	7
Sodium	34	34

[a]RDA for a 19-year-old, moderately active, person of average height and weight.
[b]Fat does not have an RDA. The standard of comparison used is 30% of the energy RDA.

During withdrawal from drugs, an important aspect of treatment is the identification and correction of nutrition problems.

Alcohol The nutrition implications of alcohol use and the consequences of its abuse are described in Nutrition in Practice 8. To sum them all up, alcohol is an empty-kcalorie beverage that can displace needed nutrients from the diet while simultaneously impairing the absorption and metabolism of nutrients. Imbalances therefore occur even if nutrient intakes are adequate. People who are unable to use alcohol with moderation must abstain completely from its use if they are to maintain good health.

Cigarette Smoking Cigarette smoking causes thousands of people to suffer from cancer and diseases of the cardiovascular, digestive, and respiratory systems. Within the scope of nutrition, smoking influences hunger, body weight, and nutrient status. Links between smoking's nutrition effects and lung cancer are also known.

Smoking a cigarette eases feelings of hunger. A smoker who receives a hunger signal can quiet it with a cigarette rather than with food. Such behavior ignores body signals and postpones energy and nutrient intake. Thus smokers tend to weigh less than nonsmokers and to gain weight upon cessation of smoking.[49] Weight gain is often a concern for people contemplating giving up cigarettes. The decision to quit recognizes that the risks of smoking outweigh the disadvantages of weight gain. The message to smokers wanting to quit is to work hard to adjust diet and exercise habits so as to maintain weight while quitting and thereafter.

Nutrient intakes of smokers and nonsmokers differ. Smokers have lower intakes of dietary fiber, vitamin A, folate, and vitamin C.[50] These associations are noteworthy because the metabolism of vitamin C is altered in smokers and because vitamin A exerts a protective effect against lung cancer.

Research shows that the vitamin C requirement of smokers exceeds that of nonsmokers.[51] Smokers break down vitamin C faster and therefore require more vitamin C to achieve steady body pools. The vitamin C requirement of smokers may be as much as twice as high as that of nonsmokers. The evidence for this is so strong that it is reflected in the vitamin C RDA—at least 100 milligrams per day for smokers compared to 60 for nonsmokers.[52]

Beta-carotene, a precursor to vitamin A found in vegetables, has anticancer activity.[53] Specifically, the risk of lung cancer is greatest for smokers who have the lowest intakes of carotene. Of course, this does not mean that as long as they eat their carrots, people can safely smoke cigarettes. Smokers are ten times more likely to get lung cancer than nonsmokers. People who do smoke, however, as well as those who do not, can lower their cancer risks by eating fruits and vegetables rich in carotene.

The nutrition and lifestyle choices people make as children, teenagers, and young adults have long-term, as well as immediate, effects on their health. The challenge for parents and health professionals concerned with their well-being is to motivate them to make sound choices by modeling good habits early and then by showing them how such choices relate to their own interests.

Nutrition Assessment

Assessment of nutrition status in healthy children and teenagers can confirm that development is normal or can catch potential problems early. As with pregnant women and infants, careful histories and measures of growth are most useful. In assessing, focus on the following:

- The history should reveal whether a child is eating appropriately from all food groups (recall Table 16–1). How much is the child snacking? Are snacks nutritious? Is the child receiving adequate iron from the foods typically eaten? Is milk intake adequate? If milk must be omitted from the diet, are appropriate substitutes in use? The history should discover both home and school food intakes, as well as those in any other place where the child spends significant amounts of time. Aberrant food patterns may suggest food allergies or intolerances and a need for intervention.
- The socioeconomic history may reveal a need for food assistance programs. Are any risk factors for lead poisoning present?
- By adolescence, healthful exercise habits should be apparent. The history should also reveal any factors that might interfere with adequate food intakes such as inappropriate dieting, bizarre diets, alcohol or drug use, or smoking.
- Height and weight plotted over time will produce a smooth growth curve if development is normal. If significant obesity or underweight is apparent in children, intervention is in order. During the adolescent growth spurt, wide variations in height and weight gain patterns are expected.
- Physical examination can reveal many clues to nutrition status as shown in Table 16–3. If any signs suggest possible malnutrition, further investigation is appropriate.

Clinical conditions that may affect the health care of children and teenagers are treated in later chapters and necessitate other emphases in nutrition assessment.

■ STUDY QUESTIONS ■

1. What are the health consequences of allowing children to eat large quantities of nutrient-poor foods?
2. What is the most prevalent nutrient deficiency among children and adolescents in the United States? What dietary strategies can help prevent this deficiency?
3. Describe the relationship between iron deficiency and lead poisoning in children.
4. Explain why infants and children are so vulnerable to lead poisoning.
5. Explain what a true food allergy is. Which foods most often cause allergic reactions?
6. List some strategies for introducing new foods to young children.
7. Why is a teenaged girl more likely to develop an iron deficiency than is a boy?
8. Why do drug abusers face nutrition problems?
9. How do the nutrient intakes of smokers differ from those of nonsmokers? What impacts can those differences exert on health?

NUTRITION IN PRACTICE 16

Nutrition and Premenstrual Syndrome

For the millions of women who suffer symptoms of premenstrual syndrome (PMS), the idea that some simple remedy may bring relief is inviting. And no wonder—surveys show that as many as one in three women suffers one or more symptoms of PMS. Over 100 symptoms—including mood swings, bloating, headaches, breast tenderness, anxiety, and food cravings—have been reported.[54] In about 5 percent of women, at least one physical or psychological symptom can reach such severity as to be temporarily disabling.[55] So far, though, the prevention or alleviation of PMS remains a challenge. Many nutrition-based remedies have been advocated over the years, and new claims continue to surface. Are they valid?

How is nutrition related to menstruation and PMS?

The scientific literature on PMS and nutrition is confusing. One obstacle researchers encounter in their efforts to find a treatment is that many women with PMS respond favorably to placebo treatments (see the glossary). People's faith in medicine may ease their symptoms, even when the medicine is ineffective, and the use of placebos shows that this often happens with PMS.

Some connections between nutrition and PMS are clear, however. For example, the hormones that regulate the menstrual cycle also alter the metabolic rate, glucose tolerance, appetite, and food intake. Many women find that they are hungrier than usual during the week or two prior to menstruation. Research suggests that three things happen during that time:

- Basal metabolic rate during sleep speeds up.[56]
- Appetite and food energy intake increase.[57]
- Carbohydrate intake increases.[58]

One report found no significant changes in total energy intakes before menstruation, but noted that premenstrual women drank more sugar-containing beverages.[59] Most studies seem to indicate that women take in an average of 300 kcalories a day more during the ten days prior to menstruation than during the ten days after.

Is it wrong to eat more food prior to menstruation than after?

No, in fact, these findings suggest that eating more food prior to menstruation may be appropriate at that time, because the accelerated metabolic rate raises the energy need. If eating extra food does any harm, it comes from failing to reduce intakes after menstruation when the metabolic rate again declines. Unfortunately, many women attempt to fight the menstrual cycle in an effort to control their weight. During the two weeks *following* menstruation, eating small amounts of food may be relatively easy to do, but during the two weeks *prior* to menstruation, it may be extremely difficult; women are fighting a natural, hormone-governed increase in metabolic rate and appetite, and possibly even a built-in craving for carbohydrates. It is possible that the stress of responding inappropriately to cyclic changes in appetite and basal metabolic rate contributes to symptoms such as fatigue and tension in women prior to menstruation.

Why do some women crave sweets prior to menstruation?

Research is attempting to answer this question. In a study of women who naturally tended to eat more carbohydrates prior to menstruation, researchers fed the women a high-carbohydrate meal. An hour later, women with severe PMS reported significant alleviation of their depression, confusion, fatigue, tension, and anger.[60] The high-carbohydrate meal had no effect on women in the control

Glossary

placebo (plah-SEE-bow)**:** an inert, harmless substance that resembles medicine. Placebos are used in research to distinguish the effects of faith and hope from the effects of the medicine.

premenstrual syndrome (PMS): a cluster of physical, psychological, and behavioral symptoms that some women experience prior to menstruation; the symptoms diminish during or after menstruation.

group or on the women with PMS during their postmenstrual week. As in other PMS research, though, it is possible that the women felt better because they *expected* to (the placebo effect). In any case, the researchers suggest that instead of avoiding carbohydrates as many women do, women with PMS should eat more of them prior to menstruation—especially complex carbohydrates such as pasta, whole-grain cereals, and breads—along with vegetables and fruits. This advice squares with the *Diet and Health Recommendations* introduced in Chapter 1.

Some women who have PMS symptoms say they have "changed their diets" to help relieve their symptoms. The most common dietary changes recommended to help relieve PMS discomfort involve reducing consumption of sugar, fat, salt, alcohol, and caffeine. Diets that emphasize complex carbohydrates are generally lower in simple sugar, fat, and salt than diets that do not. For this and many other reasons, everyone—including those with PMS—is wise to eat ample complex carbohydrates every day.

You mentioned that common dietary changes recommended to relieve PMS include reducing alcohol and caffeine intake. Is there proof that these changes are beneficial?

Recommendations that women with PMS reduce their alcohol intakes are based partly on the knowledge that improvements in general health and well-being are advantageous. The case regarding alcohol is based on logic: alcohol is a depressant and can worsen depression in some women. In the case of caffeine, research shows that PMS is more prevalent and severe among women who consume caffeine than among those who do not and is worst among the highest consumers.[61]

Is there any basis for taking vitamin-mineral supplements for PMS?

No evidence supports nutrient deficiencies as a cause of PMS, and in fact, one study using biochemical tests of nutrition status found no significant difference between women with and without PMS.[62] Despite this, unproven nutrient treatments for PMS continue to be advocated. Over the years, various nutrients have captured media attention as treatments for PMS. Among the most popular nutrients proposed to treat PMS are vitamin B_6, vitamin E, and zinc.

Trials of vitamin B_6 in PMS have resulted in contradictory findings. In one study, vitamin B_6 did improve premenstrual symptoms related to autonomic reactions (such as dizziness and vomiting) and behavioral changes (such as poor performance and a tendency to withdraw from social activities), but a significant number of physical symptoms remained during the premenstrual phase.[63] In another study, women with PMS symptoms received nutrition counseling, dietary instruction, and vitamin B_6 supplements (250 milligrams per day), or nutrition counseling and dietary instruction only, to see if the diet instructions or supplements might reduce the severity of PMS symptoms.[64] The researchers found no significant improvement in symptom severity with diet modification or vitamin B_6 supplements. The researchers concluded that evidence of a significant role for vitamin B_6 in PMS is still lacking. Besides, doses of vitamin B_6 as low as 50 milligrams (a dose sometimes suggested for treatment of PMS) are potentially toxic. For these reasons, any possible benefits derived from this type of therapy must be weighed against the possible detrimental effects of megadoses.

The vitamin B_6–PMS research can be summed up by saying that the vitamin may help remedy symptoms only if a relative or absolute deficiency of the vitamin has caused them. The old lesson of basic nutrition is reinforced here: a vitamin will clear up only the symptoms that are caused by a deficiency of that vitamin.

What about Vitamin E?

Vitamin E is another popular candidate for treatment of PMS, and many extravagant claims have been made for it over the years. One condition that may sometimes be caused by Vitamin E deficiency is fibrocystic breast disease, as mentioned in Chapter 7. One creditable attempt has demonstrated that vitamin E helps relieve breast pain and tenderness, which are often experienced in PMS. The research involved 41 women in a double-blind, placebo-controlled study. The results suggested that vitamin E (400 IU) brought relief, whereas the placebo did not. Vitamin E had little effect on many other symptoms of PMS, however, and until further research is done, the evidence for vitamin E as a treatment for PMS remains inconclusive.[65] Possibly, the correct logic is that vitamin E deficiency can cause sore breasts and that the menstrual cycle can make them worse, but not that vitamin E deficiency causes PMS.

What about zinc and PMS?

Because tiny amounts of zinc help regulate the secretion of hormones involved in the menstrual cycle, researchers decided to compare blood zinc concentrations of women with and without PMS.[66] The women with PMS had significantly lower blood zinc concentrations than the women without PMS. The researchers speculate that low blood zinc might impair the secretion of menstrual hormones such as progesterone, as well as natural opiates, or endorphins, which are the body's own painkillers. If zinc deficiency does contribute to PMS, however, it may affect only some women with the condition. Zinc is toxic in excess. Women should not self-diagnose zinc deficiency or self-prescribe zinc as treatment for PMS. Further research is needed to confirm a relationship between zinc deficiency and PMS. In the meantime, women who suspect their diets may be low in zinc are advised to eat (you guessed it) zinc-rich foods such as those suggested in Chapter 8.

How would you suggest that the person with PMS manage her diet?

The same advice holds for women with PMS as for women or men with any other health problem or need. Be sure to get adequate sleep and adequate exercise. Eat well, and be sensible about intakes of sugar, caffeine, salt, alcohol, and any other "abuseable" substances. If you have reason to believe your nutrient intake is inadequate and you are unable to rectify it by eating foods, fall back on a daily supplement for a while, but avoid megadoses. Stay with the moderate amounts available in an ordinary multi-vitamin-mineral supplement (see Nutrition in Practice 7). And be skeptical. Don't trust anyone who wants to pocket your money in return for a product that will relieve your symptoms. Watch out for snake-oil salespeople; they are everywhere.

■ NOTES ■

1. S. Shea and coauthors, Variability and self-regulation of energy intake in young children in their everyday environment, *Pediatrics* 90 (1992): 542–546.
2. L. L. Birch and coauthors, The variability of young children's energy intake, *New England Journal of Medicine* 324 (1991): 232–235.
3. R. E. Klesges and coauthors, Parental influence on food selection in young children and its relationships to childhood obesity, *American Journal of Clinical Nutrition* 53 (1991): 859–864.
4. Food Research and Action Center, *Community Childhood Hunger Identification Project: A Survey of Childhood Hunger in the United States, Executive Summary* (Washington, D.C.: Food Research and Action Center, March 1991).
5. Food Research and Action Center, 1991.
6. A. F. Meyers and coauthors, School breakfast program and school performance, *American Journal of Diseases of Children* 143 (1989): 1234–1239.
7. E. Pollitt, Iron deficiency and cognitive function, *Annual Review of Nutrition* 13 (1993): 521–537.
8. J. D. Haas and M. W. Fairchild, Summary and conclusions of the International Conference on Iron Deficiency and Behavioral Development, October 10–12, 1988, *American Journal of Clinical Nutrition* 50 (1989): 703–705.
9. R. Yip, The changing characteristics of childhood iron nutritional status in the United States, in *Dietary Iron: Birth to Two Years,* ed. L. J. Filer (New York: Raven Press, 1989), pp. 37–56.
10. P. L. Splett and M. Story, Child nutrition: Objectives for the decade, *Journal of the American Dietetic Association* 91 (1991): 665–668.
11. N. S. Scrimshaw, Iron deficiency, *Scientific American,* October 1991, pp. 46-52.
12. R. Yip, The interaction of lead and iron, in *Dietary Iron: Birth to Two Years,* ed. L. J. Filer (New York: Raven Press, 1989), pp. 179–181.
13. H. Needleman and coauthors, The long-term effects of exposure to low doses of lead in childhood: An 11-year follow-up report, *New England Journal of Medicine* 322 (1990): 83–88; S. Piomelli and J. A. Wolff, Childhood lead poisoning in the '90s, *Pediatrics* 93 (1994): 508–510.
14. J. Murphy, Federal agencies gearing up for new efforts against lead, *Nation's Health,* May/June 1991, pp. 1, 23.
15. A. Greeley, Getting the lead out of just about everything, *FDA Consumer,* July/August 1991, pp. 27–31.
16. Childhood lead poisoning: A disease for the history texts (editorial), *American Journal of Public Health* 81 (1991): 685.
17. J. Raloff, Lead effects show in child's balance, *Science News* 135 (1989): 54.
18. H. A. Sampson and D. D. Metcalfe, Food allergies, *Journal of the American Medical Association* 268 (1992): 2840–2844.
19. S. A. Bock and F. M. Atkins, Patterns of food hypersensitivity challenges, *Journal of Pediatrics* 117 (1990): 561–567.
20. M. L. Arbeit and coauthors, Caffeine intakes of children

from a biracial population: The Bogalusa Heart Study, *Journal of the American Dietetic Association* 88 (1988): 466–471.
21. National Cholesterol Education Program, Report of the Expert Panel on Blood Cholesterol Levels in Children and Adolescents, The population approach: Nutrition recommendations for healthy children and adolescents, *Pediatrics* (supplement) 89 (1992): 537–544.
22. National Cholesterol Education Program, Report of the Expert Panel on Blood Cholesterol Levels in Children and Adolescents, Overview and summary, *Pediatrics* (supplement) 89 (1992): 525–527.
23. W. A. Wattigney and coauthors, Increasing impact of obesity on serum lipids and lipoproteins in young adults: The Bogalusa Heart Study, *Archives of Internal Medicine* 151 (1991): 2017–2022.
24. National Cholesterol Education Program, Report of the Expert Panel on Blood Cholesterol Levels in Children and Adolescents, Rationale for attention to cholesterol levels in children and adolescents, *Pediatrics* (supplement) 89 (1992): 528–536.
25. G. S. Berenson, S. R. Srinivasan, and L. S. Webber, Cardiovascular risk prevention in children: A challenge or a poor idea? *Nutrition, Metabolism and Cardiovascular Diseases* 4 (1994): 46–52.
26. Berenson, Srinivasan, and Webber, 1994.
27. National Cholesterol Education Program, Overview and summary, 1992.
28. Timely statement on NCEP report on children and adolescents, *Journal of the American Dietetic Association* 91 (1991): 983; S. Shea and coauthors, Is there a relationship between dietary fat and stature or growth in children three to five years of age? *Pediatrics* 92 (1993): 579–586.
29. L. L. Birch, D. W. Marlin, and J. Rotter, Eating as the "means" activity in a contingency: Effects on young children's food preference, *Child Development* 55 (1984): 431–439.
30. E. Satter, *How to Get Your Kid to Eat . . . But Not Too Much* (Palo Alto, Calif.: Bull Publishing Company, 1987), pp. 13–28.
31. W. H. Dietz and S. L. Gortmaker, Do we fatten our children at the television set? Obesity and television viewing in children and adolescents, *Pediatrics* 75 (1985): 807–812, as cited in R. C. Klesges, M. L. Shelton, and L. M. Klesges, Effects of television on metabolic rate: Potential implications for childhood obesity, *Pediatrics* 91 (1993): 281–286.
32. Klesges, Shelton, and Klesges, 1993.
33. W. H. Dietz and coauthors, Effect of sedentary activities on resting metabolic rate, *American Journal of Clinical Nutrition* 59 (1994): 556–559.
34. L. E. Underwood, Normal adolescent growth and development, *Nutrition Today,* March/April 1991, pp. 11–16.
35. Underwood, 1991.
36. National Academy of Sciences, Food and Nutrition Board, Committee on Dietary Allowances, *Recommenced Dietary Allowances,* 10th ed. (Washington, D.C.: National Academy Press, 1989), pp. 24–38.
37. A. Must and coauthors, Long-term morbidity and mortality of overweight adolescents, *New England Journal of Medicine* 327 (1992): 1350–1355.
38. T. A. Wadden and coauthors, Obesity in black adolescent girls: A controlled clinical trial of treatment by diet, behavior modification, and parental support, *Pediatrics* 85 (1990): 345–392; Wattigney and coauthors, 1991.
39. J. B. Anderson, The status of adolescent nutrition, *Nutrition Today,* March/April 1991, pp. 7–10.
40. V. Matkovic, Diet, genetics, and peak bone mass of adolescent girls, *Nutrition Today,* March/April 1991, pp. 21–24.
41. Matkovic, 1991.
42. L. D. Johnston, P. M. O'Malley, and J. G. Bachman, Psychotherapeutic, licit, and illicit use of drugs among adolescents, *Journal of Adolescent Health Care* 8 (1987): 36–51.
43. American Council on Science and Health, *Cocaine: Facts and Dangers* (New York: American Council on Science and Health, 1990).
44. U.S. Department of Health and Human Services, HHS Fact Sheet, Monitoring the future study: Drug use among 8th, 10th, and 12th graders, January 1994.
45. T. C. Wu and coauthors, Pulmonary hazards of smoking marijuana as compared with tobacco, *New England Journal of Medicine* 318 (1988): 347–351.
46. J. M. Jonas and M. S. Gold, Cocaine abuse and eating disorders, *Lancet* 1 (1986): 390–391.
47. M. A. Bozarth and R. A. Wise, Toxicity associated with long-term intravenous heroin and cocaine self-administration in the rat, *Journal of the American Medical Association* 254 (1985): 81–83.

48. American Council on Science and Health, 1990.
49. M. E. Mohs, R. R. Watson, and T. Leonard-Green, Nutritional effects of marijuana, heroin, cocaine, and nicotine, *Journal of the American Dietetic Association* 90 (1990): 1261–1267.
50. A. F. Subar, L. C. Harlan, and M. E. Mattson, Food and nutrient intake differences between smokers and non-smokers in the US, *American Journal of Public Health* 80 (1990): 1323–1329.
51. G. Schectman, J. C. Byrd, and H. W. Gruchow, The influence of smoking on vitamin C status in adults, *American Journal of Public Health* 79 (1989): 158–162.
52. National Academy of Sciences, Food and Nutrition Board, Committee on Dietary Allowances, 1989, pp. 115–124.
53. T. V. Ringer and coauthors, Beta-carotene's effects on serum lipoproteins and immunologic indices in humans, *American Journal of Clinical Nutrition* 53 (1991): 688–694.
54. B. Liebman, PMS: Proof or promises? *Nutrition Action,* May 1990, pp. 1, 5–7.
55. R. L. Reid, Premenstrual syndrome, *New England Journal of Medicine* 324 (1991): 1208–1210.
56. G. A. L. Meijer and coauthors, Sleeping metabolic rate in relation to body composition and the menstrual cycle, *American Journal of Clinical Nutrition* 55 (1992): 637–640; J. T. Bisdee, W. P. T. James, and M. A. Shaw, Changes in energy expenditure during the menstrual cycle, *British Journal of Nutrition* 61 (1989): 187–199.
57. V. Tarasuk and G. H. Beaton, Menstrual-cycle patterns in energy and macronutrient intake, *American Journal of Clinical Nutrition* 53 (1991): 442–447; E. J. Gong, D. Garrell, and D. H. Calloway, Menstrual cycle and voluntary food intake, *American Journal of Clinical Nutrition* 49 (1989): 252–258.
58. J. J. Wurtman and coauthors, Effect of nutrient intake on premenstrual depression, *American Journal of Obstetrics and Gynecology* 161 (1989): 1228–1234.
59. A. K. H. Fong and M. J. Kretsch, Changes in dietary intake, urinary nitrogen, and urinary volume across the menstrual cycle, *American Journal of Clinical Nutrition* 57 (1993): 43–46.
60. Wurtman and coauthors, 1989.
61. A. M. Rossignol and H. Bonnlander, Caffeine-containing beverages, total fluid consumption, and premenstrual syndrome, *American Journal of Public Health* 80 (1990): 1106–1110; A. M. Rossignol and coauthors, Tea and premenstrual syndrome in the People's Republic of China, *American Journal of Public Health* 79 (1989): 67–69.
62. M. Mira, P. M. Stewart, and S. F. Abraham, Vitamin and trace element status in premenstrual syndrome, *American Journal of Clinical Nutrition* 47 (1988): 636–641.
63. K. E. Kendall and P. P. Schnurr, The effects of vitamin B_6 supplementation on premenstrual symptoms, *Obstetrics and Gynecology* 2 (1987): 145–149.
64. M. K. Berman, M. L. Taylor, and E. Freeman, Vitamin B_6 and premenstrual syndrome, *Journal of the American Dietetic Association* 90 (1990): 859–861.
65. R. S. London and coauthors, Efficacy of alpha-tocopherol in the treatment of the premenstrual syndrome, *Journal of Reproductive Medicine* 32 (1987): 400–404.
66. PMS: Hints of a link to lunchtime and zinc, *Science News* 27 October 1990, p. 263.

17

Nutrition for Older Adults

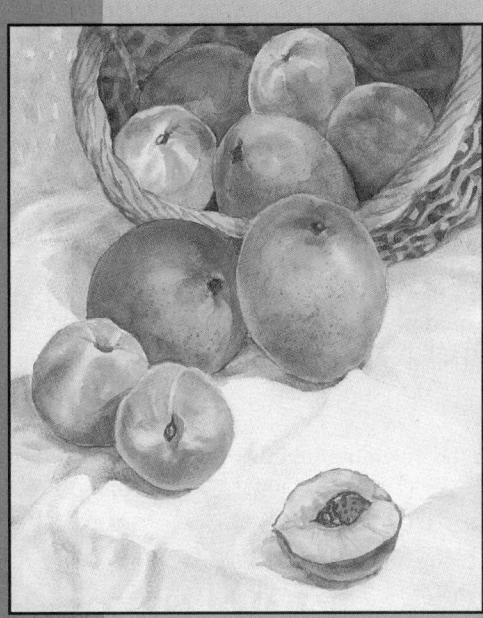

CONTENTS

The last two chapters were devoted to stages of the life cycle that require special nutrition attention: pregnancy, lactation, infancy, childhood, adolescence, and young adulthood. This chapter describes the special nutrition needs of the later adult years.

The most urgent nutrition need of older people, however, is to have made good food choices in the past! All of life's nutrition choices incur health consequences for the better or for the worse. A single day's intakes of nutrients may exert only a minute effect on body organs and their functions, but over years and decades the repeated effects accumulate to have major impacts. This being the case, it is of great importance for everyone, of every age, to pay close attention today to nutrition.

Aging and Nutrition

The majority of U.S. citizens are now middle-aged, and the ratio of old people to young is growing steadily larger, as Figure 17–1 shows. The fastest-growing age group in the United States is people over 85.[1]

life expectancy: the average number of years lived by people in a given society.

In 1992, the life expectancies for U.S. women and men were 79 years and 72 years, respectively, up from about 45 years in 1900. Advances in medical science—antibiotics and other treatments—are largely responsible for almost doubling the life expectancy in this century. Still, the biologic schedule that we call aging, which is built into human beings, cuts off life at a genetically fixed point in time. The life span (the maximum length of life possible for a species) of human beings—115 years—has not changed over the years and is probably the upper limit of human longevity.

life span: the maximum number of years of life attainable by a member of a species.

longevity: long duration of life.

The study of the aging process is one of the youngest scientific disciplines. Only in this century have human beings achieved a life expectancy worthy of a science devoted to studying it. The idea that nutrition can influence the way human bodies age is particularly appealing, since nutrition is a factor that people can control and change.

Nutrition and Longevity

What has been learned so far about the effects of nutrition and environment on longevity provides incentive for researchers to keep asking questions about how and why human beings age. Among their questions are:

- To what extent is aging inevitable? Can aging be slowed through changes in lifestyle and environment?
- What roles does nutrition play in aging, and what roles can it play in retarding aging?

With respect to the first question, it seems that aging is an inevitable, natural process, programmed into the genes at conception, but that people can adopt lifestyle habits such as physical activity and attention to work and recreational environments that will slow the process within the natural limits set by heredity. With respect to the second question, clearly, good nutrition can retard and ease the aging process in many significant ways.

Observation of Elderly People One approach researchers use to search out the secret of long life has been to study other cultures in the hope of finding an extremely long-lived group of people and then learning from them. Scientists have found people who claimed to have lived over 100 years in two different geographical areas. Further study revealed, however, that some of these people only claimed to be 100 or older because age was venerated in their societies. Still, some did prove to be not only remarkably old, but also remarkably healthy. The credit did not go to nutrition: these people did not eat according to any particular formula. The secret—the one thing they all seemed to have in common—was that they lived a physically active life and had remained active into old age. Research on longevity bears this out in this society, too; vigorous physical activity and long life seem to go together.[2] Even a moderate amount of physical activity—for example, a brisk 30-minute walk each day—is protective against early mortality.

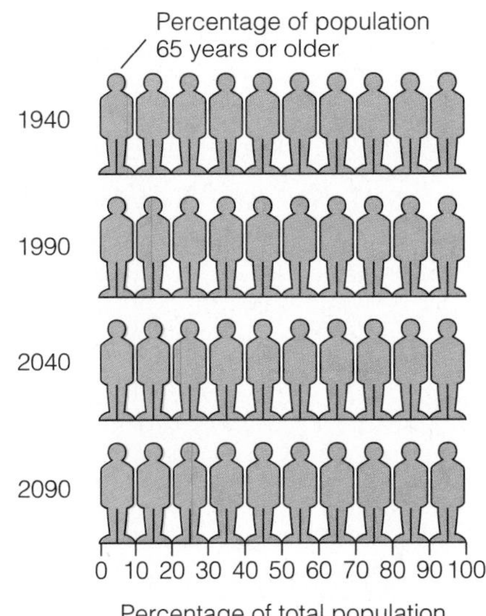

Figure 17–1
The Aging of the U.S. Population
In 1940, 6.8 percent of the population was 65 or older. In 1990, 12.7 percent of us had reached age 65; by 2040, 21.7 percent will have reached age 65; and a century from now, nearly one out of four Americans will be 65 or older. An estimated 25,000 Americans now living are 100 years old or older.

Restriction of kCalories Another approach to prevention of aging has involved manipulating animals' diets and then looking for effects on longevity. These studies have produced some interesting and suggestive findings.[3] For example, rats live longer when their food intake is restricted in the early weeks of their lives, or even when it is restricted after they are mature. Extensive research shows that it is the restriction of food energy rather than restriction of a specific nutrient that exerts the antiaging action.[4]

Several mechanisms to explain how energy restriction prolongs life in rats have been proposed but not proven. Research suggests that food restriction may extend the life span by delaying age-related diseases and preventing damaging lipid oxidation.[5]

Experiments with food restriction and longevity in rats have *not* suggested any direct applications to human nutrition, though, and the animals given restricted feedings have suffered distinct disadvantages. For example, the food restriction was so severe that half of the restricted animals died *very* early (before 300 days). The average length of life for the restricted rats was long because the few survivors lived a long time. The restricted animals that survived were retarded and malformed in a number of ways. Extreme starvation to extend life, like any extreme, is not worth the price.

One group of researchers studied the relationship between *moderate* energy restriction (80 percent of usual intake) and aging retardation in human beings.[6] Sixteen middle-aged, nonobese men were studied during ten weeks of energy restriction. Eight matched controls continued their usual diets. The energy-restricted men lost weight (mostly due to loss of fat), their blood pressures dropped significantly, and their HDL cholesterol concentrations rose significantly. Energy restriction had no adverse effects on mental and physical performance. For these men, moderate energy restriction favorably affected disease risk factors such as obesity, blood pressure, and cholesterol.

Nutrition alone, even if ideal, cannot ensure a long and robust life. Nevertheless, nutrition does clearly affect aging and longevity in human beings by way of its role in disease prevention.

Nutrition and Disease Prevention

Among the better-known relationships between nutrition and disease are the following:

- Appropriate energy intake helps prevent *obesity, diabetes,* and related *cardiovascular diseases,* such as *atherosclerosis* and *hypertension* (Chapters 9, 25, and 26), and may influence the development of some forms of *cancer* (Chapter 28).
- Adequate intakes of essential nutrients prevent *deficiency diseases* such as scurvy, goiter, anemia, and the like (Chapters 7 and 8).
- Variety in food intake, as well as ample intakes of certain vegetables, may be protective against certain types of *cancer* (Chapter 28).
- Moderation in sugar intake helps prevent *dental caries* (Nutrition in Practice 2).
- Appropriate fiber intakes help prevent malfunctions of the digestive tract such as *constipation, diverticulosis,* and possibly *colon cancer* (Chapter 2).
- Moderate sodium and adequate intakes of potassium, calcium, and other minerals help prevent *hypertension,* at least in people who are genetically predisposed to it (Chapters 8 and 26).
- An adequate calcium intake throughout life helps protect against *osteoporosis* (Chapter 8).

Other, less well established links between nutrition and disease are being discovered each day. For example, research efforts to uncover clues about the relationship between nutrition and immunity become more and more urgent as AIDS takes its toll on human life.

Cataracts The question whether nutrition is related to cataracts is under investigation. Cataracts are age-related thickenings of the lenses of the eyes that impair vision and can lead to blindness if not surgically removed. Cataracts occur even in well-nourished individuals due to injury, viral infections, toxic substances, and genetic disorders, but most cataracts are vaguely called senile cataracts—meaning "caused by aging." Cataracts become more prevalent with age. In the United States, only 5 percent of people between the ages of 52 and 64 have cataracts, compared to 46 percent of those between the ages of 75 and 85.[7]

Scientists have searched for possible roles of nutrient deficiencies, excesses, and imbalances in cataract causation. They have observed several possible (and, it should be emphasized, highly tentative) links. One link is to a high intake of galactose, derived from the sugar lactose in milk. Another link is to excess food energy intakes in people with diabetes; still another is to deficiencies of riboflavin, vitamin C, or vitamin E. An eight-year study of more than 50,000 women showed that intakes of carotene (beta-carotene and other carotenes) and vitamin A and long-term vitamin C supplementation were strongly associated with a reduced incidence of cataracts.[8]

When the researchers looked at the connections between specific foods rich in carotenes and cataracts, the results were somewhat surprising. Little or no association was found for carrots, winter squash, and sweet potatoes—foods rich in beta-carotene. However, women who ate spinach or other greens five or more times per week were up to 65 percent less likely to develop cataracts, compared to those who ate such foods less than once a month. Spinach, unlike carrots, winter squash, or sweet potatoes, is rich in the particular carotenes known as lutein and zeaxanthin. This research lends support to the notion that food choices can lower cataract risk.

Arthritis Arthritis, another disease that disables the elderly, is also suspected of having some relationships to nutrition. Arthritis is a painful swelling of the joints that troubles many people as they grow older. During movement, the ends of bones are normally protected from wear by cartilage and by small sacs of fluid that act as a lubricant; but with age, bones sometimes disintegrate, and the joints become malformed and painful to move. The cause of arthritis is unknown, but it afflicts millions around the world and is a major problem of older adults.

arthritis: a usually painful inflammation of a joint caused by many conditions, including infections, metabolic disturbances, or injury; joint structure is usually altered, with loss of function.

Unfortunately, much nutrition quackery surrounds arthritis, making it difficult to ferret out whatever valid relationships to nutrition may exist. Many bizarre diets advertise themselves as arthritis cures. Two or three new popular books on diet for arthritis come out every year, urging people to eat no meat, or drink no milk, or eat all their foods raw, or eat only "natural" foods, or avoid all additives, or—who knows what will be next? Actually, no known diet prevents, relieves, or cures arthritis, but as long as people keep buying the books that make these claims, the law of supply and demand dictates that such books will continue to be published.

Not effective against arthritis:

- Alfalfa.
- Blackstrap molasses.
- Calcium.
- Cod liver oil.
- Fruit.
- Garlic.
- Honey.
- Lecithin.
- Vitamin megadoses.
- Wheat germ oil.
- Yeast.
- 100 other substances.

One possible link between arthritis and diet is through the immune system. Researchers believe that in one type of arthritis (rheumatoid arthritis), the immune system mistakenly attacks the tissues of the bone coverings as it normally would attack an invader.[9] The integrity of the immune system depends on adequate nutrition, and a poor diet probably worsens the condition. It is also possible that for some individuals, certain foods may stimulate the immune system to attack.[10] For example, milk and milk products seem to bring on symptoms of arthritis in some people.

Another nutrient link to arthritis is the now-famous omega-3 fatty acid found in fish oil, EPA. Chapter 3 showed the links between EPA and heart health. Research shows, too, that the same diet recommended there—one low in saturated fat from red meats and dairy products and high in fish oil—can prevent the inflammation in the joints that makes arthritis so painful.[11] Researchers theorize that EPA probably interferes with the action of prostaglandins, chemicals involved in the inflammatory responses of body tissues.

A known connection between arthritis and nutrition exists in overweight persons. Weight loss is important for these people because the joints affected are often weight-bearing joints that are stressed and irritated by having to carry excess poundage. Weight-loss diets alone often relieve the worst of the pain of arthritis. Interestingly, though, weight loss often helps relieve arthritis in the hands, which are not weight bearing. Perhaps the drastic reduction in fat intake that accompanies the adoption of a kcalorie-restricted diet contributes independently to arthritis relief.

Still another nutrition connection with arthritis is through the pain-relieving drugs used to treat it. Some drugs may affect nutrient availability. When these drugs are used over long times, attention to nutrition status is mandatory. Table E-1 in Appendix E presents the nutrient interactions of many pain relievers.

These brief discussions of cataracts and arthritis show that nutrition can provide at least some protection against certain diseases commonly associated with aging. In fact, in general, it is beginning to look as if nutrition through the prime years may play a greater role than has been realized in preventing many changes once thought to be inevitable consequences of growing older.

Nutrient Needs and Nutrition Status of Older Adults

Because old age is a relatively new phenomenon, and because the ranks of senior citizens have recently been growing larger, scientists are now working out the nutrient needs of the elderly. Knowledge about the nutrient needs and nutrition status of older adults has grown considerably in the last decade or so. Still, no RDA have been set for older age groups—all people over 50 are grouped together, even though people's needs change as their bodies age. Some experts believe the knowledge gained in recent years justifies different RDA for different older age groups, at least for some nutrients.[12] One suggestion is to establish one set of RDA for those 50 to 70 years old and another for those over 70. Clearly, the need for standards is becoming more and more urgent as the bulk of the population ages.

A problem attending the setting of standards for all groups, and especially for older people, is that individual differences become more and more marked as people grow older. One person may tend to omit vegetables from his diet, and by the time he is old he will have an associated set of nutrition problems. Another may have omitted milk and milk products all her life—her nutrition problems will be different. Also, as people age, their individual health histories affect their nutrient needs: they will have suffered different diseases with different impacts. On top of all this, people start out with different genetic predispositions to faulty nutrient absorption, and the effects become magnified as the years go by. Still, some generalizations are valid, and until an improved version of the RDA is developed, the present RDA for adults is useful. The next sections give special attention to a few nutrients of concern.

Water

A large percentage of nursing home operators note that one of the biggest problems with their elderly clients is getting them to drink more water and fruit juices. Dehydration is a risk for older adults, who may not notice or pay attention to their thirst, or who are unable to obtain water because of immobility. Research shows that older adults seem to feel less thirst. In one study, despite fluid deprivation and obvious physiological need, older adults did not get thirsty or experience mouth dryness.[13] Another factor predisposing older adults to fluid imbalance is a decrease in total body water as people age. Even mild stress such as fever or a hot climate can precipitate rapid dehydration in older adults.[14] Chapter 8 described the importance of water. An intake of 6 to 8 glasses of water a day is recommended, enough to bring urine output to about 6 cups per day.

Water recommendation for adults: 1 to 1½ oz/kg actual body weight.

Energy and Energy-Yielding Nutrients

Energy needs decline with advancing age. For one thing, lean body mass diminishes as people age, slowing the basal metabolic rate. For another, as people age, they usually reduce their physical activity (although they need not do so). The lower energy expenditures of older adults mean that they require less food energy to maintain their weight. Accordingly, the energy RDA for men and women decrease slightly starting at age 51.[15] Energy intakes typically decline in parallel with needs; still, many older adults are overweight, indicating that their food intakes do not diminish enough to compensate for their reduced energy expenditure.[16]

On such limited energy allowances, people must make sure that nearly all foods they eat are nutrient dense. Little leeway exists for foods of low nutrient density such as sugars, fats, oils, or alcohol. Because overweight is well recognized as a shortener of the life span, these seem to be life-sustaining recommendations. Table 17–1 offers a daily dietary framework for older adults. Those who need additional food energy should choose extra servings from the groups of listed foods.[17]

Physical Activity The many and remarkable benefits of regular physical activity are not limited to the young. Activities of all kinds are recommended for older adults to maintain and promote health. Ideally, physical activity should be part of each day's schedule and should be intense enough to prevent muscle atrophy and to speed up the heartbeat and respiration rate for at least 20 minutes. Many older persons believe that they can't participate in strenuous exercise, but studies show that they can do more than they think they can. Studies show, too, that older people can attain health rewards equal to or greater than those attained by younger people. Some older adults fear that physical activity may cause a heart attack, but actually, sedentary life poses a greater risk: it has been shown to be the most prevalent, modifiable risk factor for heart disease.[18] Guidelines are offered in Chapter 10 for anyone who wants to become more physically active.

Table 17–1
Daily Food Plan for Older Adults

2 to 3 two-ounce servings of protein-rich food (lean meat, poultry, fish, eggs, dried beans and peas, nuts)
2 to 3 one-cup servings of milk, cheese, or yogurt[a]
6 or more servings of whole-grain breads or cereals
2 to 4 half-cup servings of fruits
3 to 5 half-cup servings of vegetables

[a] Women should aim for 3 servings of milk, cheese, or yogurt.

Source: Adapted from A. Greeley, Nutrition and the elderly, *FDA Consumer,* October 1990, pp. 25–28.

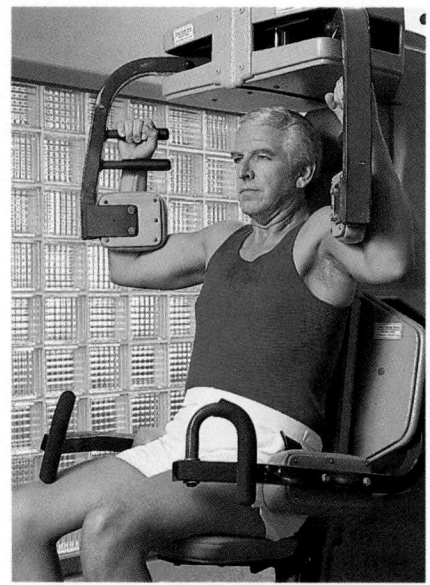
Strength training promotes strong muscles and bones and healthy appetites.

With aging, muscle mass and muscle strength decline, making older people vulnerable to falls and immobility. Many factors—including illness, aging itself, a sedentary lifestyle, and poor nutrition—contribute to muscle weakness and loss of muscle mass in older adults. Of these factors, only a sedentary lifestyle and poor nutrition are preventable or reversible. Strength training, even in frail, elderly people over 85 years of age, has been shown to improve muscle strength and mobility and to increase energy expenditure and energy intake, thereby enhancing nutrient intakes.[19]

One expert suggests the following physical activity program to maintain good health and function in older adults:[20]

- Daily: 60 minutes of physical activity, not necessarily vigorous or continuous: walking, climbing stairs, or simply moving about. This can be for 5 minutes at a time, 12 times a day; 12 minutes at a time, 5 times a day; or any combination of activity to total 60 minutes.
- Weekly: Some type of physical activity (swimming, dancing, rowing, brisk walking), for 30 to 45 minutes, 3 times a week.

Any exercise—even a ten-minute walk a day—is better than none, and with persistence, people can achieve great improvements at any age. Training not only tones, firms, and strengthens muscles, but also increases the blood flow to the brain.

Researchers studied nearly 7000 people, 65 years of age and older, to identify health behaviors that promote independence and mobility.[21] Four behaviors emerged: not smoking, low-to-moderate consumption of alcohol, maintenance of moderate body weight, and frequent physical activity. Of these behaviors, physical activity was the strongest predictor of continued mobility: moderate activity was as beneficial as more vigorous activity.

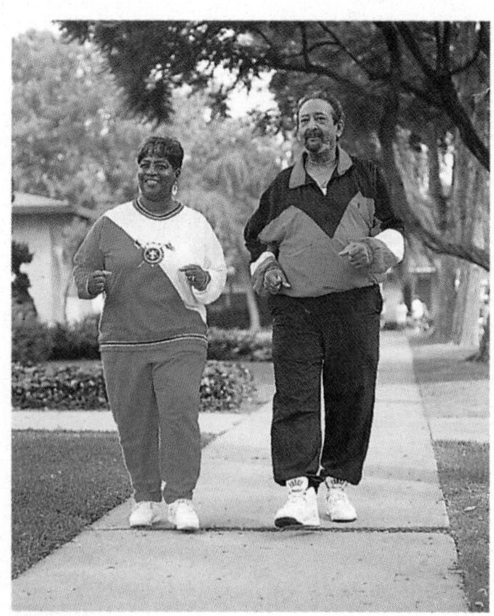
A walk in the neighborhood provides many physical benefits and a time to visit with others.

Protein The protein needs of older adults appear to be about the same as, or even greater than, those of younger people. Since energy needs decrease, however, the protein has to be obtained from low-kcalorie sources of high-quality protein. Examples of protein-rich, low-kcalorie foods include lean meats, poultry, and fish; nonfat milk; eggs; and legumes.

Carbohydrate Abundant carbohydrate is needed to protect protein from being used as an energy source. Complex carbohydrate foods such as vegetables, whole grains, and fruits are also rich in fiber and essential vitamins and minerals.

Fiber High-fiber foods can alleviate constipation—a condition prevalent among older adults, and especially among nursing home residents. Physical inactivity, scanty water intake, and heavy medication use among nursing home residents probably contribute to high rates of constipation, but lack of fiber probably does, too, in many cases. In fact, everyone's fiber intakes are lower, on average, than current recommendations (20 to 35 grams). Fiber is discussed in more detail in Chapter 2.

A reminder for those who take care of older adults in nursing homes: notice who does, and who does not, need added fiber, because both

Table 17–2
Risk Factors for Malnutrition in Older Adults

Risk Factors
Difficulties in chewing or swallowing
Difficulties in procuring or preparing food
Recent loss of spouse
Oral health problems
Poverty
Multiple drug use
Confusion or depression
Neurologic disorders
Chronic lung disease
Eating fewer than three meals per day
Anorexia
Institutionalization
Inability to self-feed
Alcoholism
Altered taste or smell
Recent surgery
Diabetes
Loneliness

Source: Adapted from R. Chernoff, Meeting the nutritional needs of the elderly in the institutional setting, *Nutrition Reviews* 52 (1994): 132–136.

extremes are always present. It has been estimated that as many as 50 percent of nursing home residents may be malnourished and underweight.[22] For these people, a diet that emphasizes fiber-rich foods such as whole grains, fruits, and vegetables may be too low in concentrated protein and energy.[23] Protein- and energy-dense snacks such as hard-boiled eggs, tuna fish and crackers, peanut butter on graham crackers, and homemade soups are valuable additions to the diets of underweight or malnourished older adults. Table 17–2 lists risk factors for malnutrition in elderly people.

Fat As is true for people of all ages, fat needs to be limited in the diet of most older adults for many reasons. Cutting fat helps cut kcalories and may also help retard the development of cancer, atherosclerosis, and other degenerative diseases. Restricting fat intakes to less than 30 percent of total energy presents a challenge for older adults, given that their limited energy allowances restrict the total kcalories they can take in daily.

Vitamins

The roles of specific vitamins in disease prevention and development and the age-related physiological changes that affect vitamin metabolism are unclear. Until more is known, vitamin recommendations for older adults remain the same as for younger adults. Vitamins A and D illustrate why research focusing on the vitamin needs of older adults deserves attention.

Vitamin A Vitamin A stands alone in that its absorption apparently *increases* with aging.[24] When the vitamin A intakes and blood retinol concentrations of healthy older adults and young adults were compared, the older people had higher blood vitamin A despite little difference in dietary intake between the two groups.[25] This research has led to a proposal to lower the vitamin A RDA for older adults. Perhaps, however, the value of the vitamin A precursor beta-carotene as a defense against oxidative damage to the body tissues and some types of cancer warrants leaving the RDA as is. Further research is needed before decisions are made.

Vitamin D Older adults face a greater risk of vitamin D deficiency than younger people do. The only food that provides significant amounts of vitamin D is vitamin D–fortified milk, yet many older adults drink little or no milk.[26] Many older adults have vitamin D intakes of less than half of the RDA.[27] Further compromising the vitamin D status of many older people, especially those in nursing homes, is their limited exposure to sunlight. Finally, age-related changes in vitamin D synthesis and metabolism increase the potential for vitamin D deficiency in older people.[28]

Some research indicates that a vitamin D intake above the RDA is necessary to prevent spinal bone mineral loss, especially in older people who are not outdoors much.[29] The results of at least one study indicate that a vitamin D supplement may be necessary to maintain vitamin D status in older adults, especially those who are housebound.[30]

Ensuring Adequate Vitamin Intakes Adequate vitamin intakes can be ensured by including foods from all food groups. Elderly people tend to eat too few vegetables, however (see Food Choices and Eating Habits of Older Adults, below).

Minerals

Among the minerals, iron deserves first mention. Iron-deficiency anemia is not as common in older adults as it is in younger people, but it still occurs in some, especially those with low food energy intakes.

Iron Aside from diet, other factors in many older people's lives make iron deficiency likely:

- Chronic blood loss from ulcers, hemorrhoids, or other disease conditions.
- Poor iron absorption due to reduced stomach acid secretion.
- Antacid use, which interferes with iron absorption.
- Use of medicines that cause blood loss, including anticoagulants, aspirin, and other arthritis medicines.

Anyone concerned with the nutrition status of an older person should not forget these possibilities.

Zinc Zinc deficiencies are common in older people. As many as 95 percent of older adults may not get the zinc they need, and many miss the mark by more than half. It is possible that improved absorption compensates for low zinc intakes, but this has not been confirmed. Some research suggests that older adults absorb zinc less efficiently than younger people do.[31] A number of different factors can impair zinc absorption or enhance its excretion and thus lead to deficiency. Chronic malabsorption diseases such as Crohn's disease impair zinc absorption. Alcohol consumption and stresses such as surgery and burns increase zinc excretion. Many medications that older adults use, both prescription and over-the-counter, either impair zinc absorption or increase excretion.[32] Older adults who do not make special efforts to eat zinc-rich foods such as meats, fish, and poultry will no doubt fail to meet the RDA for this nutrient.

It may be no coincidence that some symptoms of zinc deficiency resemble symptoms associated with aging—for example, a decline in taste acuity and dermatitis. However, it remains unclear whether the decline in taste acuity or the dermatitis associated with aging can be attributed to zinc deficiency.[33]

Calcium The importance of abundant dietary calcium throughout life, especially for women after menopause, to protect against osteoporosis was discussed in Chapter 8. The appropriate calcium intake for older adults remains controversial, however. Some researchers argue that current recommendations are too low for postmenopausal women. In one well-controlled study of more than 300 postmenopausal women, researchers found that 800 milligrams of calcium per day retarded bone loss in women whose usual calcium intakes were low (below 400 milligrams). Calcium intakes beyond 800 milligrams did not further benefit the women.[34] The Committee on Dietary Allowances contends that evidence is insufficient to warrant revising the calcium RDA upward for older women.[35]

While researchers attempt to reach agreement about the calcium requirements of older adults, especially those of women, one aspect of calcium nutrition is not controversial—calcium intakes of many people, especially women, in the United States are well below the RDA. If fresh milk causes stomach discomfort, as older people report, then dry nonfat milk can be incorporated into many foods, or lactose-free milk or other calcium-rich foods can take the place of milk.

Difficulties of Determining Mineral Requirements The determination of mineral requirements for older adults poses many challenges for researchers. Food composition tables fail to include some of the trace minerals. The accuracy of dietary intake studies is hindered when the amounts of certain nutrients present in foods are unknown. Interactions of minerals with other nutrients and drugs affect the bioavailability of the minerals, complicating the process still further. When age-related metabolic changes and disease conditions are superimposed on these problems, the task of determining mineral requirements for older people becomes increasingly difficult, but it is not impossible. The ever-growing number of older people in the world makes it imperative to learn more about how their nutrient needs differ from those of younger people and how such knowledge can enhance their health. In the meantime, people judge for themselves how to manage their nutrition, and some turn to supplements.

Supplements for Older Adults

Advertisers target older people with appeals to take supplements and eat "health foods," claiming that these products prevent disease and promote longevity. Despite this urging, and much to their credit, older adults are, for the most part, reasonable in their approaches to so-called health foods—most avoid health food stores or buy less there than others do.

Supplement Use Older adults are not always so reasonable, however, in their approaches to supplement use. About half of all women over 65 years of age take some type of nutrient supplement, while about one-fifth of older men do. Research shows that those who take supplements do not need them: they are not deficient in the nutrients being supplemented.[36] Certain diseases or health problems may necessitate the taking of supplements, but quite often, supplements have not been prescribed by a health care professional and are inappropriate.

Supplements Needed Can supplements meet the needs of older people? They probably can, at times. Calcium supplements for osteoporosis or iron for anemia, when recommended by a health care professional, may be beneficial. In most cases, though, the money people spend on supplements would be better spent on nutritious foods.

Older adults with food energy intakes less than about 1500 kcalories a day should probably take vitamin-mineral supplements—not megavitamins, but just the once-daily type of supplements. Many older adults fall into this category and should take this precaution. Physically active older adults whose energy needs remain high are an exception.

An Exercise Prescription A better choice than supplements for people with small energy allowances, however, would be to become more active and earn the right to eat more food. Food is the best source of nutrients for everybody. Supplements are just that—supplements to foods, not substitutes for them. For anyone who is motivated to obtain the best possible health, it is never too late to learn to eat well, be physically active, and adopt other lifestyle changes to facilitate the achievement of that goal, such as quitting smoking, moderating alcohol use, and the like. Table 17–3 offers strategies for growing old gracefully.

The Effects of Drugs on Nutrients

As people grow older, the use of medicines—from over-the-counter (OTC) types such as aspirins and laxatives to prescription drugs of all kinds—becomes commonplace. People over the age of 65 use more medications than any other age group; they take about 25 percent of all the over-the-counter and prescription drugs sold. Furthermore, older people often take multiple drugs simultaneously and therefore need to be particularly

Table 17–3
Strategies for Growing Old Gracefully

- Choose nutrient-dense foods.
- Maintain appropriate body weight.
- Reduce stress.
- For women, consult a physician about estrogen replacement to protect against osteoporosis.
- For people who smoke, quit.
- Expect to enjoy sex, and learn new ways of enhancing it.
- Use alcohol only moderately, if at all; use drugs only as prescribed.
- Take care to prevent accidents.
- Expect good vision and hearing throughout life; obtain glasses and hearing aids if necessary.
- Be alert to confusion as a disease symptom, and seek diagnosis.
- Control depression through activities and friendships.
- Drink 8 glasses of water every day.
- Practice mental skills. Keep on solving math problems and crossword puzzles, playing cards or other games, reading, writing, imagining, and creating.
- Make financial plans early to ensure security.
- Accept change. Work at recovering from losses; make new friends.
- Cultivate spiritual health. Cherish personal values. Make life meaningful.
- Go outside for sunshine and fresh air as often as possible.
- Be physically active. Walk, run, dance, swim, bike, row, or climb for aerobic activity. Lift weights, do calisthenics, or pursue some other activity to tone, firm, and strengthen muscles. Change activities to suit changing abilities and tastes.
- Be socially active—play bridge, join an exercise group, take a class, teach a class, eat with friends, volunteer time to help others.
- Stay interested in life—pursue a hobby, spend time with grandchildren, take a trip, read, cultivate a garden, or go to the movies.
- Enjoy life.

aware of the nutrition consequences. Most drugs interact with one or more nutrients in several ways, usually resulting in greater-than-normal needs for these nutrients. Table 12–3 in Chapter 12 lists classes of drugs that affect nutrition status, and Table 12–4 shows mechanisms and examples of food-drug interactions.

The most common drug that can affect nutrition in older people is alcohol. A recent estimate sets the incidence of alcoholism in people over 60 in our society at 2 to 10 percent. The effects of alcohol on people of all ages are explained in Nutrition in Practice 8.

Food Choices and Eating Habits of Older Adults

To provide any benefit, strategies and interventions to improve people's nutrition status must be based on knowledge of their food preferences and eating patterns. Menus and feeding programs for older adults must take into consideration not only the food likes and dislikes, but also the living conditions, economic status, and medical conditions of this diverse group of people. It is essential to know what foods they will eat, in what settings they like to eat these foods, and whether they can buy and prepare meals, if nutrition intervention is to be successful.

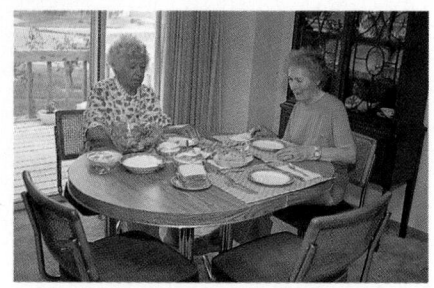

Shared meals can brighten the day and enhance the appetite.

Research Needs Many factors affect food choices, eating habits, and the nutrition status of older adults. Information about specific subgroups of older people is lacking, making it difficult to interpret existing research. For instance, nutrition surveys do not always differentiate among older people living alone, those living with others, and those in institutions.

Research Findings Research shows that the settings in which people eat make significant differences in the food practices of older adults.[37] For example, men living alone are most likely to be poorly nourished.[38] Older adults who live alone do not make poorer food choices than those who live with companions; rather, they consume too little food: loneliness is directly related to inadequacies, especially of energy intakes.[39] Different subgroups of the aging population therefore appear to need programs designed to meet different specific nutrient deficiencies.

Another factor affecting food intake and appetite in older people is depression. Though not an inevitable component of aging, depression becomes more common with advancing age. Loss of appetite and motivation to cook or even to eat frequently accompany depression. An overwhelming feeling of grief and sadness at the death of a spouse, friend, or family member may leave many people, particularly elderly people, with a feeling of powerlessness to overcome the depression. The support and companionship of family and friends, especially at mealtimes, can help overcome depression and enhance appetite. The accompanying case study presents a man who has some of these problems. Use the suggestions here, and in the Nutrition in Practice that follows this chapter, to help develop solutions.

Results of national surveys give some indication of the food likes of older adults. They tend to prefer low-fat milk and cheese from the milk group; grapefruit and melon among the fruits; potatoes and tomatoes from the vegetable group; bread, biscuits, and muffins from the grain group; and ground beef from the meats.

Survey data show that older Americans seem to be making changes in their food choices consistent with recommendations to cut down on fat and eat more fiber. More older adults are choosing low-fat poultry and fish, low-fat milk and milk products, and high-fiber breads and grains. These changes, observed between 1978 and 1988, suggest that people are more motivated to avoid disease risk by cutting down on fat than to promote health by eating more fruits and vegetables. When almost 500 participants in a meal program were surveyed about their food likes and dislikes, nine of the top ten most-disliked foods were vegetables, which are often overcooked or canned when served in such programs.[40]

Potential Applications Knowledge about the kinds of foods older people prefer and the reasons why they select or reject foods can be used to develop nutrition intervention programs and acceptable food products. Most older people are independent, productive, health-conscious consumers who know what they want from the foods they purchase. Older people spend more money per person on foods to eat at home than other

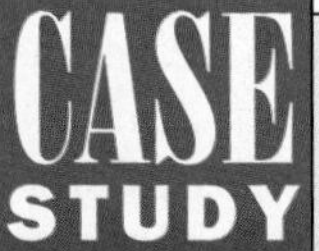

Elderly Man with a Poor Diet

Mr. Brezenoff is a 75-year-old man who lives alone. He has been losing weight slowly since his wife died a year ago. At 5 feet 8 inches tall, he currently weighs 135 pounds. His previous weight was 150 pounds. In talking with Mr. Brezenoff, you realize that he doesn't even like to talk about food, let alone eat it. "My wife always did the cooking before, and I ate well. Now I just don't feel like eating." You manage to find out that he skips breakfast, has soup and bread for lunch, and sometimes eats a cold-cut sandwich or a TV dinner for supper. He seldom sees friends or relatives. Mr. Brezenoff has also lost several teeth and doesn't eat any raw fruits or vegetables that he feels are hard to chew. He lives on a meager but adequate income.

1. What percent is Mr. Brezenoff's weight of the ideal body weight of a 75-year-old man his size (% IBW)?
2. What is his percent usual body weight (% UBW)?
3. Is his weight loss significant?
4. What factors are contributing to his poor food intake?
5. What nutrients are probably deficient in his diet?
6. Look at Mr. Brezenoff as an individual and suggest ways he can improve his diet and his lifestyle.
7. What other aspects of Mr. Brezenoff's physical and mental health should you consider in helping him to improve his food intake?

age groups and less money on food away from home. Manufacturers would be wise to cater to the preferences of older adults by providing good-tasting, nutritious foods in easy-to-open, single-serving packages with labels that are easy to read.

Researchers studying nutrition and aging are challenged by the physiological and psychosocial diversity of older adults. Many of the health problems older adults experience are currently attributed to normal, age-related processes, perhaps to the point of exaggeration. Research that focuses on how nutrition and other life factors affect aging and disease processes is vital to ensuring that more and more people can look forward to long, healthy lives.

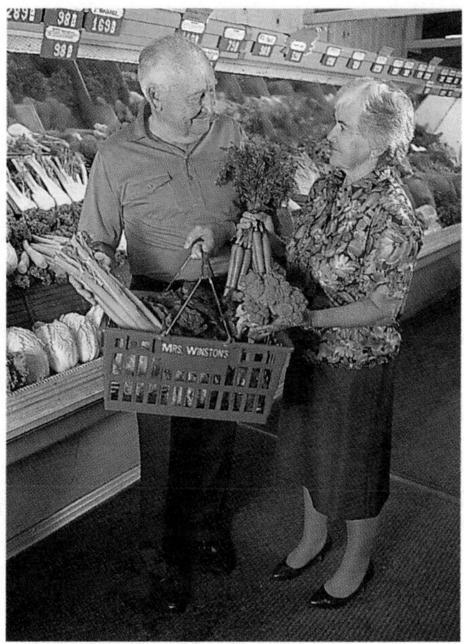

Taking time to nourish your body well is a gift you give yourself.

Nutrition Assessment

Nutrition assessment of the elderly must focus on the past as well as the present. Each person's long prior history of eating and health habits has contributed to present nutrition status.

- The history should reveal past as well as present intake habits. Of particular present interest are any habits that may jeopardize adequate nutrient intakes: Does the person skip meals or routinely exclude any food groups? Can the person procure and prepare meals?
- The drug history is usually relevant to an older person's nutrition status. What drugs does the person take, and what are each drug's effects (Appendix E)? Does the person use alcohol? How much?
- Socioeconomic factors may also be present that impact nutrition status and may imply the need for food assistance programs.

- The physical examination should be made with an eye to nutrition status. Hair, skin, and nails may offer clues to imbalances, excesses, or deficiencies. Inadequate fluid intake may be apparent from a high body temperature, a swollen tongue, reduced blood pressure, sunken eyeballs, or a reduced urine output. Are any chronic diseases, illnesses, or physical disabilities present?
- Oral health should be assessed, as it may affect food and nutrient intake. Can the person chew and swallow foods satisfactorily? Does the person have dentures, or need them? Are there any lesions in the mouth, on the lips, or on the tongue? (Problems in these areas are common in the elderly and are dealt with further in Chapter 20.)
- Anthropometric measures such as height, weight, and fatfold measures can reveal altered body composition that may indicate malnutrition. Loss of lean tissue is an early indicator of PEM. Obesity suggests a raised risk of chronic diseases.
- Biochemical measures may be used to follow up on other assessment steps as appropriate and as described in Chapter 13. These measures can confirm that PEM, iron deficiency, or other conditions are present.

Many of the chapters to come describe diseases that affect the elderly and offer details on appropriate assessment measures.

STUDY QUESTIONS

1. What roles does nutrition play in aging, and what roles can it play in retarding aging?
2. Name some factors that complicate the task of setting nutrient standards for older adults.
3. Why does the risk of dehydration increase as people age?
4. Why do energy needs usually decline with advancing age?
5. Why is the risk of vitamin D deficiency greater among older adults than younger adults?

NUTRITION IN PRACTICE 17

Food for Singles

Singles of all ages face difficulties in purchasing, storing, and preparing food. Large packages of meat and vegetables are often intended for families of four or more, and even a head of lettuce can spoil before one person can use it all. Many singles live in small dwellings and have little storage space for foods. A limited income presents additional obstacles. The following ideas can help to solve some of these problems.

My grandmother is on a fixed income. Once the rent, utilities, and other bills are paid, she doesn't have much money for groceries. What advice can I give her?

First, make sure your grandmother knows what food assistance programs she can turn to. Table 17–4 summarizes food assistance programs for the elderly.

People who have the means to shop and cook for themselves can cut their food bills just by being wise shoppers. The first decision a person with a tight grocery budget must make is where to shop. Large supermarkets are usually less expensive than independent stores, but the cost of transportation to the market is a consideration.

Next, a grocery list that includes specials and coupons will help reduce impulse buying. Specials and coupons are a bargain only when the items featured are those that the shopper needs and uses. Foods that are almost always a good buy include rice and nonfat dry milk, which can be stored on a shelf for months at room temperature; whole pieces of cheese, rather than sliced or shredded cheese; fresh produce in season; variety meats such as chicken livers; cereals that require cooking instead of ready-to-serve cereals; and dried beans and peas.

How can my grandmother buy small quantities when so many foods are packaged for families?

All singles face this problem. Packages of meat and fresh vegetables often come already wrapped in large servings. Even a half-gallon of milk can spoil before one person can use it all. People living alone can try these hints.

First, in the milk and milk product category, buy fresh milk in the size best suited for you. If your grocer doesn't carry pints or half-pints, try a nearby service station or convenience store. Pint-size and even cup-size boxes of heat-treated milk are also available and can be stored unopened on a shelf for up to three months without refrigeration. Dry powdered milk can be stored for months before it is reconstituted. You can use only the amount you need and store the rest.

Next, among the meats and meat alternates, buy only what you will use. Ask the grocer to break open a package of wrapped meat and rewrap the portion that you need. Buy eggs by the half-dozen—break the carton of a dozen eggs in half. Eggs do keep for long periods, though, if stored in the refrigerator and are such a good source of high-quality protein that you will probably use a dozen before they lose their freshness. Dried beans and peas offer high-quality protein, fiber, and many other nutrients for practically pennies and have a long shelf life.

If you have ample freezer space, you can buy large packages of meat, such as pork chops, ground beef, or chicken, when they are on sale. Then, immediately divide the package into individual servings. Wrap them in aluminum foil, not freezer paper: the foil can become the liner for the pan in which you bake or broil the meat, thus saving work over the sink. Don't label these individually; just put them all in a brown bag marked "hamburger" or "chicken thighs" or whatever, along with the date. The bag is easy to locate in the freezer, and you'll know when your supply is running low.

Among fruits and vegetables, purchase fresh ones individually. Buy only three pieces of each kind of fresh fruit: a ripe one, a semi-ripe one, and a green one. Eat the first right away, the second soon after, and let the last one ripen on your windowsill. If vegetables are packaged in large quantities, ask the grocer to break open the package so you can buy what you need. Buy small cans of fruits and vegetables even though they cost more per unit. Remember, it is expensive to buy a regular-size can and let the unused portion spoil in the refrigerator. If you have space in your freezer, buy frozen vegetables in large bags rather than in small boxes. You can take out the exact amount you need and close the bag tightly with a rubber band. If you return the package quickly to the freezer each time, the vegetables will stay fresh for a long time.

Finally, breads and cereals usually must be purchased in larger quantities. When you buy bread,

Table 17–4
Food Assistance Programs for Older Adults

TITLE IIIC NUTRITION PROGRAM FOR OLDER AMERICANS

- *Funding:* U.S. Department of Health and Human Services.
- *Services:* Congregate and home-delivered meals, therapeutic diets. Supportive services include transportation to congregate meal sites; shopping assistance; information and referral; and to some extent, nutrition counseling and education.
- *Impact:* The Title IIIc program improves the nutrient content of high-risk older adults' diets and offers socialization and recreation. Many of the nutrition programs around the country go above and beyond federal requirements of congregate and home meals by offering lunch clubs, ethnic meals, acceptance of food stamps for meal payment, and meals for older homeless people.

FOOD STAMPS

- *Funding:* U.S. Department of Agriculture.
- *Services:* Income supplement to low-income households in the form of coupons to purchase food.
- *Impact:* Some research results suggest that food stamps serve more as an income supplement to elderly participants than as a device to improve nutrition status.[a] Other research indicates that food stamp participants' nutrient intakes are higher than those of nonparticipants with similar incomes.[b]

MEALS ON WHEELS

- *Funding:* Private funding to supplement the Title IIIc program; an example of a private and public sector partnership responding to the needs of the growing numbers of older adults.
- *Services:* Direct meal delivery to the homebound elderly, integrated into the meal delivery services provided by the Title IIIc program.
- *Impact:* Meals on Wheels focuses on filling the need for weekend and holiday meals for homebound elderly people, a service that is limited in the Title IIIc program.

[a] J.S. Butler, J. C. Ohls, and B. M. Posner. The effect of the food stamp program on the nutrient intake of the eligible elderly, *Journal of Nutrition for the Elderly* 4 (1985): 25–51, as cited in M. B. Kohrs, Effectiveness of nutrition intervention programs for the elderly, in *Nutrition and Aging,* eds. M. L. Hutchinson and H. N. Munro (New York: Academic Press, 1986), pp. 139–167.
[b] J. S. Akin and coauthors, The impact of federal transfer programs on the nutrient intake of elderly individuals, *Journal of Human Resources* 20 (1985): 382–404, as cited in B. M. Posner and E. Levine, Nutrition services for older Americans, in *Geriatric Nutrition: The Health Professional's Handbook,* ed. R. Chernoff (Gaithersburg, Md.: Aspen Publishers, 1991), pp. 415–447.

Source: Adapted from B. M. Posner and E. Levine, Nutrition services for older Americans, in *Geriatric Nutrition: The Health Professional's Handbook,* ed. R. Chernoff (Gaithersburg, Md.: Aspen Publishers, 1991), pp. 415–447.

take out the amount you will use in a few days and store the rest in the freezer. Cereal grains (rice, barley, oatmeal) and pastas, like the dried beans mentioned earlier, generally have a long shelf life if you keep them sealed in jars.

For times when you have to buy more food than you can use, here are a few hints. Make mixtures of leftovers and serve them again. A thick stew prepared from leftover green beans, carrots, cauliflower, broccoli, and any meat with added onion, pepper, celery, and potatoes makes a complete and balanced meal—except for milk, but then you can add powdered milk to your stew.

Set aside a place in your kitchen for rows of glass jars containing shelf staple items—rice, tapioca, lentils or other dry beans, flour, cornmeal, nonfat dry milk, macaroni, cereal, and the like. Freeze each filled jar for one night first to kill any insect eggs that might be present. The jars will then keep bugs out of the food indefinitely. They make an attractive display and will remind you of different choices you can make to vary your menus. Cut the directions-for-use labels from the packages and store them in the jars.

Think up various ways to use a vegetable when you must buy more than you can use at a time. For example, divide a head of cauliflower into thirds. Cook one-third and eat it hot. Put the other two-thirds into a vinegar and oil marinade for use in a salad.

Also, when you cook a lot of food, invite someone to share it with you. Next thing you know, that person will invite you back, and you'll get to enjoy a meal you wouldn't have thought to cook for yourself.

Sometimes my grandmother doesn't feel like cooking a meal for herself. I'm afraid that she may not be getting the nutrients she needs.

When your grandmother does feel like cooking, she can cook several meals at a time. For example, she can boil three potatoes with skins. She can eat one hot with margarine and chives. She can use one to make a potato-cheese casserole to bake for the next evening's meal. Then she can slice

the third one into a covered bowl and pour the juice from pickles over it. The pickled potato can be used later in a salad.

Depending on her freezer space, she can make double or even six portions of a dish that takes time to prepare: a casserole, vegetable pie, or meatloaf. The little aluminum trays from frozen foods can be saved and used to freeze the extra servings. The work will seem worthwhile when several meals are prepared at once.

An occasional frozen TV dinner can also be useful—although expensive—if it makes the difference between a person's eating and not eating. Many such dinners that are now available are low in kcalories and nutritious. Adding a fresh salad, a whole-wheat roll, and a glass of milk can make a nice meal.

But encourage her to socialize, too. Sometimes, simple isolation can impair a person's motivation to cook appetizing meals.

My grandmother never drinks milk. What can I suggest?

She can try using nonfat dry milk. It is the greatest convenience food there is. Dry milk can be used in just about everything: hamburgers, gravies, soups, casseroles, sauces, and beverages, such as iced coffee. The taste is negligible, but 5 heaping tablespoons would be the equivalent of a cup of fresh milk. Weight Watchers has many recipes for delicious milkshakes and "ice cream" using nonfat dry milk. The recipes are for single servings.

Your grandmother can also increase her calcium intake by making soup stock from pork and chicken bones soaked in vinegar. The bones release their calcium into the acid medium, and the vinegar boils off when the stock is boiled. One tablespoon of such stock may contain over 100 milligrams of calcium. Something can then be cooked in this stock every day: vegetables, rice, and stews. And, of course, this stock can be used as a soup base.

One more suggestion for those who are alone at mealtime is this: make it a special occasion. One way to do this is to set the table with a tablecloth, a napkin, a full set of utensils, and fresh flowers. Set a pot of stew or homemade soup with vegetables and fresh herbs on low heat to cook, and make a salad. Get comfortable in a stuffed chair, and enjoy a book or some soothing music until the rich aroma of your simmering dinner beckons. After serving your plate, light a candle, dim the lights, savor the food, and relish some of the best company you will ever have—your own.

■ NOTES ■

1. R. Chernoff, Demographics of aging, in *Geriatric Nutrition: The Health Professional's Handbook,* ed. R. Chernoff (Gaithersburg, Md.: Aspen Publishers, 1991), pp. 1–9.
2. R. S. Paffenbarger and coauthors, The association of changes in physical activity level and other lifestyle characteristics with mortality among men, *New England Journal of Medicine* 328 (1993): 538–545.
3. E. J. Masoro, Retardation of aging processes by food restriction: An experimental tool, *American Journal of Clinical Nutrition* (supplement) 55 (1992): 1250–1252.
4. Masoro, 1992.
5. Masoro, 1992.
6. E. J. M. Velthuis-te Wierik and coauthors, Energy restriction, a useful intervention to retard human ageing? Results of a feasibility study, *European Journal of Clinical Nutrition* 48 (1994): 138–148.
7. G. E. Bunce, J. Kinoshits, and J. Horwitz, Nutritional factors in cataract, *Annual Review of Nutrition* 10 (1990): 233–254.
8. S. E. Hankinson and coauthors, Nutrient intake and cataract extraction in women: A prospective study, *British Medical Journal* 305 (1992): 335–339, as cited in G. E. Bunce, Antioxidant nutrition and cataract in women: A prospective study, *Nutrition Reviews* 51 (1993): 84–86.
9. E. D. Harris, Rheumatoid arthritis: Pathophysiology and implications for therapy, *New England Journal of Medicine* 322 (1990): 1277–1289.
10. Rheumatoid arthritis and food, *Health Gazette,* February 1989, p. 3.
11. J. M. Kremer and coauthors, Fish-oil fatty acid supplementation in active rheumatoid arthritis: A double-blind, controlled crossover study, *Annals of Internal Medicine* 106 (1987): 497–503.
12. R. M. Russell and P. M. Suter, Vitamin requirements of elderly people: An update, *American Journal of Clinical Nutrition* 58 (1993): 4–14.
13. B. J. Rolls and P. A. Phillips, Aging and disturbances of thirst and fluid balance, *Nutrition Reviews* 48 (1990): 137–144.
14. R. Chernoff, Physiologic aging and nutritional status, *Nutrition in Clinical Practice,* February 1990, pp. 5–8.
15. National Academy of Sciences, Food and Nutrition Board, Committee on Dietary Allowances, *Recommended Dietary Allowances,* 10th ed. (Washington, D.C.: National Academy Press, 1989).

16. E. T. Poehlman and E. S. Horton, Regulation of energy expenditure in aging humans, *Annual Review of Nutrition* 10 (1990): 255–275.
17. A Greeley, Nutrition and the elderly, *FDA Consumer,* October 1990, pp. 25–28.
18. Coronary heart disease attributable to sedentary lifestyle—selected states, 1988, *Journal of the American Medical Association* 264 (1990): 1390–1392, as cited in P. Astrand, Physical activity and fitness, *American Journal of Clinical Nutrition* (supplement) 55 (1992): 1231–1236.
19. M. A. Fiatarone and coauthors, Exercise training and nutritional supplementation for physical frailty in very elderly people, *New England Journal of Medicine* 330 (1994): 1769–1775; W. W. Campbell and coauthors, Increased energy requirements and changes in body composition with resistance training in older adults, *American Journal of Clinical Nutrition* 60 (1994): 167–175.
20. Astrand, 1992.
21. L. Breslow and N. Breslow, Health practices and disability: Some evidence from Almeda County, *Preventive Medicine* 22 (1993): 86–95.
22. A. A. Abbase and D. Rudman, Undernutrition in the nursing home: Prevalence, consequences, causes and prevention, *Nutrition Reviews* 52 (1994): 113–122.
23. R. Andres and J. Hallfrisch, Nutrient intake recommendations for the older American, *Journal of the American Dietetic Association* 89 (1989): 1739–1741.
24. Processing of dietary retinoids is slowed in the elderly, *Nutrition Reviews* 49 (1991): 116–118.
25. P. J. Garry and coauthors, Vitamin A intake and plasma retinol levels in healthy elderly men and women, *American Journal of Clinical Nutrition* 46 (1987): 989–994.
26. Chernoff, 1990.
27. E. E. Delvin, A. Imbach, and M. Copti, Vitamin D nutritional status and related biochemical indices in an autonomous elderly population, *American Journal of Clinical Nutrition* 48 (1988): 373–378; H. Payette and K. Gray-Donald, Dietary intake and biochemical indices of nutritional status in an elderly population with estimates of the precision of the 7-day food record, *American Journal of Clinical Nutrition* 54 (1991): 478–488.
28. Chernoff, 1990.
29. B. Dawson-Hughes and coauthors, Effect of vitamin D supplementation on wintertime and overall bone loss in healthy, postmenopausal women, *Annals of Internal Medicine* 115 (1991): 505–512, as cited in R. M. Russell, Micronutrient requirements of the elderly, *Nutrition Reviews* 50 (1992): 463–466.
30. A. R. Webb, An evaluation of the relative contributions of exposure to sunlight and of diet to the circulating concentrations of 25-hydroxy vitamin D in an elderly nursing home population in Boston, *American Journal of Clinical Nutrition* 51 (1990): 1075–1081.
31. R. J. Cousins and J. M. Hempe, Zinc, in *Present Knowledge in Nutrition,* 6th ed., ed. M. L. Brown (Washington, D.C.: International Life Sciences Institute—Nutrition Foundation, 1990), pp. 251–260.
32. G. J. Fosmire, Trace mineral requirements, in *Geriatric Nutrition: The Health Professional's Handbook,* ed. R. Chernoff (Gaithersburg, Md.: Aspen Publishers, 1991), pp. 77–105.
33. Fosmire, 1991.
34. B. Dawson-Hughes and coauthors, A controlled trial of the effect of calcium supplementation on bone density in postmenopausal women, *New England Journal of Medicine* 323 (1990): 878–883.
35. National Academy of Sciences, Food and Nutrition Board, Committee on Dietary Allowances, 1989, pp. 174–184.
36. H. Payette and K. Gray-Donald, Do vitamin and mineral supplements improve the dietary intake of elderly Canadians? *Canadian Journal of Public Health* 82 (1993): 58–60.
37. J. V. White and coauthors, Consensus of the Nutrition Screening Initiative: Risk factors and indicators of poor nutritional status in older Americans, *Journal of the American Dietetic Association* 91 (1991): 783–787.
38. I. Darnton-Hill, Psychosocial aspects of nutrition and aging, *Nutrition Reviews* 50 (1992): 476–479.
39. D. Walker and R. E. Beauchene, The relationship of loneliness, social isolation, and physical health to dietary adequacy of independently living elderly, *Journal of the American Dietetic Association* 91 (1991): 300–304.
40. V. Holt, J. Nordstrom, and M. B. Kohrs, Food preferences of older adults (abstract), *Journal of the American Dietetic Association* 87 (1987): 1597.

18

Nutrition in Severe Stress

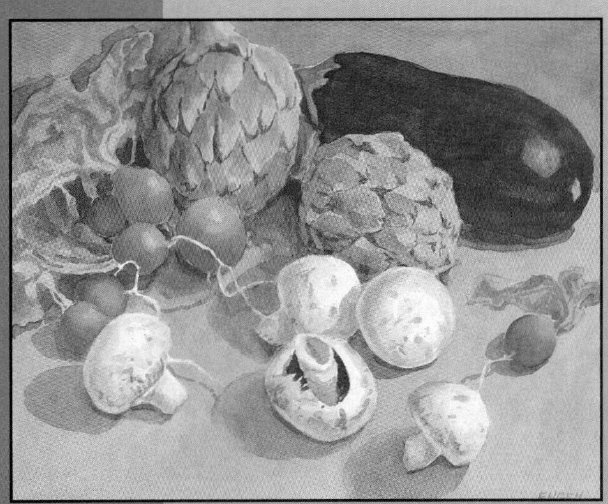

CONTENTS

This chapter examines the demands imposed by especially severe stresses. The body responds to these stresses with an arsenal of hormonal, metabolic, and immunologic changes that serve to make necessary repairs, limit further damage, and restore balance. To bolster this system of defenses against severe illnesses, nutrition is especially important.

The Body's Responses to Severe Stresses

stress: any threat to a person's physical well-being. Some stresses fall within the body's normal and healthy functioning and are known as **physiological stress.** Outside these limits, additional stresses imposed by disease or bodily insults, such as infections, surgery, or burns, can overwhelm the body; such stress is **pathological stress,** referred to here as **severe stress.** One type of pathological stress is *trauma.*

trauma: physical injury to the body, such as a broken bone, a gunshot wound, or surgery.

hypermetabolism: accelerated metabolism, a part of the body's response to stress.

Severe stresses include major infections, major trauma, surgery, and burns. In response to severe stresses, the body speeds up its metabolic rate (hypermetabolism) and mobilizes nutrients into amino acid and glucose pools, so that it can synthesize the special factors it needs to limit and repair damage. Hormonal changes and immune system factors mediate these metabolic responses.

The exact factors the body makes in response to stress depend on the type of stress. Mending a broken bone requires different factors than does healing a wound or fighting an infection. The next sections describe the general metabolic and immune responses to severe stress. As you read, keep in mind that the events being described occur in all severely stressed people: those with infections, injuries, burns, and all illnesses that speed metabolism. Details of the different reactions to these specific stresses are the subject of the next chapter.

Metabolic Responses to Severe Stress

The hypermetabolism caused by severe stress creates a demand for extra energy. To meet that demand, the body draws on its stored carbohydrate, fat, and protein in much the same way as it does when responding to fasting or starvation (see pp. 123–126).

Carbohydrate To fuel the accelerated metabolic activity brought on by stress, the body breaks down its liver glycogen (the available stored form of carbohydrate) to maintain blood glucose. Glycogen stores are limited, however, and this source of glucose is rapidly depleted.

Fat Meanwhile, the body mobilizes its fatty acids to provide fuel. In contrast to glycogen stores, fatty acid stores are plentiful. However, some of the body's cells (such as the brain cells) depend on glucose for fuel, and the body cannot convert fatty acids into glucose. Only the glycerol in each triglyceride can be used to make glucose, and this represents only about 5 percent of a typical triglyceride's kcalories. The other 95 percent, the fatty acids, are converted to ketones or other substances or broken down. Consequently, to obtain glucose, the body turns to its protein.

Most important in glucose production at first are alanine and glutamine. The liver synthesizes these amino acids from branched-chain amino acids released from muscle protein.

Protein Unlike glucose and fat, protein is not stored in case the body needs it. All of the body's proteins are already in use as skeletal muscle, cell structures, enzymes, hormones, immune system factors, and other blood proteins and body components. During the stress response,

Table 18–1
Metabolic Responses to Simple Fasting and Severe Stress Compared

METABOLIC RESPONSE	SIMPLE FASTING	SEVERE STRESS
Depletion of glycogen	Gradual	Rapid
Mobilization of fatty acids	Gradual	Rapid
Breakdown of protein tissue	Rapid, then slowed	Rapid
Total energy needs	Below normal	Greater than normal

the body must therefore break down functioning tissue to make glucose. The body also has to make special proteins to mount the stress response. The body preferentially breaks down skeletal muscle to provide the amino acids it needs, thereby preserving its vital organs for as long as possible.[1] This is why you so often see muscle wasting in stressed clients.

If the stress is severe or long lasting, however, protein from vital organs is also used, as well as functioning blood and lymph proteins such as albumin and immune factors. This redirection of vital proteins compromises the function of the heart, lungs, and GI tract and can weaken the immune response. In the worst cases, the end result is multiple organ failure.[2] Typically, respiratory failure comes first, and is followed by liver failure and kidney failure. Once this cascade of events is under way, recovery is unlikely.

Other Nutrients During this whole process, vitamins and minerals serve as cofactors in the metabolic reactions that are occurring. Depletion of these nutrients can interfere with the body's ability to mount a successful stress response and can hinder the ability of vital organs to operate.

Responses to Fasting versus Stress An important distinction between the body's responses to simple fasting and to severe stress is that in fasting, the body *slows* its initial rapid metabolism, thus conserving vital proteins, whereas during severe stress it does not. Instead, the metabolic rate remains rapid, and the body continues to deplete its fuel supplies and to rapidly break down protein tissue. Table 18–1 sums up the contrasts.

Immune Response to Severe Stress

The body's natural system of defense against pathogens—the immune system—enables the body to fight off infectious diseases. The immune system defends the body so alertly and silently that most healthy people are unaware of the thousands of enemy attacks that are mounted against them every day. Occasionally, though, an infection may succeed in making a person ill temporarily, and the immune system must then mount an emergency counterattack. Of all severe stresses, serious infections most intensely tax the immune system, and if the system fails, death follows.

In severe stresses other than infection, the immune system plays a vital, although less obvious, role. Traumas such as surgical incisions, wounds, and burns render the body vulnerable to organisms invading

Glossary of Immunity Terms

Reminder: An *antibody* is an immunoglobulin produced by the B-cells in response to the invasion of an antigen. An *antigen* is a foreign substance that induces the formation of antibodies.

acquired immunity: immunity directed at specific organisms (also called **specific immunity**). The lymphocytes mediate this type of immunity, which depends on prior exposure, recognition, and reaction to invading organisms. Two types of specific immunity are **cell-mediated immunity** and **humoral immunity.**

B-cells: lymphocytes that produce antibodies.

cell-mediated immunity: immunity conferred by the reaction of T-cells to an invading organism.

cytokines: proteins secreted by phagocytes that activate metabolic and immune responses to infections.

humoral immunity: immunity conferred by antibodies secreted by B-cells and carried to the invaded area by way of body fluids.
humor = fluid

immune system: the body's natural defense system against foreign materials that have penetrated the skin or mucous membranes.

immunity: the body's ability to recognize and eliminate foreign materials.

immunoglobulin: a protein capable of acting as an antibody.

leucocytes: white blood cells. These include the phagocytes and the lymphocytes.

lymphocytes: white blood cells that participate in acquired immunity; *B-cells* and *T-cells.*

nonspecific immunity: immunity directed at many kinds of organisms. Phagocytosis, the skin, and mucous membranes confer this type of immunity.

phagocytes: white blood cells that have the ability to ingest and destroy foreign substances.
phagein = to eat
kytos = cell

phagocytosis (FAG-oh-sigh-TOE-sis): the process by which phagocytes engulf and destroy foreign materials.
osis = intensive

T-cells: lymphocytes that attack antigens.

through breaks in the skin or internal organs or through altered circulation, and the immune system vigilantly defends against them. The body's resources are limited, however. Severe stresses can tax nutrient stores to such a degree that the synthesis of immune factors may be compromised. Severe stress is a time of great vulnerability to infectious disease.

The immune system resides in no single organ, but depends on the interactions and secretions of various organs and white blood cells (the accompanying glossary defines related terms). The body's first lines of defense against foreign substances—the skin, the mucous membranes, and the GI tract—normally deter invaders. When these shields fail, the cells of the immune system are called into play.

Reminder: *Mucus* is the noun, *mucous* is the adjective.

The Skin and Mucous Membranes The skin is thick and coated with protective waxes. It is constantly shedding its outermost layers, and its associated glands secrete sweat and oily secretions that are toxic to some types of bacteria. The mucous membranes line all of the body's openings—the eyes, nose, mouth, lungs, GI tract, and genitourinary tract—and their cells secrete a protective coating of mucus. Mucus forms a slippery coating that makes it difficult for microbes to attach to the cells; instead, microbes are trapped and expelled as mucus continuously flows out of the body. Moreover, mucus contains antimicrobial chemicals and enzymes that are lethal to invading organisms.

The Intestines Recall from Chapter 5 that the absorptive surface of the intestine is lined with fingerlike projections called villi. Healthy villi are crowded so close together that they form a physical barrier. Interspersed among the villi are cells that serve important immune functions (see Figure 18–1). To appreciate the major role of the intestine in immunity, consider that of all the body's immunologic-secreting cells, 70 to 80 percent are located within the intestine.[3] Goblet cells secrete mucus, and lymph tissue in the intestine houses phagocytes and other immune system cells. Other GI secretions (saliva, gastric acid, bile) also prevent harmful substances from entering the body.[4]

The GI tract rarely allows microorganisms to pass into the body, even though over 500 species of bacteria normally reside in the intestines.[5] The bacterial population actually helps prevent the growth of harmful bacteria in the intestine. The beneficial bacteria use the available nutrients and

Reminder: The bacterial inhabitants of the GI tract are known as the *intestinal flora.*

Figure 18–1
Immune Cells That Protect the Intestinal Villi

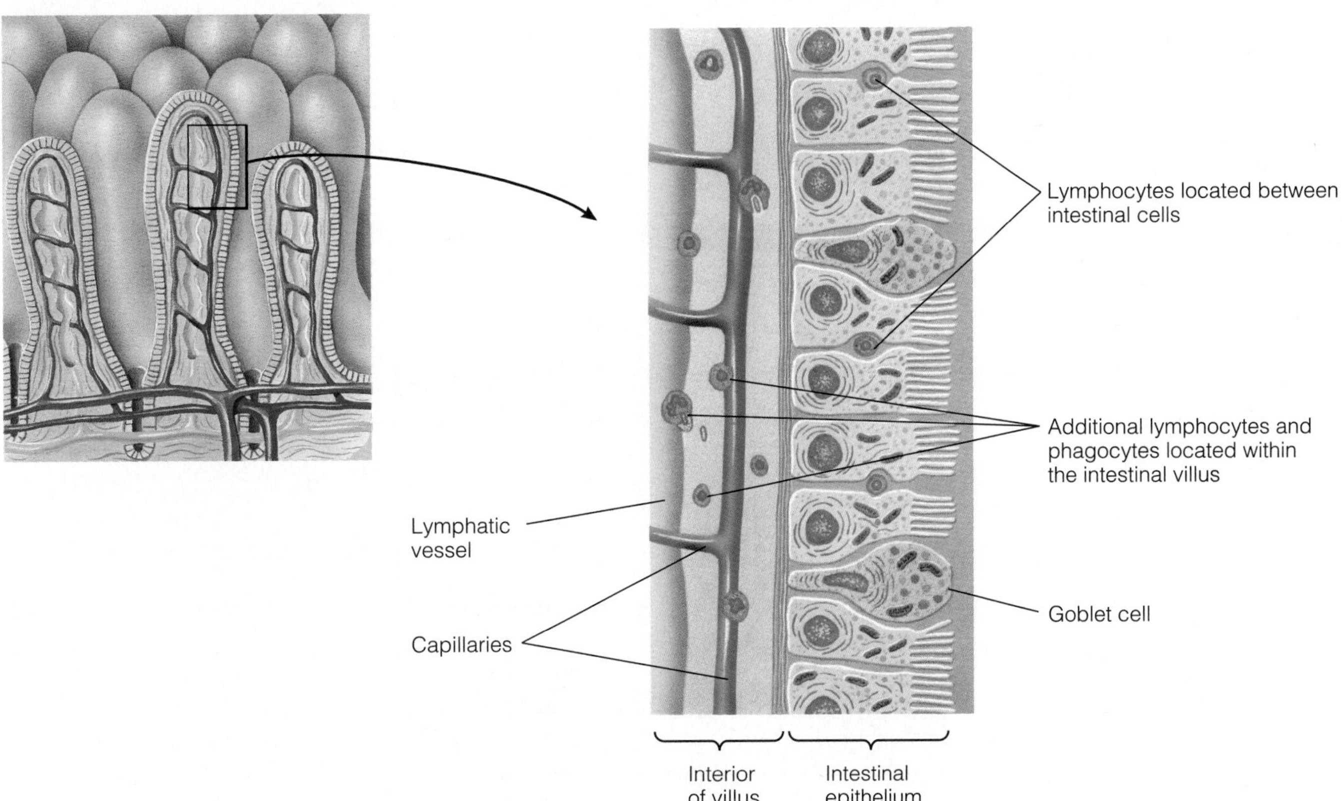

space, thereby making it hard for unwanted invaders to become established. They also produce short-chain fatty acids that prevent harmful microbes from sticking to the intestinal surface.

The only way that substances can pass from the intestine to the inside of the body is by evading the intestine's arsenal of defenses. Clearly, to help a stressed client fight infection, it is important to support the GI tract's integrity. (Nutrition in Practice 18 examines nutrition strategies designed for this purpose.) If an invader does gain entry into the body, then the body calls on its next line of defenses.

Cells of the Immune System The internal immune system consists primarily of the white blood cells (see Figure 18–2). The three types of white blood cells, the phagocytes and two types of lymphocytes, travel over the entire body, but their primary residence is the lymph tissue—the

Figure 18–2
Immune System Cells, Actions, and Results

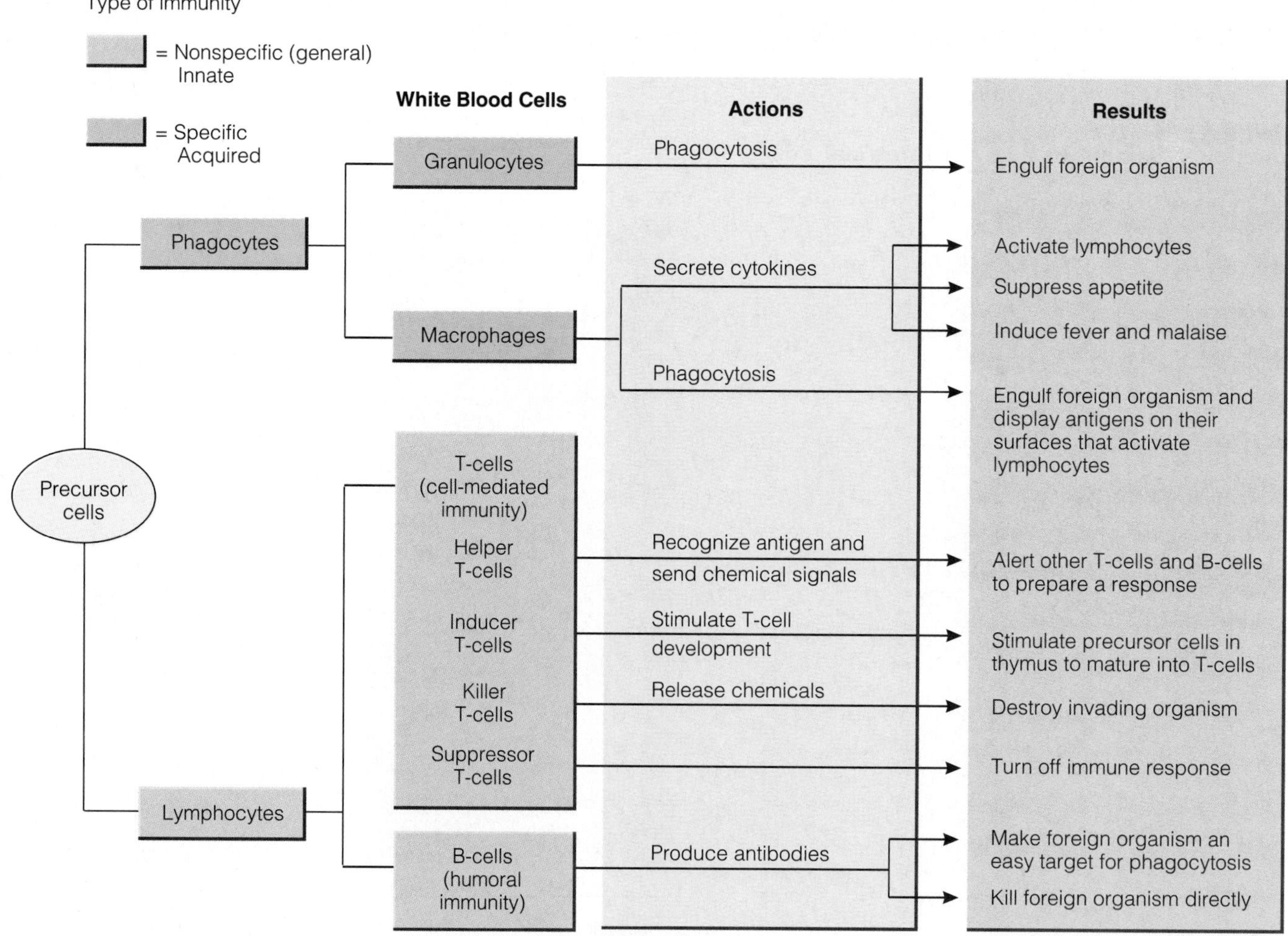

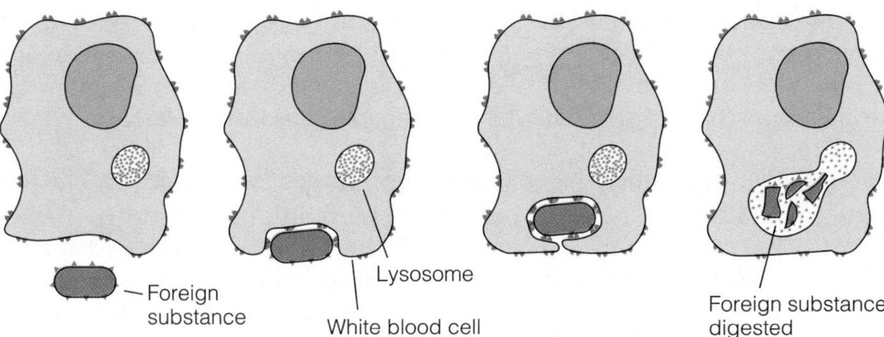

Figure 18–3
Phagocytosis
During phagocytosis, a white blood cell engulfs a foreign substance and eventually surrounds and digests it.

thymus, lymph nodes, spleen, bone marrow, and areas lining the GI tract. Of the 100 trillion cells that make up the human body, one in every hundred is a white blood cell.

Nonspecific Immunity: Phagocytes Phagocytes, the scavengers of the immune system, are the first to arrive on the scene if an invader gains entry. When a phagocyte recognizes a substance as foreign, it engulfs and digests that substance, if it can, in a process called phagocytosis (see Figure 18–3). Phagocytes also secrete proteins called cytokines that activate the metabolic and immune responses to infection.

Among the phagocytes are some that perform the special task of facilitating recognition, the hallmark of immunity. Immunity depends on these cells to recognize foreign materials and destroy or otherwise neutralize them. As a phagocyte engulfs an invading organism, it detaches a portion of the invading antigen and displays that portion on its own cell surface. This display calls a special group of lymphocytes into action. This way, if the phagocytes cannot work fast enough to rid the body of the invader, lymphocytes will be ready to aid in the body's defense.

Specific Immunity: The Lymphocytes The lymphocytes are of two distinct types: T-cells and B-cells. Unlike the phagocytes, which are capable of inactivating many different types of invaders, lymphocytes are highly specific. Each lymphocyte can attack only one type of antigen. This specificity is remarkable, for nature creates millions of antigens. After making enough cells to destroy a particular antigen, some lymphocytes retain the necessary information to serve as memory cells so that the immune system can produce the same type of lymphocytes again should the identical infection reoccur.

T stands for the thymus gland, where the T-cells are stored for a while. *B* stands for bursa, an organ in the chicken in which B-cells were first identified.

Cell-Mediated Immunity: T-Cells The T-cells participate in cell-mediated immunity, so named because the cells themselves go directly to the invasion site to battle the foreign organisms. Once there, the T-cells release powerful chemicals to destroy all foreign particles that have the specific antigen displayed on their surfaces. As the T-cells begin to win the battle against infection, they release signals to slow down the immune response.

T-cells actively defend the body against fungi, viruses, parasites, and a few types of bacteria; they can also destroy cancer cells. T-cells participate in the rejection of newly transplanted tissues, which is why physicians use drugs to inactivate them when tissue transplantation is necessary.

Humoral Immunity: B Cells and Antibodies The B-cells are important in a different type of immunity, humoral immunity, so named because the cells' secretions, not the cells themselves, mount the defensive effort. B-cells respond to infection by rapidly dividing and then producing large proteins known as antibodies. Antibodies travel in the bloodstream to the site of the infection. There they stick to the surfaces of the foreign particles and kill or otherwise inactivate them, making the foreign particles easy for the phagocytes to engulf. B-cells play a bigger role in resistance to infection than do T-cells.

The Immune System as a Whole In summary, the body's first lines of defense against foreign materials are the skin, the mucous membranes, and the GI tract. If a microorganism or other illness-causing agent gets past these barriers, the immune system calls the phagocytes into play. The phagocytes then stimulate the T-cells to recognize and destroy the foreign substances. At the same time, the B-cells secrete specific antibodies that kill invaders or weaken them to permit defeat by the phagocytes. These changes enable the immune system to respond quickly and forcefully to future exposures.

Nutrients fuel the immune response and other responses to various stresses. One of the ways in which severe stress damages the body is by leading to malnutrition. Conversely, excellent nutrition status supports strong defenses against severe stress.

Nutrition, Stress, and Immunity

The metabolic and immune responses to stress cause significant changes in the body's normal balances: anorexia, elevated blood glucose (hyperglycemia), negative nitrogen balance, increased retention of fluid and sodium, and increased excretion of potassium. As draining as these alterations may sound, medical researchers believe that the initial metabolic changes perform a valuable service. These changes help to prevent further injury and infection, repair damaged tissues, and maintain vital organ function. They facilitate the body's mobilization of its resources so that it can regain homeostasis.

Such metabolic changes constitute an adaptation that is sustained for as long as necessary or until exhaustion leads to death. Following a successful stress response, blood glucose, nitrogen and electrolyte balances, and the rate of catabolism gradually return to normal. Figure 18–4 illustrates the phases of the stress response. The following sections describe the many ways that nutrition influences the stress response and show that, clearly, the better nourished people are at the onset of stress, the better able they will be to carry the metabolic burdens imposed.

The **acute,** or **flow, phase** of the stress response is the catabolic period immediately following the onset of stress. During the **adaptive phase,** the body adjusts to the stress to minimize losses. If adaptation succeeds, **recovery** follows. If adaptation fails, **exhaustion** follows.

Figure 18–4
The Phases of the Stress Response

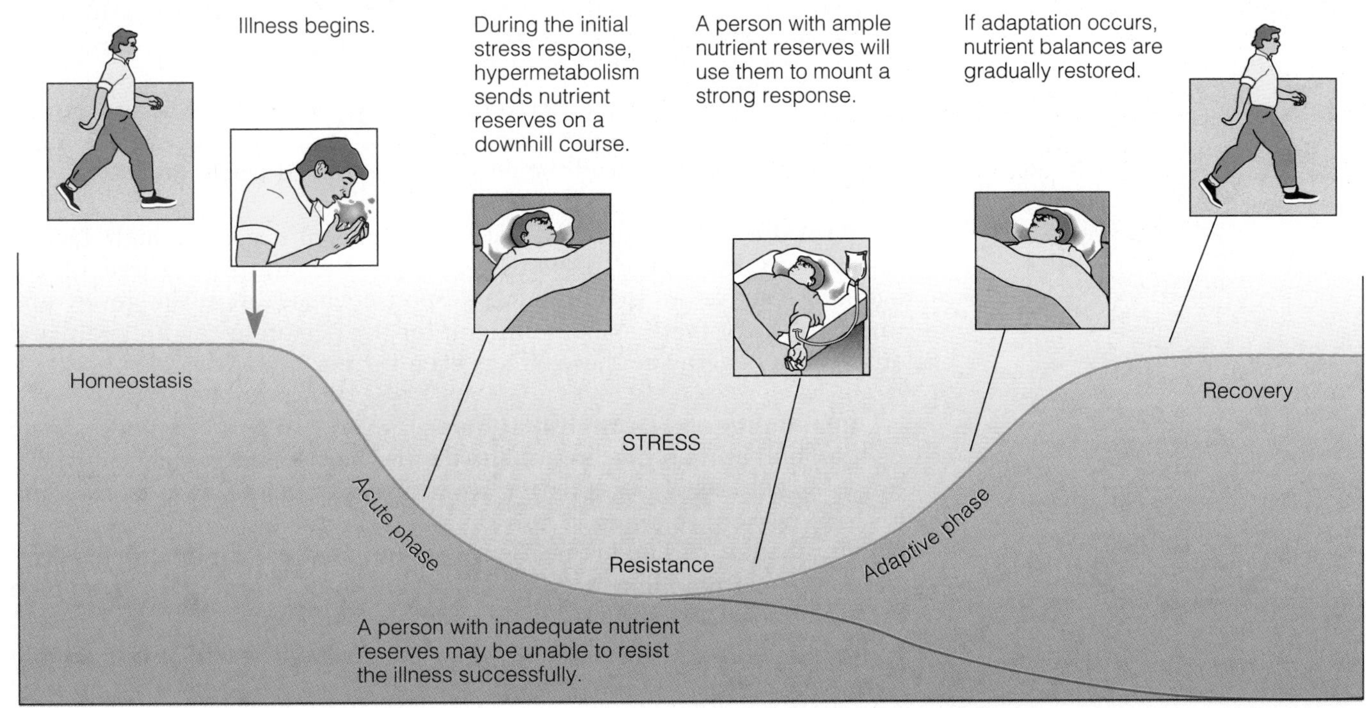

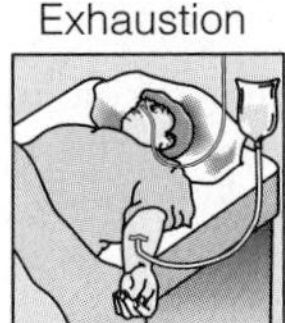

Illness begins.

A person with ample nutrient reserves will use them to mount a strong response.
If adaptation occurs, nutrient balances are gradually restored.

If depleted of nutrients, the person will be unable to make the uphill trip and may not recover (exhaustion).

Interrelationships between Nutrition and Stress

Hypermetabolic illnesses deplete energy reserves and break down protein tissues. As a result, they can lead to protein-energy malnutrition (PEM). PEM and stress then interact in a deadly cycle: stress worsens PEM, and PEM hinders the stress response. When the stress interacting with malnutrition is a severe infection, the combination is especially deadly (see Figure 18–5 on p. 446). Note, too, that malnutrition impairs every component of the immune system (Table 18–2 on p. 446). Again, this shows how crucial nutrition is to recovery.

Energy and Protein Needs The body's ability to respond to severe stress depends, to a large extent, on available energy and protein reserves. The well-nourished person can tolerate the protein-losing period (the period of negative nitrogen balance) because sufficient protein remains to support vital functions. However, protein losses can threaten the life of the person who has preexisting malnutrition. Think about the effects of protein loss on a malnourished accident victim who sustains multiple

To understand the relationship of protein-energy malnutrition to serious illness, think of energy stores and protein status as money in the bank. Illness can be compared to a major expense that arises unexpectedly. The person who has saved enough money can pay off the expense without too much difficulty. However, if more and more expenses arise, the money may run out. The person with scanty or no savings is unable to pay even a small expense.

Figure 18–5
Illness, Malnutrition, and Immunity

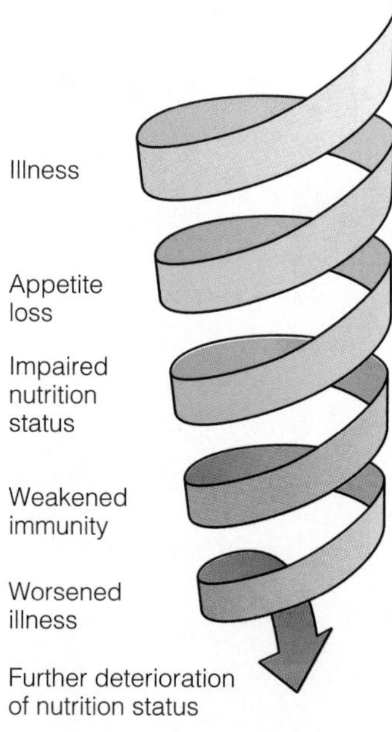

Malnutrition, illness, and impaired immunity worsen each other.

The cytokine **interleukin-1** (in-ter-LOO-kin) activates lymphocytes and is also partly responsible for the fever-induced anorexia that commonly accompanies stress. The cytokine **cachectin** (ka-KEK-tin) also induces anorexia. The cytokine **gamma-interferon** (in-ter-FEAR-on) induces the fever and malaise that frequently occur during an infection.

decubitus (dee-CUE-bih-tus) **ulcers:** the breakdown of skin and underlying tissues caused by constant pressure on and lack of oxygen to that area of the skin; often called **pressure sores** or bedsores.
de = down
cumbere = to lie

fractures and burns. What if the protein losses reflect breakdown of lung cells and too little protein remains available to synthesize immune factors? The loss of lung cells combined with reduced synthesis of immune factors invites lung infections. The result: pneumonia—on top of multiple fractures and burns.

At the same time, the person confronted with severe stress experiences anorexia, and GI tract motility decreases. These effects make it difficult or impossible to feed the person using the GI tract.

Appetite Unfortunately, just when nutrient needs are high, factors involved in the stress response suppress the appetite. Three of the cytokines active in the immune response cause anorexia, fever, and malaise.[6] All of these make it difficult for the person to eat, and pain and anxiety may aggravate these effects even further.

Immobility and Decubitus Ulcers Severe stresses often necessitate bed rest and immobility. Immobility further harms nutritional health. The immobilized body loses nitrogen from muscles and calcium from bones because without the muscle tension and weight load incurred by normal activity, the muscles and bones are not stimulated to maintain themselves. In prolonged immobilization, blood and urinary calcium may rise so high that calcium stones form in the bladder and kidneys.

An additional consequence of immobility is decubitus ulcers, which form wherever there is constant pressure on the skin. These ulcers can be extremely painful and are an open invitation for infections. Infections can further tax nutrient stores.

People with PEM, whether they are underweight or overweight, are especially vulnerable to decubitus ulcers.[7] Those who are severely underweight risk developing these ulcers because they have too little fat to cushion their bones. Those who are overweight develop ulcers because of the pressure of their weight on their skin. The elderly, people with an

Table 18–2
Malnutrition's Effects on the Immune System

IMMUNE SYSTEM COMPONENT	EFFECTS OF MALNUTRITION
Skin	Thinned, with less connective tissue
Mucous membranes	Microvilli flattened; antibody secretions reduced
GI tract	Compounded likelihood of bacterial translocation when intestines are injured
Lymph tissues	Thymus gland, lymph nodes, and spleen reduced in size; T-cell areas depleted of lymphocytes
Phagocytosis	Kill time delayed
Cell-mediated immunity	Circulating T-cells reduced
Humoral immunity	Circulating immunoglobulin levels normal; antibody response possibly impaired

impaired sense of touch, people who are unable to change position, and people who are not fully conscious also are prone to developing decubitus ulcers.

GI Tract Function Organs that undergo rapid cell replacement—such as the GI tract—are among the first to suffer the consequences of PEM. The intestinal microvilli shrink and become nonfunctional; up to 90 percent of them can be lost. GI tract motility slows. Then, even with adequate nourishment, the GI tract will have serious difficulty absorbing nutrients. Consequently, PEM may worsen, and the body may have further difficulty obtaining the extra energy and protein it needs to fight the stress.

The GI tract's immune function can also be seriously impaired by changes in the intestinal villi, changes that compromise the body's ability to protect itself against harmful microbes. An especially serious result of impaired GI tract immunity is translocation of bacteria into the body. Any condition that damages the structure of the intestinal villi, interferes with the function of the lymph tissue, or disrupts the normal intestinal flora can allow translocation.[8]

translocation: the passage of microorganisms from the interior of the intestines to the inside of the body.

Some translocation may stimulate immune defenses, because once foreign agents have entered the body, the immune system "sees" them and goes into action. However, extensive translocation can trigger infection, accelerate hypermetabolism, and ultimately lead to multiple organ failure.[9] Two conditions that frequently occur in severe stress significantly raise the risk of extensive translocation. One is reduced blood flow to the intestine (stress aggravates this); the other is having no nutrients in the intestinal tract (not feeding, or traditional feeding by vein causes this). Together these conditions can rapidly lead to atrophy of the intestinal cells and loss of their barrier function. Burn injuries, malnutrition, immunosuppressive drugs, and antibiotics that alter the intestinal bacterial flora also increase the likelihood of translocation.

Drug Therapy as a Stress Drug therapy plays an important role in the treatment of many illnesses, but it also constitutes a stress and may tax nutrition status. When people are given drugs, especially multiple drugs, the likelihood of drug-nutrient interactions is real, and serious deficiencies may result. The person who is malnourished and has few nutrient reserves may well develop nutrient deficiencies as a result of drug therapy. Furthermore, malnutrition causes atrophy of the intestinal cells, which can hinder the absorption of drugs as well as nutrients, worsening the person's medical condition.

PEM can also interfere with the metabolism and excretion of drugs. Many drugs are transported in the blood bound to blood proteins such as albumin, and one symptom of PEM is low blood albumin levels. Without sufficient carriers, drugs may reach their sites of action very slowly. Once drugs do reach their target cells, the lack of carriers may delay the drugs' transport to the liver and kidneys, where many drugs are detoxified and excreted. Thus, as a result of malnutrition, drugs may take a long time to work and then may remain active for too long, making side effects likely—another stress.

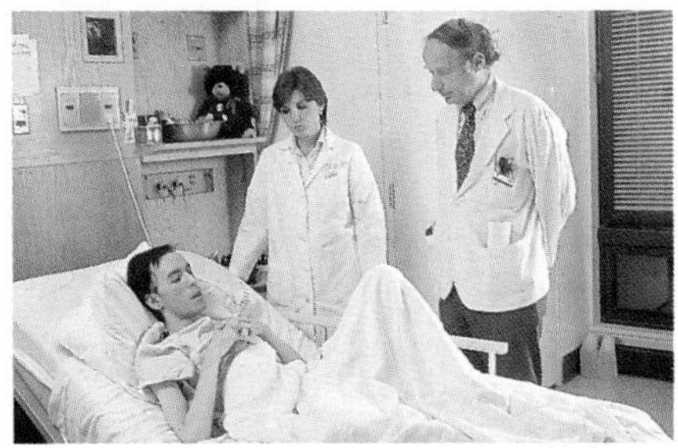

A person who looks malnourished may be showing the outward signs of a successful adaptation to stress.

Types of PEM and Stress

Chapter 4 described two types of PEM seen in developing countries: marasmus and kwashiorkor. Clinicians sometimes use these same terms to describe the PEM associated with illness; alternatively, they use the terms *chronic* and *acute* malnutrition. Whatever names are used, distinguishing between these types of malnutrition is a clinical skill that enables health care professionals to administer the nutrition therapy most likely to rehabilitate clients in each case. The person with chronic malnutrition or marasmus has lost body fat and muscle, but retained internal organ function, blood proteins, and immune function. In contrast, the person with acute malnutrition or kwashiorkor may have normal or even excess body fat and muscle, but compromised organ function, depleted blood proteins, and defective immune responses. Table 13-6 on p. 332 contrasts these two forms of malnutrition.

Chronic Malnutrition/Marasmus The individual with chronic malnutrition may look very thin, but that is because the person has *adapted* to prolonged limited energy and protein intake by conserving lean body mass to the greatest extent possible and has depended largely on fat stores for energy. Appropriate diet therapy is often successful in reversing chronic malnutrition because the vital organs have retained enough function to use nutrients as they are supplied. Overzealous feeding of the person with advanced malnutrition, however, places undue stress on organ systems and can lead to the refeeding syndrome (see pp. 453–454). Infection or stress on top of chronic malnutrition can precipitate the transition into acute malnutrition.

In place of the terms *acute malnutrition* or *kwashiorkor,* some clinicians prefer the more descriptive term *hypoalbuminemic PEM,* which emphasizes the loss of blood proteins seen as this condition sets in.

Acute Malnutrition/Kwashiorkor Acute malnutrition typically develops in the person with marginal protein status who suffers sudden, severe infection or other stress and is no longer able to cover protein needs adequately. The hormonal and immune system changes that accompany stress result in depleted blood proteins and compromised immune function; compromised organ function may soon follow.

Unlike the person with chronic malnutrition who has adapted to starvation, the person with acute malnutrition cannot adapt. Reversing protein losses through diet therapy is therefore difficult. A further danger is that this condition is easy to miss because sometimes the person has ample body fat and may not appear malnourished.

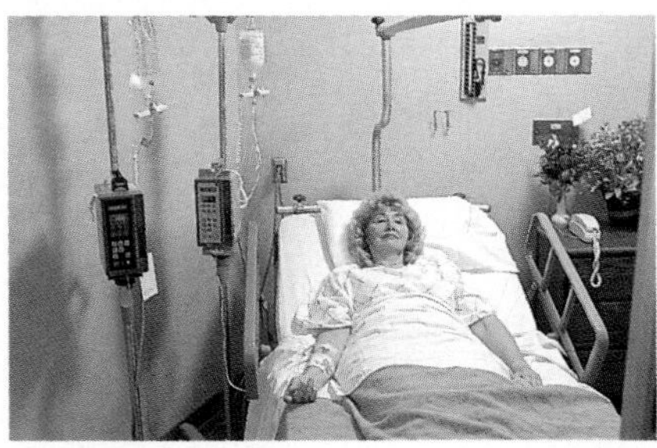

A person who has ample fat may still have kwashiorkor, a state of acute malnutrition in which the internal organs are compromised. This form of malnutrition can be dangerous and hard to treat and is easy to miss because the outward signs are misleading.

Transition to Acute Malnutrition The person who is progressing from the chronic to the acute state due to advanced malnutrition, infection, or both has all of the deficits of both conditions. Table 13–6 on p. 332 shows the anthropometric and biochemical distinctions among these types of malnutrition.

Effects of Recovery from Stress More research remains to be done, but preliminary studies suggest that the person with kwashiorkor may be more likely to develop infections and die while hospitalized than people suffering stress who do not develop kwashiorkor.[10] Marasmus alone does not appear to affect the risk of hospital infections or dying, provided that appropriate nutrition therapy is given in time. The combination, marasmus-kwashiorkor mix, may be as severe as kwashiorkor; it lengthens hospital stays and raises the cost of nutrition therapy. The studies that have revealed these serious impacts of malnutrition on illness specifically alert clinicians to the severe consequences of kwashiorkor.

Nutrition Support during Severe Stress

To rehabilitate a malnourished person who is not otherwise stressed, nutrition therapy has two simple goals: restore lean body mass and promote weight gain. In the severely stressed individual, however, the hormonal changes that drive the initial stress response make it impossible to restore nutrient deficits at first. Weight gain and positive nitrogen balance are not possible during the hypermetabolic period of severe stress. In fact, overfeeding at this time can do harm, especially in people with PEM. For these reasons, the appropriate nutrition goals for the severely stressed person are: to minimize nutrient losses, to preserve vital organs, and to maintain immune function. Generally, hypermetabolism peaks at 3 to 4 days and subsides in 7 to 10 days.[11] Thereafter, continued nutrition support restores nutrient balances.

Drug-nutrient interactions and their effects on nutrient needs must be kept in mind at all times. The margin shows some categories of drugs that are commonly used in people with severe stresses. Tables E-1A and E-1B in Appendix E list the possible impacts of these drugs on nutrition status. The next two sections deal, first, with the majority of stressed clients needing renourishment and, then, with the case of stressed malnourished clients in whom the refeeding syndrome is a problem.

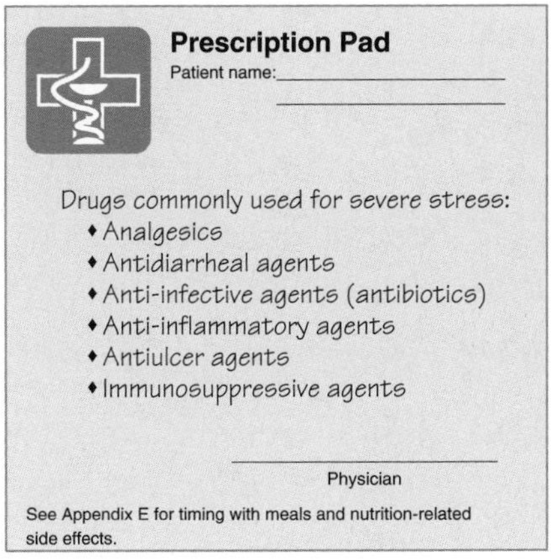

Prescription Pad
Patient name:
Drugs commonly used for severe stress:
• Analgesics
• Antidiarrheal agents
• Anti-infective agents (antibiotics)
• Anti-inflammatory agents
• Antiulcer agents
• Immunosuppressive agents
Physician
See Appendix E for timing with meals and nutrition-related side effects.

Providing Nutrients and Energy

Health professionals caring for severely stressed individuals face the challenge of providing just the right balance of fluids and electrolytes, energy, protein, lipids, and all other nutrients. Supplying too much energy can overwork the heart and lungs and lead to metabolic complications, but supplying too little energy compromises the body's ability to heal wounds, fight infections, maintain organ function, and recover.

Fluids and Electrolytes The most immediate nutrition task for the medical team following severe stress is to stabilize the body's fluid and electrolyte balance. This is critical in preventing dehydration and shock, for without adequate fluids, organ systems cannot function properly, oxygen and nutrients cannot be delivered to the cells, and waste products cannot be eliminated from the body. Intravenous fluids and electrolytes compensate for fluids and electrolytes lost through blood, wounds, vomiting, diarrhea, and fever. The physician determines the person's fluid needs based on clinical measures such as blood pressure, urinary output, level of consciousness, breathing patterns, and body temperature. Serum electrolytes are closely monitored and replaced as necessary.

shock: a sudden drop in the blood volume that disrupts the return of blood to the heart and the supply of oxygen to the tissues. Many events can lead to shock, including severe bleeding from trauma or surgery and severe dehydration.

Table 18–3
Estimation of Energy Needs Using the Harris-Benedict Equation

Harris-Benedict equation for estimating basal energy expenditure (BEE):[a]

Women:

BEE = 655 + (9.6 × wt in kg[b]) + (1.7 × ht in cm[b]) – (4.7 × age in years)

Men:

BEE = 66 + (13.7 × wt in kg[b]) + (5 × ht in cm[b]) – (6.8 × age in years)

Add to BEE for activity:

20% Sedentary

35% Moderately active

50% Active

Add to BEE for stress:

10–15% Uncomplicated elective surgery

20–40% Complicated surgery or fractures

50–100% Major burn

Add to BEE for fever (if present):

13% per degree centigrade over normal body temperature (37°C)[b]

Add to BEE to promote weight gain (if necessary):

5% if weight loss is moderate

10–15% if weight loss is severe

For people with a %IBW greater than 125, adjust the weight used in the BEE equation by following this equation:[c]

(Actual body weight – IBW) × 25%[d] + IBW = Adjusted body weight

[a]Basal metabolic rate (BMR, described on pp. 127-128) and BEE express the same thing: basal energy need. The equation for BMR is traditionally used in physiology and fitness laboratories; that for BEE, in hospitals. The two equations yield slightly different results, each suitable for the purposes intended. Adjustments for activity used in the hospital differ from those on p. 129 for similar reasons. All are approximations; all require judgment in their application.

[b]See Appendix G for equations to convert pounds to kilograms, inches to centimeters, and degrees Fahrenheit to degrees centigrade.

[c]From J. M. Karkeck, Adjustment for obesity, *American Dietetic Association Renal Practice Group Newsletter,* Winter 1984.

[d]Approximately 25 percent of body fat tissue is metabolically active.

Energy Needs Energy needs during severe stress are highly variable and depend on the type of stress, its severity, and the individual's prior nutrition status. Indirect calorimetry provides the most accurate assessment of energy needs in severe stress, but most facilities lack the equipment necessary to perform this measurement. In these cases, formulas such as the Harris-Benedict equation (see Table 18–3) provide estimates of energy needs. Alternatively, some clinicians simply provide 25 to 30 *nonprotein* kcalories per kilogram of body weight per day. No consensus has been reached on the best formula to estimate energy needs, and it is important to remember that formulas yield estimates only. Clinical judgment and continual monitoring of weight changes are always necessary to confirm that energy needs are being met.

Several studies suggest that the Harris-Benedict equation overestimates energy needs during severe stress. Therefore, it should be used with good clinical judgment.

Abbreviations:

- 1 degree centigrade is 1°C. The scientific name for the centigrade temperature scale is Celsius, also abbreviated C.
- 1 degree Fahrenheit is 1°F.

Conversion equations are provided in Appendix G.

Fever, a frequent accompaniment of stress, speeds up the basal metabolic rate (BMR). The BMR of a person with 4°F of fever—that is, a tem-

fatty acids may hold particular promise in preserving immune function.[14] Accordingly, products containing these nutrients, among others, are currently being marketed for maintaining immune function in severely stressed people. Whether these formulas will be successful, though, remains to be seen. Nutrition in Practice 18 explores further the relationships of nutrients to intestinal function.

The Refeeding Syndrome

It is urgent that people with PEM receive a high-kcalorie, high-protein diet, but a gradual approach is imperative. If nutrients are reintroduced too rapidly, severe complications, including malabsorption, cardiac insufficiency, respiratory distress, congestive heart failure, convulsions, coma, and even death, can result. Collectively, these complications have been called the refeeding syndrome.

refeeding syndrome: a set of physiological and metabolic complications associated with reintroducing adequate nutrition too rapidly for a person with severe PEM. These complications can include malabsorption, cardiac insufficiency, respiratory distress, congestive heart failure, convulsions, coma, and possibly death.

GI Tract Effects It may seem difficult to believe that simply feeding a malnourished individual can have such dire consequences. Recall, however, that malnutrition entails the loss of GI motility, as well as atrophy of intestinal villi and markedly reduced concentrations of digestive enzymes. Thus, when given food, the person with PEM often experiences nausea, vomiting, diarrhea, and malabsorption until the cells of the GI tract regenerate. Once the initial hurdle is over, though, this adaptation normally occurs fairly quickly.

Lung and Heart Effects During starvation, the body attempts to protect its lean body mass by slowing its metabolism. Then, when nutrients are reintroduced, the basal metabolic rate increases, and with it, the use of oxygen and production of carbon dioxide. Then, the lung and heart muscles, already weakened by malnutrition, must work harder to keep the body's gases in balance. Obviously, overfeeding during this critical period can overstress the lungs and heart.

Metabolic Effects Metabolic complications associated with the refeeding syndrome also occur as the body shifts from a fasting state to a fed state. Glucose again becomes the body's primary energy source, and the body immediately begins rebuilding lost tissue. As glucose and amino acids move into cells for this rebuilding process, electrolytes (potassium, phosphorus, magnesium, and calcium) move into the cells as well. As these electrolytes shift into the intracellular fluid, circulating levels can plummet, resulting in life-threatening complications.

Although the reason is unclear, a high carbohydrate intake seems to result in sodium and fluid retention. Sodium itself can increase fluid retention as well, so even simple glucose and salts, if administered too rapidly, can stress the heart and circulatory system.

Preventing the Refeeding Syndrome To prevent the refeeding syndrome, the reintroduction of nutrients to the severely malnourished individual must proceed slowly with vigilant monitoring of medical and metabolic status. Fluids and electrolytes are gradually repleted. Early feedings are low-kcalorie, moderate-carbohydrate, low-sodium, lactose-free formulas.[15] (Chapters 22 and 23 provide more information about such formulas.) Physicians and other members of the nutrition support team conscientiously monitor fluid status, electrolyte balances, and indices of organ function. Vitamin supplements are routinely provided.

When feeding begins after a long period of GI tract disuse (such as when nutrients must be provided by vein), diarrhea should be expected. It generally resolves within a few days. Feeding stimulates the rapid restoration of intestinal enzyme activity, although lactose intolerance may persist.

Delivery of Nutrients during Stress

Selecting the appropriate amounts and types of nutrients to help people recover from stress is only part of diet therapy. The nutrients must also be provided in a form and by a route the body can handle.

Importance of GI Tract Motility Feeding via the GI tract has to wait until motility is restored. The risks of feeding in the absence of peristalsis include two potentially fatal complications. One is distention with possible perforation of the bowel. The other is regurgitation of foods or formula into the lungs. Both of these conditions can result in life-threatening infections.

Early Enteral Feeding In the past, only intravenous fluids were used to deliver nutrients in the immediate poststress period because it was thought that the entire GI tract remained immobile during this time. Current studies suggest, however, that although the motility of the entire GI tract is slowed by stress, peristalsis returns much earlier in the small intestine than in the stomach and large intestine. Therefore, feeding formula directly into the small intestine through a tube is not only possible, but may be advantageous.[16] Early feeding into the small intestine protects the integrity of the GI tract and may minimize hypermetabolism and help prevent translocation.[17] Studies of animals show a higher rate of translocation when animals are fed entirely by vein.[18] Studies of human beings report significantly lower rates of infection in people with trauma injuries who receive enteral nutrition instead of intravenous feedings, even when the enteral feedings do not meet all nutrient needs.[19]

Early enteral feeding, however, is not possible in all cases. Clients with conditions that severely limit blood flow to the intestine must often be fed by vein.

Although the practice remains controversial, many health care professionals now advocate the early use of enteral feedings following severe stress.[20] Then, when bowel activity returns, oral diets can often be tolerated.

Feeding by Vein Clients who are malnourished, those who are not expected to be able to eat foods orally within a short time, and those with multiple stresses cannot go without nutrients in the immediate poststress period. When enteral nutrition is not initiated, these clients receive the nutrients they need by vein (intravenously).

Once it is medically safe, most individuals fed by vein gradually return to eating oral food. Chapter 23 explains intravenous nutrition and how clients are reintroduced to oral diets.

Oral Diets Well-nourished clients who are expected to be able to eat within a few days following stress receive simple intravenous solutions (see Chapter 23) designed to maintain fluid and electrolyte balance. Once bowel activity returns to normal, they begin to eat foods orally. Generally, the diets progress from clear liquids to full liquids and on to low-fiber foods and then regular foods as tolerated until all nutrient needs are met.

The general progression of diets from clear liquids to full liquids to low-fiber foods to regular foods is collectively called a **progressive diet.**

Dealing with Lactose Intolerance Lactose intolerance is common in people under stress, especially if they have not taken food for a while, or if they have developed PEM, or both. Giving milk or milk products can cause cramps, gas, diarrhea, and pain. The longer the lactose intolerance persists, the more important it is to find ways to deliver the nutrients of milk in a form the body can assimilate. The box in Chapter 8 entitled "How to Add Calcium to Daily Meals" offers ways to get around lactose intolerance until it resolves.

Severe stresses place tremendous demands on the body. The body uses all its resources to fight the battle to survive and regain health. Recovery depends, in part, on the body's receiving the energy and nutrients required to mount a defense, repair damaged tissues, and replenish nutrient reserves. The next chapter offers details on specific nutrient needs related to specific types of stress: infections, surgery, and burns.

STUDY QUESTIONS

1. What is the stress response, and what does it achieve?
2. How does the immune system defend the body against disease-causing organisms?
3. What special roles does the GI tract play in immune defenses?
4. Describe the effect of nutrition status on the body's ability to respond to stress.
5. How do the different types of PEM relate to stress?
6. Describe how nutrient needs change during severe stress.
7. What is the refeeding syndrome, and how can it be prevented?
8. Why may enteral nutrition be preferable to feeding by vein, even after severe stress?

CLINICAL APPLICATIONS QUESTIONS

1. Consider the case of Mrs. Gonzales, an 85-year-old woman hospitalized after suffering major injuries in a car accident. She has been NPO for three days. Mrs. Gonzales also suffers from the chronic disorders diabetes mellitus and heart disease. The health care team has recommended that she begin eating foods again. What data should be collected to determine Mrs. Gonzales's nutrition status? What steps should be taken to ensure that she begins to eat adequate amounts of food? What factors in the brief history provided suggest that drug-nutrient interactions should be considered for any drugs Mrs. Gonzales is given?
2. Bennie is a well-nourished seven-year-old who develops the flu and has a fever of 101°F for two days. Describe how this stress could temporarily impact his nutrition status. How would your concerns differ if Bennie were a seven-year-old in a hospital who had not eaten in several days?

NUTRITION IN PRACTICE 18

Fuels to Support the Intestine under Stress

What is the most appropriate mixture of nutrients to support the GI tract during stress and recovery? This discussion focuses on an area of study that has recently attracted much attention: the roles of specific nutrients in supporting GI function. Controversies surround this area, partly because much of the research has been conducted on animals and partly because studies on human beings require further elucidation and confirmation. Nevertheless, from what is known it seems clear that specific dietary constituents may be important to the health of intestinal cells. Among these dietary constituents are glutamine, short-chain fatty acids, and dietary fiber.

What is glutamine?

Glutamine is an amino acid abundant in food and the most abundant amino acid in the blood. Glutamine provides fuel for rapidly dividing cells and is the major fuel for the intestinal cells. After the intestinal cells have metabolized glutamine, the liver uses the end products, alanine and ammonia, to make glucose and urea, respectively. Glutamine is also important for the replication of all body cells, which use it to make purines, pyrimidines, and nucleotides, as well as other amino acids that they need.

In healthy individuals, glutamine is a nonessential amino acid. If food sources fail to meet the body's needs, the body can synthesize more glutamine from the branched-chain amino acids of skeletal muscle. During severe stress, however, oral intake may be interrupted, and the body may need more glutamine than it can synthesize. For these reasons, it has been suggested that glutamine becomes conditionally essential during stress.[21]

Intravenous feeding solutions traditionally do not contain glutamine, and standard enteral formulas contain only small amounts. One reason for leaving it out of feeding solutions has been its designation as a nonessential amino acid; another reason is that it is highly unstable in intravenous solutions.[22] Technological advances have made it possible to add glutamine to both intravenous and enteral feeding solutions, however.

Various animal studies show that adding glutamine to either intravenous or enteral feeding solutions helps to maintain the structure and support the function of the intestinal cells and also inhibits bacterial translocation across the intestinal barrier.[23] Glutamine may stimulate these actions by promoting protein synthesis in the intestinal cells.[24] Studies of human beings undergoing bone marrow transplants suggest that, in comparison to standard intravenous feeding solutions, glutamine-supplemented solutions improve nitrogen balance, reduce the incidence of infection, and help shorten hospital stays.[25]

Clearly, studies of the possible role of glutamine in severe stress are promising. Recommendations to select formulas based solely on their glutamine contents, however, cannot be made until further investigations confirm the safety and effectiveness of glutamine-supplemented feeding solutions.[26]

Why would short-chain fatty acids be a useful fuel for people under stress?

Short-chain fatty acids are a primary source of energy for the cells of the colon. These fatty acids, which are two to four carbons long, are produced by bacteria in the GI tract from the metabolism of dietary fiber, shed intestinal cells, and mucus. Short-chain fatty acids provide energy, stimulate intestinal cell growth, enhance intestinal blood flow, bolster secretion of pancreatic enzymes, and promote sodium and water absorption in the colon.[27]

Short-chain fatty acids may also hasten healing after intestinal surgery. After a portion of the intestine has been removed (bowel resection), reducing the absorptive surface of the intestine, the remaining intestine adapts by getting larger. This adaptation helps the body to continue absorbing nutrients. Short-chain fatty acids stimulate intestinal cell growth in rats after bowel resections.[28] Another study of rats showed that short-chain fatty acids given in addition to intravenous feeding helped maintain the size of intestinal cells.[29] Again, little is known as yet regarding the role of short-chain fatty acids in preventing translocation.

Fibers probably help by enhancing GI tract motility, right?

Yes, but that is not all that fibers do. They help to provide fuel for the intestinal cells in the colon, because the intestinal bacteria metabolize fibers to yield short-chain fatty acids. They also help directly to maintain the structure and function of the intestinal cells.

Some types of fibers exert these effects more readily than others. Soy polysaccharide, the most common type of fiber used in enteral formulas, is readily metabolized by short-chain fatty acids in the colon. These effects may help maintain bowel function and prevent intestinal cell atrophy.

Pectin and guar gums are soluble fibers that slow the rate at which the stomach empties, limit the rise in blood glucose following a meal, and support the growth of bacteria in the intestine.[30] In rats, when large portions of the small bowel have been resected, pectin added to an enteral diet helps the GI tract to adapt and the resection site to heal faster.[31]

A study of rats compared fiber-free liquid formulas to liquid formulas supplemented with either soy polysaccharide or pectin to see what effects these diets might have on absorption in the colon.[32] Both fiber-supplemented formulas improved absorption compared with the fiber-free formulas, suggesting that fiber improved colon cell function. The researchers also measured the weight, DNA content, and protein content of the colon cells. They found no significant differences in these parameters, suggesting that fiber had little effect on cell structure. Unlike other studies, this study did not find that fiber improved cell structure, but it did show that fiber improved cell functions and that soy polysaccharides and pectins were equally effective.

Do fibers help prevent translocation?

Researchers anticipate giving a "Yes" answer here. Limited studies using animals suggest that the fibers known as bulking agents may do so. Bulking agents are fibers that absorb and retain water, and water in the stool helps increase stool volume. This seems to help preserve the integrity of the GI tract and thus may help limit translocation. Studies of mice maintained on glutamine-free feeding solutions were undertaken to see what effects bulking agents might have on bacterial translocation. The mice receiving the bulking agents (cellulose and kaolin) had significantly less bacterial translocation than mice given either pectin supplements or no supplements.[33] This study suggests a role for bulking agents in preventing translocation.

Don't fibers help prevent diarrhea and constipation, too?

It is not yet clear whether fiber can prevent diarrhea in severely stressed people on liquid formula diets.[34] Some of the factors that cause diarrhea are unrelated to diet and, therefore, are not responsive to dietary changes. Regarding constipation, however, results are clearer. People maintained on liquid formulas for long periods of time or those who are paralyzed, sedated, and not severely stressed may benefit from the addition of soy polysaccharide to formulas to help prevent constipation.[35] Future studies may help identify other groups of people who may benefit from fiber-supplemented diets and may also define the best dosages and techniques for administering such diets.

Evidence to support the theory that a breach in the intestinal barrier can be a significant source of infection in severe stress is mounting, and findings to support the use of specific dietary constituents to maintain GI tract integrity are encouraging. The temptation to use what is currently known and hope for studies to confirm the benefits of this knowledge is great, but that would be premature at this time. More work must be done to determine whether a breakdown of the intestinal barrier is truly a major route of infection during stress and whether specific dietary constituents are of greater use than an ordinary well-balanced diet. Carefully controlled studies in human beings are lacking, and little work has been done to determine conditions under which specific intestinal fuels might be valuable and what doses might be safe and effective. The prospects of supporting the immune system and preventing further decline in already stressed people are inviting, and the potential benefits may prove to be life-saving.

■ NOTES ■

1. J. D. Anderson, F. A. Moore, and E. E. Moore, Enteral feeding in the critically injured patient, *Nutrition in Clinical Practice* 7 (1992): 117–122.
2. R. H. Bower, Nutritional and metabolic support of critically ill patients, *Journal of Parenteral and Enteral Nutrition* (supplement) 14 (1990): 257–259.
3. P. Brandtzaeg and coauthors, Immunobiology and immunopathology of human gut mucosa: Humoral immunity and intraepithelial lymphocytes, *Gastro-enterology* 97 (1989):; 1562–1584; M. F. Kagnoff, Immunology of the digestive system, in *Physiology of the Gastrointestinal Tract,* 2nd ed., ed. L. R. Johnson (New York: Raven Press, 1987).
4. B. Langkamp-Henken, J. A. Glezer, and K. A. Kudsk, Immunologic structure and function of the gastrointestinal tract, *Nutrition in Clinical Practice* 7 (1992): 100–108.

5. J. W. Alexander, Nutrition and translocation, *Journal of Parenteral and Enteral Nutrition* (supplement) 14 (1990): 170–174.
6. T. C. Hardin, Cytokine mediators of malnutrition: Clinical implications, *Nutrition in Clinical Practice* 8 (1993): 55–59.
7. G. Pinchocofsky-Devin, Hazards of immobility and poly-pharmacy, *Support Line* 14 (1992): 5–7.
8. J. C. Alverdy, Effects of glutamine-supplemented diets on immunology of the gut, *Journal of Parenteral and Enteral Nutrition* (supplement) 14 (1990): 109–113.
9. Alexander, 1990.
10. S. A. McClave and coauthors, Differentiating subtypes (hypoalbuminemic vs. marasmic) of protein-calorie malnutrition: Inci-dence and clinical significance in a university hospital setting, *Journal of Parenteral and Enteral Nutrition* 16 (1992): 337–342.
11. Anderson, Moore, and Moore, 1992.
12. M. M. Gottschlich, Selection of optimal lipid sources in enteral and parenteral nutrition, *Nutrition in Clinical Practice* 7 (1992): 152–165; Bower, 1990; G. L. Blackburn, In search of the "preferred fuel," *Nutrition in Clinical Practice* 4 (1989): 3–5; F. Negro and F. Cerra, Nutritional monitoring in the ICU: Rational and practical application, *Critical Care Clinics* 4 (1988): 34–47.
13. Gottschlich, 1992.
14. A. Barbul, Arginine and immune function, *Nutrition* (supplement) 6 (1989): 53–58; F. B. Rudolph and coauthors, Role of RNA as a dietary source of pyrimidines and purines in immune function, *Nutrition* (supplement) 6 (1989): 45–52; J. E. Kinsella and coauthors, Dietary polyunsaturated fatty acids and eicosanoids: Potential effects on the modulation of inflammatory and immune cells—An overview, *Nutrition* (supplement) 6 (1989): 24–44.
15. S. M. Solomon and D. F. Kirby, The refeeding syndrome: A review, *Journal of Parenteral and Enteral Nutrition* 14 (1990): 90–97; T. Havala and E. Shronts, Managing the complications associated with refeeding, *Nutrition in Clinical Practice* 5 (1990): 23–29.
16. E. H. Livingston and E. P. Pasaro, Postoperative ileus, *Digestive Diseases and Science* 35 (1990): 121–132; D. R. Wagner and coauthors, Combined parenteral and enteral nutrition in severe trauma, *Nutrition in Clinical Practice* 7 (1992): 113–116; Anderson, Moore, and Moore, 1992; Bower, 1990.
17. Anderson, Moore, and Moore, 1992.
18. J. C. Alverdy, E. Aoys, and G. S. Moss, Total parenteral nutrition promotes bacterial translocation from the gut, *Surgery* 124 (1988): 185–190.
19. F. A. Moore and coauthors, TEN versus TPN following major abdominal trauma: Reduced septic morbidity, *Journal of Trauma* 29 (1989): 916–923.
20. Anderson, Moore, and Moore, 1992; F. B. Cerra, How nutrition changes what getting sick means, *Journal of Parenteral and Enteral Nutrition* (supplement) 14 (1990): 164–169; D. Schroeder and coauthors, Effects of immediate postoperative enteral nutrition on body composition, muscle function, and wound healing, *Journal of Parenteral and Enteral Nutrition* 15 (1991): 376–383.
21. S. Mobrahan, Glutamine: A conditionally essential nutrient or another nutritional puzzle, *Nutrition Reviews* 50 (1992): 331–333; R. J. Smith, Glutamine metabolism and its physiologic importance, *Journal of Parenteral and Enteral Nutrition* (supplement) 14 (1990): 40–44.
22. Glutamine in parenteral solutions enhances intestinal mucosal immune function in rats, *Nutrition Reviews* 50 (1993): 152–155.
23. D. Burke and coauthors, Glutamine-supplemented total parenteral nutrition improves gut immune function, *Archives of Surgery* 124 (1989): 1396–1399; J. P. Grant and P. J. Snyder, Use of L-glutamine in total parenteral nutrition, *Journal of Surgical Research* 44 (1988): 506–513; J. L. Rombeau, A review of the effects of glutamine-enriched diets on experimentally induced enterocolitis, *Journal of Parenteral and Enteral Nutrition* 14 (1990): 100–105; V. S. Klimberg and coauthors, Prophylactic glutamine protects the intestinal mucosa from radiation injury, *Cancer* 66 (1990): 62–68; W. W. Souba and coauthors, Oral glutamine reduces bacterial translocation following abdominal radiation, *Journal of Surgical Research* 48 (1990): 1–5.
24. T. Higashiguchi and coauthors, Effect of glutamine on protein synthesis in isolated intestinal cells, *Journal of Parenteral and Enteral Nutrition* 17 (1993): 307–314.
25. T. R. Ziegler and coauthors, Clinical and metabolic efficacy of glutamine-supplemented parenteral nutrition after bone marrow transplantation: A randomized, double-blind, controlled study, *Annals of Internal Medicine* 116 (1992): 821–828.
26. M. A. Evans and E. P. Shronts, Intestinal fuels: Glutamine,

short-chain fatty acids, and dietary fiber, *Journal of the American Dietetic Association* 92 (1992): 1239–1246.

27. Gottschlich, 1992.
28. S. A. Kripke and coauthors, Stimulation of intestinal mucosal growth with intra-colonic infusion of short-chain fatty acids, *Journal of Parenteral and Enteral Nutrition* 13 (1989): 109–116.
29. M. J. Koruda and coauthors, Effect of parenteral nutrition supplemented with short-chain fatty acids on adaptation to massive small bowel resection, *Gastro-enterology* 95 (1988): 715–720.
30. W. Scheppach and coauthors, Addition of dietary fiber to liquid formula diets: The pros and cons, *Journal of Parenteral and Enteral Nutriton* 14 (1990): 204–209.
31. M. J. Koruda and coauthors, The effect of a pectin-supplemented elemental diet on intestinal adaptation to massive small bowel resection, *Journal of Parenteral and Enteral Nutrition* 10 (1986): 343–350; R. H. Rolandelli and coauthors, The effect of enteral feedings supplemented with pectin on the healing of colonic anastomoses in the rat, *Surgery* 99 (1986): 703–708.
32. G. M. Levine and J. Rosenthal, Effects of fiber-containing liquid diets on colonic structure and function in the rat, *Journal of Parenteral and Enteral Nutrition* 15 (1991): 526–529.
33. G. Spaeth and coauthors, Bulk prevents bacterial translocation induced by the oral administration of total parenteral nutrition solution, *Journal of Parenteral and Enteral Nutrition* 14 (1990): 442–447.
34. D. C. Frankenfield and P. L. Beyer, Dietary fiber and bowel function in tube-fed patients, *Journal of the American Dietetic Association* 91 (1991): 590–596.
35. J. C. Palacio and J. L. Rombeau, Dietary fiber: A brief overview and potential application to enteral nutrition, *Nutrition in Clinical Practice* 5 (1990): 99–106.

19

Nutrition for Infections, Surgery, and Burns

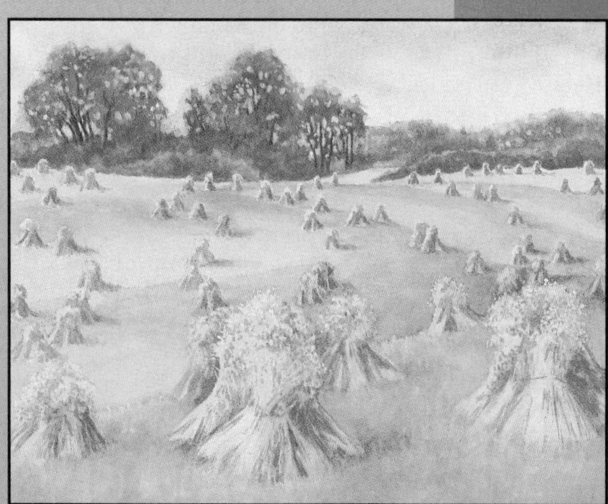

CONTENTS

As Chapter 18 described, severe stresses in general pose numerous problems for the body. This chapter goes on to describe some of the specific nutrition implications of various stresses.

Infections

Infections develop whenever disease-causing microorganisms invade the body. The infections may remain localized, or they may invade the bloodstream and spread throughout the body (sepsis). Critically ill people who develop sepsis may experience progressive failure of multiple organ systems, which frequently leads to death.

Infections spread easily in people already weakened by the stresses of malnutrition, illness, other infections, surgery, or other injury. Besides placing demands on nutrient stores, infections can also lead to fever, anorexia, nausea, vomiting, or diarrhea, further draining nutrient reserves.

During an **infection,** the body is invaded by disease-causing microorganisms, or viruses. An infection may remain localized in one area (for example, a patch of skin) or may invade the bloodstream and, thereby, the whole body.

sepsis or **septicemia** (sep-tih-SEE-me-ah)**:** the presence of microorganisms or their poisonous by-products within the bloodstream.

Drug-Nutrient Interactions The primary task in caring for the infected person is to identify and eliminate the invading organism. Often physicians prescribe anti-infective agents. These drugs may alter nutrient status; nutrients may also interfere with drug effectiveness (see Tables E–1A and E–1B in Appendix E).

anti-infective agents: drugs that kill microorganisms or interfere with their growth; also called **antimicrobials.** The major classes of anti-infective agents are **antibiotics,** which kill bacteria; **antiviral agents,** which kill viruses, and **antifungal agents,** which kill fungi.

Fluid Needs Health care professionals must closely monitor people with infections to ensure that fluid needs are met. Dehydration is usually not a problem unless a person has diarrhea, vomiting, or excessive sweating; but when these losses do occur, fluid needs may be as high as 3 to 4 liters per day. It is also possible that the infected person will retain fluids due to the hormonal changes that accompany fever. Giving excessive fluids in these cases can cause fluid overload.

anemia of infection: a condition in which iron moves from the blood to the liver. Reduced blood iron hinders the growth of infective organisms and so helps fight infection, but the storage of iron also results in a decline in hemoglobin synthesis and so causes anemia.

Anemia of Infection People with infections may develop a type of anemia referred to as the anemia of infection. At the onset of an infection, blood iron rapidly declines as iron moves into the liver for storage. This shift helps fight the infection by depriving the infecting microorganisms of the body's iron, which they require for their metabolism. However, iron in storage is also unavailable to make new hemoglobin, so anemia develops. This anemia reflects the body's *normal* physiological response to infection and does not respond to iron, folate, or vitamin B_{12} supplements, or to any other dietary or medical treatment. In fact, providing large doses of oral or intravenous iron can worsen the infection.[1] Without medical intervention, the liver will return iron to the blood as the infection resolves.

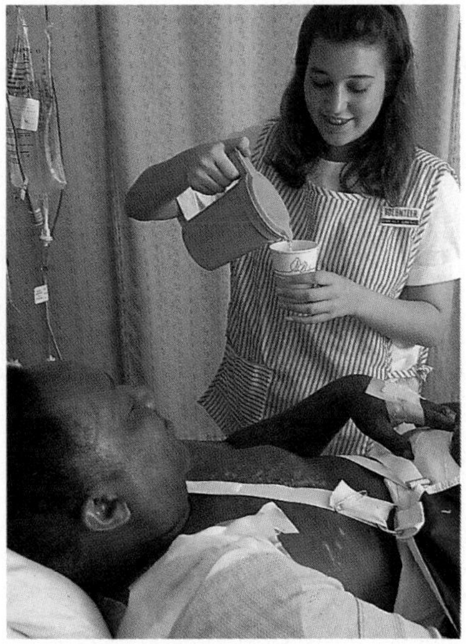

A person with an infection may need up to 4 liters of fluid a day.

Trauma and Surgery

The term *trauma* refers to any kind of injury; surgery is one instance of trauma. This section concentrates on the nutrition needs of people undergoing general surgery, including organ transplantation. Later chapters discuss nutrition needs associated with specific surgeries wherever appropriate.

Nutrition before Surgery

Surgery is an intentional trauma; clients and their caretakers often have time to prepare for it. One of the most valuable aspects of preparation is a well-designed defensive nutrition strategy.

Ideally, all clients enter surgery at appropriate weight, with full nutrient reserves, but this ideal is not always possible. Illness or stress prior to surgery may interfere with a person's food intake or use of nutrients. The person may also have to fast or follow a nutrient-poor liquid diet before undergoing diagnostic and laboratory tests, further taxing nutrition status. The caretaker who appreciates nutrition's vital support in resistance and recovery will watch for signs of nutrition risk and encourage clients to eat as well as possible.

Regular Diets for Well-Nourished Clients Before surgery, a well-nourished client who is expected to have an uncomplicated recovery usually receives a regular diet, one that provides ample food energy and protein. With this preparation, the person can withstand short-term starvation and some degree of protein catabolism without serious consequences.

Special Diets for Malnourished Clients Malnourished people undergoing surgery risk postoperative infection, delayed wound healing, morbidity, and mortality.[2] These people require diets high in energy and protein prior to surgery. Such diets generally provide about 1000 kcalories more than the person would need just to maintain weight and about 1.5 grams protein per kilogram of body weight daily. Most hospitals give malnourished clients high-kcalorie and high-protein supplements and snacks between meals; clients who understand their importance may be motivated to accept them.

For people with functioning GI tracts who cannot eat enough food orally, tube feedings may be indicated. (Specifics on tube feedings, also known as enteral nutrition, are provided in Chapter 22.) Again, those who understand the need may accept them willingly. When use of the GI tract is contraindicated, clients may receive all nutrients intravenously before surgery to maintain or boost nutrition status. (Delivering nutrients by vein is parenteral nutrition, and details are given in Chapter 23.) Although it has not been proven conclusively, preoperative nutrition support may reduce the incidence of postsurgical complications and mortality in malnourished clients.[3] Health care professionals can perform valuable services by explaining to clients how nutrition supports resistance and recovery and by helping them to relax so that anxiety will interfere as little as possible with their bodies' digestion, absorption, and storage of nutrients prior to surgery.

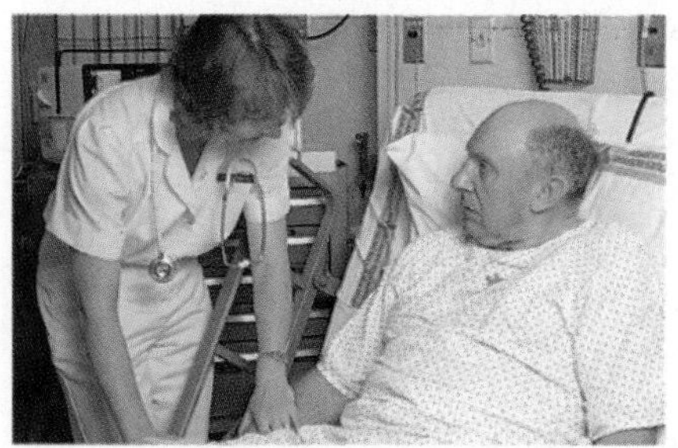

To help clients prepare nutritionally for surgery, explain the highly supportive role nutrition plays in resistance and recovery—and help them to relax, so that they can eat.

Physicians may order vitamins, minerals, and trace elements according to clients' individual needs. For example, a person with anemia caused by iron deficiency receives iron supplementation before elective surgery.

Immediate Pre-surgery Diet Physicians generally order all foods and fluid withheld for at least eight hours before surgery. This helps to prevent regurgitation and aspiration, which can occur during anesthesia or recovery. For people undergoing surgery on the GI tract, liquid diets or foods low in residue are given for two or three days before surgery. These diets minimize the amount of fecal material in the tract and help prevent distention after surgery. People restricted to liquid diets may receive residue-free liquid supplements by tube to meet their nutrient needs. A person who receives these diets accepts them best if the nurse or other caregiver explains the reasons for them.

Chapters 20 and 21 describe GI surgery.

residue: the total amount of material in the colon; it includes dietary fiber and also undigested food, intestinal secretions, bacterial cell bodies, and cells shed from the intestinal mucosa.

Nutrition after Surgery

In the immediate postsurgical period, the first and most important nutrition-related task for the medical team is to maintain fluid and electrolyte balance. Clients lose blood, fluid, and electrolytes during surgery, and thereafter, they may lose additional fluids from fever, draining wounds, vomiting, or diarrhea. The second task is to reintroduce solid foods as soon as GI tract activity resumes. A well-nourished person who can tolerate table food is ready for a progressive diet. People with depleted nutrient stores, those undergoing extensive surgical procedures, and people with postsurgical complications need the high-kcalorie, high-protein diets described earlier.

Depending on the type of surgery and the quality of the diet, some supplements may be necessary. The need for many of the B vitamins increases when energy and protein intakes increase. Vitamin C helps form collagen, which plays an important role in wound healing. Zinc also participates in wound healing. Vitamin K helps the blood to clot. Carefully selected foods and formulas high in energy and protein are rich in other nutrients as well; thus the person who consumes a variety of nutritious foods or a complete formula needs no supplements. Keep an eye open for signs of deficiencies, however, and keep in mind the possible need for supplements.

People being fed by tube or by vein before surgery usually continue receiving such feedings until they are able to eat adequately. Using the GI tract for feeding is always preferred to intravenous nutrition. A surgeon who anticipates that a person may have difficulty resuming eating may construct a feeding gastrostomy or jejunostomy during surgery so that tube feedings can bypass the mouth and be continued until oral intake is adequate.

feeding gastrostomy: a surgical opening made in the stomach through which a feeding tube can be passed. For a **feeding jejunostomy,** the surgical opening is made in the jejunum. Both of these feeding sites are discussed in Chapter 22.

Progressive Diets

As soon as clients can take foods by mouth following stress, they follow progressive diets. Liquid diets are often the first step. There are two classes of liquid diets: clear and full.

Clear-Liquid Diets Clear-liquid diets serve the primary purpose of providing fluids and electrolytes to prevent dehydration. As you might expect, they consist of foods that are relatively transparent or light, such as gelatin, tea, broth, and clear juices. They are liquid at body temperature, although they may be semisolid when cool (as gelatin is). The body digests and absorbs these liquids easily, and they contribute little or no residue in the GI tract. Table 19–1 lists the foods allowed on clear-liquid

Table 19–1
Foods Included on Liquid Diets

CLEAR-LIQUID DIETS	FULL-LIQUID DIETS
Bouillon	All clear liquids
Broth, clear	Butter
Carbonated beverages	Cheese, cottage[a]
Coffee, regular and decaffeinated	Commercially prepared liquid formulas (all)
Commercially prepared clear-liquid formulas	Cooked cereals, strained
Fruit drinks	Cream
Fruit ices	Custard
Fruit juices, strained	Egg, soft cooked or scrambled[a]
Gelatin	Flavorings
Hard candy	Ice cream, plain
Honey	Instant breakfast drinks
Lemonade	Margarine
Popsicles	Milk, all types
Salt	Potatoes, mashed and diluted in cream soups
Salt substitutes	Pudding
Sugar	Sherbet
Sugar substitutes	Soups, strained vegetable, meat, or cream
Tea, regular and decaffeinated	Sour cream
	Vegetable juices, strained
	Vegetable purees, diluted in cream soups
	Yogurt

[a]As tolerated.

diets, and the accompanying sample menu shows an example of a day's meals.

If you take a closer look at the foods allowed on a clear-liquid diet, you will see why many people find these foods unappetizing and boring. Worse, clear-liquid diets are deficient in energy and most nutrients, especially in relation to the high energy and nutrient requirements of a stressed person. No one should stay on a standard clear-liquid diet for more than a day or two, and the aware health care professional will make sure that regular food is offered as soon as possible.

Full-Liquid Diets A full-liquid diet includes both clear and opaque liquid foods. Table 19–1 lists the foods allowed on full-liquid diets, and the accompanying sample menu shows an example of a day's meals. As with clear-liquid diets, meeting nutrient needs can be difficult with a full-liquid diet.

Liquid Diet Formulas To meet the energy and nutrient needs of stressed people who must stay on liquid diets for more than a few days, health care professionals use formulas. Some hospitals routinely use these formulas following surgery to prevent the severe energy and protein

Sample Clear-Liquid Diet Menu

MENU

BREAKFAST	LUNCH	SUPPER
Strained orange juice	Bouillon	Bouillon
Flavored gelatin	Apple juice	Cranberry juice
Ginger ale	Flavored gelatin	Fruit ice
Coffee or tea	Coffee or tea	Flavored gelatin
Sugar	Sugar	Coffee or tea
		Sugar

BETWEEN MEALS

Soft drinks
Gelatin
Fruit juices

deficits incurred by incomplete liquid diets. Formulas have a consistent nutrient composition and they offer other advantages. For one, formulas of a specific osmolality can be selected to reduce the likelihood of GI problems. For another, most formulas are lactose-free, which accommodates the loss of lactose tolerance often seen in GI dysfunction. For these

osmolality: the number of molecular and ionic particles (measured in osmoles) per kilogram of water in a solution.

Sample Full-Liquid Diet Menu

MENU

BREAKFAST	LUNCH	SUPPER
Orange juice	Apricot nectar	Apple juice
Strained oatmeal	Yogurt, plain	Creamed soup
Egg, scrambled	Pudding	Custard
Milk	Milk	Milk
Sugar	Coffee or tea	Coffee or tea
Margarine	Sugar	Sugar

BETWEEN MEALS

Milkshakes (made with plain ice cream), ice cream, eggnog, pudding, custard, or gelatin

reasons, individuals who need liquid diets for more than a day or so can benefit from formulas.

Solid Foods Clients may better tolerate the shift from liquid diets to standard diets if they receive low-fiber diets during the transition. Low-fiber diets provide foods that are easy to chew, swallow, digest, and absorb. (Chapter 22 describes low-fiber diets in more detail.) Foods are often provided in small, frequent meals at first. Standard diets provide the full spectrum of nutrients and include all foods.

Diet as Tolerated Often the postsurgical diet order simply says "diet as tolerated." It is up to the nurse or dietitian to keep track of the client's tolerance and readiness to advance from liquids to solid foods. Nausea, vomiting, diarrhea, cramping, or other GI upsets indicate intolerance. At each progressive step, a client may be intolerant to a particular food (orange juice or milk, for example), rather than to the diet itself. In such a case, the offending food is withheld until food tolerance improves.

Sometimes the physician or other health care professional forgets to advance the diet; the alert nurse will then make the recommendation. Other times a person truly cannot tolerate foods other than clear liquids; in such cases, liquid formulas, tube feedings, or intravenous nutrition may be necessary. If stressed individuals must stay on liquid diets for several days, alert the dietitian or suggest to the physician that a supplemental formula be considered.

The restoration of adequate nutrition during severe stress is especially complicated in people with PEM. Although it is urgent for these individuals to receive high-kcalorie, high-protein diets right away, the refeeding syndrome may make this impossible in some cases. PEM may have incurred such severe physiological and metabolic consequences that only a gradual approach will succeed in reversing a client's debilitated state. The accompanying case study reviews the nutrition needs of a young woman undergoing surgery for appendicitis.

Organ Transplants

Organ transplants are a special case of surgery because the immune system is intentionally suppressed when they are performed. Recall that the immune response begins when the immune system cells recognize a foreign body. In an organ transplant, if the recipient's immune system identifies the antigens on the transplanted tissue as foreign, it destroys the transplant.

The destruction of healthy donor cells by the recipient is called **graft-versus-host disease.**

Medical researchers have discovered that a few specific antigens evoke a greater rejection response than others. To minimize the chances of rejection, these specific antigens from the donor and recipient are matched for compatibility. Transplants using well-matched organs are more successful than those using organs with antigen mismatches.

Drug-Nutrient Interactions In addition to antigen compatibility, drug therapy greatly improves the outcome of organ transplants.[4]

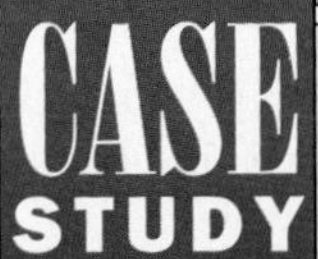

Prelaw Student with Appendicitis

Sally, a 20-year-old prelaw student, went to the university hospital complaining of nausea, fever (101°F), and severe pain in the lower right portion of her abdomen. The diagnosis was appendicitis, and Sally was taken to surgery for an appendectomy (removal of the appendix). Sally's height on admission was 5 feet 7 inches, and she weighed 132 pounds. She had experienced a 5-pound weight loss in the past month, which the dietitian attributed to irregular eating habits during a heavy work schedule.

1. From the limited information about Sally's nutrition history presented here, what can you say about her nutrition status?
2. Can you detect any nutrition risk factors?
3. What other data would be useful in evaluating her nutrition status?
4. Because Sally had emergency surgery, nothing could be done to improve her nutrition status before surgery. If surgery had been anticipated, what advice would you have given Sally about her diet?
5. Specifically, what kind of diet would you have recommended?
6. Calculate Sally's energy and protein needs, and describe what kind of diet would be most appropriate for her after surgery.
7. Would a regular diet best meet her energy, protein, vitamin, and mineral needs?
8. Consider Sally's nutrition-education needs. What type of nutrition advice could benefit Sally?
9. Who could best provide this advice?

Immunosuppressive drugs prevent rejection by inducing a generalized suppression of the recipient's immune response. Such drug therapy carries risks, of course. With the immune system suppressed, infections develop easily. Table E–1B in Appendix E provides a summary of common immunosuppressant drug side effects that may influence nutrient status.

immunosuppressants: drugs that suppress the immune response.

Nutrition Support Nutrition support during the immediate posttransplant phase follows the guidelines for postsurgical nutrition. The diet is designed to provide sufficient kcalories and protein both to promote wound healing and to enable the client to withstand the stress of possible rejection and infection, while at the same time not taxing the body's assimilative systems by overfeeding. As mentioned earlier, overfeeding can place intolerable stress on vital organs and hinder recovery. Long-term nutrition support focuses on the needs surrounding the specific organ that was transplanted (for example, in heart transplant clients, a diet to lower blood lipids and blood pressure). Of course, immunosuppressive complications such as infection require ongoing attention and management.

Prevention of Food-Borne Infection People with suppressed immune systems are unusually vulnerable to food-borne illnesses and must take extra precautions against them. They can benefit from following the same food-safety tips that travelers follow: see the box in Chapter 11 (p. 280). You may want to review Chapter 11 for other details regarding food-borne illnesses and their prevention.

Burns

An extensive burn is a second- or third-degree burn covering more than 20 percent of the body surface area (BSA) (see Figure 19–1). It is an extreme form of trauma.

Caring for Burn Victims

A burn is sometimes called a **thermal injury.**

Early care aims to assess the extent and severity of the burn wound and maintain vital organ function. Medical management focuses on fluid and electrolyte balance, prevention and control of infections, early closure of the burn wound, and nutrition support.

The fluid containing plasma proteins and electrolytes that leaks out through the capillaries is called the **exudate** (EX-you-date).
exsudare = sweat out

Reminder: The swelling caused by fluids leaking from blood vessels into interstitial spaces is *edema.*

Fluid and Electrolyte Balance Attention to fluid and electrolyte balance is critical. In the time immediately following a burn, dramatic changes take place in the circulatory system. Plasma proteins (mainly albumin) and electrolytes leak through the capillaries into the interstitial space and the burned area. The accumulation of fluid in the interstitial space around the burn site causes considerable edema, which, in turn, can compromise blood flow, lead to tissue death, and open the way for infection. Plasma volume can decline to less than one-half of normal in people with major burns.

If enough fluid, electrolytes, and albumin can be provided, they will maintain circulatory volume and prevent shock. When the burn is greater

Figure 19–1
Different Degrees of Burn Wounds

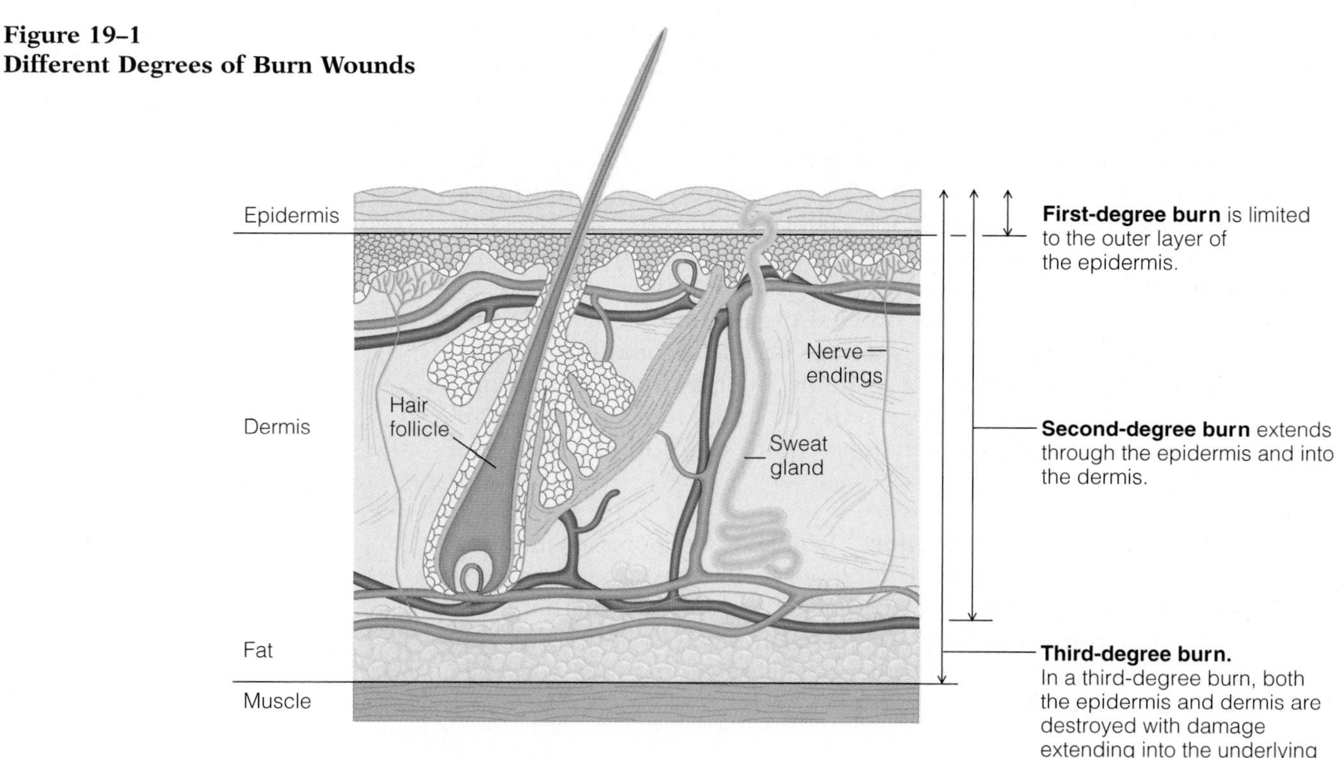
Epidermis
Dermis
Fat
Muscle
Hair follicle
Nerve endings
Sweat gland
First-degree burn is limited to the outer layer of the epidermis.
Second-degree burn extends through the epidermis and into the dermis.
Third-degree burn.
In a third-degree burn, both the epidermis and dermis are destroyed with damage extending into the underlying tissues.

than 20 percent of the body surface area, isotonic fluids are given intravenously because the person generally cannot take fluids by mouth. Clients receive sufficient quantities of fluid to maintain urinary output at about 500 milliliters per hour. On average, a burned person requires 3 to 5 liters of fluid daily to replace losses; however, some clients may require over 10 liters per day. In the period following fluid replacement, normal bowel activity usually returns, eating becomes possible, and attention to adequate nutrition now takes high priority.

isotonic: having the same concentration of solute and therefore the same osmotic pressure as human body fluid. The saline (salt) solutions used in the hospital are made isotonic to human blood.
iso = equal

Long-Term Care Nutrition needs of the burn victim are intense. Hypermetabolism follows a severe burn and causes a rapid loss of body mass. The person quickly uses all energy and protein reserves in the effort to survive. Surgery is often needed to cover the burn wound with healthy skin. The burn injury itself may make eating difficult because of the associated pain or the burn's physical location (for example, the hands). Immobilization and lack of exercise further intensify the catabolic decline. Moreover, most people with burns experience anorexia and depression, leading to poor food intake and further deterioration of nutrition status. For all of these reasons, many people with extensive burns need aggressive nutrition support. Some people with burns of less than 20 percent of the body surface area, if well nourished, can do well on regular diets. Dietitians continuously assess people with extensive burns and those in poor nutrition status to ensure appropriate nutrition support.

Providing Nutrition Support

As with other severe stresses, the goal of diet therapy for the person with an extensive burn is to minimize protein losses and to spare protein to support organ function. Burns may double the basal metabolic rate, and it is not unusual for adults with extensive burns to require about 4000 kcalories per day.

Energy Needs Numerous formulas have been used to estimate energy needs for burns.* Studies have demonstrated a large variability of energy needs in people with burns, though, even when burn injuries are similar.[5] Because of this variability, measurement of energy expenditure using indirect calorimetry provides a more reliable estimate of energy needs than the formulas. Research suggests that when indirect calorimetry is unavailable, energy needs for adults can be estimated using the Harris-Benedict equation (see p. 450).[6] An alert health care professional will adjust energy intake according to changes in the client's body weight or complications such as infection. The box on the next page shows how to estimate the energy needs of an adult with burns.

indirect calorimetry: an estimation of energy output based on measures of oxygen consumption and carbon dioxide elimination. By comparison, **direct calorimetry** estimates energy output based on measures of heat output.

*One formula, the Curreri formula, is still widely used, but numerous studies have concluded that it significantly overestimates energy needs. C. S. Ireton-Jones and C. R. Baxter, Nutrition for adult burn patients: A review, *Nutrition in Clinical Practice* 6 (1991): 3–7; J. P. Allard and coauthors, Validation of a new formula for calculating the energy requirements of burn patients, *Journal of Parenteral and Enteral Nutrition* 14 (1990): 115–118; J. J. Cunningham, Factors contributing to increased energy expenditure in thermal injury: A review of studies employing indirect calorimetry, *Journal of Parenteral and Enteral Nutrition* 14 (1990): 649–655.

HOW TO Determine Energy Needs for a Burn

The following example shows how to determine the energy needs of Bernadette, a 39-year-old female, who is 5 feet 3 inches tall, weighs 130 pounds, and recently sustained an extensive burn. Her energy needs can be estimated using the Harris-Benedict equation (see Table 18–3 on p. 450), which states that basal energy expenditure (BEE) for women is:

BEE = 655 + (9.6 × wt in kg) + (1.7 × ht in cm) – (4.7 × age in years).

Add to BEE for activity:

- 20% BEE for sedentary lifestyle.
- 35% BEE for moderately active lifestyle.
- 50% BEE for active lifestyle.

Add to BEE for burn: 50 to 100 percent BEE.
To determine Bernadette's energy needs using BEE:

$$655 + \left(9.6 \times \frac{130}{2.2}\,\text{kg}\right) + (1.7 \times 160\ \text{cm}) - (4.7 \times 39) =$$

655 + 567 + 272 – 183 = 1311 kcal.

Add 20 percent to account for sedentary activity:

1311 kcal × 0.20 = 262 kcal.

Add 100 percent to account for a severe burn: 1311 kcalories. Add BEE, activity, and burn values to arrive at the total:

1311 + 262 + 1311 kcal = 2844 kcal.

Bernadette requires nearly 2900 kcalories per day.

For children with burns, energy intake must support anticipated growth as well as healing, but without overfeeding. Burned children often tolerate nutrient excesses poorly.[7] In general, providing kcalories at twice the resting metabolic rate adequately meets energy needs.[8]

Protein To maintain nitrogen balance following a burn, adults need to receive 1.5 to 3 grams of protein per kilogram of body weight per day.[9] Typically, this translates to about 200 grams of protein per day. (In the case of Bernadette in the How-to box, 89 to 177 grams of protein would be sufficient.) Children may need from two to three times the protein RDA (as appropriate for age) per day.

Vitamins and Minerals Medical researchers assume that vitamin and mineral requirements increase along with energy and protein needs in people with burns, and many physicians prescribe supplements for their burn clients.[10] Specific vitamin and mineral requirements for people with burns have not been established, however. Researchers reviewing the current literature on micronutrient needs of burned people suggest that only vitamin C and vitamin A need to be supplemented at amounts above the RDA.[11] Other supplements are provided as appropriate.

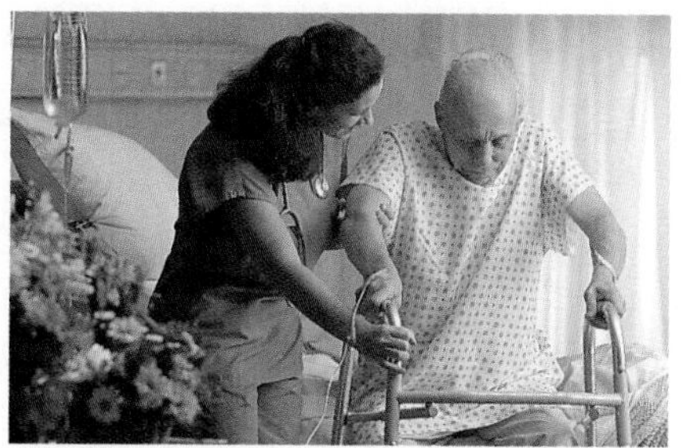

Encourage the client to get up and walk around as soon as possible. This prevents catabolism, improves morale, and stimulates the appetite.

Goals for Meeting Nutrient Needs Traditionally, health care professionals encourage clients with burns to eat as soon as GI tract motility is restored, usually in about two days. Studies of animals suggest, however, that tube feedings begun within a few hours after a burn injury limit weight loss, moderate the hypermetabolic response, and reduce the risk of translocation.[12] Feeding either orally or by tube helps to maintain the normal size and function of intestinal cells. For clients who cannot or will not eat adequate food by mouth, tube feedings or intravenous feedings should be initiated without delay.

Occasionally, people with extensive burns develop deep ulcers, usually in the duodenum, called Curling's ulcers, which can bleed profusely. A person with such ulcers cannot be fed orally, and physicians may prescribe intravenous feedings.

Solving Eating-Related Problems To encourage the individual with a burn to eat, remember to offer emotional support. Understandably, food may seem unappealing to the person who faces a lengthy hospital stay, a great deal of pain, and fear of permanent disfigurement. In addition, burn therapy involves whirlpool baths and the painful cutting away of dead skin and tissue. If possible, schedule these treatments so they will not interfere with mealtimes. Give pain medications prior to meals so that mealtimes can be enjoyable.

A client may feel awkward about eating when the location of a burn interferes with self-feeding. An occupational therapist may be able to adapt feeding utensils to assist the client. Encourage the client to get up and walk around and begin physical therapy as soon as possible. This measure helps prevent further catabolism associated with injury, improve morale, and may help to stimulate the appetite.

The next case study presents the nutrition concerns for a burn client. Use your investigative skills to answer questions about this client's nutrition needs.

To cleanse the burn wound and help loosen the eschar, the person is placed in a large whirlpool tub, where the wounds are gently cleansed with special soap that helps prevent infections. This is called **hydrotherapy** or **tanking.**

Dead, burned skin is called **eschar** (es-CAR). As the eschar becomes loose, it is removed so that the burn wound can close as soon as possible. The removal of the eschar is called **debridement** (day-breed-MON [French] or, more commonly, dee-BREED-ment).
eschara = scab

Physical therapy is important for preventing **contractures,** or loss of joint function, in people with burns. As the burn wound heals, the new skin is very tight, and it may pull the area surrounding a joint into a nonfunctional position.

Nutrition Assessment

Of course, all of the parameters of nutrition assessment discussed in Chapters 12 and 13 apply to individuals undergoing surgery or recovering from infections or burns. However, some important aspects of assessment deserve emphasis here:

- An accurate assessment of the person's *preinjury* nutrition status will help to determine nutrient needs and risks of complication.
- Careful and continuous monitoring of nutrition status will help to ensure that the diet meets nutrient needs. Remember that nutrient stores can become depleted rapidly.
- For people on oral diets, a careful history of food likes and dislikes will

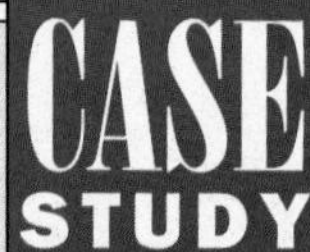

Journalist with Burn Wounds

Mr. Sampson, a 48-year-old journalist, has been admitted to the emergency room. He suffered a third-degree, 40 percent BSA burn when he was trapped in a burning building. His height on admission was 6 feet, and he weighed 175 pounds. The physician ordered lab work, including serum proteins; the results are not back yet.

1. Identify Mr. Sampson's immediate postinjury needs. How can these needs be met?
2. Do you have enough information to determine Mr. Sampson's preinjury, preburn nutrition status? If not, what information would be useful?
3. Is information about preburn nutrition status important in this case? Why or why not?
4. Calculate Mr. Sampson's energy and protein needs to support burn healing. Discuss what other nutrients must be considered.
5. Discuss some general guidelines for meeting Mr. Sampson's nutrient needs.
6. What physical and emotional factors must be considered?
7. If Mr. Sampson cannot eat enough food to obtain adequate nutrients orally after several days, how should he be fed?
8. If he develops major GI bleeding, how can he be fed?
9. Describe the roles of physical therapy and exercise in Mr. Sampson's treatment.

be invaluable as a basis for planning meals to encourage adequate oral intake.

- For people on medications, a careful evaluation of possible drug-nutrient interactions may prevent imbalances.
- Anthropometrics must be interpreted cautiously in the period immediately following the injury. Weights may be misleading because people may be retaining or losing body fluids. Also, the location of wounds may make anthropometric measurements impossible.
- In all stressed individuals, serum albumin and transferrin concentrations may be low for a while. Levels that remain depressed even after nitrogen balance has been achieved probably do not reflect nutrition status.[13] Remember that plasma proteins leak through the capillaries and into the interstitial fluid around the burn wound.
- Results from antigen skin tests remain negative for at least 10 days following trauma.[14] Therefore, skin tests cannot be used to determine protein nutrition status during this period.

While severely stressed clients are being supported with all of the equipment, attention, and procedures that modern medicine can deliver, costs mount. And when attempts are made to control costs, some aspects of care may be caught in the squeeze. The Nutrition in Practice that follows this chapter discusses the implications cost containment may have for nutrition care.

■ STUDY QUESTIONS ■

1. Describe infections and discuss how nutrient needs are altered during the course of an infection.
2. What are some factors that can lead to poor nutrition status prior to surgery? What types of diets should be eaten in the days before and after surgery? What diet modifications are made right before and after surgery, and why?
3. What nutrition-related concerns are associated with organ transplants? How are these concerns dealt with?
4. Describe the changes in body fluids that occur immediately after a person suffers an extreme burn. What is the primary concern during this period? How are these needs met?
5. What metabolic events occur during a burn injury, and how do they affect nutrient needs? When can a person be fed by mouth after a burn?
6. Discuss some major factors to keep in mind when you assess the nutrition status of a person with severe stress or trauma.

■ CLINICAL APPLICATION QUESTIONS ■

1. Using the Harris-Benedict equation (p. 450), calculate the energy needs of a 28-year-old man who is 6 feet tall, weighs 180 pounds, and has a temperature of 103°F.
2. Jana Krashow is a 28-year-old woman admitted to the hospital following a car accident in which she broke several bones, ruptured a portion of her small intestine, and suffered a third-degree 20 percent BSA burn. Aside from the nutrient needs imposed by these stresses, describe how the following factors can impair her nutrition status:
   - Jana's injuries are painful.
   - Her medications cause extreme drowsiness.
   - She is depressed.
   - She is often out of her room for X rays and other diagnostic tests when her food trays arrive.
   - Her food intake is often restricted for diagnostic tests she must have.

   How might each of these problems be resolved to improve Jana's ability to eat?

NUTRITION IN PRACTICE 19

Health Care Reform and and Cost Containment

Few issues in the United States today arouse as much debate as health care reform. Virtually everyone including politicians, health care professionals, employers, insurers, and consumers agree that spiraling health care costs in the United States have made quality health care unaffordable for many citizens. And although all agree that something must be done to ease the crisis, the agreement ends there. The plan adopted to tackle the problem will affect everyone in the country, both directly and indirectly. A multitude of special interest groups have taken stands on the issues and are actively lobbying to ensure that their concerns are addressed. Controversies abound as the country searches for a cure for its ailing health care system.

The issues pertinent to health care reform include reasons why health care costs have skyrocketed; ways health care reform might impact businesses, consumers, and health care professionals; health care interests of many groups of people; and the feasibility of various plans. This Nutrition in Practice focuses on *nutrition* services, and specifically on how nutrition services might be impacted by cost control measures. Attention to nutrition might help reduce health care costs and assure better health at the same time.

Why does the health care system need reform?

Anyone who has paid an insurance premium or needed medical attention recently knows that health care costs are sky high. The rising prices of U.S. health services have significantly outpaced the costs of other service industries. We spend more money on health care than any other nation, and yet some citizens go without needed care and some pay a very steep price for it.

Health care reform seeks to achieve three goals: to make health care accessible to all U.S. citizens; to control costs; and to ensure high quality. The control of costs may be the first goal to pursue. Cost control could help make health care more affordable and therefore accessible to many. The challenge is to ensure that quality and health are not sacrificed in the process.

How can costs be brought under control?

One major effort to control costs has involved changing the way Medicare (a form of government insurance for the elderly and disabled) benefits are paid. Prior to 1983, Medicare, like private insurance, operated on a *fee-for-service* basis. This system enabled hospitals to collect payment for any expenses incurred, so hospitals had little incentive to control costs. This system contributed to the out-of-control rise in health care costs.

To help put the brakes on the system, the U.S. government introduced the *prospective payment system* to cover people's Medicare bills. This system, in effect, gives the hospital a budget for each case. The hospital receives specified amounts for delivering care for specified disorders—so much for gallbladder surgery, so much for treating a broken arm, and so on. The diagnoses that qualify for a given amount of money are grouped together; hence the term *diagnosis-related group,* or *DRG,* for the categories of care funded by the system.

How does the DRG system motivate hospitals to cut costs?

The hospital receives a fixed payment for a given treatment, regardless of the actual costs incurred. Therefore, if the hospital can care for a client in fewer days with fewer tests than the DRG system allows, the hospital makes money. If, on the other hand, a client must remain in the hospital longer or if physicians request more tests than the system will pay for, the hospital may lose money.

That seems awfully rigid. Can the hospital apply for exceptions to these limits?

Yes. If a client must be hospitalized for much longer than normal or incurs much higher costs than a particular DRG allows, the hos-

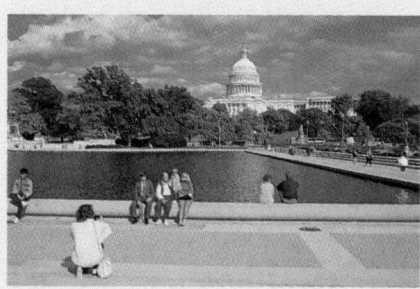

The search for a cure for the ailing U.S. health care system commands the attention of consumers, businesses, and health care professionals.

pital may receive additional support for the case. Still, in most of these cases, called *outliers,* the hospital's costs exceed what it receives in reimbursement, and the hospital loses money.

The DRG system must have helped to reduce health care costs.

Unfortunately, it has not helped as much as was hoped. The DRG system has helped keep down Medicare costs for hospital services, but not total health care costs. Private insurance companies still operate on a fee-for-service basis, rather than on a prospective payment system like the DRG system. When clients with private insurance have long hospital stays or receive extra services or tests, the insurance payments expand hospital revenues. This may help limit the losses a hospital incurs under the DRG system, but it places an additional financial burden on other consumers and their insurers. Between 1982 and 1988, Medicare expenditures under the DRG system were limited so successfully that by 1987 and 1988 they were rising by less than 1 percent per year. During this same period, however, non-Medicare increases amounted to over 9 percent per year.[15] Thus private insurers are carrying a ever-higher cost burden, and this burden is passed on to consumers as higher private insurance premiums.

The prospective payment system has also caused another problem. It has given the hospitals an incentive to discharge people as early as possible, sometimes too early. Early release from the hospital necessitates more extensive care at home. Therapies traditionally reserved for the hospital have been adapted for delivery at home.[16] Consequently, although less money is being spent on hospital care, more money is being spent on home care.

Might this not affect quality of care? Is it possible that in the effort to reduce hospital costs, clients will not receive full medical care? Will physicians hesitate to order tests that might be helpful to clients? Will clients be discharged from the hospital before they should be?

So far, these concerns appear to be unwarranted. The Prospective Payment Assessment Commission, created by Congress to oversee the DRG system, has found no evidence that the system has lowered the quality of care.[17] Hospitals and their staffs exist to treat disease and to relieve suffering and pain. The combination of a commitment to quality care, competition among hospitals for clients, and the threat of malpractice suits balances the situation.

What about effects on accessibility to health care?

The shift of costs from Medicare to private insurers and their clients has made health care less available. Because costs are passed on to consumers, insurance premiums or direct payments for medical services have become too expensive for many people to afford. In addition, private insurers hesitate to provide coverage for people with disorders that may incur substantial health care costs. Thus, medical care has become inaccessible to more people.

How do nutrition services affect costs and care?

Nutrition professionals believe that quality health care must include nutrition services as an integral part of both preventive and therapeutic efforts.[18] No one disputes that nutrition can contribute significantly to quality health care. In the climate of spiraling health care costs, though, an important question to ask is "do nutrition's contributions justify the expenses they entail?"

To answer this question, the American Dietetic Association has collected information from registered dietitians documenting the cost-effectiveness of nutrition services. Based on these data, the association estimates a cost savings of $3.25 for every $1 spent on nutrition assessment and therapy.[19] In representing the interests of dietetic professionals, the American Dietetic Association seeks to ensure that registered dietitians will be identified as qualified providers of reimbursable nutrition services.[20] The unique education and skills of registered dietitians enable them to detect nutrition problems early and to institute appropriate therapy, saving money and improving health. Consider these examples:

- Following a dietitian's assessment and development of an individualized diet plan, a woman with gestational diabetes is able to control her blood glucose and gain appropriate weight without the need for insulin. By eliminating the need for insulin during pregnancy, this nutrition care saved $2265.
- In another case, a dietitian's assessment and implementation of an appropriate nutrition care plan allowed an 83-year-old person with end-stage renal disease and heart disease to switch from intravenously administered feedings (parenteral nutrition) to a combination of an oral diet and tube feedings (enteral nutrition). Cost savings were over $2400 per month.[21]

As these examples show, real cost savings can be achieved with appropriate nutrition intervention.

Are all nutrition approaches appropriate to use? Some are quite expensive, aren't they?

Yes, and parenteral nutrition support is especially expensive. The average cost of parenteral nutrition runs about $365 per day.[22] Since the average person requiring parenteral nutrition needs the therapy for about 21 days, the cost of the nutrition alone during an average hospitalization exceeds $7600.

By comparison, enteral nutrition is far less expensive. On the average, enteral nutrition costs about $30 per day and is required for about 19 days.[23] Using these figures, the average cost of enteral nutrition during a typical hospitalization runs about $570, $7000 less.

Studies suggest that appropriate nutrition support lowers mortality rates, results in fewer complications, and shortens hospital stays. Common sense dictates that no recovery process is hastened by starvation. The degree to which nutrition support alleviates disease or promotes recovery, however, is difficult to quantify. Malnourished people who need specialized nutrition support are usually quite ill. Their diseases may lead to further complications or even death, regardless of their nutrition status. Furthermore, the severity of a given disease and the degree of malnutrition differ from case to case, and when one person recovers faster than another, health care providers cannot prove that a single factor such as nutrition was directly responsible for the difference.

Studies have clearly shown that aggressive nutrition support can improve nutrition status, but again few studies have been able to document that nutrition support affects outcome and thus saves money. The evidence shows that parenteral nutrition is most effective in the highest risk groups—that is, in people who are severely malnourished.[24] Thus careful selection of people to receive parenteral nutrition can help control costs. The same can be said for enteral nutrition. Tube feedings should be reserved for people who cannot eat adequate diets orally. Parenteral nutrition should be reserved for people who cannot tolerate tube feedings.

Other significant benefits of nutrition support are difficult to justify in terms of costs. Unfortunately, subjective improvements, such as energy level and quality of life, do not come with a dollar value. It may be cheaper to keep a person in the hospital for an extra day or two than to give several days of nutrition support, but at what price? How can the individual's comfort, desire to go home, or ability to function independently be accounted for? If nutrition support reduces the risk of relapse, what dollar value does that have? All of these factors are difficult to quantify fairly in a context where cost containment is a high priority.

Clearly, health care professionals need to work within the health care system to provide cost-effective nutrition care without sacrificing quality. Some suggestions for providing cost-saving, yet appropriate, nutrition care include:

- Use a qualified professional (registered dietitian) to complete a nutrition assessment and determine the most appropriate nutrition care plan for each person.
- Document how nutrition services that identify nutrition problems can have positive effects and general cost savings in the prevention and treatment of disease.
- Recommend the most cost-effective method of feeding people (oral, enteral, or parenteral).

Whatever the final direction of the health care reform plan, one thing is certain. Health care professionals must continue to provide high-quality nutrition care in a cost-effective manner. In so doing, they do their part in ensuring that quality, affordable health care will be available to all.

NOTES

1. N. S. Scrimshaw, Effect of infection on nutrient requirements, *Journal of Parenteral and Enteral Nutrition* 15 (1991): 589–600.
2. G. P. Buzby, Perioperative nutrition support, *Journal of Parenteral and Enteral Nutrition* (supplement) 14 (1900): 197–199.
3. A. C. Campos and M. M. Meguid, A critical appraisal of the usefulness of perioperative nutritional support, *American Journal of Clinical Nutrition* 55 (1992): 117–130.
4. O. Salvanthierra, Jr., Optimal use of organs for transplantation, *New England Journal of Medicine* 318 (1988): 1329–1331.
5. J. J. Cunningham, Factors contributing to increased energy expenditure in thermal injury: A review of studies employing indirect calorimetry, *Journal of Parenteral and Enteral Nutrition* 14 (1990): 649–655.

6. Cunningham, 1990.
7. D. A. Hutsler, Nutritional monitoring of a pediatric burn patient, *Nutrition in Clinical Practice* 6 (1991): 11–17.
8. Georgia Dietetic Association, *Diet Manual* (Atlanta, Ga.: Georgia Dietetic Association, 1987).
9. J. J. Cunningham, M. K. Lydon, and W. E. Russell, Calorie and protein provision for recovery from severe burns in infants and young children, *American Journal of Clinical Nutrition* 51 (1990): 553–557; S. J. Bell and J. Wyatt, Nutrition guidelines for burned patients, *Journal of the American Dietetic Association* 86 (1986): 648–653.
10. R. L. Shippee, S. W. Wilson, and N. King, Trace mineral supplementation of burn patients: A national survey, *Journal of the American Dietetic Association* 87 (1987): 300–303.
11. M. M. Gottschlich and G. D. Warden, Vitamin supplementation in the patient with burns, *Journal of Burn Care and Rehabilitation* 11 (1990): 275–279.
12. S. Inque and coauthors, Prevention of yeast translocation across the gut by a single enteral feeding after burn injury, *Journal of Parenteral and Enteral Nutrition* 13 (1989): 565–571; H. Saito and coauthors, The effect of route of nutrient administration on nutritional state, catabolic hormone secretion, and gut mucosal injury after burn injury, *Journal of Parenteral and Enteral Nutrition* 11 (1987): 1–7.
13. F. B. Serra, How nutrition intervention changes what getting sick means, *Journal of Parenteral and Enteral Nutrition* (supplement) 14 (1990): 164–169.
14. R. P. Bynoe, Nutrition support in trauma patients, *Nutrition in Clinical Practice* 3 (1988): 137–144.
15. W. B. Schwartz and D. N. Mendelson, Hospital cost containment in the 1980s, *New England Journal of Medicine* 324 (1991): 1037–1042.
16. K. S. Crocker, Current status of home infusion therapy, *Nutrition in Clinical Practice* 7 (1992): 256–263.
17. American Society for Parenteral and Enteral Nutrition, PENline (newsletter discussing the DRG system), February 1987.
18. American Dietetic Association, Position of the American Dietetic Association: Affordable and accessible health care services, *Journal of the American Dietetic Association* 92 (1992): 746–748.
19. American Dietetic Association, President's page: Health care reform—where the ADA stands, *Journal of the American Dietetic Association* 93 (1993): 1043–1044.
20. American Dietetic Association, White paper on health care reform, *Journal of the American Dietetic Association* 92 (1992): 749.
21. American Dietetic Association, 1993.
22. M. Regenstein, Reimbursement for nutrition support, *Nutrition in Clinical Practice* 4 (1989): 194–202.
23. Regenstein, 1989.
24. J. M. Daly, H. P. Redmond, and H. Gallagher, Perioperative nutrition in cancer patients, *Journal of Parenteral and Enteral Nutrition* (supplement) 16 (1992): 100–105; J. M. Eisenberg and coauthors, Does perioperative total parenteral nutrition reduce medical care costs? *Journal of Parenteral and Enteral Nutrition* 17 (1993): 201–209; Veterans Affairs Total Parenteral Nutrition Cooperative Study Group, Perioperative total parenteral nutrition in surgical patients, *New England Journal of Medicine* 325 (1991): 525–532.

20

Nutrition and Upper GI Disorders

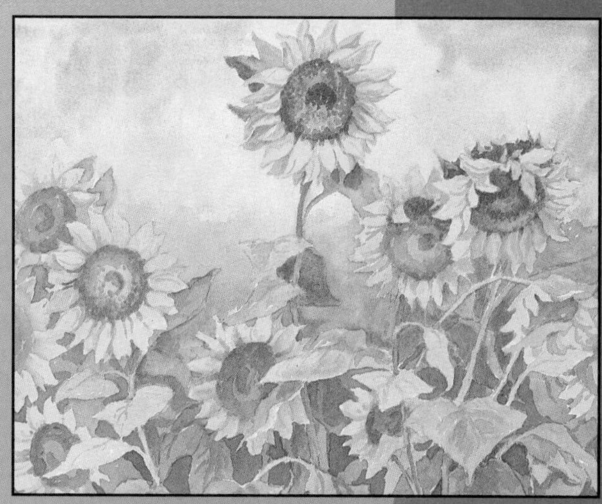

CONTENTS

The remarkable GI tract serves as a conduit from the external world to the internal body environment. When healthy, the GI tract allows the body to ingest, digest, and absorb nutrients, but in people with physical or emotional disorders, the GI tract can fail to accomplish any or all of these tasks, seriously impairing health. This chapter describes some common upper GI tract disorders and their nutrition implications. (The next chapter does the same for the lower GI tract.)

Disorders of the Mouth and Esophagus

The upper GI tract consists of the mouth, throat, esophagus, and stomach. These organs accomplish feats that people rarely think about: chewing, swallowing, and the first steps of digestion. When things go wrong, however, major health problems can ensue.

Difficulties Chewing

Many conditions can temporarily or permanently interfere with chewing, from injuries, surgery, or infections of the mouth to missing teeth, ill-fitting dentures, or strokes. People with these conditions may eat too little, lose too much weight, and suffer the consequences of deteriorating nutrition status. To prevent malnutrition, the diet needs adjustment.

The process of chewing is sometimes called **mastication.**

Time Limit on Liquids If a person can tolerate only liquids and will not be able to eat solid food again soon, the person should be given nutritionally complete formulas. A person who cannot drink enough liquids to meet nutrient needs should be fed by tube; otherwise nutrition status can deteriorate rapidly. Careful assessment may correctly indicate, however, that many people can manage foods.

Diet Adjustment Adjustment of the diet to a mechanical soft diet can often help ease problems with chewing. A mechanical soft diet is a regular diet modified to eliminate all foods that a person cannot easily chew. All foods and seasonings are permitted on mechanical soft diets, but are prepared in liquid, chopped, tender-cooked, or pureed form. Drinking plenty of fluids along with meals can often ease chewing and swallowing. Some people find it helpful to suck fluids through a straw after taking each mouthful of food. Health care professionals should work closely with clients, family members, and caregivers to make needed adjustments and should encourage clients to eat foods as similar as possible to those of a regular diet. This strategy enhances appetite and minimizes the likelihood of nutrient deficiencies.

mechanical soft diet (also called a **dental soft diet**): a diet in which all foods are easy to chew and swallow.

Pureed Foods Until the diet has been individualized, clients on a mechanical soft diet are often given baby foods. While baby foods offer nutrients, their blandness may create a psychological block to eating, and malnutrition can follow. Whenever possible, pureed adult foods should be served in preference to baby foods. Better still are chopped or soft foods, when manageable.

Figure 20–1
Make Pureed Foods Appetizing
A dinner of baked chicken, boiled potatoes, and green beans may look appetizing, but when it is pureed to white mush, more white mush, and a green blob, it may be unacceptable. To enhance the eye appeal of such a meal, foodservice staff can substitute more colorful foods, arrange and shape them attractively on the plate, and add garnishes for color.

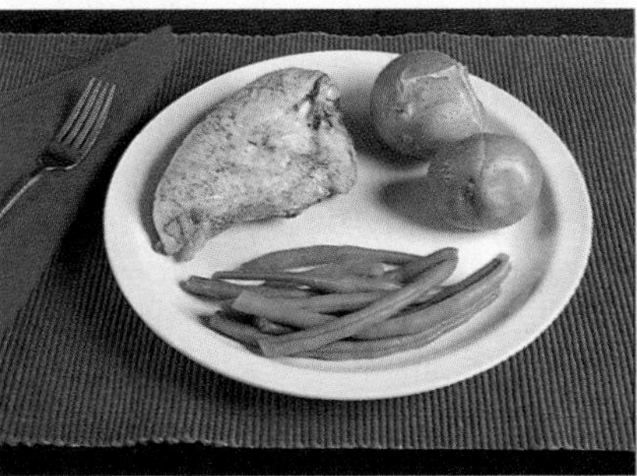

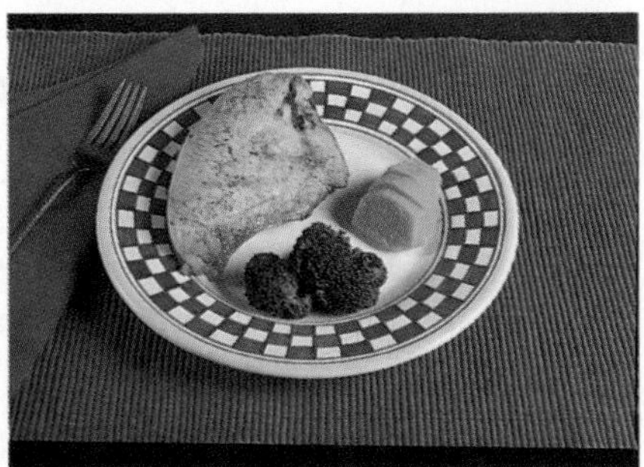

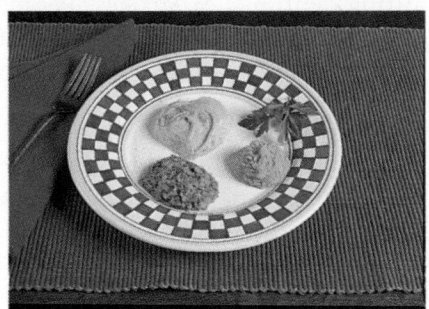

This meal may look appetizing, but when pureed, it loses its appeal:

These foods make a more attractive meal when pureed:

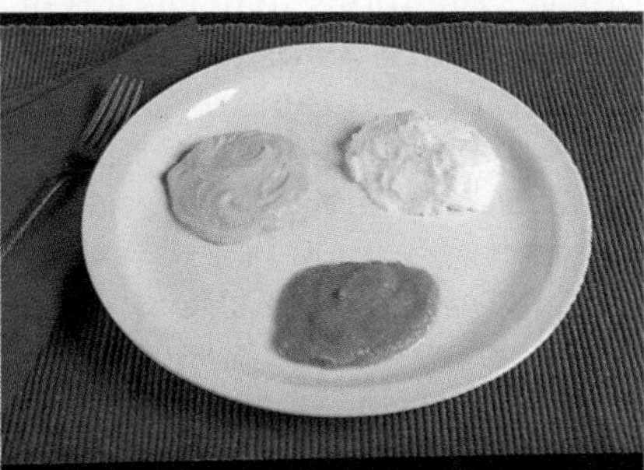

If pureed foods are necessary, help the person select well-balanced, colorful, appetizing meals (see Figure 20–1). For example, in place of plain, mashed white potatoes, substitute seasoned, mashed sweet potatoes. Serve foods attractively and at the right temperature. Commercial products can be used to thicken and shape pureed foods to look like the real thing.

Exclude seasonings and spices only if it hurts to eat them (see "Mouth Pain," next) or if some other valid reason forbids their use. Pureed foods should be smooth and thick, not watery and thin. If a client consistently refuses pureed foods, confer with the administrative dietitian or foodservice manager.

mouth ulcers: lesions or sores in the lining of the mouth.

Mouth Pain People with mouth ulcers or inflammation of the mouth or lips may find spicy or acidic foods (such as citrus fruits and tomatoes) too painful to eat. In addition, nuts or seeds in foods (such as sesame or poppy seeds in breads) can become trapped in mouth ulcers and cause discomfort. Heat hurts, too, and clients with mouth ulcers often prefer foods served at room temperature or cold.

Reduced Flow of Saliva People with dry mouths can often stimulate their saliva secretion by sucking on sour candy or chewing gum. Encourage these clients to practice good oral hygiene; when salivary flow is reduced, the mouth is poorly defended against dental caries. Drugs that stimulate the flow of saliva are also available.

Difficulties Swallowing

Problems in swallowing are known as dysphagia. Dysphagia can arise from many causes; ordinary aging, nervous system diseases, injuries, surgery, developmental disabilities, or strokes. A person with dysphagia may be unable to initiate swallowing, to chew foods and mix them with saliva, or to push foods to the back of the throat and into the esophagus. Some forms of dysphagia specifically interfere with the muscular contractions of the esophagus.

dysphagia (dis-FAY-gee-ah)**:** difficulty in swallowing.
dys = bad
phagein = to eat

Subtle and Dangerous Dysphagia often goes undiagnosed, especially when caused by aging, because symptoms are not always obvious. Everybody "catches food in their throat" at one time or another, and if this gradually becomes a more and more frequent event, it may be considered normal and go unnoticed. The person may gradually stop eating and develop nutrient deficiencies.

Dysphagia can be dangerous. Foods that move into the throat may enter the trachea and pass into the lungs (aspiration), carrying bacteria with them and causing pneumonia. In healthy people, the presence of food in the trachea elicits a coughing response, which prevents food from entering the lungs, but some people with dysphagia fail to cough when food slips into the trachea. Such "silent" aspiration, which can occur in people following strokes, carries with it the risk of serious pneumonia and death.[1]

aspiration: the inhaling of food or liquid into the lungs.

Signs of Dysphagia Health care professionals should be alert to subtle symptoms of dysphagia including an unexplained decline in food intake or even repeated bouts of pneumonia.[2] Other symptoms include pain on swallowing, weight loss, a fear of eating certain foods or any food at all, a feeling that food is sticking in the throat, a tendency to hold food in the mouth or to cough or choke during meals, frequent throat clearing, drooling, or a "wet" sound to the voice.

Diet for Dysphagia Because of the dangers just described, the diet for dysphagia leaves little room for error or experimentation.[3] Speech pathologists, dietitians, physicians, and nurses work together to assess a person's swallowing abilities and design an individualized diet. A mechanical soft diet is often appropriate, because often the person can handle only semisolid foods or thickened liquids that flow slowly enough to allow time to coordinate swallowing movements. Smooth solids such as puddings and smooth yogurts are good choices; commercial thickeners, tapioca pudding, or baby cereal can be used to thicken liquids. Health care workers should never feed people with syringes into the throat; people

Table 20–1
Substances That Weaken the Cardiac Sphincter

Alcohol
Anticholinergic agents
Atropine
Caffeine-containing beverages
Chocolate
Cigarette smoking
Cinnamon
Fat
Garlic
Onions
Peppermint and spearmint oils

who cannot swallow for themselves need tube feedings to ensure that food goes to the stomach, not into the lungs.

With time, in some cases, swallowing function improves. The health care team constantly monitors the person and expands the diet to include additional food consistencies as tolerated. Ideally, the diet is progressed to a regular, solid-food diet, although this is not always possible.

Tube Feedings As always, tube feedings are used only if attempts to feed the person orally are unsuccessful. Tube feedings may be particularly beneficial for severely malnourished individuals who are unable to take adequate nourishment orally and those whose swallowing function continues to deteriorate. Tube feedings delivered into the stomach may be contraindicated, however, due to the high risk of aspiration pneumonia.[4] Feedings into the intestine often provide a safer alternative. (Chapter 22 provides the details of gastric and intestinal tube feedings.)

Reflux Esophagitis

reflux esophagitis (eh-sof-ah-JYE-tis): the backflow or regurgitation of gastric contents from the stomach into the esophagus, causing inflammation of the esophagus.

In reflux esophagitis, the cardiac sphincter fails to close tightly. Highly acidic fluids from the stomach can splash backward into the esophagus and irritate the esophageal mucosa. Reflux esophagitis can occur whenever the cardiac sphincter is too weak to stay closed. It frequently develops as a consequence of aging. A common cause of reflux esophagitis is hiatal hernia (discussed later).

Chronic Esophagitis When esophagitis becomes chronic, inflammation and scarring may damage the inside of the esophagus, reducing its inner diameter. Then dysphagia can result, together with the potential complications already described. Chronic esophagitis can also produce ulcers in the esophagus.

Scarring of the esophageal mucosa, which narrows the diameter of the esophagus, is known as **esophageal stricture.**

heartburn: a burning sensation felt behind the sternum caused by stomach acid splashing back up into the esophagus.

Heartburn The burning pain of heartburn, a symptom of reflux esophagitis, is caused by stomach acid burning the esophagus. At times, the pain may be so severe as to awaken a sleeping person. Heartburn usually hurts behind the sternum (see Figure 20–2), often spreading in waves into the neck and back of the throat. Because heartburn occurs when pressure in the stomach exceeds pressure in the esophagus, it tends to flare up when a person lies down or bends over.

Dietary Prevention and Treatment The best treatment for reflux esophagitis is prevention. First, encourage clients to relax and try to enjoy their meals. Then, instruct them to avoid substances and activities that compromise the strength of the cardiac sphincter (see Table 20–1). Treatment for active reflux esophagitis aims at reducing gastric acidity and the irritation of an already inflamed esophagus. In addition, physicians may prescribe antacids or other drugs to neutralize gastric acidity. Generally, these measures can control esophagitis. If medical management fails, however, surgery may be indicated. The box (see p. 484) offers diet advice.

For a listing of antacids and other drugs that reduce gastric acidity, see "Peptic Ulcers," later in this chapter.

Figure 20–2 Effect of Gastric Pressure on Reflux
Overeating and overdrinking can increase the pressure in the stomach. Whenever the pressure in the stomach exceeds the pressure in the esophagus, the chances of reflux increase.

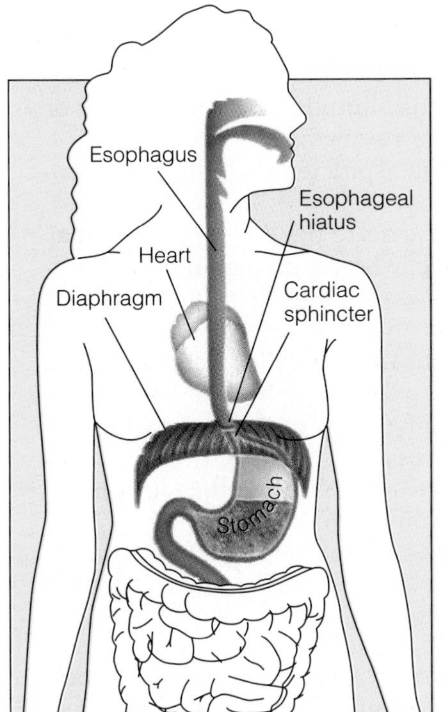

NORMAL
The stomach lies below the diaphragm, and the esophagus passes through the esophageal hiatus. The cardiac sphincter prevents reflux of stomach contents.

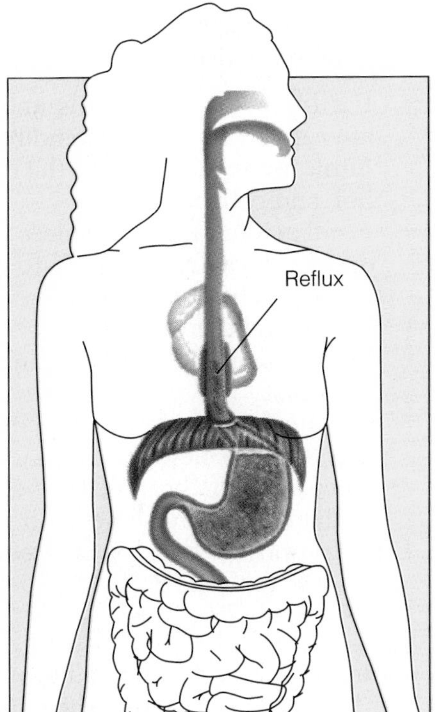

REFLUX
Overeating and overdrinking can increase pressure in the stomach. Whenever the pressure in the stomach exceeds the pressure in the esophagus, the chance of reflux increases. The resulting "heartburn" is so-named because it is felt in the area of the heart.

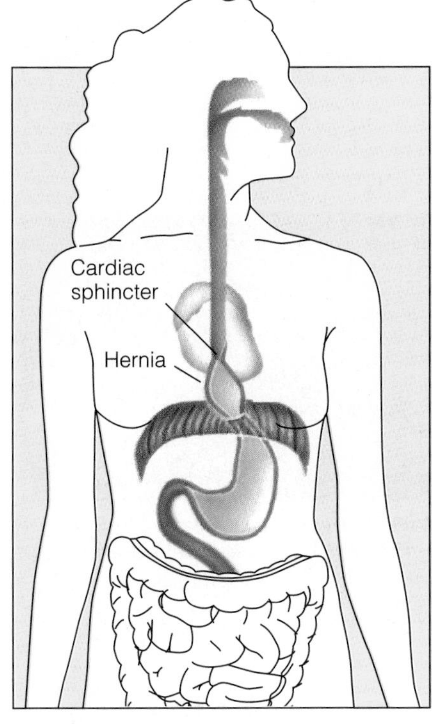

SLIDING HIATAL HERNIA
A sliding hiatal hernia results when part of the stomach, with the cardiac sphincter, slips through the diaphragm. This type of hiatal hernia is the most common.

Hiatal Hernia

The esophagus joins the stomach at the cardiac sphincter, and normally this sphincter sits right in the hiatus in the diaphragm and is reinforced by it. Normally, then, the esophagus lies completely above, and the stomach completely below, the diaphragm. Sometimes, however, the hiatus enlarges or weakens, so that a portion of the stomach can slide up through it, an abnormality called a hiatal hernia. Figure 20–2 shows the relationship of the upper GI tract to the diaphragm and the changes that occur when a hernia is present.

esophageal hiatus (high-AY-tus)**:** the opening in the diaphragm through which the esophagus passes.

hiatal hernia: protrusion of a portion of the stomach up through the esophageal hiatus of the diaphragm. There are several types of hiatal hernias, but the *sliding hiatal hernia* is the most common (see Figure 20–2).
hiatus = to yawn

Symptoms Once a hiatal hernia has formed, the cardiac sphincter, which holds food in the stomach, no longer is reinforced by the sur-

HOW TO Prevent and Treat Reflux Esophagitis

To prevent and treat reflux esophagitis and its associated discomfort, instruct clients to:

- Eat frequent small meals and drink liquids one hour before or after meals to avoid distending the stomach.
- Limit foods that weaken the cardiac spincter, including fat, alcohol, and caffeine.
- Avoid acidic foods and juices that irritate the esophagus, such as orange, grapefruit, or tomato juice, when experiencing the symptoms of reflux esophagitis.
- Lose weight, if overweight.
- Refrain from wearing clothing that fits tightly, especially around the waist.
- Refrain from lying down or bending over, particularly after eating, to avoid elevating stomach pressure.
- Sleep with the head of the bed elevated. Keeping the chest higher than the stomach helps to prevent reflux.
- Refrain from smoking cigarettes.

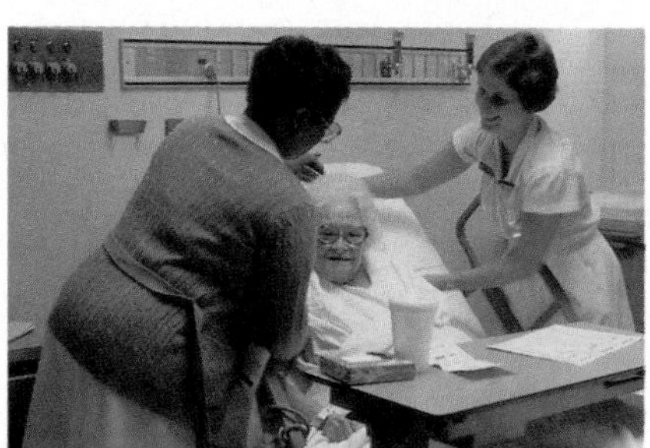

Elevate the head of the bed to minimize the likelihood of reflux from the stomach to the esophagus.

rounding diaphragm, and it becomes easy for acidic gastric juices to reflux into the esophagus. Then the symptoms of hiatal hernia result, notably, esophagitis with its associated inflammation and pain.

Nutrition Care The goals of nutrition care for hiatal hernia are the same as for esophagitis: to prevent reflux, neutralize gastric acidity, and eliminate foods that irritate the esophagus. The accompanying case study provides questions that review the diet modifications needed by a client with a hiatal hernia.

Disorders of the Stomach

Turn on the television set and quite likely you will see several advertisements touting cures for indigestion and stomach upset. These common GI discomforts are not diseases, but symptoms that occur for many reasons.

Indigestion

dyspepsia: vague abdominal discomfort; a symptom, not a disease.
dys = bad
peptein = to digest

Indigestion, or dyspepsia, is a vague term used to describe any discomfort in the GI tract. Although it refers most often to the stomach, it can also be a symptom of disorders involving the intestines or other organs. Oftentimes, emotional tension triggers indigestion. You may hear a person comment that "I have a nervous stomach," or "I'm so mad my stomach is tied in knots." In addition to emotional factors, indigestion can be caused by malnutrition, disease, eating too much, eating too rapidly, or chewing too briefly.

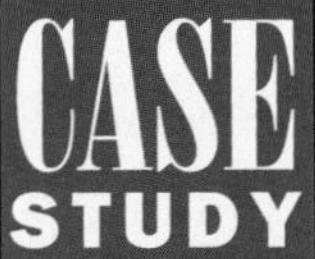

Accountant with a Hiatal Hernia

Mrs. Scarlatti, a 49-year-old accountant, recently underwent a complete physical examination. She told her physician that she had been feeling fairly well, except for heartburn, which had been occurring with increasing frequency. The attacks usually occurred after she had eaten a large meal, particularly if she lay down after eating. She told the doctor that her life was pretty hectic these days, this being the middle of the tax season.

Mrs. Scarlatti's past medical history shows no signs of significant health problems. The physician did advise her to stop smoking cigarettes and to lose 20 pounds during her last physical, which she has yet to do. A diet history taken by the nurse shows that Mrs. Scarlatti usually skips breakfast, eats lunch hurriedly at her desk, and eats a large dinner around 8:00 P.M.. She generally enjoys one or two alcoholic beverages in the evening before going to sleep. She drinks 6 to 8 cups of coffee during the day. Her current height and weight are 5 feet 6 inches and 170 pounds. The physician diagnosed a sliding hiatal hernia after using a long tube equipped with a special optical device called a gastroscope to inspect the interior of the esophagus, stomach, and duodenum.

1. Can you explain to Mrs. Scarlatti what a sliding hiatal hernia is and how it leads to heartburn?
2. Describe the care plan you would develop for Mrs. Scarlatti.
3. What suggestions can you give her to help relieve the symptoms associated with the hernia?
4. What other therapy might her physician prescribe?

Dietary Interventions for Indigestion A temporary bout of indigestion requires no dietary intervention; simple changes in eating habits may help. Persistent indigestion, however, suggests underlying medical problems, such as lactose intolerance, other intolerances, gastritis, or peptic ulcers, which should be identified. Persistent indigestion may lead to loss of appetite and malnutrition. The next box (p. 486) offers diet advice to help control persistent indigestion.

A person with indigestion may benefit from a low-fiber or soft diet, and may want to exclude gas-forming foods. Table 20–2 (p. 487) lists foods included in, and excluded from, a low-fiber diet, and the sample menu shows a day's food intakes for a person on a low-fiber diet. (Table 21–2 in the next chapter lists foods that commonly cause gas.)

low-fiber diet: a diet that consists of foods that are low in fiber. A low-fiber diet is the same as a *soft diet*.

Antacids In addition to dietary changes, antacids may provide relief, but they must be used with caution. Antacids can mask ulcer symptoms and create nutrient imbalances if used continuously for long periods. Antacids may contain sodium (in sodium bicarbonate), calcium (in calcium bicarbonate), or aluminum (in aluminum hydroxide), not bad for healthy individuals, but harmful in some medical conditions. Sodium can aggravate hypertension; calcium can contribute to kidney stones; and aluminum can lead to phosphorus depletion and bone disease. (More information about antacids' nutrient interactions is provided in Tables E–1A and E–1B in Appendix E.)

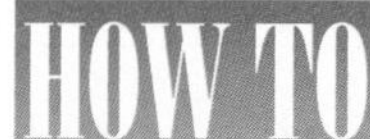

Prevent Indigestion

To prevent indigestion, take these steps:

- Eat at regular times and in a relaxed atmosphere.
- Eat slowly and chew food thoroughly.
- Eat small meals.
- Avoid gas-forming foods. Remember that milk may be one of these foods, if lactose intolerance is present. (There is more on lactose intolerance in the next chapter.)
- Avoid excessive amounts of fats, alcohol, and caffeine-containing foods and beverages.
- Avoid any food known to cause indigestion.

Nausea and Vomiting

nausea (NAW-zee-ah)**:** the inclination to vomit.

Nausea is another vague term; it describes the feeling that one is about to vomit. Many medical conditions, certain odors or motions, or even disturbing sights can trigger nausea. Nausea makes it hard to eat, and when persistent, may cause malnutrition. Tips to alleviate morning sickness during early pregnancy were given on p. 370 of Chapter 15. General dietary interventions to prevent nausea are provided in the next box (p. 488).

Vomiting in Adults If nausea leads to vomiting, other concerns may arise. As Nutrition in Practice 5 describes, simple vomiting is certainly

Sample Low-Fiber Diet Menu

MENU

BREAKFAST	LUNCH	SUPPER
Orange juice	Baked fish	Roast beef
Soft-cooked egg	White rice	Mashed potatoes
Puffed rice cereal	Green beans	Cooked carrots
White bread toast	Small banana	Canned peaches
Coffee or tea	Roll	Roll
Milk for cereal	Margarine	Margarine
Creamer	Coffee or tea	Coffee or tea
	Sugar	Sugar
	Creamer	Creamer

Table 20–2
Low-Fiber Diet

FOODS ALLOWED	FOODS AVOIDED
Meats and Meat Alternates	
Baked, broiled, or roasted beef, fish, lamb, liver, poultry, or veal; crisp bacon; hard- or soft-cooked eggs	Fried poultry or meats, cold cuts, sardines, fried eggs, or peanut butter
Milk and Milk Products	
Whole, nonfat, or low-fat milk; yogurt; mild cheeses	Milk drinks or yogurt containing whole fruits or berries, seeds, or skins; strongly flavored cheeses
Fruits and Vegetables	
Cooked or canned fruits without seeds and skins; ripe bananas, orange sections, grapefruit sections; all fruit juices; cooked asparagus tips, beets, broccoli, carrots, green beans, tomato juice, wax beans, winter squash; strained peas, spinach, summer squash, or potatoes	Berries; avocado; prune juice; raw fruits except those listed; legumes, raw vegetables, and all other vegetables except those listed
Grains	
Refined, enriched white bread; plain muffins or rolls; white flour crackers (saltines, melba toast, zwieback); refined, ready-to-eat, or cooked cereals; noodles; macaroni; spaghetti; strained oatmeal	Whole-grain breads and cereals or those containing nuts, bran, or seeds; fried breads such as doughnuts
Miscellaneous	
Tea, coffee, fruit drinks, carbonated beverages, butter, cream, margarine, mayonnaise	Any dishes made with foods to be avoided; coconut

unpleasant and wearying, but is not cause for alarm. Prolonged vomiting, however, can be serious enough to require professional medical care because large quantities of fluid are lost from the GI tract. If possible, fluids and electrolytes are replaced orally using clear liquids (see p. 464). If the person cannot keep oral liquids down, IV feedings of saline and glucose with added electrolytes are necessary until the physician diagnoses the cause of the vomiting and institutes corrective therapy. When vomiting continues for a long time, more complete feedings by peripheral or central vein may be indicated; these are described in Chapter 23.

See Nutrition in Practice 5 for information on simple vomiting and its consequences.

Vomiting in Infants and Children Single episodes of vomiting in otherwise healthy children are not unusual and are generally not a problem. The recommended treatment is to withhold all foods and fluids for one to three hours after a vomiting episode and then introduce sips of clear fluid or cracked ice or popsicles, progressing to other liquids and foods as tolerated. The goal is to prevent dehydration, which can quickly become serious in an infant or child, while allowing time for the condition to resolve. Should vomiting persist beyond 24 to 36 hours, then medical attention is needed.

HOW TO Help Prevent Nausea

To help prevent nausea, try the following ideas:

- In the morning, eat dry, carbohydrate-rich foods, such as toast or cereal without milk.
- Eat small meals frequently; keep something in your stomach.
- Avoid spicy and high-fat foods; avoid foods with odors that trigger nausea.
- Save liquids for between meals; sip clear liquids slowly.
- Suck popsicles or ice cubes made from a favorite juice or soft drink.
- Loosen tight clothes and seek fresh air.

Gastritis

gastritis: inflammation of the stomach lining.

Gastritis is a common disorder in which the mucosal lining of the stomach becomes inflamed and painful. The person with gastritis may complain of anorexia, nausea, vomiting, belching, and a feeling of fullness.

Reminder: A disease or condition that develops slowly, shows little change, and lasts a long time is said to be *chronic*. The term *acute* describes diseases or conditions that develop rapidly, exhibit severe symptoms, and are of short duration.

Acute Gastritis Acute gastritis most often follows the taking of aspirin or other drugs that irritate the gastric mucosa. Alcohol abuse, food irritants, food allergies, food poisoning, radiation therapy, stress, and infections can also cause gastritis. The dietary management of acute gastritis rests on two principles: eliminating irritating foods and reducing gastric acidity.

bland diet: a diet that excludes gastric irritants such as alcohol and caffeine and foods according to individual tolerances.

For the person with gastritis who cannot eat because of nausea or vomiting, foods and fluids are generally withheld for a day or two. Then, the diet progresses from liquids to a bland diet as tolerated. A bland diet is a highly individualized diet that eliminates foods that stimulate gastric acid secretions or irritate the gastric mucosa, such as those listed in Table 20–3. Antacids may also be given temporarily.

Table 20–3
The Bland Diet

A bland diet provides three meals a day and includes all foods except those that irritate the gastric mucosa. Substances generally contraindicated on a bland diet include:

- Any foods an individual identifies as irritating to the GI tract.
- Alcohol.
- Caffeine and caffeine-containing beverages (including cola beverages, cocoa, coffee, and tea).
- Decaffeinated coffee.
- Pepper and spicy foods except as tolerated.

Note: The bland diet shown here has replaced the earlier diet for gastritis and ulcers known as the "traditional bland diet," which was invalidated by research.

Chronic Gastritis Chronic gastritis presents the same symptoms as acute gastritis, but persists for a longer time. Chronic gastritis may accompany chronic diseases of the stomach or liver or may have no known cause. Chronic gastritis is common in the elderly. As gastritis progresses, the gastric cells atrophy, gastric secretions decline, and production of intrinsic factor is reduced.

Chronic gastritis requires diagnosis and treatment before damage and debilitation have progressed too far. Interventions need to begin early enough to prevent secondary conditions such as dehydration, malnutrition, or esophageal damage. An individualized bland diet seems to relieve GI symptoms in some cases.

Gastritis can result in vitamin B_{12} malabsorption, which may lead to pernicious anemia. Vitamin B_{12} is given by injection, when necessary, to bypass the need for absorption.

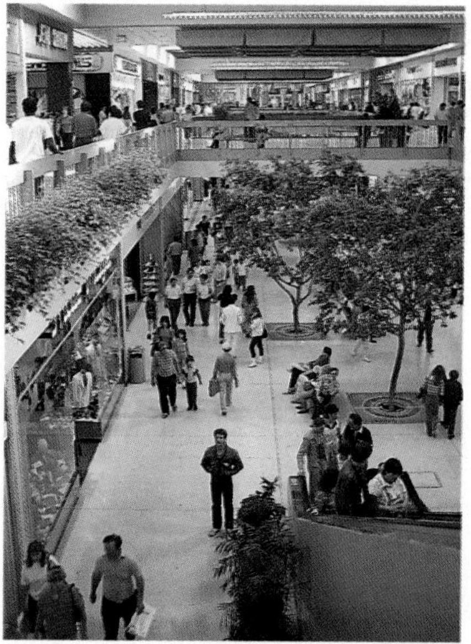

Stereotypes of people with ulcers are changing as dramatically as the treatment for ulcers itself. Any of these people could have an ulcer.

Peptic Ulcers

The term *ulcers* brings to mind the image of a frantic businessman rushing through the day with coffee cup in hand, gulping down high-fat, spicy foods, and working until midnight while suppressing the pain of bleeding sores caused by excessive acid in his stomach. But like other aspects of ulcer prevention and treatment, this stereotype has fallen by the wayside. Neither a stressful lifestyle nor male gender typifies the person with ulcers; ulcers occur in stressed and unstressed men and women alike.

Ulcers can develop both inside and outside the body, but the term *ulcer* used alone generally refers to a *peptic ulcer*—an erosion of the top layer of cells from the GI tract lining. This erosion leaves the underlying layers of cells exposed to gastric juices. When the gastric juices reach the capillaries, the ulcer bleeds, and when they reach the nerves, they cause pain.

peptic ulcer: an erosion of the top layer of cells from the mucosa of the stomach **(gastric ulcer)** or duodenum **(duodenal ulcer)**. Ulcers may develop in the mouth and esophagus, and on the skin, too.

Causes of Ulcers Three major causes of ulcers have been identified: bacterial infection, the use of certain anti-inflammatory drugs, and disorders that cause excessive gastric acid secretion.[5] Treatment aims at relieving pain, healing the ulcer, and minimizing the likelihood of recurrence.

The bacterial infection frequently associated with ulcers is caused by *Helicobacter pylori.* The drugs associated with ulcers are nonsteroidal anti-inflammatory agents such as ibuprofen and naproxen.

Drug Therapy Drug therapy plays the primary role in the treatment of ulcers. The specific type of drug depends on the cause of the ulcer. Antibiotics are used to treat bacterial infections. Other drugs may be used to neutralize acid, reduce acid secretion, or otherwise protect the stomach and duodenal wall from erosion by acid. Nutrition side effects of antiulcer drugs are shown in Table E–1B in Appendix E.

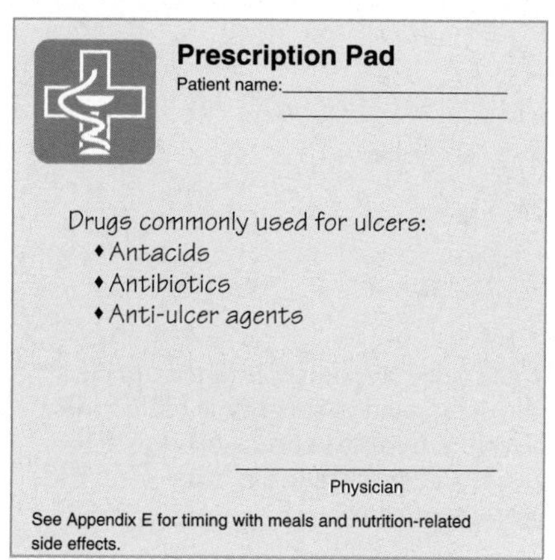

Prescription Pad
Patient name:
Drugs commonly used for ulcers:
♦ Antacids
♦ Antibiotics
♦ Anti-ulcer agents
Physician
See Appendix E for timing with meals and nutrition-related side effects.

Changing Diet Advice Diet therapy once played a major role in ulcer treatment, but current practice is simple: (1) eliminate any food that routinely causes indigestion or pain; (2) avoid caffeine-containing beverages and *all* coffee and tea, even decaffeinated; and (3) avoid alcohol-containing beverages. Research has shown that it is not the caffeine in coffee and tea that stimulates gastric acid secretion. *Decaffeinated* coffee and tea stimulate gastric acid secretion to the same degree as the caffeinated versions; therefore, all coffee and tea are restricted.

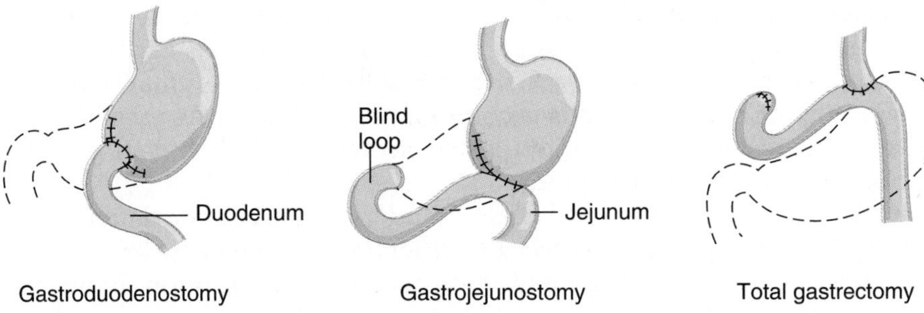

Figure 20–3
Typical Surgeries Involving Total or Partial Removal of the Stomach (Gastric Resections)
The dotted areas show where a structure was removed.

Gastric Surgery and Dumping Syndrome

Gastric surgery may be used to remove gastric cancer or repair bleeding ulcers or injuries. Figure 20–3 illustrates several common procedures. Of course, the general nutrition care for surgical clients described in Chapter 19 applies to those undergoing gastric surgery, but additional nutrition concerns also arise.

After gastric surgery, people may lose large amounts of weight due to limited food intake, malabsorption, increased metabolic requirements, or any combination of these. Some people have trouble regaining their preoperative weights; some people develop specific nutrient deficiencies.

dumping syndrome: the symptoms that result from the rapid emptying of undigested food into the jejunum: sweating, weakness, and diarrhea shortly after eating and hypoglycemia later.

Dumping Syndrome One problem that may occur when a significant portion of the stomach has been removed is dumping syndrome. A typical scenario goes something like this: Mrs. Clark had a fairly extensive gastric resection about a week ago and has just begun to eat solid foods. She swallows the food and about 15 minutes later begins to feel weak and dizzy. She looks pale, her heart beats rapidly, and she breaks out in a sweat. Shortly thereafter, she develops diarrhea. What causes this sequence of events?

Mrs. Clark has lost an important function of her stomach: its control of the rate at which food empties into the intestine. Now food gets "dumped" rapidly into the jejunum. (The duodenum is short, and even if it is not bypassed by surgery, food still passes quickly through it into the jejunum.) As the mass of food is digested all at once, the intestinal contents rapidly become concentrated. Water from the body moves into the intestinal lumen to dilute the concentration. Consequently, the volume of circulating blood diminishes rapidly, causing weakness, dizziness, and a rapid heartbeat. The large volume of hypertonic fluid and unabsorbed material in the jejunum causes pain and hyperpersistalsis; cramping and diarrhea result. Figure 20–4 illustrates the sequence of events that occurs in dumping syndrome.

The type of hypoglycemia that occurs following gastric surgery is called **alimentary hypoglycemia** (al-ih-MEN-tah-ree) or **postgastrectomy hypoglycemia.**

Two to three hours later, Mrs. Clark experiences many of the same symptoms again: dizziness, fainting, nausea, and sweating. This time the cause is different. She digested and absorbed the carbohydrates from her meal so rapidly that her blood glucose rose quickly. Her pancreas responded by overproducing insulin, which made her blood glucose *fall* quickly. Now, hypoglycemia is causing the symptoms.

Figure 20–4
Dumping Syndrome
When partially digested food rapidly enters the jejunum, it creates a hyperosmolar load. Fluid from the intestinal capillaries enters the jejunum, diminishing blood volume and stimulating peristalsis. The result: low blood pressure and diarrhea.

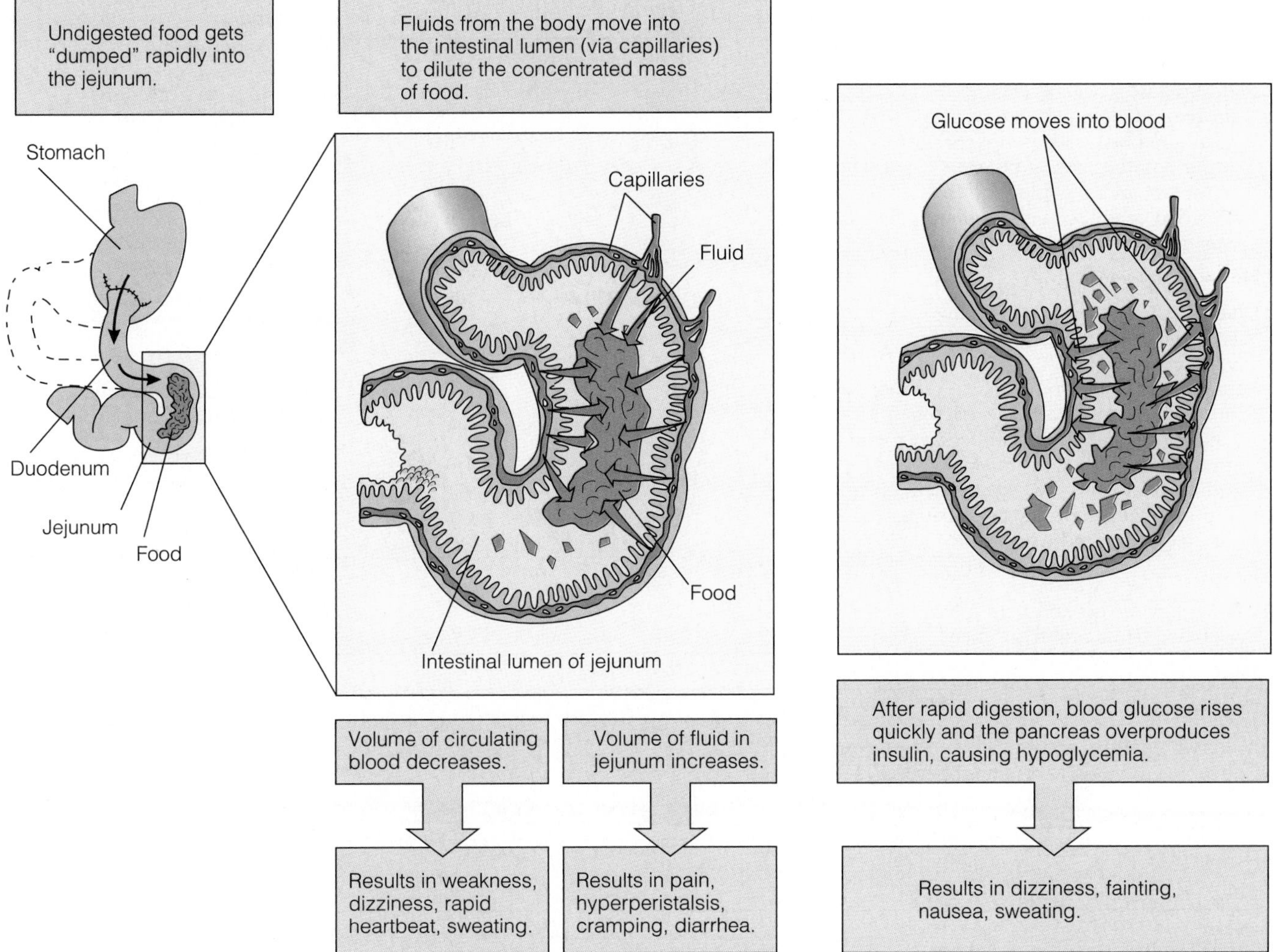

Not all people with gastrectomies experience the diarrhea of dumping syndrome. Even fewer develop hypoglycemia. Many people who initially experience dumping syndrome gradually adapt to a fairly normal diet. However, a special diet benefits clients during the immediate postsurgical period and in prolonged or severe cases. Along with diet, health care professionals monitor fluid and electrolyte balances carefully, correcting any imbalances that occur.

postgastrectomy diet: a carbohydrate-controlled diet given to prevent the symptoms of dumping syndrome and hypoglycemia that sometimes follow gastric surgery.

The Postgastrectomy Diet The postgastrectomy diet limits carbohydrates and especially concentrated sweets, in order to alleviate the symptoms of dumping syndrome. It emphasizes foods containing protein

Table 20–4
Postgastrectomy Diet

FOOD ITEM	ALLOWED	EXCLUDED	COMMENTS
Meats/meat alternates	X		Any type
Grains/starchy vegetables			
Plain breads, crackers, rolls, unsweetened cereal, rice, pasta, corn, lima beans, parsnips, peas, white potatoes, sweet potatoes, pumpkin, yams, winter squash	X		Limit to 5 servings daily
Sweetened cereal; cereal containing dates, raisins, or brown sugar		X	
Nonstarchy vegetables			
Chicory, Chinese cabbage, endive, escarole, lettuce, parsley, radishes, watercress	X		As desired
Asparagus, bean sprouts, beets, broccoli, brussels sprouts, cabbage, carrots, cauliflower, celery, cucumbers, eggplant, green pepper, greens, mushrooms, okra, onions, rhubarb, sauerkraut, string beans, summer squash, tomatoes, turnips, zucchini	X		Limit to two ½ c servings daily; individual tolerances will vary
Vegetables prepared with sugar		X	
Fruits			
Unsweetened fruit and fruit juices	X		Limit to 3 servings daily
Sweetened fruits and fruit juices		X	
Fats	X		Any type
Beverages			
Milk (whole milk, nonfat milk, or buttermilk)	X		If tolerated
Coffee, tea, dietetic carbonated beverages	X		
Alcohol, carbonated beverages, sweetened milk, cocoa, fruit drinks		X	
Desserts			
Cakes, cookies, ice cream, sherbet		X	
Other			
Honey, jam, jelly, syrup, sugar		X	

and fat, which are digested more slowly than carbohydrates and therefore do not attract fluid as rapidly as carbohydrates do. Table 20–4 lists foods included on, and excluded from, the postgastrectomy diet. A sample postgastrectomy diet menu is also provided. Diet advice to offer with the postgastrectomy diet is provided in the accompanying box.

Dietitians carefully tailor the postgastrectomy diet to meet the person's needs. Initially, visits to the client after each meal uncover and deal with food intolerances. Gradually, a person may become able to tolerate small amounts of concentrated sweets, larger quantities of foods, and some liquids with meals. Sometimes adding pectin and guar gum (types

Sample Postgastrectomy Diet Menu

MENU

BREAKFAST
1 scrambled egg
1 slice toast
1 tsp butter
1/2 c milk (take 30–60 minutes after meal)

LUNCH
2 oz hamburger patty
1/4 c mashed potatoes
1 tsp margarine
1/2 small banana
1/2 c milk (take 30–60 minutes after meal)

SUPPER
2 oz boiled ham
1/4 c rice
1/2 c carrots
2 tsp butter
1/4 c unsweetened peach slices
1/2 c milk (take 30–60 minutes after meal)

MIDMORNING SNACK
1/4 c cottage cheese
1 graham cracker

MIDAFTERNOON SNACK
2 tbs peanut butter
3 saltine crackers

EVENING SNACK
1/4 c tuna
1 tsp mayonnaise
1 slice bread

of dietary fiber) to the diet can help prevent dumping syndrome. Unfortunately, diet does not correct the symptoms of dumping syndrome for everyone. When all dietary measures fail, additional surgery may be necessary to resolve the problem.

HOW TO Adjust to Meals after Gastric Surgery

After a person has had a gastrectomy, advise the person as follows:

- Eat no concentrated sweets (sugar, cookies, cakes, pies, or soft drinks) because the body digests these carbohydrates most rapidly.
- Take frequent small meals to fit the reduced storage capacity of the stomach.
- Drink liquids about 45 minutes before or after meals, not with them. This precaution helps slow the rate of food's passage from the stomach to the intestine and prevents overloading the stomach's reduced storage capacity.
- Lie down immediately after eating to help slow the transit of food to the intestine.
- Be aware that lactose intolerance may develop and produce discomfort in response to milk and milk products. Discontinue use of those products until recovery is under way. Then try them with caution.

Anemia Other nutrition concerns arise in people with gastrectomies. For example, clients may develop iron-deficiency anemia. Blood loss from surgery, accompanied by inadequate nutrition and poor iron absorption, contributes to the problem. Iron is usually changed to its absorbable form in the stomach. Also, 50 percent of iron absorption normally takes place in the duodenum, and now the transit time through the duodenum may be rapid, or the duodenum may be bypassed altogether. An iron supplement helps to correct the deficiency.

Anemia can also be caused by a deficiency of vitamin B_{12} or folate. Vitamin B_{12} cannot be absorbed without the intrinsic factor, which is synthesized in the stomach. Depending on the location and extent of the gastric resection, intrinsic factor production may be minimal or absent, and clients may need to receive vitamin B_{12} by injection (to bypass the need for absorption) and supplemental folate orally.

stasis (STAY-sis)**:** standing still. Normal actions of the intestines keep a steady stream of secretions flowing through them. Stasis in a blind loop allows bacteria to flourish.

The problems of fat malabsorption and vitamin B_{12} and folate deficiencies that result from the overgrowth of bacteria in a bypassed segment of the intestine are called **blind loop syndrome.**

steatorrhea (stee-ah-toe-REE-ah)**:** the fatty diarrhea characteristic of fat malabsorption; stools are foamy, greasy, malodorous, and float in the toilet.
steatos = fat
rhea = flow

Blind Loop Syndrome In some types of gastric resections, a portion of the small intestine is also bypassed, making that portion nonfunctional. The bypassed portion is called a blind loop. (Figure 20–3 illustrated such a gastric resection.)

Stasis occurs in the blind loop, and bacteria normally not present in that part of the intestine may begin to flourish. The bacteria compete with the body for vitamin B_{12} and folate, limiting the available supply. The bacteria also partly dismantle bile salts, hampering fat digestion and absorption. Figure 20–5 repeats the figure from Chapter 5 (p. 105) that shows how bile prepares fat for digestion, this time illustrating how bacteria interfere with that process. The bacterial overgrowth that occurs in a blind loop leads to fat malabsorption and steatorrhea as well as vitamin B_{12} and folate deficiencies. To correct these problems, clients receive fat-restricted diets, parenteral vitamin B_{12}, and oral folate supplements.

Figure 20–5
Steatorrhea

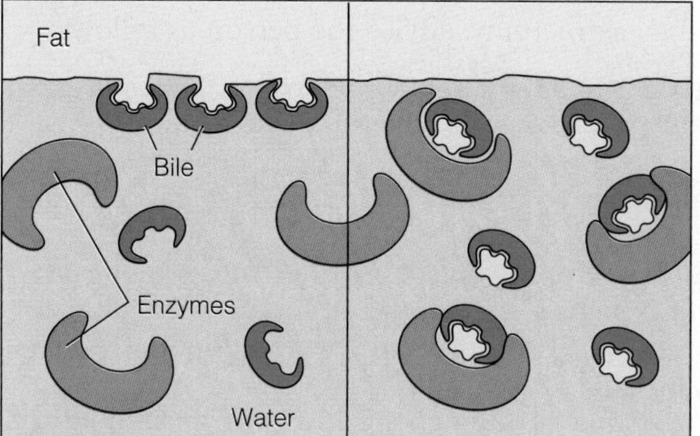

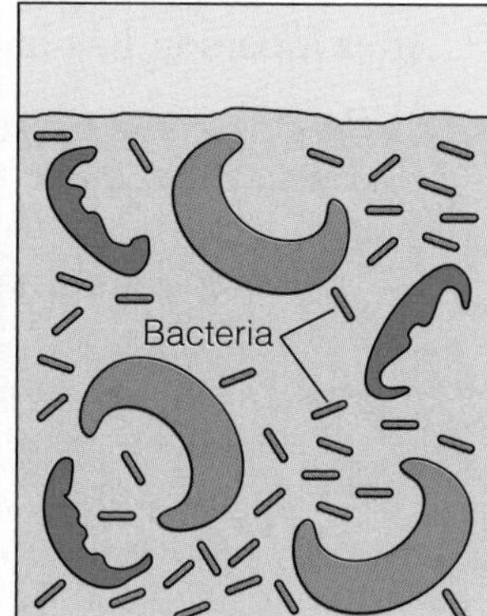

Impaired bile action
Bacteria
In blind loop syndrome, bacteria damage the bile, so that it is ineffective in fat digestion and absorption.
The result is fat malabsorption and steatorrhea.

Physicians also prescribe antibiotics to inhibit bacterial growth. Sometimes the blind loop must be removed surgically.

Malabsorption Malabsorption occurs in many disorders; much of the next chapter is devoted to it. Malabsorption occurs whenever food passes rapidly through the GI tract and is an especially common problem for any client who has had a total gastrectomy or whose stomach is surgically connected directly to the jejunum. Normally, food entering the duodenum triggers the release of the hormones secretin and cholecystokinin, which mediate the secretion of digestive enzymes and bile into the duodenum. When the duodenum is bypassed, these hormones cannot aid fat digestion and absorption as usual. The next case study facilitates review of the needs of a client following gastric surgery.

Gastric Partitioning

Another use for gastric surgery is to treat clinically severe obesity. Two gastric partitioning procedures have gained wide acceptance and are illustrated in Figure 20–6 (p. 496).[6] Both procedures effectively limit food intake by reducing the size of the stomach. Both also reduce the size of the outlet, so as to delay the passage of food from the stomach into the intestine and thereby ease digestion and absorption.

clinically severe obesity: obesity defined by a BMI of 40 or greater or 100 pounds or more overweight for an average adult. A less preferred term used to describe the same condition is **morbid obesity.**

gastric partitioning: a surgical procedure used to treat clinically severe obesity. The operation limits food intake by limiting the size of the stomach and delays gastric emptying by restricting the outlet.

Diet Following Surgery The long-term safety and effectiveness of gastric partitioning depend, in large part, on the client's compliance with dietary instructions. Poor dietary habits may prevent weight loss, rupture staples, or obstruct the small passage into the lower stomach. Common postsurgical complications include infections, nausea, vomiting, dehydra-

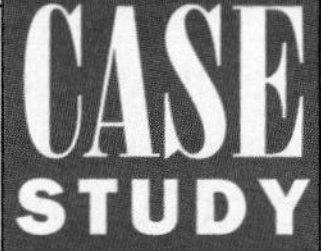

Commercial Artist Requiring Gastric Surgery

Mr. Miyamotto, a 42-year-old commercial artist, was admitted to the emergency room in serious condition after suffering severe abdominal injuries in a car accident. After his initial examination, a surgeon was consulted, and Mr. Miyamoto was taken to surgery immediately. A gastrojejunostomy (see Figure 20–3) was performed. Mr. Miyamoto was sent to the intensive care unit following surgery and is recovering as expected. The health care team members anticipate nutrition-related problems, and they are taking measures to prevent them.

1. Review Figure 20–3 to understand the procedure that Mr. Miyamoto underwent. Consider the possibilities that he might develop dumping syndrome, blind loop syndrome, and general malabsorption. Explain why and how these conditions might occur.
2. What diet will the physician prescribe for Mr. Miyamoto after he begins eating orally? Describe the diet and how it progresses.
3. What advice can you give Mr. Miyamoto to prevent dumping syndrome?
4. Discuss the nutrition-related concerns associated with blind loop syndrome. How can these concerns be handled?

Figure 20–6
Surgical Procedures to Control Obesity
The shaded areas highlight the flow of food through the GI tract. Notice that the first procedure maintains the normal flow whereas the second one bypasses most of the stomach, all of the duodenum, and some of the jejunum. The white areas indicate the sections that have been bypassed.

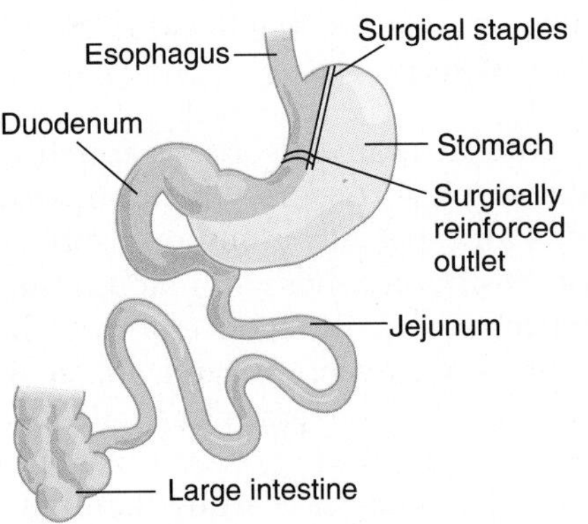

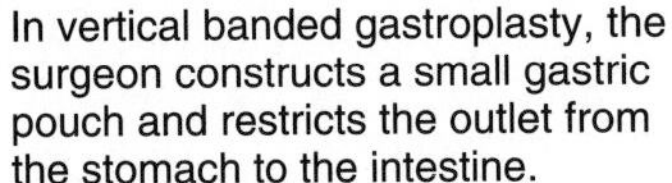
In vertical banded gastroplasty, the surgeon constructs a small gastric pouch and restricts the outlet from the stomach to the intestine.

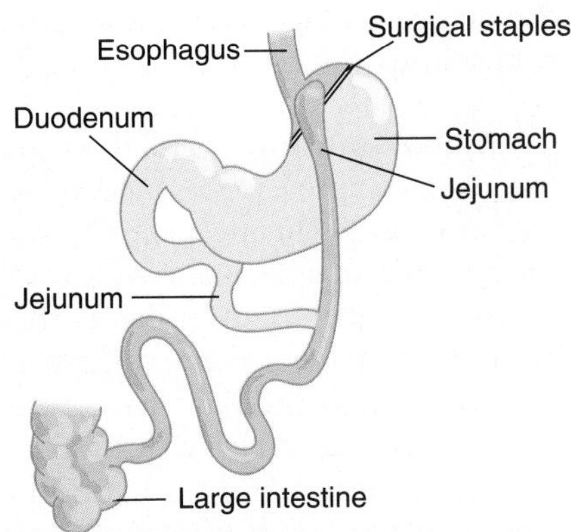

In gastric bypass, the surgeon constructs a small gastric pouch and creates an outlet directly to the jejunum.

tion, dumping syndrome, esophageal reflux, and, as a result of all this and more, depression.

Short-Term Diet For about eight weeks after surgery, clients follow a liquid diet to minimize the risk of disrupting the line of surgical staples. Liquids flow easily through the opening to the lower stomach (or jejunum). Clients can tolerate only small amounts of liquids at one time because of the stomach's small size. Overeating or overdrinking can cause vomiting.

Long-Term Diet After about two months, the person can gradually begin to eat soft or pureed foods, but still only small amounts of food at a time. Later, the person can add solid foods as tolerated, but must continue to eat small meals. Clients must understand that their selections of foods and beverages influence the extent of their weight loss. (If they drink high-kcalorie liquids or eat high-kcalorie foods all the time, even if only in small quantities, they will not lose weight.) Their selections also affect the nutritional quality of their diets. Deficiencies, particularly of vitamin B_{12}, folate, and iron, are common after gastric bypass surgery. Careful planning, diligent compliance with the prescribed diet, and supplements are necessary to ensure the adequacy of energy-restricted diets that demand small intakes.[7]

Nutrition Assessment

This chapter has shown how disorders of the upper GI tract can limit food intake and impair nutrition status. When you assess the nutrition status of people who have these disorders, keep these special points in mind:

- Obtain a thorough diet history. People who have difficulties chewing or swallowing may have poor intakes of one or several nutrients. Other disorders such as nausea, indigestion, gastritis, or peptic ulcers sometimes cause intolerances to certain foods. A food intake record can help to pinpoint offending foods so that they can be avoided. For the person who has undergone gastric partitioning, use the diet history to assess energy intake and eating habits.

- Monitor body weight regularly. Disorders of the upper GI tract often lead to weight loss due to either poor food intake or malabsorption of nutrients. Conversely, excessive eating and weight gain can interfere with efforts to control the symptoms of reflux esophagitis and can loosen or dislodge gastric staples.
- Assess biochemical parameters with an awareness that people with severe vomiting or those with dumping syndrome may be dehydrated, making lab values appear deceptively elevated.

This chapter has dealt with problems of the upper GI tract. The next chapter examines problems of the lower GI tract.

■ STUDY QUESTIONS ■

1. Describe some conditions of the mouth that can affect food intake. What diet modifications would you advise in these cases? How should the diet be planned?
2. What is dysphagia, and how is it managed? Why does dysphagia often go unrecognized? What are the potential consequences of dysphagia?
3. What is a hiatal hernia? What causes the symptoms associated with a hiatal hernia? What advice can you give the person with a hiatal hernia to prevent and treat these symptoms?
4. Under what circumstances can indigestion, nausea, and vomiting present a risk to nutrition status?
5. Explain the basis for the diet therapy used to help treat peptic ulcers.
6. Describe the events associated with dumping syndrome. What diet modifications might help to prevent these symptoms?
7. What is blind loop syndrome? What are the nutrition consequences? How are these problems avoided or corrected?
8. Discuss the dietary recommendations, and the rationale behind them, for a person who undergoes gastric surgery for clinically severe obesity.

■ CLINICAL APPLICATION QUESTIONS ■

1. People on mechanical soft diets differ in the kinds of foods they can handle, in the lengths of time that diet modifications remain necessary, and in the kinds of help they need from health care professionals. Think about the difference between a person who has had no teeth for years and a person who has recently had mouth surgery and is just beginning to eat again. Describe some nutrition-related concerns you might have for the person who has been following a mechanical soft diet for years. How would these concerns differ for a person who needs the mechanical soft diet only temporarily? Contrast the amounts of time a nurse or dietitian might need to spend with the two types of clients.
2. Many of the diets described in this chapter are highly individualized. A particular food may give one person indigestion and have no effect on another. One person with a gastrectomy may experience lactose intolerance, while another may not. Describe practical ways to keep track of food intolerances.

NUTRITION IN PRACTICE 20

Caffeine—Addictive Drug? Beneficial Drug?

Caffeine is one of the most widely used nonnutrient substances in the world. Defined as a drug—that is, a substance that alters one or more of the body's functions—caffeine occurs naturally in many plant-based foods and beverages. Nearly every human culture has adopted one or another of these plants as a dietary staple. Coffee, tea, chocolate, and cola beverages all are popular and widely used for their stimulant effect and flavor.

What does caffeine do to the body?

Pharmacologically, caffeine is classed as a mild stimulant. It stimulates the digestive tract, promoting efficient elimination, and it "wakes up" the central nervous system, a well-known and valued effect. Curiously, caffeine also raises brain serotonin concentrations, which are generally associated with drowsiness.[8]

Caffeine also stimulates thermogenesis, the body's heat production. The dose in 1 cup of coffee speeds metabolism slightly for an hour or two, leading at least one group of researchers to speculate that caffeine may reduce body fat stores.[9] If a person wanting to lose weight could refrain from making up this energy deficit with food, the small changes in the metabolic rate (75 to 100 kcalories per day) could theoretically lead to weight loss of nearly a pound a month.[10]

That sounds wonderful. But does it work and is it safe?

The usefulness of caffeine in the treatment of obesity is unsubstantiated. But caffeine is not, for most people, a dangerous drug. The Food and Drug Administration (FDA) lists it as a multipurpose GRAS (generally recognized as safe) substance that may be added to foods and beverages. Drug industries in developed countries use caffeine in many kinds of drugs: stimulants, pain relievers, cold remedies, diuretics, and weight-loss aids.

How does the body handle caffeine?

The adult body quickly absorbs caffeine and circulates it to all tissues within 15 to 45 minutes depending on the source, dose, and individual. The liver breaks down caffeine, and the kidneys excrete most of it. Clearance times vary depending in part on prior caffeine use, to which the body is conditioned. Clearance may be slowed by liver disease, pregnancy, and oral contraceptive use; accelerated by smoking; and either slowed or accelerated by various other drugs.[11]

I've heard that people need more and more caffeine to get the same effect. Is that true?

Yes, most people develop caffeine tolerance rather quickly, as their bodies adapt to chronic consumption. Researchers speculate that the body develops an enhanced sensitivity to its own internally made compound adenosine, which blunts caffeine's effects. Caffeine raises blood pressure and stimulates urine output, central nervous system activity, lipid breakdown, and intestinal peristalsis. Adenosine exerts the opposite effects.

Doesn't that mean that caffeine is an addictive drug?

Yes, caffeine is addictive; the body adapts to its presence. Sudden abstinence after long use (even moderate use), cutting down from a high to a low dose, or switching to decaffeinated products causes characteristic withdrawal symptoms—headaches, drowsiness, and fatigue. Caffeine withdrawal headaches are so common that many pain relievers include caffeine in their formulas, even though caffeine is not a pain reliever.

Does long-term caffeine use do any harm to the body?

Caffeine has been loosely associated with a variety of conditions and diseases, but never pinpointed as the cause of any of them. For the most part, caffeine seems to be relatively harmless when used by healthy adults in moderate doses (the equivalent of, say, 2 to 3 average-sized cups of coffee a day).

What is the harm in drinking too much caffeine?

In large amounts, caffeine can produce reactions that are just like anxiety attacks. People who drink between 8 and 15 cups of coffee a day, for example, have been known to seek help from physicians for complaints such as dizziness, agitation, restlessness, recurring headaches, intestinal discomfort, and sleep difficulties. Before recommending tranquilizers or expensive therapies, physicians would do well to inquire about their clients' caffeine intakes.

How much caffeine is too much?

It depends on the individual. Younger people can tolerate more than older people, and caffeine taken in the morning is less likely to disrupt sleep than that taken late in the day. Even 1 cup of coffee late in the day can disrupt normal sleep patterns, most often delaying sleep or leaving a person feeling tired after a night's sleep. People who have trouble sleeping should avoid caffeine-containing beverages within four hours of bedtime. As is true of many other substances, moderation in the use of caffeine-containing foods and beverages is advisable. To reduce or eliminate caffeine without withdrawal symptoms, cut down gradually.

How does caffeine affect the stomach? Does it cause ulcers or heartburn?

Both regular and decaffeinated coffee and tea stimulate stomach acid secretion and so aggravate *existing* ulcers. This effect occurs in response to the beverage and not to caffeine per se. Other compounds resembling caffeine, known as xanthines, occur in coffee and other caffeine-containing beverages; and one or more of these must contribute to this effect. Studies have not shown that coffee consumption raises the risk of *developing* ulcers, but caffeine-containing drugs may stimulate stomach acid secretion in some people, causing nausea and GI distress.[12]

As this chapter explained, heartburn occurs when the cardiac sphincter relaxes and allows stomach acid to splash back up into the esophagus. Therefore, anything that relaxes the cardiac sphincter can cause heartburn; caffeine itself does not seem to have this effect, but coffee does in some people, and by stimulating gastric acid secretion, coffee may accentuate the pain caused by reflux. People who experience heartburn should pay attention to whether coffee aggravates it and act accordingly.

What about caffeine and heart disease?

For 40 years, studies on caffeine's relationships with heart disease have produced various findings, but no study indicates that moderate caffeine intake causes cardiovascular disease. Some studies suggest that coffee raises heart rate, blood pressure, and blood lipids; some do not. Some, comparing decaffeinated brews with coffee, suggest that a component other than caffeine is responsible for the effects seen.

Limited caffeine consumption is often advised for those who have suffered heart attacks. The increased metabolic rate and the possibility of an anxiety attack associated with excess caffeine use can aggravate stress.

Furthermore, although caffeine may not cause heart disease directly, it may mask the warning signs. During times of overexertion, a diseased heart hurts, and the resulting chest pain is well known as a prime symptom of heart disease and a signal to slow down. The pain has been traced to an effect of the compound adenosine, which opposes caffeine's effects.[13] Caffeine opposes adenosine's actions, and so may blunt the sensation of pain and override adenosine's warnings.

I've heard that caffeine causes breast disease. Is that true?

The relationship between caffeine consumption and fibrocystic breast disease is tenuous at best. Some women may benefit slightly from caffeine abstinence, but for the most part changes are clinically insignificant.

Is it OK for pregnant women to use caffeine?

During pregnancy, caffeine readily crosses the placenta to enter the fetal bloodstream, but the fetus cannot metabolize it. In animal studies, large caffeine doses lead to birth defects, but human studies have established no such association. Limited evidence suggests that moderate-to-heavy use of coffee correlates with low infant birthweights.[14] Common sense dictates that women limit their caffeine intakes during pregnancy, but data are insufficient to set a specific limit.

Breastfeeding mothers are discouraged from drinking large quantities of coffee or other caffeine-containing beverages, but limited caffeine consumption (the equivalent of 1 to 2 cups of coffee daily) is thought unlikely to impair milk production or harm nursing infants.[15] Larger doses of coffee may interfere with the iron availability from breast milk and impair the infant's iron status.

Does caffeine affect nutrition?

Some studies suggest that caffeine may hinder the availability of certain nutrients such as calcium and iron. Evidence is sparse and inconsistent but worthy of brief mention here.

Concerning calcium, caffeine has been considered a possible risk factor for the development of osteoporosis, but evidence is inconclusive.[16] Some studies indicate that caffeine accelerates calcium excretion; other studies have found no significant effects.[17] The effects of caffeine on calcium bal-

Table 20–5
Caffeine Content of Beverages, Foods, and Over-the-Counter Drugs

	AVERAGE (mg)	RANGE (mg)
Beverages and Foods		
Coffee (5 oz cup)		
Brewed, drip method	115	60–180
Brewed, percolator	80	40–170
Instant	65	30–120
Decaffeinated, brewed or instant	3	1–5
Tea (5 oz cup)		
Brewed, major U.S. brands	40	20–90
Brewed, imported brands	60	25–110
Instant	30	25–50
Iced (12 oz glass)	70	67–76
Soft drinks (12 oz can)		
Dr. Pepper		15–23
Colas and cherry cola		
Regular		30–46
Diet		0–35
Caffeine-free		0–trace
Jolt		72
Mountain Dew, Mello Yello		52
Fresca, Hires Root Beer, 7-Up, Sprite, Squirt, Sunkist Orange		0
Cocoa beverage (5 oz cup)	4	2–20
Chocolate milk beverage (8 oz)	5	2–7
Milk chocolate candy (1 oz)	6	1–15
Dark chocolate, semisweet (1 oz)	20	5–35
Baker's chocolate (1 oz)	26	26
Chocolate-flavored syrup (1 oz)	4	4
Drugs[a]		
Cold remedies (standard dose)		
Dristan		0
Coryban-D, Triaminicin		30
Diuretics (standard dose)		
Aqua-ban, Permathene H_2Off		200
Pre-Mens Forte		100
Pain relievers (standard dose)		
Excedrin		130
Midol, Anacin		65
Aspirin, plain (any brand)		0
Stimulants		
Caffedrin, NoDoz, Vivarin		200
Weight-control aids (daily dose)		
Prolamine		280
Dexatrim, Dietac		200

Note: A pharmacologically active dose of caffeine is defined as 200 milligrams.
[a]Because products change, contact the manufacturer for an update on products you use regularly.

Source: Data from International Food Information Council, Caffeine and health: Clarifying the controversies, *IFIC Review,* May 1993; C.W. Lecos, Caffeine jitters: Some safety questions remain, *FDA Consumer,* January 1988, pp. 22–27.

ance may be harmful only when calcium intake is low.

Regarding iron, both coffee and tea inhibit iron absorption. Most likely, though, this effect is due to the polyphenol and tannic acid content, not to the caffeine content.

How can I tell how much caffeine is in the foods and beverages I choose?

Table 20–5 shows that, in general, a cup of coffee contains the most caffeine; a cup of tea, less than half as much; and cocoa or chocolate, less still. As for cola beverages, they are made from kola nuts, which contain caffeine, but most of their caffeine is added, using the purified compound obtained from decaffeinated coffee beans. Don't forget that many drugs contain caffeine; see the table.

Is decaffeinated coffee a safe alternative to regular coffee?

Whether a person drinks regular or decaffeinated beverages seems to be of little, if any, significance. In every disease or condition men-

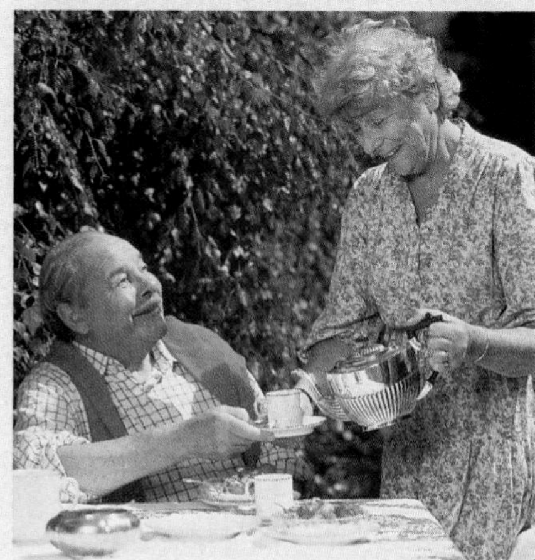

In moderate amounts, caffeine-containing beverages can add pleasure to the day without harming health.

tioned earlier, other factors weigh far more heavily on a person's health than caffeine does. A woman threatened with osteoporosis would do well to exercise and consume more calcium. A person trying to ease the pain of an ulcer would benefit most from drug therapy. A person wanting to lower the risk of heart disease should limit fat intake. A woman wanting to foster a healthy pregnancy should abstain from smoking and drug use. For most people, then, caffeine-containing beverages can find a place in a healthy diet; it just can't be a very large place.

■ NOTES ■

1. J. Horner and E. W. Massey, Silent aspiration following stroke, *Neurology* 38 (1988): 317–319.
2. E. M. Pardoe, Development of a multistage diet for dysphagia, *Journal of the American Dietetic Association* 93 (1993): 568–571.
3. Pardoe, 1993.
4. J. V. Sizmann, Nutritional support of the dysphagic patient: Methods, risks, and complications of therapy, *Journal of Parenteral and Enteral Nutrition* 14 (1990): 60–63.
5. D. Y. Graham, *Helicobacter pylori:* Its epidemiology and its role in duodenal ulcer disease, *Journal of Gastroenterology and Hepatology* 6 (1991): 105–113.
6. Gastrointestinal surgery for severe obesity: National Institutes of Health Consensus Development Conference statement, *American Journal of Clinical Nutrition* 55 (1992): 615S–619S.
7. T. Andersen and U. Larsen, Dietary outcome in obese patients treated with gastroplasty program, *American Journal of Clinical Nutrition* 50 (1989): 1328–1340.
8. Caffeine can increase brain serotonin levels, *Nutrition Reviews* 46 (1988): 366–367.
9. A. Astrup and coauthors, Caffeine: A double-blind, placebo-controlled study of its thermogenic, metabolic, and cardiovascular effects in healthy volunteers, *American Journal of Clinical Nutrition* 51 (1990): 759–767.
10. A. G. Dulloo and coauthors, Normal caffeine consumption: Influence on thermogenesis and daily energy expenditure in lean and postobese human volunteers, *American Journal of Clinical Nutrition* 49 (1989): 44–50.
11. T. K. Leonard, R. R. Watson, and M. E. Mohs, The effects of caffeine on various body systems: A review, *Journal of the American Dietetic Association* 87 (1987): 1048–1053.
12. D. E. Powers and A. O. Moore, *Food Medication Interactions*, 6th ed. (Phoenix, Ariz.: Food Medication Interactions, 1989).
13. Dr. Luiz Belardinelli, professor of medicine at the University of Florida Medical School, as cited in Caffeine may mask angina, *Tallahassee Democrat*, April 11, 1991.
14. Food and Nutrition Board, *Nutrition during Pregnancy* (Washington, D.C.: National Academy Press, 1990), p. 399.
15. Food and Nutrition Board, *Nutrition during Lactation* (Washington, D.C.: National Academy Press, 1991), p. 176.
16. C. D. Arnaud and S. D. Sanchez, The role of calcium in osteoporosis, *Annual Review of Nutrition* 10 (1990): 397–414.
17. M. J. Barger-Lux, R. P. Heaney, and M. R. Stegman, Effects of moderate caffeine intake on the calcium economy of premenopausal women, *American Journal of Clinical Nutrition* 52 (1990): 722–725.

21

Nutrition and Lower GI Disorders

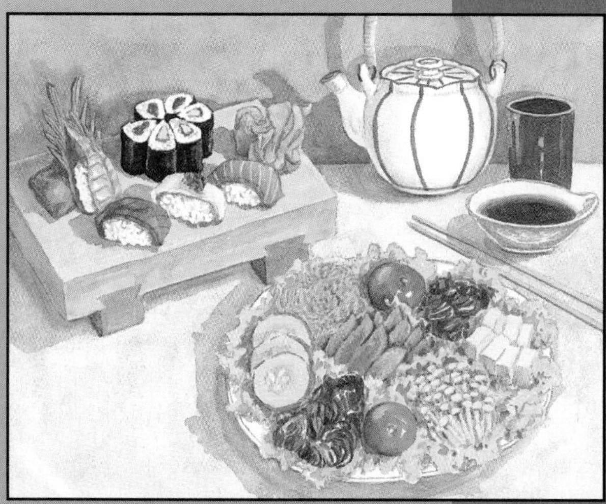

CONTENTS

As Chapter 5 observed, the intestine is "the" organ of digestion. Any disorder of the intestine, particularly if it results in malabsorption, can seriously impair nutrition status. This chapter describes disorders of the lower GI tract that influence nutrition status or are affected by diet. It begins with motility disorders, then takes up disorders of the pancreas and intestine that cause malabsorption, then those of the colon. (Some common digestive problems, such as gas, short bouts of diarrhea, and constipation, that do not seriously impact nutrition status were already discussed in Nutrition in Practice 5.)

Diarrhea and Irritable Bowel Syndrome

Diarrhea and irritable bowel syndrome are both motility disorders of the GI tract. Their causes may not always be known, but nutrition support may help alleviate their symptoms while a diagnosis is being sought.

Severe Diarrhea and Dehydration

Diarrhea occurs either when fluids are drawn from the GI tract lining and added to the food residue, or when the intestinal contents move so quickly through the GI tract that fluids are not absorbed. In both cases, the result is frequent, watery bowel movements.

Diarrhea that results from an accelerated movement of fluids and electrolytes from the intestinal capillaries into the lumen of the intestine is called **secretory diarrhea.** Diarrhea that results from unabsorbed water and electrolytes increasing the osmolarity of the intestinal contents is called **osmotic diarrhea.** Unabsorbed fat that is excreted in the stools causes steatorrhea, defined earlier. Severe, chronic diarrhea that does not respond to treatment attempts is often called **intractable diarrhea.**

Causes of Diarrhea Many things can trigger diarrhea: emotional stress, food allergies, overeating, food contaminated with infectious bacteria, bacterial overgrowth in the gut, GI disorders that lead to malabsorption, and malnutrition. So can many drugs and radiation treatments that irritate the GI tract. Infants, children, and severely stressed adults frequently develop diarrhea when given formulas that their GI tracts cannot tolerate. Lactose intolerance is another frequent cause. A person with severe, persistent diarrhea may rapidly become dehydrated, lose weight, and develop multiple nutrient deficiencies. It is urgent to start nutrition support before severe depletion occurs.

Dehydration Dehydration can be life-threatening. An average-sized adult producing a large volume of watery stools can lose more than 1 liter of fluid and electrolytes per hour—a fluid loss that can be fatal in six hours or less. A child or infant can lose proportionately more fluid and die of dehydration in a still shorter time. Table 21–1 on the next page lists findings associated with dehydration.

oral rehydration therapy (ORT): a mixture of water, glucose, and a combination of sodium and potassium salts used to prevent or treat dehydration associated with diarrhea. **ORT formulas** contain these ingredients already mixed.

Oral Rehydration Therapy (ORT) In many cases, all it takes to replace the fluids and solutes lost in diarrhea is a simple mixture of water, salts, and sugar known as oral rehydration therapy, or ORT. Some public health agencies make recipes available so that people in remote areas can prepare this mixture at home; an example is shown in the margin.[1] Ready-made formulas are also available. ORT formulas can successfully reverse dehydration in some cases of severe diarrhea, and given early enough, can sometimes eliminate the need for hospitalization.

The World Health Organization recipe for rehydration in diarrheal disease: in 1 liter of water, dissolve 3.5 g sodium chloride, 2.5 g sodium bicarbonate, 1.5 g potassium chloride, and 20 g glucose (or 40 g sucrose).

Table 21–1
Physical and Laboratory Indices of Dehydration

Physical signs
Sunken eyes
Hollow cheeks
Stunned facial expression
Dry mucous membranes
Deep, gasping respirations
Weak, rapid pulse
Low blood pressure
Skin that lacks elasticity when pinched (may not be a valid finding in the elderly)
Weak cry (infants)
Depression of anterior fontanel (infants)
Laboratory findings
Serum sodium, potassium, and chloride elevated
Blood urea nitrogen (BUN) elevated
Hemoglobin and hematocrit elevated

Note: Laboratory indices can vary depending on the cause of dehydration.

Bowel Rest Often, especially in seriously ill individuals, it becomes necessary to stop placing demands on the GI tract and let it rest while investigating the cause of diarrhea. All foods and beverages may be withheld for 24 to 48 hours, during which time treatment primarily focuses on maintaining fluid and electrolyte balances intravenously.

Progressive Diets After a day or so of bowel rest, the person tries a clear-liquid diet and then progresses, as tolerance permits, to a full-liquid diet; then a low-fat, low-fiber diet; and finally a regular diet. Frequent small meals may be easiest to manage at first. The diet temporarily excludes lactose and any food believed to have irritated the GI tract. Applesauce or scraped raw apples may be given every two to four hours because they contain pectin, which sequesters water and helps solidify the stools. Permanent dietary changes are necessary for diarrhea caused by food sensitivities or allergies.

Alternate Feedings If the diarrhea worsens as the diet progresses, then alternate feeding programs are appropriate. Easy-to-digest formulas given by tube (enteral formulas) are preferred, but for people with chronic diarrhea who cannot tolerate enteral feeding, special feedings by vein (parenteral nutrition) are indicated. The next two chapters are devoted to enteral and parenteral nutrition.

enteral: by way of the stomach or intestine; a term that technically refers to both oral and tube feedings, but usually used to refer to tube feedings.

parenteral: not into the intestine; a term used to describe nutrition given by vein.

Other Measures The exact treatment plan depends on the cause of the diarrhea. If a drug is responsible for diarrhea, a different drug or drug form (injectable versus oral, for example) may alleviate the problem. Drugs can also be used to treat diarrhea, often by slowing intestinal motility. Diarrhea caused by infectious agents is treated with antimicrobial drugs.

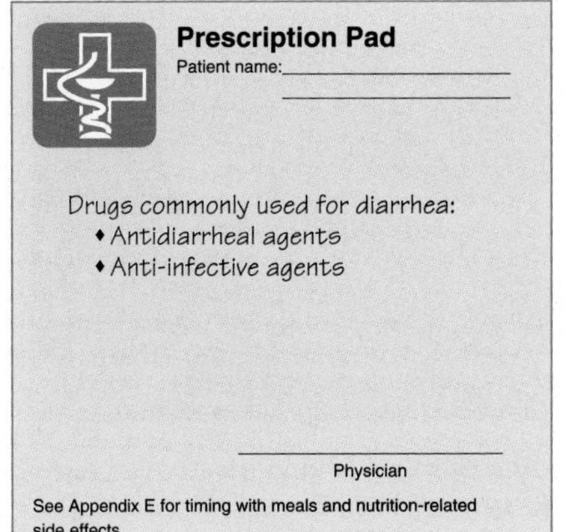
Prescription Pad
Patient name:

Drugs commonly used for diarrhea:
- Antidiarrheal agents
- Anti-infective agents

Physician

See Appendix E for timing with meals and nutrition-related side effects.

Irritable Bowel Syndrome

Like diarrhea, irritable bowel syndrome is a common disorder involving GI tract motility. In this syndrome, however, constipation may alternate with the diarrhea. The person with irritable bowel syndrome may have indigestion, nausea, abdominal pain, gas, diarrhea, constipation, or alternating diarrhea and constipation. The dietary treatment depends on the symptoms.

Diet Treatments A high-fiber, low-fat diet is frequently recommended for the person with irritable bowel syndrome. High-fiber diets may also cause gas and abdominal pain, however, so it is important to add fiber gradually. When the client experiences gas and abdominal pain, it may be helpful to avoid the foods and ingredients listed in Table 21–2.

Table 21–2
Foods and Food Ingredients That May Produce Gas

Apples	Fried foods
Artichokes, Chinese	Garlic
Asparagus	Gravy
Barley	High-fat meats
Beans	Honey
Beer	Kohlrabi
Bran	Legumes
Broccoli	Mannitol
Brussels sprouts	Milk
Cabbage	Molasses
Carbonated beverages	Nuts
Cauliflower	Onions
Celery	Pastries
Cherries	Prunes
Coconut	Radishes
Cream sauces	Raisins
Cucumber	Sorbitol
Eggplant	Soybeans
Eggs	Wheat
Figs	Yeast
Fish	

Note: Many of these are high-fiber foods that pass undigested and unabsorbed into the colon where bacteria metabolize them, producing gas in the process. High-fat foods cause gas for many people, as do large amounts of fructose and the artificial sweeteners, sorbitol and mannitol. Milk, milk products, and other lactose-containing products may cause gas if lactose intolerance is present. Beer and carbonated beverages may cause gas in people with ostomies.

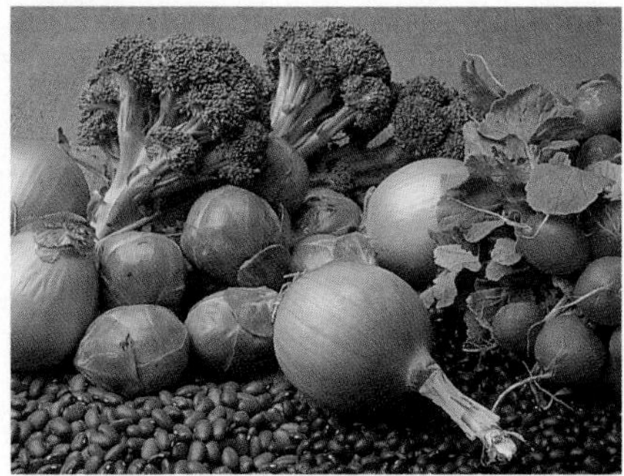

Some people with irritable bowel syndrome may need to exercise moderation in eating foods that produce gas.

hydrophilic colloid: a type of laxative that attracts water in the intestine to form a bulky stool, which then stimulates peristalsis. (Metamucil and Fiberall are examples of hydrophilic colloids.)

Other foods that may cause intolerances must also be identified and eliminated.

Bran People can add bran or hydrophilic colloids to their meals to help relieve constipation. If the bran causes gas, though, they should use the colloids only.

Akin to diarrhea and irritable bowel syndrome, which may cause water loss and dehydration, are many disorders involving malabsorption. In the case of malabsorption, however, fat is often the focus of concern.

Malabsorption

Several disorders that lead to malabsorption are discussed throughout the remainder of this chapter, but whatever the cause, malnutrition always threatens. Table 21–3 lists the ways that malabsorption can lead to malnutrition.

Fat Malabsorption Malabsorption of any nutrient is possible, but most commonly, it is fat that is malabsorbed. The excretion of unabsorbed fat in the stools causes the type of diarrhea known as steatorrhea. The effects of fat malabsorption can be severe (see Figure 21–1). The loss of fat in the stools means that valuable food energy, fat-soluble vitamins, and some minerals are lost as well. Fat-soluble vitamins normally travel and are absorbed with fat, so fat-soluble vitamins are lost as a consequence of steatorrhea. Minerals normally are absorbed in the colon, but when malabsorption occurs, unabsorbed fatty acids form soaps with minerals such as calcium and magnesium and carry them out of the body in steatorrhea. Vitamin D losses further aggravate calcium malabsorption.

Table 21–3
Causes of Poor Nutrition Status in Malabsorption

REDUCED INTAKE	EXCESSIVE NUTRIENT LOSSES	RAISED NUTRIENT NEEDS
Abdominal pain	Bacterial overgrowth of the small intestine	Drug therapy
Anorexia	Diarrhea	High basal energy expenditure
Bowel rest	Drug therapy	Infection
Drug therapy	Fistulas	Surgery
Emotional stress	General malabsorption	
Food intolerance	Intestinal losses of serum proteins	
Indigestion	Short bowel syndrome	
Nausea	Steatorrhea	
Obstructions	Vomiting	

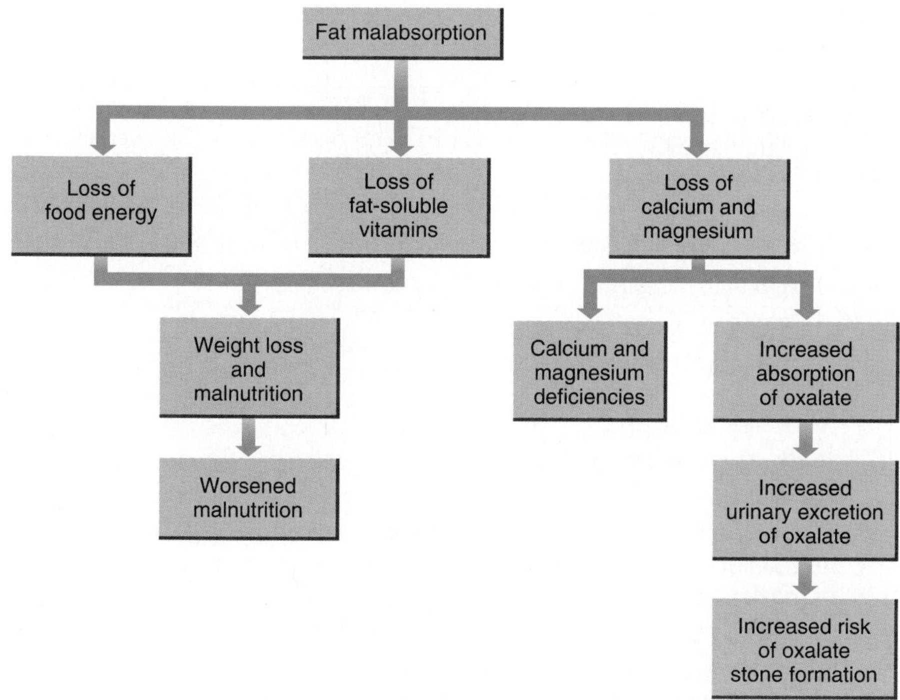

Figure 21–1
The Effects of Fat Malabsorption

Oxalate Stones The binding of calcium to fatty acids can cause another problem. Oxalate, which is present in some foods, normally binds with some of the calcium in the gut and is excreted with it. But when fatty acids bind calcium, the oxalate remains unbound and the intestine absorbs it. The body cannot metabolize oxalate, however, so it must excrete more oxalate in the urine. High urinary oxalate favors the formation of kidney stones (see Nutrition in Practice 27).

These diet principles are common to fat-restricted diets for malabsorption:

- MCT may supply part of the fat allowance.
- Fat-soluble vitamins may be given in a water-miscible form when malabsorption is severe.
- Fat is tolerated best when given in frequent small doses.

Fat-Restricted Diets

To treat steatorrhea successfully, the underlying disorder must be diagnosed and treated. Along with this treatment, dietary fat is restricted, and fat-soluble vitamins are supplemented in a water-miscible form that facilitates absorption. Tolerance to fat improves if fat is provided in frequent small meals. Often the person with malabsorption initially receives a fat-restricted diet (shown in Table 21–4 on p. 508); a sample fat-restricted diet menu is also shown.

water-miscible (MISS-ih-bul) **vitamins:** fat-soluble vitamins in a form that readily mixes with water and can be absorbed without fat.

Medium-Chain Triglycerides People on fat-restricted diets may find it difficult to get enough food energy. In such cases, products made from medium-chain triglycerides (MCT) can add energy to meals. MCT oil and formulas containing MCT provide as many kcalories as regular fats, but people who cannot digest and absorb LCT can digest and absorb MCT easily. MCT does not contain essential fatty acids, however, so the diet must include some LCT.

Recall that most naturally occurring fats are *long-chain triglycerides (LCT);* they have fatty acid chains with at least 14 carbon atoms, and they require lipase and bile for absorption. In contrast, *medium-chain triglycerides (MCT)* contain fatty acid chains with only 8 to 12 carbon atoms and they can be absorbed without lipase and bile.

MCT oil can replace regular oil in salad dressings; can be added to beverages, desserts, and other dishes; and can be used in cooking and bak-

Table 21–4
Fat-Restricted Diet (35 grams)

Use

1. Nonfat milk, nonfat-milk cheeses, yogurt made from nonfat milk, sherbet, and fruit ices.
2. Low-fat egg substitutes and up to three regular eggs per week.
3. Up to 6 oz of lean meats and poultry *without skin* daily.
4. Up to 3 servings of fat daily. One serving is any one of the following:

   1 tsp butter, margarine, shortening, oil, or mayonnaise.

   1 strip crisp bacon.

   1 tbs heavy cream or Italian or French dressing.

   ⅛ avocado.

   2 tbs light cream.

   6 small nuts.

   5 small olives.

   If fat is used to cook or season food, it must be taken from this allowance.
5. All vegetables prepared without fat.
6. All fruits prepared without fat.
7. Plain white or whole-grain bread; nonfat cereals, pasta, rice, noodles, and macaroni.
8. Clear soups and cream soups made with nonfat milk.
9. Angel-food cake and fruit whips made with gelatin, sugar, and egg-white meringues.
10. Jelly, jam, honey, gumdrops, jelly beans, and marshmallows.

Do not use

1. Whole milk, chocolate milk, whole-milk cheeses, and ice cream.
2. Pastries, cakes, pies, sweet rolls, or breads made with fat.
3. More than one egg a day, fried or fatty meats (sausage, luncheon meats, spareribs, frankfurters), duck, goose, or tuna packed in oil (unless well drained).
4. More than 3 servings of fat per day.
5. Desserts, candy, or anything made with chocolate or nuts.
6. Creamed soups made with whole milk.
7. Fried foods (except those fried with cooking sprays).

Suggestions

1. To make the diet still lower in fat, reduce the fat and meat (and egg) servings.
2. To raise the fat content, give additional fat or meat servings.
3. To improve acceptance of the diet, check the fat content of a well-liked food and allow that food if possible. Use the exchange system fat list for alternate suggestions for fat servings.

ing. Clients can obtain MCT from pharmacies without a prescription, but they are expensive.

Oxalate-Restricted Diet To reduce the risk of oxalate stones, clients with fat malabsorption may be advised to limit foods high in oxalate. Foods notable for their high oxalate content include spinach, rhubarb, beets, nuts, chocolate, tea, wheat bran, and strawberries.

Sample Fat-Restricted Diet Menu
All foods are prepared without added fat.

MENU

BREAKFAST	LUNCH	SUPPER
1 soft-cooked egg	3 oz broiled chicken	3 oz lean roast beef
1/2 c dry cereal	1/2 c rice	1/2 c mashed potatoes
4 oz orange juice	1/2 c green beans	1/2 c peas
Coffee, sugar	Tossed salad	1 slice bread
1 slice whole-wheat toast	1 tbs low-fat French dressing	1 tsp margarine
1/2 tsp margarine	Fresh apple	Peaches
Nonfat milk	Iced tea, sugar	Nonfat milk
	1 tsp margarine	**SNACK**
		Fruit ice

Tips for Fat-Restricted Diets A fat-restricted diet can be difficult to follow. Fats give flavors to foods—flavors that some people may miss. Chapter 3 offers suggestions in the box entitled "How to Lower Fat Intake—by Food Group" (p. 70), and also provides information on fat substitutes that can help to make the diet more palatable. In addition, both low-kcalorie and low-fat cookbooks feature recipes low in fat. New fat-free products appear on market shelves daily, and most people like these products. People who use MCT products should be advised to add them to the diet gradually. Nausea, vomiting, diarrhea, abdominal pain, and distention can result if a person takes too much MCT all at once.

Pancreatitis

In pancreatitis, the cause of malabsorption is impaired digestion. Pancreatic secretions contain many enzymes necessary for the digestion of protein, fat, and carbohydrate, together with bicarbonate-rich juices that provide the optimal pH necessary to activate these enzymes. By impairing digestion, pancreatic disorders impair absorption and nutrition status.

pancreatitis: inflammation of the pancreas.

Pancreatic Damage Biliary tract disease, surgery of the stomach or biliary tract, and alcoholism most often precipitate pancreatitis. The damaged pancreas retains pancreatic secretions, including digestive enzymes, and these begin to digest the pancreas itself, causing severe pain, nausea, and vomiting. In some cases, death of the pancreatic tissue leads to serious complications including fistulas and abscesses.

fistula (FIS-too-lah): an abnormal opening between two organs or from an organ to the skin.
fistula = pipe

abscess: an accumulation of pus, caused by a local infection, that builds up and may eventually burst.

Treatment of Pancreatitis Initial therapy aims to suppress pancreatic secretions. Food is withheld, since food stimulates pancreatic activity. A tube is inserted to suction out the stomach's secretions, so as to further reduce stimulation of the pancreas. Intravenous fluids are given to maintain fluid and electrolyte balance. Blood tests for pancreatic enzymes such as amylase are used to monitor progress. Falling enzyme levels indicate that pancreatitis is resolving.

Mild to Moderate Pancreatitis Mild to moderate pancreatitis often lasts for less than a week; in such cases, no special nutrition support is needed. The person can begin oral intake when abdominal pain subsides and serum amylase returns to normal or near normal. The diet progresses from a clear-liquid diet to a low-fat diet and, finally, to a regular diet as tolerated. If food intake causes pain, or if serum amylase rises, food is withheld; when these signs and symptoms subside, food can again be reintroduced.

Severe Pancreatitis If pancreatitis is severe, and if oral food intake fails to meet nutrient needs for more than a week, special nutrition support is indicated.[2] Enteral feeding is preferred, but if it worsens abdominal pain, edema, or drainage from fistulas, or if vomiting is a problem, then total nutrition by vein is the feeding of choice (see Chapter 23).

Chronic Pancreatitis If an acute episode of pancreatitis doesn't subside, or if episodes recur at frequent intervals, the pancreatic cells can be permanently destroyed, leading to chronic pancreatitis. With extensive degeneration of the pancreas, digestion, especially of fat, becomes permanently impaired. Abdominal pain is often severe and unrelenting, vomiting is frequent, and severe weight loss is common.

Moderate Fat-Restricted Diet Health care professionals recommend a moderate fat-restricted diet for chronic pancreatitis; restricting fat too severely may make it difficult for the person to gain or maintain weight. Enzyme replacements taken with meals help the person digest and absorb protein and fat. Small meals may be easiest to digest. Absolutely no alcohol is permitted.

enzyme replacements: extracts of pork or beef pancreatic enzymes that can be taken as supplements to help with digestion.

Vitamin Supplements and MCT If steatorrhea is severe, physicians prescribe fat-soluble vitamins in a water-miscible form. Vitamin B_{12} absorption may be reduced, so injections of vitamin B_{12} may be necessary. The person who needs extra food energy may benefit from products containing MCT. During active attacks of pancreatitis, diet therapy reverts to that described earlier for acute pancreatitis.

Diabetes-like Symptoms Sometimes pancreatitis damages the cells that produce insulin and its opposing hormone, glucagon. In these cases, clients become glucose intolerant, as in diabetes (see Chapter 25), and must use a diabetic meal pattern in addition to the diet restrictions already mentioned. Maintaining blood glucose in clients with chronic

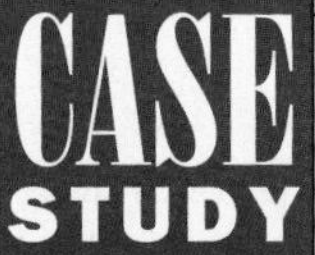

Homemaker with Pancreatitis

Mrs. Corey is a 52-year-old homemaker who was admitted to the hospital with severe abdominal pain, nausea, and vomiting. Laboratory tests reveal very high serum amylase, low serum albumin, and red blood cell indexes consistent with folate-deficiency anemia. Mrs. Corey is diagnosed as having pancreatitis. She is 5 feet 3 inches tall and weighs 100 pounds. Mrs. Corey's family has told her physician that she may have a problem with alcohol abuse. The health care team is concerned not only with the diagnosis of pancreatitis, but also with Mrs. Corey's nutrition status and possible alcohol abuse.

1. How would you describe pancreatitis to Mrs. Corey?
2. Why is her serum amylase elevated?
3. How can pancreatitis lead to poor nutrition status?
4. Discuss factors in Mrs. Corey's medical history that put her at risk for poor nutrition status. (Assume alcohol abuse for the purposes of this question and review the description in Nutrition in Practice 8 of how alcohol impairs nutrition status.)
5. Describe when and how Mrs. Corey should be fed.
6. What factors would determine the need for tube feedings or parenteral nutrition?
7. If Mrs. Corey develops chronic pancreatitis, how should her food intake be modified?
8. What other measures should be taken to ensure adequate digestion and absorption?
9. Make up a teaching plan that you would use for Mrs. Corey.

pancreatitis is often complicated by hypoglycemia, which may occur more often than in others with diabetes due to a deficiency of glucagon. The accompanying case study provides a review of pancreatitis and its treatment.

Cystic Fibrosis

Cystic fibrosis is the most common fatal genetic disorder in North America.[3] It usually starts in infancy or early childhood when nutrient needs are high. It may affect many organs, including the pancreas, lungs, liver, heart, gallbladder, and small intestine. People with cystic fibrosis often have three major symptoms: chronic lung disease, pancreatic insufficiency (which causes malabsorption), and abnormally high electrolyte concentrations in the sweat.

cystic fibrosis: a hereditary disorder characterized by the production of thick mucus that affects many organs, including the pancreas, lungs, liver, heart, gallbladder, and small intestine.

In cystic fibrosis, glands throughout the body produce a thick, sticky mucus. The airways in the lungs become plugged with mucus, making breathing labored. As the thick mucus stagnates in the bronchial tubes, bacteria multiply in it. Lung infections are the usual cause of death in people with cystic fibrosis.

Cystic fibrosis affects the pancreas in 80 to 85 percent of cases. The thick mucus obstructs the small pancreatic ducts and interferes with the secretion of digestive enzymes and pancreatic juices. It can also damage the cells that produce insulin, resulting in diabetes. Malabsorption of many nutrients, including fat, protein, vitamins, and minerals, often leads to malnutrition.

Energy and Nutrient Needs Frequent infections, rapid turnover of protein and essential fatty acids, intense protein catabolism, and high basal energy expenditure, as well as nutrient losses through malabsorption and electrolyte losses through sweat, all contribute to making energy and nutrient needs high in the person with cystic fibrosis.[4] Extra energy is needed simply to breathe. Loss of appetite with a diminished food intake is common and is aggravated by chronic infections and emotional stress. Coughing to clear the lungs may trigger vomiting or reflux of foods from the stomach. No wonder the person with cystic fibrosis finds it difficult to take in enough food energy and protein to meet needs.

Enzyme Replacements With such high energy needs, fat restriction is inappropriate; rather, enzyme replacements are used to control steatorrhea. People with cystic fibrosis who experience persistent steatorrhea, gas, and abdominal distention may find relief from these symptoms by taking larger doses of enzyme replacements.[5]

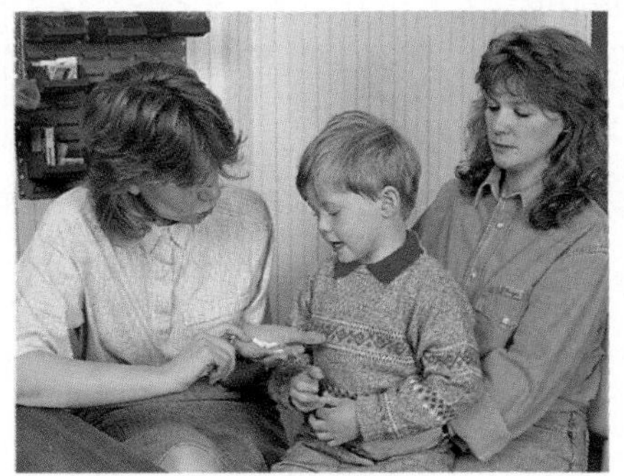

Children with cystic fibrosis may need to learn to take enzyme replacements.

Vitamin Supplementation Multivitamin supplements are prescribed to help meet the high vitamin requirements that high energy, high protein intakes demand. As the disorder progresses, extra fat-soluble vitamins are often given as well as multivitamin supplements. For people with severe steatorrhea, the water-miscible form is appropriate.

Feeding Infants For some infants, breastfeeding can sustain normal growth if enzyme replacements are given.[6] These infants must be closely monitored, however, to ensure that they meet their high energy and nutrient needs.[7] Breastfed infants with cystic fibrosis need the daily addition of ⅛ to ¼ teaspoon of table salt, given in water, to replace sweat-induced electrolyte losses.

Infants who cannot be breastfed can usually tolerate regular infant formula. Energy can be added to infant formulas by adding carbohydrate and fat, including MCT oil (see Appendix H). Infants intolerant to regular formulas often receive special, easy-to-digest formulas. Regardless of the type of feeding—human milk, standard infant formula, or special formula—enzyme replacements are always given as well.

Children and Adults A child with cystic fibrosis is weaned from breast milk or infant formula to a high-kcalorie, nutritionally balanced diet carefully tailored to the child's tolerances. Nutrition assessments repeated at regular intervals determine if nutrient intakes are adequate or if further dietary interventions are necessary. Height and weight measurements are particularly relevant. Every effort should be made to maintain each child at greater than 90 percent of weight appropriate for height, gender, and age.[8] If weight falls below 85 percent of standard weight, tube feeding is indicated.[9] Weight below 75 percent indicates advanced malnutrition that necessitates tube feeding or parenteral nutrition. For adults, the goal is to maintain a healthy weight for height.

Home parenteral and enteral nutrition programs (see Nutrition in Practice 23) may help clients meet the high nutrient needs imposed by cystic fibrosis. Clients may benefit from regular diets during waking hours and tube feedings or parenteral nutrition at night.

Emotional Support Nutrition support programs offer promise, but people with cystic fibrosis and their caregivers must deal with practical difficulties and emotional demands. The person with cystic fibrosis faces repeated hospitalizations and oftentimes an early death. The child's guardians must deal with complex emotional problems such as guilt in addition to the many aspects of care important to survival, of which nutrition is only one. The client or caregivers must ensure that daily respiratory therapy treatments, enzyme replacements, and often antibiotics are given, to say nothing of managing emotional adjustment, social life, and work or schoolwork. The accompanying case study discusses the needs of a client with cystic fibrosis.

Crohn's Disease

The two most prevalent disorders that inflame the bowel are Crohn's disease and ulcerative colitis. The two disorders share some clinical features but are thought to be distinct conditions. Their causes remain unknown.

In Crohn's disease, cracklike ulcers and many granulomas accompany inflammation of the GI tract, most often in the ileum and colon. No medical cure exists, and even if acute symptoms resolve, recurrences are likely. Chronic inflammation can cause fistulas and abscesses to develop. Scarring may narrow the intestine, sometimes obstructing it. The intestine may also rupture and cause a severe, and sometimes fatal, infection (peritonitis). These complications may necessitate surgical removal of

Crohn's disease: inflammation and ulceration along the length of the GI tract, often with granulomas; also called **regional ileitis** (ILL-ee-EYE-tis).

granulomas (gran-you-LOH-mahs): granular tumors or growths.
granulum = little grain
oma = tumor

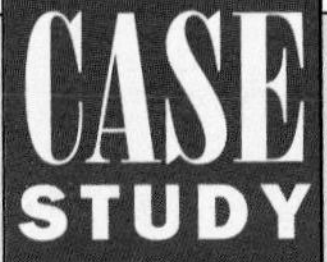

Boy with Cystic Fibrosis

Ryan is a 7-year-old boy diagnosed with cystic fibrosis. Symptoms of steatorrhea and failure to gain weight during infancy prompted tests that led to the diagnosis. Ryan is currently in the hospital to treat a respiratory infection. He has a temperature of 102°F. He is 43½ inches tall and weighs 38 pounds.

1. Describe cystic fibrosis.
2. Why are growth failure and repeated respiratory infections hallmarks of the disorder?
3. Look at the growth chart appropriate for Ryan's age and sex in Appendix E. Plot Ryan's height and weight. What does the growth chart tell you about his growth?
4. What type of diet should Ryan follow?
5. How can enzyme replacements be used effectively?
6. What important measure should be taken to ensure that Ryan's diet is adequate?
7. Formulate a teaching plan for Ryan and his parents.
8. How can people who are caring for Ryan and his family offer emotional support?

parts of the intestine. This may offer relief, but does not prevent recurrences.

The intestinal loss of serum proteins is called **protein-losing enteropathy.**

Nutrition Status Nutrition status is severely threatened in Crohn's disease. The person with Crohn's disease often experiences emotional stress, anorexia, weight loss, fever, diarrhea, malabsorption, and cramping abdominal pain—all of which can lead to nutrient deficiencies. In addition, bleeding from the ulcers can lead to anemia, and inflammation can cause the secretion and loss of serum proteins, with resulting hypoalbuminemia.[10] The accompanying drug therapy can also impair nutrition status. If the person requires surgery or develops an infection, nutrient needs become even greater. Because surgery removes a portion of the bowel, the procedure itself contributes to malabsorption (see "Malabsorption Caused by Intestinal Surgery" later in this chapter).

In children with Crohn's disease, who already need additional nutrients for growth and maturation, nutrition problems are compounded. Growth failure is common. Restoring and maintaining nutrition status for the person with Crohn's disease is therefore a challenging task. PEM and deficiencies of calcium, magnesium, zinc, iron, vitamin B_{12}, folate, vitamin C, and fat-soluble vitamins are commonly reported. Low serum albumin and multiple nutrient deficiencies threaten immune function and may reduce the effectiveness of drug therapy.

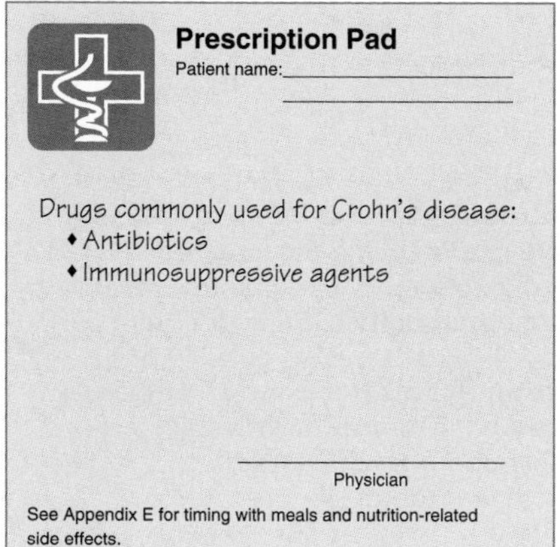

Prescription Pad
Patient name:
Drugs commonly used for Crohn's disease:
• Antibiotics
• Immunosuppressive agents
Physician
See Appendix E for timing with meals and nutrition-related side effects.

Specialized Nutrition Support In most cases, people with active Crohn's disease benefit from enteral formulas or total parenteral nutrition.[11] Enteral nutrition is the preferred feeding route, and special, easy-to-digest formulas may offer some advantages over standard formulas or table food.[12] If people cannot take these formulas orally, tube feedings are employed. In some cases, feeding tubes can be placed so as to bypass fistulas or partial obstructions, allowing enteral feeding without adding to the risk of complications. When enteral nutrition aggravates pain and diarrhea, when the bowel is obstructed or the risk of obstruction is present, when complete bowel rest might help a fistula to close, or when enteral nutrition cannot meet nutrient requirements, the IV route can be used to deliver nutrients (see Chapter 23).

Oral Diets As the acute stage of Crohn's disease resolves, the person gradually progresses, as tolerance permits, to an oral diet, often a high-kcalorie, high-protein diet. A fat-restricted diet is necessary for people with fat malabsorption. Low-fiber diets are recommended for those with partial obstructions of the intestine. Clients may be intolerant to specific foods or food components, including lactose, and these substances should be identified and eliminated from the diet. Supplemental vitamin-mineral preparations are frequently prescribed. Clients need encouragement to eat nutrient-rich, well-balanced meals. Frequent reassessment of nutrition status is needed to ensure that nutrient needs are being met. Clients who cannot maintain nutrition status on oral diets can benefit from special nutrition taken at home, as described in Nutrition in Practice 23. A Crohn's disease case study is presented to illustrate these principles.

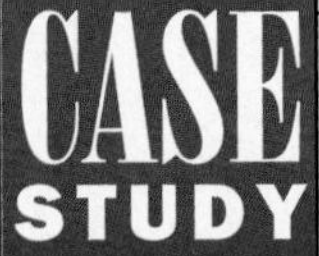

Respiratory Therapist with Crohn's Disease

Lilinoe, a 27-year-old respiratory therapist, was first diagnosed with Crohn's disease when she was 18 years old. At that time, she weighed 120 pounds and was 5 feet 7 inches tall. Her normal weight had been 130 pounds until the disease symptoms began to appear. Since then, she has been hospitalized several times for recurrent attacks of Crohn's disease. As anticipated from her weight-loss history, Lilinoe's nutrition assessment shows that she is suffering from severe PEM. In talking with Lilinoe, you discover that she is very particular about the foods she eats and often simply does not eat. Her physician has ordered a special formula diet to be fed to Lilinoe through a tube.

1. Review Lilinoe's weight history. What is her ideal body weight?
2. What measures could have been taken to avoid weight loss?
3. What possible benefits might a special formula diet offer Lilinoe?
4. Why might the physician prefer tube rather than oral feedings for Lilinoe?
5. Consider Lilinoe's long-term dietary management. What type of diet should she eventually follow?
6. What if an oral diet fails to meet her needs?
7. What goals should be set for weight gain?
8. Why is it important to reassess her nutrition status regularly?
9. Given Lilinoe's age and stage of development, what emotional concerns may she be experiencing?
10. What interventions might be planned to enhance her sense of hope, self-esteem, and well-being?

Ulcerative Colitis

Unlike Crohn's disease, which can occur anywhere along the GI tract, ulcerative colitis develops only in the large intestine. It causes severe diarrhea, rectal bleeding, cramping, abdominal pain, anorexia, and weight loss. Diarrhea can be almost continuous, resulting in poor absorption of nutrients in the upper small intestine and great losses of fluids and electrolytes. Anemia may develop due to the bleeding and nutrient losses. For people with active ulcerative colitis who fail to respond to medical therapy, surgery to remove the colon and rectum is recommended. Unlike intestinal surgery for Crohn's disease, which fails to cure the disorder, removal of the colon and rectum does cure ulcerative colitis.

ulcerative colitis (ko-LYE-tis): inflammation and ulceration of the colon.

Special Nutrition Support For people with active ulcerative colitis, no dietary interventions seem to lessen disease activity. People with severe abdominal pain and diarrhea need complete bowel rest with no enteral stimulation. Total nutrition by vein can help to maintain nutrition status, especially when surgery is anticipated.[13] Meanwhile, drugs can help to control disease symptoms.

Oral Diets Many of the dietary principles outlined for Crohn's disease apply to ulcerative colitis. A primary concern is to ensure adequate intake of fluids and electrolytes. The diet includes high-kcalorie, high-protein foods and restricts fat if the client has symptoms of fat malabsorption. Individual tolerances determine if other foods should be restricted. A low-residue or low-fiber diet is necessary for some clients; others may tolerate a regular diet. Milk and milk products may need to be eliminated if lactose intolerance is present. Supplemental vitamins and minerals may be necessary.

Malabsorption Caused by Intestinal Surgery

Surgery of the intestine may be necessary for people with inflammatory bowel diseases, cancer of the intestine, obstruction, diverticulitis, or impaired blood supply to the intestine. Diarrhea, protein and fat malabsorption, weight loss, muscle wasting, hypocalcemia, hypomagnesemia, and anemia can result. When several of these conditions occur at the same time, they are collectively called the *short bowel* or *short gut syndrome.* The actual absorption of nutrients after a small intestine resection depends on three factors:

short bowel syndrome or **short gut syndrome:** a complex of symptoms that may include diarrhea, weight loss, malabsorption, hypocalcemia, hypomagnesemia, and anemia; it can occur whenever the absorptive surface of the small bowel is reduced.

- The extent and location of the resection.
- The presence or absence of the ileocecal valve.
- The adaptive ability of the remaining bowel.

Extent and Location of the Resection Generally, up to 50 percent of the small intestine can be resected without serious nutrition consequences. Remarkably, even resections of up to 80 percent may be well tolerated, provided that the terminal ileum, the ileocecal valve, and the colon remain intact.[14] When the ileum has been resected, however, the absorption of fat, protein, carbohydrates, fat-soluble vitamins, vitamin B_{12}, calcium, and magnesium can be impaired. The ileum is also where bile salts are normally reabsorbed. Without bile salt reabsorption, a smaller body pool of bile salts is available, and this intensifies fat malabsorption (see Figure 21–2).

The Ileocecal Valve The ileocecal valve controls the rate at which the intestinal contents move from the small to the large intestine. Without the valve, transit time through the small intestine is rapid, the time available for nutrient absorption is limited, and the colon receives large volumes of fluids, electrolytes, and bile salts. Thus, nutrient absorption is impaired and severe diarrhea results. If the colon is resected as well, severe fluid and electrolyte imbalances threaten health.

Adaptation After a small intestinal resection, a remarkable adaptive response occurs in the portion of the intestine that remains: it gets longer, thicker, and wider, and it either absorbs nutrients more efficiently or begins to absorb nutrients. When the jejunum is resected, for example, the ileum begins to absorb nutrients formerly absorbed in the jejunum. The presence of nutrients appears to stimulate this adaptation—an argument for using oral or enteral nutrition whenever possible. Specific dietary constituents, namely glutamine, short-chain fatty acids, and fiber may also aid in this adaptation (recall Nutrition in Practice 18). With an extensive bowel resection, however, even adaptation will fail to compen-

Figure 21–2 Nutrient Absorption in the GI Tract
About 90 to 95 percent of nutrient absorption takes place in the first half of the small intestine. After a resection, nutrient absorption is altered.

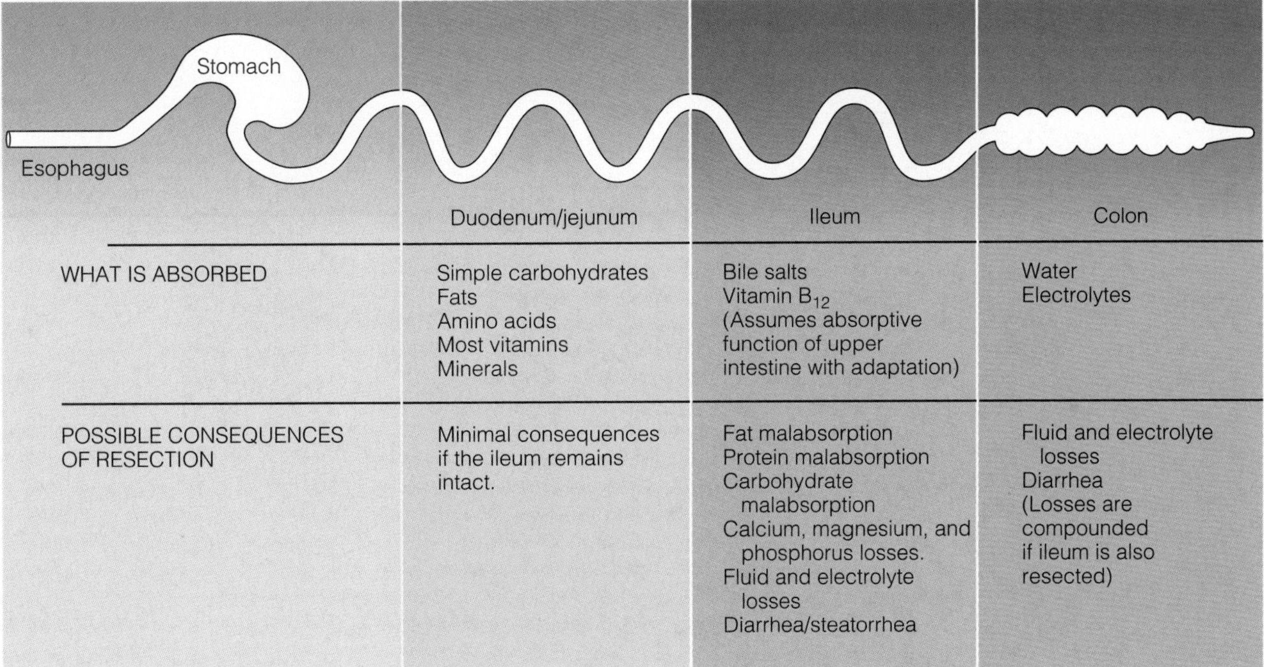

sate for the reduced surface area. People who become malnourished despite all preventive efforts require permanent parenteral nutrition support.

Stomach
Esophagus
Duodenum/jejunum
Ileum
Colon
WHAT IS ABSORBED
Simple carbohydrates
Fats
Amino acids
Most vitamins
Minerals
Bile salts
Vitamin B12
(Assumes absorptive function of upper intestine with adaptation)
Water
Electrolytes
POSSIBLE CONSEQUENCES OF RESECTION
Minimal consequences if the ileum remains intact.
Fat malabsorption
Protein malabsorption
Carbohydrate malabsorption
Calcium, magnesium, and phosphorus losses.
Fluid and electrolyte losses
Diarrhea/steatorrhea
Fluid and electrolyte losses
Diarrhea
(Losses are compounded if ileum is also resected)

Nutrition Support Immediately after surgery, the primary nutrition concern is to replace fluids and electrolytes. TPN is provided initially to meet energy and protein needs until adaptation has occurred.[15] Enteral nutrition (usually by tube feeding) is initiated in limited amounts as early as possible to stimulate adaptation. People gradually progress to oral, high-kcalorie, high-protein, fat-restricted diets, as tolerance permits. If additional energy is needed, fat intake can be increased. If fat precipitates steatorrhea, MCT can replace some of the fat to provide needed food energy. If the ileum has been resected, vitamin B_{12} cannot be absorbed and must be supplemented parenterally.

Resections of the Large Intestine Resections of the large intestine are less likely to create nutrient deficiencies than resections of the small intestine, because most nutrients are absorbed before the intestinal contents reach the colon. However, fluids and electrolytes are normally reabsorbed in the colon and losses can be severe after partial removal of the colon.

In an ileostomy, the ileum becomes the terminal GI segment. The entire colon and rectum are removed, and the ileum is then brought out

Figure 21–3 Ileostomy and Colostomy
The dotted areas show the removed section.

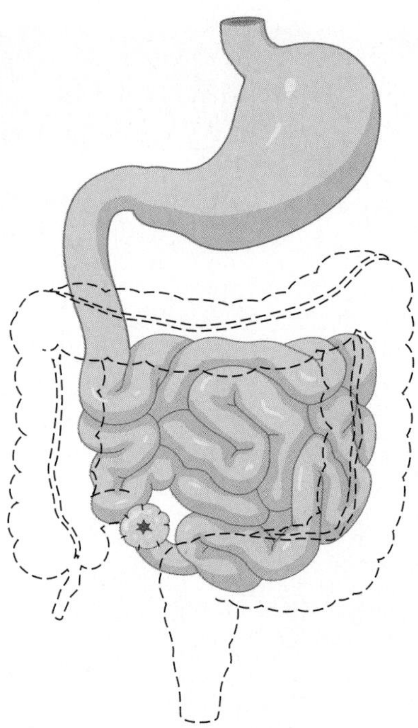

In an ileostomy, the entire colon, rectum, and anus are removed, and the stoma is formed from the ileum.

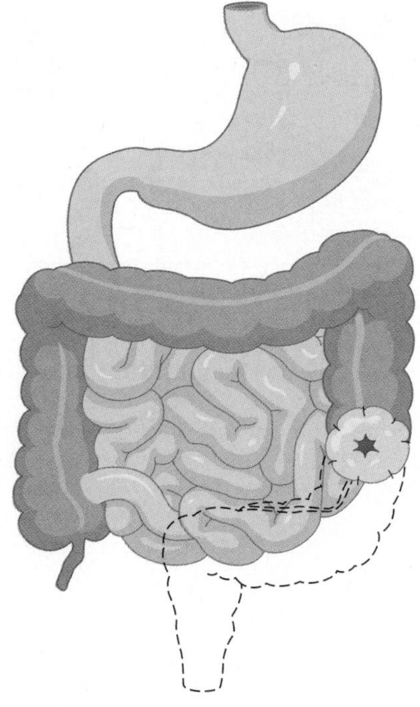

In a colostomy, the rectum and anus are removed, and the stoma is formed from the remaining colon.

stoma (STOH-ma): a surgically formed opening. After an ileostomy or colostomy, a stoma is formed as the cutoff end of the intestine is brought out through the abdominal wall, rerouting the excretion of wastes.
stoma = window

ostomate (OSS-toe-mate): a person who has a surgically formed opening from the bowel to the outside of the body, bypassing the anus. An **ileostomate** (ILL-ee-OSS-toe-mate) has an **ileostomy;** a **colostomate** (ko-LOSS-toe-mate) has a **colostomy.**

through the abdomen via a stoma to allow for defecation (see Figure 21–3). Watery stools result from ileostomies because the entire colon, which is the GI tract's water-retrieval site, has been removed. In a colostomy, part of the colon remains and is attached to the stoma; only the rectum and anus are removed. The stools resulting from colostomies are more formed because some colon remains to absorb water into the body.

Nutrition Support for Ostomates When oral intake is permitted following surgery, people who have undergone ileostomies or colostomies generally receive low-fiber diets to prevent obstructions, help promote healing of the stoma, and relieve GI upsets. However, clients need encouragement to try regular foods as soon as possible. They should add foods one at a time and in small amounts so that their effects can be assessed. If they have problems with a new food, they can try it again in a few weeks or months.

Encouraging Fluids Ostomates need extra fluid because they are absorbing less. They may tend to restrict their fluid intakes, however, for fear of aggravating diarrhea. Caregivers should explain to them that fluids help prevent dehydration and constipation, and reassure them that excess fluids taken above and beyond the amount lost through the ostomy will be absorbed and excreted by the kidneys and will not aggravate diarrhea.

Controlling Diarrhea Ostomates may benefit from foods that thicken the stool and help control diarrhea. These foods include applesauce, bananas, cheese, creamy peanut butter, and starchy foods such as breads, rice, and potatoes. Foods that may aggravate diarrhea include apple juice, grape juice, and prune juice; highly seasoned foods; and caffeine. Different individuals respond differently to these and other foods, so each person has to determine tolerances by trial and error.

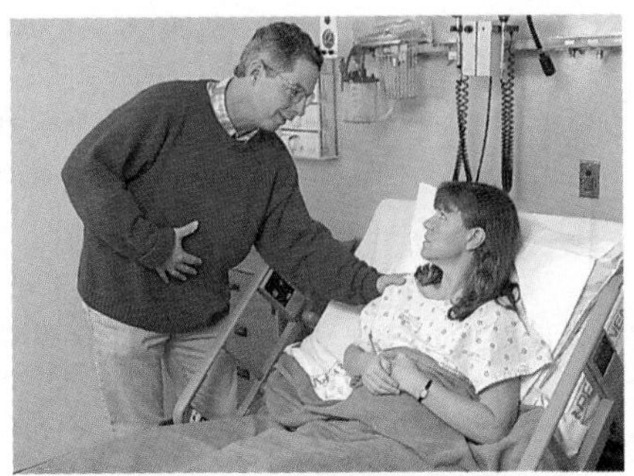

A person who has adjusted to an ostomy can greatly encourage a new ostomy client.

Reducing Gas and Odors Ostomates are often concerned about gas and odors associated with foods. Gas-forming foods in general were listed in Table 21-2, but certain particular foods seem to cause problems in ostomates: asparagus, beans, beer, broccoli, brussels sprouts, cabbage, carbonated beverages, cauliflower, eggs, fish, garlic, and onions. Foods thought to reduce odors include buttermilk, cranberry juice, parsley, and yogurt.

Preventing Obstructions Caused by Foods Some foods are more likely than others to remain incompletely digested and cause obstructions for ostomates. These include stringy foods such as celery, spinach, and bean sprouts; foods with tough skins such as dried fruits, raw apples, and corn; foods with seeds; mushrooms; and nuts. Practitioners report that some of these foods can be used if the client cuts them into small pieces and chews them thoroughly. An undigested mushroom, for example, may act as a plug and obstruct an ostomy, but if it is cut into small pieces, it may be tolerated.

Providing Emotional Support Emotional support for ostomates is best begun before surgery. They will have many adjustments to make after surgery. They often feel they have lost control over a basic and private function. The retraining required to care for the ostomy and maintain bowel function may be difficult. Ostomates may also be worried that loved ones, particularly spouses, may find them unattractive. The health care team must work closely with each person and the family to help everyone make the necessary adjustments and resume normal activities (see the case study on ileostomy on p. 520). Most communities have ostomy support groups that meet regularly to discuss mutual concerns.

A health care professional specially educated to assist ostomates in learning the proper methods of caring for ostomy sites and adjusting to the ostomy is an **enterostomal** (en-ter-oh-STOME-al) **therapist (E.T.).**

Celiac Disease

Celiac disease is a hereditary disorder with an incidence of about 1 in every 2000 to 3000 births. It arises when changes in the intestinal mucosal cells lead to malabsorption. The cells become sensitive to gluten, a protein found in wheat, oats, rye, and barley. A fraction of the gluten protein, gliadin, acts as a toxic substance, causing the intestinal villi to atrophy and seriously reducing the absorptive surface of the intestinal tract. The disaccharidases (including lactase) and the carrier molecules normally found on the villi disappear. The result is malabsorption of many nutri-

celiac (SEE-lee-ack) **disease:** a sensitivity to gliadin that causes flattening of the intestinal villi and generalized malabsorption; also called **gluten-sensitive enteropathy** (EN-ter-OP-ah-thee) or **celiac sprue.**

gluten (GLUE-ten): a vegetable protein found in wheat, oats, rye, and barley.

gliadin (GLIGH-ah-din): a fraction of the gluten protein.

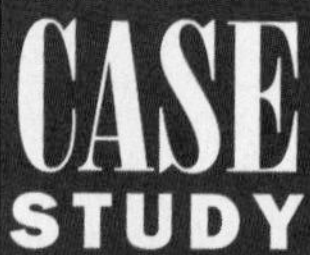

Accountant Who Underwent an Ileostomy

Tim is a 24-year-old accountant who recently developed a severe small bowel obstruction secondary to recurrent bouts of Crohn's disease. Medical and dietary management failed, and Tim underwent an ileostomy in which the ileocecal valve remained intact. Tim was malnourished on admission, and he began receiving nutrition by vein in the immediate postoperative period. After several days, he began receiving small amounts of formula through a tube.

1. Describe the alterations in nutrient absorption that will occur due to Tim's surgery.
2. Why is enteral nutrition important after a small bowel resection?
3. Tim will be coping with many fears and concerns associated with his ileostomy. How can health care professionals help him make the necessary adjustments?
4. Remember that diet is only a small part of that adjustment. What type of diet will be appropriate for Tim once he is on an oral diet?
5. How can he keep track of foods that give him problems?
6. How will his diet change in the weeks to come?

ents, including fat, protein, carbohydrate, fat-soluble vitamins, iron, calcium, magnesium, zinc, and some water-soluble vitamins.

The person with celiac disease often experiences steatorrhea, diarrhea, weight loss, and malnutrition. Anemia may occur as a result of iron, folate, or vitamin B_{12} deficiency. Because protein is malabsorbed, serum protein can decline dramatically, inducing edema. The person may develop a vitamin K deficiency and bleed easily due to clotting abnormalities. Calcium deficiency may cause tetany and bone pain.

Fortunately, when gluten is removed from the diet, the intestinal changes reverse almost completely. Generally, improvement occurs within a few weeks of strict adherence to the diet guidelines. However, lactase deficiency and lactose intolerance may be permanent. If the person fails to exclude gluten, the symptoms will return.

Remember "WORB" to identify the grains that must be restricted in celiac disease:

- **W**heat.
- **O**ats.
- **R**ye.
- **B**arley.

Gluten-Restricted Diets The treatment for celiac disease sounds deceptively simple: eliminate gluten. Such a diet prescription is easier to describe than to follow, for wheat, oats, rye, and barley are common in many foods, as you can see from Table 21–5. Processed foods such as ice cream, salad dressings, and canned foods often use wheat flour as an extender. People with celiac disease and those who care for them need help understanding what foods to avoid. They need prompting to read food labels and help in figuring out how to find foods they can eat.

Suggestions Health care professionals can suggest the use of arrowroot, corn, potato, rice, and soybean flours as substitutes for wheat flour in recipes. A low-gluten wheat starch flour is also available. Those who are lactose intolerant will also need to limit milk and milk products and find

Table 21–5
Gluten-Restricted Diet

MEAT AND MEAT ALTERNATES
Any allowed except those that are breaded, prepared with bread crumbs, or creamed.
MILK AND MILK PRODUCTS
Any allowed except milk mixed with Ovaltine, commercial chocolate milk with a cereal additive, pudding thickened with wheat flour, or ice cream or sherbet containing gluten stabilizers.
FRUITS AND VEGETABLES
Any allowed except those that are breaded, prepared with bread crumbs, or creamed.
GRAINS
Allowed: Bread, cereal, or dessert products made from arrowroot, cornmeal, soybean flour, rice flour, potato flour, and gluten-free starch; gluten-free macaroni and porridge; tapioca; cornmeal, cornflakes, popcorn, and hominy; rice, cream of rice, puffed rice, and rice flakes; potato chips. *Not allowed:* Bread, cereal, or dessert products made from wheat, oats, rye, or barley; commercially prepared mixes for biscuits, cornbread, muffins, pancakes, buckwheat pancakes, cakes, cookies, or waffles; bran; pasta; malt; pretzels; wheat germ; doughnuts; ice cream cones; matzo.
OTHER
Not allowed: Beer; ale; certain whiskeys (Canadian rye); cereal beverages (Postum); root beer; commercial salad dressings that contain gluten stabilizers; soups containing any ingredient not allowed (such as barley or noodles).

substitutes that deliver the nutrients in these foods. Any family with a member who has celiac disease needs energetic encouragement from the health care team and may benefit from attending support groups. Books, recipes, and addresses of support groups and suppliers of special food products are available and should be shared with the family.

Diverticular Disease of the Colon

Sometimes pouches of the intestinal wall (called diverticula) bulge out through the muscles surrounding the large intestine, often at points where blood vessels enter the muscles (see Figure 21–4). Evidence suggests that the pouches result from intense pressure in the intestinal lumen combined with weakness of the supporting muscles in the intestinal wall. Strong intestinal contractions pinch off segments of the intestine; pressure then builds in the segments and forces parts of the membrane of the intestine to balloon outward through the muscle layer.

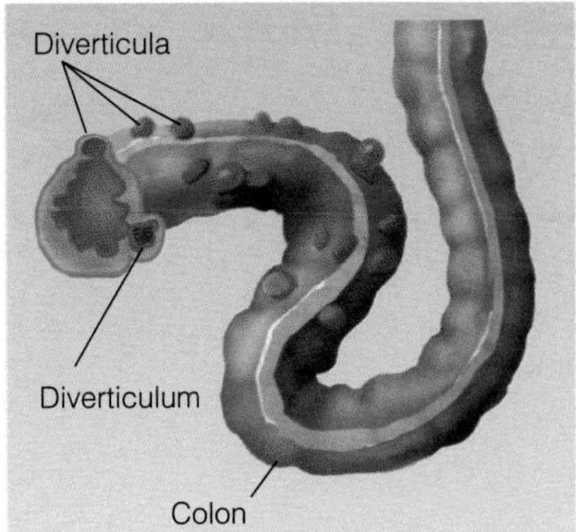

Figure 21–4 Diverticula
Outpocketings of intestinal linings that balloon through weakened muscles of the intestinal wall are known as **diverticula** (dye-ver-TIC-you-la); the singular is *diverticulum*.

diverticulosis: the condition of having diverticula.

diverticulitis: the condition of having infected diverticula.

Diverticulosis and Diverticulitis People with diverticulosis are frequently symptom-free and unaware of the disorder. In some people, however, fecal material gets trapped in the diverticula, causing inflammation and infection, a condition called diverticulitis. People with diverticulitis may suffer from cramps, alternating diarrhea and constipation, dyspepsia, gas, and abdominal swelling. Occasionally, a diverticulum ruptures, causing a life-threatening infection. If the diverticula become inflamed repeatedly, the intestinal wall can thicken, narrowing or even obstructing the intestine. An inflamed bowel segment can also stick to other pelvic organs, forming a fistula.

High-Fiber Diets For many years, health care professionals advised people with diverticulosis to adopt low-fiber diets, believing that fiber tended to become trapped in the diverticula and cause irritation. However, this advice has changed dramatically. Now health care professionals believe a high-fiber diet may actually reduce the incidence of diverticulosis by stimulating normal GI action and maintenance. Many people with established diverticular disease have been observed to remain symptom-free while following a high-fiber diet. They may, however, need to avoid foods with seeds such as okra and strawberries; the seeds may get trapped in the diverticula and cause irritation.

A high-fiber diet includes generous servings of plant foods: grains, fruits, and vegetables. It is easy to construct by following the Daily Food Guide presented in Chapter 1. Besides including the recommended servings of grains, fruits, and vegetables, the person should emphasize foods identified with the fiber symbol in Appendix C. Tips for adapting to a high fiber intake are summed up in the accompanying box; a sample high-fiber diet menu is also shown.

With help, clients can make the necessary adjustments and avoid unpleasant symptoms. During periods of active diverticulitis, a low-fiber diet is appropriate. To review your knowledge of diverticular disease, read the case study (p. 524).

Nutrition Assessment

This chapter has shown that diseases of the GI tract can impair nutrition status by interfering with food intake or the absorption of nutrients or by raising nutrient needs. Remember to keep these points in mind when you interpret nutrition assessment data:

- Review Table 21–3, which shows how malabsorption syndromes lead to poor nutrition status. Compare these factors with the client's history.
- Obtain a history of weight fluctuations, food intolerances, and chronic drug use. Weight loss commonly occurs in GI tract disorders, and PEM is a risk. Likewise, the chronic drug use often necessary to treat GI tract disorders can contribute to malnutrition.
- A history of food intolerances will be helpful in planning a diet that will cause the least discomfort. For people with malabsorption, the diet history offers the opportunity to estimate tolerance for fat. People with

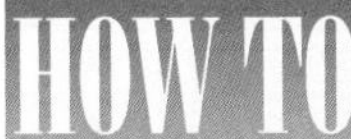

Adapt to a High-Fiber Intake

During the first few weeks on a high-fiber diet, a person may feel bloated, pass gas frequently, or experience heartburn. These suggestions may help.

1. *Motivate.* People with diverticulosis who were previously advised to adopt low-fiber diets may be skeptical about switching to high-fiber foods. To help them accept the diet change, explain the rationale for including high-fiber foods and stress the positive effects of adding these foods. Point out to them that high-fiber diets foster weight control, support GI health, help prevent colon cancer, and may lower blood cholesterol.
2. *Go slow.* Add high-fiber foods gradually, and in small portions at first. Enlarge portion sizes and add foods as tolerated.
3. *Add fluids.* Fiber attracts water as it moves through the intestine.
4. *Experiment.* Try small servings of various fiber-containing foods at first and adopt those that are most pleasing.
5. *Mix high-fiber foods with other foods.* Sprinkle bran or bran flakes on salads or applesauce. Add bran or mashed legumes to meatloaf. Add legumes and other high-fiber vegetables to soups.
6. *Use high-fiber foods rather than fiber supplements.* Supplements are associated with harmful side effects and do not provide the balance of nutrients that foods do.

Sample High-Fiber Diet Menu

MENU

BREAKFAST	LUNCH	SUPPER
1 c multigrain cereal	1 c black bean soup	3 oz baked fish
1/2 banana	3 oz broiled chicken	1 baked potato with skin
1 c nonfat milk	1/2 c steamed broccoli	1/2 c peas
1/2 grapefruit	1/2 c baked sweet potatoes	1 whole-wheat dinner roll
2 slices whole-wheat toast	1 fresh pear	2 tsp margarine
2 tbs peanut butter	1 whole-wheat dinner roll	1 piece carrot cake
1 c coffee	1 tsp margarine	1 c nonfat milk

SNACK

3 c popcorn

1 c tomato juice

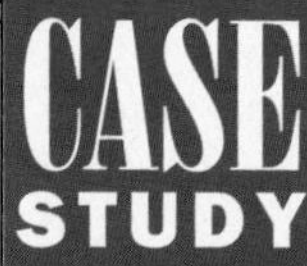

Retired Schoolteacher with Diverticular Disease

Mr. Stavros is a 69-year-old retired schoolteacher. He recently told his doctor that he had been experiencing severe cramps. He also described a change in bowel function: he is frequently constipated, although he occasionally experiences diarrhea. He further complained of indigestion and a bloated feeling. Mr. Stavros was admitted to the hospital. After an examination that included X rays of the intestine, the physician made a diagnosis of diverticulitis, for which Mr. Stavros was treated. No food or drink was allowed by mouth, and a tube was inserted to suction gastric contents. Intravenous (IV) feeding was started to prevent fluid and electrolyte imbalances. Antibiotics were also given to treat the infection. After several days, suction was discontinued, and oral intake was initiated. Once Mr. Stavros was tolerating adequate liquids orally, the IV was discontinued. He is now symptom-free and ready for discharge from the hospital.

1. Describe diverticular disease to Mr. Stavros. Be sure to distinguish between diverticulosis and diverticulitis.
2. How do diverticula form, and what consequences may follow?
3. Are Mr. Stavros's symptoms typical of people with diverticulitis?
4. Do all people with diverticular disease have such symptoms?
5. What diet would you recommend Mr. Stavros follow to treat the diverticular disease?
6. What advice can you give him about adjusting to such a diet?
7. Given his age, what may be the most difficult problem he may face?
8. How would you assess his understanding of, and compliance with, the diet?

ostomies often benefit from keeping food records to help them adjust their diets.

- Interpret anthropometric measurements cautiously because they will be affected by the state of hydration. Keep in mind that anthropometric measurements, including weight, may be deceptive in people who have edema. Remember that people with low serum albumin (as occurs in malabsorption and weight loss) often have edema.
- Evaluate results from laboratory tests. Table 21–6 lists laboratory tests used to identify various types of malabsorption syndromes.

Table 21–6
Laboratory Tests Useful in Assessing Malabsorption Syndromes

- Direct stool examination: Stool checked for weight (greater than normal weight suggests malabsorption) and oily materials (excess fat in stool suggests steatorrhea).
- Chemical analysis of fecal fat: Fecal fat of greater than 7 g/day when the diet includes 100 g of fat/day indicates fat malabsorption..
- Serum carotene: Low serum levels accompany steatorrhea.
- Serum calcium: Low levels seen in calcium or vitamin D malabsorption. (Recall that steatorrhea can lead to calcium malabsorption.)
- D-xylose test: Test of carbohydrate absorption.
- Chemical analysis of fecal nitrogen: Normal fecal nitrogen is less than 2 g/day.
- Schilling test: Usual test for identifying vitamin B_{12} malabsorption.

- Consider that biochemical measurements may be falsely elevated in dehydration. Serum albumin in people with Crohn's disease correlates with the severity of the disease rather than with nutrition status. Dehydration is a possibility in anyone who is experiencing severe diarrhea or vomiting (review Table 21–1).
- Look for signs of individual nutrient deficiencies, particularly in people with long-standing problems with malabsorption.

This chapter has shown how diseases of the intestine can seriously impair nutrition status. With careful attention to diet and medical intervention, many people can recover from such diseases and regain health.

STUDY QUESTIONS

1. Describe the dietary treatment of diarrhea. When is diarrhea a cause for alarm?
2. What are the signs of dehydration? Why is it dangerous? What are the first steps taken to remedy it?
3. What is irritable bowel syndrome, and how is diet used to control its symptoms?
4. Discuss various conditions that can lead to malabsorption. Why does fat most frequently cause problems for people with malabsorption? What are the effects of fat malabsorption? What dietary modifications can be useful in treating fat malabsorption?
5. Recommend ways to ease acceptance of a fat-restricted diet.
6. How can pancreatitis lead to the malabsorption of nutrients? Contrast the dietary treatment of a person with acute pancreatitis with the dietary treatment of a person with chronic pancreatitis.
7. What are the nutrition needs of the child with cystic fibrosis? How can the infant with cystic fibrosis be fed? What is the optimal diet for the child or adult with cystic fibrosis? How and why are enzyme replacements used in the treatment of cystic fibrosis?
8. What are inflammatory bowel diseases? Distinguish between Crohn's disease and ulcerative colitis. How can inflammatory bowel diseases lead to malabsorption?
9. Describe the diet therapy for a person with Crohn's disease.
10. What is the recommended diet for the person with ulcerative colitis?
11. What factors affect absorption after small bowel surgery? Describe short bowel syndrome and its effect on nutrition status.
12. Describe the adaptive process that occurs in the remaining intestine after a portion of the intestine is resected. What diet is most useful following intestinal resections?
13. What is an ileostomy? What is a colostomy? What diet, if any, can benefit the person who has undergone one of these procedures?
14. What protein and protein fraction are of particular concern in the person with celiac disease? What diet is useful in the treatment of celiac disease? Discuss the difficulties involved in following the diet.
15. What theory explains the development of diverticula in the intestine? What dangers are associated with diverticular disease? What diet is useful for treating diverticular disease? What precautions should the person trying a high-fiber diet for the first time take?

CLINICAL APPLICATION QUESTIONS

1. Using Table 21–4 as a guide, plan a day's menus for a diet containing 35 grams of fat. Take care to make the meals both palatable and nutritious. How can the menus be improved using the suggestions shown on p. 70?
2. With the information presented in this chapter, you can see why Crohn's disease can lead to long-term or permanent problems with the absorption of nutrients enterally. Explain why permanent feeding problems are common in people with Crohn's disease. Think about and describe the time, commitment, costs, and emotional stress that may have to go into the long-term medical and nutrition management of Crohn's disease.
3. As stated in this chapter, treatment of celiac disease is deceptively simple—eliminate gluten. Take a trip to the grocery store and randomly select 20 to 25 of your favorite snack foods and convenience foods. Check the labels of these products and see if they are allowed on a gluten-restricted diet. Find acceptable substitutes for the products that are not allowed. (Warning: This may be a tough exercise.)

NUTRITION IN PRACTICE 21

Nutrition and Diagnostic Tests

This and later chapters of this book mention many tests used in the diagnosis of clients' disorders. Nutrition can influence diagnostic test results. Some blood tests, for example, require that a person fast overnight; some require the consumption of a specific substance; and some are not affected by diet. The purpose of this Nutrition in Practice is to describe dietary precautions that relate to diagnostic tests and their interpretation.

Why must a person sometimes fast before a blood test?

Meals change the concentrations of nutrients in the blood, and this may affect test results. For example, vitamin and mineral tests often reflect recent intakes. In other cases, nutrients interfere with testing procedures. Shortly after a meal, for example, blood triglycerides rise, causing the blood to become cloudy and interfering with many metabolic reactions. Thus, if a test to ascertain blood lipids were performed after a meal, it would reflect these elevated levels, not the average blood levels of triglycerides.

In some cases, the test is designed to test the effect of a food or nutrient on a lab value. For example, tests for fat malabsorption require that a certain amount of fat be eaten prior to and during testing. Similarly, glucose tolerance tests for diabetes require a high carbohydrate intake before measurements are taken.

What test is used to diagnose fat malabsorption?

The test requires that the person's stools be collected for 48 to 72 hours while the person is on a diet that provides about 100 grams of fat per day. More than 7 grams of fat in the stools indicates fat malabsorption.

Is it safe to give a person so much fat?

Providing 900 kcalories from fat goes against traditional nutrition wisdom, but the diet is temporary, so the risk is minimal. Some people simply cannot eat that much fat, however, particularly when they are ill. In such cases, diets can be planned to include from 60 to 80 grams of fat, and different standards are used to determine malabsorption. To ensure that the data will be useful, it is essential not only to present the client with a high-fat diet, but also to monitor the actual fat intake.

When must foods be restricted so that a test will be valid?

Several tests require dietary restrictions in order to obtain valid results. One example is a test for cancer of the colon, which looks for GI bleeding. The person can take this test at home. For 48 to 72 hours before the test, and then during the three test days, in which stools are collected, the person should follow a high-fiber diet and eat no red meats, poultry, fish, turnips, or horseradish. The high-fiber foods speed up intestinal transit time and maximize the likelihood of detecting significant blood loss if it is present. Omitting red meats and other foods listed above helps prevent false positive results—that is, results that suggest significant GI blood loss, when in fact there is none.

Vitamin C and iron supplements are also restricted before and during the test. Vitamin C supplements (more than 500 milligrams per day) can produce false normal test results, even when significant GI bleeding is taking place. In contrast, iron supplements may produce some GI bleeding, even though there is no lesion.

Another test, used to detect certain tumors, also requires that certain foods be excluded. The test looks for a compound called 5-HIAA in the urine. If present, 5-HIAA signifies abnormal production of the neurotransmitter serotonin. Some foods contain significant amounts of serotonin and can interfere with test results. Diet rules for the 24 hours preceding the test are:

- *Alcohol.* Abstain completely.
- *Fruits.* Eat no avocados, bananas, kiwis, pineapples, plantains, or plums.
- *Vegetables.* Eat no eggplants or tomatoes.
- *Nuts.* Eat no butternuts, pecans, or walnuts.

Even breath tests can be affected by diet. An analysis of hydrogen in the breath is used to diagnose lactose intolerance. Foods the person eats the day before the test can influence this test's results. Breads and pastas made from wheat flour and legumes can contribute significant breath hydrogen, so the person is instructed not to eat those foods the evening before the test. The person fasts beginning at midnight. Then breath hydrogen is collected to obtain a background level, and the person takes an oral dose of lactose. Breath hydrogen is measured thereafter at intervals.

Who is responsible for making sure the diet rules are followed?

This is an important question. Like so many elements of client care, the tests require cooperation and communication between various health care professionals. First, the physician ordering the test must also order the test diet. The diet order may read simply, "diet for breath hydrogen test." In a hospital, the dietary department is then responsible for sending the appropriate diet, which is specified in the diet manual. The nurse working with the client can check the diet manual to see what the diet entails and instruct the client about the diet, making clear how long it will last. The laboratory analyzing the test may also provide information about testing precautions.

For tests that require ingestion of a measured amount of a nutrient, such as the fat malabsorption tests, nurses and dietitians frequently share responsibility for monitoring and recording the client's intake. The dietitian is often responsible for calculating expected fecal fat excretion. Nurses are responsible for stool and urine collections; laboratory technicians draw blood for blood tests.

Extra care must be taken when clients are being tested in an outpatient setting. Clients who are at home during the test period have free access to a wide variety of foods, nutrient supplements, and drugs. Often the dietitian or nurse will ask them to keep food and drug records, so that their actual intakes can be assessed.

Do drugs ever interfere with test results?

Yes, and you are wise to be alert to the potential for such interactions. Test instructions given to clients include warnings about possible drug-test interactions. Health care professionals must be aware of potential problems and give clients clear instructions about any drug use.

Finally, it is important to note that laboratory procedures change from time to time. When new and better tests are developed, precautions needed earlier may no longer apply. Regular communication between the laboratory, the physician, the nursing service, and the dietary department can help keep everyone up to date.

■ NOTES ■

1. M. E. Avery and J. D. Snyder, Oral therapy for acute diarrhea: The underused simple solution, *New England Journal of Medicine* 323 (1990): 891–894; Dietitians urged to educate parents about preventing diarrheal dehydration in children, *Journal of the American Dietetic Association* 90 (1990): 1550.
2. A.S.P.E.N. Board of Directors, Practice guidelines: Pancreatitis, *Journal of Parenteral and Enteral Nutrition* (supplement) 17 (1993): 16.
3. Determinants of energy utilization in patients with cystic fibrosis, *Nutrition Reviews* 50 (1992): 202–203.
4. J. D. Lloyd-Still, A. E. Smith, and H. U. Wesses, Fat intake is low in cystic fibrosis despite unrestricted dietary practices, *Journal of Parenteral and Enteral Nutrition* 13 (1989): 296–298.
5. M. S. Brady, Effectiveness of enteric coated pancreatic enzymes given before meals in reducing steatorrhea in children with cystic fibrosis, *Journal of the American Dietetic Association* 92 (1992): 813–817.
6. B. W. Ramsey, P. M. Farrell, and P. Pencharz and the Consensus Committee, Nutritional assessment and management in cystic fibrosis: A consensus report, *American Journal of Clinical Nutrition* 55 (1992): 108–116.
7. P. C. Cannella and coauthors, Feeding practices and nutrition recommendations for infants with cystic fibrosis, *Journal of the American Dietetic Association* 93 (1993): 297–300.
8. Ramsey and coauthors, 1992.
9. A.S.P.E.N. Board of Directors, Practice guidelines: Cystic fibrosis—Pediatric, *Journal of Parenteral and Enteral Nutrition* (supplement) 17 (1993): 44.
10. M. D. Sitrin, Nutrition support in inflammatory bowel disease, *Nutrition in Clinical Practice* 7 (1992): 53–60.
11. A.S.P.E.N. Board of Directors, Practice guidelines: Inflammatory bowel disease, *Journal of Parenteral and Enteral Nutrition* (supplement) 17 (1993): 18–19.
12. M. H. Giaffer, G. North, and C. D. Holdsworth, Controlled trial of polymeric versus elemental diet in treatment of active Crohn's disease, *Lancet* 335 (1990): 816–819; S. Klein, Elemental versus polymeric feeding in patients with Crohn's disease—Is there really a winner? *Gastroenterology* 99 (1990): 893–894; A.S.P.E.N. Board of Directors, 1993, pp. 18-19.

13. A.S.P.E.N. Board of Directors, 1993, pp. 18-19.
14. Presented by W. D. Heizer, Short bowel syndrome: Treatment strategies, *Fourth Annual Advances and Controversies in Clinical Nutrition,* sponsored by the Mayo Clinic, Jacksonville, FL, April 18, 1994.
15. P. P. Purdum and D. F. Kirby, Short-bowel syndrome: A review of the role of nutrition support, *Journal of Parenteral and Enteral Nutrition* 15 (1991): 93–101.

22

Specialized Nutrition Support: Enteral Nutrition

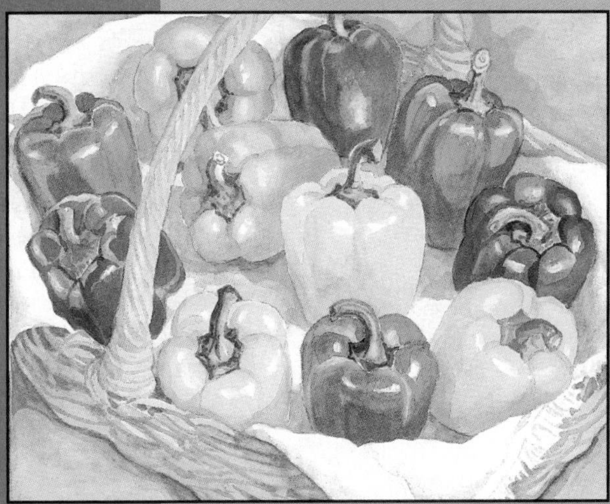

CONTENTS

To meet nutrient needs, a person must be able to eat, digest, and absorb nutrients in the amounts necessary to satisfy metabolic demands. Most people, whether healthy or ill, can meet these needs with conventional foods. As Chapters 19, 20, and 21 showed, however, some illnesses interfere with eating, digestion, absorption, or metabolism to such a degree that conventional foods fail to deliver necessary nutrients. If poor appetite is the primary nutrition problem, health care professionals diligently encourage clients to eat (see the suggestions for helping clients to eat on pp. 353–354). Alternatively, clients may benefit from meals in liquid form—that is, formulas. These can be given orally if the clients can drink them in sufficient amounts.

For clients who cannot eat or drink, it may be necessary to deliver food by tube or even by vein. Feedings by tube or mouth are *enteral* ("into the intestine") feedings, the subject of this chapter. Feedings into a vein are *parenteral* ("around" or "bypassing the intestine"), the subject of the next chapter. Actually, even for people who can take food by mouth, enteral formulas may be useful as supplemental feedings between meals. They can nourish all people whose GI tracts are working and who can digest food. Parenteral nutrition is an alternative for people whose GI tracts cannot digest and absorb nutrients from foods or enteral formulas. Figure 22–1 summarizes some of the factors involved in deciding the most appropriate way to feed a client.

enteral formulas: liquid formulas intended for oral use or for tube feedings.
enteron = intestine

Figure 22–1
Selection of a Feeding Method

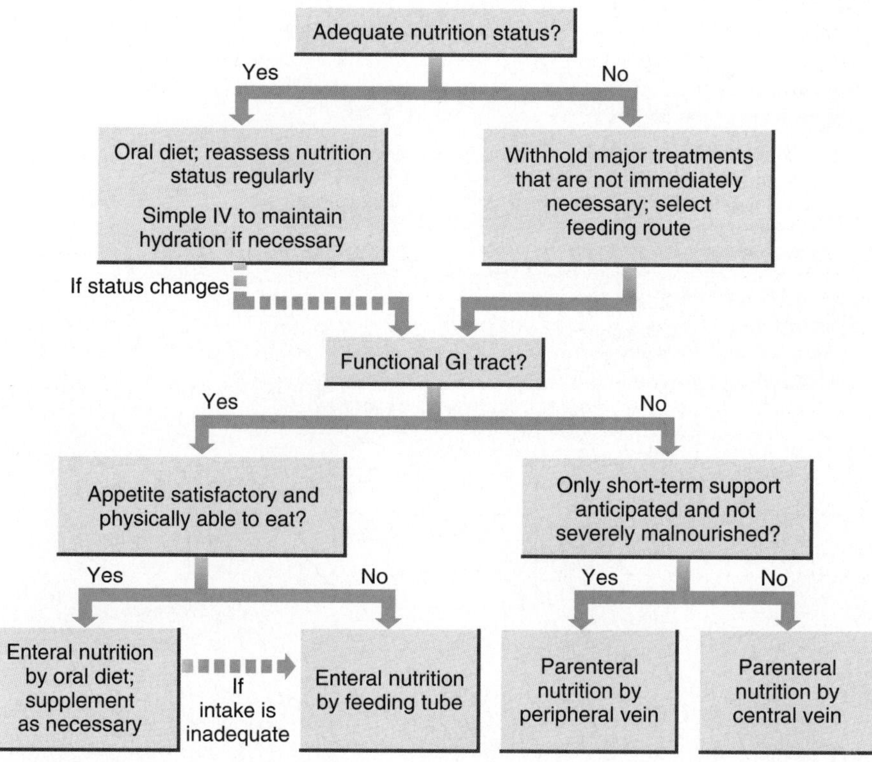

Enteral Formulas

The number of enteral formulas available is staggering (some are listed in Appendix H). Formulas are available in ready-to-use liquid form, as concentrates, or in powdered form. They are designed to meet a variety of medical and nutrition needs and can be used alone or modified with other supplements to meet an even wider range of needs. The client's specific needs, identified through a careful medical and nutrition assessment, determine the most appropriate formula for a tube feeding. Nutrition in Practice 22 describes some concerns regarding the marketing and use of formulas.

Complete formulas, when given in appropriate amounts, supply all the nutrients a client needs. Complete formulas should always be used whenever clients are receiving nothing but tube feedings or oral liquid diets for more than a few days. Complete formulas can also be (and often are) used in smaller quantities to supplement regular diets.

complete formula: a liquid formula that supplies all the nutrients needed when given in sufficient volume.

Types of Formulas

Formulas are classified in many ways, but for purposes of this book, it is reasonable to think of two major kinds categorized by the type of protein. Intact formulas contain complete proteins, whereas hydrolyzed formulas contain small fragments of proteins (including free amino acids, dipeptides, and tripeptides).

Intact Formulas Intact formulas are appropriate for people who are able to digest and absorb nutrients without difficulty; they come as either protein isolate formulas or blenderized formulas. A protein isolate formula contains a purified protein. Blenderized formulas usually contain pureed meat, vegetables, fruits, milk, and starches with vitamins and minerals added as necessary; they can be made in a blender or purchased commercially.

intact formula: a liquid diet that contains complete molecules of protein; also called a **polymeric formula.**

protein isolate: a protein that has been separated from a food such as milk. Examples include casein and albumin.

Hydrolyzed Formulas To simplify the body's digestive work, a complete protein can be partially broken down to yield small peptides. Alternatively, a formula can be made from free amino acids. In this text we call both of these types of formulas *hydrolyzed* for simplicity. Both need only minimal digestion. People who cannot digest or absorb nutrients well may benefit from hydrolyzed formulas.

hydrolyzed formula: a liquid diet that contains broken-down molecules of protein such as amino acids and short peptide chains; also called a **monomeric formula.**

Modular Formulas A few formulas, called modular formulas, are made by combining specific nutrients (protein, fat, or carbohydrate). Modules can be conventional table foods (such as vegetable oils), intravenous nutrients, or commercial formulas (see Appendix H). Modules can be added to formulas to alter their composition (for example, to add protein), or they can be mixed to construct special combinations. Modular formulas are particularly useful when clients have unusual nutrient needs. Designing a formula that will meet all of an individual's nutrient needs is a challenge that requires an in-depth knowledge of nutrition. A committed nutrition support team ensures that modular formulas are designed, prepared, and delivered in a way that meets the client's needs, which may change rapidly as medical status changes.[1]

modular formula: a formula made by combining several prepared mixtures or modules.

Nutrient Composition Formulas differ in both the amounts and types of nutrients they contain. The variations allow clinicians to select specific formulas that meet the specific needs of people with different disorders.

For practical purposes, 1 ml (milliliter) is equivalent to 1 cc (cubic centimeter).

Standard formulas provide about 1 kcalorie per milliliter. Formulas containing 1.5 to 2.0 kcalories per milliliter and more protein than standard formulas meet energy and protein needs in a smaller volume. One formula may provide a higher percentage of energy from fat, another from carbohydrate. Percentages of vitamins and minerals may also vary from one formula to the next.

Formulas also derive their nutrients from different sources. Some contain intact proteins; others hydrolyzed proteins. Some formulas provide all of their fat as long-chain triglycerides (LCT); others provide varying amounts of medium-chain triglycerides (MCT) in addition to LCT. Sources of carbohydrate also differ. One formula derives part of its carbohydrate from lactose, another from fiber. The client with lactose intolerance needs a lactose-free formula. For a client with constipation, a fiber-containing formula might help to stimulate gastric motility.

Reminder: *Residue* is the total amount of material in the colon. It includes dietary fiber and also undigested food, intestinal secretions, bacterial cell bodies, and cells shed from the intestinal mucosa.

Residue and Fiber The contribution a formula makes to fecal bulk is related to the digestibility of the formula. The total amount of material in the colon, or residue, includes intestinal secretions, bacteria, and shed mucosal cells, as well as undigested food and fiber. Low-residue formulas are well tolerated and are useful in the treatment of some GI tract disorders, for many surgeries of the GI tract, and as early feedings after GI tract disuse. Since hydrolyzed formulas are almost completely absorbed, they leave little residue in the GI tract. Many protein isolate formulas have a low to moderate residue content.

Blenderized diets contain fiber; other formulas have fiber added. Adding fiber to a formula necessarily adds residue because dietary fibers cannot be digested by enzymes in the human digestive tract. High-fiber formulas can cause gas and GI upsets in some people, but they benefit people who can tolerate them by helping to maintain GI tract integrity.[2] Because tube feedings are usually used for relatively short periods, it is not yet clear how to determine which people on tube feedings will benefit from fiber-enriched formulas.[3] Some research suggests that fiber may benefit persons with diarrhea or constipation and those who must have tube feedings for long periods.[4] Furthermore, certain fibers (pectins) may be beneficial when they are digested by bacteria in the intestine to short-chain fatty acids (see Nutrition in Practice 18).

Reminder: *Fiber* is the portion of the intestinal contents that remains in the colon because people don't have the enzymes to digest it—mostly plant fibers such as cellulose, lignin, and pectin.

Formula Osmolality Some formulas resemble blood serum in containing the same number of particles per unit of water. These are called *isotonic* formulas. Some formulas are more concentrated and are called *hypertonic* formulas. Most formulas are either isotonic or only moderately hypertonic, and people tolerate them well. Many people can also tolerate more concentrated formulas, but in some, they cause cramping and diarrhea.

Reminder: The concentration of particles in a solution is its *osmolality* and is expressed as the number of milliosmoles (mOsm) per liter. The osmolality of normal blood serum is about 300 mOsm/liter. Formula concentrations vary from about 250 to 800 mOsm/liter.

Cost Costs vary greatly for individual products in different parts of the country and for different hospitals. As a general rule, however, hydrolyzed formulas are more expensive than intact formulas because they require more commercial modification.

Despite the differences, many formulas fit into general categories, and some can be used interchangeably. For example, several intact formulas are isotonic and provide similar amounts of energy, protein, carbohydrate, fat, and other nutrients. They may derive their protein from different sources, but the sources are all high-quality proteins. One formula may provide more vitamins in a smaller volume, but that may be of little consequence to the person who is receiving a large volume of formula or a person who needs the formula only to boost energy and protein intake. In some cases, however, such differences can be significant. For example, an individual who is receiving a formula as the sole source of nutrients and who must also limit fluid intake benefits from a formula with high nutrient density.

Formula Selection

Choosing a formula can be a complicated process. Dietitians and physicians can use a logical approach to simplify decision making; Figure 22–2 shows some of the considerations involved. In a nutshell, the formula that meets the client's medical and nutrient needs with the lowest risk of complications and at the lowest cost is the best choice. If no formula can be found that meets all the client's nutrient needs, then modules can be used to create an appropriate formula (as described earlier in the discussion of modular formulas).

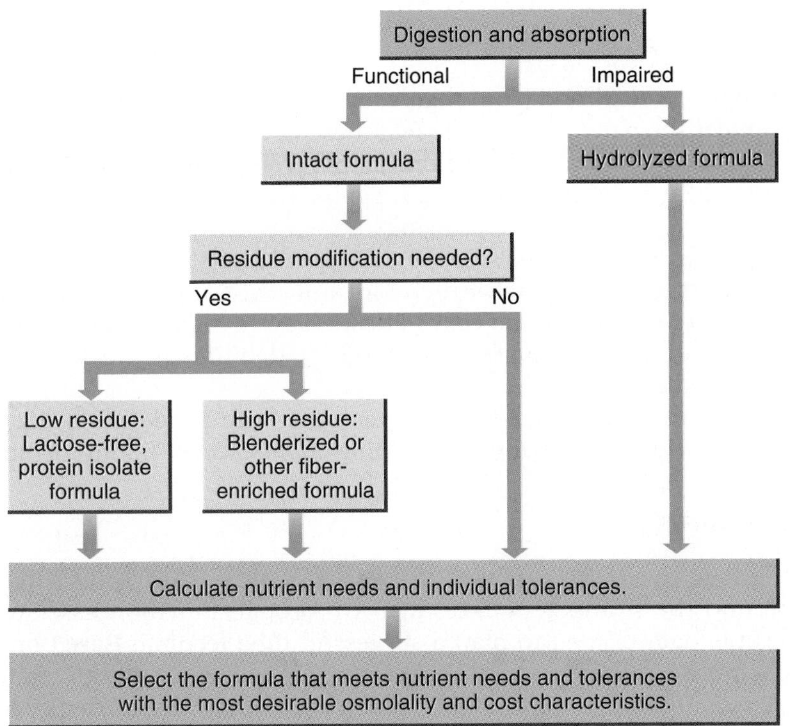

Figure 22–2
Selection of Formulas

Factors to consider in selecting a formula include:

- *The client's digestive and absorptive function.* A person whose GI tract is not functioning is not a candidate for an oral or tube feeding. People with minimal GI function, however, may be able to benefit from hydrolyzed formulas.
- *Nutrient requirements.* Nutrient requirements are estimated based on a careful nutrition assessment. The client's age, medical condition, nutrition status, and metabolic rate are all important considerations in estimating nutrient requirements. If a nutrient must be restricted, a formula must be selected that delivers just the prescribed amount of that nutrient per day.
- *Individual tolerances (food allergies and sensitivities).* Lactose-free formulas are frequently selected because temporary and permanent lactose intolerances are common problems following surgery, stress, or long periods of GI tract disuse.

For more information about lactose intolerance, see Chapter 18 (p. 455).

- *Residue or fiber modifications.* The choice of formulas is narrowed when a person needs a low-residue or high-fiber diet.
- *Availability.* Health care facilities cannot stock all formulas, so formula selection is usually limited by the local availability.

In the final analysis, the dietitian or physician can, at best, make only an educated guess about the best formula for an individual. Health care professionals monitor each person's nutrition status and tolerance to the formula and are prepared to make or recommend changes to help ensure that individual needs are being met.

Formulas Used as Supplements

supplemental nutrition: foods or oral formulas used to augment nutrient intake.

Some people can eat food from regular meals, but not in sufficient quantities to meet their nutrient needs. For these people, supplemental nutrition formulas are useful to make up the difference. Supplements can be any foods given in addition to meals, such as sandwiches at bedtime or milkshakes or instant breakfast drinks between meals. Many people do well with such supplements, and they are particularly valuable in adding energy and protein to the diet. Enteral formulas are often used as supplements; they are nutritious and easy to drink. Psychologically, liquids seem less filling, and they are easier than food for debilitated, weak, or tired people to handle.

When used as an oral diet, formulas must taste good. The accompanying box provides suggestions for helping clients accept liquid formulas.

Tube Feedings

tube feeding: feeding a nutrient solution via a tube into the stomach or intestine.

Tube feedings, or enteral nutrition, are simply complete formulas delivered by tube into the stomach or intestine. A thorough nutrition assessment provides the data needed to plan a successful tube feeding. Based on the assessment, the health care team can evaluate the client's need for a tube feeding, select the formula that will best meet the client's nutrient needs,

HOW TO Help Clients Accept Oral Formulas

People on liquid formulas are often quite ill and frequently have poor appetites. Even when a person enjoys a liquid supplement, palatability becomes a problem after long-term use. Hydrolyzed formulas are often less palatable than intact formulas, and clients may find them hard to accept. Caring health care professionals can help by using the following suggestions:

1. Ask the dietitian to let the client try different formulas appropriate for the client's needs, and select the one the client likes best.
2. Serve formulas attractively and remind clients to drink them. Formulas offered in a glass are far more appealing than those served from a can with an unfamiliar name. Some people find the smell of liquid formulas unappealing. Covering the top of the glass with plastic wrap or lid, leaving just enough room for a straw, can help.
3. Provide easy access. Keep formula close to the client's bed where little effort is required to reach it, and within sight, to remind the client to drink it. Clients who are very ill may lack the motivation even to reach for formula, let alone drink it. In such cases, offer the formula ready to drink and in small amounts, frequently during the day.
4. Keep formula in an ice bath, so that it will be cool and refreshing when the client drinks it.
5. Ask the dietitian for help if the client stops drinking the formula after a while. The dietitian may be able to recommend different flavors or a different formula to help relieve boredom.

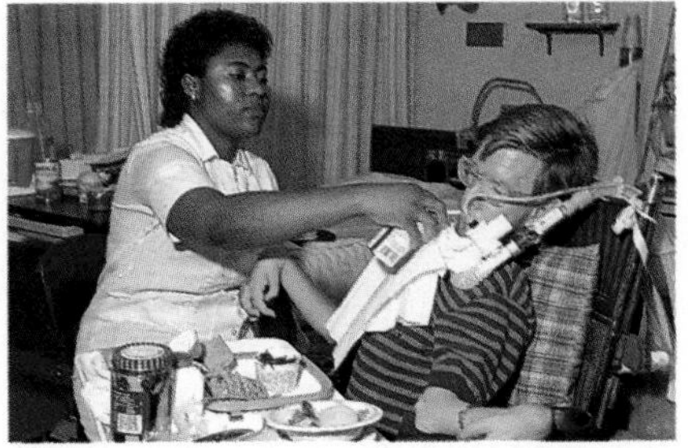

Health care professionals encourage clients to drink liquid supplements.

and choose the method that will deliver nutrients most successfully. Dietitians, uniquely attuned to the influence of age and medical conditions on nutrient requirements, assume a primary role in the management of people on tube feedings.

Reminder: Technically, both oral diets and tube feedings are types of enteral nutrition. The term *enteral nutrition* is frequently used interchangeably with *tube feeding,* however, and is often used in that sense in this book.

Candidates for Tube Feedings An individual who has a functioning GI tract but is unable to ingest enough (or the appropriate type) nutrients by mouth to meet present needs is a candidate for a tube feeding. Such a person may have medical problems that make chewing and swallowing difficult, have no appetite for an extended time, have an obstruction or altered motility in the upper GI tract, be in a coma, or have very high nutrient requirements. Table 22-1 (p. 536) lists indications and contraindications for feeding people by tube.

Advantages of Tube Feedings Tube feedings are always preferred to parenteral nutrition because, as emphasized in Chapter 18, enteral nutrition helps maintain normal GI tract function. Enteral nutrition is also associated with fewer serious complications than feeding by vein and is far less costly. In addition, enteral feedings may prevent the translocation of

Table 22–1
Indications and Contraindications for the Use of Tube Feedings

INDICATIONS
Protein-energy malnutrition with inadequate oral nutrient intake for 5 or more days
Less than 50% of required nutrient intake orally for 7–10 days
Severe dysphagia (difficulty swallowing)
Major bowel resections (see Chapter 21) when used along with parenteral nutrition
Low-output enterocutaneous fistulas (abnormal openings between an internal organ and the skin)
CONTRAINDICATIONS
Intestinal obstruction that prohibits use of the intestine
Paralytic ileus (paralysis of the intestine)
Intractable vomiting
Severe diarrhea
High-output enterocutaneous fistulas
Severe acute pancreatitis

Source: Adapted from A.S.P.E.N. Board of Directors, Guidelines for the use of enteral nutrition in the adult patient, *Journal of Parenteral and Enteral Nutrition* 11 (1987): 435, 439.

intestinal bacteria from the gut to the portal vein and lymphatic system, a recognized source of sepsis in people who are critically ill.[5] (Chapter 18 describes translocation.)

Feeding Tube Placement

Feeding tubes are inserted into different locations along the GI tract depending on the client's medical problems and estimated length of time on tube feedings. The accompanying glossary describes various feeding tube placement sites and Figure 22–3 illustrates them.

The technique for creating an opening for a tube feeding into the stomach without surgery is called **percutaneous endoscopic gastrostomy (PEG).** When the feeding tube is passed from such an opening in the stomach to the jejunum, the procedure is called a **percutaneous endoscopic jejunostomy (PEJ).** When the opening is made directly into the jejunum, the procedure is called a **direct endoscopic jejunostomy (DEJ).**

Tube Insertion When clients are not expected to be on tube feedings for more than about six weeks, feeding tubes are frequently inserted through the nose and passed into the stomach or intestine.[6] For longer feedings, or when a feeding tube cannot be passed through the nose, esophagus, or stomach due to an obstruction or for other medical reasons, an opening can be made into the stomach or jejunum. These openings can be made either surgically or nonsurgically using local anesthesia. Table 22–2 (p. 538) compares some of the features of these sites, and the box suggests ways to reduce anxiety for a client beginning a tube feeding.

Feeding Tubes Feeding tubes in wide use today are soft, flexible, and small in diameter. They come in a variety of diameters and lengths, and many have special characteristics that make them desirable for spe-

Glossary of Feeding Tube Placement Sites

These terms are listed roughly in order of the digestive tract organs.

transnasal: through the nose. A **transnasal feeding tube** is one that is passed through the nose.
naso = nose

nasogastric (NG): from the nose to the stomach.

nasoenteric: from the nose to the stomach or intestine. *Nasoenteric feedings* include nasogastric, nasoduodenal, and nasojejunal feedings. Some clinicians use *nasoenteric* to refer to nasoduodenal and nasojejunal feedings only.

nasoduodenal (ND): from the nose to the duodenum.

nasojejunal (NJ): from the nose to the jejunum.

orogastric: from the mouth to the stomach. This method is used to feed infants because they breathe through their noses and tubes inserted through the nose can make breathing difficult. The tube is inserted before each feeding and removed afterwards.

gastrostomy (gas-TROSS-toe-mee): an opening in the stomach made surgically or under local anesthesia through which a feeding tube can be passed.

jejunostomy (JEE-ju-NOSS-toe-mee): an opening in the jejunum made surgically or under local anesthesia through which a feeding tube can be passed. A **duodenostomy** (DEW-odd-eh-NOSS-toe-mee) is not used as a feeding site because the duodenum swings toward the back of the body and is not easily accessible.

cific purposes. Which feeding tube is appropriate depends on how the tube will be placed (for example, nasogastric or gastrostomy) and where it will be placed (stomach or intestine), as well as on its inner diameter. Once the appropriate length is selected, the smallest tube through which the formula will flow readily is best, but it is important that the tube not be so small that it becomes clogged. Unclogging a tube is a difficult pro-

Figure 22–3
Feeding Tube Placement Sites

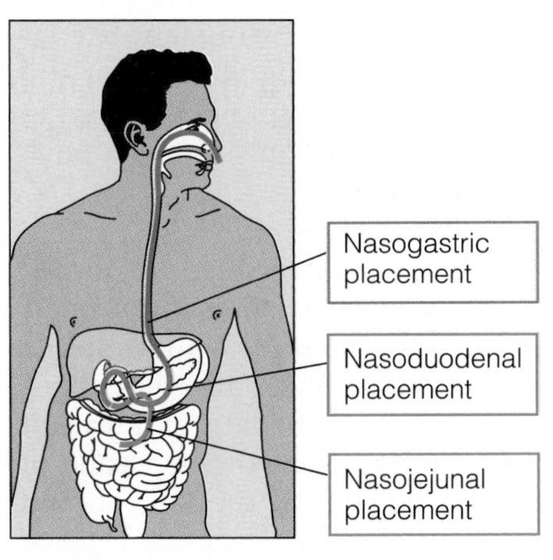

Transnasal feeding tube placements

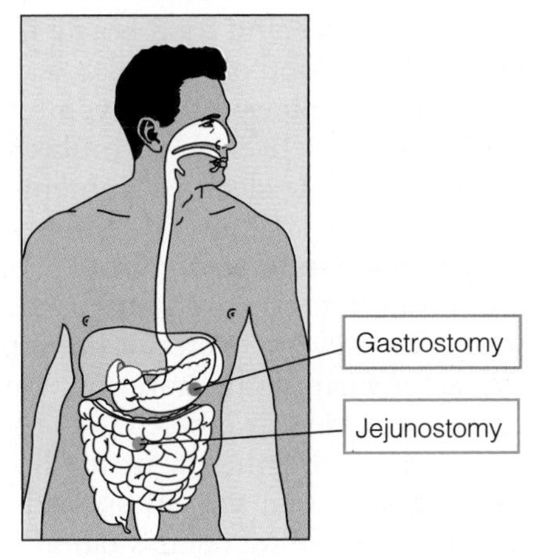

Ostomies (artificial openings in the abdominal wall)

Table 22–2
Features of Feeding Tube Sites

SITE	INSERTION	POTENTIAL IRRITATIONS	RISK OF REGURGITATION[a]	LONG-TERM TOLERANCE	CHANCE OF REMOVAL BY UNCOOPERATIVE CLIENT
Nasogastric	Nonsurgical	Nasal passages, esophagus	High	Fair[b]	Likely
Nasoduodenal	Nonsurgical	Nasal passages, esophagus	Low	Fair[b]	Likely
Nasojejunal	Nonsurgical	Nasal passages, esophagus	Low	Fair[b]	Likely
Gastrostomy	Surgery may be required	Skin irritation	Moderate	Good	Unlikely
Jejunostomy	Surgery may be required	Skin irritation	Low	Good	Unlikely

[a] Relative to the other feeding sites. The absolute risk of regurgitation depends on the person's medical condition.
[b] When the appropriate type and size of tube are used.

The inner open space of a tube or hollow organ is called the **lumen.**

cedure that interrupts the feeding schedule and is frequently unsuccessful.[7] Insertion of a new tube can cause undue stress and anxiety.

After a formula is selected for tube feeding, it must be prepared and given at intervals or continuously. Thereafter, faithful and frequent monitoring of each person helps ensure the success of the feeding.

Formula Preparation

Many people on tube feedings are severely ill, and many are likely to develop infections. People with suppressed immune systems are particularly vulnerable and food-borne illness is a threat.[8] Unfortunately, bacterial contamination of formulas occurs frequently, opening the way for still more serious illness. To prevent contamination, all personnel involved in preparing or delivering formulas should handle them only in clean environments, using clean equipment and clean hands.

At the Preparation Site Formulas that must be mixed or diluted are most often prepared and packaged in the dietary department or pharmacy. To prevent bacterial contamination, some institutions use sterile water for formula preparation. Once a formula has been mixed or diluted, the container is labeled with the client's name, room, date, and time of preparation and then sent to the nursing station. Ready-to-use cans of formula are often sent unopened to the nursing station; they too should be labeled with the client's name and room number.

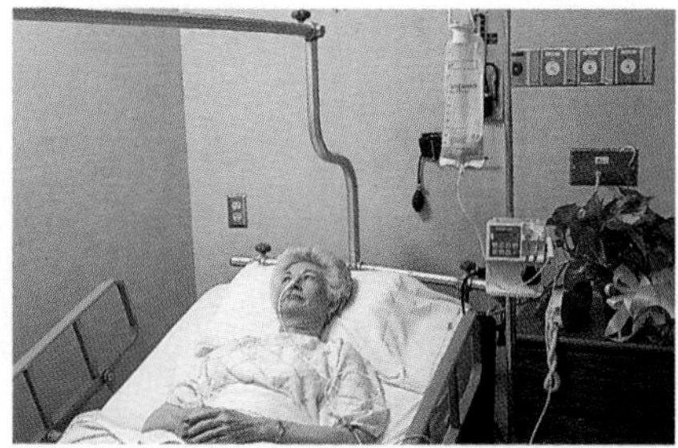

Feeding tubes provide access to the stomach and intestine for clients who cannot eat oral diets.

HOW TO Help Clients Cope with Tube Feedings

The thought of being "force-fed" is frightening to many people. One person may picture a large feeding tube and fear that the procedure will be extremely painful. Another has heard about tube feedings only from the popular press and associates a feeding tube with an irreversible coma. This person may fear that the tube feeding will be needed for a very long time. Clients who understand the strategic role that nutrition plays in recovery from disease are most likely to accept tube feedings. These pointers can help health care professionals prepare clients for transnasal tube feedings:

1. Show the client the feeding tube. Because feeding tubes are soft and narrow (only about half the diameter of a pencil), allowing the client to see and touch the tube before it is inserted eases fears.
2. Explain that the client remains fully alert during the procedure and helps pass the tube by swallowing. Health care professionals spray the back of the throat with a numbing solution to minimize discomfort and prevent gagging while the tube is being inserted.
3. Tell the client that once the tube has been inserted, most people become accustomed to its presence within only a few hours. In most cases, the client can easily swallow foods and liquids with the tube in place. If permitted, favorite foods or drinks can still be taken by mouth and enjoyed.
4. Assure the client that tube feedings are usually temporary.

Although the thought of a tube feeding is frightening for some, for others it is a relief. People who understand that they should eat, but have lost the desire, may be relieved to know they can benefit from sound nutrition without making any effort. As they feel better and begin to eat again, the tube feeding can be discontinued.

Some people feel self-conscious about how the feeding tube looks; others feel tied down by the equipment. A few simple measures can help:

- Show clients how to manipulate the feeding equipment so that they can get out of bed and move around.
- Encourage clients to walk around and socialize with other clients.
- Recommend that clients keep busy with activities they enjoy.

The more complex the procedure that a health care professional is responsible for, the more tempting it becomes to focus on the procedure and forget about the client's feelings. No matter how many technicalities you have to keep in mind, remember to stay focused on the person who is the object of your care.

At the Nursing Station Once a formula reaches the nursing station, the nursing staff assumes responsibility for its safe handling. Mixed, diluted, or open cans of formulas should be promptly refrigerated. In addition, the following steps reduce the likelihood of formula contamination:

- Before opening a can of ready-to-use formula and adding it to the feeding bag, carefully clean the can lid. If you do not add the entire can at one time, label the can with the time it was opened, cover the remaining formula or store it in a closed container, and promptly refrigerate it.
- Discard unlabeled or improperly labeled containers and all opened cans of formula not used within 24 hours.

At the Bedside Safeguard formulas delivered to the client by following these precautions:

- Before adding formula to the feeding bag or bottle, rinse the feeding container and the tubing attached to it with water and allow them to air dry. Never add fresh formula to formula still in the container.
- Flush the feeding tube with water before and after each use.
- Change the feeding bag or bottle and the tubing attached to it (except the feeding tube itself) every 12 to 24 hours.

Tube feedings sometimes come prepackaged in closed containers that can be connected directly to the feeding tube without having to be transferred to another feeding container. Such systems save nursing time and significantly reduce the risk of bacterial contamination.[9]

Formula Administration

Most people can receive undiluted formula (either isotonic or hypertonic) at the start of a feeding.[10] People under severe stress or those who have not eaten for several weeks, however, may not be able to tolerate large volumes of hypertonic formulas. In such cases, formulas are given slowly at first, at about 30 to 50 milliliters per hour. If the person tolerates the formula, the rate of feeding can be increased by 20 to 25 milliliters per hour every 6 hours (see the margin note). If the new rate is not tolerated, back up and proceed more slowly, giving the person more time to adapt.

As an example of volume progression for a tube feeding, start the feeding at 50 ml/hour at full strength and then progress the feeding as follows:

- After 6 hours: 75 ml/hour.
- After 12 hours: 100 ml/hour.
- After 18 hours: 125 ml/hour.

In addition to the formula itself, water can also be provided through the feeding tube. Using water to flush the feeding tube before and after a feeding or when the feeding apparatus is being changed not only helps prevent the feeding tube from becoming clogged but also helps keep the client hydrated. (Water can also be given orally if the person can drink it.) Supplemental water is often needed to meet the client's daily fluid requirements. Fever, excessive sweating, severe vomiting, diarrhea, blood loss, burns, and some types of kidney disease raise water requirements. In other types of kidney diseases, as well as in liver and heart diseases, total water may need to be restricted.

Formulas themselves contain considerable amounts of water. A standard formula (1.0 kcal/ml) contains about 850 ml of water per liter of formula. Higher-kcalorie formulas contain less water: formulas that contain 1.5 kcal/ml or 2.0 kcal/ml provide about 775 ml and 600 ml of water per liter of formula respectively.

Attention to indicators of body water balance can help determine how much free water an individual needs in addition to formula. In alert adults, thirst is a good regulator of water needs; a person complaining of thirst generally needs water. In elderly people, however, thirst may be slow to develop in response to dehydration. Other clues to dehydration include unexplained weight loss, high serum electrolytes or hematocrit, and low blood pressure.

Formula Delivery Techniques

When people are receiving formula, they should not be lying flat; the risk of aspiration is too great. Whatever method is used to deliver a formula, elevate the client's upper body to at least a 30-degree angle during the feeding and for 30 minutes after an intermittent feeding, whenever possible.

A day's volume of a formula can be given either intermittently (for example, four to eight times daily) or continuously over a period of 8 to 24 hours. Each method has specific uses, advantages, and disadvantages.

Intermittent Feedings Intermittent feedings are best tolerated when no more than 250 milliliters is given in 20 to 30 minutes. The larger the volume of formula needed to meet nutrient needs, the more frequently feedings are delivered. (People with very high nutrient needs who need large volumes of formula often receive feedings continuously.) Delivering formulas in larger volumes or more rapidly—called bolus feeding—often leads to complaints of abdominal discomfort, nausea, fullness, and cramping. This makes sense. After all, you do not gobble down a meal in just a few minutes, especially when you are not feeling well.

Intermittent feedings work well for clients able to tolerate them. Such feedings mimic the usual pattern of eating, allow the client freedom of movement between meals, and require less nursing time, making them less costly. Individuals on long-term tube feedings may gradually adapt to larger volumes of formula given over shorter periods of time.

Delivery of no more than 250 ml of formula over 20 to 30 minutes is sometimes called an **intermittent feeding by slow drip.** Delivery of up to 400 milliliters of formula within 10 minutes or less is called **bolus feeding.**

A can of ready-to-feed formula typically contains 240 ml of formula, and feedings are often divided so that one can of formula can be given at each feeding.

Continuous Feedings Continuous feedings are delivered slowly and in constant amounts over a period of 8 to 24 hours. Such feedings benefit people who cannot tolerate large volumes of formula. People who have received no food through the GI tract for a long time, those who are hypermetabolic, or those receiving jejunal feedings often benefit from continuous feedings. Infusion pumps (such as the one shown in the photo on p. 538) help ensure accurate and constant flow rates. The next box (p. 542) explains several ways to program tube feedings.

Delivery of a formula continuously over a period of 8 to 24 hours is called a **continuous feeding.**

Prevention of Tube-Feeding Complications

When formulas are correctly selected, prepared, and administered, and problems are quickly identified and corrected, chances are good that tube feedings will successfully support nutritional health. However, continuous monitoring of clients is necessary to prevent and eliminate problems. Table 22–3 (p. 543) provides a monitoring schedule that ensures early detection of problems.

If mechanical problems, such as a clogged feeding tube or a malfunctioning feeding pump, interrupt the feeding schedule, the client may fail to receive needed nutrients. Problems must be corrected promptly. Complications related to the formula or its administration can result in such GI complaints as nausea, vomiting, diarrhea, cramps, constipation,

Formula left in the stomach from a previous feeding is known as **gastric residual** and it is measured by gently withdrawing the gastric contents through the tube using a syringe. For intermittent feedings, the gastric residual is measured before each feeding and should not exceed 100 ml. With continuous drip administration, residual is measured every 4 to 8 hours and the measured residual should not exceed the amount of formula administered during the preceding two hours.

HOW TO Plan a Tube Feeding Schedule

To establish a tube feeding schedule, the planner needs to know how much formula a person needs in a day to meet nutrient needs. Consider, for example, a client who needs 2000 milliliters of formula per day to meet his nutrient requirements. If the client is to receive the formula intermittently six times a day, he needs about 330 milliliters at each feeding. Alternatively, if he is to receive the same volume of formula eight times a day, then he needs 250 milliliters (or about one can of ready-to-feed formula) at each feeding. He will probably tolerate this volume of formula best if it is given to him over 20 to 30 minutes or more at each feeding.

If the client is to receive the formula continuously over 24 hours, he needs 85 milliliters of formula each hour (2000 ml ÷ 24 hours = 83 ml/hour).

delayed gastric emptying, and abdominal distention. Metabolic complications such as dehydration, electrolyte imbalance, and elevated blood glucose can also occur. Table 22–4 (pp. 544–545) summarizes problems associated with tube feedings, their causes, and ways to prevent them.

Drug Administration through Feeding Tubes

Advances in our understanding of nutrition and the availability of many new formulas have supported a dramatic increase in the use of tube feedings. The method is widely used for people who are seriously ill—people who are likely to be receiving numerous medications. Often these medicines are delivered through the feeding tube, and in some cases, undesirable interactions can occur.

Keep in mind that tube-feeding formulas can interact with drugs in the same ways that ordinary foods can (see Appendix E). The effects of drug therapy should be carefully considered by the person calculating nutrient requirements.

Drugs that may clog feeding tubes include:*

- Dyazide.
- Ibuprofen.
- Magnesium oxide.
- Metamucil.
- Micro K.
- Theodur Sprinkles.

Prevent Clogged Feeding Tubes It is a common, but unwise, practice to crush tablets and mix them with water so that they will flow through the feeding tube. The particles are often too large for the lumen of the feeding tube, and if they clog the tube, this may necessitate reinsertion with considerable discomfort to the client. Even liquid medications, if they are thick and sticky, can clog feeding tubes.

Some drugs are not compatible with feeding solutions. Common examples are highly acidic drugs that thicken and clump formulas, which, in turn, clog feeding tubes. Following any of these suggestions may help minimize the likelihood of clogged feeding tubes:

---

*Source: M. L. Gora, M. M. Tschampel, and J. A. Visconti, Considerations of drug therapy in patients receiving enteral nutrition, *Nutrition in Clinical Practice* 4 (1989): 105–110.

Table 22–3
Checklist for Monitoring Clients on Tube Feedings

Before starting a new or intermittent feeding:	Complete a nutrition assessment.
	Check tube placement.
	Check gastric residual.
Every half-hour:	Check gravity drip rate, when applicable.
Every hour:	Check pump drip rate, when applicable.
Every 4 to 8 hours of continuous feeding	Check gastric residual
Every 4 hours:	Check vital signs, including blood pressure, temperature, pulse, and respiration.
Every 6 hours:	Refill feeding container.
	Check blood glucose; monitoring glucose can be discontinued after 48 hours if test results are consistently negative in a non-diabetic client.
Every 8 hours:	Check intake and output.
	Check specific gravity of urine.
	Chart client's total intake of, acceptance of, and tolerance to tube feeding.
Every day:	Weigh client.
	Change feeding bag and tubing.
	Check electrolytes, blood urea nitrogen, and blood glucose until stabilized.
Every 7 to 10 days:	Check all laboratory findings.
	Reassess nutrition status.
As needed:	Observe client for any undesirable responses to tube feeding: for example, nausea, vomiting, or diarrhea.
	Check nasogastric tube placement.
	Check nitrogen balance.
	Check laboratory data.
	Check feeding equipment.
	Chart significant details.

- Give medications orally whenever possible.
- If feasible, use an injectable or intravenous form of the drug.
- Flush the feeding tube with at least 30 milliliters of warm water or saline before and after giving any form of medicine through it.
- Deliver liquid medication through the tube using a syringe, if possible.
- Before administering thick or sticky liquid medications, dilute them with water.
- If tablets are the only form in which a medicine is available, crush them *finely* and mix them with water before administering them.[11]

Some drugs that are known to be incompatible with formulas are listed in Table 22–5 (p. 545).

Avoid Drug-Formula Interactions Medications should never be added directly to formula and allowed to hang together, because too little

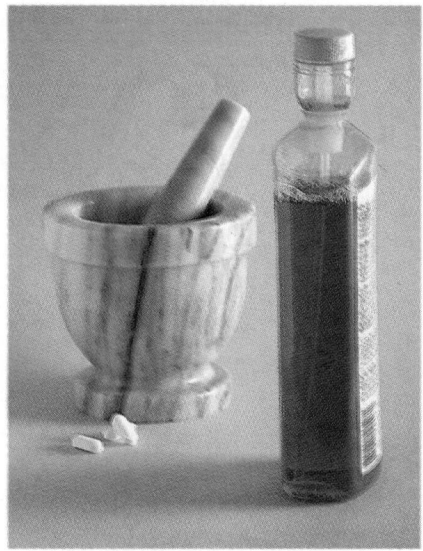

Use liquid medicines when available for delivery through feeding tubes; otherwise, finely crush the tablets and mix them with water.

Table 22–4
Causes and Prevention or Correction of Tube-Feeding Complications

COMPLICATION	POSSIBLE CAUSES	PREVENTIVE/CORRECTIVE MEASURES
Aspiration pneumonia	Regurgitation of formula, which is subsequently inhaled into lungs	Use nasoenteric, gastrostomy, or jejunostomy feedings in high-risk clients; use small-diameter transnasal tube; elevate head of bed during and 30 minutes after feeding; use continuous drip method of delivery; check gastric residual.
Clogged feeding tube	Formula too thick for tube	Select appropriate tube size; dilute formula with water; flush tubing with water before and after giving formula.
	Medications given through tube inadequately crushed or incompatible with formula	Use liquid or injectable medications whenever possible; dilute thick or sticky liquid medications with water before administering; crush tablets finely and mix with water; flush tubing with water before and after medicines are given; give medicine individually; do not mix medication with formula.
Constipation	Low-fiber formula	Provide additional fluids; use high-fiber formula; give laxatives or enemas if necessary.
	Lack of exercise	Encourage walking and other activities, if appropriate.
	Drug therapy	Change drug therapy if possible; use laxatives if indicated.
Dehydration and electrolyte imbalance[a]	Excessive diarrhea	See items under *Diarrhea.*
	Inadequate fluid intake	Provide additional fluid.
	Carbohydrate intolerance	Use continuous drip administration of formula; monitor glucose levels in blood and urine; consider administering insulin; change amount or type of carbohydrate.
Diarrhea, cramps, distention	Excessive protein intake	Monitor blood electrolyte levels; reduce protein intake.
	Bacterial contamination	Use fresh formula every 24 hours; store opened or mixed formula in a refrigerator; rinse feeding bag and tubing before adding fresh formula; change feeding bag every 24 hours; prepare formula with clean hands using clean equipment in a clean environment.
	Lactose intolerance	Use lactose-free formula in lactose-intolerant and high risk clients.
	Hypertonic formula	Use small volume of formula and increase volume gradually; use isotonic formula.
	Rapid formula administration	Use continuous drip administration of formula.
	Malnutrition/low serum albumin	Use small volume of dilute formula and increase volume and concentration gradually.
	Drug therapy	Use antidiarrheal agents; change drug therapy if possible.
	Low-fiber formula	Provide high-fiber formula.

[a] This cluster of symptoms is sometimes called the tube-feeding syndrome. Imbalances of any electrolytes are possible, and corrective measures would vary.

Table 22–4 *(continued)*

COMPLICATION	POSSIBLE CAUSES	PREVENTIVE/CORRECTIVE MEASURES
Hyperglycemia	Diabetes, hypermetabolism, drug therapy	Check glucose in blood and urine; slow administration rate; provide adequate fluids; limit type or amount of carbohydrate; consider hypoglycemic drug therapy.
Nausea and vomiting	Obstruction	Discontinue tube feeding.
	Delayed gastric emptying	Check gastric residual; use continuous drip method of administration.
	Intolerance to concentration or volume of formula	Use small volume of dilute formula and increase volume and concentration gradually; use continuous drip method of administration.
	Drug therapy	Change drug therapy if possible; use anti-nausea and antiemetic drugs.
	Psychological reaction to tube feeding	Address client's concerns.
Skin irritation around feeding ostomy site	Leakage of GI secretions and friction caused by the tube	Keep site clean; inspect area for redness, tenderness, and drainage; use protective skin cream.

Note: Many of the complications presented here can be caused by the client's primary disorder rather than the tube feeding itself. In such a case, the corrective measure would include treatment of the disorder.

is known about drug-formula interactions. Instead, deliver medications orally, by injection, intravenously, or through the feeding tube using a syringe.

Do not mix drugs together; give each drug individually, and flush the feeding tube with water after each one. This measure reduces the likelihood of both drug-formula and drug-drug interactions.

Table 22–5
Selected Drugs That Are Incompatible with Some Formulas

Chlorpromazine concentrate	Mellaril concentrate
Cibalith-S syrup	Mellaril oral solution
Dimetane elixir	Neo-Calglucon syrup
Dimetapp elixir	Paregoric elixir
Feosol elixir	Potassium chloride
Fleet's phosphosoda	Reglan syrup
Gevrabon liquid	Robitussin expectorant
Klorvess syrup	Sudafed syrup
Mandelamine Forte suspension	Thorazine concentrate
MCT oil	Zinc sulfate capsules

Note: These substances may be compatible with some formulas and not others.

Source: P. E. Burns, L. McCall, and R. Wirsching, Physical compatibility of enteral formulas with various common medications, *Journal of the American Dietetic Association* 88 (1988): 1094–1096; A. J. Cutle, E. Altman, and L. Lenkel, Compatibility of enteral products with commonly employed drug additives, *Journal of Parenteral and Enteral Nutrition* 7 (1983): 186–191.

The location of the feeding (whether gastric or intestinal) is also relevant to drug administration. Some drugs are designed to dissolve in the stomach's acidic environment. Delivered directly to the duodenum or jejunum, such drugs may not be readily absorbed. Similarly, a drug that is optimally absorbed in the duodenum may be poorly absorbed in the jejunum. In such cases, oral, intravenous, or injectable forms of the drug are appropriate.

Some types of tablets and capsules are intended to release their contents slowly. These types of medicine should not be crushed, or the person may be exposed to too much of the drug at one time.

Consider Drug-Nutrient Interactions Any drug-nutrient interaction that occurs between conventional foods and drugs can occur between formulas and drugs as well. In some cases, formulas pose special problems. One example is phenytoin (a drug used to control seizures). Absorption of phenytoin may be markedly reduced for a person who is on continuous feedings. Stop the tube feeding for two hours before and two hours after giving phenytoin whenever possible.

Limit GI Intolerances Drugs can trigger GI side effects similar to those associated with tube feedings. Nausea, vomiting, diarrhea, and electrolyte disturbances are a few of the possible complications. When tube feedings are being given, side effects of drugs should be considered as a possible source of problems. In some cases, a substitute drug with similar pharmaceutical action, but without the side effects, can be used to reduce GI problems.

An important consideration in preventing GI intolerance is the medication's concentration. Highly concentrated medications given too rapidly cause the same undesirable side effects as hypertonic formulas. To avoid problems, dilute drugs with water and administer them slowly. Then rinse the feeding tube before resuming the feeding. The physician may also consider using injectable forms of the drugs or giving smaller doses of the drug more frequently.[12]

Diarrhea is a common complication of tube feedings, and drug therapy is frequently the culprit. In addition, liquid preparations delivered through feeding tubes often contain sorbitol, a sugar alcohol that causes diarrhea if given in large doses. This is particularly likely when an adult receives a liquid pediatric preparation in high doses.

What to Chart

Chapter 14 emphasized the importance of the medical record as a communication tool. Document this information about tube feeding:

- Estimated nutrient needs.
- Type of feeding tube.
- Tube placement.
- Client's response to tube insertion.
- Administration schedule (concentration and rate).
- Method of delivery (intermittent or continuous).

- Client's tolerance to tube feeding (note any complications and any corrective actions taken).
- Client's response to tube feeding.
- Actual amount of formula the client receives.
- Reasons (if necessary) that a tube feeding was interrupted or could not be delivered as ordered.
- Drugs, drug form, and problems noted when drugs are delivered through feeding tubes.
- Education about feeding received by the client.

The dietitian records the nutrient content of the selected formula. If a person on a tube feeding does not seem to be responding adequately, investigate to see if the feeding has been delivered as intended. Some questions to consider include:

- Is the client receiving the prescribed formula?
- Is the client receiving the amount of formula that has been ordered? If not, why not? (When changing the feeding bag or adding fresh formula to a bag that has been rinsed with water, check and record the amount of formula left from the previous feeding.)
- Is the formula being delivered at the correct flow rate? If a pump is being used, is it working correctly?

Charting problems and finding solutions can help ensure that nutrient needs are met. A study of 35 people on tube feedings found that only 16 received 100 percent of their estimated energy needs on *any* day during the period they were tube fed.[13] Average intakes were only 61 percent of estimated energy needs. The major reasons cited for the failure to meet energy needs included inadvertent removal of the feeding tube, GI intolerances, intentional discontinuation of the feeding in order to perform medical procedures, and difficulty in positioning the tube in the appropriate feeding site (duodenum, jejunum). Furthermore, the study found that physicians typically ordered only 75 percent of their clients' calculated energy needs. Some of these problems can be prevented, others can be corrected. In any case, appropriate charting helps all members of the health care team to deliver optimal care.

From Tube Feedings to Table Foods

Once the problem causing the need for a tube feeding resolves, the client can gradually shift to an oral diet as the volume of formula is tapered off. The client should be eating adequate food by mouth before the tube feeding is discontinued. The person with a gastrostomy or jejunostomy can eat foods without difficulty. The person with a transnasal tube can eat orally with the tube in place. In many cases, the person can drink the same formula that was earlier given by tube. Some people cannot make the transition to oral intake for medical reasons and go home on tube feedings. (Nutrition in Practice 23 discusses how these home feedings work.) The case study on the next page helps you to consider the many factors involved in tube feedings.

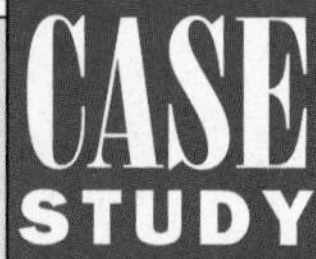

Graphics Designer Needing Enteral Nutrition

Ms. Innis is a 24-year-old graphics designer who fell from a cliff while hiking. She suffered multiple fractures. She has been in the hospital for seven days and has no appetite. Ms. Innis has lost 6 pounds over the course of hospitalization. Due to the nature of her injuries, Ms. Innis is in traction and is immobile, although the head of her bed can be elevated to 30 degrees. From the history, the dietitian determined that Ms. Innis's nutrition status was adequate prior to hospitalization. The health care team agrees that a nasoduodenal tube feeding should be instituted before nutrition status deteriorates. The intact formula selected for the feeding is lactose-free, and Ms. Innis's nutrient requirements can be met with 2500 milliliters of the formula per day.

1. What steps can the health care team take to prepare Ms. Innis for tube feeding?
2. Based on the limited information available, is the choice of formula appropriate?
3. The physician's orders specified that the feeding should be given continuously over 18 hours. Develop a tube-feeding schedule for Ms. Innis.
4. What parameters should be monitored to ensure that Ms. Innis's fluid needs are being met?
5. How can additional fluids be given?
6. Describe precautions that should be taken if Ms. Innis is to receive medications through the feeding tube.
7. After three days of feeding, Ms. Innis develops diarrhea. Look at Table 22–4 to determine the possible causes.
8. What measures can be taken to correct the various causes of diarrhea?
9. What should be charted in the medical record about Ms. Innis's tube-feeding program?
10. When Ms. Innis is ready to eat table foods again, what steps will the health care team take?

In many situations, tube feedings are a practical solution to feeding a person who is unable to consume adequate nutrients by mouth. However, a person without a functional GI tract cannot benefit from a tube feeding. In such a case, intravenous nutrition (the subject of the next chapter) can be a lifesaving treatment option.

■ STUDY QUESTIONS ■

1. Describe complete formulas, intact formulas, hydrolyzed formulas, and modular formulas, explaining the characteristics of each and how they differ.
2. What factors are considered in selecting an appropriate formula for an oral or tube feeding? How does the digestive and absorptive function of the client narrow the formula choice? How do nutrient needs affect formula selection? How does the feeding route influence formula selection? How do individual tolerances limit the choice of formula?
3. What is supplemental nutrition, and how are enteral formulas used in supplemental nutrition?
4. What are tube feedings? How are feeding tubes placed?
5. Discuss the ways in which tube feedings can be administered to clients.
6. What are the major complications of tube feedings? What are their causes? How are they prevented or corrected?
7. Describe the problems that can occur when drugs are delivered through feeding tubes. What guidelines can be used to help prevent these problems?
8. Discuss ways to help clients make the transition from tube feedings to an oral diet.

CLINICAL APPLICATION QUESTIONS

1. Complex procedures, such as those necessary to deliver enteral nutrition, require attention to many technical details, making it easy to focus on the procedure and forget about the person who is the object of your care. Consider how a person who needs a transnasal tube feeding might feel. How might she react to the insertion procedure as well as to the feeding itself? What things would she miss about eating table foods? Think of ways you might help a client on a tube feeding deal with these feelings.
2. Take a look at the checklist for monitoring people on tube feedings (Table 22–3). You can see that the person on a tube feeding requires a great deal of care. Discuss the advantages of a nutrition support team in monitoring clients on tube feedings. What contributions might various members of the team make in working with tube-fed clients (see Nutrition in Practice 14)? How can the team influence health care costs (Nutrition in Practice 19)?
3. The development of technologies for feeding people by tube and by vein has expanded our knowledge in a variety of fields and has raised important issues as well. Specifically, special nutrition support techniques have:
   - Sparked an understanding of the role of nutrition in the stress response (Chapter 18).
   - Enlightened medical professionals about the importance of the GI tract during stress (Nutrition in Practice 18).
   - Spurred progress in the home health care industry (Nutrition in Practice 23).

   Issues raised by these techniques include:

   - Formula safety and efficacy. How should formulas be regulated so that their safe use can be assured (Nutrition in Practice 22)?
   - Ethics. When are special feedings appropriate (Nutrition in Practice 28)?
   - Cost containment. Do the benefits of specialized nutrition support techniques justify their costs (Nutrition in Practice 19)?

   Reflect on Chapter 18 and its Nutrition in Practice and consider how special nutrition support contributed to knowledge of the stress response and the role of the GI tract during this response. As you read the remaining chapters, notice how special nutrition support influences medical care.

NUTRITION IN PRACTICE 22

Enteral Formulas: Who's Minding the Market?

The medical marketplace offers an astounding array of enteral formulas. New products appear regularly, paralleling the trend that favors the use of enteral over parenteral nutrition to feed people who cannot meet their nutrient needs orally. Some of these formulas contain nutrients or other dietary constituents in types or amounts that differ considerably from those found in standard diets. These formulas are a cross-breed between foods and drugs. Yet enteral formulas are exempt from the testing for safety and effectiveness that drugs must go through before they can be marketed. This Nutrition in Practice addresses the concerns health care professionals may have about the expanding enteral formula market and its regulation.

I don't understand how enteral formulas can be a cross-breed between foods and drugs. Can you explain?

The constituents of foods are delivered to the body in physiological doses—that is, doses to which the body is adapted. Physiological doses of nutrients are appropriate to sustain metabolism. The constituents of drugs are delivered to the body in pharmacological doses—that is, doses that *alter* metabolism. Even ordinary nutrients, if given in high enough doses, can have pharmacological effects.

Standard enteral formulas mimic regular diets in their sources of nutrients and proportions of protein, carbohydrate, and fat. Thus these formulas are nutritionally similar to traditional foods.

Other formulas, designed for use in specific medical situations, differ from standard formulas in either the types or amounts of nutrients they supply. Hydrolyzed formulas are special because they supply free amino acids rather than intact proteins; they are also much lower in fat than standard formulas. Other special formulas may go a step further—for example, they may provide exceptionally high doses of certain essential amino acids and low doses of others. Still other formulas may contain added amounts of dietary constituents that are not known to be essential. Formulas designed to stimulate immune function have added nucleotides, omega-3 fatty acids, and the nonessential amino acid arginine. When such formulas are used, are the dietary constituents acting as nutrients or drugs? Are the formulas being used to sustain normal physiological processes or to alter them? Finally, if the formulas alter metabolism, do the benefits outweigh the risks?

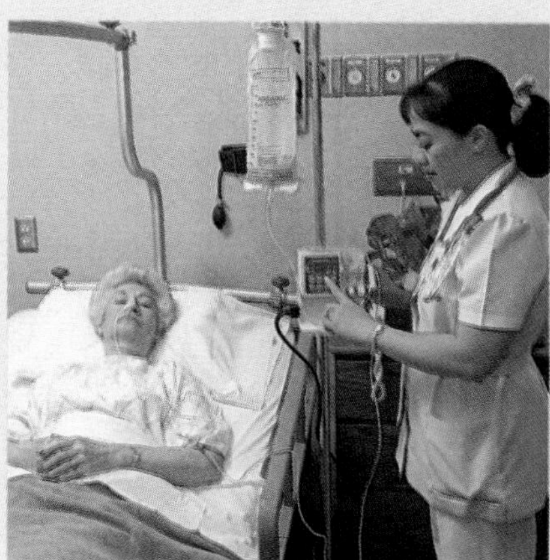

Conscientious health care professionals assume the ultimate responsibility for ensuring the safety of the enteral formulas they recommend for clients.

How are enteral formulas currently regulated?

In the United states, enteral formulas are currently regulated as "medical foods." The Food and Drug Administration (FDA) defines a *medical food* as "a food which is formulated to be consumed or administered enterally under the supervision of a physician and which is intended for the specific dietary management of a disease or condition for which distinctive nutritional requirements, based on recognized scientific principles, are established by medical evaluation."[14]

As medical foods, enteral formulas must conform to the manufacturing standards applied to all foods. These standards ensure that products are prepared in a sanitary environment and are free of contamination. They also require that the formulas contain ingredients in the amounts stated on their labels. The FDA requires manufacturers to submit evidence of the safety and suitability of medical foods for their intended purposes. Manufacturers, motivated to protect their reputations and limit their legal liabilities, generally conduct clinical trials before marketing their products and maintain high quality control standards.[15] The FDA monitors the safety and suitability of medical foods by evaluating the clinical studies submitted by manufacturers.

If clinical trials are being conducted to ensure a formula's safety, isn't that a secure guarantee of safety?

No. The research conducted to ensure the safety of formulas is far less extensive than the research drugs must undergo before they can be marketed. Most people receiving special formulas are quite ill, and they are depending on formulas as their sole source of nutrients. Their physiological processes are already altered by disease. Little is known about nutrient requirements and nutrient interactions in specific medical conditions. Do higher-than-normal amounts of one nutrient consistently benefit a client with a particular medical condition? Does the addition of this nutrient cause other nutrient deficiencies, or does it stress various organ systems to a degree that creates new medical problems? Even though questions such as these may be unanswered, manufacturers are permitted to develop formulas for specific medical conditions and to market the formulas before fully documenting their safety and effectiveness.

Can you give me an example?

Preliminary studies suggest that glutamine, a nonessential amino acid, may help protect the integrity of the GI tract during severe stress (see Nutrition in Practice 18). Because the body may not be able to make enough glutamine to meet its needs, researchers are examining whether supplemental glutamine might be a safe and effective therapy. Spurred by these potentially important studies, formulas with added glutamine have been quickly developed and marketed. The potential benefits and risks of these products, however, have not been satisfactorily documented. Consider some of these unanswered questions:

- Is glutamine a conditionally essential amino acid during stress?
- How are glutamine needs during stress affected by the type and degree of stress or by the person's age, gender, or other medical conditions?
- At what level should glutamine be supplemented?
- Is there a measurable benefit from using a glutamine-enriched formula over a standard formula provided in appropriate amounts?
- Are any risks associated with providing too much glutamine?

These questions are still to be answered. An example of a potential risk associated with glutamine-enriched formulas involves their use in people with compromised liver and kidney function. (Recall that organ function may deteriorate as a result of severe stress.) End products of glutamine metabolism include ammonia and urea, substances that can be toxic to people with inadequate liver and kidney function, respectively. Because an enteral formula often represents the sole source of nutrients for the person who needs it, and who may be quite ill, there may be little leeway for errors that could hinder recovery.

Why isn't clinical research completed before formulas are marketed?

Although clinical trials could help to refine the art of selecting and administering enteral formulas, conducting truly adequate clinical trials in human beings is extremely difficult, particularly in people with severe stresses. The type and degree of stress, individual responses to stress, prior nutrition status, age, preexisting medical conditions, and varying techniques for providing care are but a few of many factors that complicate clinical studies and limit their application to other clinical situations. Therefore, when there is evidence that a product may be beneficial, clinicians must weigh the potential benefits of the product against the potential risk of using the product for the particular client. In the example given above, a clinician may decide to use a glutamine-enriched formula for a stressed client, if the formula meets all the client's other nutrient needs and the client shows no signs of liver or kidney impairment.

Have there been any major problems with enteral formulas under current regulations?

Fortunately, no. Medical food manufacturers have an excellent record; no crises have arisen. Although clinicians hold the ultimate responsibility for using enteral products that are safe for their clients, the FDA recognizes that problems may arise as the enteral formula market expands rapidly and new manufacturers with unproven track records enter the market.

What new regulations are being proposed?

Since the 1970s, the FDA has considered proposals for medical food regulations, although none have been approved to date. Specifically, the FDA wants to clarify the definition of medical foods and incorporate it into labeling laws. The FDA notes that to qualify as medical foods, products must meet the following criteria:

- They must be designed for oral or tube feeding.
- They must be labeled for the dietary management of a disor-

der that has distinctive nutrient requirements.

- They must be intended for use with medical supervision.
- They must be specifically formulated and processed, as opposed to a naturally occurring food used in a natural state.

Products that do not qualify as medical foods include parenteral nutrients, single-nutrient preparations, weight-loss products, and foods recommended by physicians or other health care professionals as part of an overall diet to reduce the risk of a medical disease.[16]

The FDA's proposed rules further note that labeling regulations for medical foods might include:

- Labeling of nutrient content and substantiation of label claims in a different, perhaps more detailed, manner than for table foods.
- Provisions for the inclusion of adequate directions for use.
- Assurances of product quality.

As of this writing, the FDA is in the process of reviewing comments on the proposed regulations. Following the review, the FDA intends to develop final regulations. Regardless of the final regulations that govern enteral formulas, health care professionals hold the final responsibility for the safe use of these products.

What guidelines can health care professionals use to meet their responsibilities with respect to enteral formulas?

First of all, most clients on tube feedings are on standard formulas that have been used safely for many years. The benefits of these formulas outweigh the risks of starving or subsisting on nutrient-deficient intakes.

Special formulas should be thoroughly investigated by the nutrition support team or by a skilled dietitian or physician. The investigation should involve evaluating clinical studies, reviewing product literature, and determining the values of different formulas for their intended uses. Sound medical judgment that weighs the expected benefits against the potential risks of different formulas will factor heavily in the final selection of new products. Conscientious professionals know that availability of an enteral formula does not ensure safety and effectiveness. These professionals will keep abreast of new regulations and consider how these regulations will affect formula development and selection.

■ NOTES ■

1. D. K. Bernard, J. Mandt, and E. P. Shronts, Creation of a unique modular enteral feeding system, *Support Line* 15 (1993): 10–14.
2. D. C. Frankenfield and P. L. Beyer, Dietary fiber and bowel function in tube-fed patients, *Journal of the American Dietetic Association* 91 (1991): 590–596.
3. J. Slavin, Commercially available enteral formulas with fiber and bowel function measures, *Nutrition in Clinical Practice* 5 (1990): 247–250; Frankenfield and Beyer, 1991.
4. J. C. Palacios and J. L. Rombeau, Dietary fiber: A brief review and potential application to enteral nutrition, *Nutrition in Clinical Practice* 5 (1990): 99–106; K. Shankardass and coauthors, Bowel function of long-term tube-fed patients consuming formulae with or without dietary fiber, *Journal of Parenteral and Enteral Nutrition* 14 (1990): 508–512.
5. B. Langkamp-Henken, J. A. Glezer, and K. A. Kudsk, Immunologic structure and function of the gastrointestinal tract, *Nutrition in Clinical Practice* 7 (1992): 100–108; J. W. Alexander, Nutrition and translocation, *Journal of Parenteral and Enteral Nutrition* (supplement) 14 (1990): 170–174.
6. R. S. DeChicco and L. E. Matarese, Selection of nutrition support regimens, *Nutrition in Clinical Practice* 7 (1992): 239–245.
7. S. P. Marcuard, K. L. Stegall, and S. Trogdon, Clearing obstructed feeding tubes, *Journal of Parenteral and Enteral Nutrition* 13 (1989): 81–83.
8. G. Moe, Enteral feeding and infection in the immunocompromised patient, *Nutrition in Clinical Practice* 6 (1991): 55–64.
9. L. Vaughan, M. Manore, and D. Wilson, Bacterial safety of a closed-administration system for enteral nutrition solutions, *Journal of the American Dietetic Association* 88 (1988): 35–37.
10. G. P. Zaloga, Enteral nutrition in hospitalized patients: A summary, in *Enteral Nutrition Support for the 1990s: Innovations in Nutrition, Technology, and Techniques*, Report of the Twelfth Ross Roundtable on Medical Issues, Ross Laboratories, 1992.
11. M. L. Gora, M. M. Tschampel, and J. A. Visconti, Considerations of drug therapy in patients receiving enteral nutrition, *Nutrition in Clinical Practice* 4 (1989): 105–110.
12. C. Thomson and C. Rollins, Enteral feeding and medication

incompatibilities, *Support Line* 13 (1991): 9–12.

13. G. B. Abernathy and coauthors, Efficacy of tube feedings in supplying estimated energy requirements of hospitalized patients, *Journal of Parenteral and Enteral Nutrition* 13 (1989): 387–391.
14. Medical Foods, *Federal Register,* November 27, 1991, pp. 60377–60378.
15. I. S. Bass, A legal overview of the status of medical foods in the United States, *Food Drug Cosmetic Law Journal* 44 (1989): 467–477.
16. F. E. Scarbrough, Medical foods: An introduction, *Food Drug Cosmetic Law Journal* 44 (1989): 463–466.

23

Specialized Nutrition Support: Parenteral Nutrition

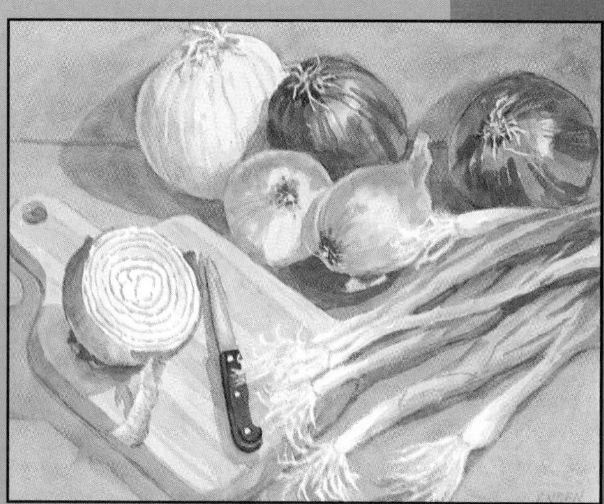

CONTENTS

As Chapter 22 described, it is best to deliver nutrition through the GI tract. Health care professionals first make every effort to feed clients an oral diet of conventional foods, supplements (including enteral formulas), or a combination. When a person with a functional GI tract cannot, will not, or should not eat an oral diet, tube feedings are given. Only when people cannot meet their nutrient requirements using the enteral route should they receive parenteral or intravenous (IV) nutrition.

parenteral nutrition: the delivery of nutrients directly through a vein, bypassing the intestines; also called **intravenous (IV) nutrition.**
para = outside
enteron = intestine
intra = within
vena = vein

Intravenous Nutrition

Although total parenteral nutrition is a lifesaving option for people with nonfunctional GI tracts, it carries a greater risk of serious complications, is more expensive, and fails to maintain GI tract integrity as well as enteral nutrition does. On the other hand, parenteral nutrition offers some practical advantages that make its use appealing to many practitioners. Because GI tolerance is not a factor in parenteral nutrition, food intolerances need not be considered in meeting nutrient needs by vein. Also, IV feedings do not have to be stopped for medical procedures and tests, whereas enteral feedings often do.

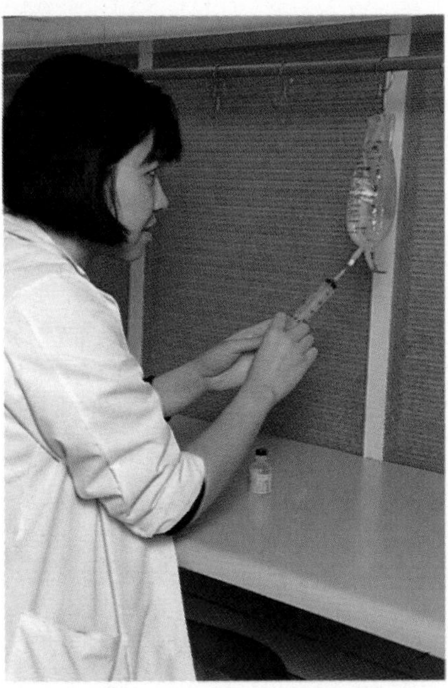

Pharmacists prepare IV solutions for each individual under sterile conditions.

Intravenous Solutions

A variety of nutrient solutions can be administered by vein to people who are unable to eat or drink. These IV solutions contain any or all of the essential nutrients: water, amino acids, carbohydrate, fat, vitamins, and minerals. The box on the next page describes how to read IV solution abbreviations.

Amino Acids Standard IV amino acid solutions contain both essential and nonessential amino acids to meet the body's need for protein. Special products that contain essential amino acids only or have large amounts of certain amino acids and small amounts of others are also available for specific medical conditions. Products designed for people with liver failure, for example, may contain more branched-chain amino acids and less aromatic amino acids because this disorder alters amino acid metabolism (see Chapter 24).

Carbohydrate Standard IV solutions provide carbohydrate as dextrose, a form of glucose that is especially soluble in water. Whereas glucose provides 4.0 kcalories per gram, dextrose provides only 3.4 kcalories per gram because it contains some water.

Fat Intravenous fat emulsions are the vehicle for fat in IV solutions. Intravenous fats are provided either daily or periodically (once or twice a week). If provided daily, IV fat can serve as a concentrated source of energy; if offered less often, it serves primarily as a source of essential fatty acids. Ten percent fat emulsions provide 1.1 kcalories per milliliter, and 20 percent fat emulsions provide 2.0 kcalories per milliliter.

A 500-milliliter bottle of a 10% IV fat emulsion provides 550 kcalories; a 500-milliliter bottle of a 20% IV fat emulsion provides 1000 kcalories.

HOW TO Read IV Solution Abbreviations

The labels of IV solutions use several abbreviations, including:

- **D:** dextrose.
- **W:** water.
- **NS:** normal saline (0.9 percent sodium chloride solution).

Interpret these abbreviations as follows:

- **D_5W:** Read as 5 percent dextrose in water (the subscript following the *D* tells you the percentage of dextrose in the solution).
- **D_{10}W:** Read as 10 percent dextrose in water.
- **D_5½ NS:** Read as 5 percent dextrose in a ½ normal saline solution (0.45 percent sodium chloride).

How would you read D_{50}W?

Intravenous fat can safely provide about 50 percent of the total daily energy requirement for many clients who are not severely stressed.[1] For clients under stress, clinicians frequently provide up to 30 percent of the total daily energy need as fat.[2]

The source of lipid in IV fat emulsions may be important.[3] Currently available IV fat emulsions, which are made from egg phospholipids and plant-derived oils, are rich sources of omega-6 fatty acids. When given in excess, these fatty acids may impair immune function, a threat to critically ill people. Alternate lipid sources are currently under investigation. Among the possible alternates are fish oils (a rich source of omega-3 fatty acids) and triglycerides chemically modified to contain both long- and medium-chain fatty acids.

Intravenous fat emulsions are contraindicated for some individuals. Examples include newborns with markedly elevated bilirubin levels, people with severe liver disease, people with some types of hyperlipidemias, and those with severe egg allergies. Cautious use of IV fats is recommended for people with atherosclerosis, moderate liver disease, blood coagulation disorders, pancreatitis, and some types of lung problems.

bilirubin: a pigment in the bile whose concentration in the blood may become elevated as a result of some disorders.

Liver disease is the subject of Chapter 24. Hyperlipidemias and atherosclerosis are discussed in Chapter 26.

Occasionally, people experience adverse reactions to IV fat emulsions, particularly when the fats are given in large doses or administered too rapidly. Immediate reactions may include fever, warmth, chills, backache, chest pain, allergic reactions, palpitations, rapid breathing, wheezing, cyanosis, nausea, and an unpleasant taste in the mouth. Irritation and inflammation of the vein are also possible. After long-term administration, brown pigments may accumulate in certain liver cells, but these pigments disappear after parenteral therapy is stopped, and their effects on liver function are unknown. Other effects of prolonged IV fat use may include an enlarged liver and spleen and a decline in the number of blood platelets and white blood cells, suggesting a possible impairment of immune function.

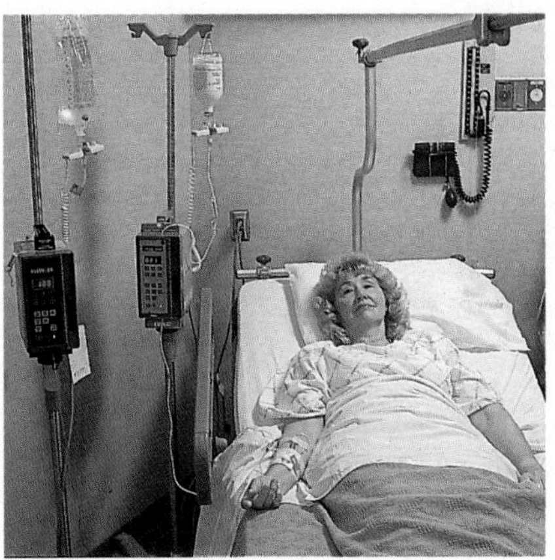

Intravenous fat emulsions provide energy and essential fatty acids and can be recognized by their milky white color.

Micronutrients Vitamins, electrolytes (minerals), and trace elements may be used in IV solutions. Currently available IV multivitamin solutions for adults meet the recommendations of an American Medical Association nutrition advisory group and do not include vitamin K; this vitamin is added separately if needed.[4] Pediatric multivitamin solutions contain vitamin K.

Some electrolytes (particularly calcium and phosphorus) can precipitate with other IV solution components. As an indication of the seriousness of this problem, the Food and Drug Administration (FDA) recently warned health care professionals that a precipitate of calcium phosphate might have been responsible for two deaths and at least two cases of respiratory distress in one institution.[5] A skilled pharmacist knows how to mix solutions to minimize the risk of precipitation.

Other Additives Medications are sometimes added to IV solutions. Common examples include heparin, insulin, cimetidine, ranitidine, and famotidine.

Intravenous Feeding Methods

Intravenous solutions can be delivered in different ways. The method used depends on the person's nutrition status, anticipated length of time on IV nutrition support, and nutrition needs.

Simple IV Solutions Simple IV solutions are used routinely in hospitals to provide water, dextrose, and electrolytes, and they help to maintain or restore the fluid-and-electrolyte and acid-base balances. For the well-nourished person who is expected to eat within a few days following surgery or trauma, simple IV solutions are very useful.

People who cannot use their GI tracts for a long time, those who are malnourished, and those who have high nutrient requirements need more complete solutions than a simple IV offers, however. The next box (p. 558) explains how to calculate the nutrient content of IV solutions. Highly concentrated nutrient solutions cannot be infused by simple IV delivery because the small-diameter peripheral veins, such as those in the forearm and on the back of the hand, become irritated and eventually collapse. To deliver all the needed nutrients by less-concentrated solutions would require 12 to 15 liters of solution a day, a volume far greater than the body could safely handle. Instead, the required nutrients are provided by complete parenteral nutrition.

peripheral veins: the small-diameter veins that bring blood to the extremities (arms and legs).

Peripheral Total Parenteral Nutrition (Peripheral TPN) The delivery of IV fat, amino acids, dextrose, vitamins, minerals, and trace elements by peripheral vein to meet all nutrient needs is peripheral total parenteral nutrition (peripheral TPN). A typical peripheral TPN solution

peripheral total parenteral nutrition (peripheral TPN): the provision of a nutrient solution that meets nutrient needs by peripheral vein.

HOW TO Calculate the Nutrient Content of IV Solutions

You can have confidence in IV solutions if you know what is in them. The basic thing to remember is that the percentage of a substance in solution tells you how many grams of that substance are present in 100 milliliters. For example, a 5 percent dextrose solution contains 5 grams of dextrose per 100 milliliters. A 3.5 percent amino acid solution contains 3.5 grams of amino acids (protein equivalents) per 100 milliliters. A 0.9 percent normal saline solution contains 0.9 grams of sodium chloride per 100 milliliters.

Suppose a person is receiving 1500 milliliters of 50 percent dextrose and 1500 milliliters of 7 percent amino acid solution. For dextrose, the person would get:

$$\frac{50 \text{ g dextrose}}{100 \text{ ml}} = \frac{x \text{ g dextrose.}}{1500 \text{ ml}}$$

$$\frac{50 \text{ g dextrose} \times 1500 \text{ ml}}{100 \text{ ml}} = 750 \text{ g dextrose.}$$

And for amino acids:

$$\frac{7 \text{ g amino acids}}{100 \text{ ml}} = \frac{x \text{ g amino acids.}}{1500 \text{ ml}}$$

$$\frac{7 \text{ g amino acids} \times 1500 \text{ ml}}{100 \text{ ml}} = 105 \text{ g amino acids.}$$

To calculate the total kcalories in the mixture, simply multiply by kcalories per gram:

$$750 \text{ g dextrose} \times 3.4 \text{ kcal/g} = 2550 \text{ kcal}$$

$$105 \text{ g amino acids} \times 4.0 \text{ kcal/g} = 420 \text{ kcal}$$

$$\text{Total} = 2970 \text{ kcal}$$

delivers about 2500 kcalories per day and provides about 150 grams of amino acids; IV fat contributes more than half of the total kcalories. Intravenous fat emulsions are isotonic to blood and do not irritate the veins the way hypertonic glucose and amino acid solutions do.

One liter of a typical peripheral TPN solution contains 10% dextrose and 5% amino acids. Often 3 liters of the solution are given daily along with 1 500-milliliter bottle of 20% IV fat emulsion.

Peripheral TPN best suits people who need only short-term nutrition support (about 7 to 14 days), people with normal renal function who do not have excessive energy requirements, people who are allowed unrestricted fluids, people in whom inserting an IV catheter into a central vein might be difficult, and people on oral or tube feedings who need additional nutrients temporarily.[6] People with weak peripheral veins that collapse easily or those with fluid restrictions are not candidates for peripheral TPN.

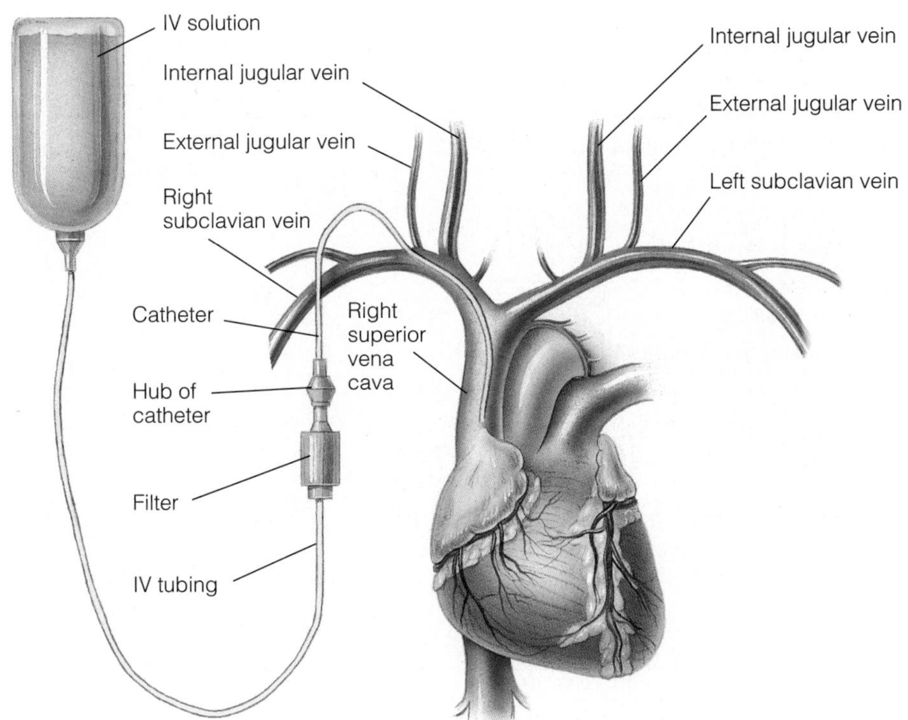

Figure 23-1
The Central Veins Used for TPN
Most often, TPN catheters enter the circulation at the right subclavian vein and are threaded into the superior vena cava with the tip of the catheter lying close to the heart. Less often, catheters are threaded into the superior vena cava from the left subclavian vein, the internal jugular veins, or the external jugular veins.

TPN by Central Vein Another method used to meet all nutrient needs by vein is TPN by central vein. This method is sometimes called central total parenteral nutrition, but it is usually abbreviated simply TPN. In TPN, the IV catheter is placed in a large-diameter central vein (see Figure 23-1). Almost a gallon of blood rushes through one such vein, the right superior vena cava, each minute, so highly concentrated solutions quickly become diluted. By the time these solutions reach the peripheral veins, they are diluted and, therefore, not irritating.

TPN is indicated whenever the GI tract cannot be used, long-term parenteral nutrition will be required, and nutrient needs are high. Some specific conditions that may necessitate its use are listed in Table 23-1 (p. 560). Ideally, the person should not reach a severely depleted state before TPN is initiated. It is much easier to maintain nutrition status than to try to replenish lost nutrient stores with TPN.

The actual concentrations of amino acids and dextrose that compose the TPN solution are determined by each person's unique medical and nutrient needs. TPN solutions meet energy needs primarily from dextrose or a combination of dextrose and fat. Current practice is to use IV fat emulsions frequently so that they can serve as a daily energy source. People with severe stress may become intolerant to high glucose loads. Providing fat allows glucose intake to be reduced, thus helping to alleviate this problem. Providing more energy from fat may also be beneficial for people in respiratory failure, because fat oxidation produces less carbon dioxide than glu-

central veins: the large-diameter veins located close to the heart (see Figure 23–1).

central total parenteral nutrition (TPN): a method of meeting all nutrient needs by infusing formulas into large-diameter central veins.

IV catheter: a thin tube inserted into a vein through which nutrient solutions or medications can be given directly.

One liter of a typical central TPN solution contains 25% dextrose and 3.5% amino acids. Often 3 liters of the solution are given daily and provide 3000 kcalories and 105 g protein.

Table 23–1
Possible Indications for TPN by Central Vein

Extensive small bowel resections
Radiation enteritis (inflammation of intestine caused by radiation)
Severe diarrhea
Intractable vomiting
GI obstructions
Bone marrow transplants
Inflammatory bowel disease (see Chapter 21)
Severe acute pancreatitis
Severe malnutrition when GI tract is nonfunctional
Hypermetabolic disorders, or major surgery, when it is anticipated that the GI tract will be unusable for more than 2 weeks
Enterocutaneous fistulas
Severe nausea and vomiting associated with pregnancy (hyperemesis gravidarum) when it lasts for more than 14 days
Severe malnutrition if surgical or intensive medical intervention is necessary
When it is anticipated that adequate enteral nutrition cannot be established within 14 days of hospitalization

respiratory acidosis: a condition of too much acid in the blood caused by failure of the lungs to ventilate properly. Excess acids are normally released from the lungs during exhalation; diseased lungs, however, are unable to perform this function rapidly enough.

cose oxidation does. Carbon dioxide dissolved in the blood becomes carbonic acid, and excesses can lead to respiratory acidosis.

Intravenous Nutrition Techniques

Intravenous formulas are like tube feedings in that careful attention to formula selection, preparation, and delivery helps minimize the risks of complications. The risks associated with IV nutrition are more serious than those associated with enteral nutrition.

Insertion and Care of the TPN Catheter

Insertion of a catheter for peripheral TPN is the same as for simple IV solutions, but for central TPN it often requires a surgical procedure. A qualified physician may insert the catheter at bedside, however, rather than in an operating room. The client generally is awake but is given a local anesthetic. Unnecessary apprehension can be avoided by explaining the procedure to the client.

Maintaining the integrity of peripheral veins is often a problem for peripheral TPN. Veins may become inflamed (phlebitis) and sometimes infected. Often the infusion catheter must be removed and reinserted at a new site; consequently, long-term feedings are difficult and rarely indicated.

Reminder: The presence of disease-causing bacteria in the blood is *sepsis*. Sepsis is a major complication of TPN.

Infections can develop at the catheter site in both peripheral TPN and central TPN. Compared with peripheral TPN, though, central TPN presents a greater risk of introducing disease-causing microorganisms into the bloodstream because the catheter is inserted so near the heart. Health care workers must inspect the catheter site regularly and change the dressing frequently to keep the site clean.

Administration of the TPN Solution

Just as a tube feeding is started slowly to allow the GI tract to adapt to the formula, a central TPN feeding is started slowly to give the person time to adapt to the high glucose concentration and osmolality of the TPN solution. Typically, 1 liter of TPN solution is infused by continuous drip during the first 24 hours. An infusion pump is used to ensure an accurate delivery rate. Electrolytes and blood glucose are monitored periodically. If tests indicate electrolyte imbalances or unacceptably high blood glucose, the causes are investigated and treated. After the first 24 hours, the infusion rate is often increased by 1 liter a day until the desired volume of solution is being given every 24 hours.

Rapid changes in the infusion rate can cause significant hypoglycemia or hyperglycemia, which can lead to coma, convulsions, and even death, so all changes must be made gradually and carefully. When the administration of solution gets behind or ahead of schedule, the drip rate should be adjusted to the correct hourly infusion rate, but no attempt should be made to speed up or slow down the rate to meet the originally ordered volume. When a person is being taken off TPN, the infusion rate of the solution must be tapered off gradually; otherwise, hypoglycemia can occur. Table 23-2 (p. 562) lists the many types of complications associated with TPN, and Table 23-3 (p. 563) provides guidelines for monitoring clients on TPN.

Peripheral TPN Infusion Unlike central TPN solutions, peripheral TPN does not have to be increased gradually when feedings are initiated or tapered off gradually when feedings are discontinued. Peripheral TPN solutions do not have such high nutrient concentrations and do not present the associated problems.

TPN solutions that contain all nutrients, including fat, are called *total nutrient admixtures, three-in-one admixtures,* or *all-in-one admixtures.*

IV Fat Infusion Traditionally, amino acids, dextrose, and micronutrients are mixed together to form the base TPN solution. Intravenous fat emulsions are then infused separately from the base solution. In periodic IV fat administration, usually a 500-milliliter bottle of IV fat is infused over 6 to 8 hours, two to three times per week. When the IV fat is used as an energy source, the IV fat emulsion is sometimes added directly to the base TPN solution.

Cyclic Infusion Another way of administering TPN is called cyclic parenteral nutrition. A person on cyclic parenteral nutrition receives a TPN solution consisting of dextrose, amino acids, and fat for 8 to 12 hours a day. The infusion can be given during the night to allow freedom for normal daytime activities and is often used for long-term support.

cyclic parenteral nutrition: the periodic administration of standard TPN solutions.

Administering TPN solutions in this way may help prevent a problem that has been observed when TPN is given continuously: when a person receives a TPN solution by continuous drip, insulin levels stay high. As a result, the person cannot mobilize fat stores for energy or to free up essen-

Table 23–2
Complications Associated with TPN

CATHETER- OR CARE-RELATED COMPLICATIONS
Fluid in the chest (hydrothorax)
Air or gas in the chest (pneumothorax)
Blood in the chest (hemothorax)
Catheter tip broken off, obstructing blood flow (catheter embolism)
Air leaking into catheter, obstructing blood flow (air embolism)
Hole or tear made in heart by catheter tip (myocardial perforation)
Catheter inadvertently placed in subclavian artery (arterial puncture)
Improperly positioned catheter tip
Sepsis
Blood clot (thrombosis)
METABOLIC COMPLICATIONS
Elevated blood glucose (hyperglycemia)
Low blood glucose (hypoglycemia)
Dehydration
Coma from excessive glucose load (hyperosmolar, hyperglycemic, or nonketotic coma)
Low blood magnesium (hypomagnesemia)
Low blood calcium (hypocalcemia)
High blood phosphorus (hyperphosphatemia)
Low blood phosphorus (hypophosphatemia)
Low blood potassium (hypokalemia)
Essential fatty acid deficiency
Trace element deficiencies
High blood ammonia levels (hyperammonemia)
Acid-base imbalances
Elevated liver enzymes

tial fatty acids, and eventually fat may be deposited in the liver. Cyclic TPN reverses these problems.[7] Additionally, fewer kcalories seem to be necessary to maintain nitrogen balance, probably because the person uses body fat for energy. Some people, however, cannot tolerate large volumes of solutions delivered in shorter periods of time.

From Parenteral to Enteral Feedings

Once the problem causing the need for IV nutrition resolves, the client can gradually shift to an enteral diet while the volume of the IV feeding is tapered off. This transition requires careful planning. During long periods of disuse, the intestinal villi shrink and lose some of their function. The return to enteral nutrition must be gradual to avoid problems of malabsorption and other GI discomforts. Reintroducing nutrients to the GI

Table 23-3
Guidelines for Monitoring People on TPN

Every 4 to 6 hours:	Check blood glucose. Monitor vital signs (respiration, pulse, temperature).
Daily:	Monitor weight changes. Record intake and output carefully. Check urine specific gravity.
Daily until stable, and then two or three times weekly:	Monitor serum electrolytes. Monitor blood urea nitrogen.
Weekly:	Conduct a nutrition assessment. Monitor serum protein. Monitor serum calcium. Monitor serum phosphorus. Monitor serum ammonia. Monitor complete blood count.

tract at the appropriate rate and volume will stimulate the progressive restoration of the villi's normal structure and function.

Transitional Feedings The transition from IV feeding to an enteral diet can be accomplished in different ways and often involves a combination of feeding methods. One way is to start an oral diet while the person is still on IV nutrition. The diet is often progressive, beginning with liquids, and given in small amounts. If the person cannot eat enough food to meet at least 50 percent of daily nutrient needs within a few days, and intake does not seem to be improving, tube feedings should be considered.[8]

Whether a person is given a tube feeding initially or provided an oral diet and then switched to a tube feeding, the volume of the IV solution is reduced as the volume of tube feeding is increased. The person who cannot tolerate large volumes of tube feeding can still rely on TPN to meet nutrient needs. Parenteral nutrition can be discontinued when at least 60 percent of estimated energy needs are being met by oral intake, tube feeding, or a combination of the two.[9] (Chapter 22 described the transition from tube feedings to table foods.)

Psychological Effects Returning to oral intake after having been fed either intravenously or by tube can have a variety of psychological effects. Some people may be extremely eager to eat again, and food can be an important morale booster. Others may be apprehensive about eating, particularly if they have had extensive GI problems. Appetite may be slow to return for some. In such circumstances, all members of the health care team can support the successful reintroduction of food. Recognize each person's concerns, and provide reassurances that you will be there to help throughout the process. The many decisions surrounding the provision of TPN require careful consideration. The case study on the next page presents an example for review.

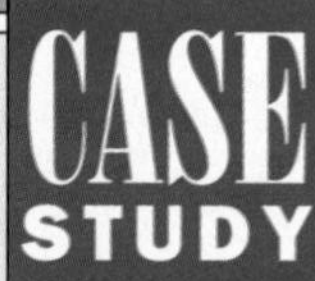

Mail Carrier Needing Parenteral and Transitional Nutrition

Mr. Rossi, a 37-year-old mail carrier, has been admitted to the hospital for Crohn's disease (see Chapter 21). He has been steadily losing weight and appears emaciated. A thorough examination indicates that Mr. Rossi needs surgery as soon as possible to remove a portion of his small intestine. The nutrition assessment reveals severe protein-energy malnutrition.

Mr. Rossi is placed on central TPN before surgery. He progresses well, gains weight, and undergoes surgery about one week after admission.

1. What factors in Mr. Rossi's history indicate the need for central TPN?
2. How would you explain the need for TPN to Mr. Rossi?
3. Describe the components of a typical TPN solution.
4. Calculate the energy and protein that would be supplied by 1 liter of the solution you described.
5. Consider some of the physiological and psychological problems Mr. Rossi might face when enteral nutrition is reintroduced.
6. How will the health care team know when it will be safe to take Mr. Rossi off central TPN?
7. Describe different ways the transition from TPN can be accomplished.

■ STUDY QUESTIONS ■

1. Describe the differences between simple IV solutions, peripheral TPN solutions, and central TPN solutions. When would each type be used?
2. How have IV fat emulsions made it possible to meet energy requirements by peripheral vein? When is IV fat preferable to IV glucose for meeting energy needs?
3. What are the components of a typical TPN solution? What other additives may be present?
4. How are TPN catheters inserted? How is a TPN feeding initiated? Stopped? Why must care be taken in starting or discontinuing a TPN solution.
5. Why is cyclic feeding of TPN solutions possibly preferable to continuous feeding?
6. Describe some ways in which a person on parenteral nutrition can be weaned to ordinary table foods.

■ CLINICAL APPLICATION QUESTIONS ■

1. Calculate the kcalorie and protein intake of a person on peripheral TPN who receives 3 liters of the solution described in the margin note on p. 558. Be sure to include the kcalories from one bottle of 20% fat emulsion (p. 555 margin).
2. One liter of a TPN solution contains 500 milliliters of 50 percent dextrose and 500 milliliters of 8.5 percent amino acids. Determine the daily kcalorie and protein intake of a person who receives 2 liters of such a TPN solution. Calculate the average daily energy intake if the person also receives 500 milliliters of a 20 percent fat emulsion three times a week.

NUTRITION IN PRACTICE 23

Tube Feedings and IV Nutrition at Home

Occasionally, a client's primary medical condition has stabilized, but ongoing tube or IV feedings are necessary to deliver nutrition support. In such a case, it may be the need for special nutrition support rather than the need for intensive medical care that keeps the person in the hospital. An option for such people is to continue the nutrition support at home.

Wouldn't it be much easier to stay in the hospital?

Nutrition support at home has a great advantage: it permits a person to receive nutrition care in familiar surroundings. If you have ever been in the hospital, or for that matter, just taken a long trip, you probably remember the comfort you experienced when you returned to your own bed, knew where things were, and could get things when you needed them. Often, people who receive nutrition support at home can resume many activities, such as going to work, driving, and playing sports.

Does it cost less to continue nutrition at home, too?

The savings gained from home nutrition support can be dramatic when the responsibilities formerly performed by hospital staff are assumed by the client or caregiver. One institution reports a cost savings of $1.5 million a year for ten clients maintained on home TPN versus TPN in the hospital.[10]

The costs of home programs are rising, however. The home health care industry is strictly regulated. Home health care workers are required to be highly trained and to give more time than in the past because of the increasingly complex care available for home clients.[11]

The number of people benefiting from home programs is growing, and health care professionals who work with these programs are gaining skill. Many medical supply companies now provide the equipment, formulas, and service necessary to support home nutrition care.

Isn't it hard for people to manage their own nutrition s'upport at home?

Yes, and home programs are not for everyone. The nutrition support team most frequently decides whether a client is a candidate for home enteral or parenteral nutrition. Among the factors to consider: the candidate for home nutrition support and the caregivers must have rational, stable personalities so they can successfully handle the problems that arise. They must be capable of learning the necessary techniques and of dealing with complications. They must also have adequate financial resources and access to the equipment, supplies, and professional support that are integral components of a successful home program.

How do health care professionals function in relation to home programs?

Once a home nutrition program is initiated, a nurse visits the client at home, and the person also sees a physician at regular intervals. In some programs, dietitians also make home visits. A qualified nurse, dietitian, or physician must be available to answer questions and handle problems as they arise.

How are tube feedings and IV feedings managed at home?

For tube feedings, gastrostomies (see Chapter 22), and sometimes jejunostomies, usually provide access to the GI tract for long-term tube feedings. Some people learn to use transnasal tubes, which they insert at each feeding. Others have transnasal tubes inserted as described in Chapter 22. When possible, intermittent feeding schedules are arranged so that clients are free to move around between meals. Sometimes, feedings are given only at night. Clients on continuous feedings who must use pumps can obtain small pumps that are easily concealed in clothing and allow freedom of movement.

The person on a home program usually purchases commercially prepared, premixed formulas. Most clients prefer these, and such formulas should certainly be used whenever a person's ability to mix the formula safely and appropriately is questionable.

What about people on home TPN?

Several different types of home TPN programs are currently in use. Ideally, clients are given as much responsibility for their own care as they can handle. For example, a client who is capable of changing the catheter dressings is trained to do so. Typically, caregivers also learn the techniques so that they can assist as needed.

Special catheters designed for long-term use often are inserted for home TPN. The day's volume of TPN solution is frequently

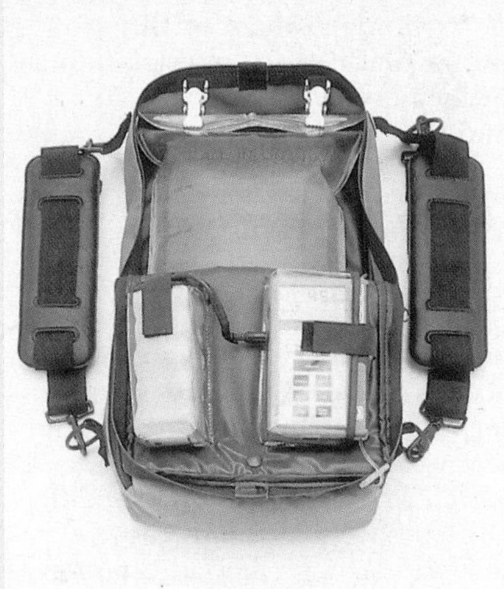

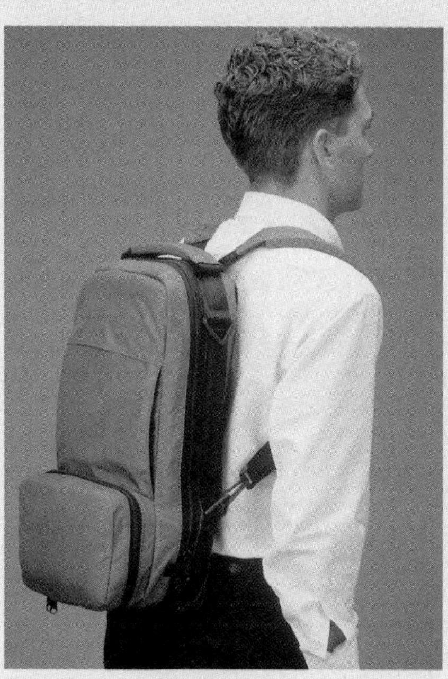

Portable pumps and convenient carrying cases for IV solutions allow home TPN clients to move about freely.

delivered within 8 to 12 hours using an infusion pump. The client infuses the solution while sleeping or at some other convenient time and thus is free to move about unencumbered for much of the day.

For people who cannot tolerate an 8- to 12-hour infusion rate, nutrients are infused over 24 hours. Those who are ambulatory can benefit from a lightweight carrying case that holds a small pump and IV bags. This system allows the client to move around freely with little inconvenience.

Unquestionably, special nutrition support provides a lifesaving alternative for nourishing people who cannot eat traditional diets. Such support can be adapted for use in virtually any medical disorder, including the severe liver diseases described in the next chapter.

NOTES

1. *Intravenous Fat Emulsion,* Drug Evaluation Monographs, vol. 73 (Denver, Colo.: Micromedex, 1992).
2. R. G. Barton, Nutrition support in critical illness, *Nutrition in Clinical Practice* 9 (1994): 127–139.
3. M. Gottschlich, Selection of optimal lipid sources in enteral and parenteral nutrition, *Nutrition in Clinical Practice* 7 (1992): 152–165.
4. J. D. Anderson, Components and compounding of total parenteral nutrition, *Support Line,* February 1993, pp. 12–15.
5. Food and Drug Administration, FDA Safety Alert: Hazards of Precipitation Associated with Parenteral Nutrition (a letter sent to health care professionals), April 18, 1994.
6. M. A. Stokes and G. L. Hill, Peripheral parenteral nutrition: A preliminary report on its efficacy and safety, *Journal of Parenteral and Enteral Nutrition* 17 (1993): 145–147.
7. L. M. Gramlich and B. Bistrian, Cyclic parenteral nutrition: Considerations of carbohydrate and lipid metabolism, *Nutrition in Clinical Practice* 9 (1994): 49–50.
8. R. S. DeChicco and L. E. Matarese, Selection of nutrition support regimens, *Nutrition in Clinical Practice* 7 (1992): 239–245.
9. M. F. Winkler and coauthors, Transitional feeding: The relationship between nutritional intake and plasma protein components, *Journal of the American Dietetic Association* 89 (1989): 969–970.
10. E. T. Herfinal and coauthors, Survey of home nutritional support patients, *Journal of Parenteral and Enteral Nutrition* 13 (1989): 255–261.
11. K. S. Crocker, Current status of home infusion therapy, *Nutrition in Clinical Practice* 7 (1992): 256–263.

Nutrition and Liver Disorders

24

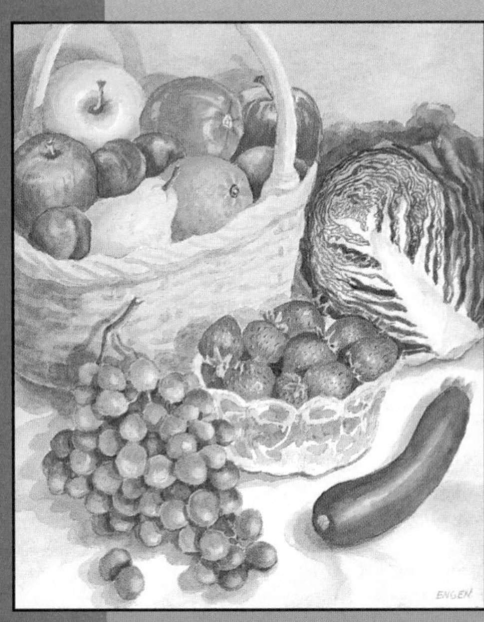

CONTENTS

The liver is the metabolic crossroads of the body, and its health is crucial to every body function. The liver receives nutrients and metabolizes, packages, stores, or ships them out for use by other organs. It metabolizes and stores most vitamins and many minerals. It manufactures bile, which the body uses in emulsifying fat so it can be digested and absorbed. The liver detoxifies drugs, prepares waste products for excretion, and participates in iron recycling and blood cell manufacture. It also makes clotting factors. No wonder, then, that hepatic disorders profoundly affect both nutrition and general health status.

hepatic (he-PAT-ik): of, like, or pertaining to the liver.

A variety of conditions can lead to liver disease: alcohol abuse, congenital disorders, poisoning, infections, gallbladder and bile duct obstructions, heart disease, and others. This chapter describes several types of liver disorders for which dietary management is appropriate.

Fatty Liver and Hepatitis

Two of the more common disorders of the liver are fatty liver and hepatitis. Diet, in particular, alcohol consumption, can play a role in the development of both disorders, although both may also arise from other causes. Similarly, diet management may play a role in the treatment of both disorders.

Fatty Liver

Reminder: A *fatty liver* is an early sign of liver deterioration seen in several diseases, including kwashiorkor and alcoholic liver disease. Fatty liver is characterized by an accumulation of fat in the liver cells.

Fatty liver is also called **hepatic steatosis** (STEE-ah-TOE-sis).

Fatty liver develops when the liver either synthesizes too much fat, oxidizes too little, takes up too much from the blood, releases too little back to the blood, or any combination of these errors. In fatty liver, triglycerides accumulate in the liver and cause it to enlarge.

Causes of Fatty Liver Most commonly, fatty liver develops from the liver's exposure to toxic substances such as alcohol (described in Nutrition in Practice 8), from an inadequate intake of protein (as in kwashiorkor), or as the result of an infection or malignant disease. Fatty liver can also develop as a complication of drug therapy (such as therapy with corticosteroids or tetracycline), obesity, TPN, or small bowel bypass surgery.

Normal Course Fatty liver alone usually causes no harm and remits without incident. The liver's accumulation of fat, however, suggests the presence of an underlying primary disorder that can become more serious if not corrected.

Therapy for Fatty Liver Quite often, the appropriate therapy for fatty liver focuses on eliminating the cause and reversing its effects. Fatty liver caused by malnutrition demands a diet adequate in protein, energy, and all other nutrients. Fatty liver due to alcohol abuse requires abstinence from alcohol and an adequate diet to replenish nutrient stores. Fatty liver caused by drug therapy requires alternative drugs or other therapies. Fatty liver caused by TPN can sometimes be reversed as Chapter 23 described, by use of cylic infusion. Otherwise, no specific treatment is recommended for fatty liver.

Fatty liver generally resolves with proper attention. In contrast, hepatitis poses major problems that can lead to death if treatment fails.

Hepatitis

In hepatitis, the liver becomes inflamed. Inflammation may occur when any of several viruses (known as the hepatitis A, B, and C viruses) attack the liver cells or when excessive or chronic ingestion of alcohol, drugs, or toxins damages the liver cells.

hepatitis: inflammation of the liver caused by a virus, alcohol, a drug, or other toxin. Hepatitis can progress to cirrhosis.
hepat = liver
itis = inflammation

Symptoms of Hepatitis During the early stages of hepatitis, the person may develop fatigue, joint and muscle pain, anorexia, nausea, vomiting, diarrhea or constipation, and low-grade fever. As hepatitis progresses, yellow bile pigments accumulate in the diseased liver and spill into the blood, causing jaundice and producing a dark urine. In the later stages of hepatitis, the liver enlarges and becomes tender. In severe cases, hepatitis can lead to liver failure and hepatic coma (described later).

Reminder: *Jaundice* is the yellowing of the skin caused by bile pigments (bilirubin) from the liver spilling into the bloodstream.

Consequences of Hepatitis The origin of hepatitis, the extent of liver damage, and the person's response to treatment all determine how seriously the disease will affect health. For example, hepatitis A can be so mild as to go unnoticed; hepatitis B can be so severe as to be fatal; and hepatitis C may become chronic and then flare up periodically even after long, symptom-free periods.[1]

Excess bilirubin in the blood is called **hyperbilirubinemia.**

Anorexia, nausea, vomiting, and fever may accompany hepatitis, and result in malnutrition. People with alcohol-related hepatitis have an especially high risk of nutrient deficiencies.

Therapy for Hepatitis Liver cells need nutrients to help them recover from hepatitis. Abstinence from alcohol is important to recovery. The person with hepatitis who is in good nutrition status receives a regular, well-balanced diet. The malnourished person with hepatitis receives a high-kcalorie, high-protein diet to replenish nutrient stores. For the person with mild anorexia, suggest frequent small meals, liquid supplements, or both. Persistent anorexia, nausea, or severe malnutrition may make tube feedings necessary. For the person who experiences persistent vomiting, parenteral nutrition is an alternative.

When fatty liver or hepatitis go unresolved, cirrhosis can develop. Cirrhosis is not only the most serious type of liver injury, but is also irreversible.

Cirrhosis

Cirrhosis begins when liver cells become filled with fat or are damaged by inflammation. The liver cells die, and scar tissue invades the liver. Chronic alcohol abuse is the most common cause of cirrhosis in the United States, although not all people with cirrhosis are alcohol abusers, and not all alcohol abusers develop cirrhosis. Other causes of cirrhosis include infections, biliary obstructions, heart disease, and exposure to toxic chemicals.

cirrhosis: an advanced form of liver disease, in which liver cells turn orange, die, and harden, permanently losing their function.

The type of cirrhosis associated with alcohol abuse and malnutrition is called **Laennec's** (lay-eh-NECK'S) **cirrhosis**.

In fact, any cause that leads to either fatty liver or hepatitis can progress to cirrhosis.

Consequences of Cirrhosis

Unlike healthy liver tissue, which is soft and flexible, scar tissue is unyielding. This difference leads to major consequences, including portal hypertension, varicose veins in the esophagus, ascites (described later), altered blood chemistry, and loss of consciousness.

Reminder: The *portal vein* is the blood vessel that carries nutrients from the GI tract to the liver. The *hepatic vein* returns blood from the liver to the heart. The *hepatic artery* delivers oxygen-rich blood from the heart back to the liver.

portal hypertension: elevated blood pressure in the portal vein caused by obstructed blood flow through the liver.

Portal Hypertension The portal vein and the hepatic artery carry 1½ quarts of blood every minute through miles of intermeshed capillaries within the liver. This huge volume of blood cannot pulse easily through the scarred tissue of a cirrhotic liver, so it backs up into the portal vein. Consequently, blood pressure in the portal vein rises sharply, causing portal hypertension. Figure 24–1 provides a diagram of the liver's circulatory system.

Esophageal Varices With normal blood flow through the liver blocked, pressure forces some of the blood to take a detour through smaller vessels around the liver and out to the rest of the body. These collater-

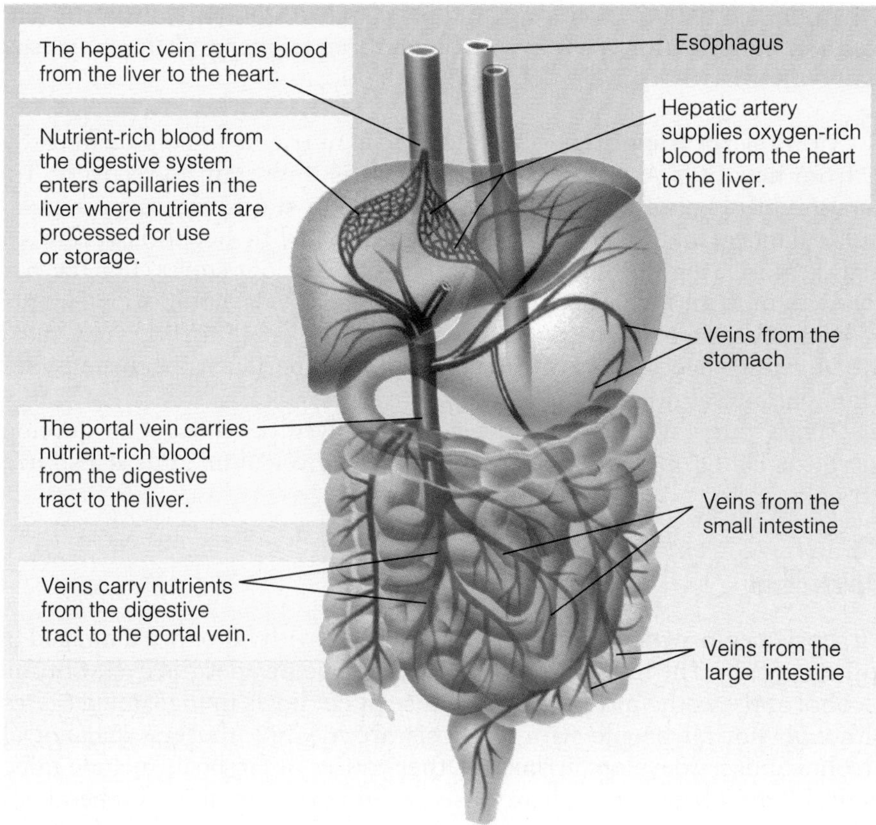
The hepatic vein returns blood from the liver to the heart.
Esophagus
Nutrient-rich blood from the digestive system enters capillaries in the liver where nutrients are processed for use or storage.
Hepatic artery supplies oxygen-rich blood from the heart to the liver.
Veins from the stomach
The portal vein carries nutrient-rich blood from the digestive tract to the liver.
Veins from the small intestine
Veins carry nutrients from the digestive tract to the portal vein.
Veins from the large intestine

Figure 24–1
The Liver's Circulatory System
Note that poor circulation in the liver can raise blood pressure in the portal vein, causing portal hypertension. Pressure builds up and affects the veins surrounding the intestinal system, including the esophagus. These veins may enlarge, grow weak, and burst.

als, or shunts, often develop in the area around the esophagus. Frequently, high pressure enlarges the collaterals so that they bulge into the lumen of the esophagus, creating esophageal varices in much the same way that high pressure in the legs causes varicose veins. Eventually, the thin lining of the esophagus that covers the varices wears away, and massive bleeding follows. Bleeding esophageal varices tend to recur, and people can bleed to death.

collaterals: small blood vessels that develop to divert blood flow away from an obstructed organ; also called **shunts**.
shunt = to avoid

esophageal varices (ee-SOFF-ah-GEE-al VAIR-ih-seez): tangles of distended blood vessels that protrude into the esophagus.

Ascites The rising pressure in the portal vein forces plasma out of the liver's blood vessels into the abdominal cavity, causing the abdomen to swell. This accumulation of fluid in the abdominal cavity is called ascites. Ascites tends to be a self-aggravating condition. Because less blood reaches the kidneys, they call for more aldosterone, the hormone that makes the body retain sodium and water. Then more fluid leaks out, the ascites grows worse, and edema spreads to other parts of the body. To make matters worse, the diseased liver cannot dispose of aldosterone efficiently, so aldosterone levels remain high. Figure 24–2 summarizes the sequence of events leading to ascites.

ascites (ah-SIGH-teez): a type of edema characterized by the accumulation of fluid in the abdominal cavity.

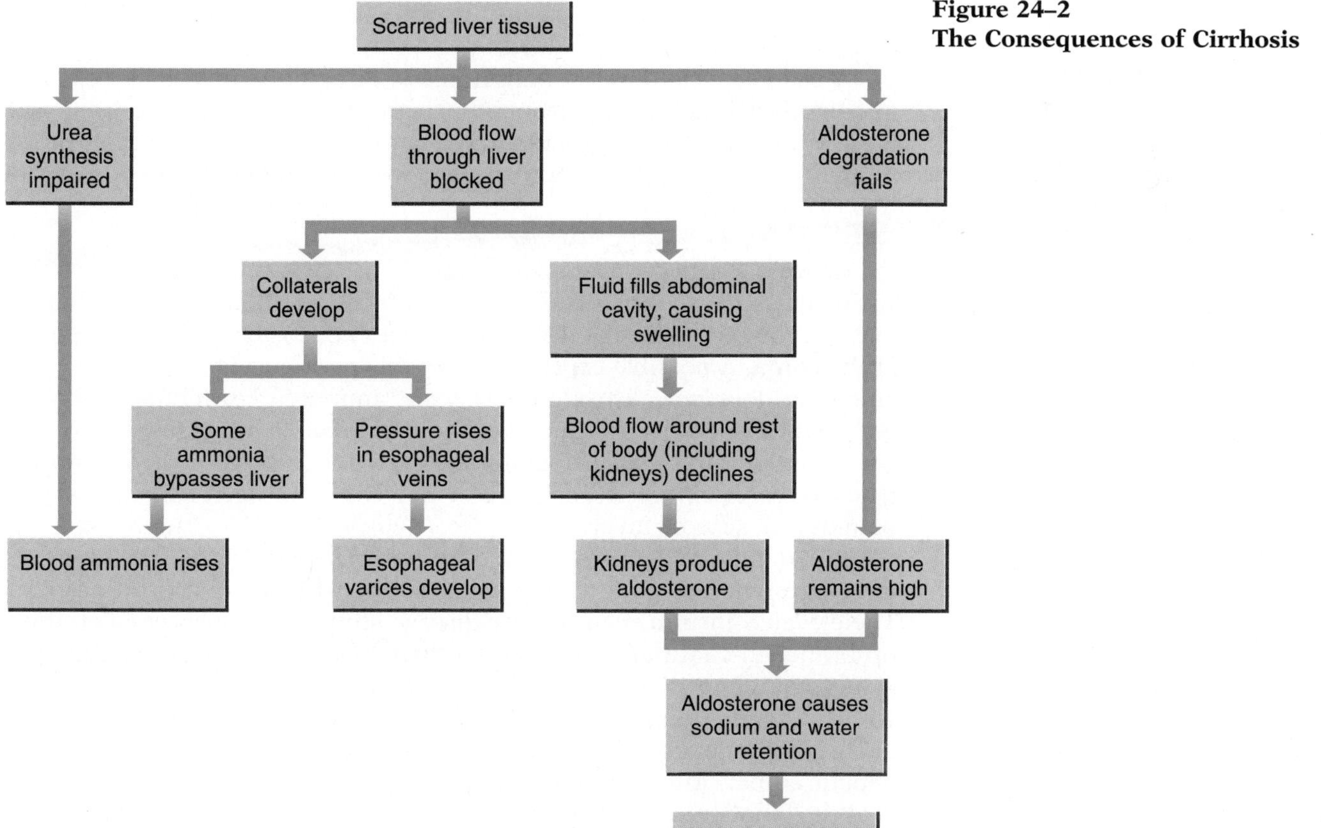

Figure 24–2
The Consequences of Cirrhosis

Figure 24–3
Ammonia Production in the Body

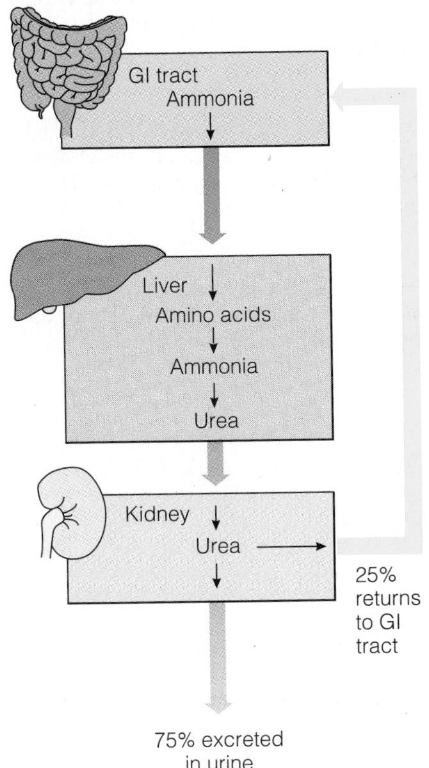

An elevated blood ammonia level is called **hyperammonemia**. Normal blood ammonia levels range from 80 to 110 µg/100 ml.

hepatic coma: a state of unconsciousness that results from severe liver disease; also called **hepatic encephalopathy** or **portal systemic encephalopathy.**

Elevated Blood Ammonia Levels Normally, the healthy liver removes ammonia from circulation and converts it to urea, but a severely diseased liver fails at this task, and blood ammonia rises. Even if the liver does handle the ammonia it receives, some ammonia-laden blood bypasses the liver by way of the collaterals. Elevated blood ammonia disrupts central nervous system function, compounding the risk of hepatic coma. Therapy therefore has to turn to controlling ammonia production.

Ammonia Production As Figure 24–3 shows, blood ammonia comes from several sources. Principally, ammonia comes from the GI tract: intestinal bacteria produce ammonia, and digestive enzymes generate ammonia as they dismantle protein. Also, recall that amino acids contain amino groups (NH_2). These amino groups generate small but significant quantities of ammonia (NH_3) during metabolic processes. Therapy designed to reduce blood ammonia therefore aims at eliminating ammonia-producing bacteria and at reducing the amount of protein present in the GI tract.

Limiting the intake of dietary protein will help to meet the goal of reducing protein in the GI tract. Even without dietary protein to digest, though, the enzymes in the GI tract have access to protein from the many cells that are constantly shed from the GI lumen. Moreover, if the person has GI bleeding from gastritis, ulcers, or esophageal varices, the blood serves as an additional source of protein. These three protein sources in the GI tract—food, shed mucosal cells, and blood—account for about two-thirds of the ammonia that finds its way into the blood. The GI tract bacteria produce the other third.

A vicious cycle develops: ammonia is directly toxic to liver cells and impairs liver function; consequently, the liver metabolizes less ammonia, blood ammonia rises further, and liver function deteriorates even more. Many drugs used to treat liver disease work in the intestines to prevent this vicious cycle.

Hepatic Coma Hepatic coma is a dangerous complication of cirrhosis. Its exact cause remains elusive; high blood ammonia plays an important role, but the degree of the elevation does not correlate with the severity of the coma. A possible explanation for this poor correlation is that *blood* ammonia does not always parallel *brain* ammonia concentration. When brain ammonia is high, the body produces greater quantities of two substances (glutamine and ketoglutarate), and the degree of their elevation tends to correlate with the degree of coma. Other nitrogen-containing compounds may also be involved.

Blood amino acid patterns also change in hepatic coma. The liver fails to break down aromatic amino acids, so their blood concentrations rise. The elevated insulin seen in liver disease stimulates muscle cells to take up branched-chain amino acids, so their blood concentrations fall. The resulting high ratio of aromatic to branched-chain amino acids interferes with the formation of certain neurotransmitters (dopamine and norepinephrine), but causes the production of substances that may contribute to hepatic coma.[2] Altered amino acid metabolism also adds ammonia directly to the blood. Figure 24–4 provides examples of aromatic and branched-chain amino acid structures.

Typically, the person with impending hepatic coma exhibits mental disturbances such as changes in judgment, personality, or mood. Sometimes sleep patterns change. The person may be unable to draw even a simple shape, such as a star. A sweet, musty, or pungent odor may develop on the breath. Flapping tremor may also develop in the precoma state. Just before passing into a coma, the person becomes very difficult to arouse.

flapping tremor: uncontrolled movement of the muscle group that causes the outstretched arm and hand to flap like a wing; occurs in hepatic coma and other diseases that cause encephalopathy; also called **asterixis**.

Diet Therapy for Cirrhosis

Diet therapy for cirrhosis presents a dilemma. The diet must provide enough protein to maintain nutrition status, allow the liver cells to regenerate, and prevent infections, but not enough to aggravate ammonia buildup and induce hepatic coma. A diet adequate in energy and restricted, but not low in protein sets the cornerstone for cirrhosis treatment.

Energy and Protein In providing diet therapy for cirrhosis, health care professionals must pay attention to clients' intakes of energy, protein, and, in many cases, sodium and fluid. To maintain positive nitrogen balance, clients need a diet that provides adequate energy and protein. Table 24–1 provides dietary guidelines for liver disease. Note that protein needs for people with liver disease who do not show signs of hepatic coma are higher than the RDA (0.8 grams per kilogram per day).

A person who shows signs of impending coma requires additional dietary modifications. Protein intake must be restricted to 40 to 60 grams of high-quality protein per day. Although this limited protein may reduce the risk of coma, it may not maintain protein status. If clinicians want to provide additional protein, they may use special enteral and parenteral formulas that are low in aromatic amino acids and high in branched-chain amino acids. If coma ensues, some people may be able to tolerate special formulas; for others, both dietary protein and special formulas may be restricted.[3] Clients also receive drugs to rid the body of excess ammonia. As a client's neurological status improves, protein can be gradually increased.

Figure 24–4
Examples of Aromatic and Branched-Chain Amino Acids

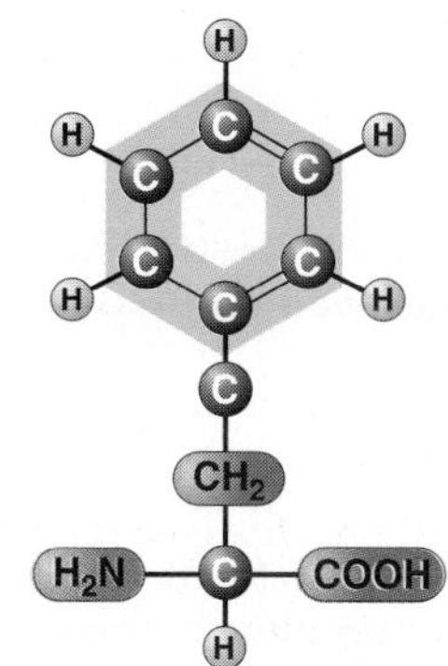

Phenylalanine

Aromatic amino acids are characterized by a ring structure. Other aromatic amino acids are tyrosine and tryptophan.

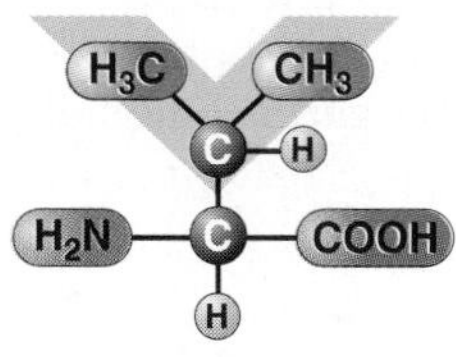

Valine

Branched-chain amino acids are characterized by a branched structure. Other branched-chain amino acids are leucine and isoleucine.

Table 24–1
Dietary Guidelines for Liver Disease

In general, the diet should provide:

Energy: 35 to 45 kcalories per kilogram actual body weight.

Protein in cirrhosis: 1.0 to 1.5 grams per kilogram body weight.

Protein in impending coma: 40 to 60 grams per day from foods; additional protein to meet needs can be supplied from special formulas.

Protein in severe hepatic coma: protein from all sources may need to be restricted. Tolerances are determined individually; protein intake is gradually increased as the condition improves.

Sodium and fluids: restrict sodium to 1000 to 2000 milligrams per day and fluids to 1500 to 2000 milliliters per day if ascites has developed; then increase intake as liver function improves.

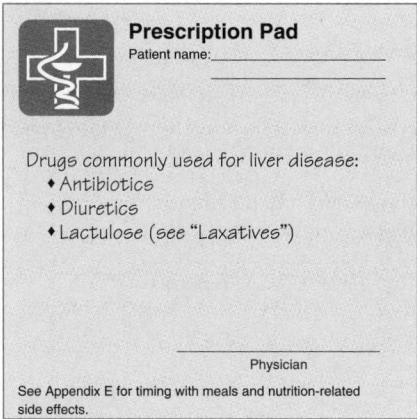

Prescription Pad

Patient name:__________

Drugs commonly used for liver disease:

- Antibiotics
- Diuretics
- Lactulose (see "Laxatives")

Physician

See Appendix E for timing with meals and nutrition-related side effects.

Table E–1B in Appendix E lists the nutrition-related side effects of diuretics.

People with liver disease may tolerate vegetable and dairy proteins better than meat protein, perhaps because nonmeat protein contains fewer ammonia-forming components and aromatic amino acids and more branched-chain amino acids than do meats. In addition, diets high in plant foods contain more fiber, which speeds up intestinal transit, thereby reducing the time available for the production and absorption of ammonia in the gut.

Fat Because fat helps make foods appetizing and delivers energy efficiently, it serves an important role in the diet of a person with cirrhosis. Fat needs to be restricted only if the cirrhotic person develops steatorrhea, a clear sign of fat malabsorption. Even then, the body can usually handle MCT fat.

Fluid and Sodium When physicians prescribe diuretics for people with ascites, they also restrict fluid and sodium intakes. To assess changes in fluid balance, weigh the person *daily*. Rapid weight gain indicates fluid retention; sudden weight loss, in contrast, indicates successful fluid excretion. Table 24–2 shows diet patterns for various levels of sodium restriction. The accompanying menu illustrates sample protein-restricted, sodium-restricted meals.

Alcohol To protect the liver from further injury, clients with cirrhosis must completely abstain from alcohol use. A cirrhotic liver continually exposed to alcohol cannot manufacture the lipoproteins needed to rid itself of accumulated lipids. Without alcohol, and with just enough protein to serve as new raw material, the cirrhotic liver seems to manage

Sample Protein-Restricted (60 g), Sodium-Restricted (1000 mg) Diet Menu

Foods on this low-sodium menu are cooked without salt. To raise sodium intake, add salt to foods. To reduce sodium, use unsalted margarine and milk. The kcalories provided by this menu depend on how much fat is used in cooking. To raise energy intake, if needed, encourage the liberal use of fats and sugars from foods that do not contain protein (for example, margarine and table sugar).

MENU

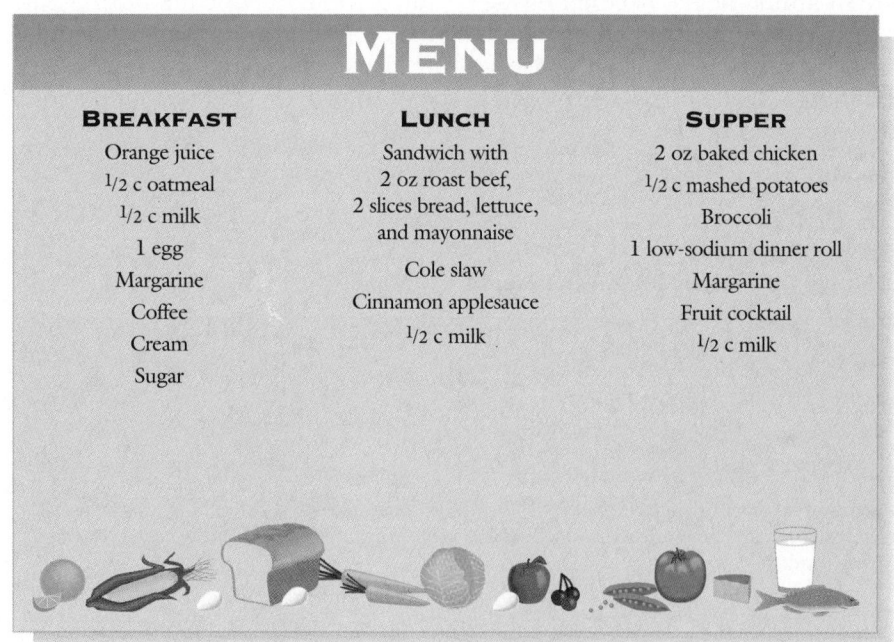

Breakfast	Lunch	Supper
Orange juice	Sandwich with 2 oz roast beef, 2 slices bread, lettuce, and mayonnaise	2 oz baked chicken
1/2 c oatmeal	Cole slaw	1/2 c mashed potatoes
1/2 c milk	Cinnamon applesauce	Broccoli
1 egg	1/2 c milk	1 low-sodium dinner roll
Margarine		Margarine
Coffee		Fruit cocktail
Cream		1/2 c milk
Sugar		

Table 24-2
One–and Two–Gram Sodium–Restricted Diets

FOODS RESTRICTED	SODIUM RESTRICTION		SERVING SIZE	SODIUM PER SERVING (mg)
	1 Gram (1000 mg)	2 Gram (2000 mg)		
Regular breads and cooked cereals	3	4	1 slice	125
Fresh, frozen, or canned vegetables without salt: artichokes; beets; carrots; celery; beet, collard, dandelion, mustard, and turnip greens; kale; swiss chard; white turnips; low-sodium vegetable juice	3 per week	Avoid excessive use	½ cup	50
Canned or frozen vegetables with salt; frozen corn, lima beans, mixed vegetables, and peas	0	2	½ cup	250
Regular nonfat, whole, and evaporated milk and milk products	2	2	1 cup	120
Fresh and fresh frozen meats, poultry, and freshwater fish; low-sodium canned meats and fish, peanut butter, cheese; unsalted soybeans, textured vegetable protein, and cottage cheese	8	8	1 oz	25
Eggs	1	1	1	70
Regular butter and margarine	0	6	1 tsp	50

FOODS ALLOWED

1. Low-sodium breads, bread products, and cereals; bread products made without salt and with low-sodium baking powder; puffed rice and wheat and shredded wheat cereals; rice; pasta.
2. Fresh, unsalted frozen, and low-sodium canned vegetables (except those listed above); low-sodium tomato juice.
3. All fruits and fruit juices.
4. Unsalted butter, margarine, nuts, and gravy; low-sodium salad dressings and mayonnaise; shortening.
5. Low-sodium catsup, mustard, and tabasco sauce.
6. Soups, casseroles, and recipes made with allowed foods and food ingredients.

FOODS NOT ALLOWED (Unless Calculated into the Diet)

1. Table, celery, garlic, and onion salts; reduced-sodium salts; regular catsup, mustard, and tabasco sauce; monosodium glutamate; Worcestershire, barbeque, and soy sauces; baking power and soda.
2. Instant and quick-cooking hot cereals; commercial bread products made from self-rising flour or cornmeal, salt, baking powder, or baking soda; salted snack foods such as potato chips, corn chips, tortilla chips, popcorn, and pretzels.
3. Sauerkraut, pickles, and salted vegetable juices.
4. Maraschino cherries; crystallized or glazed fruits, and dried fruits with sodium sulfite added.
5. Buttermilk, chocolate milk, instant milk mixes, regular cheeses, and prepared pudding mixes; commercial ice cream, sherbet, and frozen desserts.
6. Cured, canned, salted, or smoked meats, poultry, and fish such as bacon, luncheon meats, corned beef, kosher meats, and canned tuna and salmon; imitation fish products; salted textured vegetable protein; regular peanut butter; salted nuts.
7. Salt pork and bacon fat; commercial salad dressings and mayonnaise; olives; regular gravy.
8. Regular canned soups and bouillon.

lipids well enough. (Nutrition in Practice 24 addresses the vital nature of alcohol abstinence in treating liver disease.)

Vitamins Recall from Chapter 7 how the B vitamins serve as coenzymes for the liver's many metabolic reactions and repair work. In liver disease, deficiencies of thiamin, vitamin B_6, riboflavin, and folate are likely. Virtually all people with advanced liver disease require supplements of some vitamins, as well as minerals and trace elements. Physicians determine which micronutrients to supplement by monitoring serum nutrients and checking for clinical signs of deficiencies. Often, clients receive supplements of water-soluble vitamins in large amounts.

Fat-soluble vitamins may be malabsorbed when steatorrhea develops. Body tissues may not receive the vitamin A they need if the diseased liver fails to synthesize adequate amounts of retinol-binding protein.

Reminder: *Retinol-binding protein,* or *RBP,* is the protein made in the liver that carries vitamin A through the blood to the tissues that need it.

Vitamin D nutrition status may suffer if the diseased liver fails to activate vitamin D for the body's use. Because liver disease can prolong the time blood takes to clot, clients may also need vitamin K supplements.

The time blood takes to clot is called the **prothrombin time.** Both vitamin K deficiency and liver disease can prolong prothrombin time.

Minerals Calcium deficiencies can develop from three causes: steatorrhea, low serum albumin (albumin, which carries calcium in the blood, is manufactured in the liver), and impaired vitamin D metabolism. Iron deficiencies can develop from the GI bleeding that occurs with liver disease. Fluid and electrolyte imbalances and ascites may necessitate the use of diuretics, and these may lead to losses of the minerals potassium, magnesium, and zinc.

Solving Diet-Related Problems Dietitians face a challenge in devising a diet low in sodium that delivers adequate protein and also stimulates the appetite. Many high-protein foods (for example, eggs, meat, and milk) contain too much sodium to be allowed. To circumvent this problem, planners use special low-sodium supplements and milk products. Diet offers critical support in the recovery from cirrhosis, and health care professionals should make every effort to solve diet-related problems.

Specialized Nutrition Support If the person with cirrhosis cannot take enough food by mouth, health care professionals should promptly begin tube feedings or TPN. A person who has bleeding esophageal varices is unable to take food by mouth and is often given a simple IV solution to maintain fluid and electrolyte balance. If the person is malnourished or unable to resume oral intake for an extended time, peripheral or central TPN should be considered.

The accompanying case study deals with cirrhosis. Use your clinical knowledge and judgment to answer the questions.

Liver Transplantation

When liver disease becomes severe and irreversible, liver transplantation may become an option. Surgeons remove the diseased liver and replace it with a donor liver, reconnecting the blood vessels and the biliary tract. In

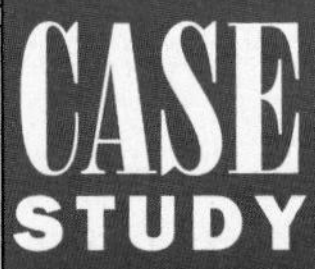

Carpenter with Cirrhosis

Mr. Sloan, a 48-year-old carpenter, has been in he hospital many times. He recognizes his problem with alcohol abuse and has entered alcohol rehabilitation programs several times over the last few years. Nevertheless, he is still drinking. Mr. Sloan was recently admitted to the hospital, and a diagnosis of alcoholic cirrhosis has been confirmed. At 5 feet 7 inches tall, Mr. Sloan, who once weighed 150 pounds, now weighs 120 pounds. He looks thin, although his abdomen is distended with ascites, and his skin is yellow. His liver disease is advanced, and he is showing signs of impending hepatic coma. Laboratory findings include:

- AST, 295 U/ml.
- Alkaline phosphatase, 13 Bodansky units.
- BUN, 8 mg/100 ml.
- Blood ammonia, 125 µg/100 ml.

1. Check these findings against Table 24–3. Are they consistent with liver disease?
2. Explain to Mr. Sloan what cirrhosis is and what its consequences are.
3. From the limited information available, what can you determine about Mr. Sloan's nutrition status?
4. Calculate his %IBW and %UBW (see p. 325 in Chapter 13).
5. What dietary changes do clients with cirrhosis generally receive?
6. How will Mr. Sloan's diet be altered now that he is in a precoma state?
7. Why is Mr. Sloan's abdomen distended?
8. Explain the development of ascites in liver disease and how diet is adjusted.
9. Would you expect Mr. Sloan's blood ammonia levels to be high? Why or why not?
10. Describe portal hypertension, jaundice, and esophageal varices.
11. How would Mr. Sloan's diet be changed if he were found to have esophageal varices?

Table 24–3
Standards for Tests Commonly Used to Diagnose Liver Disease

TEST	NORMAL VALUES	VALUES IN LIVER DISEASE
Albumin	4–6 g/100 ml	Decreased
Alkaline phosphatase	2.0–4.5 Bodansky units	Elevated
Ammonia	10–80 µg/100 ml	Elevated
AST (formerly SGOT)[a]	0–35 U/ml	Elevated
Bilirubin	0.1–1.0 mg/100 ml	Elevated
BUN[a]	8–18 mg/100 ml	Normal
Prothrombin time		Slow

Note: To convert albumin (g/100 ml) to standard international units (g/L), multiply by 10; to convert ammonia (µg/100 ml) to standard international units, multiply by 0.5872; to convert bilirubin (mg/100 ml) to standard international units (µmol/L) multiply by 17.10; to convert BUN (mg/100 ml) to standard international units (mmol/L urea), multiply by 0.3570; to convert AST (U/ml) to standard international units (µkat), multiply by 0.01667).

[a]AST = aspartate transaminase; SGOT = serum glutamic oxalacetic transaminase; BUN = blood urea nitrogen.

10 to 20 percent of liver transplant cases, the graft fails to function, and retransplantation is necessary to forestall an otherwise inevitable death.

Nutrition before Transplantation In severe liver failure, malnutrition may have progressed for some time. One clinician reports malnutrition in 70 percent of liver transplant recipients.[4] A liver transplant candidate must often wait for a liver donor before surgery is possible. Wise health care professionals use this time to identify and correct nutrient imbalances whenever possible. The person equipped with adequate nutrient stores faces the transplant prepared to fight infections, heal wounds, and mount a stress response.

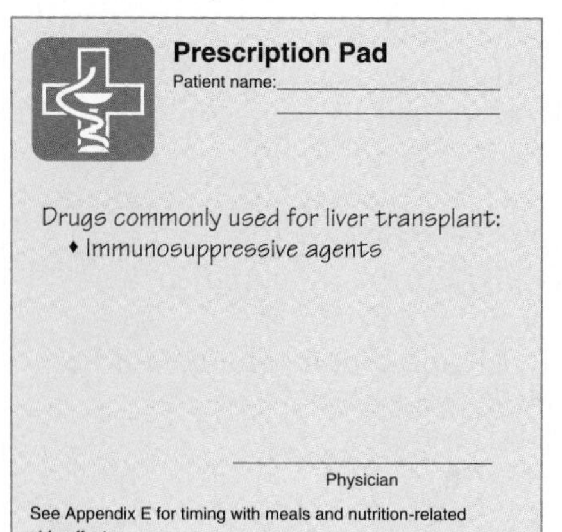

Prescription Pad
Patient name:
Drugs commonly used for liver transplant:
• Immunosuppressive agents
Physician
See Appendix E for timing with meals and nutrition-related side effects.

Nutrition Following Transplantation Following liver transplantation, liver function determines nutrient needs. All people are hypermetabolic after surgery, and in liver transplant recipients, energy needs are especially high. Moreover, drugs given to transplant recipients to prevent tissue rejection further contribute to nutrient imbalances. The nutrition support team often uses indirect calorimetry to estimate energy needs and carefully monitors clinical and laboratory data to make specific nutrient recommendations.

Nutrition Assessment

When you assess the nutrition status of people with disorders of the liver, keep several points in mind:

- People with diseases of the liver (especially those who abuse alcohol) are often malnourished. Obtain an accurate diet history to calculate nutrient requirements and identify inadequate nutrient intakes.
- Careful diet histories can help pinpoint protein tolerance for people with advanced liver disease.
- People who habitually abuse alcohol derive much of their energy from it. Because alcohol is not allowed in the hospital, special care must be taken to ensure that the diet is adequate to meet energy needs. Routinely reassess nutrition status to check energy adequacy.
- The person with cirrhosis may retain enough fluids to affect weight measurements significantly. Generalized edema may also alter arm anthropometrics and laboratory results. Under these circumstances, weight measures become meaningless as an indicator of body tissue gains and losses, but do reflect whether the person is mobilizing fluids or not. Weight loss is a good sign that some liver function is returning.
- An assessment strategy useful in treating people with ascites is to measure abdominal girth. Place a tape measure around the back and over the person's abdomen directly over the umbilicus. Repeat the measurement periodically. A decreasing abdominal girth indicates fluid mobilization. In contrast, an increasing girth signifies that the ascites is becoming worse.
- In people with advanced liver disease, the metabolic effects of liver disease and malnutrition are difficult to distinguish. Laboratory tests, including serum albumin, often reflect liver function rather than nutri-

tion status. Supplying extra amino acids will not help if the liver cannot function well enough to synthesize albumin from them.

The recovery of people with disorders of the liver depends in large part on attention to nutrition and nutrition assessment parameters.

Liver disorders wreak havoc on the body's metabolic work. Equally disturbing to homeostasis are disorders that alter blood glucose concentrations, the topic of the next chapter.

■ STUDY QUESTIONS ■

1. What is fatty liver, and what causes it? What diet modifications, if any, are useful for the treatment of fatty liver?
2. What is hepatitis, and what nutrition concerns arise in the person suffering from hepatitis?
3. Describe cirrhosis, and explain how it leads to portal hypertension, esophageal varices, formation of collaterals, ascites, and elevated blood ammonia.
4. Describe the dietary treatment of the person with cirrhosis and hepatic coma. Consider special dietary concerns of the person with ascites and esophageal varices.
5. How does nutrition status influence recovery from a liver transplant?
6. Why is it difficult to assess nutrition status in people with severe liver disease?

■ CLINICAL APPLICATION QUESTIONS ■

1. Think about the problems a person might encounter in following an 1800-kcalorie diet with protein restricted to 40 grams. On such a diet, the total protein allowance could be spent on just one scrambled egg, 3 ounces of meat, a cup of milk, and two slices of bread. Using Figure 6-6 (pp. 134–135) for reference, write down which exchange lists contain no protein, and add enough of these foods to the diet to meet energy needs.

   Now compare the result with the Daily Food Guide on pp. 14–15. Which food groups have you offered in the recommended quantities? Which food groups are in short supply on such a diet? Which nutrients might be low? How might fats and sugars be useful in such a diet?
2. The more restrictive a diet, the more difficulty a person usually has complying with it. The person given the diet in question 1, for example, may miss eating large amounts of meat or meat alternates, breads and grains, or milk and dairy products. What effect might additional restrictions, such as fluid and sodium restrictions, have on dietary compliance? Consider how much more difficult compliance might be for an alcohol abuser, who must also abstain from alcohol.

NUTRITION IN PRACTICE 24

Therapeutic Diets in Perspective

The clinical chapters of this book describe how health care providers use modified diets to help treat various disorders. You may have the impression that symptoms X, Y, and Z will appear when a person has disorder A, and that the person will recover when given diet Q. In reality, nothing could be less true. Diet therapy is only one part of treatment. Prescribed diets may be critical to recovery, they may help only a little or not at all, or they may even be contraindicated. Also, clients comply with and benefit from diet therapy to different degrees. At one extreme, a client may comply perfectly and the diet may seem to work wonders. At the other extreme, a client may refuse to comply at all and you may never have the chance to see if the diet would have worked. This discussion contains a few facts and many judgments—much like real clinical situations that health care professionals face.

Are you saying that it is not always appropriate to energetically advocate a therapeutic diet for a disorder?

Yes. To decide how hard to push a diet, first ask what you can realistically expect from it. Consider the following questions:

- What are the proven benefits of the diet in question?
- What are the negative effects of the diet?
- What are the proven risks of *not* following the diet?

The decision also depends on your sense of how the client will respond to diet instructions.

Give me some examples.

Take the case of Marion, for example. Marion's chart reads "fatty liver" and "underweight," but let's say that you know she is an alcohol abuser. Marion has been advised to abstain from alcohol permanently and to eat a high-protein, high-kcalorie diet until she has reached the appropriate weight for her height.

Marion smiles and nods when you discuss diet with her, and, of course, she has to comply while in the hospital, but when she returns home, you have reason to believe she will resume abusing alcohol. She has followed this pattern several times in the past. How hard should you try to persuade her to comply with the diet instructions? The answer depends largely on her motivation, which a psychiatrist, psychologist, or social worker might be best able to assess.

In cases that involve alcoholism, abstinence from alcohol is crucial to recovery, and motivation is crucial to abstinence. It is proper to teach Marion how alcohol can damage her liver and how important healthy liver function is to her overall health. It is also proper to help her figure out how to comply with the diet orders. It is equally important, though, to assist her in establishing connections with a counselor who can help her get the support she needs to keep her on track.

What about someone without a major mental health problem? Is diet compliance easier to achieve?

Not necessarily. Take the case of Ted, a busy executive who leads a hectic life and has just found out that he has reflux esophagitis. His doctor has prescribed six small meals a day; no food at bedtime; limited fat, alcohol, and caffeine intake; and antacids between meals.

After you win his trust, Ted confides that he has no intention of following the diet. He barely has time to eat three meals a day, let alone six. He insists on having his morning coffee and is irate about having to give up his evening cocktails and bedtime snack.

In such a case, should the diet adviser just give up?

No, but you might decide to discuss Ted's attitude with the physician, and if the physician approves, you might work out an alternative approach. You might try instructing Ted to eat three small meals a day with two snacks in between and no food at bedtime. This plan would recommend no change in policy regarding the coffee and alcohol. In talking to Ted, you should reemphasize that these beverages are not recommended, and explain why. Use some common sense and add that if he does not experience pain when he drinks these beverages, it is okay to have them on occasion, but not to drink them on an empty stomach.

Suppose Ted still balks. He says he can't squeeze two extra snacks into his day and objects to giving up his evening cocktail and bedtime snack. Then what should the diet adviser do?

Don't give up on him. Realize that he needs to better understand the benefits of the diet, and explain further.

You may succeed in convincing Ted that your diet advice is worth following. If so, then you can help him think through the changes he needs to make in his daily life. If not, you can try again in a few weeks, or let Ted know that you care about his health and ask him to call if he would like advice. It is up to Ted to make the choice between changing his lifestyle or accepting the pain and consequences of reflux esophagitis.

It sounds as though you should bend the rules when people don't want to follow diet advice. Is that always okay?

No, sometimes the rules must be obeyed. Consider Conchita, a healthy young woman of 25, who was born with phenylketonuria (PKU). Fortunately, it was diagnosed within three days, and her parents instituted the PKU diet immediately to promote Conchita's normal development. Conchita followed the diet until she had stopped growing. Then, when the restrictions were no longer crucial to her development, she switched to a regular diet. She has led a fairly normal life since then.

Now Conchita wants to get pregnant. Her doctor has told her she must resume the PKU diet prior to conception and follow it through the pregnancy to prevent her baby from developing mental retardation. Conchita resents the necessity of following the diet's rules and buying its expensive special products. She remembers that the diet cramped her lifestyle and kept her from participating fully in many social activities. (Nutrition in Practice 25 describes how difficult the diet is to follow.)

What should I say to Conchita?

First, consult the facts. As Nutrition in Practice 25 points out, when a woman goes off the PKU diet as an adult, her blood concentration of harmful by-products soars. In adults, these by-products do not cause the irreversible brain damage evident in young children, but during pregnancy, they are devastatingly harmful to fetal development. Disobeying the doctor's orders in this case poses intolerable risks to Conchita's unborn infant. Conchita's refusal to follow the diet would make severe disability inevitable.

Present Conchita with the facts, and make sure that she receives meticulous instructions about the intricacies of the diet. She will make her own decision, but you cannot in good conscience support her if she chooses not to comply with the doctor's orders. Inform the other members of the health care team about Conchita's feelings so that all of you can work together to help her make the difficult adjustment.

Are any other diets as critically important as the PKU diet?

Yes, diets for liver failure, renal failure, and diabetes, among others, bring about life-sustaining changes in metabolism. All efforts should focus on ensuring compliance with these diets.

A person's complaint that a diet is restrictive does not make it all right to abandon the diet. The complaint is a signal to look for options. Most diets can be planned to accommodate people's lifestyles and preferences.

Most foods can be worked into therapeutic diets on occasion with careful planning. An occasional lapse from the diet rules will not be fatal. However, "forbidden" foods should be used only infrequently, in limited amounts, and when planned. When addiction to alcohol is involved, total abstinence is advised.

Nurses and dietitians who care enough to provide the best nutrition therapy for their clients work hard to develop skill in tailoring diet advice to individuals. They don't give the same diet advice to everyone who has the same "label." Furthermore, because research in diet therapy moves fast, health care professionals must keep their eyes and ears open for new information on the benefits and risks of diet therapies. They develop their clinical judgment, as all good judges do, by allowing each new fact and each new case to find its proper place in decision making.

With each client, you will encounter a variety of unique circumstances. You may find that this uniqueness makes your job difficult at times, but meeting the challenge will also make it rewarding.

■ NOTES ■

1. M. J. Alter, The natural history of community-acquired hepatitis C in the United States, *New England Journal of Medicine* 327 (1992): 1899–1905.
2. J. E. Fischer, Branched-chain-enriched amino acid solutions in patients with liver failure: An early example of nutritional pharmacology, *Journal of Parenteral and Enteral Nutrition* (supplement) 14 (1990): 249–256.
3. A.S.P.E.N. Board of Directors, Practice guidelines: Liver failure, *Journal of Parenteral and Enteral Nutrition* (supplement) 17 (1993): 14–15; E. P. Shronts and coauthors, Nutrition support of the adult liver transplant candidate, *Journal of the American Dietetic Association* 87 (1987): 441–451.
4. J. Hasse, Nutrition and transplantation, *Nutrition in Clinical Practice* 8 (1993): 3–4.

25

Nutrition and Disorders of Glucose Metabolism

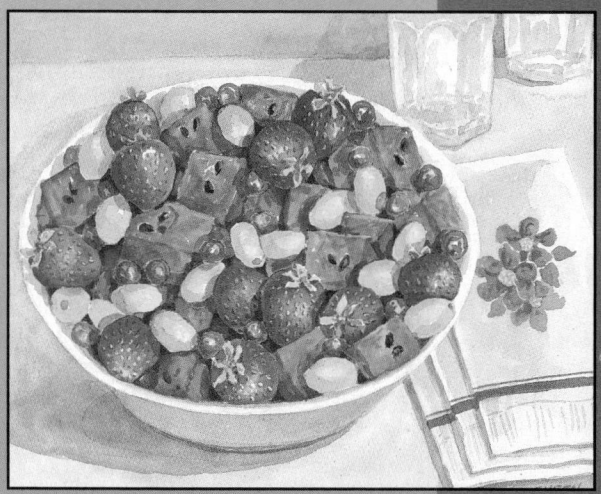

CONTENTS

The body's metabolic activities are so vital that disturbances of metabolism are often severe and even fatal, but some are responsive to dietary control. This chapter is devoted to disorders of glucose metabolism, in which diet therapy is of major importance.

Glucose is an indispensable fuel for the brain and other tissues. To regulate it, the body produces insulin to drive glucose into cells for use or storage; and glucagon, epinephrine, and other hormones to bring glucose out of storage again. Diabetes mellitus and hypoglycemia reflect two extremes of glucose imbalance: diabetes is characterized by high blood glucose and hypoglycemia by low blood glucose.

Diabetes Mellitus

Some 5 to 6 million people in the United States have diabetes, and about half of these people do not know they have it.[1] Many more have the first signs indicating that they will develop the condition later; the prevalence of diabetes increases with age.

Excessive thirst and hunger and frequent urination are common early symptoms of diabetes. People who experience these symptoms should be tested.

An Overview of Diabetes

The only common conditions called diabetes that most people hear of are the two forms of *diabetes mellitus* described here. Another form, *diabetes insipidus,* is treated with medication, not with nutrition therapy, and so is not described here.

Diabetes ranks among the leading causes of death in the United States. It is a major cause of blindness, kidney failure, infections necessitating leg amputations, and birth defects. In addition, people with diabetes are twice as likely to develop atherosclerosis and hypertension (see Chapter 26) as those without diabetes.

diabetes (DYE-uh-BEET-eez) **mellitus** (MELL-ih-tus or mell-EYE-tus): a metabolic disorder characterized by altered blood glucose regulation and utilization usually caused by insufficient or relatively ineffective insulin.

Screening for Diabetes Routine blood or urine tests help identify people with diabetes or impaired glucose tolerance so that prompt treatment can begin. A high fasting blood glucose suggests diabetes; a second similar test result confirms the diagnosis. Fasting blood glucose that is higher than normal but not high enough to confirm diabetes indicates impaired glucose tolerance. People with impaired glucose tolerance are retested regularly, and health care professionals often recommend that clients begin diet therapy for diabetes. People with normal fasting blood glucose should be retested every three years. Some physicians prefer to test a person's fasting blood glucose, then give a dose of glucose, and then retest several times more—a procedure called a glucose tolerance test.

Fasting blood glucose:
>140 mg/100 ml—diabetes
115–140 mg/100 ml—impaired glucose tolerance
<115 mg/100 ml—normal

glucose tolerance: the ability of the body to adjust to doses of dietary carbohydrate by bringing its blood glucose back down to normal.

In some cases, physicians detect the first hint of diabetes from routine urine tests. High urinary ketones and glucose indirectly reflect high blood glucose and suggest the need for a follow-up blood test.

Reminder: *Insulin* is the hormone that, among other things, enables cells to take up glucose from the blood.

Insulin-Dependent Diabetes Mellitus (IDDM) Table 25–1 (p. 584) summarizes the distinguishing features of the two main forms of diabetes. In insulin-dependent diabetes mellitus (IDDM), which occurs in about 5 to 10 percent of all cases, the pancreas becomes competely unable to synthesize insulin. When a person with IDDM eats carbohydrate and absorbs the glucose from it, the glucose remains in the blood, even though the body's cells may be starved for it. The person must inject insulin regularly to assist the cells in taking up the needed glucose; hence the descriptive term *insulin-dependent*. The insulin must be injected; it cannot be taken orally

insulin-dependent diabetes mellitus (IDDM): the less common type of diabetes in which the person produces no insulin at all; also known as **type I diabetes** or **juvenile-onset diabetes** (because it frequently develops in childhood), although some cases arise in adulthood.

Table 25–1
Features of IDDM and NIDDM

	IDDM	NIDDM
Other names	Type I diabetes Juvenile-onset diabetes Ketosis-prone diabetes Brittle diabetes	Type II diabetes Adult-onset diabetes Ketosis-resistant diabetes Lipoplethoric diabetes Stable diabetes
Age of onset	<20 (mean age, 12)	>40
Associated conditions	Viral infection	Obesity
Insulin required?	Yes	Sometimes
Cell response to insulin	Normal	Usually resistant
Symptoms	Relatively severe	Relatively moderate

because insulin is a protein and the GI tract enzymes would digest it. IDDM most frequently develops in people younger than 20.

noninsulin-dependent diabetes mellitus (NIDDM): the predominant type of diabetes in which the cells fail to respond effectively to insulin; also called **type II diabetes** or **adult-onset diabetes.** NIDDM is usually milder than IDDM, and it progresses more slowly. A type of NIDDM that develops during the teen years has been termed **maturity-onset diabetes in the young (MODY).**

insulin resistance: the condition in which a normal amount of insulin produces a subnormal effect; a metabolic consequence of obesity.

Noninsulin-Dependent Diabetes Mellitus (NIDDM) In 90 to 95 percent of all cases, diabetes mellitus is noninsulin dependent (NIDDM). The pancreas produces insulin, and the cells respond to it, but less sensitively. As in IDDM, blood glucose rises too high. The pancreas responds by making more insulin, which may rise very high, but glucose uptake is still inadequate to meet the cells' needs. Over time, the pancreas produces less insulin. NIDDM develops most often in people over 40 and is nearly always associated with obesity. Obesity aggravates insulin resistance: as body fat increases, adipose and muscle tissues become more and more unable to take up glucose. Hunger and overeating are common, and this worsens the obesity. Unlike IDDM, which necessitates insulin injections, NIDDM may be controlled by diet, oral drugs, insulin injections, or some combination of these.

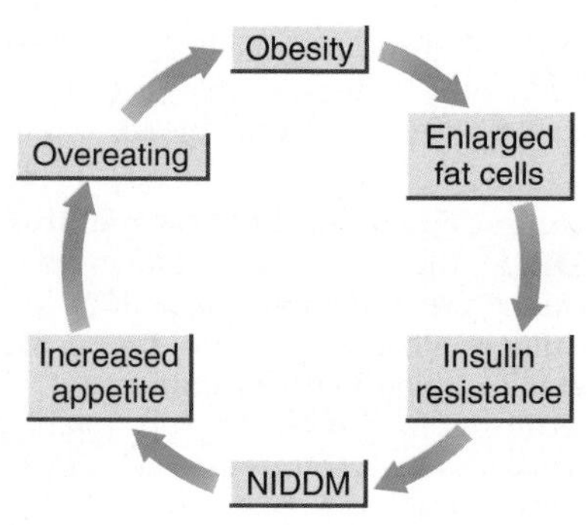

Complications of Diabetes Both forms of diabetes mellitus described here are characterized by high blood glucose and either insufficient or ineffective insulin. To appreciate the problems this causes, recall that after meals, insulin normally enhances cellular uptake of glucose, amino acids, and fatty acids and stimulates protein synthesis, glycogen synthesis, and fat synthesis. Disruption of energy metabolism and exposure of the tissues to high glucose concentrations results in both acute and chronic complications.

Acute Complications of Diabetes

Figure 25–1 provides an overview of the metabolic changes that occur in uncontrolled diabetes. Notice that in NIDDM some glucose enters the cells, so many of the symptoms of IDDM do not appear.

Figure 25–1
Metabolic Consequences of Untreated IDDM and NIDDM
As you can see, when glucose cannot enter the cells, a cascade of metabolic changes follows. In NIDDM, some glucose enters the cells. Because the cells are not "starved" for glucose, the body does not shift into the metabolism of fasting (losing weight and producing ketones).

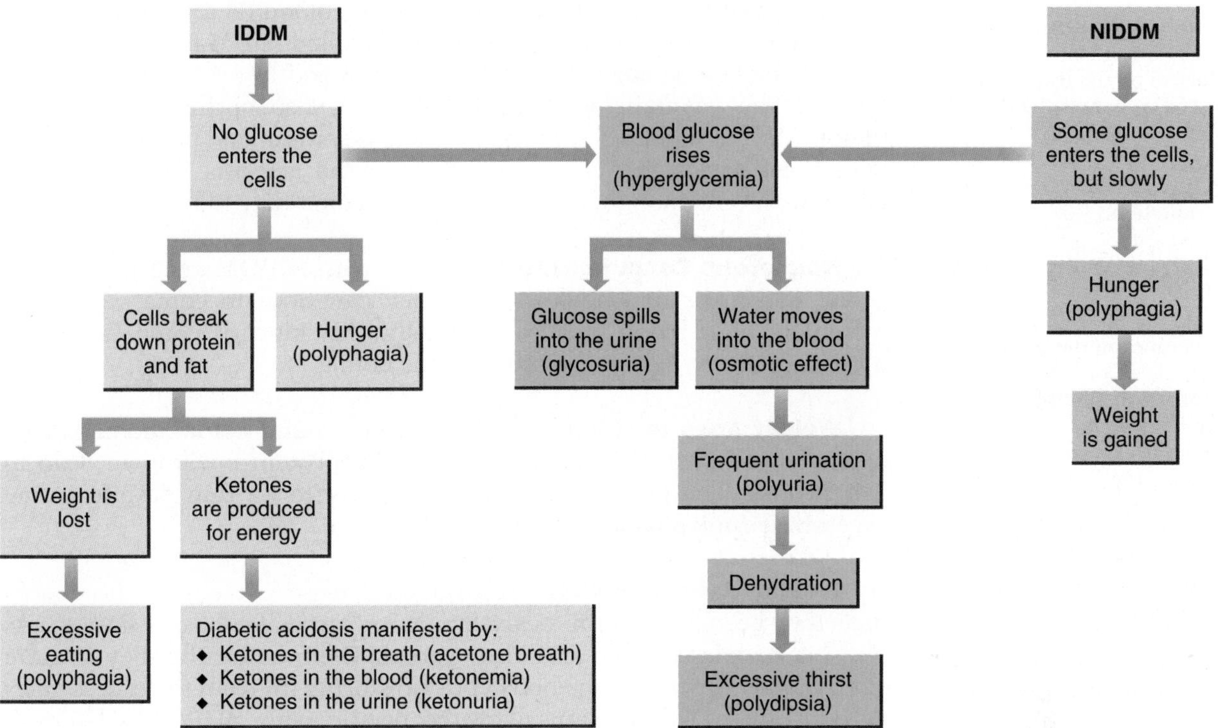

Blood and Urine Glucose As blood glucose rises, hyperglycemia results; its symptoms are listed in the margin. Normally, the kidneys retain all glucose, but when blood glucose rises above a certain threshold, the excess "spills" into the urine. Glycosuria generally occurs when blood glucose exceeds 180 milligrams per 100 milliliters.

Hyperglycemia occurs in untreated diabetes or when people with diabetes do not have enough insulin to meet their needs—for example, when they have eaten too much or eaten at the wrong time. People with diabetes who are ill quickly develop serious hyperglycemia (recall that stress causes hyperglycemia in any person). Ironically, taking too much insulin can also cause hyperglycemia: it may cause blood glucose to fall so rapidly that it triggers the liver to release counterregulatory hormones (insulin antagonists). These hormones may raise blood glucose higher than the available insulin can handle. Hyperglycemia can also occur early in the morning as the liver's natural response to an overnight fast. Hyperglycemia is serious and sometimes fatal.

hyperglycemia: an abnormally high blood glucose concentration, often a symptom of both types of diabetes.
hyper = too much
glyce = sweet (glucose)
emia = in the blood

Symptoms of hyperglycemia:
- Acetone breath.
- Confusion.
- Glycosuria.
- Intense thirst.
- Labored breathing.
- Nausea.
- Vomiting.

glycosuria (GLY-ko-SUE-ree-ah): an abnormal amount of glucose in the urine; also known as **glucosuria** (GLUE-ko-SUE-ree-ah).

Dehydration As glucose builds up in the blood, it attracts fluids from the tissues. Then, glucose and the accompanying fluids spill into the urine, causing dehydration. Excessive urine (polyuria) and excessive thirst (polydipsia) are symptoms of uncontrolled diabetes.

Ketosis and Coma in IDDM Because IDDM continuously deprives cells of the energy fuels they need, the cells mobilize their own stored protein and fat for energy. As the cells release fatty acids, the liver responds by making ketones, which accumulate in the blood (ketonemia). A fruity odor on the breath of a person with uncontrolled IDDM reflects the presence of the ketone acetone. Ketones in the blood lower its pH (acidosis) because they contain acid groups. Ketones also appear in the urine (ketonuria). In addition, the kidneys excrete sodium and potassium along with the ketones in a way that worsens the acidosis. When acidosis becomes severe enough, a potentially fatal coma may follow.

Nonketotic Coma in NIDDM People with NIDDM generally are not prone to ketosis and acidosis, but they can develop coma caused by extremely high blood glucose. Logically, this kind of coma is termed hyperosmolar hyperglycemic nonketotic coma.

Weight Loss in IDDM Losses of glucose and ketone bodies (both energy sources) in the urine, together with protein breakdown, lead to weight loss. The person with IDDM is likely to be thin despite eating excessively (polyphagia).

Weight Gain in NIDDM NIDDM also deprives cells of the energy fuels they need, not continuously, but enough to make the cells hungry. As a result, people with NIDDM also overeat. Then the insulin they do have slowly takes effect, and the body ends up storing fat from the excess energy consumed. This explains why the person with NIDDM is likely to remain overweight and also why ketones do not build up in the blood and urine.

Hypoglycemia Hypoglycemia is a consequence, not of untreated diabetes, but rather of inappropriate management: it is a reaction to oral drugs that lower blood glucose or to insulin. Hypoglycemia can result from taking too much insulin, strenuous physical activity, skipping meals, delaying meals, eating too little, vomiting, or severe diarrhea. It is most likely in people who practice intensive insulin therapy in an attempt to tightly control their blood glucose.[2]

Left untreated, hypoglycemia can lead to seizures, loss of consciousness, coma, and death. Mental confusion and shakiness may make it difficult for the person to recognize the symptoms of hypoglycemia (see the list in the margin) and to take corrective measures. Furthermore, adults who have had diabetes for a long time risk severe hypoglycemia because the warning signs become less noticeable with time. Symptoms can also occur while the person is sleeping, making hypoglycemia difficult to detect.

The person with hypoglycemia may appear to be intoxicated. If the true problem goes unrecognized, the person may die. To prevent such a

Hyperglycemia that results from excessive secretion of counterregulatory hormones (glucagon, epinephrine, and glucocorticoids) in response to excessive administration of insulin is called **rebound hyperglycemia** or the **Somogyi** (so-MOAG-yee) **effect.**

Early morning hyperglycemia that develops in IDDM in response to the release of glucose by the liver after an overnight fast is known as the **dawn phenomenon.**

polyuria (POLL-ee-YOU-ree-ah): excessive urine production.

polydipsia (POLL-ee-DIP-see-ah): excessive thirst.

ketonemia: ketones in the blood.

acetone breath: a distinctive, fruity odor that can be detected on the breath of a person who is experiencing ketosis. Acetone is a simple ketone.

ketonuria: ketones in the urine.

diabetic coma: unconsciousness precipitated by ketosis in uncontrolled diabetes.

hyperosmolar hyperglycemic nonketotic coma: a coma that occurs in uncontrolled NIDDM precipitated by the presence of hypertonic blood and dehydration.

polyphagia (POLL-ee-FAY-gee-ah): excessive eating.

insulin reaction: hypoglycemia that results from an overdose of insulin, strenuous physical activity, skipped meals, or inadequate intake of food; also called **insulin shock.**

Symptoms of hypoglycemia:
- Dizziness.
- Double vision.
- Nervousness.
- Shallow breathing.
- Sweating.
- Weakness.

mistake, advise every person with IDDM to wear identification in the form of a bracelet or necklace and to carry some form of easy-to-absorb carbohydrate (a later section provides the details).

Hypoglycemia that occurs while a person is sleeping is called **nocturnal hypoglycemia.**

Chronic Complications of Diabetes

Over the long term, the person with diabetes suffers not only from the acute complications just described, but also from its chronic effects. Chronic hyperglycemia affects the structures of the blood vessels and nerves, leading to poor circulation and loss of nerve function. Poor circulation and glucose-rich blood and urine increase the likelihood of infections, which may go undetected when nerve function is also impaired. For these reasons, people with diabetes must pay special attention to hygiene and must learn to stay on the lookout for early signs of infection.

Cardiovascular Diseases Atherosclerosis tends to develop early in people with diabetes. As Chapter 26 describes, blockage of the arteries that feed the heart and brain can lead to heart attacks or strokes. If nerve function is impaired, the person may have a heart attack and not even realize it. In people with NIDDM, who are often obese and may also have hypertension, cardiovascular disease is a major cause of death.

A heart attack that goes unnoticed is called a **silent heart attack.**

Microangiopathies Disorders of the small blood vessels (capillaries), called microangiopathies, may also develop and lead to loss of kidney function and retinal degeneration with loss of vision. About 85 percent of people with diabetes have nephropathy, retinopathy, or both. Consequently, as mentioned in the introduction, diabetes is a leading cause of both kidney failure and blindness.

microangiopathies (MY-crow-ANN-gee-OP-ah-thees): disorders of the capillaries, often seen in diabetes: **nephropathy** (nee-FROP-ah-thee) is a type of microangiopathy affecting the capillaries of the kidney; **retinopathy** (RET-in-OP-ah-thee) affects the capillaries of the eye.
- *micro* = tiny
- *angio* = blood vessel
- *pathy* = disease
- *retino* = of the retina
- *nephro* = of the kidney

Neuropathy Nerve tissues may also deteriorate, resulting in neuropathy. Neuropathy may express itself at first as a painful prickling sensation, often in the arms and legs. Later, the person loses sensation in the hands and feet. Thereafter, injuries to these areas may go unnoticed, and infections can progress rapidly. With loss of both circulation and nerve function, undetected injury and infection may lead to death of tissue (gangrene), necessitating amputation of the limbs (usually the legs and feet). People with neuropathy are warned to take conscientious care of their feet.

neuropathy (new-ROP-ah-thee): any disease of the nerves.

Neuropathy can also delay gastric emptying. When the stomach empties slowly after a meal, the person may experience a premature feeling of fullness, bloating, nausea, vomiting, weight loss, and poor blood glucose control due to irregular nutrient absorption.

Delayed gastric emptying is **gastroparesis.**

Treatment of Insulin-Dependent Diabetes Mellitus (IDDM)

A diagnosis of IDDM can be devastating. The parents of a young child with IDDM may feel overwhelmed, angry, anxious, and even guilty. A teenager may feel that it is the end of the world. A person of any age may fear the prospect of daily insulin injections, possible complications, and the new diet. However, to control blood glucose successfully, the person must master the complex task of coordinating diet, insulin, and physical activity. Only with this mastery can a person lead an active and full life.

The goals of medical and nutrition therapy for diabetes are to maintain blood glucose within a fairly normal range, achieve optimal blood lipid levels (see Chapter 26), control blood pressure (see Chapter 26), support health and well-being, and treat complications. The most important of these goals is blood glucose control, as demonstrated by a major multicenter clinical trial (the Diabetes Control and Complications Trial, or DCCT). This trial showed that tightly controlling blood glucose to keep it within a fairly normal range can reduce the risks of onset and progression of retinopathy, nephropathy, and neuropathy by about 50 percent. Tight blood glucose control can also lower elevated blood cholesterol.[3] Tight control is now possible, thanks to improved and widely available technology for monitoring blood glucose at home.

Insulin for IDDM

Because people with IDDM cannot make their own insulin, they must receive it by injection. Insulin is available in many types that act with different timing, called rapid-acting, intermediate-acting, and long-acting insulins; Table 25–2 lists examples. Insulin delivery is timed to mimic the body's normal insulin action as closely as possible. Normally, the body secretes a constant, baseline amount of insulin at all times and more after meals. The person with IDDM needs insulin both to meet baseline needs and to process energy nutrients after meals. The physician initially prescribes the types and dosages of insulin based on individual needs. The health care team teaches people with IDDM to adjust their insulin doses to accommodate changes in their eating patterns, physical activity, or health status, as decribed later.

Table 25–2
Actions of Some Types of Insulin

TYPE	DURATION OF ACTIVITY (HOURS)	PEAK OF ACTION (HOURS)
Rapid acting (regular)		
Human	3 to 6	2 to 3
Animal	4 to 6	3 to 4
Intermediate acting		
Human	10 to 18	4 to 12
Animal	16 to 20	8 to 14
Long acting		
Human	18 to 20	uncertain
Animal	24 to 36	minimal

Insulin Delivery People with IDDM inject insulin or use pumps to deliver the insulin they need. The person with IDDM who chooses injections often receives a mixture of two or more types of insulin, two or more times daily; single injections are seldom effective. Intensive therapy requires multiple daily injections or the use of a pump.

multiple daily injections (MDI): delivery of insulin by injection three or more times daily.

External pumps, about the size of a beeper, hold enough insulin to meet needs for two to three days. Tubing carries the insulin from the pump to a needle that has been inserted into the abdominal area. Pumps deliver a constant, baseline level of insulin, and the client releases extra insulin to cover meals. Personal preferences and financial considerations guide each client in deciding which delivery system will work best.

The Honeymoon Phase Some clients experience a temporary remission of diabetes after their initial treatment with insulin—a time referred to as the "honeymoon phase." Why this honeymoon occurs remains a bit of a mystery. Perhaps with insulin treatment and relief from the constant hyperglycemia of uncontrolled diabetes, the insulin-producing cells of the pancreas become able to function normally again—but only temporarily. Tight control of blood glucose—whether by diet, insulin, or hypoglycemic agents—helps prolong the honeymoon.

Diet and Activity in IDDM

The diabetic diet parallels a healthy diet for all people in both amounts and types of nutrients. It differs from a regular diet, however, in that carbohydrate intake must be consistent from day to day and at each meal and snack. The concept is simple, but putting it into practice requires a lifelong commitment to a lifestyle that includes a carefully orchestrated diet, physical activity plan, and insulin program.

Assessment is important here: an accurate history enables the health care team to work out an acceptable daily diet, activity, and insulin treatment program. The program teaches clients to make adjustments for their lifestyles and health status, rather than to alter their lifestyles to accommodate their disease.

Diet-related behaviors that may improve blood glucose control include:

- Adherence to the meal plan.
- Appropriate treatment of hypoglycemia.
- Prompt treatment of hyperglycemia.
- Consistent and appropriate bedtime snacking.[4]

Later sections provide more detailed information about these and other diet-related behaviors useful in the treatment of diabetes.

Meal Planning Strategies Dietitians depend on a variety of strategies to help people with diabetes plan their diets; adequate blood glucose control can be achieved in many ways.[5] Dietitians teach the diet in stages, starting first with simple concepts and progressing to more difficult ones as the client's abilities and needs dictate.

Some diet strategies teach clients to use food guides or simple menus to plan diets. Other strategies focus mainly on the carbohydrate content of foods. Traditionally, however, diet planners use the exchange patterns described in Nutrition in Practice 6 (pp.132–137) for planning diabetic diets. The foods in each of the exchange system's six groups are similar in food energy and in carbohydrate, protein, and fat per portion. The person with diabetes learns that the food portions on any one list can be exchanged freely for one another. For example, "a starch/bread exchange" is any portion of grain or starchy vegetable that contains about 80 kcalories of food energy, 15 grams of carbohydrate, 3 grams of protein, and trace amounts of fat. One slice of most breads, one small potato, or ⅓ cup of rice all fit that description, so these items can be exchanged for each other in meal planning. Besides the starch/bread list, the exchange system includes a milk list, a meat list, a fruit list, a vegetable list, and a fat list. Appendix C provides additional details of the exchange lists, and the box that follows (p. 592) shows how dietitians use them to plan a diet.

Energy The diet for IDDM first focuses on providing adequate food energy to achieve or maintain a healthy and realistic body weight and to support growth in children and pregnant women. To determine whether energy intake is appropriate, the planner uses the energy RDA as a guide, takes height and weight measures periodically, and adjusts the diet as necessary.

Carbohydrate In IDDM, carbohydrate-containing foods act not just as an energy source but as blood glucose regulators, together with insulin and exercise. The diet for IDDM does not restrict carbohydrate intake. In fact, the carbohydrate content of the diet is fairly high, and the foods eaten at meals and snacks keep an even flow of glucose available. The exact amounts of carbohydrate included in the diet are determined through careful nutrition assessment and analysis of eating habits. Typically, carbohydrates contribute from 45 to 60 percent of the total kcalories.

Encourage clients to select foods rich in complex carbohydrates: whole-grain breads and cereals, legumes, fruits, and vegetables. These foods provide fiber, and diets high in fiber offer many health benefits (see p. 44–45).

Traditionally, concentrated sweets were strictly excluded from the diabetic diet, but now they are restricted only to the same extent as they are for all people. Health care professionals recognize that the total amount of carbohydrate is of greater concern in diabetes than the type of carbohydrate.[6] The person with diabetes can consume concentrated sweets as part of a healthy diet, with meals, and in limited amounts as long as they are counted as part of the carbohydrate allowance. Artificially sweetened beverages and artificial sweeteners can be used freely.

Recall that authorities recommend 20 to 35 of dietary fiber a day.

Reminder: Sweeteners that are used to take the place of sugar (sucrose) are called *alternative sweeteners*. They are of two types. The *nonnutritive sweeteners*, or *artificial sweeteners* (aspartame and saccharin), contain negligible kcalories. The *nutritive sweeteners* (fructose, sorbitol, and xylitol) contain the same number of kcalories as an equivalent amount of sugar (see Chapter 2).

Protein Protein provides about 10 to 20 percent of the total kcalories in the diabetic diet. Providing adequate but not excessive protein helps control intakes of total fat and saturated fat and may protect kidney function, important measures for individuals prone to cardiovascular and kidney diseases. At the first sign of kidney disease, people with diabetes may need to restrict protein to 0.8 grams per kilogram of body weight (that is, the RDA).[7]

An early sign of impending kidney disease is the appearance of greater-than-normal amounts of albumin in the urine or **microalbuminuria.**

Fat People with diabetes and normal blood lipids benefit from a fat intake consistent with the *Diet and Health* recommendations (30 percent or less of total kcalories from fat and less than 10 percent from saturated fat). Those who need to lose weight may need to restrict fat intake further. People with diabetes and elevated LDL may need to restrict saturated fat to 7 percent or less of total kcalories and cholesterol to less than 200 milligrams daily. Encourage the use of low-fat milk, nonfat milk, and lean meats to lower fat and cholesterol intakes.

Sodium People with diabetes frequently develop hypertension and are likely to be salt sensitive (see p. 622 in Chapter 26). Many practitioners advise all clients with diabetes to limit their sodium intakes. For diabetics with hypertension, sodium is often restricted to 2400 milligrams (6 grams of salt, or about 1¼ teaspoons) or less per day.

Alcohol The person whose blood glucose is well controlled can usually include some alcoholic beverages with the consent of the physician. However, alcohol can cause hypoglycemia in any person, and the person with hypoglycemia may appear to be intoxicated, too. The consumption of alcohol adds confusion to a potentially dangerous situation.

Most people with IDDM can consume alcohol in moderate amounts (no more than two drinks per day), with meals, and in addition to the usual meal plan. Alcohol intake is discouraged for people with a history of alcohol abuse; those with pancreatitis, abnormal blood lipids, or neuropathy; and pregnant women. For people who are overweight there is little room in the diet for empty-kcalorie foods; if alcohol is used, it is substituted for fat exchanges. Drinks that contain carbohydrate (drinks made with mixers, sweet wines, and liqueurs) are best avoided. If they are used, the planner must also count their carbohydrate contents. Whiskey, gin, vodka, and rum contain no carbohydrate.

Alcohol for Diabetic Diets: When counting kcalories, 1 drink = 2 fat exchanges. One drink is defined as 1½ oz liquor, 5 oz wine, or 12 oz beer. Light beer contains the same amount of alcohol as regular beer, with half the carbohydrate.

Timing and Composition of Meals and Snacks In IDDM, consistent timing and composition of meals and snacks from day to day can help improve glucose control. An evening snack is especially important, because it must sustain the person's blood glucose through the night. A person with a regular physical activity program who takes a prescribed dose of insulin at a set time and then eats about the same amount of carbohydrate at about the same time each day knows that insulin will be available when needed. Meal patterns that change from day to day require careful blood glucose monitoring, described later, to help maintain control. People who have difficulty maintaining a set meal plan learn how to adjust their insulin doses to cover their food intakes.

Missed Meals A person with IDDM who misses a meal needs to eat some 15 to 30 grams of complex carbohydrate to forestall hypoglycemia.

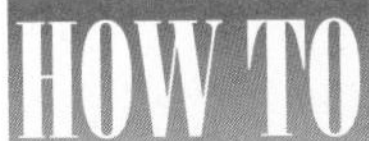

Plan a Diet Using Exchange Lists

Dietitians carefully assess the individual's diet history and educational level to select the appropriate diet strategy and design a realistic diet plan. When exchange lists are to be used, some calculating is required.

At first, using exchange lists to plan diets may take hours. With practice, however, dietitians can prepare complete diet plans in a matter of minutes by using a few shortcuts. This diet plan follows the shortcut steps.

1. *Estimate desirable body weight.*
   Adults: Refer to Table 9-1 (p. 215).
   Children: Refer to the growth charts in Appendix E.

This example uses a woman whose actual weight is 160 pounds and whose appropriate weight is 140 pounds.

By comparing the person's actual weight to her appropriate weight, you can determine whether she needs a weight-loss or weight-maintenance diet. For the person in our example, a weight-loss diet is in order.

2. *Calculate energy needs in kcalories.* Multiply appropriate body weight by 15 for men and active women; by 13 for most women, sedentary men, and adults over age 55; and by 10 for sedentary women, obese people, and sedentary adults over age 55.[a]

Children require about 1000 kcalories a day for the first year of life. Add 100 kcalories per year, up to 2000 kcalories at age 11. From age 12 to 15, add 100 kcalories per year for girls and 200 kcalories per year for boys. Re-member, this is an estimate, and children's needs depend more on size than on age.

In this example, the woman is sedentary and needs the following number of kcalories:

$$140 \text{ lb} \times 10 \text{ kcal/lb} = 1400 \text{ kcal.}$$

Note: The Harris-Benedict equation shown in Table 18–3 on p. 450 can also be used to determine energy requirements.

3. *Determine the grams of carbohydrate, fat, and protein.*
   45 to 60 percent of the kcalories from carbohydrate.
   Less than 30 percent of the kcalories from fat.
   10 to 20 percent of the kcalories from protein.

For 1400 kcalories, this division of kcalories translates into nutrients as follows:

Carbohydrate:

$$45\% \times 1400 \text{ kcal} = 630 \text{ kcal.} \qquad 630 \text{ kcal} \div 4 \text{ kcal/g} = 158 \text{ g.}$$
$$60\% \times 1400 \text{ kcal} = 840 \text{ kcal.} \qquad 840 \text{ kcal} \div 4 \text{ kcal/g} = 210 \text{ g.}$$

The woman needs between 158 and 210 grams of carbohydrate.

[a]M.J. Franz, Diabetes and nutrition: State of the science and the art, *Topics in Clinical Nutrition* 3 (1988): 1–16

How To (continued)

Table 25–3
A Day's Exchanges for a Sample 1400-kCalorie Diet

EXCHANGE ITEM	NUMBER OF EXCHANGES	CARBOHYDRATE (g)	PROTEIN (g)	FAT (g)	ENERGY (kcal)
Starch/bread	6	90	18	—	480
Meat (lean)	4	—	28	12	220
Vegetable	4	20	8	—	100
Fruit	4	60	—	—	240
Milk (nonfat)	2	24	16	—	180
Fat	4	—	—	20	180
		194	70	32	1400

Note: This diet supplies 55 percent of the energy as carbohydrate, 20 percent as protein, and 21 percent as fat. The percentages do not add up to 100 percent because the kcalorie values used in the exchange system are approximations, and percentages are rounded off.

Fat:

30% x 1400 kcal = 420 kcal. 420 kcal ÷ 9 kcal/g = 47 g.

The woman needs less than 47 grams of fat.

Protein:

10% × 1400 kcal = 140 kcal. 140 kcal ÷ 4 kcal/g = 35 g.

20% × 1400 kcal = 280 kcal. 280 kcal ÷ 4 kcal/g = 70 g.

The woman needs between 35 and 70 grams of protein.

4. *Translate the diet prescription into a meal plan.* Table 6–5 (on p. 137) provides examples of diet patterns for different energy intakes. Using that table as a guide, a dietitian might select the pattern of exchanges shown in Table 25–3, columns 1 and 2. The dietitian could then calculate the grams of energy nutrients by referring to Table 6–3 (on p. 133) and come up with the next three columns in Table 25–3. Total energy and percentages of kcalories contributed by each nutrient are shown at the bottom of the table. As you can see, the diet delivers 55 percent of its energy from carbohydrate, 20 percent from protein, and 21 percent from fat, a balance that meets recommended standards.

With this information in hand, the dietitian and client can begin to fill in the plan with real foods to create a menu (see Appendix C). Developing menus takes time and patience; it is a matter of trial and error until the actual plan comes "close enough" to the goals. Finally, the client tries the plan, identifies problems (if any), and consults the dietitian to make adjustments (if necessary).

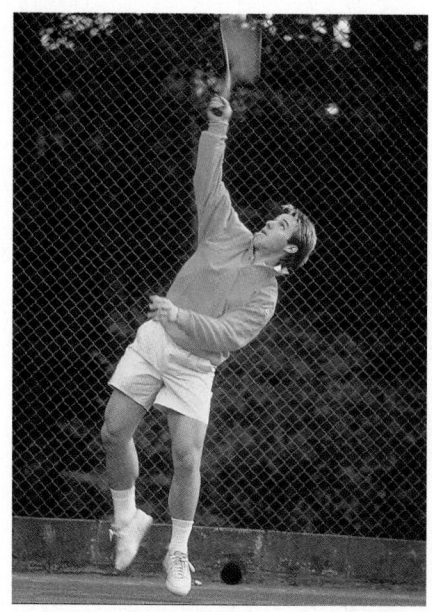

Physical activity plays an important role in the management of diabetes.

If appetite is poor, juice, flavored gelatin, soft drinks, or frozen fruit juice bars can meet needs for carbohydrates. In the hospital, if a person with IDDM misses a meal, different procedures may be employed. One procedure provides at least half the prescribed carbohydrate and kcalories within three hours of the missed meal. If this cannot be done, the physician may change the insulin schedule, give IV dextrose, or change the diet prescription to include more simple carbohydrates.

Tube Feedings and TPN When people with IDDM require tube feedings or TPN, adjustments may need to be made for the abundant carbohydrate the formulas contain. Often health care professionals adjust insulin doses to meet the higher carbohydrate load.[8] Even with additional insulin, some people may be unable to tolerate the carbohydrates in TPN. For these people, the glucose in the formula may have to be reduced and some of its energy delivered by IV fat emulsions instead (see Chapter 23). People who cannot tolerate the carbohydrates in standard tube feedings may benefit from specially designed formulas that contain less total carbohydrate.

Physical Activity and Blood Glucose Fitness programs confer benefits on the cardiovascular system that people with diabetes especially need. (See Chapter 10 for more on the benefits of physical activity.) For nondiabetic people, blood glucose generally varies little during physical activity unless the activity is intense and of very long duration, such as marathon racing. However, blood glucose can vary markedly when people with IDDM exercise. Those with mild hyperglycemia may experience a *fall* in blood glucose during physical activity, whereas those with marked hyperglycemia may have the opposite reaction, experiencing a still greater *rise* in blood glucose. For this reason, people with IDDM check their blood glucose prior to exercise and refrain from vigorous physical activity if it is too high.

Physical Activity and Food Intake The person with IDDM may need to eat before, during, and after vigorous physical activity. Especially important is carbohydrate, which is readily available from fruits, fruit juices, yogurt, crackers, and other starches. As a general guideline, the exerciser should have about 10 to 15 grams of additional carbohydrate before moderate activity or about 20 to 30 grams of carbohydrate before vigorous activity. The best way to determine the appropriate course of action is to check blood glucose 30 minutes before and 1 hour after exercise. Table 25–4 lists general guidelines for providing additional carbohydrate for varying activity intensities and blood glucose concentrations.

Physical Activity and Insulin Dosages Generally, insulin should be taken more than an hour before physical activity.[9] Vigorous exercise and warm temperatures set the stage for a hypoglycemic reaction, which may even occur after several hours. Reducing the insulin doses both before and after the activity by up to 30, or even 50 percent, can help to prevent this sequence of events.

Table 25–4
Guidelines for Providing Additional Carbohydrate for Activity in IDDM

EXERCISE INTENSITY	BLOOD GLUCOSE (mg/100ml)	ADDITIONAL CARBOHYDRATE TO PROVIDE (g)
Low	<100	10–15
	>100	none
Moderate	<100	15–20
	100–180	10–15
	180–300	none
Strenuous	<100	35-40
	100–180	25–50
	180–300	10–15

Note: These values are estimates only. The individual should monitor blood glucose to determine specific needs more accurately.

Source: Adapted from M. J. Franz, Exercise and the management of diabetes mellitus, *Journal of the American Dietetic Association* 87 (1987): 872-880.

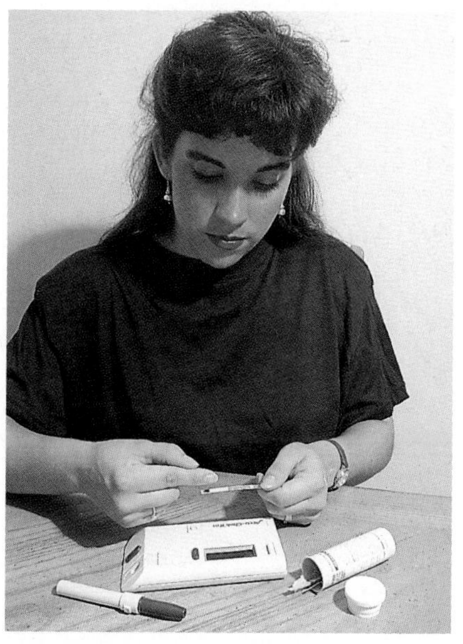

Blood glucose monitoring allows people to maintain blood glucose in a safe range.

Coordinating Therapy

The health care team evaluates the client with IDDM and, based on this evaluation, provides an initial diet and insulin treatment plan. To see if the plan is working and to make any adjustments, clients learn to monitor their own blood glucose. To make sense of blood glucose results, evaluators (both clients and health care professionals) need records of insulin administration, food intake, physical activity, and illness.

Blood Glucose Monitoring Ideally, until blood glucose is under control, the person performs blood tests seven times a day: before each meal, two hours after each meal, and at bedtime. As people learn how their blood glucose responds to food intake and physical activity, they can test less often—say, four times daily. Once the client's routine is established and control is good, two tests a day may suffice for monitoring.

To monitor blood glucose, the client pricks a finger and touches the blood to a paper strip. The paper strip changes to different colors, depending on the blood glucose concentration. Meters that provide more accurate readouts of actual glucose concentrations are also available, but the disposable strips that are used with them are expensive.

Another test used to monitor blood glucose control measures *glycated hemoglobin*. This test is "cheat-proof." Urine and blood glucose tests permit "cheating" because they reflect diabetes control only just prior to the test, but glycated hemoglobin enables the physician to determine how successful diabetes control has been over the past two to four months.

Urine Monitoring Health care professionals often recommend that clients monitor urinary ketones when blood glucose is over 250 milligrams per 100 milliliters. As described earlier, high blood glucose may predispose the person to ketosis and coma. Such a course is especially likely during illness.

Diet and Activity Records At medical appointments, health care team members review clients' records of food intake and physical activity in relation to blood glucose. Then they can offer suggestions for adjusting the day's meals, physical activity, or insulin doses. Table 25–5 provides some examples of how problems might be solved.

Illness During illness, even a minor illness such as a cold or flu, blood glucose may rise dramatically and raise insulin requirements. Thus

Table 25–5
Blood Glucose Monitoring and Problem Solving

PROBLEM	POSSIBLE SOLUTIONS[a]
Hyperglycemia	
Before breakfast	▸ Adjust dose of intermediate-acting insulin at bedtime.[b]
Before lunch	▸ Adjust morning dose of rapid-acting insulin.[b] ▸ Reduce amount of carbohydrate at breakfast. ▸ Reduce or omit midmorning snack. ▸ Change time of breakfast or midmorning snack.
Before dinner	▸ Adjust afternoon dose of rapid-acting insulin.[b] ▸ Reduce carbohydrate at lunch. ▸ Reduce or omit midafternoon snack. ▸ Change time of lunch or midafternoon snack.
At bedtime	▸ Adjust insulin dose before dinner.[b] ▸ Reduce amount of carbohydrate at dinner. ▸ Reduce amount of carbohydrate at evening snack.
Hypoglycemia	
Before breakfast	▸ Adjust dose of intermediate- or long-acting insulin at bedtime.[b] ▸ Add carbohydrate at evening snack. ▸ Omit strenuous activity late in the day.
Before lunch	▸ Adjust morning dose of rapid-acting insulin.[b] ▸ Add carbohydrate at breakfast. ▸ Add a morning snack. ▸ Change time of breakfast or morning snack.
Before dinner	▸ Adjust afternoon dose of rapid-acting insulin.[b] ▸ Add carbohydrate at lunch. ▸ Change time of lunch or afternoon snack. ▸ Add an afternoon snack. ▸ Adjust physical activity schedule.
At bedtime	▸ Adjust evening insulin dose.[b] ▸ Add carbohydrate at dinner. ▸ Add an evening snack. ▸ Change time of dinner or evening snack.

[a] Skilled health care professionals gather additional data to find the best solution for problems with blood glucose control. Is the problem an isolated occurrence or a pattern? Has food intake changed? If yes, why? Has the activity level changed? Has illness been a problem? Whenever possible, the diet is maintained, and insulin is adjusted to correct problems.
[b] Adjust doses in amount or time or both.

a record of illness helps evaluators make sense of blood glucose test results. During such precarious times, clients with diabetes should monitor blood glucose and urinary ketones vigilantly and follow insulin and dietary instructions especially carefully. Physicians may advise clients to reduce total energy and carbohydrate intakes slightly, in order to limit the need for extra insulin. A major concern is to prevent starvation, dehydration, and vomiting.

Treating Hyperglycemia A pattern of hyperglycemia before lunch or dinner in a person with a consistent carbohydrate intake clues the health care professional to look back to the previous meal and make corrections. (Recall that it takes time for food to be digested and absorbed before blood glucose rises.) Treatment may involve adjusting the dose of regular insulin, reducing the amount of carbohydrate at the previous meal, or spacing the meals so that the available insulin has time to work. The client's lifestyle and preferences dictate which course is best. Early morning hyperglycemia often requires adjusting the dose or timing of the intermediate-acting insulin given at bedtime. Rebound hyperglycemia is treated by reducing the insulin dose.

Severe Hyperglycemia and Ketoacidosis Severe hyperglycemia and ketoacidosis can occur in untreated IDDM, or when the person with IDDM fails to recognize and treat hyperglycemia or suffers a stress (infection, trauma) that causes blood glucose to rise. Severe hyperglycemia with ketoacidosis is a serious medical condition that can lead to coma and death. Prevention is the best treatment. Educating the client to follow the treatment plan (including regular blood glucose monitoring) is critical. When prevention fails, a physician treats hyperglycemia and ketoacidosis by carefully administering insulin and correcting fluid and electrolyte and acid-base balances, using IV fluids.

Hyperglycemia symptoms are on p. 585.

Treating Hypoglycemia People with IDDM and those who spend time with them need to learn to recognize the symptoms of hypoglycemia. As soon as the symptoms are observed, the person needs 10 to 15 grams of easy-to-absorb glucose—½ cup of orange juice, for example. Blood glucose is then checked within 15 to 20 minutes to see if it has risen to an acceptable level. If not, an additional 10 to 15 grams of carbohydrate is given, and blood glucose is rechecked. The procedure continues until blood glucose returns to an acceptable range.

It is important not to overtreat hypoglycemia because blood glucose can rise too high. Advise individuals with IDDM to carry concentrated sweets, such as glucose tablets or gel, sugar cubes or hard candy, or tubes of cake frosting so that they can act immediately when hypoglycemic symptoms occur. Consistent hypoglycemia before meals suggests the need to lower the insulin dose, increase the carbohydrate intake at the previous meal, or eat the next meal earlier. Again, the best step to take depends on the person's preferences and lifestyle. People prone to nocturnal hypoglycemia may be advised to wake up during the night and test their blood glucose. Engaging in consistent bedtime snacking or undertaking strenuous activity earlier in the day can help eliminate the problem.

Hypoglycemia symptoms are on p. 586.

Severe Hypoglycemia In severe cases, the person may be unable to safely swallow and may need to receive IV glucose, the hormone glucagon, or both to counteract an insulin reaction. Without treatment, the person may lapse into coma and die.

Children and Teens with IDDM

The energy and nutrient needs of children keep changing throughout the growing years. Children's appetites and activities vary widely from day to day. A child may eat like a horse one day and like a mouse the next day. A teen may spend hours walking around the mall one day, and spend the next day watching TV. Growth and activity influence their needs for food and insulin. Diabetes management for children and teens must adjust to meet their needs.

Meal Plans To support growth and development, children with IDDM need balanced meals and snacks that offer wide varieties of foods from each of the six exchange lists. Energy needs depend on age, gender, activity level, and growth status. Allow concentrated sweets within the context of a healthy diet. Dietitians often emphasize the carbohydrate-containing exchanges and teach appropriate substitutions. Caretakers should not force children to finish meals, but should encourage them not to skip meals either, since hypoglycemia can result. Meals and snacks are best taken at approximately the same times each day, and children should eat the same foods as the rest of the family. Children need to learn strategies for dealing with foods at school and at parties, as well as at home.

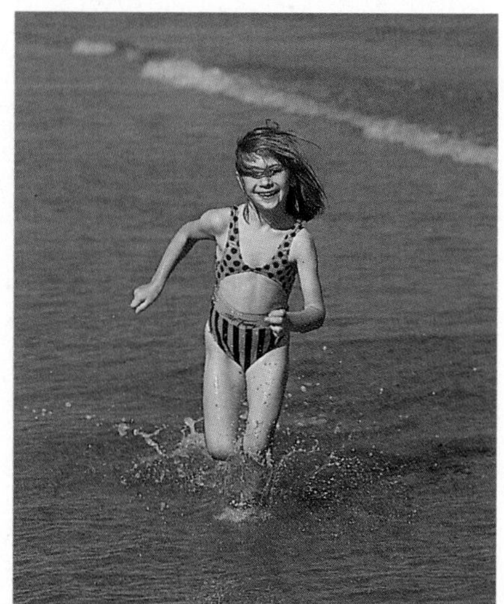

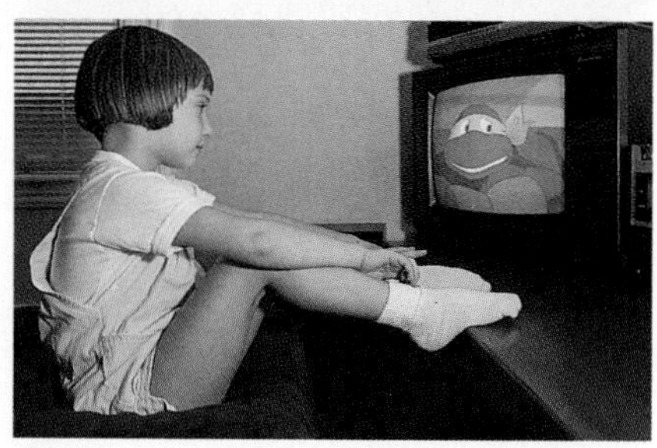

Because a child's activities vary from day to day, food and insulin needs may also change.

Camps for Children Children can combine diabetes education and summer vacation by attending camps designed especially for them. At these camps, children "live" the lifestyle under supervision. They learn to describe their meals and snacks in terms of exchange lists. They trade snack ideas, try new recipes, and get involved in preparing meals. Older children assist younger ones, and both groups benefit. The accompanying case study offers an opportunity to review the principles involved in helping children deal with diabetes.

Teenagers Initially, teenagers often have intense trouble accepting a diagnosis of diabetes. At a time when they are striving to develop their identity with a group and to be as similar to their peers as possible, they may deny their diagnosis and refuse to cooperate. Yet they must learn to manage their food, insulin, and exercise appropriately, for their lives are at stake. The person who appreciates a teen's special views on life is best prepared to help with the adjustment. Teens especially need to know that they can manage the disease themselves—that it won't turn them back into dependent children.

Family Members Parents and other family members also face the challenge of living with diabetes. The intensity of their emotional reactions to the diagnosis can either reinforce or disrupt family unity. Parents

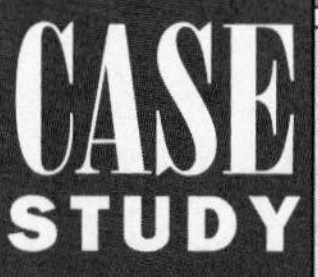

Child with IDDM

One year ago, Yusuf, a 12-year-old boy, was diagnosed with IDDM. The initial diagnosis was made after Yusuf's parents became concerned when he began to lose weight, to urinate excessively, and to complain of thirst. Aware of a family history of diabetes, Yusuf's parents quickly sought medical help. Since that time Yusuf's diabetes has been well controlled. Recently, however, Yusuf was admitted to the emergency room, complaining of nausea, vomiting, and intense thirst. His blood glucose monitoring records from the previous day showed that he had a fever and that his blood glucose was high throughout the day. The physician observed that Yusuf was confused and breathing with difficulty and also noted the smell of acetone on his breath. Urine tests were positive for glycosuria and ketonuria, and his blood glucose was 400 milligrams/100 milliliters. The diagnosis was diabetic ketoacidosis.

1. Describe the metabolic events that led to the symptoms associated with diabetes (before diagnosis), as well as those associated with diabetic ketoacidosis.
2. Were Yusuf's physical symptoms and laboratory tests consistent with this diagnosis?
3. How can you distinguish between diabetic ketoacidosis and an insulin reaction?
4. When Yusuf recovers, what advice can you offer him in order to prevent future incidents of ketoacidosis? Assume that he has never had diabetic diet instructions. What dietary modifications would you advise him to follow?
5. Think about and discuss the influence of Yusuf's age on his outlook and ability to cope with diabetes. What problems does his age pose? Consider some ways you might help him deal with these problems.
6. Regarding his future, describe the possible role of diet in preventing the vascular complications of diabetes.

may resent the demands of caring for a child with a chronic illness; at the same time, they may feel guilty for having selfish feelings. They may feel anxiety about allowing their child to follow the diabetes care regimen without their constant assistance. Especially in the case of an older child, they may press their care and control on a child who needs to develop autonomy and self-care. Parents may also become emotionally upset when they see their child feeling anxious, depressed, or withdrawn. Parents may benefit from attending meetings with other parents of children with diabetes to share feelings, ideas, and frustrations. Sometimes just knowing that you're not alone helps.

Family Lifestyles Successful diet management incorporates prescribed meals into existing family lifestyles and eating patterns. Depending on insulin administration and personal preferences, children generally receive three meals and two to three snacks a day. Snacks before bedtime may help prevent nocturnal hypoglycemia, especially if the child engages in strenuous activity late in the day. Caretakers should vary snacks to prevent boredom, provide enough to share with friends, and avoid identifying foods as "good" or "bad." Such connotations create unrealistic expectations or fears and invite the development of manipulative eating behaviors.

Treatment of Noninsulin-Dependent Diabetes Mellitus (NIDDM)

The onset and severity of symptoms are less dramatic for NIDDM than for IDDM. Similarly, the treatment regimen for NIDDM, though still important, is more flexible.

Goals of NIDDM Therapy The goals of therapy for NIDDM mimic those for IDDM, namely:

- To maintain blood glucose within a near-normal range.
- To achieve and maintain appropriate blood lipid levels.
- To prevent the acute and chronic complications associated with diabetes.
- To promote quality of life by encouraging people with NIDDM to resume the activities they enjoy with the best possible health.

The treatment needed to attain these goals is different, however, because NIDDM develops from a resistance to, and an impaired secretion of, insulin rather than from lack of it.

People with NIDDM may have higher than normal levels of insulin (hyperinsulinemia) early in the course of their disease. Later, insulin secretion declines.

Diet in NIDDM The diet for NIDDM provides for a balanced nutrient intake with carbohydrates spaced evenly throughout the day. As in IDDM, many approaches can be used to plan diets in NIDDM. The composition of the diet for people with NIDDM parallels recommendations for healthy eating for all people and is the same as for people with IDDM.

Weight Control Weight loss is often prescribed in NIDDM. Even moderate weight loss (10 to 20 pounds) can help reverse insulin resistance, improve blood lipids, and reduce blood pressure. Physical activity helps to control weight, and the combination of weight loss and physical activity is especially effective. Weight-reduction diets that provide at least 10 kcalories per pound of body weight allow a safe and gradual weight loss. The person at a healthy weight may not need to limit energy intake but still needs to follow the principles of diet for diabetes.

Timing and Distribution of Meals Timing and distribution of meals are not as critical in NIDDM as in IDDM because carbohydrate does not have to be coordinated with insulin delivery. Carbohydrates should be evenly spaced throughout the day, however. Giving too much carbohydrate at one time can raise blood glucose too high, stressing the already compromised insulin-producing cells. People taking drugs to control blood glucose need some carbohydrate to prevent hypoglycemia.

Alcohol The guidelines for alcohol use in NIDDM are the same as in IDDM (see p. 591). Forewarn clients on oral drugs (described later) that the combination of alcohol and oral hypoglycemic agents can cause flushing of the skin and a rapid heartbeat in some people.

Physical Activity A program of moderate physical activity offers many benefits, but its greatest value is its contribution to weight loss.

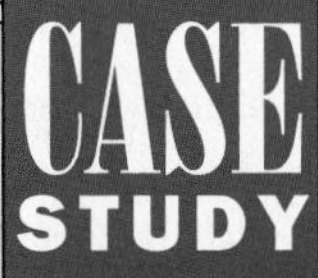
CASE
STUDY

Truck Driver with NIDDM

Mr. Evans, a truck driver, was 52 years old when he was first diagnosed with NIDDM. He visited his physician after experiencing excessive thirst, excessive urination, and excessive appetite. Mr. Evans, who stands 5 feet 11 inches tall and currently weighs 200 pounds, experienced a 30-pound weight gain over the past two years. His fasting blood glucose is 235 milligrams/100 milliliters.

The health care team members have evaluated Mr. Evans's case. They are eager to help him achieve the first goal of diabetes management—that is, to bring his blood glucose under control.

Mr. Evans is concerned about his health. He is worried that he may need insulin injections, and overwhelmed by all the information he has been given over the past few days.

1. Can you explain to Mr. Evans how NIDDM differs from IDDM?
2. Describe what factors in Mr. Evans's history might have predisposed him to NIDDM.
3. What will be the primary objective of the diet therapy for Mr. Evans?
4. Determine Mr. Evans's ideal body weight, and plan a diet for him. (Use the information on exchange lists in the box on pp. 592–593.)
5. Can NIDDM usually be controlled by diet alone? What other measure might help Mr. Evans bring his blood glucose under control?
6. What alternative treatments might Mr. Evans's physician consider if diet alone fails?
7. Consider Mr. Evans's emotional health. How can the health care team help him during his difficult period?

Many clinicians believe that most people with NIDDM who are overweight can achieve metabolic control if they follow a kcalorie-restricted diet combined with a physical activity program of moderate intensity. Furthermore, studies suggest that vigorous physical activity may delay or prevent the onset of NIDDM.[10] The accompanying case study offers an example of a person with NIDDM.

Drug Therapy People with NIDDM can sometimes control their blood glucose through diet and physical activity alone. When these measures fail, oral drugs may be started. Oral hypoglycemic agents appear to stimulate the release of insulin from the pancreas, reduce insulin resistance, and suppress glucose release from the liver. Oral agents have a maximum dose; if blood glucose cannot be controlled at the maximum dose, physicians prescribe insulin therapy or a combination of oral hypoglycemic agents and insulin. A person diagnosed with NIDDM who receives insulin therapy is thereafter treated as having IDDM. Drugs do not replace diet and physical activity; remind clients to continue these therapies as instructed.

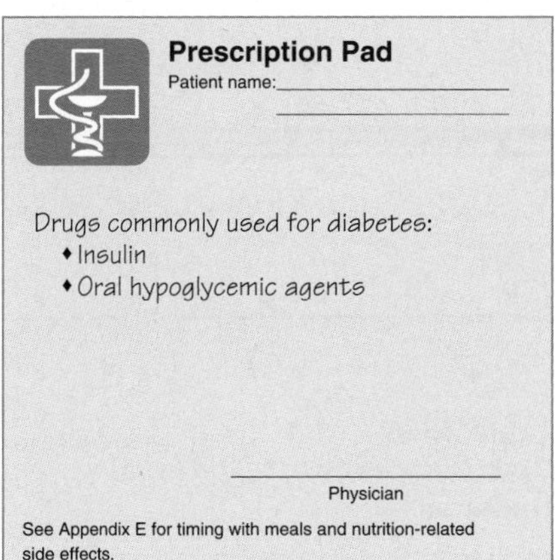
Prescription Pad
Patient name:
Drugs commonly used for diabetes:
• Insulin
• Oral hypoglycemic agents
Physician
See Appendix E for timing with meals and nutrition-related side effects.

oral hypoglycemic agents: drugs that can be taken by mouth to lower blood glucose in NIDDM; these drugs are ineffective in IDDM.

Diabetes in Pregnancy and Later Life

Special considerations apply when a person with diabetes is a pregnant woman or an elderly person. A section on each follows.

Diabetes Management in Pregnancy

Pregnancy in all women elevates blood insulin and alters insulin resistance. Blood insulin begins to rise soon after conception, and the cells respond by storing energy nutrients to provide for the developing fetus. Later in pregnancy, insulin remains high, but the cells become insulin resistant. Hormones that act antagonistically to insulin rise. This hormonal shift signals the body to stop storing energy fuels and to begin allowing the fetus to extract energy nutrients rapidly during the mother's fasting times. Because pregnancy stresses the glucose-regulatory system in these ways, women with diabetes should expect control to become more difficult during pregnancy.

The hormones that antagonize the action of insulin during late pregnancy are placental lactogen, cortisol, prolactin, and progesterone.

Risks of Diabetes during Pregnancy Women with diabetes who are contemplating pregnancy should know that uncontrolled diabetes presents risks for both mother and infant. Women face a high infertility rate and those who do conceive may experience episodes of severe hypoglycemia or hyperglycemia, spontaneous abortion, and pregnancy-induced hypertension. Infants may suffer increased mortality and morbidity, congenital abnormalities, and other complications such as severe hypoglycemia or respiratory distress, both of which can be fatal.

Reminder: High blood pressure that develops in pregnancy is known as *pregnancy-induced hypertension* and may signal the onset of other complications (see pp. 369-370).

respiratory distress: a disorder of the lung membranes that results in delayed onset of respiration at birth and difficulty in breathing after birth.

Gestational Diabetes Previously nondiabetic women may also develop diabetes during pregnancy (gestational diabetes). It usually appears late in pregnancy when the tissues become insulin resistant. Health care professionals evaluate a woman's potential for gestational diabetes by checking the risk factors listed in Table 25–6 during the first prenatal examination. As added insurance against problems with diabetes, all pregnant women have urine tests for glucose and ketones at each checkup. Many physicians give glucose tolerance tests routinely between 24 and 28 weeks of gestation.

Reminder: Abnormal glucose tolerance during pregnancy, with a subsequent return to normal glucose tolerance postpartum is *gestational diabetes*.

Blood Glucose Monitoring Obstetricians recommend blood glucose monitoring for all pregnant women with any type of diabetes. Establishing blood glucose control is important to the health of both mother and infant. Pregnant women with diabetes may also need to monitor their urine for ketones because ketosis in early pregnancy can lead to congenital malformations, central nervous system disorders, and low measures of intelligence in infants.

Table 25–6
Risk Factors for Gestational Diabetes

- Previous gestational diabetes.
- History of large infant (9 pounds or more).
- Family history of diabetes.
- Symptoms of diabetes and glycosuria.
- Obesity or excessive weight gain.
- Recurrent urinary tract infections.
- History of spontaneous abortions.
- Previous unexplained stillbirth.

Diet For the pregnant woman with diabetes, the diabetic diet, tailored to meet the increased nutrient demands of pregnancy, and carefully coordinated with insulin therapy when necessary, is central to therapy. The diet plan aims to provide adequate, but not excessive, kcalories to prevent excessive weight gain. A bedtime snack is recommended to prevent nocturnal hypoglycemia in the mother, and to provide fuel and prevent the buildup of ketones in the developing fetus.

Preventive Measures for Gestational Diabetes Almost one-third of all women who have gestational diabetes develop NIDDM within five years. The risk of developing NIDDM or glucose intolerance after childbirth increases with each pregnancy.[11] Research indicates that the incidence of NIDDM in women with previous gestational diabetes is twice as high in those who are 20 percent or more overweight, compared with those of normal weight. Therefore, health care professionals encourage clients with gestational diabetes not to gain excessive weight during pregnancy, and to lose weight (if necessary) and pay careful attention to diet following pregnancy.

Treatment of Elderly People with Diabetes

The elderly face special problems in dealing with diabetes. They have a greater risk of hyperglycemia and hypoglycemia because of reduced appetite, altered thirst regulation, altered kidney and liver function, depression or mental deterioration, multiple medications, and coexisting medical conditions. The elderly may also lack the financial resources or social support necessary to help them cope with their diabetes. Caring health professionals address these problems and help elderly clients find solutions.

To meet all the goals of diabetes education requires support from the diabetes care team—physicians, nurses, dietitians, counselors, and exercise specialists. Each member of the team coordinates instructions with other team members so that clients receive consistent advice that will not overwhelm or confuse them

People with diabetes and those who work with them need to realize that the learning process takes time. After their initial introduction to the world of diabetes, clients benefit from education programs and frequent follow-up visits to address problems, expand their knowledge and promote independence.[12]

Hypoglycemia

Strictly speaking, the term *hypoglycemia* simply means "low blood glucose." It is not a disease but a symptom of altered carbohydrate metabolism. In normal metabolism, blood glucose rises after eating and then gradually declines while the cells begin to store fuels. As blood glucose falls, the liver starts to release glucose from stored glycogen for the body's use. Throughout, blood glucose remains in the normal range, and the transition occurs without notice. In some people, however, hypoglycemia occurs as the body shifts from the fed to the fasting state. Hypoglycemia may or may not be accompanied by other symptoms, and the symptoms may or may not be uncomfortable. There are two major types of hypoglycemia, reactive and fasting.

hypoglycemia: an abnormally low blood glucose concentration, a condition that may indicate any of several diseases, including early diabetes (NIDDM).

Reactive Hypoglycemia Reactive hypoglycemia occurs within an hour or two after eating and is related to the release of the hormone epinephrine, triggered by rapidly falling blood glucose. The symptoms of reactive hypoglycemia are like those of an anxiety attack: weakness, rapid heartbeat, sweating, anxiety, hunger, and trembling.

reactive hypoglycemia: hypoglycemia experienced simultaneously with epinephrine-release symptoms one to three hours after a meal; also called **postprandial hypoglycemia.**

In most cases, the reason why blood glucose falls rapidly is unknown. In some cases, though, another medical problem leads to reactive hypoglycemia—for example, in the person who has dumping syndrome after gastric surgery, when central TPN solutions are discontinued too quickly (described in Chapters 20 and 23), or early in NIDDM.

Diagnosis of Reactive Hypoglycemia True reactive hypoglycemia can be identified by directly testing the blood glucose concentration at intervals after a meal.[13] The finding that a person has reactive hypoglycemia requires two simultaneous observations: (1) low blood glucose and (2) the simultaneous presence of symptoms. True reactive hypoglycemia is rare, although it is often misdiagnosed, and has been the subject of much misguided advice.

Diet for Reactive Hypoglycemia For persons who experience reactive hypoglycemia, a carbohydrate-modified diet may bring needed relief. Avoidance of low-carbohydrate dieting and of sudden large sugar doses may be all that is required. People need to avoid concentrated sweets, eat regularly, and eat balanced meals. If several average-sized meals fail to relieve symptoms, a person may benefit by eating smaller meals more frequently. A diet adviser develops a diet similar to the diet for diabetes, which is appropriate to achieve or maintain a healthy body weight; the exchange lists may be used for instruction.

Fasting Hypoglycemia A person who has symptoms while well advanced into the fasting state (for example, overnight) is experiencing a different kind of hypoglycemia. This condition arises from medically diverse disorders that interfere with normal blood glucose regulation, such as diabetes or tumors of the pancreas or liver. Table 25–7 lists the major distinguishing characteristics of reactive and fasting hypoglycemia. The symptoms of fasting hypoglycemia differ from those of reactive hypoglycemia because they are not related to epinephrine. Instead, blood glu-

fasting hypoglycemia: hypoglycemia that sets in gradually and primarily affects the brain and central nervous system.

Table 25–7
Characteristics of Reactive and Fasting Hypoglycemia

	REACTIVE TYPE	FASTING TYPE
Onset of symptoms	Sudden; occurs 1 to 3 hours after meals	Gradual; occurs after fasting
Type of symptoms	Weakness, rapid heartbeat sweating, anxiety, hunger, trembling	Headache, mental dullness, fatigue, confusion, amnesia, seizures, unconsciousness
Duration of symptoms	Transient	Persistent
Possible causes	Early NIDDM, gastric surgery, TPN	Hormonal imbalance, diabetes, drugs, tumors
Clinical course	Less serious; treat with diet	Can be serious; treat underlying problems
Other names	Alimentary, postprandial, idiopathic, functional	—

cose falls gradually, affecting the brain and central nervous system. The symptoms include: headache, mental dullness, fatigue, confusion, amnesia, and even seizures and unconsciousness. Treatment of fasting hypoglycemia depends on the underlying cause.

Diet for Fasting Hypoglycemia Earlier sections of this chapter described how an evenly spaced and consistent carbohydrate intake can help prevent and treat fasting hypoglycemia in people with diabetes. Surgery is the primary treatment of fasting hypoglycemia caused by tumors, although carbohydrate-modified diets (as described for reactive hypoglycemia) may be used temporarily.

Nonhypoglycemia Many dishonest or ill-informed practitioners "diagnose" hypoglycemia on the basis of their clients' verbal reports alone and prescribe all sorts of "remedies" for it with transparently thin rationale. People also "diagnose" themselves so commonly that physicians have identified a special category for their condition: *non*hypoglycemia. Word-of-mouth reports that a person has hypoglycemia, unaccompanied by valid test results to back them up, warrant no concern for a person's physical health, but may require tactful handling and referral.

nonhypoglycemia: a term used when people think they have hypoglycemia but don't.

Nutrition Assessment

Keep these points in mind when assessing the nutrition status of people with disorders of glucose metabolism:

- Obtain an accurate assessment of both current and appropriate weight. In treating IDDM, doses of insulin are based on body weight, as are the calculations of total daily food energy intakes. On reassessment, energy intake may need to be adjusted frequently, particularly in the growing child.
- Obtain an accurate diet and physical activity history from the person with diabetes. This step is instrumental in planning an acceptable diet, as well as in identifying possible nutrient deficiencies. During reassessment, use food intake records along with records of blood glucose monitoring to check compliance with the treatment plan and to help the client make necessary adjustments. Food records for people with hypoglycemia help pinpoint food habits associated with unwanted symptoms.
- Arm anthropometrics may be difficult to obtain and interpret in some people with IDDM, especially when the midarm area has hypertrophied due to repeated insulin injections. Fat measurements can be taken using other areas of the body in these cases.
- Monitor blood glucose, blood lipids, and blood pressure regularly in people with diabetes. Also check tests of renal function periodically.

Diet therapy is of major importance in the treatment of metabolic disorders, and conscientious attention to diet brings great rewards. The Nutrition in Practice that follows shows that diet can be crucial in preventing complications of inborn errors of metabolism, including mental retardation.

STUDY QUESTIONS

1. What biochemical tests are used to diagnose diabetes?
2. Name the two major types of diabetes. Which type is more common? Describe some differences between the two types.
3. Describe the basic problem in diabetes, and tell how it leads to these symptoms: hyperglycemia, glycosuria, dehydration, polyuria, polydipsia, weight loss, polyphagia, acetone breath, ketosis, and ketonuria.
4. What is hyperosmolar hyperglycemic nonketotic coma? How is it different from the diabetic coma that develops from severe hyperglycemia in the person with IDDM?
5. What types of chronic complications can arise as a result of diabetes?
6. What are the goals of therapy for all people with diabetes? Name the three aspects of lifestyle that must be coordinated for the person with IDDM.
7. What two types of insulin requirements do our bodies have, and how is commercially available insulin given to simulate these requirements? Why is insulin not taken orally? How do insulin needs change with body weight?
8. What is the recommended distribution of nutrients in the diet used to treat IDDM? How does this recommendation compare to the healthy diet recommended for all people?
9. Describe some general guidelines for the use of alcohol in the diabetic diet.
10. Why are the timing and composition of meals important considerations in planning a diet for a person with IDDM?
11. How are the carbohydrate content of the diet and insulin adjusted for physical activity? How is the diet adjusted if a person misses meals?
12. What methods can the person with diabetes use to monitor blood glucose? What is glycated hemoglobin, and what is the advantage of measuring it in the blood?
13. Describe ways that diet and insulin are adjusted for people with IDDM who experience hyperglycemia or hypoglycemia.
14. What is the primary goal of diet therapy for the person with NIDDM? How does diet therapy differ from that for IDDM?
15. Consider some of the special needs of children who have diabetes. How is the diet adjusted to meet these needs?
16. What events occur in all pregnancies that may interfere with the control of blood glucose in the pregnant woman with diabetes? How is the pregnant woman with IDDM managed? How is the pregnant woman with NIDDM managed?
17. What is gestational diabetes? How is it managed?
18. What special concerns arise in elderly people with diabetes?
19. Besides diabetes, what are some other causes of hypoglycemia? What is the recommended treatment for reactive hypoglycemia?

CLINICAL APPLICATION QUESTIONS

1. Using the box on pp. 592–593, plan a diet using the exchange lists for a sedentary woman with IDDM who is 5 feet 9 inches tall and weighs 160 pounds. Round off kcalories and develop a sample diet pattern.
2. An important part of learning is being able to apply knowledge and guidelines to real-life situations. Using Table 25–5 as a guide, think about the possible remedies for either hyperglycemia or hypoglycemia. Describe at least one situation when it might be preferable to alter the insulin dose and one when it might be preferable to alter the carbohydrate intake.
3. Visit a pharmacy and price these items: blood glucose meter, glucose test strips, lancets, insulin, and syringes. Determine the approximate costs of insulin for a person who uses 14 units of regular insulin and 26 units of NPH insulin in three injections daily. Then estimate the cost of testing blood glucose four times daily. How do the costs of glucose test strips differ when used with or without a meter? How are the costs associated with diabetes affected by the need for a well-balanced diet? Consider how an external pump might affect the total cost of managing diabetes.

NUTRITION IN PRACTICE 25

Inborn Errors of Metabolism

The preceding chapter has shown how devastating disorders of metabolism can be and how important diet can be to their control. Inborn errors of metabolism extend those themes further. Each inborn error affects metabolism in a unique way and has specific implications for diet.

What is an inborn error of metabolism?

An inborn error is a genetic error that causes a protein to be made in an insufficient quantity or to have an abnormal structure. When a protein is abnormal, some body function such as a metabolic reaction or a transport process that depends on that protein cannot proceed. For example, if an enzyme is missing or malfunctioning in the metabolic pathway that converts compound A to compound B, then compound A accumulates and compound B becomes deficient. Both the excess of compound A and the lack of compound B can lead to a variety of problems and, in many cases, can cause death. Furthermore, high concentrations of compound A become available for use in other metabolic pathways, while low concentrations of compound B make it less available. This may in turn create excesses and deficiencies of other compounds that present another array of problems. The accompanying glossary defines related terms.

Do all inborn errors cause severe illness or death?

No, many do not. In some instances, the accumulated compound is not toxic and the deficient compound is not essential, so individuals experience no problem. They may not even know about the error. In other cases, however, inborn errors have severe consequences; many of them may cause mental retardation or prove lethal, but some may be treated by diet. As with most medical disorders, the earlier the diagnosis and treatment, the better the prognosis.

How are inborn errors treated?

The primary treatment for many inborn errors is nutrition. With an understanding of the biochemical pathway involved, a clinician can often manipulate the diet to compensate for excesses and inadequacies. Management involves restricting precursors that occur prior to the error in the metabolic pathway, replacing needed products that fail to be produced, or both. The goals of therapy are to:

- Prevent the accumulation of toxic compounds.
- Replace essential nutrients that become deficient as a result of the defective metabolic pathway.

Glossary of Terms Related to Inborn Errors of Metabolism

carrier: an individual who possesses one dominant and one recessive gene for a recessive trait, such as an inborn error of metabolism. Such a person may show no signs of the trait but can pass it on.

dominant gene: a gene that has an observable effect on an organism. Most of the time, normal genes are dominant over abnormal genes. An abnormal gene can, however, sometimes exert an observable effect even when it is paired with a normal gene. See also *recessive gene.*

galactosemia: an inborn error of metabolism in which galactose cannot be metabolized normally to compounds the body can handle and an alternative metabolite accumulates in the tissues, causing damage.

genes: the basic units of hereditary information, made of DNA, that are passed from parent to offspring in the chromosomes. Each gene codes for a protein.

inborn error of metabolism: an inherited flaw evident as a metabolic disorder or disease present from birth.

mutation: an alteration in a gene such that an altered protein is produced.
muta = change

phenylketonuria (PKU): an inborn error of metabolism in which phenylalanine, an essential amino acid, cannot be converted to tyrosine. Alternative metabolites of phenylalanine (phenylketones) accumulate in the tissues, causing damage, and overflow into the urine.

recessive gene: a gene that has no observable effect on an organism as long as it is paired with a normal gene that can produce a normal product. In this case, the normal gene is said to be *dominant.*

- Provide a diet that supports normal growth, development, and maintenance.

Meeting these three goals is a major challenge that was unattainable until earlier in this century. New knowledge about the body's many biochemical pathways, coupled with current technology for synthesizing formulas of specific nutrient compositions, has greatly enhanced the treatment of inborn errors.

Can you give a specific example of a typical inborn error?

A classic example that illustrates the principles of treatment is the most common inborn error of metabolism: phenylketonuria (PKU). PKU is one of many inborn errors that affect amino acid metabolism. Other disorders affect not only amino acid metabolism but also carbohydrate, lipid, and vitamin metabolism.

PKU affects approximately 1 out of every 10,000 newborns in the United States. The ability to detect and treat PKU has saved and significantly improved the lives of many people and provides an example that offers hope to those suffering from other inborn errors.

What causes PKU?

Classic PKU results from a deficiency of an enzyme that converts the essential amino acid phenylalanine to tyrosine (see Figure 25–2). Without the enzyme, abnormally high concentrations of phenylalanine and other related compounds accumulate and damage the developing nervous system. Simultaneously, the body cannot make the amino acid tyrosine or other compounds (such as the hormone epinephrine) that normally derive from it. Under these conditions, tyrosine becomes an essential amino acid; that is, the body cannot make it, so the diet must supply it.

How is PKU diagnosed?

PKU is a hidden disease that cannot be seen at birth, yet diagnosis and treatment beginning in the first few days of life can prevent its devastating effects. For these reasons, and because PKU is the most common inborn error of metabolism, all newborns in the United States receive a screening test, conducted after they have received several feedings containing protein (usually after one to seven days). Before screening became routine in the 1960s, an infant with PKU would suffer the dire consequences of uncorrected high phenylalanine concentrations. At first, the only signs are a skin rash and light skin pigmentation. Between three and six months, signs of developmental delay begin to appear. The infant becomes irritable, unable to sleep restfully, and frantic. By one year, irreversible brain damage is clearly evident.

What is the dietary treatment for PKU?

Essentially, the diet restricts phenylalanine and supplements

Figure 25–2
The Biochemical Pathway in PKU

Normal:
Normally, the amino acid phenylalanine follows two pathways, one in the liver, the other in the kidneys. In the liver, the enzyme phenylalanine hydroxylase adds a hydroxyl group (OH) to produce the amino acid tyrosine. Tyrosine, in turn, produces melanin, the pigmented compound found in skin and brain cells; the neurotransmitters epinephrine and norepinephrine; and the hormone thyroxine. In the kidneys, enzymes convert phenylalanine to by-products that are excreted.

In the liver:

Phenylalanine (an amino acid) → [Phenylalanine hydroxylase (an enzyme)] → Tyrosine (an amino acid) → Melanin (a pigment); Epinephrine (a neurotransmitter); Norepinephrine (a neurotransmitter); Thyroxine (a hormone)

In the kidneys:

Phenylalanine → Phenylpyruvic acid (a ketone) → Other phenyl acids

In PKU:
Individuals with PKU lack the liver enzyme phenylalanine hydroxylase, impairing conversion of phenylalanine to tyrosine. Phenylalanine accumulates in the liver and blood, reaching the kidneys in abnormally high concentrations. In the kidneys, an enzyme converts phenylalanine to the ketone phenylpyruvic acid,which spills into the urine—thus the name phenylketonuria.

In the liver:

Phenylalanine (accumulates) → [Phenylalanine hydroxylase (deficient)] → Tyrosine (deficient)

In the kidneys:

Phenylalanine (accumulates) → Phenylpyruvic acid (accumulates) → Other phenyl acids (accumulate)

tyrosine to levels that maintain blood concentrations within safe ranges. Its effectiveness is remarkable: in almost every case, it can prevent the devastating array of symptoms described. As most dietitians can attest, though, the diet is more easily described than designed.

Because phenylalanine is an essential amino acid, the diet cannot exclude it completely. If phenylalanine intake is too low, children suffer bone, skin, and blood disorders; growth and mental retardation; and death. Therefore, the diet must strike a balance, providing enough phenylalanine to support normal growth and health but not enough to cause harm. The problem is not that children with PKU require less phenylalanine than other children, but that they cannot handle excesses without detrimental effects. To ensure that blood phenylalanine and tyrosine concentrations remain within safe ranges, children with PKU receive blood tests periodically and alterations in their diets when necessary. With a controlled phenylalanine intake, children with PKU can lead normal, happy lives.

Special low-phenylalanine formulas are the primary source of energy and protein for children with PKU. The diet excludes high-protein foods such as meat, fish, poultry, cheese, eggs, milk, nuts, dried beans, and peas. Also excluded are commercial breads and pastries made from regular flour, which has a high phenylalanine content. Basically, the diet allows foods that contain some phenylalanine, such as fruits, vegetables, and cereals, and those that contain none, such as fats, sugars, jellies, and some candies. Clearly, it is impossible to create such a diet using only whole, natural foods, and children who depend primarily on a formula for their nourishment risk multiple trace mineral deficiencies.[14] The accompanying menu provides a sample phenylalanine-restricted diet for a child with PKU.

Sample PKU Menu for a Child

MENU

Breakfast	Lunch	Supper
2 tbs raisins 5 tbs cream of rice 2 tsp sugar 8 oz Lofenalac	1/2 small banana 2 tbs tomato soup (without milk) 3 tbs rice 1 1/2 tsp margarine 8 oz Lofenalac	2 tbs instant potatoes (without milk) 3 tbs green beans 4 tbs vegetable and beef broth 1 1/2 tsp margarine 3/4 c sliced peaches 8 oz Lofenalac

Midmorning Snack	Afternoon Snack	Bedtime Snack
4 oz orange juice	4 oz Lofenalac 5 round butter crackers	2 tbs raisins 4 oz Lofenalac

*Lofenalac is a special PKU formula that is low in phenylanine.

Do people with PKU have to stay on the diet for life?

The answer to that question is unclear. During the early years of central nervous system development, the diet is clearly critical to preventing irreversible mental retardation. Less clear is the length of time the nervous system is vulnerable to the PKU defect.

Until the late 1970s, researchers assumed that the child with PKU could abandon the special diet after the first few years of life when the central nervous system had completed its development. Unfortunately, however, even though the damage is less severe than at an earlier age, elevated phenylalanine concentrations in the older child do cause problems such as short attention span, poor short-term memory, and poor eye-to-hand coordination. A child with PKU who has discontinued the controlled diet may experience problems in school performance, mood, and behavior. For these reasons, clinicians now encourage children to continue the low-phenylalanine diet indefinitely. Reinstituting the phenylalanine-restricted diet in adolescents or adults after several years of unrestricted diets requires intense education and reinforcement, and even then it is quite often unsuccessful. Reinstitution of a controlled diet, if successful, does improve blood phenylalanine concentrations, behavior, and measures of intelligence.

Therapy for PKU and other inborn errors goes beyond nutrition to include psychological counseling for the people who are

genetic disorder is a lifelong problem that affects the entire family. All family members are at high risk for being carriers, and they inevitably become involved in the care and management of the person with the inborn error. Therefore, families must learn how to handle the impact such a diagnosis has on their relationships. Some family members may be PKU carriers, and for women who wish to conceive, it is important to know and deal with that fact.

What is a carrier?

A carrier is a person who inherits one defective gene and one normal gene. PKU, like all inborn errors, is a recessive disorder; that is, it appears only when a person inherits two defective genes—one from each parent. This can occur even if neither parent has PKU because both may be carriers (see Figure 25–3). The carriers may be unaware they have the defective gene, for the symptoms are usually mild or absent. The chance that two people with PKU may meet and conceive a child is not unlikely because of their many contacts with each other through PKU clinics and support groups.

If a woman with PKU becomes pregnant, how does the disorder affect her fetus?

Her high blood phenylalanine presents a hostile environment to fetal development. The fetus's blood concentrations rise even higher than hers, and she may experience a spontaneous abortion; or her infant may suffer mental retardation, microcephaly, congenital heart disease, and low birthweight.[15] For these reasons, women with elevated phenylalanine concentrations need counseling *prior* to pregnancy on the problems their condition may create for their children.

Dietary control of maternal PKU may protect the fetus, at least in part, if implemented early enough. Dietary control does not ensure a successful outcome of pregnancy, but the children of

Figure 25–3
The Inheritance of PKU

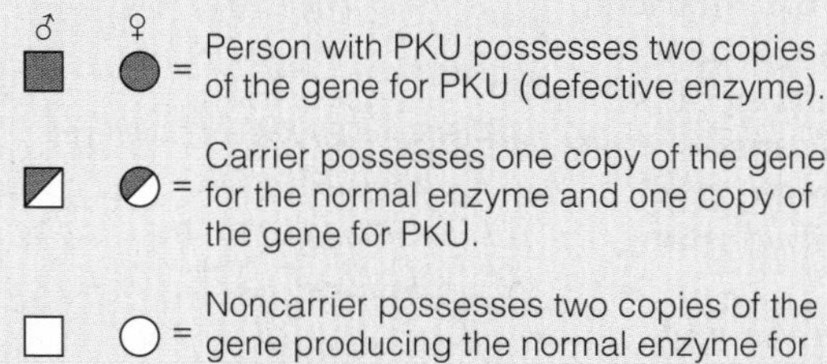
♂ ♀
= Person with PKU possesses two copies of the gene for PKU (defective enzyme).
= Carrier possesses one copy of the gene for the normal enzyme and one copy of the gene for PKU.
= Noncarrier possesses two copies of the gene producing the normal enzyme for processing phenylalanine

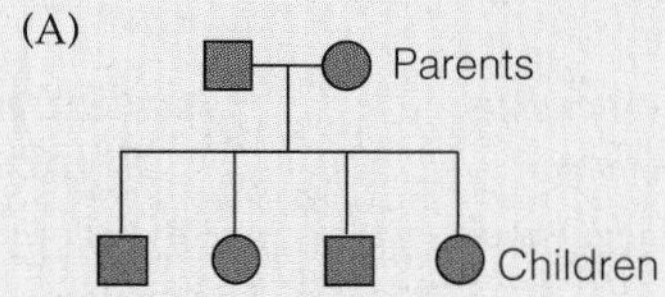
(A)
Parents
Children

When two people with PKU mate, all of their children will have PKU.

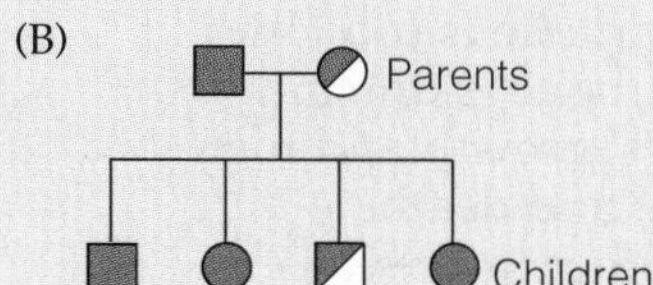
(B)
Parents
Children

When a person with PKU mates with a carrier, their children will have a 50% chance of either having PKU or being a carrier.

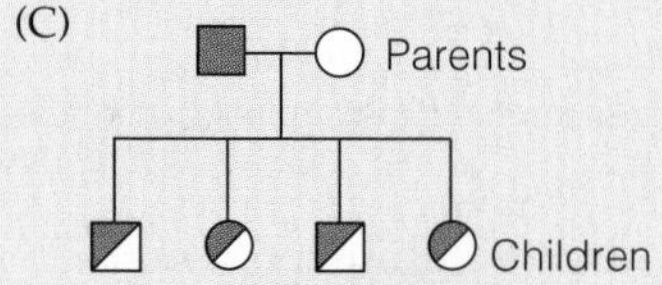
(C)
Parents
Children

When a person with PKU mates with a noncarrier, all of their children will be carriers.

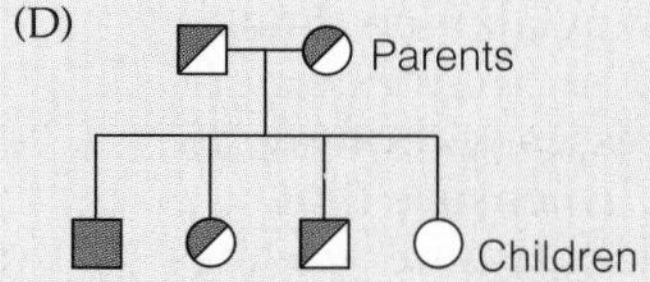
(D)
Parents
Children

When two carriers mate, they can pass on either the gene for the normal enzyme, or the gene for PKU. For each birth, there is one chance in four that the child will have PKU, two chances that the child will be a carrier, and one chance that the child will be PKU-free.

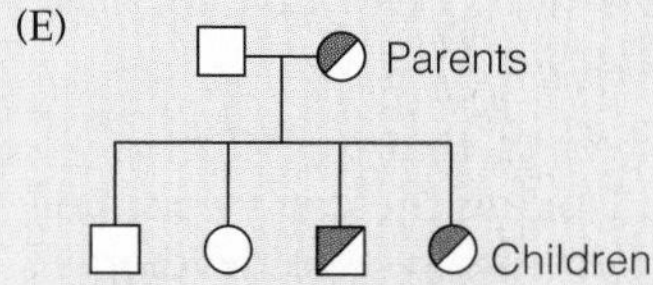
(E)
Parents
Children

When a noncarrier mates with a carrier, none of the children will have PKU. The parents may not even know that the gene for PKU is present, but half of their children (on average) will be carriers. This is how the gene for PKU "hides" in the general population.

women who follow a low-phenylalanine diet from before conception and throughout pregnancy are more likely to have higher birthweights, larger head circumferences, fewer malformations, and higher scores on intelligence tests than the children of women who begin diet therapy during their pregnancies or not at all.[16]

As mentioned, many physicians recommend adherence to a restricted diet throughout life anyway, but if a PKU woman has departed from her restricted diet as a child, she must resume the low-phenylalanine diet at least one to two months prior to conception and maintain it throughout her pregnancy.[17] Special formulas for pregnant women with PKU that meet the energy, protein, vitamin, and mineral needs of pregnancy are now available. Still, resuming a low-phenylalanine diet is not easy.

Are all inborn errors managed the same way as PKU?

In some ways, all are similar, but in other ways each is different. As an example, galactosemia is an inborn error of carbohydrate metabolism in which an enzyme that converts galactose to glucose is missing or defective. When infants with galactosemia are given milk (which contains a galactose unit in each molecule of lactose), they vomit and have diarrhea. The abnormal metabolism causes growth failure, liver enlargement, and other neurological abnormalities that lead to coma and death. Early introduction of a galactose-restricted diet prevents or minimizes most of these symptoms.

Dietary adjustment in galactosemia is simpler than in PKU for two reasons. First, unlike phenylalanine, galactose is not an essential nutrient. The galactosemia diet needs only to exclude galactose, not to provide a perfectly calculated dose. Second, since galactose occurs primarily in lactose (the sugar in milk), treatment depends chiefly on the careful restriction of all milk and milk products. Although lactose is found in many foods, it is less widespread in the diet than the amino acid phenylalanine, which appears in all proteins.

As scientific understanding of human genetics and biochemistry increases, more and more inborn errors affecting enzyme function are being recognized. Understanding the roles of enzymes in metabolism sometimes makes it possible to compensate for these defects, which otherwise would destroy the quality of life. In such cases, diet can make a dramatic difference in people's lives.

■ NOTES ■

1. M. J. Franz, Practice guidelines for nutrition care by dietetics practitioners for outpatients with non-insulin-dependent diabetes mellitus: Consensus statement, *Journal of the American Dietetic Association* 92 (1992): 1136–1139.
2. R. B. Lyon and D. M. Vinci, Nutrition management of insulin-dependent diabetes mellitus in adults: Review by the Diabetes Care and Education dietetic practice group, *Journal of the American Dietetic Association* 93 (1993): 309–314, 317.
3. As cited in the DCCT Research Group, Expanded role of the dietitian in the Diabetes Control and Complications Trial: Implications for clinical practice, *Journal of the American Dietetic Association* 93 (1993): 758–764, 767.
4. American Diabetes Association, Nutrition recommendations and principles for people with diabetes mellitus, *Diabetes Care* 17 (1994): 519–552.
5. Diabetes Care and Education Dietetic Practice Group of the American Dietetic Association, *Meal Planning Approaches for Diabetes Management* (Chicago, Ill.: American Dietetic Association, 1994).
6. American Diabetes Association, 1994.
7. American Diabetes Association, 1994.
8. P. J. Charney, Nutrition support in patients with diabetes mellitus, *Support Line* 15 (1993): 1–4.
9. A. G. Scrimgeour and J. T. Devlin, Prescribing exercise for patients with IDDM, *Internal Medicine* 12 (1991): 56–58, 63–65, 69–70.
10. J. Manson and coauthors, A prospective study of exercise and incidence of diabetes among U.S. male physicians, *Journal of the American Medical Association* 268 (1992): 63–67; S. P. Helmrich and coauthors. Physical activity and reduced occurrence of non-insulin-dependent diabetes mellitus, *New England Journal of Medicine* 325 (1991): 147–152.
11. D. K. Silverstein, E. B. Connor, and D. L. Wingard, The effect of parity on the later development of non-insulin-dependent diabetes mellitus or impaired glucose tolerance, *New England Journal of Medicine* 321 (1989): 1214–1219.
12. G. L. Grossan and M. L. Uster, Islet pilots—An educational program for children with diabetes, *Journal of the American Dietetic Association* 88 (1988): 471.
13. J. Palardy and coauthors, Blood glucose measurements during symptomatic episodes in patients with suspected postprandial hypoglycemia, *New England Journal of Medicine* 321 (1989): 1421–1425.
14. C. Reilly and coauthors, Trace

element nutrition status and dietary intake of children with phenylketonuria, *American Journal of Clinical Nutrition* 52 (1990): 159–165; S. Stepnick-Gropper and coauthors, Trace element status of children with PKU and normal children, *Journal of the American Dietetic Association* 88 (1988): 459–465.

15. P. B. Acosta, Phenylketonuria—Impact of nutrition support on reproductive outcomes, *Nutrition Today,* January/February 1991, pp. 43–47.
16. Committee on Genetics, Maternal phenylketonuria, *Pediatrics* 88 (1991): 1284–1285. Acosta, 1991.
17. P. B. Acosta, Maternal PKU. Address presented at the conference Nutrition for Pregnancy, Lactation, and Infancy, Gainesville, Florida, February 13, 1987.

26

Nutrition and Disorders of the Blood Vessels, Heart, and Lungs

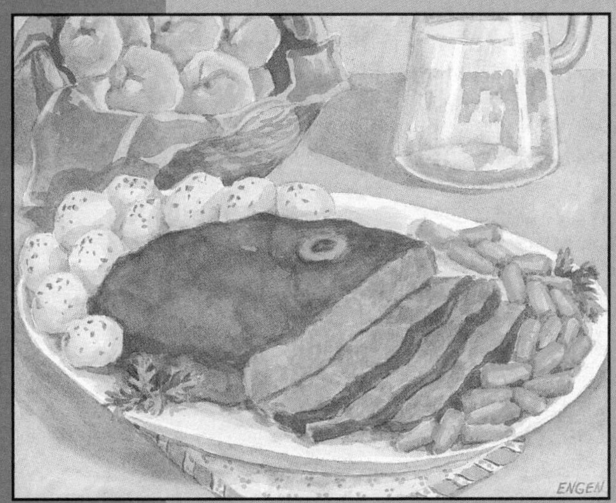

CONTENTS

Reminder: *Cardiovascular disease (CVD)* is a general term for all diseases of the heart and blood vessels. The main form of CVD is atherosclerosis, arterial blockage caused by plaques. When atherosclerosis damages the arteries that feed the heart, and the heart muscle begins to deteriorate, it is **coronary heart disease (CHD)**. When people speak of heart disease, it is usually coronary heart disease they are referring to.

Reminder: *Atherosclerosis* is characterized by plaques along the inner walls of the arteries. (The related term *arteriosclerosis* refers to all conditions in which the arteries lose elasticity, including some rare diseases.)

hypertension: high blood pressure.

heart attacks: blockages of vessels that feed the heart muscle, which cause sudden tissue death, also called **myocardial infarctions (MI).**
myo = muscle
cardial = heart
infarct = tissue death

strokes: events in which the blood flow to a part of the brain is suddenly cut off.

plaques (PLACKS): mounds of lipid material, mixed with smooth muscle cells and calcium, which develop in the artery walls in atherosclerosis. This type of plaque is known as an **atheromatous** plaque.
placken = patch or plate

platelets: tiny, disc-shaped bodies in the blood, important in blood clot formation.

thrombosis: the formation or development of a *thrombus*, a blood clot that may obstruct a blood vessel or the heart cavity, causing gradual death of tissue. A *coronary thrombosis* is the blockage of a vessel that feeds the heart muscle. A *cerebral thrombosis* is the blockage of a vessel that feeds the brain.
thrombo = clot

Cardiovascular disease (CVD) is the leading cause of death around the world today.[1] Heart disease and strokes rank first and third, respectively, as causes of death in men and women.[2] The rate of CVD has fallen steadily in the United States since 1950, as people have learned to improve their lifestyles to reduce their risks. Nevertheless, the rate is still high and is rising in other parts of the world.

Most CVD involves both atherosclerosis and hypertension. Each of these conditions has its own set of risk factors, listed later. Each makes the other worse.

This chapter examines the factors that lead to atherosclerosis and hypertension. Then it describes the major consequences of ignoring these conditions—heart attacks and strokes. It continues with discussions on related disorders: congestive heart failure and disorders of the lungs.

Atherosclerosis and Coronary Heart Disease

No one is free of the fatty streaks that gradually become the fibrous plaques of atherosclerosis. For most adults, the question is not whether you have plaques, but how far advanced they are and what you can do to retard or reverse their progression.

How Atherosclerosis Develops

Atherosclerosis usually begins with damage to the inner arterial walls followed by the accumulation of soft fatty streaks, especially at branch points (see Figure 26–1). These fatty streaks gradually enlarge and become hardened with minerals, forming plaques. Plaques stiffen the arteries and obstruct the flow of blood through them. Most people have well-developed plaques by the age of 30.

Plaques in the coronary arteries limit oxygen delivery and blood flow to the heart muscle, leading to coronary heart disease (CHD). Surgery may be required to bypass clogged arteries if they are conveying too little blood to the heart.

Blood Pressure Rises Normally, the arteries expand with each heartbeat to accommodate the pulses of blood that flow through them. Arteries stiffened and narrowed by plaques cannot expand, and so the blood pressure rises. This damages the artery walls further. Plaques are especially likely to form at damage points; thus the development of atherosclerosis is a self-accelerating process.

Blood Clots Form Small, cell-like bodies in the blood, known as platelets, cause clots to form whenever they encounter injuries in blood vessels. Clots normally form and dissolve in the blood all the time, but in atherosclerosis, clots form faster than they dissolve because the platelets "see" the plaques as injuries.

Thrombosis and Embolism Abnormal blood clotting can trigger life-threatening events. A blood clot may stick to a plaque and gradually grow large enough to close off a blood vessel (thrombosis), or a clot may

Figure 26–1
The Formation of Plaques in Atherosclerosis
When plaques have covered 60 percent of the coronary artery walls, the critical phase of heart disease begins.

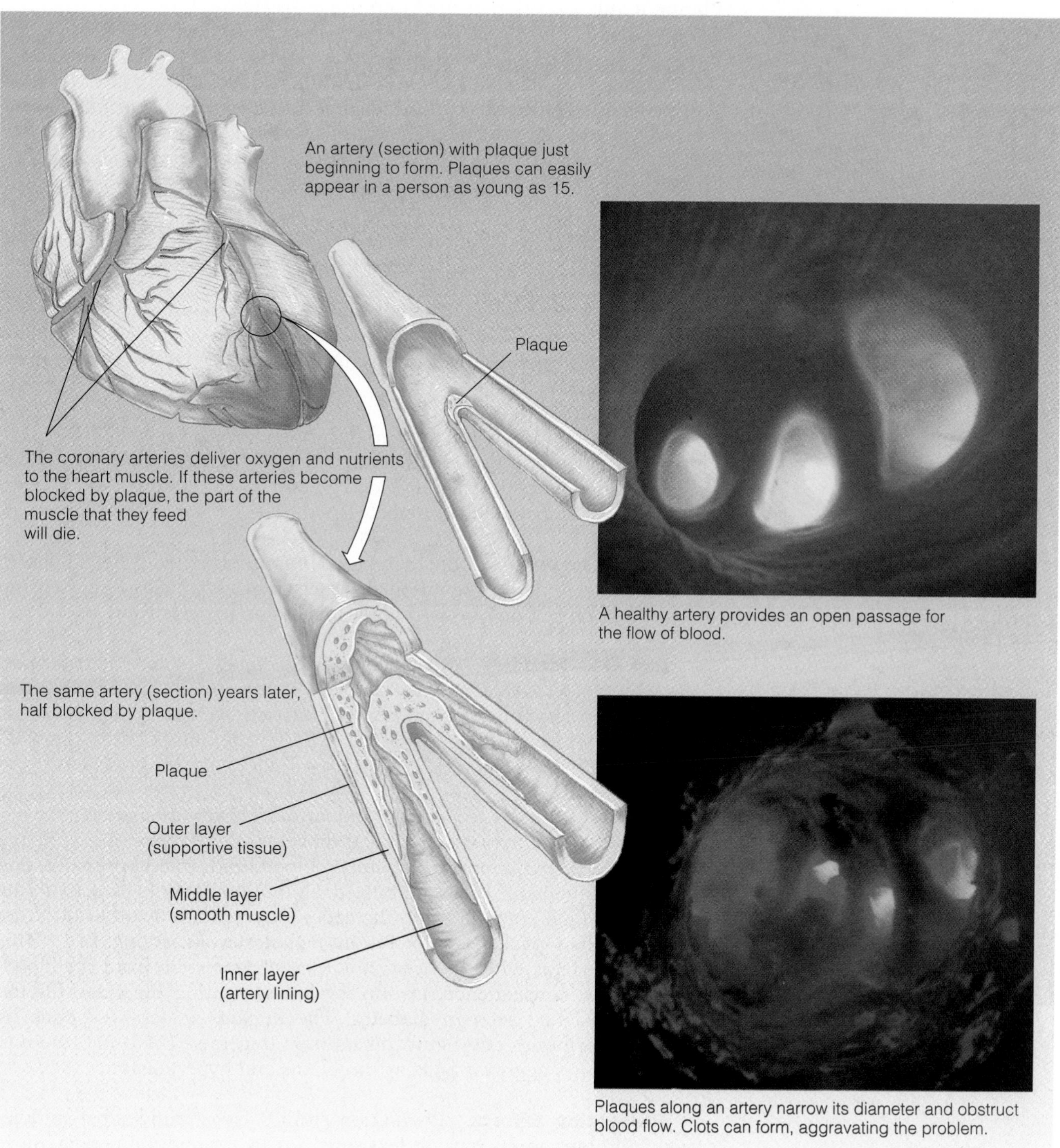
An artery (section) with plaque just beginning to form. Plaques can easily appear in a person as young as 15.
Plaque
The coronary arteries deliver oxygen and nutrients to the heart muscle. If these arteries become blocked by plaque, the part of the muscle that they feed will die.
A healthy artery provides an open passage for the flow of blood.
The same artery (section) years later, half blocked by plaque.
Plaque
Outer layer (supportive tissue)
Middle layer (smooth muscle)
Inner layer (artery lining)
Plaques along an artery narrow its diameter and obstruct blood flow. Clots can form, aggravating the problem.

embolism: the obstruction of a blood vessel by a traveling clot, causing sudden death of tissue.
embol = to insert, plug

break loose and travel the circulatory system until it lodges in a small artery and suddenly shuts off the blood flow to an area (embolism). Such a clot lodged in an artery of the heart causes sudden death of part of the heart muscle—a heart attack. When the clot lodges in an artery of the brain, it kills a portion of the brain tissue—a stroke.

Risk Factors for CHD

Reminder: Factors that are associated with an elevated frequency of a disease are *risk factors*. Some risk factors, such as diet and physical activity, are *modifiable*, meaning that they can be changed; others, such as genetics, cannot be changed.

Major risk factors for CHD:

- High LDL cholesterol.
- Male gender with age 45 years or older.
- Female gender with age 55 years or older, or with premature menopause and not on estrogen replacement therapy.
- Low HDL cholesterol.
- Hypertension.
- Smoking.
- Diabetes mellitus.
- Family history of heart attacks or sudden death prior to age 55 in a male parent or sibling or prior to age 65 in a female parent or sibling.
- Subtract 1 risk factor if HDL cholesterol ≥ 60 mg/dL.

Although atherosclerosis can invade any blood vessel, the coronary arteries are most often affected. The margin lists the major risk factors for CHD.[3] Organizations such as the American Heart Association add obesity and lack of physical activity to this list, as factors that significantly modify the major risk factors without being risk factors themselves. The criteria for defining blood lipids, blood pressure, and obesity in relation to CHD risk are shown in Table 26–1 and Table 26–2.

Reminder: Cholesterol is carried in several lipoproteins, chief among them LDL and HDL (see Chapter 3 for details). Remember them this way:

- **HDL** = **H**igh-density lipoproteins = **H**ealthy.
- **LDL** = **L**ow-density lipoproteins = **L**ess healthy.

High blood cholesterol carried in LDL correlates *directly* with heart disease, whereas high blood cholesterol in HDL correlates *inversely* with risk.

Blood Cholesterol and Other Lipids The blood cholesterol linked to atherosclerosis risk is LDL cholesterol. HDL also carry cholesterol, but raised HDL represent cholesterol returning from the arteries to the liver and thus indicate a *reduced* risk.[4] Therapy therefore focuses on reducing LDL cholesterol.

To a lesser extent, elevated triglycerides have been linked to CHD, although they are not yet considered a risk factor. Elevated triglycerides are associated with high fasting blood glucose levels and low HDL and are often evident in people with diabetes or those who are overweight.

Hypertension Chronic high blood pressure frequently accompanies atherosclerosis, and as mentioned, atherosclerosis makes hypertension worse. A later section of this chapter focuses on hypertension.

Diabetes Mellitus Most people with diabetes (more than 80 percent) die of CVD. Women with diabetes are especially at risk; diabetes doubles the risk of death from heart disease in women. Diabetes, too, is associated with high LDL, low HDL, hypertension, and obesity (particularly abdominal obesity).

Obesity Obesity, especially abdominal obesity, is associated with high blood lipids, hypertension, and diabetes. Researchers are studying the links between abdominal fat stores, blood lipids, blood pressure, and glucose metabolism.[5] When mobilized, abdominal fat goes directly to the liver rather than emptying into the general circulation as other fat does. The liver then packages this fat into cholesterol-carrying LDL. This process interferes with the liver's ability to clear insulin from the bloodstream. As a consequence, insulin levels rise, setting the stage for the insulin resistance seen in diabetes. The nervous system responds by releasing hormones and neurotransmitters that raise the heart rate and blood pressure, aggravating heart problems and hypertension.

Prevention Efforts Population studies have found most middle-aged and older adults have at least one risk factor and many have more

Table 26–1
Standards for CHD Risk Factors

LDL CHOLESTEROL	TOTAL CHOLESTEROL [b]
<130 mg/dL = desirable[a] 130–159 mg/dL = borderline high ≥160 mg/dL = high	<200 mg/dL = desirable 200–239 mg/dL = borderline high ≥240 mg/dL = high
HDL CHOLESTEROL	**TRIGLYCERIDES (FASTING)[d]**
HDL ≤35 mg/dL indicates risk[c] LDL-to-HDL ratio: Men: > 5.0 indicates risk Women: > 4.5 indicates risk	<200 mg/dL = desirable 200–400 mg/dL = borderline high 400–1000 mg/dL = high >1000 mg/dL = very high
HYPERTENSION	**OBESITY**
Diastolic pressure:[e] <85 = normal 80–89 = high-normal 90–99 = mild 100–109 = moderate 110–119 = severe >120 = very severe	Body mass index: Men: >27.8 Women: >27.3

[a]For people with existing CHD, desirable LDL cholesterol values are lower (≤ 100 mg/dL).
[b]To convert cholesterol (mg/dL) to standard international units (mmol/L), multiply by 0.02586. For cholesterol values for children and adolescents, see Table 26–2.
[c]This HDL value may be too low for women; no alternative value has yet been proposed. NIH Consensus Development Panel on Triglyceride, High-Density Lipoprotein, and Coronary Heart Disease, Triglyceride, high-density lipoprotein, and coronary heart disease, *Journal of the American Medical Association* 269 (1993): 505–510.
[d]High triglycerides alone normally do not indicate *direct* risk, but may reflect lipoprotein abnormalities associated with CHD. The risk of CHD increases as triglyceride levels increase in people with other risk factors. High triglycerides also occur in conditions such as kidney disease and diabetes, which suggest a high CHD risk.
[e]Diastolic pressure is the lower of the numbers in the blood pressure reading—for example, the 70 in 105/70. Blood pressure is measured in millimeters of mercury (mm Hg), a standard unit for the measurement of pressure.

Sources: Blood lipid standards adapted from The Expert Panel, Summary of the second report of the National Cholesterol Education Program (NCEP) Expert Panel on Detection, Evaluation, and Treatment of High Blood Cholesterol in Adults (Adult Treatment Panel II), *Journal of the American Medical Association* 269 (1993): 3015–3023; hypertension standards adapted from the Fifth Report of the Joint National Committee on Detection, Evaluation, and Treatment of High Blood Pressure, National High Blood Pressure Education Program, National Heart, Lung, and Blood Institute, National Institutes of Health, October 30, 1992, p. 5.

Table 26–2
Cholesterol Values for Children and Adolescents

	TOTAL CHOLESTEROL (mg/dL)	LDL CHOLESTEROL (mg/dL)
Acceptable	<170	<110
Borderline	170–199	110–129
High	≥200	≥130

than one. As a result, both the United States and Canada have developed a population approach to prevention; and both also screen to find individuals at high risk so as to offer special preventive efforts and treatment.

It befits a nutrition book to focus on diet and exercise strategies to reduce CHD risk. Several of the major risk factors can be modified by diet and

The **population approach** to diet advice aims to lower disease risks among all people through population-wide changes in eating patterns. The **individual approach** aims to identify and treat only people who are at the greatest risk of disease development.

activity: high LDL cholesterol, low HDL cholesterol, hypertension, and diabetes mellitus.

Diet Therapy for Atherosclerosis

Diet can modify several of the risk factors for atherosclerosis. Note, however, that diet is not itself a major risk factor and may not reduce risk factors as successfully as other interventions do. The extent to which changes in diet reduce CHD risk has been the subject of much debate.

Therapy to Normalize Blood Lipids Therapy for improving blood lipids may involve dietary measures, drug therapy, or both. Diet therapy is preferred; drug therapy is reserved for those who cannot adequately normalize blood lipids using diet alone. When high LDL or related abnormalities develop as a result of another disorder such as diabetes, treatment of the disorder often helps normalize blood lipids.

Therapy aims to reduce LDL cholesterol to different degrees, depending on whether the person has existing CHD or other risk factors. Table 26–3 shows the goals of diet therapy based on LDL cholesterol.

Two-Step Plan To implement diet therapy, a review panel of experts recommends a two-step plan, shown in Table 26–4.[6] The Step 1 diet was originally designed for people with borderline-high or high LDL cholesterol, but because atherosclerotic disease is so common, many experts advocate the diet for everyone. If Step 1 lowers blood cholesterol, good; if not, the therapy goes on to Step 2. An exception to this guideline is made for people with existing CHD; they are immediately placed on the Step 2 diet.

Control Weight Dietary plans to reduce LDL cholesterol include attention to weight reduction or weight maintenance (see Chapter 9). When overweight people lose weight, their heart disease risk factors improve.[7] Weight loss also improves insulin resistance in people with diabetes.

Table 26–3
Dietary Treatment Guidelines Based on LDL Cholesterol

RISK FACTOR STATUS	CHOLESTEROL VALUES WHEN DIET THERAPY SHOULD BEGIN	GOALS FOR CHOLESTEROL VALUES WITH DIET THERAPY
▸ Without existing CHD and with one other risk factor	≥160 mg/dL[a]	<160 mg/dL
▸ Without existing CHD and with two or more risk factors	≥130 mg/dL[b]	<130 mg/dL
▸ With existing CHD	>100 mg/dL	≤100 mg/dL

[a]Note that ≥160 mg/dL indicates high risk.
[b]Note that ≥130 mg/dL indicates borderline-high risk.

Source: Adapted from The Expert Panel, Summary of the second report of the National Cholesterol Education Program (NCEP) Expert Panel on Detection, Evaluation, and Treatment of High Blood Cholesterol in Adults (Adult Treatment Panel II), *Journal of the American Medical Association* 269 (1993): 3015–3023.

Table 26–4
Characteristics of Diets to Reduce Elevated LDL Cholesterol

	STEP 1	STEP 2
Energy[a]	Adequate	Adequate
Total fat[b]	<30%	<30%
Saturated fat[b]	8–10%	<7%
Polyunsaturated fat[b]	Up to 10%	Up to 10%
Monounsaturated fat[b]	10–15%	10–15%
Cholesterol	<300 mg/day	<200 mg/day

[a]Total food energy intake should be adequate to achieve and maintain desirable weight.
[b]All but cholesterol are expressed as percentages of total food energy.

Source: Adapted from N.D. Ernst and coauthors, The National Cholesterol Education Program: Implications for dietetic practitioners from the Adult Treatment Panel Recommendations, *Journal of the American Dietetic Association* 88 (1988): 1401–1411.

Reduce Fat, Especially Saturated Fat In addition to limiting total energy intake, the Step 1 diet recommends a total fat intake of less than 30 percent of total kcalories, with saturated fat no more than one-third of that and dietary cholesterol less than 300 milligrams a day. Chapter 3 (pp. 67–71) provides practical suggestions for reducing fat and saturated fats in the diet.

The Step 1 diet eliminates obvious sources of saturated fat and cholesterol from the diet. These changes can be made without radically modifying the diet. Step 2 reduces saturated fat and cholesterol further, as shown. A registered dietitian can help clients with these diets, particularly with the Step 2 diet.

Notice that the fat-restricted diet described here restricts both the amount and the types of fat. By comparison, the fat-restricted diet described in Chapter 21's discussion of malabsorption syndromes concentrates on simply limiting total fat.

Antioxidant Nutrients and LDL A tentative finding connecting diet with CVD is that LDL promote the formation of plaques only after undergoing oxidation by free radicals inside the artery wall.[8] Research shows that vitamin E plays a predominant role in protecting LDL against oxidation. Large doses of vitamin E supplements are associated with a reduced risk, and the association remains strong when other coronary risk factors and other dietary antioxidants are ruled out.[9] The researchers emphasize that unknown factors could be responsible for the findings and advise people to eat healthy diets and to exercise, rather than rely on vitamin pills to protect against heart disease. The susceptibility of LDL to oxidation may also depend on the concentrations of the other antioxidant nutrients, beta-carotene and vitamin C. The best way to ensure ample intakes of the antioxidant nutrients is to eat generous servings of fruits and vegetables, especially citrus fruits and green and yellow vegetables.

Physical Activity Physical activity deserves attention in any program to reduce CHD risk. Physical activity can ease weight loss, raise HDL, lower LDL, reduce hypertension, and improve glucose tolerance. Frequent and sustained *aerobic* activity may be most effective. Some evi-

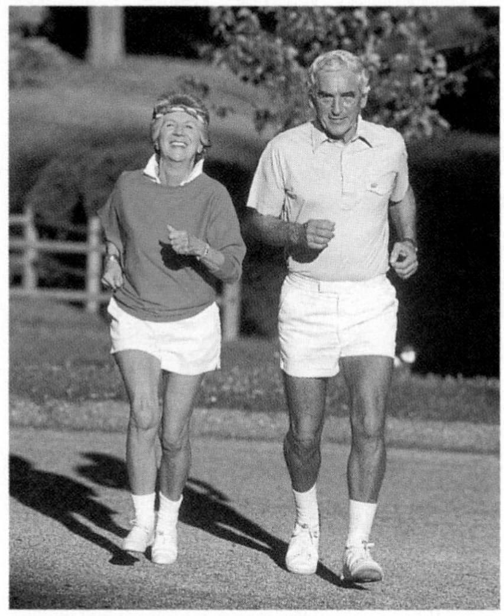

Regular aerobic exercise can help to defend against heart disease by strengthening the heart muscle, promoting weight loss, and improving blood lipid and blood glucose regulation.

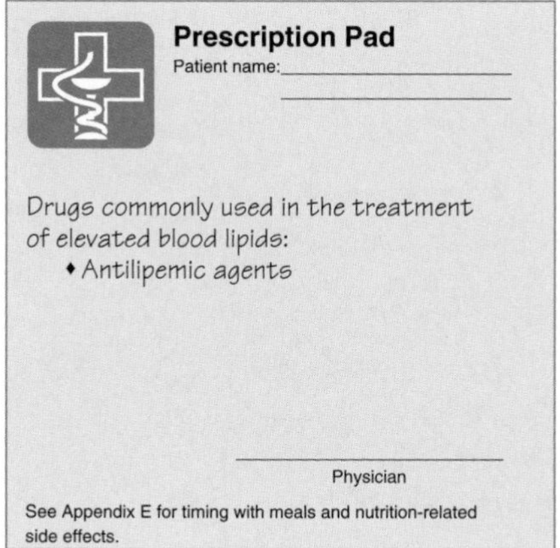

Prescription Pad

Patient name:

Drugs commonly used in the treatment of elevated blood lipids:

- Antilipemic agents

Physician

See Appendix E for timing with meals and nutrition-related side effects.

dence suggests that weight training can also raise HDL somewhat if undertaken regularly.[10]

If heart and artery disease has already set in, a monitored program of physical activity may actually help to reverse it.[11] Diet helps a little, physical activity helps a little, and the combination is better still. People with CHD have been able to reduce plaque buildup in their arteries by following a comprehensive plan combining a low-fat vegetarian diet, no cigarette smoking, stress management training, and moderate exercise.[12] Without such a program, atherosclerosis would most likely have progressed; instead, it regressed and did so without lipid-lowering drugs.

Alcohol In moderate doses, alcohol been associated with a reduced risk of heart disease in both men and women. However, alcohol has many negative effects on body systems, as Nutrition in Practice 8 described. Excessive alcohol use aggravates the risk of liver disease and death from accidents, and some individuals are prone to alcohol abuse. Whatever benefits alcohol may confer on cardiovascular health, they seldom outweigh the negative effects.

Drug Therapy As a rule, physicians do not prescribe drugs until after a six-month trial of intensive diet therapy has proven unsuccessful in lowering blood lipid concentrations.[13] For people with very high LDL cholesterol (greater than 220 milligrams per deciliter), a shorter diet trial may be considered. Drugs, including aspirin and anticoagulants, may also be used to prevent clot formation. Some research suggests that lipid-lowering drugs may reduce the risk of CHD, but may be associated with higher mortality from other causes. All of these drugs are also associated with nutrition-related side effects, as shown in Appendix E. The risk of side effects is especially high in CHD because drug therapy usually continues for many years or even for life.

Hypertension

Chronic elevated blood pressure, or hypertension, a major risk factor for CHD, is believed to affect more than a third of the entire U.S. adult population.[14] Hypertension contributes to over a million heart attacks and half a million strokes each year. The higher the blood pressure is above normal, the greater the risk. (Low blood pressure, on the other hand, is generally a sign of long life expectancy and low risk.) People cannot feel high blood pressure, but it can impair life's quality and end life prematurely.

How Hypertension Develops

The blood pressure ensures that the cells receive a constant supply of nutrients and oxygen. The heart's pumping action must create enough pressure to push the blood through the major arteries into smaller arteries and finally into tiny capillaries. The nervous system and kidneys help maintain the blood pressure by adjusting the size of the blood vessels, setting in motion mechanisms that change blood volume, and influencing the heart's pumping action. The narrower the blood vessels or the greater the volume of blood in the circulatory system, the harder the heart must pump (and the more pressure the heart must create) to feed the tissues. As described earlier, atherosclerosis contributes to hypertension by narrowing and stiffening the arteries.

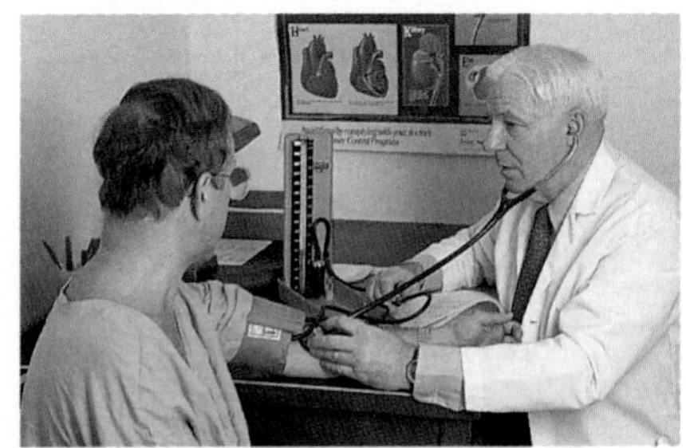

Screening people for high blood pressure is a first step in reducing CHD risk from hypertension.

Complications When the heart must constantly sustain a high blood pressure, strain on the heart's pump, the left ventricle, can enlarge and weaken it, until finally it fails (heart failure). Constant high pressure in the aorta may cause it to balloon out and burst (aneurysm), which can lead to massive bleeding and death. Pressure in the small arteries of the brain may make them burst and bleed (stroke). The kidneys, which are expecially sensitive to the blood flow, can be damaged when the heart is unable to adequately pump blood through them (kidney failure).

Prevention and Risk Factors The most effective single step people can take against hypertension is to find out whether they have it: know your blood pressure. A major national effort to identify and treat hypertension is currently underway. Even mild hypertension can be serious.[15] Treatment produces better health and a higher-quality, longer life. The major risk factors that predict the development of hypertension are those listed in the margin.

Major risk factors for hypertension:

- *Age.* Blood pressure increase with age; most people who develop hypertension do so in their 50s and 60s.
- *Heredity.* A family history of hypertension and heart disease raises the risk of developing hypertension two to five times.
- *Obesity.* Obese people are more likely to develop hypertension.
- *Race.* Hypertension is twice as common among blacks as among whites; it also tends to develop earlier and become more severe.

Diet Therapy for Hypertension

Among diet-related factors that affect blood pressure, most people blame salt (or sodium), but research has disappointed investigators who were looking for a single answer. Many other factors are suspected as well.

Weight Control Excess body fat, especially abdominal fat, can precipitate hypertension and thus raise risks of heart attack and stroke. Weight reduction in people with high-normal diastolic blood pressure (80 to 90) is an effective strategy for lowering blood pressure.[16] Those who are using drugs to control their blood pressure can often reduce or discontinue the drugs if they lose weight. Even a weight loss of 10 pounds may significantly lower blood pressure.[17] Thus weight loss alone is one of the most effective nondrug treatments for hypertension.

Physical Activity Physical activity helps with weight control, and moderate aerobic activity also helps to lower blood pressure directly. Those who engage in regular aerobic activity may not need medication for mild hypertension.[18] The higher the blood pressure and the less active the person to begin with, the greater the likelihood that exercise will be effective in reducing blood pressure.[19]

Recall that aerobic, endurance activity, such as brisk walking, undertaken faithfully as a daily or every-other-day routine can also improve cardiovascular health in several ways. It strengthens the heart and blood vessels; alters body composition in favor of lean over fat tissue; expands the volume of oxygen the heart can deliver to the tissues at each beat, reducing its workload; changes the body's hormonal climate so as to lower

Chapter 10 describes exercise for cardiorespiratory endurance.

blood pressure; and redistributes body water, easing transit of blood through the peripheral arteries.

Sodium/Salt Restriction Salt clearly has something to do with blood pressure. In fact, for years, research on populations seemed to indicate that a high *sodium* intake was "the" factor responsible for high blood pressure. Much of the early research implicating sodium in hypertension's causation, however, may have unwittingly uncovered the combined effects of both sodium and chloride, so now we talk in terms of salt (sodium chloride).[20] Salt has a greater effect on blood pressure than either sodium or chloride alone or in combination with other ions.[21] Furthermore, since most dietary sodium comes from salt, a diet that restricts either one invariably limits the other.

The salt concentration in the blood and other body tissues is precisely maintained by the kidneys, the adrenal glands, the pituitary gland, and other glands. Most people can therefore safely consume more salt than they need and rely on these control mechanisms to excrete the excess as needed. Some individuals, however, are genetically prone to experiencing high blood pressure from excess sodium or salt intakes. People with chronic renal disease or diabetes, those who have one or both parents with hypertension, blacks, and persons over 50 years of age are most likely to be salt sensitive. An estimated one-third of people with hypertension are salt sensitive. For salt-sensitive individuals, salt avoidance may help lower blood pressure somewhat.

Tips for Reducing Salt Many professionals believe that everyone should use salt in moderation. Salt-sensitive individuals in particular should limit their salt intakes to 5 to 6 grams per day.

The person who normally uses salt liberally may find foods unpalatable without salt. Diet compliance will probably be poor if the person is handed an instruction sheet without encouragement or guidance. The suggestions in the accompanying box may help clients make the necessary changes.

Low-Sodium Products Many low-sodium products are available, but a tasty low-sodium diet can be planned without them. Clients need to be aware that any sodium these products contain must be calculated into the diet.

Potassium Even in people without high blood pressure, a high potassium intake protects against stroke.[22] Some authorities believe that potassium might both prevent and help to correct hypertension. When researchers fed potassium-restricted diets to men with normal blood pressures, the men's blood pressures rose significantly over nine days.[23] Hypertensive men who consumed potassium-restricted diets also experienced a rise in blood pressure.[24]

When the body retains sodium, it excretes potassium. Moreover, people who eat many foods high in salt often happen to be eating fewer potassium-containing foods at the same time. Figure 8–2 in Chapter 8 showed that as a food goes through several processing steps, it loses

HOW TO Counsel Clients to Reduce Salt Intake

1. Take time, one-on-one, to explain the diet thoroughly to ensure that the client becomes familiar with hidden sources of salt (such as processed foods), as well as obvious sources (such as table salt).
2. Provide clients with a list of foods to restrict, such as the following:

- Foods prepared in brine, such as pickles, olives, and sauerkraut.
- Salty or smoked meats, such as bologna, corned or chipped beef, frankfurters, ham, luncheon meats, salt pork, sausage, and smoked tongue.
- Salty or smoked fish, such as anchovies, caviar, salted and dried cod, herring, sardines, and smoked salmon.
- Snack items such as potato chips, pretzels, salted popcorn, and salted nuts and crackers.
- Bouillon cubes; seasoned salts (including sea salt); and soy, Worcestershire, and barbecue sauces.
- Cheeses, especially processed types.
- Canned and instant soups.
- Prepared horseradish, catsup, and mustard.

3. Instruct the client to read labels and to watch for the many food ingredients that contain salt.
4. Reduce salt gradually to give the person time to adjust to the natural flavors of foods without added salt.
5. Make sure the person understands that 1 teaspoon of salt contains 2 grams of sodium. If restricted to 1 gram of sodium a day, then, the person should think in terms of half a teaspoon of salt. Since salt is present in so many foods, this would mean no salt could be used in cooking and none could be added at the table.
6. See the person regularly to adjust the salt level, give encouragement, monitor compliance, and answer questions.
7. Encourage the person to replace salt in cooking with spices and herbs, such as those listed in the margin. Cookbooks with low-sodium recipes can be a big help in preparing appetizing foods.
8. Suggest experimenting with salt substitutes. Tell the person not to heat them, because they turn bitter. Some products are half regular table salt and half salt substitute. Although these products may help make foods tasty, they do add salt to the diet. People with renal disease should not use salt substitutes that contain potassium.

A teaspoon of salt contains about 2 g of sodium.

Sodium-Free Spices and Herbs

- Allspice
- Almond extract
- Basil
- Bay leaves
- Caraway seeds
- Chives
- Cinnamon
- Curry powder
- Dill
- Garlic
- Garlic powder
- Ginger
- Green peppers
- Lemon extract
- Lemon juice
- Mace
- Maple extract
- Marjoram
- Mint
- Mustard
- Nutmeg
- Onion powder
- Onions
- Oregano
- Paprika
- Parsley
- Pepper
- Peppermint
- Pimiento
- Rosemary
- Sage
- Sesame seeds
- Tarragon
- Thyme
- Turmeric
- Vanilla extract
- Vinegar
- Walnut

potassium and gains sodium, so its potassium-sodium ratio falls dramatically. Sodium avoidance may help in two ways, then—by lowering blood pressure in salt-sensitive individuals and by indirectly raising potassium intakes in all individuals.

Sample Fat-Restricted, No-Added-Salt, High-Potassium Diet Menu
Foods for this menu are prepared with little or no salt and minimal fat. The fats used for cooking or for flavor are monounsaturated and polyunsaturated.

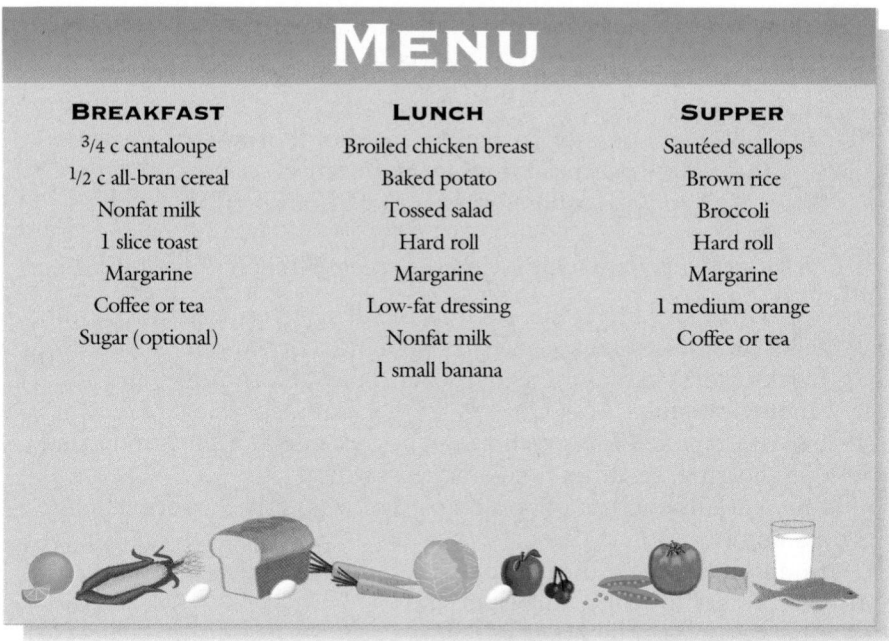

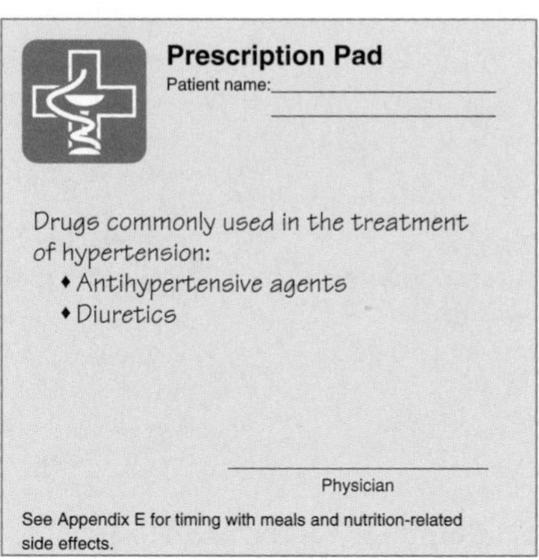

Some diuretics used to treat hypertension also promote potassium excretion. People taking such diuretics must be particularly careful to include good sources of potassium in their daily diets. Their physicians may even advise them to use potassium supplements.

To promote ample potassium consumption, remind clients that whole foods of all kinds—fruits, vegetables, legumes, grains, meats, fish, and poultry—are good sources of potassium. Appendix A shows both the potassium and sodium contents of foods. Blood potassium should be monitored regularly, and clients should watch for signs of potassium deficiency, such as weakness (particularly of the legs), unexplained numbness or tingling sensations, cramps, irregular heartbeats, and excessive thirst and urination. The accompanying menu illustrates a sample fat-restricted, no-added-salt, high-potassium diet.

Fat Fat's contribution to atherosclerosis is well known, but its effects on hypertension remain uncertain despite extensive research.[25] Nevertheless, because hypertension and CHD often coexist, and because fat restriction helps with weight loss, many professionals recommend a fat-restricted diet, such as the Step 1 diet in Table 26–4 on p. 619.

Count as one drink:
- 4 to 5 oz wine.
- 10 oz wine cooler.
- 12 oz beer.
- 1¼ oz distilled liquor (80 proof).

For more information on alcohol and nutrition, see Nutrition in Practice 8.

Alcohol Alcohol is clearly associated with hypertension, and hypertension is a known risk factor for stroke. Alcohol is, in fact, associated directly with strokes independently of hypertension. The surgeon general's advice on alcohol use is straightforward: if you drink, do so in moderation. *Moderation* means no more than one drink a day for women and no more than two drinks a day for men. People who need to lose weight must consider the kcalories contributed by alcohol as well.

Other Factors Research is continuing to reveal factors linked to hypertension. Hypertension may be an insulin-resistant state, and measures preventive against diabetes may also protect against hypertension. Vitamin C also seems to be protective: studies examining the roles of antioxidant nutrients and blood pressure are finding an inverse relationship between vitamin C status and blood pressure.[26]

Endpoints: Heart Attacks, Strokes, and Congestive Heart Failure

When atherosclerosis and hypertension run their courses without treatment, the consequences can be fatal. Most often, these conditions lead to heart attacks, strokes, or congestive heart failure.

Heart Attacks

The heart receives nutrients and oxygen, not from inside its chambers, but from arteries on its surface (shown earlier in Figure 26–1). As mentioned previously, a heart attack, or myocardial infarction (MI), occurs when the supply of blood to the heart muscle is cut off, causing tissue death.

Immediate Care The first priority following a heart attack is to reduce the heart's workload. Water and food may be withheld. People commonly experience nausea and vomiting immediately after an MI, and IV infusions are used to prevent fluid and electrolyte imbalances.

Early Dietary Interventions After several hours of observation, the person can usually begin to eat (as outlined in the accompanying box).

HOW TO Manage Diet after a Myocardial Infarction (MI)

- Offer nothing by mouth immediately after an MI; give IV fluids if necessary.
- After several hours, give a 1000- to 1200-kcalorie diet progressing from liquids to low-sodium, low-fiber foods of moderate temperature in frequent, small feedings.
- After five to ten days, adjust the diet to meet individual needs, usually in three meals a day.
- Many practitioners restrict caffeine during the first few days after an MI and generally recommend a prudent caffeine restriction (no more than 3 cups of a caffeine-containing beverage per day) thereafter. (Nutrition in Practice 20 described the effects of caffeine on the cardiovascular system.)

The diet moderately restricts sodium (to about 2 grams) and food energy (to about 1000 to 1200 kcalories). Gas-forming foods, which can cause abdominal distention and stress the heart, are avoided (Table 21–2 on p. 505 lists such foods) .

Long-Term Diet Therapy After the person is out of immediate danger (in about five to ten days), the diet is tailored to meet individual needs, and to deal with existing conditions such as hypertension, obesity, diabetes, or the like. Whatever else may be necessary, a fat-restricted diet that moderately restricts sodium is appropriate for reducing the risk of further CHD and hypertension. Such a diet can be planned to provide three meals a day, but people who still have chest pain after an MI may continue to benefit from eating frequent small meals. Advise them to eat slowly and to avoid exercise immediately before and after meals.

Encourage Lifestyle Changes An MI victim eagerly applies helpful advice, so use the opportunity to offer sound and useful counsel. Continue to offer support and encouragement for as long as possible. Clients may readily return to their old habits when their symptoms disappear if they haven't fully incorporated new healthful behaviors into their lives.

Strokes

When blood flow to the brain becomes insufficient, or when blood vessels burst and blood flows into the brain, a stroke, or cerebrovascular accident (CVA), results. Most strokes occur as a consequence of atherosclerosis, hypertension, or a combination of the two.

Complications Affecting Food Intake Stroke victims may suffer a temporary or permanent impairment of the ability to communicate. This makes it difficult for them to tell health care providers about foods they can or would like to eat or about problems they may be having with meals.

Reminder: *Dysphagia* refers to an inability to coordinate swallowing safely.

Dysphagia Dysphagia (described in Chapter 20) affects many stroke victims. The stroke victim may fail to respond to the presence of food in the trachea with a coughing response, and food may enter the lungs. "Silent" aspiration has been documented in a number of people who develop dysphagia following a stroke.[27] Tube feedings may be indicated initially until the person is able to work with a speech therapist and dietitian to determine what foods can be safely handled and how to chew and swallow them.

Physical Problems Some stroke victims have problems with the physical process of eating. Such problems can include an inability to grasp utensils or coordinate movements that bring foods or liquids from the table to the mouth. Nutrition in Practice 26, which follows this chapter, describes ways to handle such problems.

Long-Term Diet Therapy Long-term diet therapy for stroke victims depends on the underlying medical condition. A diet to limit kcalories, fat, and salt is often appropriate. Food energy may need to be limited due to inactivity. Clients who must relearn how to walk or use other muscle groups can best do so if they are not overweight. Underweight can also hinder physical rehabilitation, however, so be sure the person does not become malnourished.

Congestive Heart Failure

Congestive heart failure (CHF) can arise as a result of many disorders, most commonly from CHD, hypertension, or kidney disease. In CHF, the weakened heart muscle can no longer pump enough blood through the circulatory system. Blood flow to the kidneys decreases, and this signals the kidneys to retain fluid, which in turn increases the load on the heart and further weakens it. Since the heart cannot effectively pump out the blood forcefully entering it from the veins, peripheral, and sometimes pulmonary, edema develops. The person becomes "congested" with excess fluids. The heart enlarges and beats rapidly to try to compensate for its inability to pump forcefully. CHF threatens life, particularly when accompanied by pulmonary edema. Pulmonary edema aggravates the risks of pneumonia and other respiratory infections and further stresses the heart and lungs.

congestive heart failure (CHF): a form of heart disease in which the heart can no longer adequately pump blood through the circulatory system.

pulmonary edema: fluid in the lungs.

Enlargement of the heart is **cardiomegaly** (CAR-dee-oh-MEG-ah-lee). A rapid heart rate is **tachycardia** (TACK-ee-CAR-dee-ah).

Malnutrition in CHF The person with CHF has high energy needs because the heart and lungs must work hard to deliver blood and oxygen. Because the heart fails to pump adequately, it cannot propel an adequate supply of nutrients and oxygen to the peripheral tissues. Malnutrition can result, particularly as the disorder progresses. Other factors intensify the risk of malnutrition, including anorexia, altered taste sensitivity, intolerance to food odors, physical exhaustion caused by the effort to eat or defecate, dislike of the diet used for treatment, and the long-term use of medications that interfere with nutrition status. Respiratory infections further tax nutrition status. Undernutrition in people with CHF often goes unnoticed because edema masks their underweight condition. Malnutrition, in turn, can further contribute to heart muscle weakness and precipitate or aggravate heart failure.

Chronic protein-energy malnutrition that develops as a consequence of heart disease is called **cardiac cachexia** (ka-KEKS-ee-ah). The weakened heart muscle fails to adequately pump nutrients to the peripheral tissues.

Do Not Overfeed Providing adequate nutrients to the person with CHF is important, but overfeeding stresses the heart, particularly in the severely malnourished person. In people who suffer from constipation, overfeeding can also worsen the struggle to empty the bowels and thereby add emotional stress. If refeeding occurs too rapidly, the blood volume and metabolic rate may increase to the point of overloading the already taxed heart. A gradual return to optimal intake with careful adjustment of dietary roughage is a wiser course.

Reduce Stress to the Heart Muscle Diet therapy includes measures to reduce the work required of the heart, to alleviate edema, and to correct nutrition problems. The person with CHF may be underweight and malnourished, but may also be overweight, in which case weight reduction will help to relieve stress to the heart. A sodium- and fluid-restricted diet also reduces the work required of the damaged heart by alleviating edema. The extent of sodium and fluid restriction depends on

HOW TO Manage Diet for Congestive Heart Failure (CHF)

- Restrict sodium and fluids.
- Restrict food energy if weight loss is needed.
- Provide frequent small meals of foods least likely to form gas (see Table 21-2 in Chapter 21) to ease the task of eating and to reduce abdominal distention that displaces the diaphragm toward the heart.
- Monitor elimination and take steps to ensure that constipation does not become a problem.
- Liquid formulas low in residue and high in nutrient density can be useful as an oral supplement or tube feeding to prevent or reverse severe malnutrition. In some cases, TPN may be required.
- Whether enteral or parenteral, all formulas are carefully selected and given cautiously to ensure that energy, sodium, and fluid intake will not overload the person.

the degree of heart failure. Generally, a person with a moderate degree of heart failure benefits from limiting sodium to 2 grams per day and restricting fluid to about 1½ to 2 liters daily. The accompanying box outlines the dietary guidelines for CHF.

Other Treatments The medical treatment of CHF involves the use of diuretics to promote fluid excretion and other drugs to increase the strength of heart muscle contractions. Some of these may adversely affect the appetite, especially in elderly people. Bed rest helps to reduce the workload of the heart. When not on bed rest, the person must rest frequently and avoid overexertion.

Drugs used to increase the strength of the heart's contractions are **digitalis** (DIJ-ih-TAL-is) **glycosides.**

The accompanying case study presents a man with heart disease. Your careful consideration of the questions posed will help you to review the information presented to this point in the chapter.

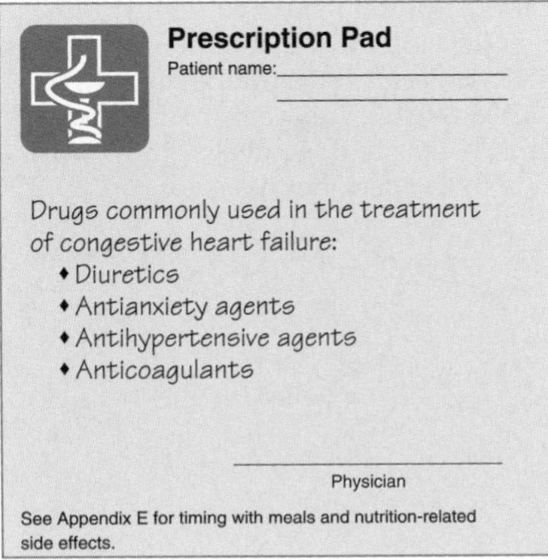
Prescription Pad
Patient name:
Drugs commonly used in the treatment of congestive heart failure:
• Diuretics
• Antianxiety agents
• Antihypertensive agents
• Anticoagulants
Physician
See Appendix E for timing with meals and nutrition-related side effects.

Disorders of the Lungs

The heart and lungs work together to ensure the delivery of oxygen to the cells of the body and to remove wastes generated by metabolic processes in these cells. Lung disorders, then, can affect nutrition status. In this section, two types of lung disorders, chronic obstructive pulmonary diseases (COPD) and respiratory failure, are described, and their nutrition implications are explained.

Chronic Obstructive Pulmonary Diseases (COPD)

Chronic obstructive pulmonary diseases (COPD) are conditions characterized by persistent obstruction of air flow through the lungs. Smoking is a primary risk factor for COPD, but heredity also plays a role. Other risk factors are exposure to environmental pollution (including exposure of nonsmokers to cigarette smoke), alcohol consumption, and, possibly,

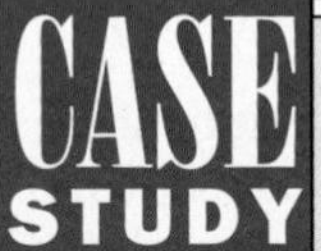

History Professor with Coronary Heart Disease

Dr. Jablonski, a history professor, age 48, has just been diagnosed with a blood lipid profile that includes elevated LDL cholesterol. He is 5 feet 7 inches tall and weighs 200 pounds. Dr. Jablonski has a family history of CHD. His diet history shows excessive intakes of food energy, cholesterol, total fat, saturated fat, and sodium. He smokes a pack of cigarettes a day, and his lifestyle leaves him little room for exercise. Dr. Jablonski also has hypertension, for which diuretics have been prescribed. He frequently forgets to take his pills, though, and his blood pressure is often quite high.

1. Name the risk factors for CHD in Dr. Jablonski's history. Which of them can he control? Which can be helped by diet?
2. What complications might you expect if his condition goes untreated?
3. What type of diet, if any, would you recommend for Dr. Jablonski's high LDL? Explain the rationale for each dietary change.
4. How will his current diet change? What types of foods should he eat?
5. What type of diet, if any, would you recommend for Dr. Jablonski's hypertension?
6. What suggestions might you offer to help him make the necessary dietary changes?
7. Are these dietary changes consistent with those you would recommend for high LDL?
8. Plan a day's menus for Dr. Jablonski based on the diet you would recommend for him.
9. What laboratory and clinical tests would you expect to see monitored regularly? Why?
10. Name at least three ways in which Dr. Jablonski could benefit from losing weight. How does exercise fit into a weight-loss plan?
11. Discuss nutrition considerations if Dr. Jablonski should have a heart attack, develop congestive heart failure, or have a stroke.
12. Describe the relationships of these disorders to atherosclerosis and hypertension.

repeated respiratory tract infections in young children. The two major types of COPD are emphysema and chronic bronchitis. (Cystic fibrosis, which was described in Chapter 21, is a less common form of COPD.)

chronic obstructive pulmonary diseases (COPD): disorders that cause blockage of the lungs' air passages and thus interfere with the exchange of gases between the air and the body.

Emphysema In emphysema, the small passages and air sacs (alveoli) within the lungs lose their elasticity. The victim can breathe air in, but has trouble exhaling it. Stale air containing an excess of carbon dioxide becomes trapped in rigid pockets in the lung, and these pockets enlarge to accommodate the increased air volume. As the air pockets in the lung expand, their walls grow thin and weak; then they tend to collapse during exhalation. Emphysema is believed to be caused by the destruction of elastin, the lungs' major structural protein.

emphysema (EM-fe-ZEE-ma): a type of COPD in which the lungs lose their elasticity and the victim has difficulty breathing.

alveoli (al-VEE-oh-lie): air sacs in the lungs; one sac is an *alveolus*.

Bronchitis In chronic bronchitis, excessive mucus clogs the air passages (bronchioles). The passages become inflamed, and this obstructs the airways further.

bronchitis (bron-KYE-tis): inflammation of the lungs' air passages.

bronchioles (BRON-key-ohls): the small air passages from the trachea to the lungs.

Consequences of COPD Regardless of the type of COPD, the lungs gradually lose surface area and strength, making it difficult for them to deliver oxygen to the blood and to remove carbon dioxide from it. Lung function becomes increasingly compromised, and pulmonary infections become more and more likely. No cure for COPD is available; treatment is aimed at relieving the symptoms. The prevalence of COPD is increasing, and the search for ways to improve the length and quality of life for people with COPD continues.

People with COPD frequently experience infection, weight loss, and PEM. People with pulmonary disease account for many cases of malnutrition in hospitals. The extent of malnutrition appears to correlate with the severity of the pulmonary disease.

Weight loss in people with COPD may be rapid and dramatic. The weight loss may occur for many reasons, including the following:

- Anorexia and poor food intake.
- High energy expenditure associated with labored breathing.
- Steroid drug therapy, which raises nutrient requirements and compromises nutrition status (see Tables E–1A and E–1B in Appendix E).
- Use of mechanical ventilators, because people who require them are in a hypermetabolic state and cannot eat.
- Repeated infections, which raise nutrient needs and cause deficiencies. These, in turn, increase the likelihood of infection, a vicious cycle.

mechanical ventilator: a machine that "breathes" for the person who can't.

As weight is lost, resting energy expenditure speeds up, especially if malnutrition is also present.[28] Heart failure and mortality rates are highest in people with COPD who lose weight.

Dietary Interventions Repleting and maintaining nutrient stores for the person with COPD can help to maintain lung function and prevent lung infections. However, overfeeding people with COPD can be as harmful as underfeeding them. Overfeeding produces high carbon dioxide levels, which the stressed lungs must work hard to expel. Clients replete nutrient stores best when refed gradually. Often they progress to a high-kcalorie, high-protein diet. A severely depleted person may require tube feedings or parenteral nutrition.

Respiratory Failure

respiratory failure: failure of the lungs to exchange gases.

In today's intensive care units, respiratory failure is a frequent cause of illness and death. Respiratory failure can result from advanced COPD, sepsis, severe stresses, and many other disorders. In respiratory failure, a person's lungs are unable to exchange gases, and the person requires mechanical ventilation until able to breathe again.

Malnutrition and Respiratory Failure Malnutrition can contribute to respiratory failure in several ways. Reduced lung muscle mass makes forceful respiratory movements difficult. Weak muscles fail to push blood through the veins, and the result is poor local circulation, which worsens local nutrition. The combination of poor respiration, poor circulation, and malnutrition makes pulmonary infections likely.

Malnutrition also leads to low concentrations of serum proteins. The osmotic pressure exerted by these proteins falls, and this contributes to pulmonary edema. Pulmonary edema increases the workload of the lungs.

Energy Needs In healthy people, breathing requires relatively little energy. People in respiratory failure, however, spend much energy in efforts to breathe. Eating or moving in any way increases the work of the lungs, so that even more energy must be expended to breathe. The person being weaned from mechanical ventilation also has high energy needs. The switch from mechanical ventilation to normal breathing is a stressful and energy-consuming process. The person's lungs were weak before mechanical support was offered, and they have become weaker with disuse. Now they must do more work as the ventilator does less of the work of breathing.

Diet Therapy Nutrition support during respiratory failure and recovery maintains lung function and helps prevent infections. High-energy, easy-to-eat foods best support such efforts, and the types of energy nutrients provided also make a difference. Protein must be supplied in amounts adequate to sustain and rebuild body cell mass.

The ratio of carbohydrate to fat affects the lungs' workload; so does total energy delivered. During metabolism, glucose generates more carbon dioxide per kcalorie delivered than does fat. Overfeeding also generates excess carbon dioxide. Therefore, carbohydrate or food energy in excess of the body's needs taxes the lungs. For this reason, authorities currently recommend that both carbohydrate and total kcalories be carefully controlled for people in respiratory failure.[29] Early reports suggested that fat should supply as much as 50 to 60 percent of the total kcalories, but high fat intakes are associated with impaired immune function. Many authorities use indirect calorimetry to determine the ratio of carbon dioxide produced to the amount of oxygen consumed and use the results to develop an individualized diet plan.

The ratio of carbon dioxide produced to oxygen consumed is the **respiratory quotient (RQ)**. Clinicians use the RQ to help them estimate energy, carbohydrate, and fat needs.

Fluids and Electrolytes People in respiratory failure often have excess fluid in their lungs. Fluid and sodium restrictions may be necessary. Controlling other electrolytes, particularly phosphorus, potassium, calcium, and magnesium, is also important. These electrolytes help maintain muscle tissue.[30]

Enteral and Parenteral Nutrition Generally, ventilator-dependent people are unable to meet their nutrient needs with an oral diet. Tube feedings are the next best alternative, when feasible. Compared with IV feedings, they are safer and less costly, and help to maintain the integrity of the GI tract better. Possibly, they support immune function better, too. Intestinal feedings are preferred over gastric feedings because they minimize the risk of aspiration—a consideration of particular importance to the person in respiratory failure. Special enteral formulas, designed for respiratory failure, are available. When enteral nutrition is contraindicated, TPN should be started without delay. Both central and parenteral solutions can be tailored to meet people's specific diet plans.

Nutrition Assessment

To help pinpoint areas of particular concern in the nutrition assessment of individuals with CVD or COPD, consider the following:

- For clients with CHD, pay particular attention to the total food energy intake and total fat intake if weight loss is needed. For clients with COPD, ensure an adequate energy intake to prevent weight loss.

- For clients with atherosclerosis, check the diet history for the cholesterol, saturated fat, and polyunsaturated fat content of the diet. Determine the dietary fiber intake as well.
- For clients with hypertension, in addition to energy and fat intake, examine the diet history for sodium and salt, potassium, and alcohol intakes.
- Diet histories will help determine which diet changes are needed and how urgent such changes may be. The medical history will identify other conditions, such as diabetes, that may alter treatment and nutrient needs.
- Generally, the only time anthropometric measurements pose a problem in people with CHD is when they have edema (such as in CHF). Weight gain, swelling in the extremities, and high blood pressure signal possible fluid retention.
- Expect abnormal lab values (for example, for albumin and transferrin) in people with CHF if they are retaining fluids. Monitor serum cholesterol in people with CHD. Monitor serum potassium in people on diuretics.

In everyone you assess, look for factors in the history that increase the risk for CHD. Based on this information, you may be able to recommend diet and other relevant lifestyle changes before problems arise.

■ STUDY QUESTIONS ■

1. What is atherosclerosis? How can atherosclerosis lead to hypertension, thrombosis, heart attacks, and strokes?
2. What risk factors for CHD can be helped by diet? What dietary measures are recommended to reduce CHD risk?
3. What is hypertension? Discuss the role of diet in hypertension. Describe some steps that people with hypertension can take to lower their blood pressure.
4. What is a myocardial infarction, and what events trigger an attack? Describe the diet therapy for a heart attack victim immediately after a heart attack, after several hours, and after a week. State the rationale for each diet modification you list.
5. Consider some of the ways in which a person's nutrition needs are affected by a stroke. How can nutrition affect the way a person responds to physical therapy?
6. What is congestive heart failure? Why is malnutrition common in the person with CHF?
7. Describe the diet recommended for the person with CHF. What is the rationale for each of the recommendations? Discuss some special concerns that must be considered when feeding the person with CHF by tube feeding or TPN.
8. Explain what COPD is and describe the two major types. What circumstances alter nutrition status in people with COPD?
9. What is respiratory failure? How can malnutrition affect the course of respiratory failure? Describe how the nutrient needs of the person with respiratory failure should be met.

■ CLINICAL APPLICATION QUESTIONS ■

1. Consider the list of risk factors for CHD and include obesity and lack of physical activity as well. Describe possible interrelationships among the factors. For example, a female over age 55 has a high risk of diabetes; a person with diabetes is also more likely to have hypertension.
2. Pull together the information you have learned about stress from Chapter 18, tube feedings from Chapter 22, parenteral nutrition from Chapter 23, and respiratory failure from this chapter. If a person suffers a major stress (a severe burn, for example) and later develops an infection and respiratory failure, many factors are influencing nutrient needs. List these factors and consider how nutrient needs might be met by tube feedings or parenteral nutrition. What would be the advantages of tube feedings for this person? The possible disadvantages? What would be the advantages of parenteral nutrition? The possible disadvantages? Describe some special problems both tube feedings and parenteral nutrition might pose for a severely stressed, infected person in respiratory failure.

NUTRITION IN PRACTICE 26

How People Live with Feeding Disabilities

This Nutrition in Practice appears here because strokes often lead to feeding disabilities. However, the information presented here has much broader applications. Thousands of people face overwhelming obstacles in the ordinary task of eating. These obstacles can arise at any time in a person's life and from any number of conditions. An infant may be born with a physical impairment such as cleft palate; an adolescent may suffer injuries in a car accident; or an older adult may struggle with the pain of arthritis. Table 26–5 introduces some of the conditions that may lead to feeding problems.

Disabilities may also have nutrition-related consequences beyond their effects on feeding. As one example, a disability may make it difficult for a person to engage in enough physical activity to support a healthy appetite. Then the person's nutrient intake may not meet nutrient needs. As another example, a person who has lost a limb to amputation has altered energy needs. Energy needs are reduced in proportion to the weight and metabolism represented by the missing limb, but may be increased if extra effort is necessary to do ordinary things—such as walking on crutches. As still another example, people with involuntary motor activity may have exceedingly high energy needs.

The nurse and occupational therapist most often become involved with feeding disabilities. They can help people achieve as much independence in eating as possible and can point out ways that caretakers can help.

How do disabilities impair eating?

When you think of the number of individual coordinated motions that are required to get food from the table to the stomach, you may be amazed. Recall how difficult it is for infants to learn to feed themselves. At first, an infant can neither sit upright nor hold a spoon. Every single little action—biting, chewing, and swallowing—requires coordinated movements. Any injury or disability that interferes with these movements in a person of any age can lead to feeding problems.

Other disabilities do not involve oral-motor skills. For example, a person who has problems with sight, or who cannot drive or walk or carry groceries, or who cannot plan meals and think through what to buy has a disability that affects eating. Disabilities of any type can cause people to have trouble maintaining adequate nutrition status.[31] Their number-one nutrition problem is inadequate food intake, which leads to malnutrition, underweight, and, in children, poor growth.[32]

On top of nutrition-related problems, people who have difficulty eating often encounter emotional and social problems. For example, children fail to receive the social training that mealtimes provide, and older people miss the social stimulation that goes with eating in the company of others.

How can health care professionals promote independent eating for people with disabilities?

The evaluation and treatment of a feeding problem requires the joint efforts of several health care professionals, possibly including a dietitian, a psychologist, an occupational therapist, a physical therapist, a speech pathologist, a dentist, and one or several nurses.[33] Table 26–6 provides a checklist of observations health

Table 26–5
Conditions Leading to Feeding Problems

The following conditions may lead to feeding problems by interfering with a person's ability to suck, bite, chew, swallow, or coordinate hand-to-mouth movements.

- Amputations
- Arthritis
- Birth defects
- Cerebral palsy
- Down's syndrome
- Head injuries
- Huntington's chorea
- Hydrocephalia
- Language, visual, or hearing impairment
- Microcephalia
- Multiple sclerosis
- Muscle weakness
- Muscular dystrophy
- Neuromotor dysfunction
- Parkinson's disease
- Polio
- Spinal cord injuries
- Stroke

Table 26–6
Feeding Evaluation

Oral ability
- Sucking
- Oral prehension
- Swallowing
- Breathing and swallowing coordinated
- Drooling
- Lips
- Tongue size, thrust, mobility
- Biting
- Munching
- Chewing
- Drinking
- Response to input

Oral structure
- Occlusion
- Teeth
- Caries
- Gingiva
- Oral hygiene
- Palate
- Pain on exam
- Hypersensitivity
- Teething stage

Body position
- General tone and movement
- Reflex activity
- Head control
- Sitting balance
- Placement of feet
- Usual feeding position

Hand use
- Palmar grasp
- Pincer grasp
- Opposition finger/thumb
- Hand-to-mouth control

Developmental feeding
- Breast ____ bottle ____ weaned _____
- Baby food ___ junior food ___ mashed table food ___ minced foods _____
- Cut table foods _____ regular table foods _____
- Closes hands in on bottle
- Hand to mouth/sucks on fingers
- Teething biscuit, holds and brings to mouth
- Finger feeds
- Opposes lips to rim of cup
- Attempts to grasp spoon
- Grasps spoon
- Dips spoon in dish
- Brings spoon to mouth
- Holds bottle and drinks independently
- Grasps cup
- Raises cup to mouth
- Lifts cup, drinks, and replaces
- Scoops well with spoon
- Feeds independently with spoon
- Drinks with straw
- Spears with fork
- Spreads with knife

Feeding environment
- Time of feedings (note number and length of feedings)
- Atmosphere of feedings (tense, pleasant, unpleasant)
- Person responsible for feeding
- Parental and/or caretaker's attitude toward feeding
- Past successful and unsuccessful methods
- Identify positive and negative reinforcing behaviors
- Behavioral problems

Diet history, including:
- Total fluid intake
- Types of foods consumed

Medications
- Type
- Dosage
- Time given
- Nutrition-related side effects

Bowel concerns
- Regular
- Constipation
- Diarrhea

Anthropometric data

Clinical data

Laboratory findings

Source: Adapted with permission from R. B. Howard, Nutritional support of the developmentally disabled child, in *Textbook of Pediatric Nutrition*, ed. R. M. Suskind (New York: Raven Press, 1981), pp. 577–582.

care professionals use to assess feeding skills. Because each case differs, it makes sense for everyone on the health care team to be familiar with all of these variables.

The dietitian assesses the client's nutrition status and plans a diet. The most valuable assessment tool is observation of clients during mealtimes. While observing feeding skills, the assessor can conduct a complete nutrition assessment and provide appropriate nutrition counseling. The dietitian must also ensure that the diet provides foods appropriate for the client's oral-motor capabilities. For example, people with swallowing problems prefer thickened liquids and pureed foods, which flow slowly enough to allow time to coordinate oral movements. To thicken liquids, add commercially available thickeners or baby cereal. To puree foods easily, use a blender or a baby food grinder. If the client's abilities to eat improve, the diet can gradually progress through all stages from pureed foods to a regular diet.[34] The planner faces many challenges in designing a diet that coordinates the client's energy and nutrient needs, stage of development, and personal preferences.[35] But seeing a client's ability to swallow improve due to a change in the diet's texture and consistency can be very rewarding.[36]

The occupational therapist evaluates oral-motor abilities and feeding skills and then develops a care plan, educates the client, and shows the caretaker, if there is one, ways to implement feeding techniques at home. It may be necessary to teach the client (or caretaker) the proper sitting position for ease of eating. The therapist may instruct the client to sit in a chair with the head and trunk in midline, the back straight and supported, the hips and knees at right angles, and the feet flat and supported on a surface.

Aren't there special implements that people can use to eat, too?

Yes (see Figure 26–2 on p. 636), and these devices can make a remarkable difference in a person's ability to eat independently. For a person who cannot grasp an ordinary fork, a special fork may be the key to future health.

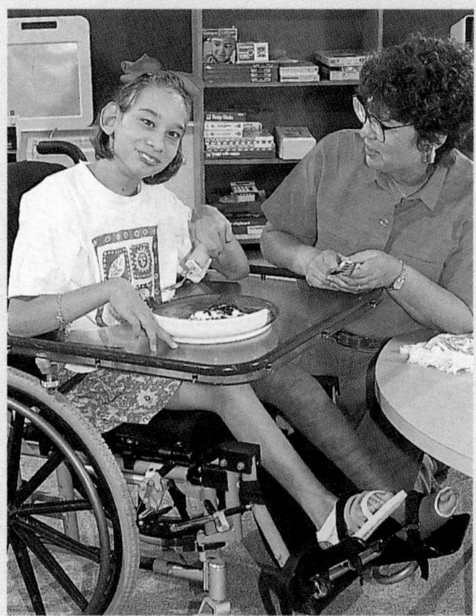

Specially designed eating utensils enable some people with feeding disabilities to be independent.

Can clients also receive behavioral training—such as practice eating sessions?

Yes, and such practice is very valuable. *Knowing how* is not enough to achieve good nutrition; *doing* is the key. Clients may need help in developing eating skills—for example, in learning to swallow. Commonly, a care plan calls for the speech therapist to step in and provide this help, for the speech therapist teaches use of the lips, tongue, and throat in speaking and eating. The dentist may also be needed to evaluate the client's dental health and provide instructions on oral hygiene.

Then all helpers can employ strategies such as those listed in Table 26–7 (on p. 637) to help clients gain skills. For example, if a hyperreactive child is overly sensitive to oral sensations, an attendant can help by desensitizing the client gradually over time. Start by gently stroking the face with a hand, washcloth, or soft pliable toy. (This can be done playfully, making a game of it.) When the child can tolerate touch on less sensitive areas of the face such as the forehead, cheeks, and lips, then slowly and firmly rub the gums, palate, and tongue.

This discussion of ways to help clients achieve independence in feeding themselves has been brief, but the principles are clear. Accurate identification of the eating-related skills that are impaired leads to appropriate treatment. The treatment can be considered a success if the client becomes independent—that is, able to prepare, serve, and eat nutritionally adequate food daily without help.

■ NOTES ■

1. A. Leaf and H. A. Hallaq, The role of nutrition in the functioning of the cardiovascular system, *Nutrition Reviews* 50 (1992): 402–406.
2. National Institutes of Health, National Heart, Lung, and Blood Institute, *The Healthy Heart Handbook for Women*, NIH Publication No. 92–2720, 1992.
3. The Expert Panel, Summary of the second report of the National Cholesterol Education Program (NCEP), Expert Panel on Detection, Evaluation, and Treatment of High Blood Cholesterol in Adults (Adult Treatment Panel II), *Journal of the American Medical Association* 269 (1993): 3015–3023.
4. D. Steinberg and coauthors, Beyond cholesterol, *New England Journal of Medicine* 320 (1989): 915–924; M. J.

Figure 26–2
Examples of Special Feeding Devices

Utensils

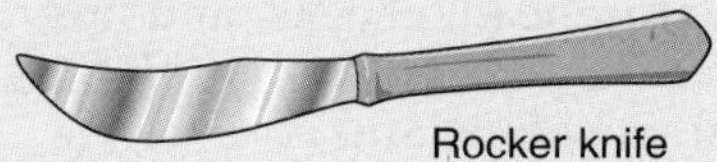

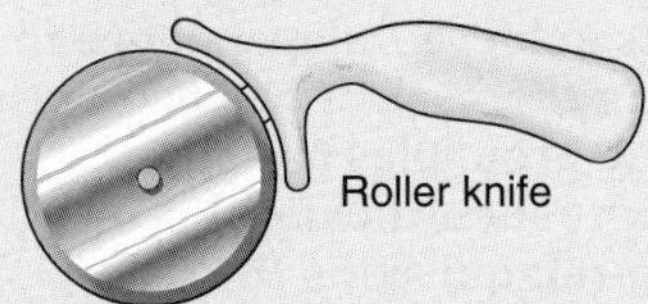

People with only one arm or hand may have difficulty cutting foods and may appreciate using a *rocker knife* or a *roller knife*.

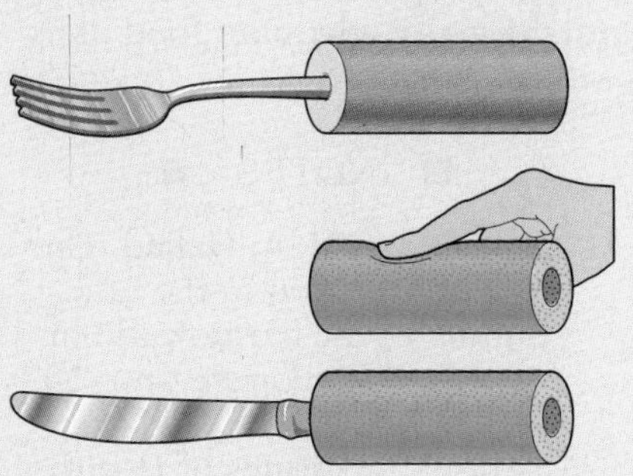

People with a limited range of motion can feed themselves better when they use *flatware with built-up handles*.

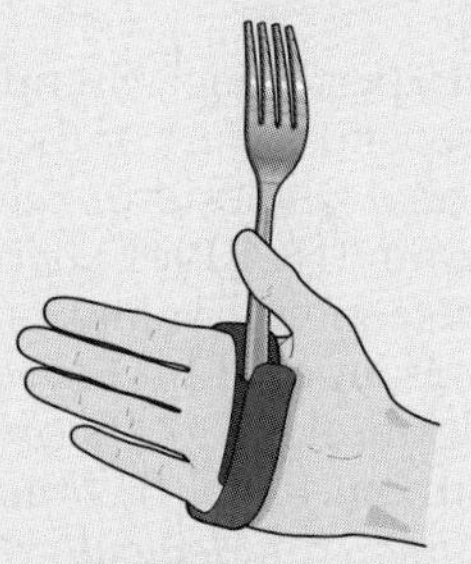

People with extreme muscle weakness may be able to eat with a *utensil holder*.

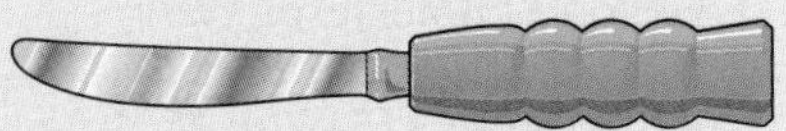

For people with tremors, spasticity, and uneven jerky movements, *weighted utensils* can aid the feeding process.

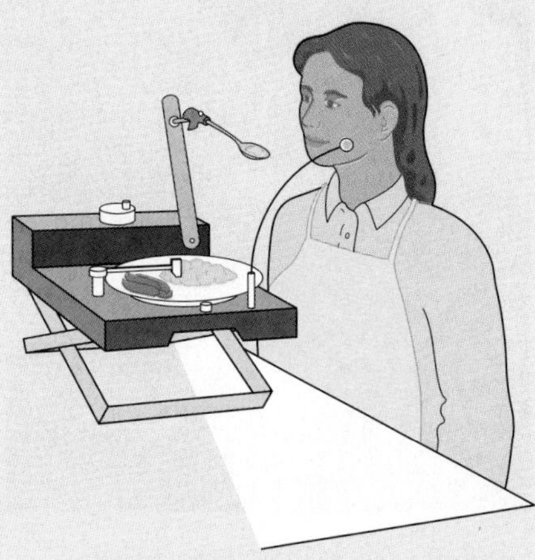

Battery-powered feeding machines enable people with severe limitations to eat with less assistance from others.

Plates

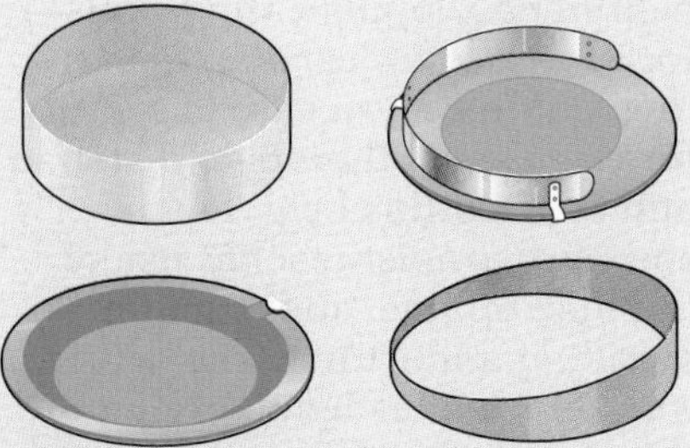

People who have limited dexterity and difficulty maneuvering food find *scoop dishes* or *food guards* useful.

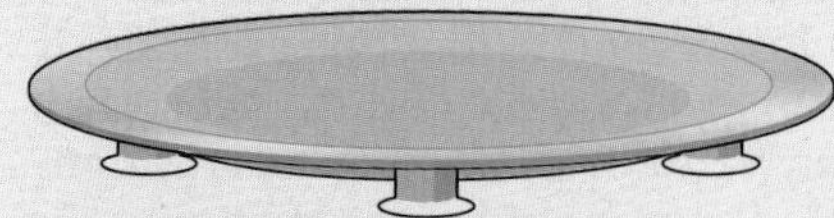

People with uncontrolled or excessive movements might move dishes around while eating and may benefit from using *unbreakable dishes with suction cups.*

Cups

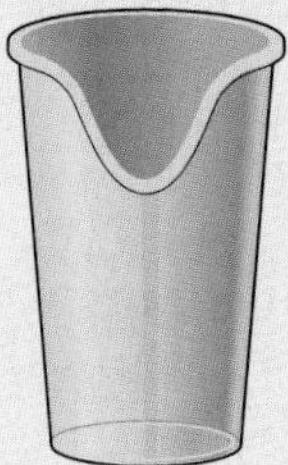

People with limited neck motion can use a *cutout plastic cup.*

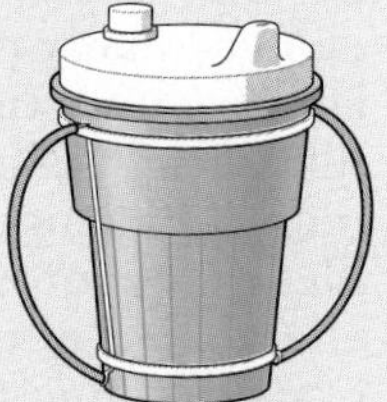

Two-handed cups enable people with moderate muscle weakness to lift a cup with two hands.

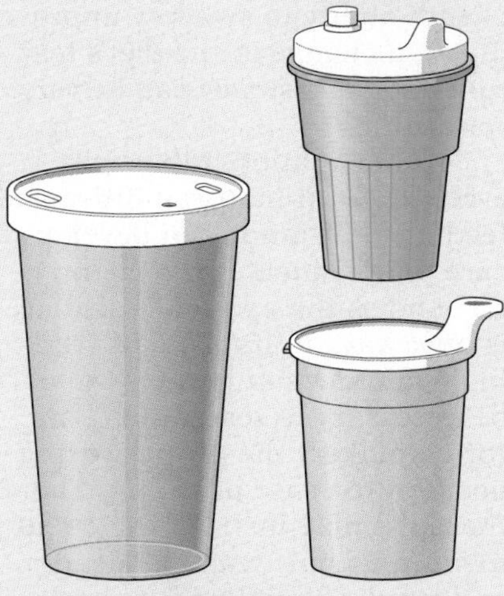

People with uncontrolled or excessive movements might prefer to drink liquids from a *covered cup* or glass with a *slotted opening* or *spout*.

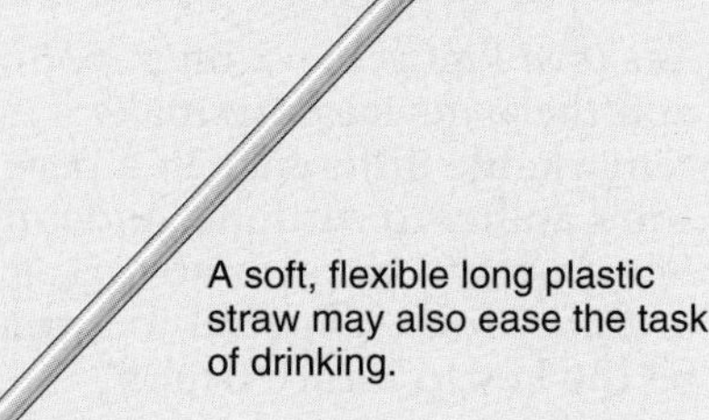

A soft, flexible long plastic straw may also ease the task of drinking.

Table 26–7
Areas of Concern and Suggested Strategies for Developing Feeding Skills

INABILITY TO SUCK
▸ Use cold substances around lips to stimulate sucking. ▸ Use a cloth soaked with water for the child to suck. ▸ Try different types of nipples. ▸ As child begins to improve in ability, change to nipple with smaller holes.
INABILITY TO CHEW
▸ Place a small amount of food between back teeth and move jaw up and down. A mirror may help demonstrate and point out various body parts. ▸ Place pureed foods such as peanut butter on lips and encourage client to wash lips with tongue. Gradually change to solid foods (sprinkle crackers in soup, etc.).
INABILITY TO SWALLOW
▸ Close jaw and lips of client together (swallowing is easiest with the mouth closed). ▸ Stroke throat upward under chin. ▸ Offer next bite of food only after client swallows. ▸ Demonstrate—let client feel *you* swallow.
INABILITY TO GRASP
▸ Allow client to finger food. ▸ Guide client in exploring mouth. ▸ Cut food into small pieces. ▸ Place your hand over client's hand and help client grasp spoon. ▸ Use adaptive equipment (plastic spoon, etc.). ▸ Make sure bowl is stabilized (suction, tape). ▸ Use plates with high straight sides, or build higher edge using aluminum foil.
POOR HAND-MOUTH COORDINATION
▸ Pour sand, etc. ▸ Exercise with ball. ▸ Exercise with push-pull objects. ▸ Study body parts with client, if appropriate.
IMPAIRED VISION
▸ Place meats and vegetables consistently in same areas of plate so client can find.
OVERWEIGHT
▸ Cut down snacks and high-kcalorie foods. ▸ Refrain from rewarding with food. ▸ Increase exercise and leisure-time activities.
UNDERWEIGHT
▸ Increase number of meals per day. ▸ Include high-kcalorie foods, especially liquid supplements. ▸ Encourage proper exercise.
LACK OF NUTRITION EDUCATION
▸ Work with families. ▸ Stress the importance of proper nutrition for *all* family members. ▸ Teach proper feeding environment (good eating habits, eating positions). ▸ Provide nutrition-instruction materials.

Source: Used with permission of Ross Products Division, Abbott Laboratories, Columbus, Ohio, from *Dietetic Currents*, 1977; 4(3): 13-18.

Stampfer and coauthors, A prospective study of cholesterol, apolipoproteins, and the risk of myocardial infarction, *New England Journal of Medicine 325* (1991): 373–381.

5. R. L. Leibel, N. K. Edens, and S. K. Fried, Physiological basis for the control of body fat distribution in humans, *Annual Review of Nutrition* 9 (1989): 417–433.
6. Expert Panel, 1993; *Diet and Health: Implications for Reducing Chronic Disease Risk*, (Washington, D.C.: National Academy Press, 1989).
7. R. R. Wing and coauthors, Change in waist-hip ratio with weight loss and its association with change in cardiovascular risk factors, *American Journal of Clinical Nutrition* 55 (1992): 1086–1092.
8. G. Luc and J. Fruchart, Oxidation of lipoproteins and atherosclerosis, *American Journal of Clinical Nutrition* (supplement) 53 (1991): 206–209; Steinberg and coauthors, 1989; M. J. Stampfer and coauthors, Vitamin E consumption and the risk of coronary disease in women, *New England Journal of Medicine* 328 (1993): 1444–1449; E. B. Rimm and coauthors, Vitamin E consumption and the risk of coronary disease in men, *New England Journal of Medicine* 328 (1993): 1450–1456; K. F. Gey and coauthors, Inverse correlation between plasma vitamin E and mortality from ischemic heart disease in cross-cultural epidemiology, *American Journal of Clinical Nutrition* (supplement) 53 (1991): 326–334.
9. Stampfer and coauthors, 1993; Rimm and coauthors, 1993.
10. I. H. Ullrich, C. M. Reid, and R. A. Yeater, Increased HDL-cholesterol levels with a weight lifting program, *Southern*

Medical Journal 80 (1987): 328–331.
11. P. D. Wood and coauthors, The effects on plasma lipoproteins of a prudent weight-reducing diet, with or without exercise in overweight men and women, *New England Journal of Medicine* 325 (1991): 461–466.
12. D. Ornish and coauthors, Can lifestyle changes reverse coronary heart disease? The Lifestyle Heart Trial, *The Lancet* 336 (1990): 129–133.
13. Expert Panel, 1993.
14. D. Farley, High blood pressure: Controlling the silent killer, *FDA Consumer,* December 1991, pp. 28–33.
15. P. R. Liebson and coauthors, Echocardiographic correlates of left ventricular structure among 844 mildly hypertensive men and women in the Treatment of Mild Hypertension Study (TOMHS), *Circulation* 87 (1993): 476.
16. Hypertension Prevention Collaborative Research Group, The effects of nonpharmacologic interventions on blood pressure of persons with high normal levels, *Journal of the American Medical Association* 267 (1992): 1213–1220.
17. S. A. Corrigan and coauthors, Weight reduction in the prevention and treatment of hypertension: A review of representative clinical trials, *American Journal of Health Promotion* 5 (1991): 208–214.
18. M. H. Keleman and coauthors, Exercise training combined with antihypertensive drug therapy: Effects on blood lipids, blood pressure, and left ventricular mass, *Journal of the American Medical Association* 263 (1990): 2766–2771.
19. B. M. Massie, To combat hypertension, increase activity, *The Physician and Sportsmedicine* 20 (1992): 89–111.
20. *Diet and Health: Implications for Reducing Chronic Disease Risk,* 1989, p. 423; T. W. Kurtz, H. A. Al-Bander, and C. Morris, "Salt-sensitive" essential hypertension in men: Is the sodium ion alone important? *New England Journal of Medicine* 317 (1987): 235–240.
21. T. A. Kotchen and J. M. Kotchen, Nutrition, diet, and hypertension, in *Modern Nutrition in Health and Disease,* 8th ed., eds. M. E. Shils, J. A. Olson, and M. Shike (Philadelphia: Lea & Febiger, 1994), pp. 1287–1297.
22. K. T. Khaw and E. Barrett-Connor, Dietary potassium and stroke-associated mortality: A 12-year prospective population study, *New England Journal of Medicine* 316 (1987): 235–240.
23. G. G. Krishna, E. Miller, and S. Kapoor, Increased blood pressure during potassium depletion in normotensive men, *New England Journal of Medicine* 320 (1989): 1177–1182.
24. G. G. Krishna and S. C. Kapoor, Potassium depletion exacerbates essential hypertension, *Annals of Internal Medicine* 115 (1991): 77–82.
25. J. T. Salonen and coauthors, Blood pressure, dietary fats, and antioxidants, *American Journal of Clinical Nutrition* 48 (1988): 1226–1232; F. M. Sacks and E. H. Kass, Low blood pressure in vegetarians: Effects of specific foods and nutrients, *American Journal of Clinical Nutrition* 48 (1989): 289–290.
26. J. P. Moran and coauthors, Plasma ascorbic acid concentrations relate inversely to blood pressure in human subjects, *American Journal of Clinical Nutrition* 57 (1993): 213–217; D. L. Trout, Vitamin C and cardiovascular risk factors, *American Journal of Clinical Nutrition* 53 (1991): 322S–325S.
27. J. Horner and E. W. Massey, Silent aspiration following stroke, *Neurology* 38 (1988): 317–319.
28. S. Goldstein and coauthors, Energy expenditure in patients with chronic obstructive pulmonary disease, *Chest* 91 (1987): 222–224; D. O. Wilson and coauthors, Metabolic rate and weight loss in chronic obstructive lung disease, *Journal of Parenteral and Enteral Nutrition* 14 (1990): 7–11.
29. A.S.P.E.N. Board of Directors, Practice guidelines: Respiratory failure, *Journal of Parenteral and Enteral Nutrition* (supplement) 17 (1993): 16–17; C. S. Ireton-Jones, K. R. Borman, and W. W. Turner, Nutrition considerations in the management of ventilator-dependent patients, *Nutrition in Clinical Practice* 8 (1993): 60–64.
30. Ireton-Jones, Borman, and Turner, 1993; R. A. Landon and E. A. Young, Role of magnesium in regulation of lung function, *Journal of the American Dietetic Association* 93 (1993): 674–677.
31. Position of the American Dietetic Association: Nutrition in comprehensive program planning for persons with developmental disabilities, *Journal of the American Dietetic Association* 92 (1992): 613–615.
32. M. Thommessen and coauthors, Energy and nutrient intakes of disabled children: Do feeding problems make a

difference? *Journal of the American Dietetic Association* 91 (1991): 1522–1525; R. K. Johnson and M. Maeda, Establishing outpatient nutrition services for children with cerebral palsy, *Journal of the American Dietetic Association* 89 (1989): 1504–1507; M. Thommessen and coauthors, Nutrition and growth retardation in 10 children with congenital deaf-blindness, *Journal of the American Dietetic Association* 89 (1989): 69–73.

33. L. A. Wodarski, An interdisciplinary nutrition assessment and intervention protocol for children with disabilities, *Journal of the American Dietetic Association* 90 (1990): 1563–1568.
34. E. M. Pardoe, Development of a multistage diet for dsyphagia, *Journal of the American Dietetic Association* 93 (1993): 568–571.
35. M. Williams, Dysphagia—The new frontier, *Nutrition Today,* May/June 1992, pp. 26–36.
36. Pardoe, 1993; B. C. Sonies and M. C. Dalakas, Dysphagia in patients with the post-polio syndrome, *New England Journal of Medicine* 324 (1991): 1162–1167.

27

Nutrition and Renal Diseases

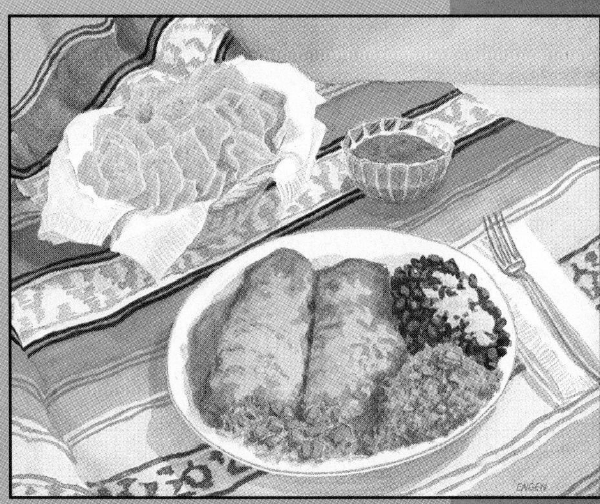

CONTENTS

The kidneys certainly illustrate the old adage that good things come in small packages. Each kidney is only about the size of a fist, yet they carry much of the responsibility for maintaining chemical homeostasis for the entire body. Probably the best way to appreciate the kidneys' vast importance is to learn first what they do normally, and then what happens when they fail.

The Kidneys

The two bean-shaped kidneys sit just above the waist on each side of the spinal column. The kidneys filter out waste products, excreting these substances in the urine. Among these substances are urea, creatinine, uric acid, and excesses of water, electrolytes, vitamins, or other metabolites. Drugs and other substances that cannot be further metabolized, such as oxalate, are also excreted. Other substances the body needs, such as plasma proteins and red blood cells, remain in the blood. Through this filtering process, the kidneys help maintain fluid, electrolyte, and acid-base balances and prevent the buildup of potentially toxic substances in the body. Figure 27–1 (on p. 642) shows the location of the kidneys and the structure of a nephron—one of the kidneys' functioning units. Note the glomerulus, a key part of the nephron, which serves as a gate through which blood passes into the nephron to be cleansed and returned to the body.

The kidneys:
- Excrete metabolic waste products and excess nutrients.
- Help maintain fluid, electrolyte, and acid-base balances.
- Help regulate blood pressure.
- Produce a hormone that stimulates red blood cell production.
- Activate vitamin D.

The Filtrate About one-quarter of the heart's total output rushes through the kidneys every minute. After being filtered, the fluid from the blood, called the filtrate, looks watery because it lacks red blood cells. The rate at which the kidneys form filtrate, known as the glomerular filtration rate (GFR), provides an index of kidney function.

As the filtrate travels through the kidneys, its composition continually changes. In the end, substances the body needs are returned to the general circulation, and waste products (including excess metabolites) leave the body in the urine. Thus the kidneys help to maintain chemical homeostasis.

filtrate: in the kidneys, the fluid that passes from the blood through the capillary walls of the glomeruli, eventually forming urine. (The *glomeruli* are the units in the kidneys that do the filtering.)

glomerular filtration rate (GFR): the rate at which the kidneys form filtrate, an index of the health of the kidneys. Normally, the GFR is between 90 and 120 ml/min.

Blood Pressure Regulation When the kidneys experience reduced blood flow, they raise the blood pressure. They secrete the enzyme renin, which triggers the adrenal glands to secrete the hormone aldosterone. Aldosterone prompts the kidneys to retain sodium and water, thereby raising the blood pressure.

Red Blood Cell Production The kidneys also produce the hormone erythropoietin in response to either oxygen depletion or anemia. Erythropoietin acts on the bone marrow to stimulate red blood cell production. Recall that red blood cells carry oxygen to the body's cells and that anemia develops when their production is impaired.

erythropoietin (eh-REE-throw-POY-eh-tin): a hormone that stimulates red blood cell production.
erythro = red (blood cell)
poiesis = creating (like poetry)

Calcium and Bone Metabolism The kidneys also convert vitamin D to its most active form. Vitamin D supports normal calcium absorption, calcium and phosphorus metabolism, and bone maintenance.

Figure 27–1
A Nephron, One of the Kidneys' Many Functioning Units

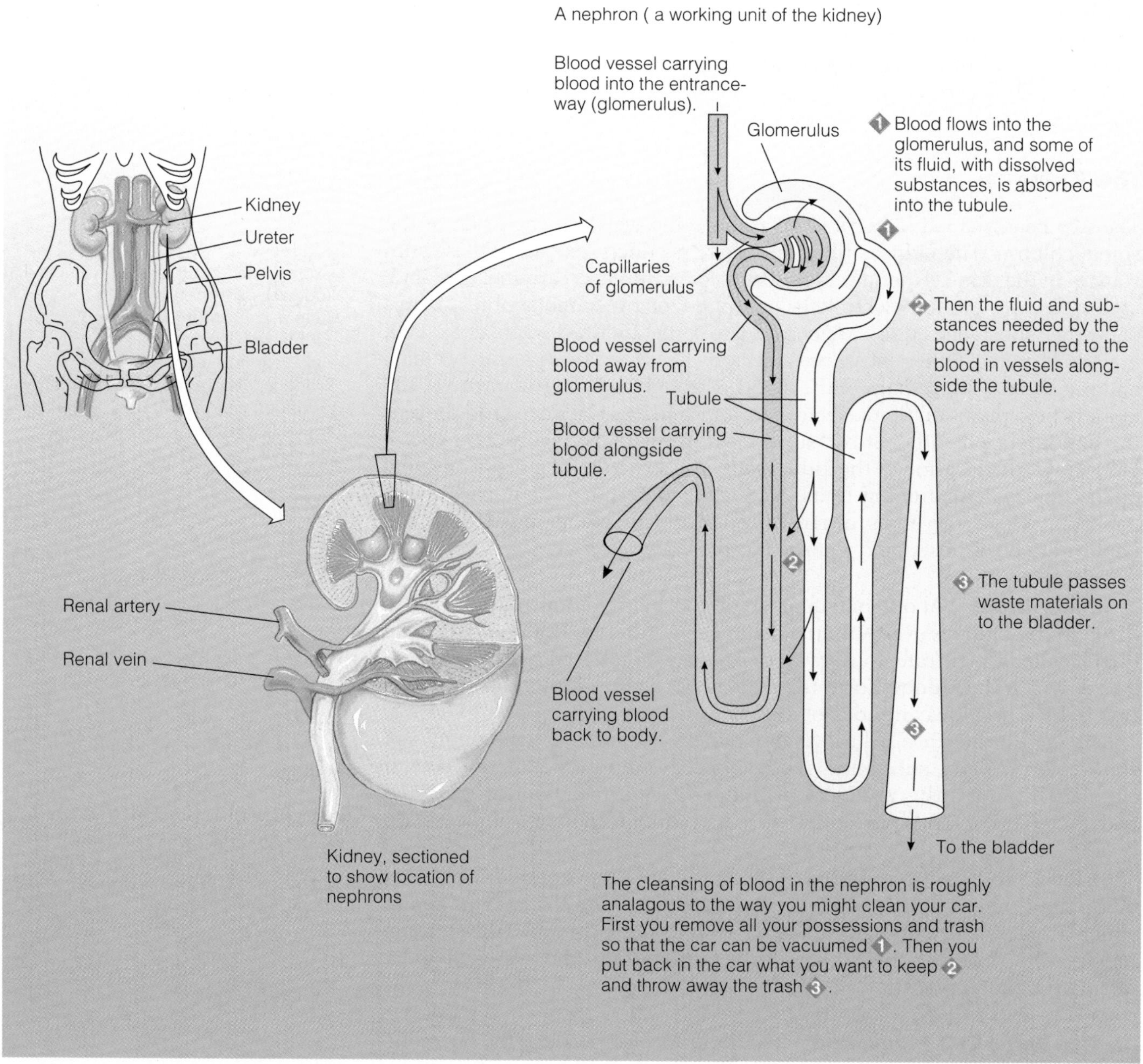

A nephron (a working unit of the kidney)
Blood vessel carrying blood into the entrance-way (glomerulus).
Glomerulus
1 Blood flows into the glomerulus, and some of its fluid, with dissolved substances, is absorbed into the tubule.
Kidney
Ureter
Pelvis
Bladder
Capillaries of glomerulus
2 Then the fluid and substances needed by the body are returned to the blood in vessels alongside the tubule.
Blood vessel carrying blood away from glomerulus.
Tubule
Blood vessel carrying blood alongside tubule.
3 The tubule passes waste materials on to the bladder.
Renal artery
Renal vein
Blood vessel carrying blood back to body.
To the bladder
Kidney, sectioned to show location of nephrons
The cleansing of blood in the nephron is roughly analagous to the way you might clean your car. First you remove all your possessions and trash so that the car can be vacuumed 1. Then you put back in the car what you want to keep 2 and throw away the trash 3.

When you consider all the vital functions the kidneys perform, it is easy to see why their failure can have serious consequences. The following sections describe renal failure.

Renal Failure

renal failure: failure of the kidneys to maintain normal function. (The term *renal* refers to the kidneys.)

Renal failure may be acute or chronic. In the acute version, healthy kidneys fail suddenly due to severe stress. In some cases, recovery follows, but in other cases, acute renal failure is irreversible. In chronic renal failure, gradual deterioration occurs with permanent damage to the kidneys.

As renal function declines, diet therapy assumes a critical role in preventing the buildup of potentially toxic metabolites. If diet can no longer control the accumulation of waste products, the person must begin dialysis to survive.

Chronic renal failure [is like] a downhill course for your patient; acute renal failure is like seeing him go over a cliff no one quite knew was there.

—J. L. Stark

Consequences of Renal Failure

As renal function deteriorates, the composition of the blood and urine changes. The body's principal nitrogen-containing metabolic waste products—blood urea nitrogen (BUN), creatinine, and uric acid—accumulate in the blood (uremia). The GFR declines. It is therefore possible to evaluate renal function by performing laboratory tests. Blood tests measure BUN, creatinine, and uric acid, and urinary clearance tests measure the GFR.

uremia (you-REE-me-ah): the buildup of toxic waste products in the blood associated with renal insufficiency.

Abnormal accumulation of nitrogen-containing substances in the blood is called **azotemia** (AZE-oh-TEE-me-ah). Normal BUN levels are 10 to 20 mg/dL. A BUN of 50 to 150 mg/dL indicates serious impairment of renal function. BUN may rise as high as 150 to 250 mg/dL in end-stage renal disease.

Renal Dialysis

The kidneys are virtually irreplaceable. No perfect substitute for one's own kidneys has been found, but dialysis benefits the person with renal failure who needs immediate help in restoring normal blood balances.

During dialysis, excess fluids and wastes flow from the blood across a semipermeable membrane into a vessel, so that they can be discarded. A solution similar in composition to normal blood plasma, called the dialysate, is placed on one side of the semipermeable membrane; the person's blood flows by on the other side. Urea and electrolytes can cross the membrane, and because they are more concentrated in the blood than in the dialysate, these substances diffuse out of the blood into the dialysate. The dialysate also contains glucose, which cannot cross the membrane, so *fluid* moves *toward* the glucose, also leaving the blood. The more glucose in the dialysate, the more fluid leaves the blood. The dialysate is then discarded.

Dialysis effectively removes excess wastes and fluids, but it does not restore the hormonal functions of the kidneys. Blood loss is likely; and infections are also a risk. Among nutrition problems, anemia is common, as are deficiencies of nutrients lost in the dialysate: vitamins, minerals, and amino acids, among others.

When the GFR falls below 4 to 5 ml/min, dialysis is usually initiated. Recall that normal GFR is between 90 and 120 ml/min.

dialysis (dye-AL-ih-sis): removal of waste from the blood using the principles of simple diffusion and osmosis through a semipermeable membrane.

The two main types of dialysis are **hemodialysis** and **peritoneal dialysis.**

In hemodialysis, a blood vessel is tapped, and the blood is routed through a dialysis machine and then returned to the body. Inside the machine, the blood flows within a semipermeable membrane which is bathed in dialysis fluid so that exchange can take place.

In peritoneal dialysis, the dialysis fluid is infused into the person's abdomen outside the peritoneal membrane, the sac that holds the intestines. Exchange takes place across this membrane, and the dialysis fluid is then withdrawn. The process is repeated a number of times until sufficient wastes have been removed.

Acute Renal Failure

Acute renal failure develops rapidly as a consequence of another medical condition. It is sometimes reversible, but it may progress to chronic renal failure. About half of all people with acute renal failure die. Recovery often depends on successful treatment of the underlying cause.

Causes of Acute Renal Failure Acute renal failure frequently develops when blood flow to the kidneys declines. Severe stresses such as heart failure, shock, or severe blood loss after surgery or an accident can all reduce blood flow to the kidneys. Less than normal amounts of blood are filtered and less urine is produced. Other causes include urinary tract obstructions and damage to the kidneys themselves due to infections, toxins, some drugs, or environmental pollutants.

Consequences of Acute Renal Failure A sudden and precipitous drop in the GFR and urine output characterizes the early stages of acute renal failure. Blood pressure shoots up, and toxic waste products begin to accumulate in the blood. Acidosis is common. Because victims of acute renal failure have frequently suffered severe stress, they are also hypercatabolic. As their bodies' cells break down, intracellular fluids release potassium and the kidneys fail to excrete it, so blood potassium rises sharply. Common clinical symptoms of acute renal failure include hiccups, anorexia, nausea, vomiting, drowsiness, agitation, and confusion. GI bleeding and diarrhea sometimes occur.

The early phase of acute renal failure, when urine volume is reduced, is the **oliguric phase;** the phase characterized by large fluid and electrolyte losses in the urine is the **diuretic phase;** the gradual return of renal function marks the **recovery phase.**

Urine volume may diminish at first, but later in the course of renal failure, the kidneys cannot conserve water, and the person begins to excrete large amounts of urine and electrolytes. If recovery occurs, kidney function gradually normalizes over a 3- to 12-month period.

Treatment of Acute Renal Failure

The primary concern in acute renal failure is to treat the underlying disorder in order to prevent permanent or further damage to the kidneys. For example, if severe blood loss is the problem, a blood transfusion is given to restore blood volume. Other measures must be taken to restore fluid and electrolyte balance and minimize blood concentrations of toxic waste products. In addition to the nutrition factors mentioned in the following paragraphs, treatment may require dialysis (to control blood urea, creatinine, and potassium) and sometimes diuretics (to mobilize fluids).

Energy As mentioned, the person in acute renal failure is often in a hypercatabolic state and suffering from another major illness. Add nausea, vomiting, and confusion, and you have a person who needs food energy but is unable to eat. Without sufficient energy, protein breakdown occurs, raising blood urea and potassium even higher and further taxing the kidneys. Problems such as impaired wound healing, infection, muscle wasting, and negative nitrogen balance, which are commonly seen in individuals with acute renal failure, often prove fatal. The person's exact energy needs depend on the rate of catabolism. Usually, 35 to 50 kcalories per kilogram of body weight will meet these needs.

Protein The protein needs of people with acute renal failure also depend on the metabolic rate and nutrition status, but no perfect way of determining them is known. Generally, the diet restricts protein to about 30 to 40 grams per day. People with high catabolic rates, and those who are malnourished may need a higher protein intake, even if it necessitates dialysis. If dialysis is instituted, a more liberal protein intake of 70 to 85 grams may be allowed.

Fluids Health care professionals must carefully control clients' total fluid intakes to avoid overhydration or dehydration. Health care professionals determine fluid requirements by carefully measuring urine output. To the measured volume of urine, they add about 400 to 500 milliliters for water lost through the skin, lungs, and perspiration. The person who is vomiting, has diarrhea, has a high fever, or otherwise loses fluids needs more. In the oliguric stage, the person needs small volumes of fluids. In the diuretic stage, up to 3 liters of urine may be lost daily, and large amounts of fluids have to be provided.

Electrolytes Sodium may be restricted (to 500 to 1000 milligrams) in the oliguric phase, but this may change as the person enters the diuretic phase. Likewise, potassium is often restricted (to less than 2 grams per day) in the oliguric phase but may need to be supplemented in the diuretic phase. Potassium is especially critical in the person with acute renal failure—hyperkalemia can be life-threatening.

hyperkalemia: an excessive amount of potassium in the blood.

Drug Treatment Drugs called exchange resins must sometimes be used to treat severe hyperkalemia. These drugs, which are placed rectally, exchange sodium for potassium in the colon, and the potassium is then excreted in the stool. Another way to temporarily reduce high potassium is to give IV dextrose and insulin. Insulin lowers blood potassium in two ways. First, as insulin moves glucose into the cells, potassium follows. Second, as an anabolic hormone, insulin minimizes tissue breakdown and, consequently, the release of potassium from cells.

Special Nutrition Support Because clients with acute renal failure are often severely stressed, they frequently receive their nutrients from tube feedings or TPN. The person with renal failure who is restricted to a certain amount of fluid has to derive a maximum of energy from a small volume; therefore, enteral and parenteral formulas designed for renal failure often meet energy, protein, and other nutrient needs in smaller volumes. Compared with standard enteral formulas, renal formulas have less protein and fewer electrolytes so that electrolytes can be added at an appropriate level for each individual (see Appendix H). TPN formulas containing mixtures of both nonessential and essential amino acids at lower concentrations than in standard TPN solutions produce favorable results. Health care professionals monitor and adjust energy, protein, and electrolytes as necessary.

Glucose intolerance and insulin resistance are common in both renal and catabolic illnesses, so insulin must often be given in coordination with feeding. Fat can be used to add kcalories, to reduce the need for carbohydrate, and to limit the glucose load.

The case study (p. 646) presents a client with acute renal failure. Take a moment to review the many parameters health care providers must consider when treating such clients.

Chronic Renal Failure

Unlike acute renal failure, which develops suddenly, chronic renal failure develops gradually. Many disorders can permanently damage the kidneys, notably nephritis; renal artery obstruction; nephrotic syndrome (described

nephritis (nef-RYE-tis): inflammation of the kidneys.

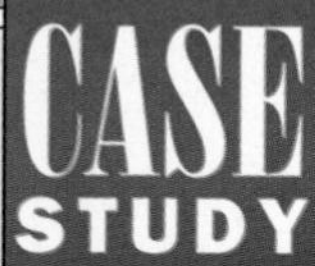

CASE STUDY: Store Manager with Acute Renal Failure

Mrs. Calley is a 35-year-old convenience store manager admitted to the hospital's intensive care unit. She was first seen in the emergency room after she sustained multiple and severe injuries in an auto accident. She had lost so much blood she almost died before reaching the hospital. Her injuries include a fractured leg, broken ribs, a collapsed lung, and internal bleeding. Following emergency surgery to uncover and correct the source of the internal bleeding and repair injuries, she has developed acute renal failure. Mrs. Calley is 5 feet 3 inches tall and weighs 125 pounds.

Mrs. Calley has a urine volume of less than 50 milliliters per day and a BUN of 75 milligrams per deciliter. A test of GFR could not be performed due to the low volume of urine she was excreting.

1. Describe the most probable reason why Mrs. Calley developed acute renal failure. What other problems can cause acute renal failure?
2. Describe the phases of acute renal failure.
3. What are Mrs. Calley's dietary needs in the early phase?
4. What waste products and electrolytes are of greatest concern? Why?
5. What factors does the dietitian have to keep in mind in determining Mrs. Calley's energy and protein needs during acute renal failure?
6. How will these needs change if dialysis is begun?
7. How will her nutrient needs change as she progresses to the second stage of acute renal failure?

later); and damage due to diabetes (Chapter 25), hypertension (Chapter 26), or atherosclerosis (Chapter 26).

The capacity of the kidneys to function despite loss of some functioning tissue is referred to as **renal reserve.**

Consequences of Chronic Renal Failure In the early stages of chronic renal failure, the body compensates for the loss of some function by enlarging the functioning parts of the kidneys. The enlarged areas work so efficiently that the kidneys can lose about 75 percent of their tissue before they fail. The GFR may fall to as low as one-tenth of the normal rate—10 to 12 milliliters per minute—before symptoms appear. This stage of renal disease is known as end-stage renal disease.

end-stage renal disease (ESRD): the severe stage of renal disease in which diet alone is no longer effective in maintaining normal kidney functions.

uremic syndrome: a complex of symptoms caused by uremia; it is seen late in renal failure.

When urea (which can be excreted through sweat) crystallizes and becomes visible on the skin, the condition is called **uremic frost.**

Buildup of Waste Products and Fluids Unable to rid itself of excess fluids, the body may begin to swell with edema as normal fluid, electrolyte, and acid-base balances are upset. As renal failure progresses, the buildup of toxic waste products in the blood (uremia) can precipitate a complex of symptoms known as the uremic syndrome. The person with uremia exhibits symptoms affecting virtually every body system: fatigue, weakness, diminished mental alertness, muscular twitches, muscle cramps, anorexia, nausea, vomiting, stomatitis, and an unpleasant taste in the mouth. The skin may itch uncomfortably, and in later stages, GI ulcers and bleeding commonly develop.

Chronic Complications Hypertension and congestive heart failure from the expanded blood volume may follow. For unknown reasons, renal disease is associated with elevated blood lipids (especially elevated triglycerides) and atherosclerosis; atherosclerosis further adds to hypertension and the risk of congestive heart failure. Elevated potassium causes the heart to enlarge and beat irregularly and can eventually contribute to heart failure and cause death. Elevated phosphorus upsets the body's balance of phosphorus and calcium, often leading to the bone disease associated with renal failure. Depressed erythropoietin synthesis by the damaged kidneys, restrictive diets, nausea and vomiting, GI blood losses, and blood losses through dialysis and from frequent blood testing often result in anemia. Growth failure and wasting are common, as described next.

The bone disorder resulting from calcium and phosphorus imbalances in renal disease is **renal osteodystrophy** (OS-tee-oh-DIS-tro-fee). One type of renal osteodystrophy that leads to a softening of the bones is called **osteomalacia** (see p. 145).

Growth Failure and Wasting Syndrome Children with renal disease often fail to grow normally, and people of any age with renal disease may have the wasting syndrome—reduced muscle mass, depleted fat tissue, and lowered blood proteins. Poor growth and wasting can occur for many reasons:

- Limited food intake due to GI distress, depression, other illnesses, or restrictive and unpalatable diets.
- Failure to excrete toxic waste products and excess fluids and electrolytes.
- Inability of the renal tubules to reabsorb many needed nutrients.
- Losses of nutrients through vomiting, diarrhea, GI bleeding, and poor absorption.
- Reduced renal inactivation of many hormones.
- Reduced synthesis of other important substances, such as erythropoietin and active vitamin D.
- Alteration of nutrient needs by other medical therapy (dialysis and drugs).

Because of these difficulties, the nutrition status of people with chronic renal failure is often compromised. Children with renal disease need nutrition intervention before the end of puberty if they are to make up growth deficits. Adults with renal disease can improve their nutrition status and quality of life by attending to diet as well.

Dietary Treatment in Chronic Renal Failure

The early stages of renal failure generally go undetected, so clients make no dietary adjustments. When treatment does begin, diet plays a significant role. The objectives of the dietary management of chronic renal failure are:

- To achieve or maintain optimal nutrition status and nitrogen balance.
- To delay the progression of renal failure.
- To prevent the buildup of toxic metabolic waste products and nutrient excesses.
- To prevent complications, such as growth failure, wasting syndrome, bone disease, hypertension, edema, and congestive heart failure.
- To foster the client's well-being.

Renal diets are highly individualized. Most often, they prescribe total kcalories, restrict protein, and carefully control phosphorus, fluids, sodi-

Table 27–1
Typical Nutrient Needs in Chronic Renal Failure

NUTRIENTS	RENAL INSUFFICIENCY PREDIALYSIS	HEMODIALYSIS	PERITONEAL DIALYSIS
Energy (kcal/kg)	35–40	30–35	33–45
Protein (g/kg)	0.6–0.8	1.1–1.4	1.2–1.5
Fluid (ml)	Typically not restricted	500–750 plus daily urine output, or 1000 if anuric	≥2000
Sodium (g)	1–3	2–3	2–4
Potassium (mg/kg)	Typically not restricted	40	Typically not restricted
Phosphorus (mg/kg)	8–12[a]	≤17[a]	≤17[a]
Supplements			
Calcium (mg)	1200–1600	As appropriate	As appropriate
Folate (mg)	1	1	1
Vitamin B_6 (mg)	5	10	10
Vitamin C (mg)	70–100	100	100
Other water-soluble vitamins	RDA	RDA	RDA
Vitamin D	As appropriate	As appropriate	As appropriate

Note: The actual amounts of these nutrients in the diet must be highly individualized based on each person's responses. For example, calcium supplementation may be as high as 3000 milligrams per day.
[a]The extent of phosphorus restriction depends on serum phosphorus. The goal is to maintain serum phosphorus between 4.5 and 6.0 milligrams per deciliter. Often phosphate binders are useful for this purpose.

Source: Adapted from Meeting the challenge of the renal diet: A preview of the 'National Renal Diet' educational series, *Journal of the American Dietetic Association* 93 (1993): 637–639.

um, and potassium. The physician prescribes each diet and regularly adjusts it based on the degree of renal insufficiency and other complications. Table 27–1 summarizes nutrient needs in chronic renal failure and shows how they change if the person is on hemodialysis or peritoneal dialysis.

Importance of Diet As you read the following sections, notice how complex the renal diet is and how critical the control of certain nutrients. Keep in mind how restrictions placed on those nutrients affect food choices. Remember, when you communicate with a client, a family member, or another health care team member, you need to know *why* nutrients such as protein must be restricted so that your instructions to clients will be backed by your conviction of their importance. You serve clients most effectively when you truly understand the disease and the necessity of dietary changes.

Energy All people with renal failure need adequate food energy to achieve or maintain a desirable body weight and to *prevent protein catabolism.* Adults need at least 35 kcalories per kilogram of body weight per day.

For children with renal disease, at the minimum, energy intake should meet the RDA.[1]

Adding fat to the diet presents a dilemma for the diet planner, however. Because the person with altered renal function often has elevated blood lipids, an ideal diet would also be fat-restricted. Adding carbohydrate presents a dilemma as well. Because renal diets often restrict electrolytes, this means limiting many foods rich in complex carbohydrates. Additionally, many people with altered renal function also have diabetes (see Chapter 25) and total carbohydrate intake is a concern. Diet planners often must accept that under such circumstances, no diet will be ideal. The need to adjust the diet for renal failure outweighs the other dietary considerations.

To raise energy intake, clients are encouraged to use high-kcalorie, zero-protein, low-electrolyte foods such as sugars (hard candy and jelly), sweet drinks, and polyunsaturated fats (margarine and oil). Special formulas containing glucose polymers can also add kcalories. The person with elevated blood lipids is advised to restrict fat and modify the type of fat as much as possible. The person with diabetes is advised to eat a consistent amount of carbohydrate at regular intervals daily, and to adjust insulin to cover carbohydrate intake.

Protein Providing the right amount of protein to the person in renal failure is like walking a tightrope. Too little protein, and the person develops malnutrition. Too much protein, and blood urea (the toxic waste product of protein metabolism) rises. Many studies spanning more than a decade of scientific work have shown that protein-restricted diets can delay or halt the progression of chronic renal failure. Clinicians frequently provide 0.6 grams of protein per kilogram of body weight per day. Most of this protein should be from high-quality sources. A combination of high-quality protein from plant and animal sources may be best; this combination complements the high quality of animal proteins with the low-saturated fat, low-cholesterol nature of plant protein sources.[2] Some clinicians prefer to use diets low in whole proteins and supplemented with essential amino acids or precursors (keto-acids). Complete vegetarian diets are also being investigated.

Once the client begins dialysis, protein restrictions are relaxed. Dialysis results in protein losses and can even cause protein deficiency.

Phosphorus The cascade of events leading to renal osteodystrophy is largely preventable through dietary control. Therapy aims to maintain blood phosphorus between 4.5 and 6.0 milligrams per deciliter using a combination of diet, drugs, and dialysis.[3] The person must limit foods particularly high in phosphorus, such as those shown in the margin photo.

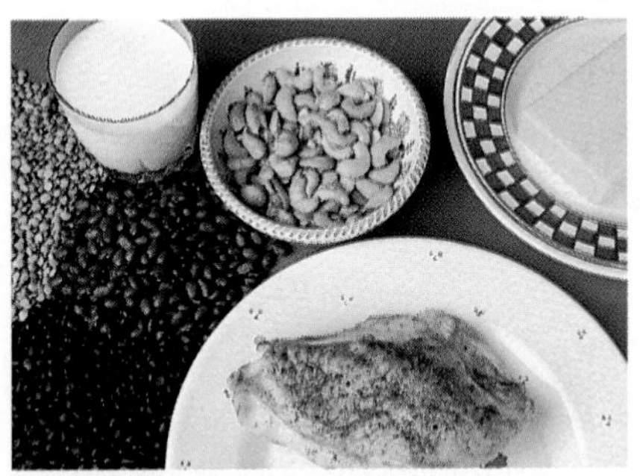

Foods such as milk and milk products, cheese, poultry, nuts, and legumes are high in phosphorus and so must be restricted in a renal diet.

The drugs used to help control serum phosphorus work by binding phosphate in the GI tract, thereby making it unavailable for absorption. Calcium salts—calcium carbonate and calcium acetate—are the preferred phosphate binders, and they are taken shortly before or with meals.[4] Aluminum salts also bind phosphate, but are used less often because they carry a risk of aluminum toxicity, which is linked to bone disorders and mental disturbances.

Calcium Supplements Impaired calcium absorption due to the lack of active vitamin D and the limited calcium intake may lead to a calcium deficiency. Most people with renal disease need calcium supplements (1000 to 3000 milligrams daily) to help prevent calcium deficiency. Calcium-containing phosphate binders can serve as calcium supplements as well. However, hypercalcemia can be a problem for people taking calcium-containing phosphate binders.[5] The renal health care team monitors serum calcium closely to prevent both low and high blood calcium.

Active vitamin D or **calcitriol** comes in oral and intravenous forms. An experimental form of active vitamin D called **22 oxa calcitriol** is associated with a less marked rise in serum calcium.

Vitamin D Supplements Supplemental vitamin D in its active form can also help maintain blood calcium and prevent the hormonal abnormalities that cause it. Both the supplement doses and the methods of administering them must be carefully tailored to individual needs to prevent hypercalcemia. Supplements are not used if serum phosphorus is high (to prevent further deterioration of renal function) or when calcium carbonate is given (to prevent hypercalcemia).

Fluids Individual needs for fluids and electrolytes vary and must be determined by carefully monitoring each person's weight, blood pressure, urine output, and blood electrolyte levels. A rapid rise in body weight and blood pressure means that the person is retaining sodium and fluid; conversely, a rapid decline in body weight and blood pressure (a desirable outcome of dialysis) suggests that sodium and fluid excretion is occurring. Daily fluid needs amount to daily urine output plus 500 milliliters for insensible water losses. Once a person is on dialysis, fluid intake is controlled to allow a weight gain of about 2 to 2½ pounds (of fluid) between dialysis treatments.

A typical renal diet provides from 500 to 3000 milliliters (about ½ to 3 quarts) of fluids daily. All beverages must be considered as part of the fluid allowance. Table 27–2 lists foods that contain considerable amounts of fluid; these must be counted as part of the fluid allowance.

Sodium Early in renal failure, the kidneys lose the ability to reabsorb sodium. Renal volume may be reduced somewhat, but the person can at first maintain sodium balance on a moderate sodium intake. As end-stage renal disease approaches, however, the person excretes less urine and cannot handle normal amounts of sodium. At this point, both sodium and water must be restricted to prevent hypertension, edema, and heart failure. A typical diet will contain from 1 to 4 grams of sodium daily.

Reminder: Minimal urine volume is *oliguria;* no urine excretion is *anuria.*

A person on dialysis who is excreting little or no urine must take extreme precautions not to exceed permitted sodium and fluid intakes. Sodium becomes of special concern for the person on peritoneal dialysis because this type of dialysis does not remove sodium as effectively as does hemodialysis.

People with renal failure must avoid low-sodium products and salt substitutes that contain potassium.

Potassium Most people with renal failure can handle normal intakes of potassium. However, if hyperkalemia develops, it can be fatal, so potassium is often moderately restricted to about 1½ to 3 grams per day. This means limiting high-potassium foods and using no special products that contain potassium, as low-sodium products or salt substitutes often do. In contrast, if a person is on potassium-wasting diuretics, potassium intake may need to be raised.

Vitamins People with renal failure frequently develop water-soluble vitamin deficiencies due to the restrictive diet, loss of vitamins in dialysis, drug therapy, and altered metabolism. For these reasons, clients receive generous amounts of vitamin B_6 (5 to 10 milligrams), vitamin C (70 to 100 milligrams), and folate (1 milligram), along with the RDA of the remaining water-soluble vitamins. Supplementation of the fat-soluble vitamins, except for vitamin D, is usually not necessary.

Iron People with chronic renal failure frequently develop iron-deficiency anemia and often receive iron supplements. In addition, those who take erythropoietin to stimulate red blood cell synthesis need adequate iron to make hemoglobin.[6]

Zinc and Magnesium People on dialysis frequently complain of anorexia and altered taste perceptions (dysgeusia), symptoms typical of zinc deficiency. Studies providing supplemental zinc to improve taste sensitivity and appetite have shown variable and inconclusive results. As for magnesium, people with renal failure should never take antacids, laxatives, or enemas high in magnesium; serious hypermagnesemia can result.

Special Nutrition Support If people with chronic renal failure become ill or otherwise unable to eat, health care professionals first try to supplement the diet orally if the GI tract is functional. Special glucose polymer powders efficiently add food energy without requiring clients to eat extra food or use their fluid allowances.[7] In addition, special enteral and parenteral formulas designed for use with renal failure are available (see Appendix H). Enteral formulas can be provided orally or by tube.

Putting It All Together No doubt you have long since arrived at the conclusion that designing renal diets is a task for a specialist. Diet planners must carefully adjust intakes of energy, protein, lipids, liquids, vitamins, and minerals—and then find food combinations that will deliver the necessary amounts of these nutrients. Not only that, these foods must be ones *the individual on the diet will accept and enjoy.* Renal dietitians face these challenges every day. Many of them use exchange systems that group foods by their protein, sodium, potassium, and phosphorus contents to develop renal diets. A sample menu is provided on p. 652.

Even with the best planning, the diet for renal failure can be extremely restrictive, unappealing, and monotonous. Loss of interest in food can lead to reduced food intake and undernutrition.[8] The next box provides suggestions to ease the task of complying with a renal diet.

To work successfully with clients, diet advisers have still another task—communicating with, and especially listening to, their clients. Inside that tangled web of grossly altered metabolic processes, dialysis lines, and toxic waste products is a person, often a frightened or discouraged one. If you have ever been on any kind of diet, you will appreciate some of the problems these people face.

Table 27–2
Beverages and Foods Controlled on Fluid-Restricted Diets

BEVERAGES	
All	
FOODS	
Frozen yogurt	Popsicles
Gelatin	Sherbet
Ice cream	Soup
Ice milk	
OTHER	
Cream	
Ice	
Liquid medications	

Note: All foods contain some water, but these foods are liquids or melt to liquids at room temperature. Because they contain considerable amounts of water, they must be considered part of the fluid allowance on a fluid-restricted diet.

Sample Renal Diet Menu
This diet menu provides 60 grams of protein and controls phosphorus, potassium, and sodium intake. To increase the kcalories in this diet, prepare food with oil or unsalted margarine (regular margarine, if allowed) and use additional sugar or syrup whenever possible. For example, canned fruit packed in heavy syrup, rather than in juice, adds kcalories.

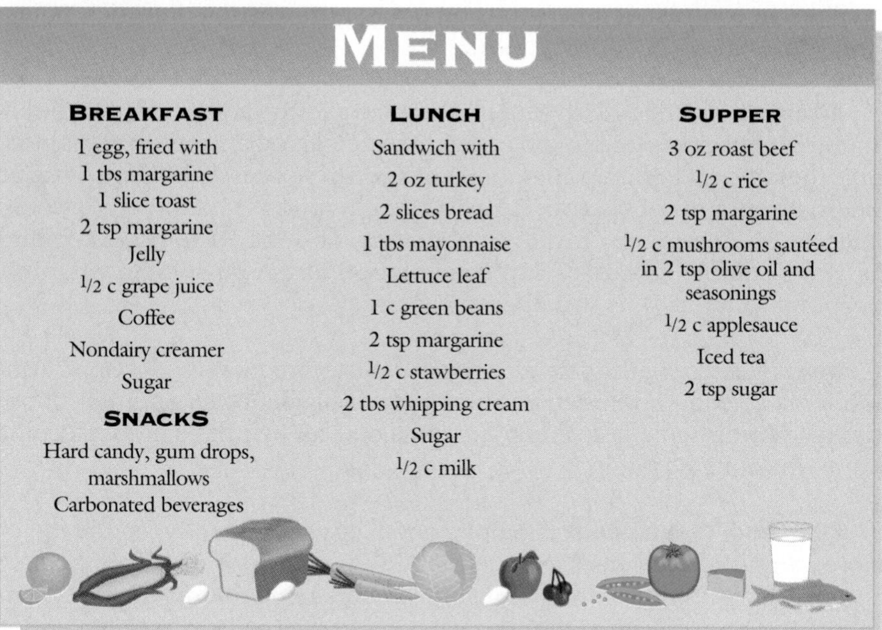

MENU
BREAKFAST
1 egg, fried with
1 tbs margarine
1 slice toast
2 tsp margarine
Jelly
1/2 c grape juice
Coffee
Nondairy creamer
Sugar
SNACKS
Hard candy, gum drops, marshmallows
Carbonated beverages
LUNCH
Sandwich with
2 oz turkey
2 slices bread
1 tbs mayonnaise
Lettuce leaf
1 c green beans
2 tsp margarine
1/2 c stawberries
2 tbs whipping cream
Sugar
1/2 c milk
SUPPER
3 oz roast beef
1/2 c rice
2 tsp margarine
1/2 c mushrooms sautéed in 2 tsp olive oil and seasonings
1/2 c applesauce
Iced tea
2 tsp sugar

HOW TO Improve Renal Diet Compliance

The following suggestions can help clients comply with the renal diet. To keep track of fluid intake:

- Fill a container with an amount of water equal to your total fluid allowance. Each time you use a liquid food or beverage, discard an equivalent amount of water from the container. The amount remaining in the container will show you how much fluid you have left for the day.
- Be sure to save enough fluid to take medications.

To help control thirst:

- Chew gum or suck hard candy.
- Freeze fluids so they take longer to consume.
- Add lemon juice to water to make it more refreshing.
- Gargle with refrigerated mouthwash.

To prevent the diet from becoming monotonous:

- Experiment with new combinations of allowed foods.
- Use favorite foods whenever possible.
- Add zest to foods by seasoning with garlic, onion, chili, curry powder, oregano, pepper, or lemon juice.
- Consult a dietitian when you want to eat restricted foods. Many restricted foods can be used occasionally in small amounts if the diet is carefully adjusted.

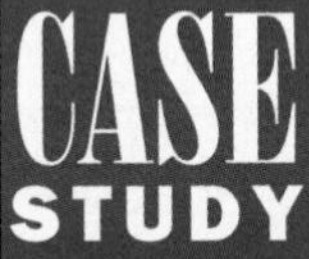

Child with Chronic Renal Failure

Mickey is a nine-year-old child who developed chronic glomerulonephritis several months after suffering from a streptococcal infection (strep throat). Mickey's renal function has declined steadily over the last three years. His mother consulted his physician because the boy had been very tired, unable to eat, and complaining of stomach cramps and unpleasant taste sensations. Laboratory tests revealed the following information:

- GFR: 4 ml/min (below normal).
- BUN: 102 mg/dL (above normal).

Mickey was admitted to the hospital, and after further testing, dialysis was instituted. A search for a suitable kidney donor was also initiated. Mickey is 4 feet 3 inches tall and weighs 55 pounds. Before coming to the hospital, Mickey was following a 30-g-protein, sodium-, potassium-, and fluid-restricted diet. His typical energy intake is 1100 kcalories per day.

1. Describe chronic renal failure. Are the symptoms Mickey complained of typical of renal failure?
2. Why did Mickey's GFR fall, and why did his BUN levels rise?
3. Look closely at Mickey's height and weight. How do they compare with the height and weight of a child his age without renal disease? (Use the growth charts in Appendix E.)
4. Discuss reasons why growth may be compromised in the child with renal failure.
5. Think about Mickey's diet before he came into the hospital. Describe the reasons why protein, sodium, and potassium were restricted.
6. Compare Mickey's energy RDA with his estimated energy intake.
7. Consider the effect of Mickey's energy intake on his growth.
8. Describe ways Mickey's nutrient needs will change when he begins hemodialysis.
9. How will his needs change if he receives a kidney transplant?
10. Discuss some diet strategies you can suggest to Mickey and his parents to help him comply with his diet.
11. Consider the impact of renal disease on Mickey and his family. How can all members of the health care team help support Mickey and his family during this difficult crisis?

The person with renal disease has to live with many frustrations. Successful treatment often hinges on compliance with diet and drug orders. All the members of the health care team need to know what is involved if they are to offer the most effective possible support. The accompanying case study helps direct your thoughts toward the special needs of a child with chronic renal failure.

Kidney Transplants and Diet

An alternative preferred to dialysis in ESRD is a kidney transplant. Kidney transplants can successfully restore kidney function and promote normal growth. For this reason, transplants are particularly desirable in children. The elderly, people with other life-threatening conditions, and people who prefer dialysis are generally not considered candidates for kidney transplants. Given a choice, many would opt to receive transplants, but suitable kidney donors cannot always be found.

Table 27–3
Dietary Guidelines after a Kidney Transplant

After a kidney transplant, a client needs:

- An energy intake in accordance with the client's need to either gain or lose weight. (Immunosuppressants can induce weight gain.)
- A daily protein intake above the RDA—between 1.2 and 1.5 grams per kilogram of body weight. Intakes may be adjusted downward to restore normal lab values or upward to counteract catabolic effects of immunosuppressants. (Immunosuppressants can induce protein catabolism and lead to negative nitrogen balance.)
- Restriction of sodium to 2 to 4 grams per day, about the same as for a person being prudent for the sake of heart disease prevention. (Hypertension and edema often accompany immunosuppressant treatment.)
- A carbohydrate intake of 40 to 50% of energy intake with an emphasis on complex carbohydrates. (Glucose intolerance can develop in people taking immunosuppressants.)
- A fat intake of 30% or less of total energy with less than 10% from saturated fat and 300 milligrams cholesterol. (Elevated lipids are common in renal disease and also as a result of immunosuppressants.)
- Adjustment of potassium intake when necessary. (Many people with renal transplants require potassium-wasting diuretics.)

Immunosuppressant Drug Therapy After receiving a new kidney, the person must take very large doses of immunosuppressant drugs to prevent rejection (see Tables E–1A and E–1B in Appendix E for nutrient-drug interactions). Muscular weakness, GI bleeding, carbohydrate intolerance, sodium retention, hypertension, and a puffy-faced appearance commonly accompany medical therapy. Infections and increased susceptibility to malignant tumors are also common. The kidney may be rejected or fail to function, in which case dialysis must be reinstituted.

Dietary Interventions The person with a successful kidney transplant may have normal renal function and can enjoy a wider choice of foods than the person on dialysis. Typical post-transplant diet modifications appear in Table 27–3.[9]

People with kidney transplants may reject their new kidneys either temporarily or permanently. During these times, they must return to the prescribed diet for renal failure. Clients may find this regression difficult to accept and need to be prepared for the possibility before it occurs.

nephrotic syndrome: the complex of symptoms that occur when glomerular function fails; it includes proteinuria and albuminuria.

The loss of protein in the urine is called **proteinuria,** and the loss of the protein albumin in the urine is called **albuminuria.** Newer laboratory methods allow clinicians to detect *microalbuminuria*, the loss of albumin in the urine at levels that are greater than normal, but less than frank albuminuria. Such tests are routinely performed in people at high risk for renal disease.

Nephrotic Syndrome

Unlike renal failure, which severely impacts many kidney functions, nephrotic syndrome is the complex of symptoms that occur when the glomerular capillaries are damaged, their permeability increases, and plasma proteins escape into the urine. Nephrotic syndrome is sometimes an early sign of progressive renal disease, especially in people with diabetes mellitus (see Chapter 25). Other disorders can lead to nephrotic syndrome, including glomerulonephritis, infections, and renal vein thrombosis.

Consequences of Nephrotic Syndrome

Low serum albumin, edema, and elevated blood lipids are the primary manifestations of the syndrome. Hypocalcemia and iron-deficiency anemia may also occur.

Blood Albumin Falls and Edema Develops As plasma proteins are lost in the urine, blood proteins fall sharply. Albumin, the major plasma protein, is also the major protein lost in the urine, and its blood level is markedly reduced. Along with other factors, low blood protein allows fluid to move into the interstitial space, and edema develops. Fluids exit from the blood, leaving the blood volume low, and the body responds by retaining sodium and fluid.

Among the blood proteins lost are transferrin, the iron-carrying protein, and immunoglobulins, important in immunity. Loss of transferrin may lead to anemia. Losses of immunoglobulins render the person prone to infection, which can compromise nutrition status further. If protein loss continues without replacement, lean body tissues break down, and malnutrition follows. Figure 27–2 illustrates these and other consequences of the nephrotic syndrome.

Blood Lipids Change Elevated cholesterol, triglycerides, LDL, and VLDL, and low HDL characterize the nephrotic syndrome for reasons that remain unclear. The altered lipid patterns may increase the likeli-

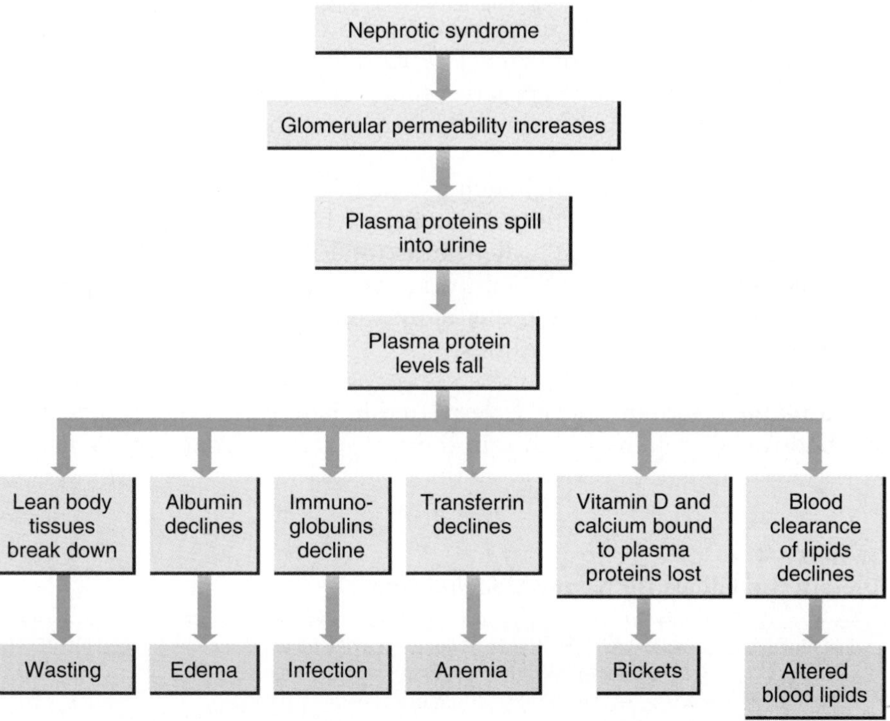

Figure 27–2
Consequences of the Nephrotic Syndrome
Note that malnutrition further depletes lean body mass and plasma proteins and raises the likelihood of edema, infection, and anemia.

hood of cardiovascular disease and stroke, as well as intensifying the risk of further kidney damage.[10]

Vitamin D Deficiency and Hypocalcemia Develop The plasma protein that binds vitamin D is also excreted in the urine along with the vitamin D it carries. Consequently, vitamin D deficiency develops, leading to hypocalcemia. Not only is calcium absorption impaired, but some calcium is lost along with albumin in the urine. Rickets may develop, particularly in children.

Dietary Interventions

Treatment of nephrotic syndrome depends largely on the underlying cause. Diet is the key to preventing protein malnutrition and alleviating edema. Table 27–4 summarizes dietary guidelines for nephrotic syndrome.

Energy A diet adequate in energy (about 35 kcalories per kilogram of body weight) is necessary to maintain weight and spare protein. Additional kcalories may be appropriate if the person loses weight or develops an infection or fever. Obese people with nephrotic syndrome may be advised to slightly reduce their energy intakes to help control blood lipids and gradually lose weight.

Protein In the past, high-protein diets (about 120 grams per day) were often prescribed for people with nephrotic syndrome, stemming from the belief that high dietary protein would compensate for urinary protein losses. Providing extra protein, however, does not correct the metabolic consequences of urinary protein loss and may accelerate renal deterioration.[11] A common practice today is to provide protein at 0.8 to 1.0 gram per kilogram of body weight—that is, about the RDA.

Fat A fat-restricted diet such as one of the plans shown in Chapter 26 (see p. 619) can help control the altered blood lipids associated with nephrotic syndrome. Such a diet limits total fat, saturated fat, and cholesterol. Often people with nephrotic syndrome are unable to control blood lipids adequately using diet alone, and physicians prescribe drugs to help correct lipid abnormalities.

Sodium Sodium must be restricted in nephrotic syndrome because the body avidly retains sodium. In the early stage of treatment, a diet low

Table 27–4
Dietary Guidelines for Nephrotic Syndrome

The diet for a person with nephrotic syndrome should supply:

- Energy: 35 kcalories per kilogram of body weight per day.
- Protein: 0.8–1.0 gram per kilogram of body weight per day.
- Fat: <30% of total kcalories, low in saturated fat and cholesterol.
- Sodium: 1500 milligrams per day.

in sodium (250 milligrams), combined with diuretics, helps the body to mobilize the fluid that has accumulated in the interstitial space.

Hidden sources of sodium can undermine severely restricted diets. If local water supplies with a high sodium content are used for preparing and cooking foods, they can significantly contribute to sodium intake. (Health departments can supply information on the sodium in local water supplies.) Medications such as antacids, antibiotics, cough medicines, laxatives, pain relievers, and sedatives may contain sodium. Some toothpastes and mouthwashes also contain large amounts of sodium; people should not swallow these compounds and should rinse thoroughly after brushing their teeth or using mouthwash. Chapters 8 and 26 provide more information on low-sodium, low-salt diets.

Once edema is resolved and sodium balance is achieved, the sodium restriction relaxes to about 1500 milligrams per day—still fairly stringent. If physicians prescribe potassium-wasting diuretics, they must advise clients to select foods rich in potassium. As a general rule, whole, unprocessed foods in all categories fit that description: meats, milk products, grains, fruits, and vegetables (see pp. 14–15 and Appendix A).

Nutrition Assessment

The person in renal failure is a likely victim of malnutrition. It therefore becomes essential that health care providers conduct nutrition assessments frequently and that problems be prevented or promptly corrected; otherwise nutrient stores will dwindle. The dietitian considers:

- Diet history, to determine the usual intakes of kcalories, protein, sodium, potassium, phosphorus, calcium, and vitamin D. Diet adjustments can then be based on the newly diagnosed person's current eating habits, thereby easing compliance with the restricted diet. For the person already following a renal diet, the diet history helps in assessing the person's understanding of, and compliance with, the diet.
- Anthropometric measurements, which will be significantly influenced by the state of hydration. The weight taken immediately after dialysis treatments will most accurately reflect the person's true weight. (This weight is sometimes called the "dry weight.") When the person is not on dialysis, weight may be deceptively normal or high because of water retention. Likewise, arm measurements may be affected by edema. Edema can be a problem for both those with nephrotic syndrome and those in renal failure.
- Weight changes and blood pressure, which are useful in assessing the state of hydration in people with renal failure. Weight gain and high blood pressure suggest fluid retention; weight loss and low blood pressure suggest dehydration.
- Weight and height in children, which must be routinely assessed to ensure that their diets are meeting the needs for growth. Remember that growth failure is common in children with renal failure. Weight loss often occurs in renal failure. Wasting is common in people with nephrotic syndrome who fail to eat enough protein.
- Albumin and transferrin levels, which may be extremely low in people with nephrotic syndrome and which rise when protein intake is adequate. People with renal failure also have lower transferrin levels than

healthy people do; and these levels are even lower when malnutrition accompanies renal disease.

- Serum electrolytes, BUN, and creatinine, which must be carefully monitored in renal failure.
- Serum lipids, which are frequently elevated in both chronic renal failure and nephrotic syndrome.

People with chronic renal failure must be carefully monitored to prevent growth failure and renal osteodystrophy. Anemia is another problem that can be partially corrected by diet.

Most of this chapter has been devoted to the consequences of renal failure and dietary treatments to help resolve them. Nutrition in Practice 27 describes the development and treatment of "stones" in the kidneys.

■ STUDY QUESTIONS ■

1. What functions do the kidneys perform? What is the role of the kidneys in maintaining chemical homeostasis?
2. What is renal failure?
3. What happens in the end stage of renal failure? Describe some of the symptoms associated with the buildup of toxic metabolic products in the blood. When is dialysis or a kidney transplant considered for the person with renal failure?
4. Describe acute renal failure and list some of its causes. What are the consequences of acute renal failure?
5. What are the nutrient needs of the person in the oliguric phase of acute renal failure? How do these needs change as the person progresses to the diuretic phase?
6. Can tube feedings and TPN be used safely in the person with renal failure? What special considerations must be made when selecting an enteral or parenteral formula for the person with acute renal failure?
7. What are the causes of chronic renal failure? Why is it often difficult to detect in the early stages? What are its consequences? Describe some factors that can lead to growth failure and wasting in people with chronic renal failure.
8. What are the objectives of dietary treatment of chronic renal failure?
9. What are the energy needs of adults with chronic renal failure? Of children? What are the consequences of providing too little energy in the diet of the person with chronic renal failure?
10. Why is the protein (nitrogen) intake of the person with chronic renal failure a particular concern? How does dialysis affect protein needs?
11. What modifications involving phosphorus, calcium, and vitamin D are made in the diet of the person with chronic renal failure? Why? What fluid and electrolyte modifications are made?
12. What other vitamins and minerals need special consideration in the diet of the person with chronic renal failure? Describe why each of the nutrients you list may be a problem.
13. Discuss the nutrient needs of the person with a kidney transplant.
14. What is nephrotic syndrome? What are its consequences? What are the energy and protein needs of the person with nephrotic syndrome? Why is a low-fat, low-cholesterol diet important in nephrotic syndrome? What are the fluid and electrolyte needs of individuals with nephrotic syndrome?

■ CLINICAL APPLICATION QUESTIONS ■

1. Chapter 18 described severe stresses and discussed how the combination of severe stress, hypermetabolism, and malnutrition can lead to multiple organ failure. The sequence of multiple organ failure often begins with respiratory failure (Chapter 26), followed by liver failure (Chapter 24), and then renal failure. On a sheet of paper make three columns, one for each disorder. Under each column, list the energy, protein, fat, fluid, and other nutrient considerations for treating each organ failure individually. Which nutrient modifications are common to all three disorders? Do some of the necessary modifications for one disorder conflict with those for another? If yes, describe how the final decision might be made for the most appropriate diet.
2. Using the box on p. 652 as a guide, give suggestions for helping people adjust to different aspects of their renal diets. Can you think of any other suggestions?

NUTRITION IN PRACTICE 27

Prevention and Treatment of Kidney Stones

Unlike renal disease, which is rare, kidney stones are common. In the United States, about one in every ten adults suffers from kidney stones, a condition that is painful, though rarely fatal. Most of these people are men over 25 years old. Stones often occur only once; recurrences may be preventable. The accompanying glossary defines terms used to describe kidney stones.

What are kidney stones made of?

The composition of kidney stones varies, but about three-fourths of them contain calcium in the form of calcium oxalate. Less commonly, stones are composed of uric acid, the amino acid cystine, or magnesium ammonium phosphate (known as struvite).

Are any causes of stone formation known?

Practitioners widely accept that kidney stones form when stone constituents become concentrated in the urine and form crystals that grow. Some practitioners believe that a deficiency of one or more naturally occurring stone *inhibitors* in the urine may contribute to stone formation. Research has yet to provide enough knowledge about these inhibitors to influence therapy. Thus risk factors for stone formation include excessive urinary excretion of stone constituents, low urine volume, or a combination of these; deficiencies of substances that normally inhibit stone formation may contribute to the problem. About half of all people with calcium oxalate stones have normal urinary calcium levels, and the other half excrete excess urinary calcium for no known underlying cause—idiopathic hypercalciuria. Uric acid stones are frequently associated with gout, a metabolic disorder that causes excessive urinary excretion of uric acid. Cystine stones form when an inherited disorder of amino acid metabolism (cystinuria) causes the abnormal excretion of cystine in the urine. Struvite stones, sometimes called "infection stones," form when the urinary tract becomes infected with a specific type of microorganism.

Table 27–5 (p. 660) summarizes some disorders associated with stone formation. Because so many disorders are associated with stone formation, treatment and prevention depend on correct diagnosis.[12] Clinicians analyze the chemical composition of urine, blood, and stones (when available) to determine the cause of stone formation. Of course, the underlying disorder and the kidney stones demand medical and dietary attention.

Glossary

cystinuria (SIS-te-NEW-ree-ah): the presence of cystine in the urine, the symptom of an inherited metabolic disorder in which large amounts of the amino acids cystine, lysine, arginine, and ornithine are excreted in the urine. Cystinuria commonly results in kidney stone formation.

dysuria (dis-YOU-ree-ah): painful or difficult urination.

gout: a metabolic disorder that results in excess uric acid in the blood and sometimes in the urine; characterized by acute arthritis and inflammation of the joints.

hematuria (HEME-at-YOU-ree-ah): blood in the urine.

hypercalciuria (HIGH-per-kal-see-YOU-ree-ah): excessive urinary excretion of calcium. When this is not related to a known underlying medical condition, it is known as **idiopathic hypercalciuria.**

hyperoxaluria (HIGH-per-ox-al-YOU-ree-ah): excessive urinary excretion of oxalate; may occur when calcium intake is insufficient to bind oxalate in the intestine, thus allowing excessive oxalate absorption. When GI diseases cause excessive oxalate absorption and subsequent excessive oxalate excretion, it is known as **enteric hyperoxaluria.**

nidus (NIGH-dus), or **nucleus:** a small bit of crystallized mineral or other material that serves as a matrix for crystallization.

renal colic: the severe pain that accompanies the movement of a kidney stone from the kidney through the ureter to the bladder.

struvite: crystals of magnesium ammonium phosphate.

supersaturation: a term that describes the concentration of a substance in a liquid at the point where the substance is too concentrated to stay in solution and begins to precipitate.

Table 27–5
Conditions Associated with Kidney Stones

Bowel diseases causing malabsorption
Cystinuria
Glucocorticoid excess
Gout
Hyperparathyroidism
Hyperthyroidism
Immobilization
Malignancies (some types)
Osteoporosis
Paget's disease
Recurrent urinary tract infections
Renal tubular acidosis
Vitamin D intoxication

Are kidney stones painful?

In most cases, no, especially when they are few and small. Small stones (less than 5 millimeters, or one-fifth of an inch, in diameter) may require no treatment. They may pass readily through the ureters and out of the body via the urine (see Figure 27–3). Larger stones cannot exit the body as easily. When a large stone or a large broken-off piece of a stone enters a ureter, the person experiences a severe, stabbing pain, called *renal colic.* Typically, the pain starts suddenly in the back, just above the bottom ribs, and intensifies as the stone follows the ureter's course down the abdomen toward the groin. The pain is intense and is often accompanied by nausea and vomiting. When the stone reaches the bladder, the pain subsides abruptly. Urinary symptoms include frequent urination, urgency of urination, dysuria, and hematuria. If a stone blocks the flow of urine, a physician often uses shock waves to break the stone into pieces small enough to pass easily through the urinary tract.

How can diet help treat kidney stones?

Dietary regimens vary according to the type of stone, but all include one bit of advice: increase fluid intake to dilute the urine and reduce the risk of stone formation. People with kidney stones need to drink enough fluid to maintain a urine volume of at least 2 liters per day. This requires an intake of about 3 to 4 liters total, taken at regular intervals throughout the day. Physically active clients, or those who live in warm climates, need additional fluids.

Other than fluids, do any dietary measures help prevent kidney stones?

Yes, but oddly enough, the advice is not always to provide low intakes of the constituents of the stone. In the case of calcium oxalate stones, for example, it might seem reasonable to strictly limit dietary calcium, but this is not a wise move. Some people with calcium oxalate stones do excrete large amounts of calcium, and calcium restriction can lower urinary excretion, but low calcium intakes are unwise. Those who follow a low-calcium diet generally excrete more calcium than they ingest, indicating that they are losing calcium from their bones. To put it simply, the low-calcium diet may lead to negative calcium balance and bone loss.

Low calcium intakes also increase urinary oxalate excretion, a problem for people who are susceptible to developing calcium oxalate stones. Instead of a low-calcium diet, then, treatment moderately limits calcium intake to up to 1 gram a day and limits oxalate intake. (Chapter 21 described why calcium oxalate stones may form as a result of fat malabsorption. Calcium restriction is not appropriate for this type of stone.)

Figure 27–3
The Urinary Tract

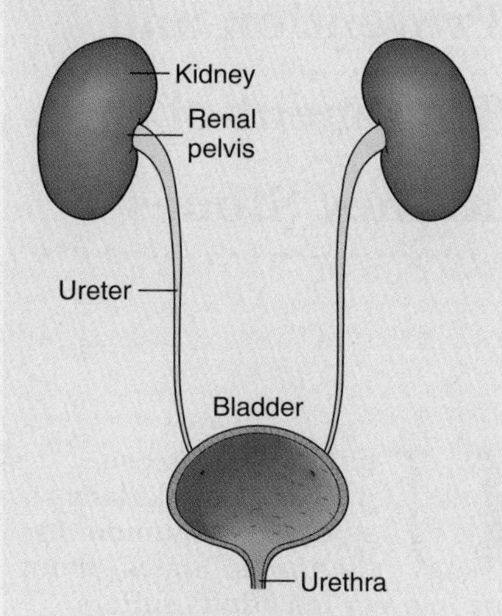

People with calcium oxalate stones are advised to limit their intakes of foods high in oxalate—spinach, rhubarb, beets, nuts, chocolate, tea, wheat bran, and strawberries.[13] Some clinicians report that for most people, only nuts (and peanut butter) need be restricted.[14] Vitamin C supplements should be avoided.

Why should vitamin C supplements be avoided?

One of the pathways of oxalate synthesis in the body begins with vitamin C. Megadoses of vitamin C over long periods raise urinary oxalate concentrations, which can aggravate stone formation in some people. People with hyperoxaluria must steer clear of vitamin C supplements.

What about treatment of other stones?

For uric acid stones, low-purine diets are commonly prescribed. A low-purine diet restricts red meats, particularly organ meats,

anchovies, sardines, and meat extracts. The benefits of such a diet are unproven, but it may be useful to limit excessive protein intake. Drug therapy is commonly prescribed to inhibit uric acid production, thus reducing both uric acid levels and urinary acidity.

For cystine stones, health care professionals prescribe a diet restricted in the amino acid methionine because the body makes cystine from methionine. Drug therapy to reduce urinary acidity may also be beneficial.

For struvite "infection" stones, no specific diet therapy is recommended. Effective treatment includes removal of the stones and antibacterial drugs.

Many connections exist between diet and kidney stones. Dramatic advances in the nonsurgical treatment of kidney stones have triggered a renewed interest in this field. Health care professionals will want to keep up with changes so that they can provide the best possible care for their clients.

■ NOTES ■

1. A.S.P.E.N. Board of Directors, Practice guidelines: Kidney failure—Pediatric, *Journal of Parenteral and Enteral Nutrition* (supplement) 17 (1993): 43.
2. L. Oldrizzi, C. Rugio, and G. Maschio, Nutrition and the kidney: How to manage patients with renal failure, *Nutrition in Clinical Practice* 9 (1994): 3–10.
3. P. Harum, Vitamin, mineral, and hormone interactions in renal bone disease, *Journal of Renal Nutrition* 3 (1993): 30–35.
4. Harum, 1993.
5. M. Emmett and coauthors, Calcium acetate control of serum phosphorus in hemodialysis patients, *American Journal of Kidney Diseases* 17 (1991): 544–550.
6. L. W. Moore and coauthors, Incidence, causes, and treatment of iron deficiency anemia in hemodialysis patients, *Journal of Renal Nutrition* 2 (1992): 105–112.
7. M. A. Allman and coauthors, Energy supplementation and the nutritional status of hemodialysis patients, *American Journal of Clinical Nutrition* 51 (1990): 558–562.
8. E. Dobell and coauthors, Food preferences and food habits of patients with chronic renal failure undergoing dialysis, *Journal of the American Dietetic Association* 93 (1993): 1129–1135.
9. M. S. Edwards and S. Doster, Renal transplant diet recommendations of a survey of renal dietitians in the United States, *Journal of the American Dietetic Association* 90 (1990): 843–846.
10. J. D. Dwyer, Vegetarian diets for treating nephrotic syndrome, *Nutrition Reviews* 51 (1993): 44–56; G. A. Kaysen, Nutritional management of nephrotic syndrome, *Journal of Renal Nutrition* 2 (1992): 50–58.
11. R. W. Davies and coauthors, Proteinuria, not altered albumin metabolism, affects hyperlipidemia in the nephrotic rat, *Journal of Clinical Investigations* 86 (1990): 600–605.
12. Kaysen, 1992.
13. L. K. Massey, H. Roman-Smith, and R. A. L. Sutton, Effect of dietary oxalate and calcium on urinary oxalate and risk of formation of calcium oxalate kidney stones, *Journal of the American Dietetic Association* 93 (1993): 901–906.
14. C. L. Smith, M. Davis, and R. O. Berkseth, Dietary factors in calcium nephrolithiasis, *Journal of Renal Nutrition* 2 (1992): 146–153.

28

Nutrition and Cancer

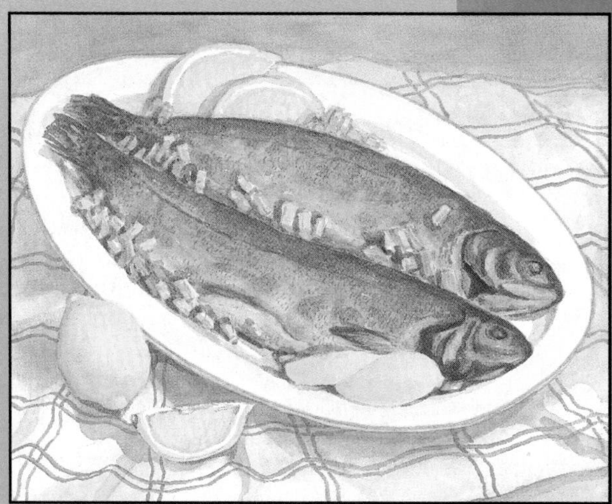

CONTENTS

Previous chapters have shown that malnutrition accompanies and complicates many disorders. Chronic liver and renal diseases and inflammatory bowel diseases, already discussed, last for long times and can eventually lead to severe protein-energy malnutrition (PEM). Cancer, discussed in this chapter, and AIDS, discussed in the next chapter, also impair nutrition status severely.

Cancer affects many organ systems, and both the disease and its treatments cause wasting. Malnutrition aggravates the symptoms, interferes with treatment, impairs life's quality, and shortens its length.

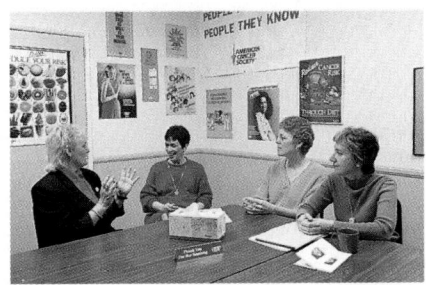

Until medical science wins the battle against cancer, people with cancer take comfort from the support of others.

Cancer

The thought of cancer often strikes fear in people. The prognosis for most people, however, is far brighter today than in the past. Some cancers are preventable and many are curable, especially when detected early. New techniques for detecting cancers early and innovative therapies to wipe out cancers offer hope and encouragement.

The word *cancer* refers to any uncontrolled growth of abnormal cells. Cancer is not a single disorder; instead, there are many different *cancers*. They have different characteristics, occur in different locations in the body, take different courses, and require different treatments.

A growing tumor, or neoplasm, interferes with the normal functioning of an organ or tissue. The growth has no built-in brakes and is supported by nutrients from the diet or body reserves. The words *malignant neoplasm, malignant tumor,* and *cancer* are synonymous and are used interchangeably to describe the unchecked growth of harmful abnormal cells.

cancer: a disease in which abnormal cells multiply out of control and disrupt the normal functioning of the body's cells or organs.

tumor: an unchecked new growth of tissue forming an abnormal mass with no function. A cancerous growth may also be called a **neoplasm** (NEE-oh-plazm). Liquid tissues such as the blood or lymph may form neoplasms (leukemia or lymphoma).

Tumors that pose no problem are called **benign** (bee-NINE); those that are harmful and require treatment are **malignant.** A cancer that spreads from one part of the body to another is said to **metastasize** (me-TAS-tah-size).
benign = mild
malignant = bad

How Cancer Develops

Cancer develops in steps. First, a carcinogen or a dose of radiation alters a cell somewhere in the body and initiates the process, probably by altering the cellular DNA. Then, promoters enhance the cancer's development so that cells begin to multiply out of control and a tumor or other malignant neoplasm forms. Because these steps take time, there are many opportunities for intervention.

Cancer is probably not often caused by initiators in foods. Instead, nutrition is most likely influential after the cancer cells are multiplying. Then, chemical promoters in foods, particularly fatty foods, may cause cancer cells to multiply more rapidly than they would otherwise. Certain foods, however, particularly vegetables, may help *prevent* initiation.

carcinogen (car-SIN-oh-jen): a cancer-initiating substance. A carcinogen is one kind of initiator; radiation is another.
carcin = cancer
gen = gives rise to

promoters: factors that favor the development of cancer once an initiating event has taken place. Other factors, **antipromoters,** oppose the development of cancer.

Prevention of Cancer

Genetic susceptibility plays a role in cancer; certain types of cancer, such as breast cancer, tend to run in families. Environmental factors such as smoking, water and air pollution, and exposure to the sun also play roles in cancer development. Dietary constituents can also be carcinogens, and the emphasis here is on these factors.

Carcinogens—Cancer Initiators Cancer risk rises with repeated exposure to carcinogens. People who wish to reduce their cancer risks can reduce their exposure to environmental and dietary factors that have been linked to cancer. Table 28–1 lists various types of cancers and the specific dietary factors that are associated with them.

Table 28–1
Dietary Factors Associated with Cancer at Specific Sites

CANCER SITES	ASSOCIATED WITH THESE FACTORS
Esophageal cancer	High alcohol use, tobacco use, and especially combined use; use of preserved foods (such as pickles); low intakes of vitamins and minerals
Stomach cancer	High intakes of salt-preserved foods (such as dried, salted fish); low intakes of fresh fruits and vegetables Protective effect of fresh fruits and vegetables
Colorectal cancer	High intakes of fat (particularly saturated fat) and alcohol (especially beer); low intakes of vegetables Protective effect of high intake of vegetables
Liver cancer	Infection with hepatitis B or aflatoxins; alcohol abuse
Pancreatic and lung cancer	No dietary risk factors have been established; correlated primarily with cigarette smoking. Findings on coffee are inconsistent. Protective effect of fruits and green and yellow vegetables rich in beta-carotene
Breast cancer	High intakes of food energy, dietary fat, and alcohol Protective effect of fruits and vegetables, especially green and yellow ones
Ovarian cancer	No dietary risk factors have been established; inversely correlated with oral contraceptive use Protective effect of fruits and vegetables, especially green and yellow ones
Endometrial cancer	No dietary risk factors have been established; associated with estrogen therapy, obesity, hypertension, and diabetes (NIDDM)
Bladder cancer	*Possible* associations with coffee, artificial sweeteners, and alcohol; associated with cigarette smoking Protective effects of fruits and vegetables, especially green and yellow ones
Prostate cancer	High fat intakes Protective effect of fruits and vegetables, especially green and yellow ones

Note: Findings based on epidemiological studies.

Sources: Diet and Health: Implications for Reducing Chronic Disease Risk (Washington, D.C.: National Academy Press, 1989), pp. 594–600; J. H. Weisburger, Nutritional approach to cancer prevention with emphasis on vitamins, antioxidants, and carotenoids, *American Journal of Clinical Nutrition* (supplement) 53 (1991): 226–237; R. G. Ziegler, Vegetables, fruits, and carotenoids and the risk of cancer, *American Journal of Clinical Nutrition* (supplement) 53 (1991): 251–259.

Dietary Carcinogens Some experts estimate that diet may contribute to a third or more of all cancer cases. Consequently, many people think they should avoid eating foods that contain carcinogens. Some people fear food additives, but this fear is irrational. Contaminants of foods—things that get into foods by accident—may be powerful carcinogens, but the additives permitted in foods are not. Additives and contaminants receive attention in Chapter 11.

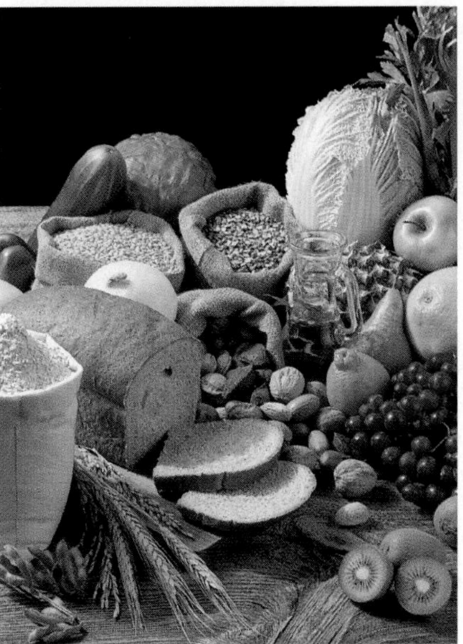

Vegetables rich in fiber and the antioxidant nutrients (beta-carotene, vitamin C, and vitamin E) help to protect against cancer.

Cancer Promoters Studies suggest that certain dietary fats, if taken in excess, may be cancer promoters. Once cancer has been initiated, these fats may cause tumors to develop earlier and in greater numbers. Linoleic acid, the polyunsaturated fatty acid of vegetable oils, is thought to be one such promoter; in contrast, omega-3 fatty acids and monounsaturated fatty acids appear not to be cancer promoters.[1]

Antipromoters Foods may also contain antipromoters and Table 28–1 includes foods that have protective effects. Dietary components and practices that may act as antipromoters include:

- *Dietary fiber.* Fiber may help to speed the transit of all materials through the colon, so that the colon walls are not exposed for long to cancer-causing substances. Perhaps more importantly, fiber may alter the chemistry of substances released by the intestinal bacteria, making them less carcinogenic.
- *Plant foods.* Extensive research supports special roles for plant foods in cancer resistance. Almost without exception, epidemiological studies—including studies of people who move from one region of the world to another—find that people who regularly eat yellow and green fruits and vegetables have fewer cancers of most types than those who rarely eat these plant foods.[2]
- *Antioxidants.* By acting as scavengers of oxygen-derived free radicals, beta-carotene, vitamin C, vitamin E, and the mineral selenium help prevent cell and tissue damage that can give rise to diseases, including cancer.[3] The anticancer activity of beta-carotene may also be partially due to its ability to support the immune system, thus bolstering tumor resistance.
- *Cruciferous vegetables.* Vegetables of the cabbage family contain nonnutrient compounds (indoles and dithiolthiones) that activate enzymes capable of destroying carcinogens.*
- *Vegetarian diets.* Vegetarians have lower mortality rates from cancer than the rest of the population, even when cancers linked to smoking and alcohol are set aside. Vegetarian diets usually contain more plant foods and fibers than do diets of meat eaters.

cruciferous vegetables: a group of vegetables that includes cauliflower, broccoli, and brussels sprouts, named for their cross-shaped blossoms. They have been shown to protect against cancer in laboratory animals.

indoles: a family of compounds with a structure resembling that of the amino acid tryptophan; mentioned here because some of those found in cruciferous vegetables have anticancer activity.

dithiolthiones: a class of compounds found in plant foods that seem to exhibit anticancer activity.

Dietary Recommendations to Reduce Cancer Risk On the basis of current knowledge and available evidence, the American Cancer Society offers the following guidelines to reduce cancer risks:

*Researchers have recently identified a chemical in broccoli called sulforaphane that stimulates the body to produce cancer-fighting enzymes.

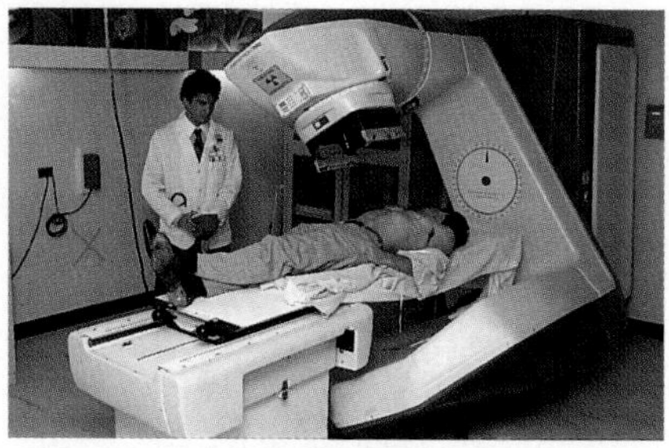

Radiation therapy is one of several weapons in the fight against cancer.

- Avoid obesity.
- Eat less total fat.
- Eat more high-fiber foods, such as whole-grain breads and cereals, vegetables, and fresh fruits.
- Eat a variety of vegetables and fruits daily.
- Avoid possible carcinogens by limiting consumption of foods preserved by salt, smoke, or nitrites.
- Limit or stop consumption of alcoholic beverages.

Cancer-prevention efforts are not always successful. When people do get cancer, early treatment can enhance recovery.

Treatments for Cancer

Unlike the treatments for diabetes, heart disease, and renal failure, in which diet plays a central role, cancer's primary treatments include radiation therapy, chemotherapy, surgery, or any combination of the three, and nutrition plays a secondary, supportive role. Ironically, though, people with cancer may be more seriously affected by the nutrition side effects of these treatments than by the cancer that necessitated them.

radiation therapy: the use of radiation to arrest or destroy cancer cells.

chemotherapy: the use of drugs to arrest or destroy cancer cells. Drugs used for chemotherapy are called **chemotherapeutic** or **antineoplastic agents.**

Radiation Therapy Radiation therapy disrupts the synthesis of new DNA, and therefore most severely damages cells that are actively dividing and making new DNA, such as malignant cells. Unfortunately, radiation also damages healthy body cells that are dividing actively, such as the cells of the blood and the GI tract.

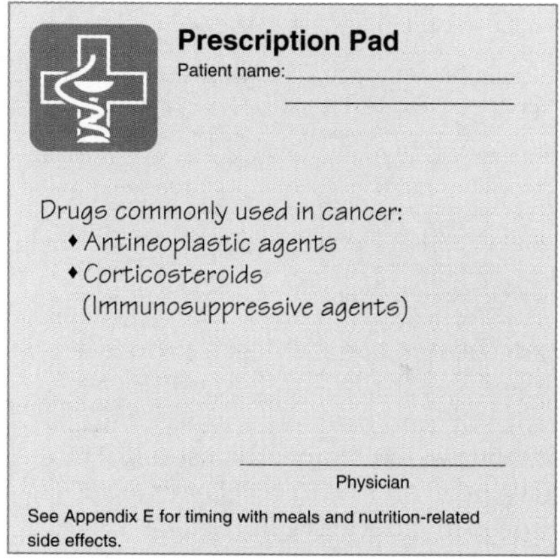
Prescription Pad
Patient name:

Drugs commonly used in cancer:
- Antineoplastic agents
- Corticosteroids (Immunosuppressive agents)

Physician

See Appendix E for timing with meals and nutrition-related side effects.

Chemotherapy Many chemotherapeutic drugs work the same way as radiation—they destroy dividing cells by interfering with DNA (or RNA) synthesis. Like radiation, these drugs also affect normal cells, especially those that divide the most rapidly.

The various types of chemotherapeutic agents include antibiotics, alkaloids, alkylating agents, antimetabolites, steroids, and others. The current trend in chemotherapy is to use high doses of several chemotherapeutic agents together in cycles. This method helps ensure that malignant cells will be destroyed. Although these treatments are often effective, they frequently intensify undesirable side effects.

Surgery Often surgery is necessary to remove a tumor. The side effects of surgery depend on the location of the tumor and its extent. Surgery is often followed by radiation or chemotherapy to prevent further tumor growth.

bone marrow transplant: the replacement of diseased bone marrow in a recipient with healthy bone marrow from a donor; used as a treatment for breast cancer, leukemia, and other blood disorders.

leukemia (loo-KEE-me-ah): cancer of the white blood cells.

Bone Marrow Transplants Bone marrow transplants are among the newer treatments for cancer; they are used to treat advanced breast cancers, leukemia, and other blood disorders. The recipient is prepared for the procedure with high doses of chemotherapy and sometimes whole-body radiation therapy. Although the preparatory procedure does effectively kill leukemic cells, it kills healthy white blood cells as well, opening the way for infection. Many of the nutrition consequences of bone marrow transplants are caused by chemotherapy, radiation, and infections.

Other Treatments Researchers continue to search for more effective ways of treating people with cancer. One such treatment, immunotherapy, provides antigens to bolster the immune system so that it can recognize and attack cancer cells. Another treatment being investigated uses specific antibodies to deliver chemotherapy directly to specific types of cancer cells, leaving nearby healthy cells unaffected. The overall effectiveness of these therapies remains to be determined.

Drug Therapy Depending on which organ systems are affected by cancer, many different drugs may be used in its treatment. Drugs commonly used to treat symptoms of cancers include antinausea agents, antidiarrheal agents, analgesic agents, and sedatives. Appendix E lists the nutrition-related side effects of many of these drugs.

Unproven Treatments People who feel they are making little progress in their fight against cancer or believe conventional medicine offers little hope of recovery may try unresearched and unproven treatments. Some unproven therapies have dangerous side effects. Others may not be dangerous in themselves, but people who delay using a prescribed therapy while trying an unproven treatment lose valuable time in fighting progression of the cancer.

Many unproven cancer therapies include nutrition components. It is beyond the scope of this text to describe unproven remedies in detail, but health care professionals should be alert to such potentially dangerous practices as:

- Discontinuing prescribed therapy to adhere to an unproven remedy.
- Following a diet that eliminates or severely restricts specific food groups.
- Taking vitamins or minerals that can be toxic in large doses.
- Using herbal preparations that may be contaminated.

As described earlier, both cancer and its treatment can impair nutrition status. The next section describes these adverse effects.

Nutrition Consequences of Cancer

The nutrition consequences of cancer may vary dramatically depending on the location of the cancer. An isolated, nonspreading type of skin cancer may be removed in a physician's office with no observable effect on nutrition status, but a pancreatic cancer can seriously impair the person's ability to digest and absorb nutrients. The following sections describe the kinds of nutrition problems that often occur in more serious cancers.

Cancer Cachexia

About two-thirds of people with cancer develop cachexia—a combination of anorexia and an accelerated, abnormal metabolism. Often cachexia is evident at the time of diagnosis.[4] The combination of poor appetite and rapid metabolism simultaneously reduces the supply of energy and nutrients and increases the demand for them.

cancer cachexia (ka-KEKS-ee-ah): a syndrome that frequently accompanies many types of cancer, characterized by anorexia, inadequate intake of food, malnutrition, accelerated metabolism and wasting, and general ill health.

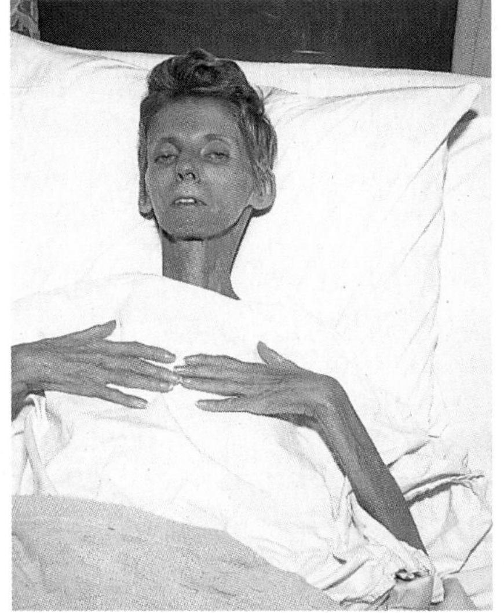

Cancer cachexia is a common and debilitating complication of many types of cancer.

Cachexia is not common to all cancers. People with advanced cancers, particularly of the GI tract, pancreas, lung, and prostate, as well as those with some types of lymph node cancers, are more likely to suffer from cachexia than those with cancer of the breast or sarcomas.

The Effects of Cachexia People who develop cachexia swiftly fall into a downward spiral. Poor food intake paired with heightened nutrient demands leads to muscle wasting and general poor health, which further contributes to inadequate nutrient intakes. The body is unable to respond to this reduced nutrient supply as it does during uncomplicated fasting, and continues to deplete its nutrient stores at an accelerated rate. The resulting malnutrition compromises the quality of life and may lead to illness and early death. Figure 28–1 summarizes some of the many known causes of cancer cachexia syndrome.

PEM is common among people with cancer. Loss of appetite, weight loss, and depletion of lean body mass and serum proteins typify cancer cachexia.

Mechanisms of Cachexia Altered metabolism begins early in tumor development, even before weight loss occurs.[5] Cachexia appears to be tumor derived; that is, the tumor itself causes the changes that lead to cachexia, and removal of the tumor can reverse the cachexia. Investigators continue to search for clues as to what tumor-related factors might be involved.

A promising area of research suggests that cytokines may be important mediators of the wasting in cancer as well as in other disorders.[6] Cytokines may induce anorexia and lead to the metabolic alterations typical of cachexia. Research efforts to clearly define the roles of various cytokines, and possibly to block their actions, hold promise for treating cachexia.

Reminder: *Cytokines* are proteins secreted by the immune system that activate the immune responses. Some of the cytokines identified as mediators of cancer cachexia include tumor necrosis factor (cachectin), interleukin-1 alpha and beta, interleukin-6, interferon-τ, and differentiation factor.

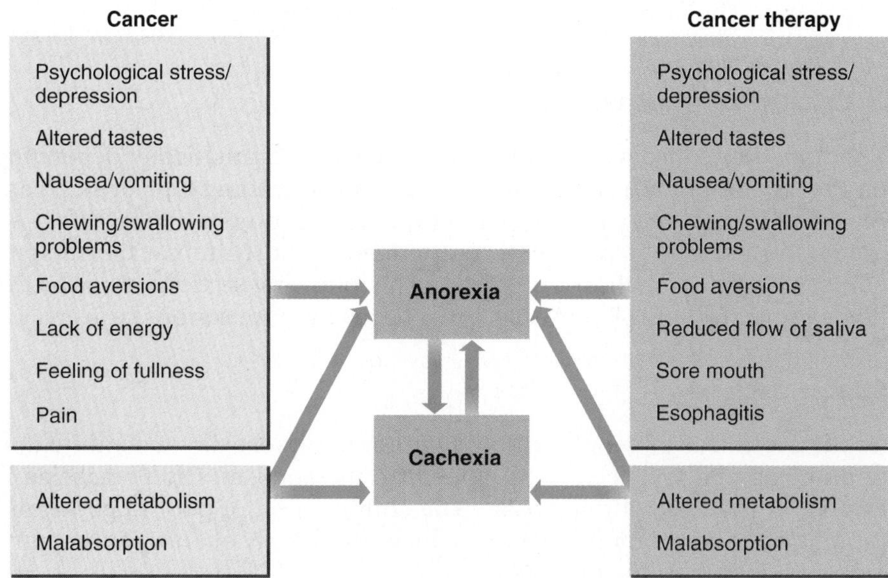

Figure 28–1
Causes of Cancer Cachexia
Anorexia and cachexia contribute to each other. Cancer makes cachexia worse, and so do cancer treatments.

Anorexia and Inadequate Nutrient Intake

Cancers often precipitate other problems that further contribute to anorexia. Some of the more important ones are listed in the margin. In addition, the treatment the person receives may itself contribute to anorexia.

Cancer can lead to anorexia by causing:
- Early satiety.
- Fatigue.
- Pain.
- Psychological stress.
- Obstructions.

Early Satiety A person with cancer sometimes experiences a premature feeling of fullness: "I feel hungry, but I take a few bites and I'm full." Animal studies suggest that one of the cytokines may delay gastric emptying, an effect that could explain the feeling of fullness.[7] In other cases, the person may feel full because a tumor is pressing against the stomach or some other part of the GI tract.

Fatigue and Pain People with cancer often tire easily. Consequently, they lack energy to prepare meals and eat. Many people with cancer feel the most energetic and the least full in the morning. As the day progresses, they become drained. Others have more energy and can eat better later in the day. Pain associated with a tumor or its treatment can cause a person to take little interest in food. Eating may make the pain worse.

Psychological Stresses Psychological stresses further contribute to anorexia. The very diagnosis of cancer can cause so much anxiety that eating becomes unimportant. People with terminal cancer may feel that eating simply isn't worth the effort. In addition, self-image may suffer from some of the treatments for cancer (for example, from a colostomy to treat colon cancer, hair loss that may accompany chemotherapy, or radical surgery that disfigures the body). The depression that follows interferes with food intake. As weight loss continues, depression may grow worse.

Obstructions Some types of cancer cause anorexia when they obstruct the GI tract. For example, a tumor of the esophagus may cause a partial or complete obstruction; the person with such a tumor is unable to eat or has difficulty swallowing. A tumor obstructing the lower GI tract may cause nausea and vomiting.

Cancer Therapy Therapy for cancer, whether chemotherapy, radiation therapy, surgery, or a bone marrow transplant, can dramatically reduce food intake and contribute to wasting. People who receive radiation or chemotherapy frequently experience anorexia, nausea, vomiting, and altered taste perceptions. Table 28–2 summarizes the effects of radiation and chemotherapy on nutrition status. The ways these treatments affect digestion, absorption, and metabolism are described later in this chapter; consider here how they affect food intake.

Cancer therapy can lead to anorexia by causing:
- Depression.
- Nausea.
- Vomiting.
- Altered taste perceptions.
- Mouth blindness.
- Dry mouth.
- Esophagitis.
- Stomatitis.
- Mouth ulcers.
- Food aversions.

Chemotherapy Chemotherapy can inflame the lining of the mouth (stomatitis) and sometimes cause mouth ulcers, making chewing and swallowing painful. Altered taste perceptions are common: clients often describe a metallic taste associated especially with red meats. The person on chemotherapy may also experience abdominal pain or develop intesti-

Table 28–2
Effects of Radiation and Chemotherapy on Nutrition Status

	REDUCED NUTRIENT INTAKE DUE TO	ACCELERATED NUTRIENT LOSSES DUE TO	ALTERED METABOLISM DUE TO
Radiation	Anorexia Damage to teeth and bones Esophagitis Nausea Reduced salivary secretions Taste alterations Thick salivary secretions Vomiting	Chronic blood loss Diarrhea Fistula formation Intestinal obstructions Malabsorption Vomiting	Secondary effects of malnutrition or infections
Chemotherapy	Abdominal pain Anorexia Intestinal ulcers Nausea Taste alterations Vomiting	Diarrhea Malabsorption Vomiting	Fluid and electrolyte imbalances Hyperglycemia Interference with vitamins or other metabolites Negative nitrogen and calcium balance Secondary effects of malnutrition or infections

nal ulcers, which interfere with food intake. Table E–1B in Appendix E describes the drug-nutrient interactions of various antineoplastic agents.

Radiation Therapy People receiving radiation therapy to the head and neck frequently experience altered taste perceptions and diminished taste sensitivities. As a result of this "mouth blindness," foods they once liked may taste unpleasant to them. An intolerance to meat, especially red meat, often develops. For some, food is just not sweet enough; for others, it is too sweet.

Radiation to the head and neck area can also reduce saliva production, and the saliva that is available is often thick, making swallowing difficult. In addition, radiation may damage the bones of the jaws and the teeth, interfering with the ability to chew and swallow. Radiation can also cause mouth ulcers to form and make eating quite painful.

Radiation to the esophagus can cause reflux esophagitis (see Chapter 20). Esophagitis often resolves when radiation therapy ends, but some people develop fibrosis or strictures, resulting in permanent swallowing problems. Fistulas can also develop, which may necessitate the use of a feeding tube or parenteral nutrition. When you consider that a person undergoing radiation therapy, particularly to the head and neck area, may suffer from several of these complications, you can see how markedly impaired nutrient intake can become.

Reminder: A *fistula* is an abnormal opening between two organs or from an organ to the skin.

Food Aversions People treated with either radiation or chemotherapy may develop a strong dislike for certain foods, tastes, and odors.

Aversions to meats, especially red meats, are most common.[8] These aversions seem to develop for foods, tastes, or odors that are associated closely in time with nausea. For example, if the person eats a certain food an hour before chemotherapy, and the chemotherapy causes nausea, the person may develop an aversion to that food. Studies suggest that, if not reinforced, aversions wane a few months after they have first developed.[9]

Surgery Surgery, of course, can also cause anorexia, nausea, and vomiting; and some types of cancer surgery have additional side effects. For example, partial or total removal of the tongue, resection of the muscles of the mouth or esophagus and salivary glands, and removal of the lower jaw invariably create extensive problems with chewing and swallowing. People with these kinds of surgery often receive tube feedings or TPN. Table 28–3 summarizes the effects some types of GI tract surgery for cancer can have on nutrition status.

Graft-versus-Host Disease People undergoing bone marrow transplants who develop graft-versus-host disease often develop anorexia, nausea, vomiting, difficulty in swallowing, mouth ulcers, taste alterations, dry mouth, and esophagitis. Bone marrow transplant recipients frequently receive nourishment parenterally until their immune status improves and adequate oral intake resumes.

Reminder: *Graft-versus-host disease* is the destruction of healthy donor white blood cells by the recipient's immune system, which sees the donor cells as foreign.

Table 28–3
Possible Effects of Surgery for Cancer on Nutrition Status

HEAD AND NECK RESECTION	
Difficulty in chewing and swallowing	Inability to chew or swallow
ESOPHAGEAL RESECTION	
Difficulty in swallowing	Inability to swallow
Reduced gastric acid secretion	Stenosis (constriction)
Reduced gastric motility	
STOMACH RESECTION	
Dumping syndrome	Vitamin B_{12} malabsorption
Hypoglycemia	General malabsorption
Lack of gastric acid	
INTESTINAL RESECTION	
General malabsorption	Hyperoxaluria
Steatorrhea	Fluid and electrolyte imbalance
Diarrhea	Blind loop syndrome
PANCREATIC RESECTION	
General malabsorption	Diabetes mellitus

Nutrient Losses

Cancer can lead to nutrient losses by causing:
- Inadequate digestion.
- Malabsorption.
- Severe vomiting or diarrhea.
- Radiation enteritis.

Excessive nutrient losses in the person with cancer can impair an already poor nutrition status. Like anorexia, nutrient losses can develop due to cancer or to the treatment for it.

Problems with Digestion and Absorption Depending on the location and type of cancer, maldigestion or malabsorption of nutrients can be a problem. For example, cancer of the pancreas may create a deficiency of pancreatic enzymes; cancer of the liver may deplete bile salts. In the Zollinger-Ellison syndrome, tumors secrete the hormone gastrin, which triggers the hypersecretion of gastric acid, thereby inactivating digestive enzymes. Tumors of the small intestine cause malabsorption, as does a tumor that obstructs the upper small intestine and creates a blind loop. (See Chapter 21 for a description of blind loop syndrome and how it causes malabsorption.)

Zollinger-Ellison syndrome: a condition caused by pancreatic tumors secreting excess gastrin, which stimulates the stomach to release large amounts of hydrochloric acid and pepsin, frequently leading to severe peptic ulcers.

Vomiting and Diarrhea Some cancers directly cause severe vomiting, diarrhea, or both, resulting in electrolyte imbalances and dehydration. For example, a tumor that obstructs the stomach or small bowel may cause vomiting. People who develop graft-versus-host disease following a bone marrow transplant may experience severe diarrhea, with diarrheal fluids in excess of 10 liters per day.

Radiation Enteritis Radiation therapy to the small bowel often interferes with normal intestinal function, resulting in vomiting and diarrhea. The radiation alters the structure of the intestinal cells (radiation enteritis). The intestinal wall becomes thick and fibrotic, and the small intestinal arteries may become so inflamed that blood flow to the bowel is cut off in some places. The lumen of the intestine may become narrow and obstructed, or a fistula may form. Radiation enteritis causes malabsorption and chronic blood loss from the intestine and bladder, leading to malnutrition and fluid and electrolyte imbalances. Intestinal function may return after radiation therapy ends, but for some people, changes may be permanent.

radiation enteritis: changes in the structure of the small intestine caused by radiation therapy.

Chemotherapy Chemotherapy may also cause diarrhea and malabsorption because it prevents the cells of the intestine from regenerating as they normally do, thus impairing nutrient absorption. As shown in Chapters 20 and 21, surgery to the GI tract can also have many ill effects on nutrition status. (These effects were summarized in Table 28–2.)

Bone Marrow Transplants Bone marrow transplants can lead to many problems that incur nutrient losses: vomiting, diarrhea, repeated infections, or pancreatitis. On top of all this, people receiving bone marrow transplants receive radiation or chemotherapy, with all the nutrition consequences of those treatments.

Thus, all these forms of cancer treatment, as well as cancer itself, point in the same direction: cachexia—the combination of anorexia, accelerated nutrient losses, and altered metabolism that leads to malnutrition. In fact, an estimated 4 to 23 percent of people with cancer die from cachexia.[10]

Metabolic Alterations

If reduced food intake were the only problem caused by cancer, then weight loss would occur largely at the expense of body fat. But much of the weight loss in cancer is due to extensive muscle wasting. Even when nutrients are supplied in apparently adequate amounts (through tube feedings or TPN), not all people with cancer maintain their weight and lean body mass. The metabolic changes that occur in cancer account for these losses.

Altered Energy Metabolism In people with cancer, metabolic changes either raise energy needs or cause the body to use energy nutrients inefficiently. Some people are hypermetabolic. Others are not, but even in the absence of hypermetabolism, metabolic pathways are altered and nutrients are used in inefficient ways that create a demand for energy.

Normal cells acquire energy mainly through a metabolic pathway that uses oxygen. This pathway (the TCA cycle) generates energy efficiently and can metabolize either glucose or fat for energy. Tumor cells, on the other hand, acquire energy mainly through a pathway that does not require oxygen. This pathway (glycolysis) produces energy inefficiently and relies primarily on glucose for its fuel.

As the tumor metabolizes glucose without oxygen, lactic acid (lactate) is produced. Lactate then returns to the liver, which reconverts it to glucose in a process that requires energy. Thus the tumor demands that the body provide energy to support its preferred metabolic pathway.

Chemotherapy and radiation therapy can alter energy and nutrient needs when they accelerate nutrient losses. Surgery and infections make energy and nutrient needs still greater (see Chapter 19).

Protein Metabolism After depleting the body's glycogen stores to provide energy, muscle cells are sacrificed to provide fuel and amino acids. The muscle mass becomes progressively depleted.

Carbohydrate Metabolism Many people with cancer develop insulin resistance; then hyperglycemia follows. The limited glucose and amino acids in the blood become even less available to the cells, so more body tissues break down to contribute materials. Also, hunger is triggered by the return of blood glucose to fasting levels, and in the person with hyperglycemia, this return may be delayed—hence the person's lack of appetite.

Lipid Metabolism Changes in lipid metabolism also occur, typically resulting in hyperlipidemia and depletion of fat stores. These changes may be due to a defect in the activity of the enzyme that helps move lipids from the blood into the fat cells for fat synthesis. People with cancer tend to mobilize their fat stores instead, and this, coupled with defective clearance of lipids from the blood, may suppress immune function.[11]

Other Metabolic Effects Vitamin antagonists are sometimes used in chemotherapy, and they can create vitamin deficiencies (see Figure 12–2 on p. 307). Anemias caused by a variety of vitamin deficiencies are frequently seen in people with cancer.

Obviously, the person with cancer risks poor nutrition status. Providing optimal nutrition care can be crucial to recovery.

Nutrition Support for People with Cancer

For many years, the deteriorating nutrition status that accompanies cancer was largely ignored. Many practitioners believed that emaciation and physical debilitation were inevitable. Others believed that if you fed the client, you also fed the tumor, so to "starve the tumor," they would almost starve the client. Another problem was that little technology was applied in the art of feeding people. The widespread use of tube feedings and TPN is a relatively recent advance.

The Scope of Nutrition Support

As mentioned earlier, nutrition cannot cure cancer; nor does it serve as a primary treatment for cancer. Nevertheless, nutrition does play a supportive role.

What Nutrition Support Can Do Weight loss and progressive malnutrition in people with cancer can weaken them and even lead to death. In contrast, attention to diet can prevent or reverse poor nutrition status so that a person with cancer:

- Feels better and functions better.
- Resists infections better.
- May tolerate cancer therapies better.
- Enjoys a better quality of life.

These benefits may be hard to quantify, but experts recognize that they are of great importance to the person with cancer.[12]

What Nutrition Support Cannot Do Although it makes sense to prevent PEM in the person with cancer, actual efforts to restore and maintain lean body mass have met with disappointing results. Despite seemingly adequate nutrition support, people with cancer cachexia often fail to replete their lean body masses. They may gain weight, but this weight often reflects fat and water rather than lean body mass. Whether nutrition support directly prolongs survival or improves tolerance for chemotherapy, radiation therapy, or surgery cannot be proven. Nutrition support may not yet be sophisticated enough to deal with the specific metabolic changes associated with cancer, and this may partially explain why studies have met with mixed results.

Possible Disadvantages of Nutrition Support As suggested earlier, some clinicians express concern that feeding the host may feed the tumor.

If this is so, then nutrition support may feed the tumor especially well. Animal studies clearly show that nutrition support stimulates tumor growth, but this effect has not been scientifically documented in people with cancer.[13] Controversies remain. Future research may reveal whether specific nutrients or nutrient combinations either stimulate or inhibit tumor growth.

Ethical Issues Every malnourished person with cancer who cannot consume an adequate diet orally is a potential candidate for special nutrition support. Before tube feeding or parenteral nutrition is undertaken, though, some important questions should be considered. What will change if the cachexia is reversed or progressive wasting is arrested? Will the person survive longer? Will quality of life improve? Will therapy be more successful? If special nutrition support can provide direct benefits, it should be undertaken. However, for the person with little hope of recovery, its yet unproven benefits may not be worth the cost and discomfort involved. Making this decision requires good clinical judgment from the health care team, and most importantly, consideration of the client's feelings about the goals of the nutrition therapy. Nutrition in Practice 28 describes these and other ethical issues that must be considered when people receive tube feedings or TPN.

Dietary Interventions

Health care professionals face an enormous challenge in helping people with cancer to maintain their nutritional health. Every bit of nutrition knowledge and interpersonal skill helps, beginning with the professional's awareness of the client's predicament. The box entitled "How to Help a Client Eat" on pp. 353-354 offers suggestions known to be effective.

Nutrient Needs Typical energy and protein needs for people with cancer are determined as shown in Table 28–4. Actual nutrient needs are highly variable depending on the type and severity of the cancer, its treatment, and the person's nutrition status. Table 28–5 shows diet modifications that may be necessary for specific types of cancer.

Vitamin and mineral needs are also highly variable depending on the specific treatment and the presence and severity of complications such as vomiting and malabsorption. Caretakers must carefully monitor each individual for early signs of nutrient deficiencies to keep them from becoming severe.

Table 28–4
Energy and Protein Needs for Cancer

- *Energy:* Calculate the basal energy expenditure (BEE) using the Harris-Benedict equation provided in Table 18–3 on p. 450. Energy needs range from 1.5 to 2.0 times the BEE.
- *Protein:* Supply 1.5 to 2.0 grams of protein per kilogram of ideal body weight.

Drug Therapy Antinausea drugs and analgesics can be useful for improving food intake. A new drug, megestrol acetate, may help relieve anorexia and promote weight gain in people with advanced cancer.[14]

Oral Diets Oral food intake can often be improved once the individual's specific problems are addressed. The next box is long and detailed, reflecting both the complexity and the importance of offering specific suggestions to deal with specific problems. The case study that

Table 28–5
Dietary Modifications for Various Cancers

LOCATION OF CANCER	DIETARY CONSIDERATIONS
Brain	Physical feeding disabilities (Nutrition in Practice 26); chewing and swallowing problems (see Chapter 20).
Head/Neck	Chewing and swallowing problems; tube feeding may be necessary (Chapter 22).
Mouth/Esophagus	Chewing and swallowing problems; if obstructed, tube feeding below the obstruction may be necessary.
Stomach	Nausea, vomiting; if obstructed, tube feeding below the obstruction may be necessary; if resection is performed, a postgastrectomy diet (see Chapter 20) may be needed; nutrient deficiencies due to blind loop syndrome (Chapter 20) may occur.
Intestine	If obstructed, tube feeding or TPN may be necessary; resections, fistulas, or inflammation may cause multiple nutrition problems (see Chapter 21); fat-restricted, lactose-restricted diet may be useful.
Liver	Protein-, sodium-, and fluid-restricted diet may be necessary (see Chapter 24).
Pancreas	Fat-restricted diet and enzyme replacements may be necessary (see Chapter 21) diabetic diet may be necessary if insulin production is affected (see Chapter 25).
Kidneys	Protein-, electrolyte-, and fluid-controlled diet may be necessary (see Chapter 27).

Note: The considerations listed here are specific to the type of cancer; they do not include the effects of treatment. Other factors described for all cancers, such as anorexia, nausea, and vomiting, are considered in addition to the interventions discussed here.

follows it (on p. 679) offers the opportunity to put some of those suggestions into practice.

Tube Feedings and TPN Studies have failed to confirm that adequate nutrition support directly benefits survival and response to cancer treatment. For this reason, tube feedings or TPN are not routinely recommended for adequately nourished or mildly malnourished people with cancer who must undergo surgery, chemotherapy, or radiation therapy.[15] Special nutrition support may be indicated, however, when anorexia persists or when a person is severely malnourished, particularly during and immediately after other cancer treatments. As always, if the GI tract is functional, tube feedings are preferred to TPN. People requiring head and neck resections may need long-term tube feedings and may need to continue tube feedings at home. People with severe radiation enteritis may require home TPN.

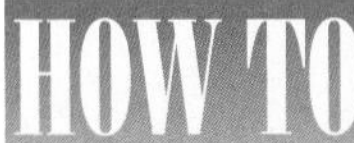

Help Clients Handle Food-Related Problems

For each problem, find a solution, using these suggestions.

1. *To improve food intake:*

- Explain why eating is important.
- Encourage clients to eat the most when they feel the best.
- Encourage people to eat extra food between chemotherapy or radiation treatments.
- Suggest that clients eat nutrient-dense foods first.
- Recommend indulging in favorite foods throughout the day.
- Encourage clients to eat with family and friends.
- Recommend smaller, more frequent meals.
- Advise clients not to drink large amounts of liquids with meals.
- Give pain or antinausea medications when they will be effective during meals.
- Provide a pleasant and relaxed environment.
- Serve foods attractively.
- Reassess clients regularly to solve problems as they arise.

2. *To save energy for eating:*

- Let others prepare foods.
- Suggest foods that are easy to prepare and eat.
- Recommend the use of time-saving appliances for food preparation.

3. *To combat bitter or metallic taste perceptions:*

- Advise clients to brush teeth or use a mouthwash before eating.
- Encourage clients to try eggs, fish, poultry, and dairy products instead of meats.
- Recommend adding sauces and seasonings to meats.
- Suggest that meats be served cold or at room temperature.
- Encourage clients to try new foods and experiment with herbs and spices.

4. *To control nausea and vomiting:*

- Give antinausea drugs before mealtimes.
- Recommend small meals.
- Advise clients to avoid spicy and high-fat foods.
- Suggest that clients avoid food odors that cause nausea. It may help to have others prepare meals, if possible.
- Encourage clients to save most liquids for after meals. Clear liquids or popsicles after meals help prevent dehydration.
- Suggest that clients get fresh air, loosen tight clothing, or rest after meals.

5. *To prevent food aversions:*

- Minimize the likelihood of learned food aversions by suggesting that clients save favorite foods for times when they are feeling relatively good.

(continued)

How To (continued)

- Advise clients not to eat their favorite foods during the times of day when they usually experience nausea or vomiting.
- Suggest to clients that they maintain a food-free "window" of an hour or so before and after treatment times, if the treatments cause nausea or vomiting.

6. *To alleviate problems with chewing and swallowing:*

- Work with clients to find the consistency of food that will be easiest to handle. Thin liquids, true solids, and sticky foods are often difficult to swallow.
- Recommend that clients add sauces and gravies to dry foods.
- Provide fluids with meals to ease chewing and swallowing.
- Advise the client with mouth sores to try foods at cooler temperatures. They are often soothing.
- Recommend that clients with mouth ulcers avoid foods that are spicy, acidic, or coarse; foods that contain seeds that can be trapped in an ulcer; or sticky foods such as peanut butter that may be difficult to swallow.
- Recommend that clients experiment with tilting the head forward and backward to see if swallowing is easier with the head positioned differently.
- Suggest a straw for drinking.
- Encourage clients who suffer from a reduced flow of saliva to rinse the mouth frequently and to avoid concentrated sweets. Artificial saliva from the pharmacy can also help. Sour candy or gum can stimulate the flow of saliva.
- Encourage good oral and dental hygiene.

7. *To add kcalories and protein:*

- Add milk powder to liquid milk, recipes, soups, puddings, and cereals.
- Add ground meats, chicken, fish, or grated cheeses to sauces, soups, casseroles, or vegetables.
- Eat peanut butter on fruit, celery, or crackers.
- Use extra butter, margarine, mayonnaise, or cream cheese whenever possible (on sandwiches or breads, potatoes, vegetables, pasta, and rice).
- Use yogurt, sour cream, or a sour cream dip with vegetables.
- Use extra mayonnaise or salad dressing on salads.
- Add whipping cream to desserts and hot chocolate, or use it to lighten coffee.
- Have snacks available at all times.
- Add nuts and dried fruits such as raisins to desserts, cereals, or salads.
- Use cream instead of milk with cereal.
- Try commercially available liquid supplements or instant breakfast mixes for milkshakes, meals, or between-meal snacks.
- Use whole milk instead of low-fat or nonfat milks.

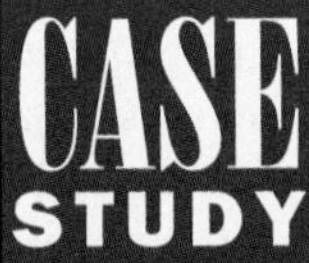

Retired Newscaster with Cancer

Mr. Bustamante is a retired newscaster who first visited his doctor when he noticed that he was losing weight rapidly and seemed to be drained of energy. He also had a lesion in his mouth that wouldn't heal. Mr. Bustamante has a history of alcohol and cigarette abuse. After he was admitted to the hospital, tests confirmed a diagnosis of cancer of the mouth. The doctor would like to prepare Mr. Bustamante nutritionally before proceeding with radiation therapy. Radical surgery is a possibility. A thorough nutrition assessment reveals that Mr. Bustamante is suffering from severe PEM that was classified as kwashiorkor-marasmus mix. His height is 5 feet 10 inches, and he weighs 125 pounds.

1. What is Mr. Bustamante's ideal weight? His %IBW?
2. What other anthropometric measurements would you expect to see affected?
3. Given his PEM status, what lab test results would you expect to find?
4. How might Mr. Bustamante's past history have affected his nutrition status before he developed cancer?
5. In what ways can cancer affect his nutrition status?
6. How can radiation therapy affect his nutrition status?
7. Discuss the possible impact of radical head and neck surgery on his nutrition status.
8. Describe cancer cachexia. What are some of its causes? What are the benefits of preventing or correcting it?
9. If Mr. Bustamante is able to take food by mouth, what suggestions will you give him for dealing with poor appetite, nausea and vomiting, dry and sore mouth, and chewing and swallowing problems?

Parenteral Nutrition after Bone Marrow Transplant As described earlier, the nutrition consequences of bone marrow transplants are those caused by extensive chemotherapy, radiation therapy, and infections. Graft-versus-host disease leads to anorexia and other problems that further interfere with food intake.

The person receiving a bone marrow transplant often receives parenteral nutrition support because the GI tract is severely compromised by the preparation procedure.[16] Appropriate nutrition helps to heal the GI tract and support the immune system. Glutamine added to the TPN solution may be particularly beneficial for people undergoing bone marrow transplants. Glutamine helps maintain the structure and function of the GI tract and may help prevent bacterial translocation across the intestine (see p. 447). Researchers have found that adding glutamine to TPN solutions results in fewer infections and shorter hospital stays for bone marrow transplant recipients.[17]

Oral Diets after Bone Marrow Transplant As GI function returns, the person begins to receive food orally, and parenteral nutrition gradually tapers off as oral intake improves. Early oral feedings often start with lactose-free, low-residue, low-fat liquids to maximize absorption and minimize the risk of nausea, vomiting, gas, and steatorrhea. Gradually, solid foods are introduced. As individual tolerances allow, fiber and lactose can be added to the diet. Additional fat is given if steatorrhea is not evident.

Because the bone marrow recipient must take immunosuppressants following the procedure, a high-protein, high-calcium diet is recommended. In addition, physicians often prescribe calcium and vitamin D supplements. Encourage people with persistent diarrhea to eat whole, minimally processed foods for their high potassium contents (see Figure 8–2 on p. 181 and the discussion on p. 182).

Nutrition Assessment

Early identification of the nutrition problems of people with cancer can enhance the quality of their lives and may improve their responses to other therapies. The following aspects of assessment are particularly useful:

- Closely examine the diet history, looking for signs of reduced food intake and pinpointing causes. Based on these factors, the dietitian can construct a viable nutrition care plan.
- Keep in mind that people with cancer, particularly those who feel they cannot benefit from therapy, are easy targets for peddlers of nutrition "cures." They may take massive doses of vitamins and minerals or follow other home remedies that may impair their nutrition status. It is important to remember to ask what supplements, and what amounts of them, clients may be taking.
- Check to see what type of therapy the person has been receiving or will receive and ascertain how it may affect nutrition status. It is important to be alert to possible drug-nutrient interactions.
- Record anthropometric measurements regularly to help determine whether energy and protein needs are being met. Monitor weight changes. Be sure to identify problems that have led to weight loss and offer solutions whenever possible. Remember that edema may be present in certain types of cancer and can affect anthropometric measurements.
- When a client has been vomiting or has diarrhea, be alert to the possibility of dehydration. Remember that biochemical parameters in dehydrated people may falsely appear to be normal.
- Total lymphocyte counts and skin testing are not useful in assessing protein status for people undergoing bone marrow transplants or those receiving radiation or chemotherapy that interferes with immune function.

PEM is a frequent complication of cancer. Health care professionals look for signs of deteriorating nutrition status and take active steps to correct problems before they become severe.

Although nutrition support is not the curative agent in cancer therapy, it is often lifesaving and is invariably crucial to the quality of life. In HIV and AIDS, discussed in the next chapter, life cannot ultimately be saved, but as in cancer, nutrition makes a major difference to life's quality.

■ STUDY QUESTIONS ■

1. What is cancer? What events are believed to lead to cancer?
2. What steps can people take to reduce their risks of cancer? Describe the dietary recommendations to reduce cancer risk.
3. What are the primary treatments for cancer, and how do they work?
4. What are the nutrition consequences of cancer? Describe how cancer contributes to each of these consequences.
5. What is cancer cachexia? What factors contribute to its development? Can nutrition intervention help prevent this problem?
6. Describe the anorexia that is associated with cancer. How does it differ from anorexia in other disease states? Discuss how cancer and its therapy contribute to anorexia.
7. What are food aversions, and how can they be handled?
8. How can cancer result in excess nutrient losses, and how do these losses contribute to the cancer cachexia syndrome?
9. Describe the metabolic changes that occur in the person with cancer, and discuss their role in the cancer cachexia syndrome.
10. What are the possible advantages of good nutrition status for the person with cancer? What *can't* nutrition do?
11. In the person with cancer, what strategies can combat anorexia? Bitter or metallic taste in the mouth? Nausea and vomiting? Problems with chewing and swallowing? Mouth ulcers? Reduced flow of saliva?
12. What are the recommended uses for tube feedings and parenteral nutrition for people with cancer?

■ CLINICAL APPLICATION QUESTIONS ■

1. Many disorders can lead to wasting. For some of these, such as renal disease, diet is a cornerstone of treatment. For others, such as cancer, nutrition plays a supportive role. What determines whether nutrition plays a major or supportive role in the treatment of a disorder?
2. When you look at the box on pp. 677–678, the suggestions for handling food-related problems may seem simple enough. The suggestions may be difficult to implement in some cases, however. What suggestions to control nausea and vomiting contradict suggestions to add kcalories and protein? What other contradictions can you find? How might a health care provider deal with such contradictions?
3. Consider problems associated with nutrition support in a 36-year-old woman with a malignant brain tumor affecting her speech center and the right side of the body. Her prognosis is poor with an expected survival time of about six months. What would be the goal of nutrition support? If she loses her ability to speak, how might her nutrition status be affected? She is right-handed; how might loss of the use of her right side affect her ability to eat?

NUTRITION IN PRACTICE 28

Ethical Issues in Nutrition Care

Enteral and parenteral feedings can meet nutrient needs and support recovery in many cases (see Chapters 22 and 23). In other cases, such support can improve the quality of a declining life. Sometimes, however, nutrition support prolongs life by merely delaying death, and the life is of low quality. When this is the case, is it morally and legally appropriate to discontinue use of nutrition support techniques? The very availability of special nutrition support forces health care professionals and society to face ethical issues such as these. Terms relating to these issues appear in the accompanying glossary.

Isn't there a moral obligation to give nutrition support whenever it will prolong life?

Not necessarily. Of course, health care professionals must never withhold nutrition support when a client has any chance of recovery, but the decision whether to feed a client becomes less clear when the client is terminally ill or in a persistent vegetative state. How do we respond to elderly or physically disabled people who want to refuse medical or special nutrition support because they feel the quality of their lives is too poor to go on? Are health care professionals morally and legally obligated to comply with, or to deny, such requests? Furthermore, when clients are incompetent and unable to speak for themselves, who, if anyone, should be allowed to make such life-and-death decisions?

Who provides the answers to questions like these?

Occasionally, these questions spark intense controversy and give rise to court cases. Then the court defines the questions clearly and lays down unambiguous rules to answer them. Sometimes hospital ethics committees work them out. Most often, though, families and physicians work out their own answers to these questions.

How does a court resolve nutrition support issues?

The case of Nancy Cruzan broke the ground on this issue more than a decade ago. Nancy Cruzan was a young woman who suffered permanent and irreversible brain damage after a car crash in 1983. For eight years, she was in a persistent vegetative state—awake but unaware. Her physicians and parents held no hope for her recovery, yet given food and water, she might have lived for another 30 years. Her parents requested permission to discontinue tube feeding, but in 1987 the Missouri Supreme Court rejected their request. The court held that Cruzan never definitively stated her "right to die" wishes, and that Cruzan's parents had no legal right to make such a request for her. The court stated that preserving life, no matter what its quality, takes precedence over all other considerations.

Cruzan's parents appealed the decision, and in 1989 the U.S. Supreme Court agreed to hear their arguments. Six major medical societies filed briefs with the Supreme Court in support of the Cruzans.[18]

The Supreme Court upheld the Missouri Supreme Court's decision and it took still another round of court battles before additional evidence convinced the Missouri Supreme Court of Nancy Cruzan's wishes. Finally, her feeding tube was removed, and she died from dehydration two weeks later.

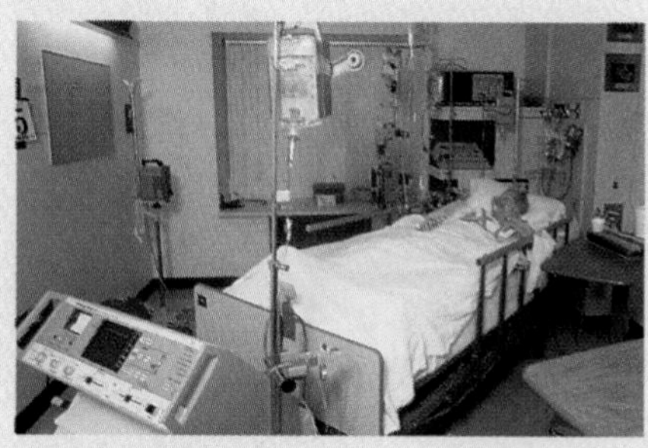

When is it morally and legally appropriate to use special nutrition support?

The cost of maintaining Cruzan must have been astronomical.

It was indeed, both financially and emotionally. In terms of money, health care costs to support her ran about $130,000 per year (paid by the state). The emotional costs are more difficult to calculate. Cruzan's parents were first faced with the initial shock of their daughter's accident. For several years they held hope that with continued care their daughter would survive and regain consciousness. Finally, they endured court battles over their child's fate—a fate that meant grief regardless of the outcome.

Are such cases unusual?

Unfortunately, no. Some 10,000 other families of people who live in a persistent vegetative state face the same dilemma. The High Court's decision has widespread implications for these people and the health professionals who take care of them. This decision touches all of us, because it influences the extent to which our society views life-sustaining treatment as optional not only for our clients, but for ourselves and our families.[19] It decides how we may be allowed to die.[20]

Does the court's decision to let Cruzan die mean that individual rights outweigh those of the state?

The emerging ethical, medical, and legal consensus seems to be tending that way. Competent individuals have a legal right to refuse medical treatment—including nourishment and hydration—even when medical experts consider that treatment necessary to sustain life. In other words, even when treatment is lifesaving and its refusal may bring an earlier death, clients' rights remain paramount. Many people seem to agree that competent adults have the right to accept or refuse medical treatment. Both Jacqueline Kennedy Onassis and Richard Nixon made such choices before they died.

How can people protect their rights to retain or refuse treatment in the event of incompetency?

Health care professionals should encourage their competent clients to express their preferences regarding medical treatments, including artificial feedings, in the event of terminal illness or coma before the situation arises. Each client's preferences should be noted in the medical records, and any health care professional who is unwilling to abide by the client's stated preferences should arrange for continuing care by another equally qualified professional and then withdraw from that client's care.[21] Clients should expect that physicians and facilities will comply with their preferences.

In addition to informing their physicians, clients can state their preferences in legal documents known as living wills (see Form 28–1). Most states have statutes governing the use of living wills; health care professionals should be aware of these regulations. Some states' laws allow withdrawal of tube feedings; others specifically prohibit it; and still others make no mention of it.[22] A living will allows a competent adult to clearly express directions regarding medical treatment in the event that the person is unable to make the necessary decisions at that time. It may specify that no extraordinary treatments be administered, or alternatively it may declare that every effort should be made to maintain life. Form 28–1 shows how a living will might begin. People should make their wishes known in writing to their attending physicians and families. Unfortunately, only one out of five adults has taken such steps.

How well do living wills hold up? Do physicians and hospitals honor them?

It is important that living wills state what should be done about food and water. Some people consider the providing of nourishment and hydration to be ordinary care. They think that withholding or withdrawing nutrition support for any reason is unjustified. For others, using arti-

Glossary of Terms Related to Ethical Issues

artificial feeding: parenteral and enteral nutrition; feeding by a route other than the normal ingestion of food.

comatose: in a state of deep unconsciousness from which the person cannot be aroused.

competent: having sufficient mental ability to understand a treatment, weigh its risks and benefits, and comprehend the consequences of refusing or accepting the treatment.

death: permanent cessation of vital functions.

durable power of attorney: a legal document in which one competent adult authorizes another competent adult to be the agent who will make decisions for her or him in the event of incapacitation. The phrase "durable power" means that the agent's authority continues when the client becomes incompetent; "attorney" refers to an attorney-in-fact (not an attorney-at-law).

ethical: in accordance with moral principles or professional standards. Socrates described *ethics* as "how we ought to live."

legal: established by law.

living will: a document signed by a competent adult that specifically states whether the person wishes any heroic measures to be taken in the event of terminal illness or irreversible coma from which the person is not expected to recover.

persistent vegetative state: exhibiting motor reflexes but without the ability to regain cognitive behavior, communicate, or interact purposefully with the environment.

terminal illness: a progressive, irreversible disease that will lead to death in the near future.

Form 28–1
An Example of a Living Will

DECLARATION TO MY FAMILY, MY PHYSICIAN, MY LAWYER, AND MY SPIRITUAL ADVISER

If the time arrives when I can no longer take part in decisions for my own future, this statement and Declaration shall stand as the expression of my wishes.

I recognize that death is as much a reality as birth, growth, maturity, and old age. It is but one phase in the cycle of life and is the only certainty. I do not fear death as much as I fear there is no reasonable expectation of my recovery from physical or mental disability, I wish to be allowed to die and not to be kept alive by artificial means or heroic measures, but wish only that drugs be mercifully administered to me for terminal suffering, even if they hasten the moment of death.

I recognize that my wishes place a heavy burden of responsibility upon you, and I therefore make the following declaration with the intention of sharing this responsibility and this decision with you and of mitigating any feelings of guilt you may have:

THIS DECLARATION is made this ______________ day of ______________, 19____.

I, ______________________________, willfully and voluntarily make known my desire that my dying not be artificially prolonged under the circumstances set forth below, and I do hereby declare:

If at any time I should have a terminal condition and if my attending physician has determined that there can be no recovery from such condition and that my death is imminent, I direct that life-prolonging procedures be withheld or withdrawn when the application of such procedures would serve only to prolong artificially the process of dying, and that I be permitted to die naturally with only the administration of medication or the performance of any medical procedures deemed necessary to provide me with comfort, care, or to alleviate pain. I desire that nutrition and hydration (food and water) be withheld or withdrawn when the application of such procedures would serve only to prolong artificially the process of dying.

In the absence of my ability to give directions regarding the use of such life-prolonging procedures, it is my intention that this declaration be honored by my family and physician as the final expression of my legal right to refuse medical or surgical treatment and to accept the consequences for such refusal.

I understand the full import of this declaration, and I am emotionally and mentally competent to make this declaration.

____
(signature)

[The form provides places for witnesses and a notary public to sign and date their signatures.]

ficial nutrition support to replace eating is no different than using a respirator to replace breathing.

Most health care professionals advocate the use of living wills and agree that clients' wishes should be honored, but actual medical care may not always reflect these beliefs. Physicians seem more likely to comply with *specific* living wills than with standard ones (see the "Attachment to the Living Will" on p. 685).[23] In practice, physicians are more likely to follow family directives concerning tube feedings and other life support than instructions written in living wills.[24]

Can people do anything else to make sure their living wills are carried out?

In many states, the durable power of attorney offers clients a way to ensure their wishes will be carried out (see Form 28–2 on p. 686). Some states have enacted statutes authorizing the use of durable powers of attorney specifically for health care.[25] A durable power of attorney allows a competent adult to designate another competent adult (usually a relative or close friend) as an agent to make health care decisions in the event of incapacitation. In essence, it says, "I give this person the right to make health care decisions on my behalf should I become unable to make them."

When you designate an agent to make life-and-death decisions for you, how can you be sure that person will do what you want?

Ideally, the person representing a client will make decisions that reflect the client's health care

Form 28–1 ***(continued)***

ATTACHMENT TO THE LIVING WILL

For each scenario listed below, please indicate your wishes with regard to measures you desire to be utilized in sustaining your life.

U= Undecided Y= Do desire

N= Do *not* desire T= Try (but discontinue if there is no clear improvement)

	COMA OR PERSISTENT VEGETATIVE STATE WITH NO CHANCE OF REGAINING AWARENESS	COMA WITH SMALL CHANCE OF RECOVERY AND GREATER CHANCE OF SURVIVING WITH BRAIN DAMAGE	IRREVERSIBLE BRAIN DAMAGE OR DISEASE	IRREVERSIBLE BRAIN DAMAGE OR DISEASE, AND TERMINAL ILLNESS
Cardiopulmonary resuscitation				
Mechanical breathing				
Artificial nutrition and hydration				
Major surgery				
Kidney dialysis				
Chemotherapy				
Minor surgery				
Invasive diagnostic tests				
Blood or blood products				
Antibiotics				
Pain medication				

I have read this attachment and have completed it after careful consideration. I reaffirm that I am competent to complete this form. This form is to be made a part of my declaration, which I have executed concurrently herewith.

The above procedures shall be considered nonexclusive. If medical procedures exist that (1) would serve artificially to prolong my life but (2) are not shown on the above matrix, then the general intent expressed in my Declaration shall still control. That is, I wish to die a natural death, uninvaded by any other extraordinary procedures not shown on this matrix.

preferences. In reality, though, when faced with hypothetical situations, clients and those who would have to decide for them agree on treatment only 70 percent of the time.[26] Such discrepancy is natural because each views the other's experience as most important when making decisions. Clients want to avoid burdening their families, and families want to provide any treatment that offers a possible cure or relief from pain. If people wish to ensure ahead of time that they receive medical care consistent with their own wishes, they need to discuss their living wills and

Form 28–2
An Example of a Durable Power of Attorney

I, __________________________________, now residing at ____ ______________________________, hereby constitute and appoint ______________________________ as my true and lawful attorney-in-fact for me and in my name, place, and stead, giving and granting unto my said attorney full power and authority to do and perform every act as fully as I might do if personally present, with full power of substitution and revocation. I hereby ratify and confirm all that my attorney shall lawfully do or cause to be done pursuant to this power.

This Power includes, but is not limited to, the right to encumber, assign, or convey realty, including homestead realty. In addition, my attorney-in-fact is authorized to arrange for and consent to medical, therapeutical, and surgical procedures for me as principal, including the administration of drugs.

I have executed this Power while in command of my faculties and with knowledge of the consequences, both legal and practical.

This durable Power of Attorney shall not be affected by my disability as principal except as provided by statute.

____
(signature)

[The form provides places for witnesses and a notary public to sign and date their signatures.]

hypothetical scenarios with family members before medical conditions arise that will necessitate others making decisions for them.

Is it unfair to lay the burden of decisions on another person?

On the contrary, the person who plans ahead for future care in the case of a terminal illness or irreversible state of unconsciousness relieves others of the guilt and some of the stress of having to make decisions. Imagine the anxiety a family member goes through in directing the health care team to stop nutrition support, knowing that doing so will hasten death. That decision is a little easier if the family member knows it is what the individual would want, or better yet, if a legal document takes the decision out of the family's hands altogether.

■ NOTES ■

1. R. A. Karmali, Fatty acid metabolism and biochemical mechanisms in cancer, in *Health Effects of Dietary Fatty Acids,* ed. G. J. Nelson (Champaign, Ill.: American Oil Chemists Society, 1991), pp. 150–156.
2. J. H. Weisburger, Nutritional approach to cancer prevention with emphasis on vitamins, antioxidants, and carotenoids, *American Journal of Clinical Nutrition* (supplement) 53 (1991): 226–237.
3. A. T. Diplock, Antioxidant nutrients and disease prevention: An overview, *American Journal of Clinical Nutrition* (supplement) 53 (1991): 189–193.
4. M. J. McNamara, R. Alexander, and J. A. Norton, Cytokines and their role in the pathophysiology of cancer cachexia, *Journal of Parenteral and Enteral Nutrition* (supplement) 16 (1992): 50–55.
5. M. M. Meguid and coauthors, The early cancer anorexia paradigm: Changes in plasma free tryptophan and feeding indexes, *Journal of Parenteral and Enteral Nutrition* (supplement) 16 (1992): 56–59.
6. T. C. Hardin, Cytokine mediators of malnutrition: Clinical implications, *Nutrition in Clinical Practice* 8 (1993): 55–59.
7. R. J. Bodnar and coauthors, Mediation of anorexia by human recombinant tumor necrosis factor through a peripheral action in the rat, *Cancer Research* 49 (1989): 6280–6284.
8. R. D. Mattes and coauthors, Clinical implications of learned food aversions in patients with cancer treated with chemotherapy or radiation therapy, *Cancer* 70 (1992): 192.
9. Mattes and coauthors, 1992.
10. As cited in F. Bozzetti, Effects of artificial nutrition on the nutritional status of cancer patients, *Journal of Parenteral and Enteral Nutrition* 13 (1989): 406–420.
11. K. A. Kern and J. A. Norton, Cancer cachexia, *Journal of Parenteral and Enteral Nutrition* 12 (1988): 286–298.
12. D. F. Cella, Overcoming difficulties in demonstrating health

outcome benefits, *Journal of Parenteral and Enteral Nutrition* (supplement) 16 (1992); 106–111.
13. M. H. Torosian, Stimulation of tumor growth by nutrition support, *Journal of Parenteral and Enteral Nutrition* (supplement) 16 (1992): 72–75.
14. N. S. Tchekmedyian, Treatment of anorexia with megestrol acetate, *Nutrition in Clinical Practice* 8 (1993): 115–118.
15. A.S.P.E.N. Board of Directors, Practice guidelines: Cancer, *Journal of Parenteral and Enteral Nutrition* (supplement) 17 (1993): 12–13.
16. V. M. Herrmann and P. J. Petruska, Nutrition support in bone marrow transplant recipients, *Nutrition in Clinical Practice* 8 (1993): 19–27.
17. T. R. Ziegler and coauthors, Clinical and metabolic efficacy of glutamine-supplemented parenteral nutrition after bone marrow transplantation, *Annals of Internal Medicine* 116 (1992): 821–828; P. R. Schloerb and M. Amare, Total parenteral nutrition with glutamine in bone marrow transplantation and other clinical applications (A randomized, double-blind study), *Journal of Parenteral and Enteral Nutrition* 17 (1993): 407–413.
18. Supreme Court of the United States Syllabus, *Cruzan, by her parents and co-guardians, Cruzan et ux. v. Director, Missouri Department of Health, et al.,* No. 88–1503. Argued December 6, 1989—decided June 25, 1990.
19. M. Angell, Prisoners of technology: The case of Nancy Cruzan, *New England Journal of Medicine* 322 (1990): 1226–1228; B. Lo, F. Rouse, and L. Dornbrand, Family decision making on trial—Who decides for incompetent patients? *New England Journal of Medicine* 322 (1990): 1228–1232.
20. The Court and Nancy Cruzan, *Hastings Center Report,* January/February 1990, pp. 38–50.
21. C. R. Gallagher-Allred, Managing ethical issues in nutrition support of terminally ill patients, *Nutrition in Clinical Practice* 6 (1991): 113–116.
22. H. Brody and M. B. Noel, Dietitians' role in decisions to withhold nutrition and hydration, *Journal of the American Dietetic Association* 91 (1991): 580–585.
23. J. W. Ely and coauthors, The physician's decision to use tube feedings: The role of the family, the living will, and the *Cruzan* decision, *Journal of the American Geriatrics Society* 40 (1992): 471–475.
24. Ely and coauthors, 1992.
25. A. M. Capron, The implications of the *Cruzan* decision for clinical nutrition teams, *Nutrition in Clinical Practice* 6 (1991): 89–94.
26. J. Hare, C. Pratt, and C. Nelson, Agreement between patients and their self-selected surrogates on difficult medical decisions, *Archives of Internal Medicine* 152 (1992): 1049–1054.

29

Nutrition, HIV Infection, and AIDS

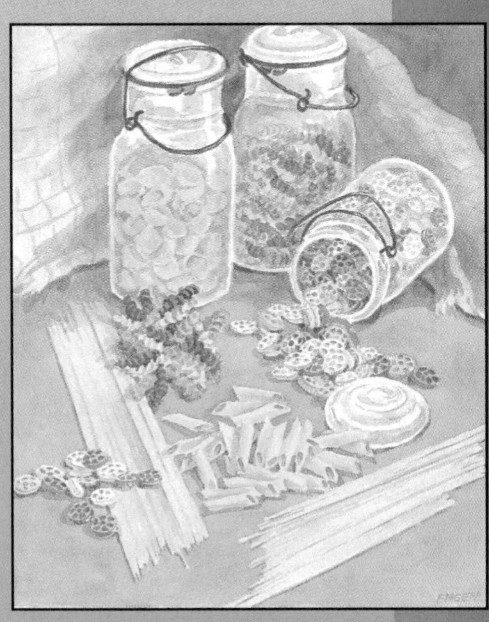

CONTENTS

Infection by the human immunodeficiency virus (HIV) eventually causes acquired immune deficiency syndrome (AIDS), a devastating, incurable, and fatal disorder. HIV infection and AIDS affect young and old, rich and poor, urban and rural dwellers, men and women—and like cancer, AIDS has a profound and severe impact on nutrition. AIDS is unlike cancer, though, in two ways. For one thing, once acquired, AIDS is incurable. The only end is death. For another, HIV infection is largely preventable. Transmission of the virus requires sexual activity, direct blood contact, or passage of the infection from a mother to her infant during pregnancy, birth, or breastfeeding. The box on p. 690 offers the guidelines everyone needs to keep in mind for prevention.

By the year 2000, an estimated 30 to 110 million adults and more than 10 million children worldwide will be infected with HIV, and some 25 million adults and several million children will have developed AIDS. As this incidence rises, prevention and treatment of HIV infection are becoming more and more critical concerns of health care professionals around the world. Because HIV infection has no cure, treatment focuses on slowing its course and controlling its symptoms to improve the victim's comfort and well-being and on prolonging life, when possible.

human immunodeficiency virus (HIV): the virus that causes AIDS. HIV is transmitted from one person to another by direct contact with contaminated body fluids, most often through sexual intercourse, through contaminated needles or blood products, or from mother to infant during pregnancy or lactation. The infection progresses to become an immune system disorder that leaves its victims defenseless against numerous infections.

acquired immune deficiency syndrome (AIDS): the end stage of HIV infection, in which severe complications are manifested. In the early, symptomless stages, the person is said to have an HIV infection.

Nutrition Consequences of HIV Infection

HIV infection attacks the immune system and leaves its victims defenseless against opportunistic infections and disorders from which most people are protected. The disorder begins with infection by the human immunodeficiency virus (HIV) and progresses in stages. At first, the HIV-infected individual is symptom-free. Later, as the infection progresses, symptoms may include fatigue, skin rashes, fevers, diarrhea, muscle pain, night sweats, weight loss, oral lesions and infections, and other opportunistic infections that are not life-threatening. In the final stages, frequent and often fatal complications arise, such as severe weight loss; tuberculosis; recurrent bacterial pneumonia; serious infections of the central nervous system, GI tract, and skin; cancers; and severe diarrhea.

opportunistic infections: infections from microorganisms that normally do not cause disease in the general population but can infect people once their immune systems are compromised (as in HIV infection).

The cluster of mild symptoms that sometimes occur early in the course of AIDS is called **AIDS-related complex (ARC).**

The HIV Wasting Syndrome

People with HIV infection frequently experience severe PEM and wasting. The wasting often begins early in the progression of the disease and becomes worse. People with AIDS may lose up to 34 percent of their ideal body weight in the four to five months before death, a degree of wasting similar to that seen in people who die from starvation.[1] Findings such as these prompt clinicians to speculate that severe wasting can by itself cause the death of some individuals with AIDS.[2] Even when other complications ultimately cause death, malnutrition appears to be an important cofactor. Studies suggest that for people with AIDS, low serum albumin and weight loss correlate strongly with a diminished survival time.[3] Also, PEM's effects on the immune system (described in Chapter 18), combined with those of HIV infection, may hasten the course of the disease.[4]

HOW TO Prevent HIV Infection

The prevention of HIV infection is not a nutrition issue, but because it is so crucial in today's world, these guidelines are offered here. To prevent the transmission of HIV infection:

- Refrain from sexual contact with anyone with HIV infection.
- Use a latex condom and a spermicidal agent if you have sexual contact with anyone whose sexual history you do not know.
- Do not share toothbrushes, razors, or other implements that could be contaminated with blood.
- Exercise caution when undergoing procedures such as acupuncture, tattooing, or ear piercing, in which needles might be contaminated.
- If you are an IV drug user, seek help for your addiction. Meanwhile, use only sterile, unused needles and dispose of them so that others will not use them. Avoid unprotected sexual contact with others.

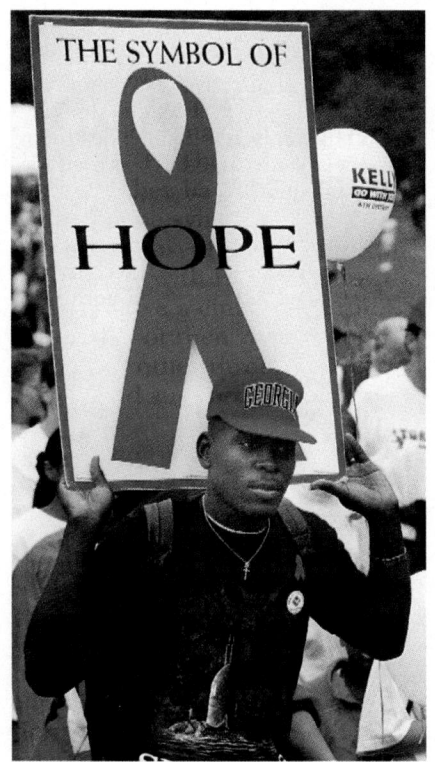

The fight against AIDS, like the fight against cancer, is bolstered by both medical science and people who refuse to give up hope.

Much as in cancer, the wasting and malnutrition associated with HIV are multifactorial: inadequate nutrient intake, excessive nutrient losses, hypermetabolism, and drug-nutrient interactions. The exact causes of wasting depend on the particular complications in each case. Repeated infections and, of course, cancer accelerate wasting dramatically. Table 29–1 illustrates the many factors that lead to progressive wasting from HIV infections.

Anorexia and Inadequate Nutrient Intake

People with HIV infections have anorexia and inadequate nutrient intakes for reasons similar to those of people with cancer. Clinicians report that the oral intakes of hospitalized people with AIDS meet only 70 percent of *basal* estimated energy needs and 65 percent of protein needs.[5] These percentages would be even lower if the *extra* energy and protein needs imposed by hypermetabolism and activity were taken into account. Clearly, HIV-infected people with additional infections do not consume adequate energy to meet their high metabolic needs.[6]

Psychological Stress Depression over the HIV diagnosis can destroy appetite even before symptoms appear. The individual who tests positive for HIV must deal with the terminal nature of the infection and the medical, personal, and financial problems that lie ahead. Understandably, people overwhelmed with such problems may lose their appetites.

Oral Candidiasis As the disorder progresses, fever, pain, and infections contribute to anorexia. In addition, people with AIDS often develop

Table 29–1
Causes of Malnutrition in HIV Infections

REDUCED FOOD INTAKE	ACCELERATED NUTRIENT LOSSES
Drug therapy	Cancer
Lack of energy to eat	Diarrhea
Pain associated with eating	Malabsorption
Fever/infection	Low serum albumin levels
Nausea and vomiting	PEM
Psychological factors such as fear, depression, and dementia	Drug therapy
Oral lesions	Related infections
Mouth blindness	
Dry mouth	
Altered taste perceptions	
Difficulty chewing/swallowing	
Esophageal lesions and obstructions	
Use of oxygen masks	
Related infections	
Cancer	
ALTERED METABOLISM	
Related infections	
Cancer	
Drug therapy	

an oral *Candida* infection (sometimes called thrush). This infection manifests itself as a thick white coating on the mouth, tongue, and sometimes the esophagus. The coating alters taste sensations, causes pain, and reduces the flow of saliva. When the esophagus becomes infected, swallowing becomes extremely painful.

candidiasis (can-did-DYE-uh-sis): a fungal infection of the mouth caused by *Candida albicans;* sometimes called **thrush.**

Herpes Virus and Kaposi's Sarcoma Oral infections caused by herpes virus, which are common in people with AIDS, lead to painful mouth ulcers and additional problems with chewing and swallowing. Kaposi's sarcoma, a cancer associated with AIDS, can cause lesions and obstructions in the esophagus that also interfere with food intake.

herpes virus: a virus that can lead to mouth lesions and may also affect the lower GI tract, causing diarrhea.

Kaposi's (cap-OH-seez) **sarcoma:** a type of cancer rare in the general population but common in people with HIV infections.

Respiratory Infections Respiratory infections such as pneumonia and tuberculosis can limit food intake in people with HIV infections. Having to use an oxygen mask (which covers the nose and mouth) may make eating difficult. Respiratory infections also cause fever and pain, which worsen anorexia.

Drug Therapy Drugs used to treat the various complications associated with HIV infections suppress appetite and reduce food intake. As in

Prescription Pad
Patient name:________________

Drugs commonly used in the treatment of HIV infections:
- Anti-infective agents
- Antineoplastic agents

____
Physician

See Appendix E for timing with meals and nutrition-related side effects.

AIDS-induced causes of nutrient losses include:
- HIV infection.
- GI tract infections.
- Malnutrition.
- Cancer.
- Cancer therapy.
- Antimicrobial drugs.
- Megadoses of vitamins.
- Home remedies for AIDS.
- Reduced gastric acid secretion.
- Bacterial overgrowth.

The diarrhea and malabsorption symptoms associated with AIDS for which no known cause has been identified are called **AIDS enteropathies.**

cancer treatment, antimicrobial drugs and chemotherapy often cause anorexia, nausea, and vomiting; food aversions associated with the side effects of drug therapy can also arise (see Table E–1B in Appendix E).

Lethargy and Dementia In the later stages of AIDS, lethargy and dementia become common problems that interfere with food intake. The individual may be chronically exhausted and may not care or even remember to eat.

Nutrient Losses

In addition to anorexia, the diarrhea and malabsorption associated with HIV infection accelerate nutrient losses. From 50 to 90 percent of people with AIDS experience chronic or recurrent diarrhea and malabsorption. Then the malnutrition itself contributes further to malabsorption and diarrhea.

GI Tract Infections Because so many people with HIV have other infections that damage the GI tract, it is difficult to determine if HIV infection alone causes malabsorption. Research suggests that it does.[7]

In some cases, the diarrhea seen in HIV cases does not respond to drug therapy, and nutrient losses continue unchecked. One common GI infection, cryptosporidia, is characterized by severe and prolonged diarrhea of 2 to 6 liters of stool per day. In rarer cases, up to 25 liters of stool per day may be excreted—possible only when a high fluid intake is provided to meet fluid needs.[8] Table 29–2 summarizes other infectious agents that can cause diarrhea and malabsorption in people with HIV infections. Some of the pathogens listed in the table come from infected foods. People with advanced HIV infections are highly susceptible to food-borne illnesses.

Reduced Gastric Acid Nutrient losses are also possible because advanced HIV infections suppress gastric acid secretion. Reduced gastric

Table 29–2
Causes of GI Infections in AIDS

Bacterial	**Protozoan**
Clostridium dificile	*Cryptosporidium* species
Mycobacterium avium-intracellulare (MAI)	*Giardia lamblia*
Mycobacterium tuberculosis	*Isosporia belli*
Salmonella species	*Microsporidium* species
Fungal	*Pneumocystitis carinii*
Candida albicans	*Toxoplasma gondii*
Cryptococcus neoformans	**Viral**
Parasitic	AIDS enteropathy
Nonpathogenic amoeba	*Cytomegalovirus* (CMV) species
Entamoeba histolytica	Epstein-Barr
	Herpes simplex

acid reduces the absorption of iron and calcium and allows bacteria to grow in the upper GI tract, promoting infections. Bacterial overgrowth can lead to the destruction of bile and malabsorption of fat, as occurs in blind loop syndrome.

Drugs and Other Therapies Drug therapies, including antimicrobial agents, can also cause diarrhea and malabsorption (see Appendix E). Cancer therapies have some effect, as do megadoses of vitamins (especially vitamin C) and other home remedies that people with HIV infections may use.

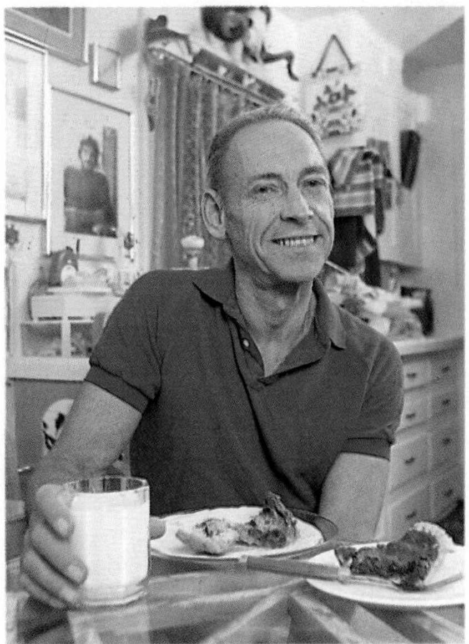

Nutrition provides an edge in maintaining quality of life and encouraging independence.

Nutrition Support for HIV Infections

Attention to nutrition cannot change the ultimate outcome of an HIV infection, but it may slow the infection's progress and improve the quality of life. At a minimum, meeting nutrient needs eliminates the additional stresses posed by malnutrition. Good nutrition status may also improve people's responses to drug therapy, shorten duration of hospital stays, and promote physical independence.[9]

Benefits of Early Nutrition Support

A positive HIV test alerts the health care professional to the need for immediate and aggressive nutrition intervention. Early intervention may detect and correct subclinical nutrient deficiencies before they become severe and helps to prepare the person for the stresses ahead. Early intervention also establishes baseline assessment parameters against which to monitor changes in nutrition status. Clinicians can begin to encourage changes in eating habits before the person becomes debilitated and the task becomes monumental. Weight loss, reduced body fat, and reduced body mass index are early signs of nutrition status deterioration in people with HIV infections.[10]

When people first learn they have HIV infections, they are susceptible to being preyed upon by the sellers of "miracle cures." Special diets or dietary supplements may be touted as offering the promise of long life or superb health, when they do not. Such practices often deplete the financial resources of people with HIV infections, and they pose other threats as well. Sometimes a person using quack remedies postpones obtaining proper medical treatment for a condition that may advance rapidly without such treatment. Sometimes, as in the case of vitamin or mineral megadoses, supplements may produce physical harm. Health care professionals should be on the lookout for unscrupulous practitioners exploiting their clients and tactfully guide clients in directions more likely to benefit them.

Dietary Interventions

Few controlled studies have as yet documented the specific nutrient needs of people with HIV infections. Instead practitioners rely on clinical experience to make recommendations, basing their judgments on the complications that arise in each case.

The discussion on pp. 450–452 in Chapter 18 describes considerations involved in estimating the energy and protein needs of people under stresses such as AIDS. As for vitamins and minerals, the exact needs of people with AIDS are not known, but they should certainly receive at least 100 percent of the RDA for these nutrients. People who cannot consume enough food to achieve adequate intakes might benefit from a supplement containing RDA amounts of the vitamins and minerals.[11] Many physicians prescribe daily *prenatal* vitamin supplements for people with HIV infections; these have slightly more than RDA amounts, but not megadoses, of all nutrients.[12]

Oral Diets For a person with AIDS, as for anyone, an oral diet is appropriate for as long as possible. The same tips that help people with cancer are useful for people with AIDS. Suggestions for alleviating anorexia, altered taste sensations, nausea and vomiting, and difficulty with chewing and swallowing were provided in the box on pp. 677-678 in Chapter 28.

Treatment of Diarrhea Treatment of HIV-associated diarrhea depends on its cause and the extent to which the intestine is affected. Although diarrhea is sometimes unresponsive to therapy, often a pathogen can be identified. Appropriate drug therapy along with the provision of adequate fluids and electrolytes is at the core of treatment. Salty broths and high-potassium foods and juices can help replace fluids and electrolytes. Often, fat-restricted, low-fiber, and lactose-restricted diets are recommended. MCT can be helpful in supplying energy from fat without aggravating malabsorption.

Susceptibility to food-borne illnesses requires that the person with HIV be given written and oral instructions on safe food handling. Foods that pose no threat for people with healthy immune systems, such as salads, may harbor organisms that will take up residence and cause serious infections in people with compromised immunity. Instructions on food handling for people with HIV infections are the same as for people who are traveling and are summed up in the box on p. 280.

Special Nutrition Support People who cannot eat enough food to prevent nutrition complications and unintentional weight loss need special nutrition support. Both enteral (oral and tube feeding) and parenteral nutrition support have been shown to be effective in repleting lean body mass and promoting weight gain in some people with AIDS.[13]

Health care professionals should not decide to institute special nutrition support in people with advanced AIDS, however, without consulting with the client and family and considering the ethical issues involved. Nutrition in Practice 28 offered some thoughts on these issues.

Enteral Nutrition As always, enteral feeding is preferred to parenteral feeding. Sometimes liquid formulas given orally with or between regular meals can help maintain or restore nutrition status; otherwise, tube feedings can be used. Tube feedings given at night can supplement oral diets during the day, especially for people at home. If pain or obstructions in the upper GI tract make nasogastric passage of the feeding tube difficult or painful, gastrostomy or jejunostomy feedings are indicated.

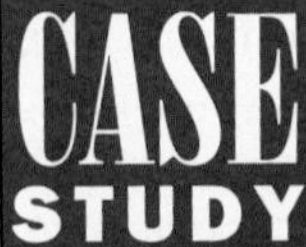

Travel Agent with HIV Infection

Mr. Sands, a travel agent, sought medical help at age 34 when he began feeling run-down and developed a painful white coating over his mouth and tongue. The presence of thrush and anemia alerted Mr. Sands' physician to the possibility of an HIV infection. When Mr. Sands tested positive for HIV, he and his family and friends were devastated by the news. Fortunately, those closest to him have supported him through this difficult time, and he has a strong desire to live out his life as independently as possible.

Four months after the diagnosis, Mr. Sands developed a serious, continuous diarrhea that required hospitalization to classify and control. Since the diagnosis, Mr. Sands has lost 10 pounds. At 6 feet tall, he currently weighs 158 pounds.

1. Describe how HIV infection can lead to reduced food intake, nutrient losses, and hypermetabolism.
2. From the limited information given here, what factors could have contributed to Mr. Sands' weight loss?
3. Discuss nutrition strategies for dealing with thrush and diarrhea.
4. Is Mr. Sands' weight loss significant?
5. What is his %IBW?
6. What steps could be effective in preventing further weight loss?

Particular care must be taken to keep tube feedings from causing diarrhea unrelated to the HIV infection. Table 22–4 on pp. 544–545 describes the causes and prevention of diarrhea associated with tube feedings. Preventing bacterial contamination of the formula is particularly important because of the susceptibility of HIV-infected individuals to GI infections.

Parenteral Nutrition Data are scarce, but seem to indicate that TPN can be used safely and effectively for people with AIDS.[14] Generally, however, TPN is used only when people need to maintain their nutrition status while undergoing a therapy that is expected to produce a real benefit. TPN may be more useful in repleting the body mass of people whose primary problems are reduced food intake or malabsorption than in supporting those who have other systemic diseases.[15] People with GI tract obstructions, severe vomiting, or GI infections affecting the entire small bowel may benefit from TPN. Home TPN is often beneficial for people with AIDS. The accompanying case study illuminates some aspects of nutrition concerns related to HIV infection and AIDS.

systemic: affecting the whole body rather than one part or organ system.

Nutrition Assessment

Early identification of the nutrition problems of people with HIV infection helps prevent severe malnutrition, improves their responses to other therapies, and enhances the quality of their lives. Anyone responsible for the nutritional health of a client with HIV should give special consideration to these aspects of nutrition status:

- Closely examine the diet history, looking for signs of reduced food intake and pinpointing causes so that the dietitian can construct a viable nutrition care plan.
- Keep in mind that people with AIDS, like people with cancer, may take

massive doses of vitamins and minerals or follow other home remedies that may impair their nutrition status. Ask what supplements clients are taking, and how much of each.

- Note what therapies the person is receiving and how they may affect nutrition status. Stay alert to possible drug-nutrient interactions.
- Record anthropometric measurements regularly to help determine whether energy and protein needs are being met. Monitor weight changes. Remember that weight loss, reduced body fat, and reduced body mass index are early signs of nutrition status deterioration in people with HIV infection. Be sure to identify problems that have led to weight loss and offer solutions whenever possible.
- When a client has been vomiting or has diarrhea, be alert to the possibility of dehydration. Remember that biochemical parameters in dehydrated people may falsely appear to be normal.
- Total lymphocyte counts and skin testing are not useful in assessing protein status in people with advanced HIV infections. HIV infection interferes with these immune system parameters independently of nutrition status.

PEM is a frequent complication of HIV infection. As with cancer, health care professionals look for signs of deteriorating nutrition status and take active steps to correct problems before they become severe.

This chapter brings to a close your introduction to normal and clinical nutrition. Congratulations! You have received an abundance of information since you first turned to page 1. The normal nutrition chapters of this text provided you with current recommendations to promote optimal health. You learned how the body transforms foods into nutrients and how those nutrients support the body's well-being. The clinical chapters addressed you as a future health care professional, concerned with the well-being of others during times of illness.

We hope this text has served you well and that you will remember, when selecting food for yourself or when making recommendations for others, to honor the body. The Nutrition in Practice that follows provides scientific reasons why you should give your own health special care by nourishing your body well.

■ STUDY QUESTIONS ■

1. What is HIV infection? What are its consequences? What is the HIV wasting syndrome?
2. Describe factors that can lead to reduced nutrient intake, excessive nutrient losses, and altered metabolism in people with HIV infections.
3. Why are people with AIDS highly susceptible to illnesses caused by uncooked foods or improperly cooked foods?
4. In what ways can good nutrition status possibly alter the course of HIV infections?

■ CLINICAL APPLICATION QUESTIONS ■

To understand why attention to nutrition is important even when it plays only a supportive role in the treatment of a disorder, review the effects of PEM on pp. 83–86 and in Chapter 18. Carefully consider how severe malnutrition can further debilitate people with HIV infections.

NUTRITION IN PRACTICE 29

Diet and Health

As this book comes to a close, it seems appropriate to put the focus back on you, the reader, and on your own health. You have just read many chapters on diseases and disorders, and on what you can do to help heal and comfort people who have these diseases. No doubt it has crossed your mind many times that it would be wonderful if people did not contract these diseases in the first place. The question asked here is, "Can diet help prevent disease?"

Clearly, for the diseases of yesterday, the answer would be no. A century ago, infectious and communicable diseases such as smallpox claimed many children's lives and limited the average life expectancy of adults. These diseases were not responsive to diet; they were caused by infectious agents—bacteria, viruses, and the like. Today, though, thanks to safe public water supplies and immunization programs in developed countries, far fewer infectious diseases threaten us.

Most people today live well into their later years, and most of the diseases that threaten their lives are not the infectious type. Today's prevalent diseases develop and become chronic due to physiological deterioration of the body induced by such factors as heredity, age, gender, lifestyle, and environment. Chronic diseases are the subject of this Nutrition in Practice. A list at the start of Chapter 17 (p. 420) itemized the many ways in which nutrition factors affect these diseases. All aspects of diet are relevant: energy balance, nutrient intakes, fiber intakes, and food choices.

What are today's major chronic diseases? Are they caused by diet?

Table 29–3 lists the ten leading causes of death in the United States.[16] Four of these causes, including the top three, have some relationship with diet: heart disease, cancers, strokes, and diabetes. Taken together, these four conditions account for two-thirds of the nation's 2 million deaths each year. Diet is not a *cause* of these diseases, but it is a *risk factor* for them.

Table 29–3
Ten Leading Causes of Death in the United States

1. **Heart disease.**
2. **Cancers.**
3. **Strokes.**
4. Chronic obstructive lung disease.
5. Unintentional injuries.
6. Pneumonia and influenza.
7. **Diabetes mellitus.**
8. Suicide.
9. HIV infection.
10. Homicide.

Note: The four causes of death that are shown in boldface type are those that are known to have some relation to diet.

What is a risk factor?

A risk factor is any aspect of a person's life that increases the person's risk of developing a chronic disease. Risk factors are identified by analyzing statistical data. A strong association between a factor and a disease means that when the factor is present, the *likelihood* of developing the disease is great. Not all people with the risk factor *will* develop the disease, nor will all people who are free of risk factors be free of the disease. On average, though, the more risk factors in a person's life, the greater that person's chances of developing the disease.

Can diet help us avoid today's chronic diseases?

Yes. Look at Figure 29–1 (on p. 698), which illustrates many relationships between diet and degenerative diseases. Note that the figure includes some risk factors, such as heredity, age, and gender, that cannot be modified, but notice how many can be.

An overweight person with a family history of diabetes cannot change his heredity, age, or gender, but clearly can benefit greatly from increasing physical activity and losing weight. Similarly, a smoker with a family history of heart disease should give up tobacco.

Note, though, that people's hereditary susceptibility to diseases and their responsiveness to dietary measures vary. Chronic diseases may be influenced by diet, but they are also influenced by genetics: they run in families. Logically, therefore, preventive efforts are most beneficial for persons with strong family histories of disease, and health care professionals should single those people out for treatment. In reality, though, such a person-by-person approach is not feasible. Instead, recommendations are aimed at the general population in the hope that all people at all levels of risk may benefit.[17] Such a strategy is similar to national efforts to vaccinate against polio, fluoridate water to prevent dental caries, and fortify grains to prevent iron deficiency.

The surgeon general's recommendations for avoiding chronic disease are shown in Table 29–4. The table also mentions the risk factors that alert people to the personally relevant diseases. Notice that the surgeon general's recommendations closely parallel those of the *Diet and Health* report in Chapter 1.

Do you think most people should follow recommendations?

Yes, the research, based on the results of over 7000 studies, seems to indicate that most people can gain some disease-prevention benefits by making dietary changes. The Committee on Diet and Health asserts that recommendations are now warranted. To wait for conclusive evidence "would be derelict"; it is time to inform people of the "likelihood of certain risks and the possible benefits of dietary modifications."[18] With these recommendations, people can begin improving their diets, and industry can begin providing new products to meet health needs.

How can people apply this information to their own lives?

To determine whether dietary recommendations may be important to you personally, examine your family history to see which diseases are common to your parents and grandparents (see Figure 29–2 on p. 700 for a hypothetical "medical family tree"). In addition to family history, personal history is also important, of course: take note of your own blood pressure, blood test results, and lifestyle habits such as smoking.

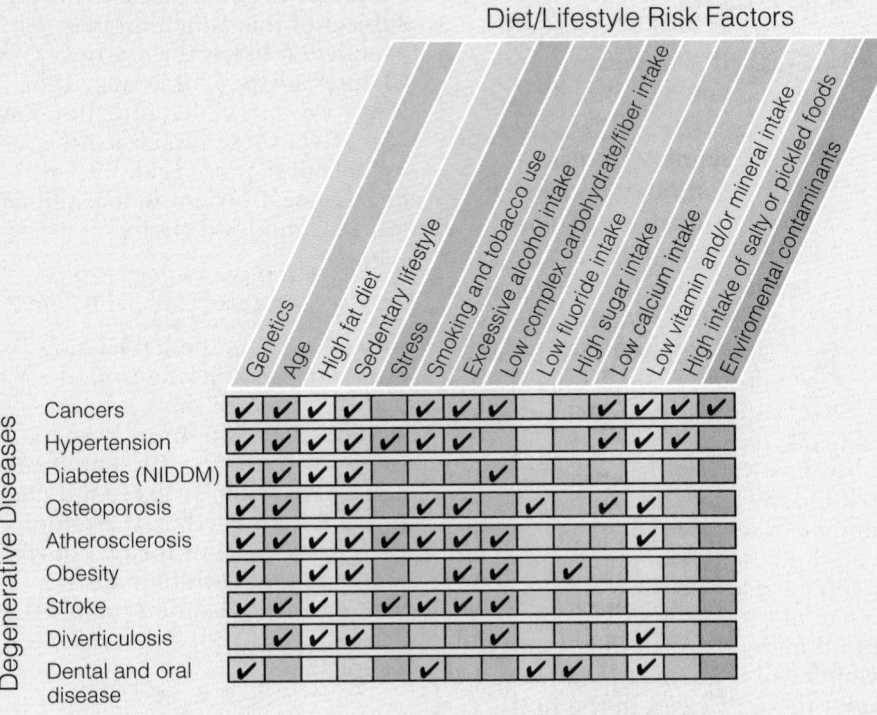

Figure 29–1
Diet/Lifestyle Risk Factors and Degenerative Diseases
Multiple risk factors have been linked to most degenerative diseases.

Diet/Lifestyle Risk Factors

Degenerative Diseases	Genetics	Age	High fat diet	Sedentary lifestyle	Stress	Smoking and tobacco use	Excessive alcohol intake	Low complex carbohydrate/fiber intake	Low fluoride intake	High sugar intake	Low calcium intake	Low vitamin and/or mineral intake	High intake of salty or pickled foods	Enviromental contaminants
Cancers	✓	✓	✓	✓		✓	✓	✓			✓	✓	✓	✓
Hypertension	✓	✓	✓	✓	✓	✓	✓				✓	✓	✓	
Diabetes (NIDDM)	✓	✓	✓	✓				✓						
Osteoporosis	✓	✓		✓		✓	✓		✓		✓	✓		
Atherosclerosis	✓	✓	✓	✓	✓	✓	✓	✓				✓		
Obesity	✓		✓	✓			✓	✓		✓				
Stroke	✓	✓	✓		✓	✓	✓	✓						
Diverticulosis		✓	✓	✓				✓				✓		
Dental and oral disease	✓					✓			✓	✓		✓		

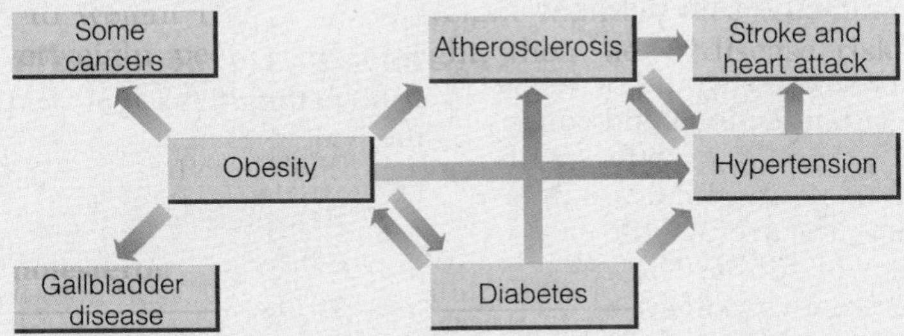

Note that obesity worsens nearly all other disease risks. Several of the recommendations are aimed at weight control: cut fat, add complex carbohydrates, and balance food intake with activity.

The problems of overweight people multiply when medical problems develop. Overweight people with diabetes (NIDDM) usually have high blood pressure and high blood cholesterol as well. Such a combination of problems may require only one treatment: lose the excess weight by adopting a healthful diet combined with regular exercise.

Dietary excesses, particularly of

Table 29–4
Recommendations from *The Surgeon General's Report on Nutrition and Health,* 1988

NUTRITION CHANGES RECOMMENDED FOR MOST PEOPLE	THIS IS ESPECIALLY IMPORTANT IF YOUR FAMILY HISTORY INDICATES:	AND/OR IF YOUR MEDICAL HISTORY INDICATES:
Energy, energy nutrients, and weight control: ▸ Achieve and maintain a healthy body weight.[a] ▸ Reduce consumption of total fat, saturated fat, and cholesterol.[b] ▸ Increase consumption of complex carbohydrates and fiber.[c]	Obesity, diabetes, cancer, or any form of cardiovascular disease.	Unhealthy weight, glucose intolerance, high blood cholesterol or triglycerides, hypertension, other cardiovascular disease
Salt/sodium: Reduce intake of salt/sodium.[d]	Hyptertension, diabetes, or any form of cardiovascular disease.	Hypertension, glucose intolerance
Alcohol: ▸ Take alcohol in moderation, if at all.[e]	Alcohol abuse, cancer, any form of cardiovascular disease, osteoporosis.	Unhealthy weight, glucose intolerance, high blood cholesterol and triglycerides, any sign of adult bone loss
▸ Abstain from alcohol.		Pregnancy, alcohol abuse, liver disease, pancreatitis
SOME ISSUES FOR SOME PEOPLE		**HIGH-RISK GROUPS**
Fluoride: Obtain adequate fluoride from community water supplies or other sources.	Osteoporosis Dental problems	Women and girls Children
Sugars: Limit the use of foods high in simple sugars.	Susceptibility to dental caries	Children
Calcium: Consume foods high in calcium.[f]	Osteoporosis	Women and girls
Iron: Consume foods high in iron.[g]		Low-income families, children, teens premenopausal women

[a]To achieve and maintain desirable body weight, choose a dietary pattern in which food energy intake matches energy expenditure. To reduce energy intake, limit foods relatively high in kcalories, fats, and sugars, and minimize alcohol consumption. Increase energy expenditure through regular and sustained physical activity.

[b]Choose foods relatively low in fats and cholesterol, such as vegetables, fruits, whole-grain foods, fish, poultry, lean meats, and low-fat dairy products. Use food preparation methods that add little or no fat.

[c]To increase consumption of complex carbohydrates and fiber, eat more whole-grain foods and cereal products, vegetables, dried beans and peas, and fruits.

[d]To reduce intake of salt/sodium, choose foods relatively low in sodium, and limit the amount of salt added in food preparation and at the table.

[e]To exercise moderation in the use of alcohol, take no more than two drinks a day. Avoid drinking any alcohol before or while driving, operating machinery, or engaging in any other activity requiring judgment.

[f]Choose low-fat milk and dairy products.

[g]Good food sources of iron are lean meats, fish, certain beans, and iron-enriched cereals and whole-grain products. This issue is of special concern for low-income families.

Source: Adapted from *The Surgeon General's Report on Nutrition and Health: Summary and Recommendations.* DHHS (PHS) publication no. 88–90211 (Washington D.C.: Government Printing Office, 1988) Table 1, p. 3.

Figure 29–2
Hypothetical Medical Family Tree
A "medical family tree" notes the types of diseases family members have had, their ages at the times of major medical events or death, and their personal medical histories.

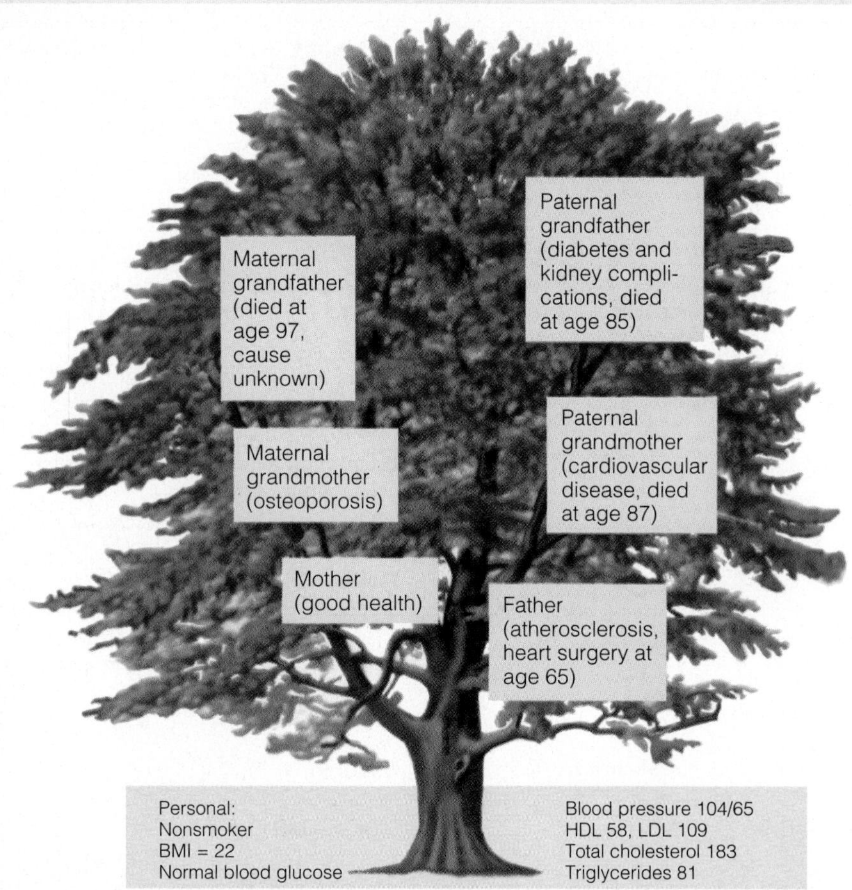

food energy and fat, make all of today's major diseases more likely. The same is true of dietary deficiencies, particularly of fiber, vitamins, and minerals. Not all diet recommendations apply equally to all of the diseases (salt has a special relationship with hypertension, for example), but fortunately for the consumer, the dietary recommendations to help prevent these diseases do not contradict one another. The surgeon general has remarked that for the two out of three Americans who do not smoke or drink excessively, "your choice of diet can influence your long-term health prospects more than any other action you might take."[19]

Indeed, thanks to the fruits of recent nutrition research, healthy adults have a great opportunity that their ancestors did not have. They can employ the benefits of a nutritious diet to help preserve their health well into their later years.

NOTES

1. D. P. Kotler and coauthors, Magnitude of body-cell-mass depletion and the timing of death from wasting in AIDS, *American Journal of Clinical Nutrition* 50 (1989): 444–447.
2. D. O. Jacobs, Bioelectrical impedance analysis: A way to assess changes in body cell mass in patients with acquired immunodeficiency syndrome? *Journal of Parenteral and Enteral Nutrition* 17 (1993): 401–402.
3. R. T. Chlebowski and coauthors, Nutritional status, gastrointestinal dysfunction and survival in patients with AIDS, *American Journal of Gastroenterology* 84 (1989): 1228–1293.
4. B. B. Timbo and L. Tollefson, Nutrition: A cofactor in HIV disease, *Journal of the American Dietetic Association* 94 (1994): 1018–1022.
5. E. B. Trujillo and coauthors, Assessment of nutritional status, nutrient intake, and nutrition support in AIDS patients, *Journal of the American Dietetic Association* 93 (1993): 477–478.
6. C. Grunefeld, M. Pange, and L. Shimizu, Resting energy expenditure, caloric intake, and short-term change in HIV infection and AIDS, *American Journal of Clinical Nutrition* 55 (1992): 455–460.
7. R. Ullrich and coauthors, Small intestinal structure and function in patients infected with human immunodeficiency virus (HIV): Evidence for HIV-induced enteropathy, *Annals of Internal Medicine* 111 (1989): 15–21.
8. P. A. Cuff, Acquired immunodeficiency syndrome and malnutrition: Role of gastrointestinal pathology, *Nutrition in Clinical Practice* 5 (1990):

43–53.
9. Federation of American Societies for Experimental Biology, Nutrition and HIV infection: A review and evaluation of the extant knowledge of the relationship between nutrition and HIV infection, *Nutrition in Clinical Practice* (supplement) 6 (1991): 46–48.
10. C. McCorkindale and coauthors, Nutritional status of HIV-infected patients during the early disease stages, *Journal of the American Dietetic Association* 90 (1990): 1236–1241.
11. Task Force on Nutrition Support in AIDS, Guidelines for nutrition support in AIDS, *Nutrition* 5 (1989): 39–46.
12. Department of Continuing Education in Health Sciences, UCLA Extension, *Nutritional Aspects of the AIDS Patient* (Los Angeles, 1989).
13. A.S.P.E.N. Board of Directors, Acquired immune deficiency syndrome, *Journal of Parenteral and Enteral Nutrition* (supplement) 17 (1993): 13–14; P. Singer and coauthors, Risks and benefits of home parenteral nutrition in the acquired immunodeficiency syndrome, *Journal of Parenteral and Enteral Nutrition* 15 (1991): 75–79.
14. Singer and coauthors, 1991.
15. D. B. Kotler and coauthors, Effect of home total parenteral nutrition on body composition in patients with acquired immunodeficiency syndrome, *Journal of Parenteral and Enteral Nutrition* 14 (1990): 454–458.
16. Centers for Disease Control, Mortality patterns—United States, 1989, *Morbidity and Mortality Weekly Report* 41 (1992): 121–125.
17. *Diet and Health: Implications for Reducing Chronic Disease Risk* (Washington, D.C.: National Academy Press, 1989), pp. 665–710.
18. *Diet and Health,* 1989.
19. *The Surgeon General's Report on Nutrition and Health: Summary and Recommendations,* DHHS (PHS) publication no. 88-50211 (Washington, D.C.: Government Printing Office, 1988).

Appendixes

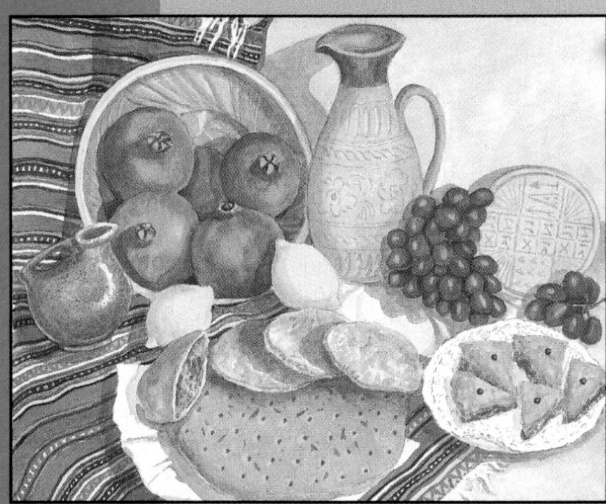

CONTENTS

APPENDIX A

TABLE OF FOOD COMPOSITION

This edition of the table of food composition contains more complete values for several nutrients than any comparable table. These include dietary fiber; saturated, monounsaturated, and polyunsaturated fat; vitamin B_6; folate; magnesium; and zinc. The table includes a wide variety of foods from all food groups and is updated yearly to reflect current food patterns. For example, this edition includes the new vegetable broccoflower, nonfat items, and new selections of frozen convenience foods and baby foods.

To achieve a complete and reliable listing of nutrients for all the foods, over 1000 sources of information are researched. Government sources are the primary base for all the data: the USDA *Handbook* series and its current supplemental data, as well as current data on baked goods, snacks, and sweets. In addition, provisional USDA information—both published and unpublished—is included. The data are refined through information obtained in many conversations with professional staff members at the USDA Human Nutrition Information Service in Hyattsville, Maryland.

Even with all the government sources available, however, some nutrient values are still missing; and as the USDA updates the various data, it sometimes reports conflicting values for the same items. To fill in the missing values and resolve discrepancies, other reliable sources of information are used. These sources include refereed journal articles, food composition tables from Canada and England, information from other nutrient data banks and publications, unpublished scientific data, and manufacturers' data.

Estimates of nutrient amounts for foods and nutrients include all possible adjustments in the interest of accuracy. When multiple values are reported for a nutrient, the numbers are averaged and weighted with consideration of the original number of samples in the separate sources. Whenever water percentages are available, estimates of nutrient amounts are adjusted for water content. When no water is given, water percentage is assumed to be that shown in the table. Whenever a reported weight appeared inconsistent (cooked eggplant and collards, for example), many kitchen tests were made, and the average weight of the typical product was given as tested.

When estimates of nutrient amounts in cooked foods are derived from reported amounts in raw foods, published retention factors are applied. Some reported data for combination foods are modified in this table to include newer data available for major ingredients. For example, since the "pies" were analyzed and reported, newer data on fruits have been published. Bakery items reflect the most current data with the new enrichment levels for certain nutrients.

Considerable effort has been made to report the most accurate data available and to eliminate missing values. The table is updated annually, and the authors welcome any suggestions or comments for future editions.

IT IS IMPORTANT TO KNOW

that many different nutrient values can be reported for foods, even by reliable sources. Many factors influence the amounts of nutrients in foods, including the mineral content of the soil, the method of processing, genetics, the diet of the animal or the fertilizer of the plant, the season of the year, methods of analysis, the difference in moisture content of the samples analyzed, the length and method of storage, and methods of cooking the food.

Although each nutrient from USDA government data is presented as a single number in some USDA publications, each number is actually an average of a range of data. The more detailed reports (Handbook 8 series) indicate the number of samples and the standard deviation of the data. One can also find different reported values for foods, as older USDA data are replaced with newer data in more recent publications. Therefore, nutrient data should be viewed and used only as a guide, a close approximation of nutrient content.

Dietary fiber deserves a special word. Estimates of dietary fiber are included for all the foods in this table. This information comes primarily from extensive published and unpublished data from the USDA Human Nutrition Information Service in Hyattsville, Maryland; *Composition of Foods by Southgate* (England); and many journal articles.

It is important to recognize that data for dietary fiber are still undergoing review in the scientific community. No doubt, these estimates will change as analytical techniques are refined and interpretations clarified.

Vitamin A is reported in retinol equivalents. The amount of this vitamin can vary by the season of the year and the maturity of the plant. Reported values in both dairy products and plants are higher in summer and early fall than in winter. The values reported here represent year-round averages. The organ meats of all animal products (liver especially) contain large amounts of vitamin A, which vary widely, depending on the background of the animal. The vitamin is also present in very small amounts in regular meat and is often reported as a trace.

Newer reported vitamin A values for some plant foods have increased significantly due to additional information and sometimes to improved plant genetics. Recent vitamin A values for canned pumpkin, for example, are 3.5 times greater than the previously reported values.

The energy and nutrients in recipes and combination foods vary widely, depending on the ingredients. The amounts of various fatty acids and cholesterol are influenced by the type of fat used (the specific type of oil, vegetable shortening, butter, margarine, etc.).

Total fats, as well as the breakdown of total fats to saturated, monounsaturated, and polyunsaturated fats, are listed in the table. The fatty acids seldom add up to the total. This discrepancy is due to rounding and to the existence of small amounts of other fatty acid components that are not included in the three basic categories, including *trans*-fatty acids and glycerol.

Niacin values are for preformed niacin and do not include additional niacin that may form in the body from the conversion of tryptophan.

The items in this table have been organized into several categories, which are listed at the head of each right-hand page. As the key shows, each group has been color-coded to make it easy to find individual items.

In an effort to conserve space, the following abbreviations have been used in the food descriptions and nutrient breakdowns:

- diam = diameter
- ea = each
- enr = enriched
- f/ = from
- g = grams
- liq = liquid
- pce = piece
- pkg = package
- w/ = with
- w/o = without
- t = trace
- 0 = zero (no nutrient value)
- — = information not available

This table has been prepared for West Publishing Company and is copyrighted by ESHA Research in Salem, Oregon—the developer and publisher of The Food Processor®, Nutrition Pro™, and Genesis™ nutrition software systems. The major sources for the data from the U.S. Department of Agriculture are supplemented by more than 1000 additional sources of information. Because the list of references is so extensive, it is not provided here, but it is available from the publisher.

A

Table A–1
Food Composition

Computer Code Number	Food Description	Measure	Wt (g)	H_2O (%)	Ener (kcal)	Prot (g)	Carb (g)	Dietary Fiber (g)	Fat (g)	Fat Breakdown (g) Sat	Mono	Poly
	BEVERAGES											
	Alcoholic:											
	Beer:											
1	Regular (12 fl oz)	1½ c	356	92	145	1	13	2	0	0	0	0
2	Light (12 fl oz)	1½ c	354	95	99[1]	1	5	1	0	0	0	0
1506	Nonalcoholic (12 fl oz)	1 ea	360	98	32	1	5	0	0	0	0	0
	Gin, rum, vodka, whiskey:											
3	80 proof	1½ fl oz	42	67	97	0	0	0	0	0	0	0
4	86 proof	1½ fl oz	42	64	105	0	<1	0	0	0	0	0
5	90 proof	1½ fl oz	42	62	110	0	0	0	0	0	0	0
	Liqueur:											
1359	Coffee liqueur, 53 proof	1½ fl oz	52	31	174	<1	24	0	<1	.1	t	.1
1360	Coffee & cream liqueur, 34 proof	1½ fl oz	47	46	153	1	10	0	7	4.5	2.1	.3
1361	Crème de menthe, 72 proof	1½ fl oz	50	28	185	0	21	0	<1	t	t	.1
	Wine:											
6	Dessert (4 fl oz)	½ c	118	72	181[2]	<1	14	0	0	0	0	0
7	Red	3½ fl oz	103	88	74	<1	2	0	0	0	0	0
8	Rosé	3½ fl oz	103	89	73	<1	1	0	0	0	0	0
9	White medium	3½ fl oz	103	90	70	<1	1	0	0	0	0	0
1592	Nonalcoholic	1 c	232	98	14	1	3	0	0	0	0	0
1593	Nonalcoholic light	1 c	251	98	15	1	3	0	0	0	0	0
1409	Wine cooler, bottle (12 fl oz)	1½ c	340	90	169	<1	20	<1	<1	0	0	t
1595	Wine cooler, cup	1 c	227	90	113	<1	13	<1	<1	0	0	t
	Carbonated:[3]											
10	Club soda (12 fl oz)	1½ c	355	100	0	0	0	0	0	0	0	0
11	Cola beverage (12 fl oz)	1½ c	370	89	151	0	38	0	<1	0	t	.1
12	Diet cola w/aspartame (12 fl oz)	1½ c	355	100	4	<1	<1	0	0	0	0	0
13	Diet cola w/saccharin (12 fl oz)	1½ c	355	100	0	0	<1	0	0	0	0	0
14	Ginger ale (12 fl oz)	1½ c	366	91	124	0	32	0	0	0	0	0
15	Grape soda (12 fl oz)	1½ c	372	89	159	0	42	0	0	0	0	0
16	Lemon-lime (12 fl oz)	1½ c	368	89	147	0	38	0	0	0	0	0
17	Orange (12 fl oz)	1½ c	372	88	178	0	46	0	0	0	0	0
18	Pepper-type soda (12 fl oz)	1½ c	368	89	150	0	38	0	<1	.3	0	0
19	Root beer (12 fl oz)	1½ c	370	89	151	0	39	0	0	0	0	0
20	Coffee,[3] brewed	1 c	240	99	5[4]	<1	1	<1	<1	t	0	t
21	Coffee,[3] prepared from instant	1 c	240	99	5[4]	<1	1	0	<1	t	0	t
	Fruit drinks, noncarbonated:[5]											
22	Fruit punch drink, canned	2 c	126	88	59	0	15	0	<1	t	t	t
1358	Gatorade	1 c	240	93	60	0	15	0	0	0	0	0
23	Grape drink, canned	2 c	125	87	62	<1	16	<1	0	0	0	0
1304	Kool-Aid, with sugar	1 c	240	90	89	0	23	0	<1	t	t	t
1356	Kool-Aid, with NutraSweet	1 c	240	95	43	0	11	0	0	0	0	0

(1)kCalories can vary from 78 to 131 for 12 fl. oz.

(2)Values are for sweet dessert wine. Dry dessert wines contain 149 kcal and 5 g of carbohydrate.

(3)Mineral content varies depending on water source.

(4)kCalorie values from USDA vary from 1 to 5 kcal per cup.

(5)Usually less than 10% fruit juice.

Chol (mg)	Calc (mg)	Iron (mg)	Magn (mg)	Phos (mg)	Pota (mg)	Sodi (mg)	Zinc (mg)	VT-A (RE)	Thia (mg)	Ribo (mg)	Niac (mg)	V-B6 (mg)	Fola (μg)	VT-C (mg)
0	18	.11	21	43	89	18	.07	0	.02	.09	1.61	.18	21	0
0	18	.14	18	42	64	11	.11	0	.03	.11	1.39	.12	14	0
0	25	.04	32	112	90	18	.04	0	.04	.11	1.62	.18	25	0
0	0	.02	0	2	1	<1	.02	0	<.01	<.01	<.01	0	0	0
0	0	.02	0	2	1	<1	.02	0	<.01	<.01	<.01	0	0	0
0	0	.02	0	2	1	<1	.02	0	<.01	<.01	<.01	0	0	0
0	1	.03	2	3	16	41	.02	0	<.01	<.01	<.07	0	0	0
7	8	.06	1	23	15	43	.07	20	0	.03	.04	.01	0	0
0	0	.03	0	0	0	2	.02	0	0	0	<.01	0	0	0
0	9	.28	11	11	108	11	.08	0	.02	.02	.25	0	<1	0
0	8	.44	13	14	115	5	.09	0	<.01	.03	.08	.03	2	0
0	8	.39	10	15	102	5	.06	0	<.01	.02	.08	.02	1	0
0	9	.33	11	14	82	5	.07	0	<.01	<.01	.07	.01	<1	0
0	21	.93	23	35	204	16	.19	0	0	.02	.23	.05	2	0
0	23	1	25	38	221	18	.2	0	0	.02	.25	.05	3	0
0	19	.92	18	22	–	29	.2	1	.03	.03	.17	.03	4	6
0	13	.61	12	15	–	19	.14	<1	.02	.02	.11	.02	3	4
0	18	.04	4	0	7	75	.35	0	0	0	0	0	0	0
0	11	.11	4	44	4	15	.04	0	0	0	0	0	0	0
0	14	.11	4	32	0	21[6]	.28	0	.02	.08	0	0	0	0
0	14	.14	4	39	7	57	.18	0	0	0	0	0	0	0
0	11	.66	4	0	4	26	.18	0	0	0	0	0	0	0
0	11	.3	4	0	4	56	.26	0	0	0	0	0	0	0
0	7	.26	4	0	4	40	.18	0	0	0	.05	0	0	0
0	19	.22	4	4	7	45	.37	0	0	0	0	0	0	0
0	11	.15	0	40	4	37	.15	0	0	0	0	0	0	0
0	18	.18	4	0	4	48	.26	0	0	0	0	0	0	0
0	5	.12	12	2	129	5	.05	0	0	0	.53	0	<1	0
0	7	.12	10	7	86	7	.07	0	0	<.01	.68	0	0	0
0	10	.27	3	1	32	28	.15	1	.03	.03	.03	0	2	37
0	0	.12	2	22	26	96	.05	0	.01	0	0	0	0	0
0	4	.12	5	5	44	1	.04	0	.01	.01	.12	.02	1	20
0	38	.12	2	48	2	34	.07	0	0	<.01	<.01	0	<1	28
0	17	.65	5	5	50	50	.26	2	.02	.05	.05	0	5	77

[6] Value for product sweetened with aspartame only; sodium is 32 mg if a blend of aspartame and sodium saccharin is used.

(For purposes of calculations, use "0" for t, <1, <.1, <.01, etc.)

Table A–1
Food Composition

Computer Code Number	Food Description	Measure	Wt (g)	H_2O (%)	Ener (kcal)	Prot (g)	Carb (g)	Dietary Fiber (g)	Fat (g)	Fat Breakdown (g) Sat	Mono	Poly
	BEVERAGES—Cont.											
	Fruit drinks, noncarbonated—Cont.											
26	Lemonade, frozen concentrate (6-oz can)	¾ c	219	52	396	1	103	1	<1	.1	t	.1
27	Lemonade, from concentrate	1 c	248	89	99	<1	26	<1	<1	t	t	t
28	Limeade, frozen concentrate (6-oz can)	¾ c	218	50	408	<1	107	1	<1	t	t	.1
29	Limeade, from concentrate	1 c	247	89	101	0	27	<1	<1	t	t	t
24	Pineapple grapefruit, canned	1 c	250	88	117	<1	29	<1	<1	t	t	.1
25	Pineapple orange, canned	1 c	250	87	125	3	29	<1	<1	t	t	t
	Fruit and vegetable juices: see Fruit and Vegetable sections											
	Slim Fast:[1]											
1612	Chocolate malt with nonfat milk	1 c	273	82	190	14	32	2	1	.3	.1	t
1613	Strawberry with nonfat milk	1 c	273	82	190	14	32	2	1	.3	.1	t
1611	Vanilla with nonfat milk	1 c	273	82	190	14	32	2	1	.3	.1	t
	Ultra Slim Fast:[1]											
1616	Chocolate with nonfat milk	1 c	278	81	200	14	36	5	1	.3	.1	t
1614	French vanilla with nonfat milk	1 c	278	81	190	14	36	4	1	.3	.1	t
1615	Strawberry Supreme with nonfat milk	1 c	278	81	190	14	36	4	1	.3	.1	t
1357	Water, bottled: Perrier (6½ fl oz)	1 ea	192	100	0	0	0	0	0	0	0	0
1594	Water, bottled: Tonic water	1½ c	366	91	124	0	32	0	0	0	0	0
	Tea:[2]											
30	Brewed, regular	1 c	240	100	2	0	1	0	<1	t	t	t
1662	Brewed, herbal	¾ c	178	100	2	0	<1	0	t	t	t	t
32	From instant, sweetened	1 c	262	91	89	<1	22	0	<1	t	t	t
31	From instant, unsweetened	1 c	237	100	2	0	<1	0	0	0	0	0
	DAIRY											
	Butter: see Fats and Oils, #158,159,160											
	Cheese, natural:											
33	Blue	1 oz	28	42	100	6	1	0	8	5.3	2.2	.2
34	Brick	1 oz	28	41	105	7	1	0	8	5.3	2.4	.2
35	Brie	1 oz	28	48	94	6	<1	0	8	4.9	2.3	.2
36	Camembert	1 oz	28	52	85	6	<1	0	7	4.3	2	.2
37	Cheddar:	1 oz	28	37	114	7	<1	0	9	6	2.7	.3
38	1" cube	1 ea	17	37	68	4	<1	0	6	3.6	1.6	.2
39	Shredded	1 c	113	37	453	28	1	0	37	23.8	10.6	1.1
	Cottage:											
1406	Low sodium, low fat	1 c	225	83	162	28	6	0	2	1.4	.6	.07
40	Creamed, large curd	1 c	225	79	232	28	6	0	10	6.4	2.9	.3
41	Creamed, small curd	1 c	210	79	216	26	6	0	9	6	2.7	.3
42	With fruit	1 c	226	72	278	22	30	0	8	4.9	2.2	.2
43	Low fat 2%	1 c	226	79	202	31	8	0	4	2.8	1.2	.1
44	Low fat 1%	1 c	226	82	163	28	6	0	2	1.5	.7	.1
45	Dry curd	1 c	145	80	122	25	3	0	1	.4	.2	t
46	Cream	1 oz	28	54	99	2	1	0	10	6.2	2.8	.4
47	Edam	1 oz	28	42	101	7	<1	0	8	5	2.3	.2
48	Feta	1 oz	28	55	75	4	1	0	6	4.2	1.3	.2
49	Gouda	1 oz	28	41	101	7	1	0	8	5	2.2	.2

(1)See Chapter 9 for healthy weight loss strategies. The formulas for these products change periodically; these data reflect nutrient values as of our publication date.

(2)Mineral content varies depending on water source.

(Computer code number is for West Diet Analysis program)

PAGE KEY: A–2 = BEV A–4 = DAIRY A–10 = EGGS A–12 = FAT/OIL A–14 = FRUIT A–24 = BAKERY A–34 = GRAIN A–40 = FISH A–44 = MEATS A–48 = POULTRY A–50 = SAUSAGE A–52 = MIXED/FAST A–60 = NUTS/SEEDS A–62 = SWEETS A–66 = VEG/LEG A–78 = MISC A–80 = SOUPS/SAUCES A–84 = FAST A–96 = FRZN ENTREE A–98 = BABY FOODS

Chol (mg)	Calc (mg)	Iron (mg)	Magn (mg)	Phos (mg)	Pota (mg)	Sodi (mg)	Zinc (mg)	VT-A (RE)	Thia (mg)	Ribo (mg)	Niac (mg)	V-B6 (mg)	Fola (µg)	VT-C (mg)
0	15	1.58	11	20	146	9	.17	22	.06	.21	.16	.05	22	39[3]
0	7	.4	5	5	37	7	.1	5	.01	.05	.04	.01	5	10[3]
0	11	.22	9	13	128	0	.09	0	.02	.02	.22	0	9	26
0	7	.07	2	2	32	5	.05	0	<.01	<.01	.05	0	2	7
0	17	.77	15	15	152	35	.15	10	.07	.04	.67	.1	26	115
0	12	.67	15	10	115	7	.15	133	.07	.05	.52	.12	27	56
4	450	6.3	140	400	690	230	5.25	350	.52	.59	7	.7	120	21
4	450	6.3	140	400	720	220	5.25	350	.52	.59	7	.7	120	21
4	450	6.31	140	401	721	220	5.24	349	.52	.59	6.99	.7	120	21
<1	450	6.3	140	400	800	230	5.25	350	.52	.59	7	.7	120	21
<1	450	6.3	140	400	730	250	5.25	350	.52	.59	7	.7	120	21
<1	450	6.3	140	400	710	250	5.25	350	.52	.59	7	.7	120	21
0	27	0	0	0	0	2	0	0	0	0	0	0	0	0
0	4	.04	0	0	0	15	.37	0	0	0	0	0	0	0
0	0	.05	7	2	89	7	.05	0	0	.03	0	0	12	0
0	4	.14	2	0	16	2	.07	0	.02	.01	0	0	1	0
0	5	.05	5	3	50	8	.08	0	0	.05	.09	<.01	10	0
0	5	.05	5	2	47	7	.07	0	0	<.01	.09	<.01	1	0
21	149	.09	6	110	73	395	.75	65	.01	.11	.29	.05	10	0
27	191	.12	7	128	39	158	.74	86	<.01	.1	.03	.02	6	0
28	52	.14	6	53	43	178	.67	52	.02	.15	.11	.07	18	0
20	110	.09	6	98	53	239	.67	71	.01	.14	.18	.06	18	0
30	204	.19	8	145	28	176	.88	86	.01	.11	.02	.02	5	0
18	122	.12	5	87	17	105	.53	51	<.01	.06	.01	.01	3	0
119	811	.77	31	577	111	701	3.51	342	.03	.43	.09	.08	21	0
9	137	.3	11	301	193	29	.8	25	.04	.36	.3	.15	27	0
33	135	.31	12	295	190	911	.83	108	.05	.37	.28	.15	27	0
31	126	.29	11	275	177	851	.78	101	.04	.34	.26	.14	26	0
25	107	.25	9	235	151	913	.65	81	.04	.29	.23	.12	22	0
19	154	.36	14	339	217	918	.95	45	.05	.42	.32	.17	30	0
10	137	.32	12	303	193	918	.86	25	.05	.37	.29	.15	28	0
10	46	.33	6	149	47	19	.68	12	.04	.21	.22	.12	21	0
31	23	.34	2	29	34	84	.15	124	<.01	.06	.03	.01	4	0
25	207	.12	8	152	53	274	1.07	72	.01	.11	.02	.02	5	0
25	139	.18	5	95	18	315	.82	36	.04	.24	.28	.12	9	0
32	198	.07	8	155	34	232	1.11	49	.01	.09	.02	.02	6	0

(3)Vitamin C can range from 5 to 72 mg in a small can of frozen concentrate, and from 1 to 18 mg in 1 c of prepared lemonade.

(For purposes of calculations, use "0" for t, <1, <.1, <.01, etc.)

A

Table A–1
Food Composition

Computer Code Number	Food Description	Measure	Wt (g)	H_2O (%)	Ener (kcal)	Prot (g)	Carb (g)	Dietary Fiber (g)	Fat (g)	Fat Breakdown (g) Sat	Mono	Poly
	DAIRY—Cont.											
	Cheese—Cont.											
50	Gruyère	1 oz	28	33	117	8	<1	0	9	5.4	2.8	.5
51	Gorgonzola	1 oz	28	39	111	7	0	0	9	5.5	2.4	.5
52	Liederkranz	1 oz	28	53	87	5	<1	0	8	5.3	2.2	.2
1676	Limburger	1 oz	28	48	93	6	<1	0	8	4.7	2.4	.1
53	Monterey Jack	1 oz	28	41	106	7	<1	0	9	5.4	2.5	.3
54	Mozzarella, whole milk	1 oz	28	54	80	5	1	0	6	3.7	1.9	.2
55	Mozzarella, part-skim milk, low moisture	1 oz	28	49	79	8	1	0	5	3.1	1.4	.1
56	Muenster	1 oz	28	42	104	7	<1	0	9	5.4	2.5	.2
1399	Nonfat (Kraft Singles)	1 oz	28	60	46	7	4	0	0	0	0	0
	Parmesan, grated:											
57	Cup, not pressed down	1 c	100	18	455	41	4	0	30	19	8.7	.7
58	Tablespoon	1 tbs	5	18	23	2	<1	0	1	.9	.4	t
59	Ounce	1 oz	28	18	129	12	1	0	9	5.4	2.5	.2
60	Provolone	1 oz	28	41	99	7	1	0	8	4.8	2.1	.2
61	Ricotta, whole milk	1 c	246	72	428	28	7	0	32	20.4	8.9	.9
62	Ricotta, part-skim milk	1 c	246	74	339	28	13	0	19	12.1	5.7	.6
63	Romano	1 oz	28	31	109	9	1	0	8	4.8	2.2	.2
64	Swiss	1 oz	28	37	106	8	1	0	8	5	2.1	.3
	Pasteurized processed cheese products:											
65	American	1 oz	28	39	106	6	<1	0	9	5.6	2.5	.3
66	Swiss	1 oz	28	42	94	7	1	0	7	4.6	2	.2
67	American cheese food, jar	1 oz	28	43	93	6	2	0	7	4.4	2	.2
68	American cheese spread	1 oz	28	48	82	5	2	0	6	3.8	1.8	.2
69	Cream, sweet:	1 c	242	81	315	7	10	0	28	17.3	8	1
	Half & half (cream & milk):											
70	Tablespoon	1 tbs	15	81	19	<1	1	0	2	1.1	.5	.1
71	Light, coffee or table:	1 c	240	74	468	6	9	0	46	28.8	13.4	1.7
72	Tablespoon	1 tbs	15	74	29	<1	1	0	3	1.8	.8	.1
73	Light whipping cream, liquid:[1]	1 c	239	63	698	5	7	0	74	46.1	21.7	2.1
74	Tablespoon	1 tbs	15	63	44	<1	<1	0	5	2.9	1.4	.1
75	Heavy whipping cream, liquid:[1]	1 c	238	58	821	5	7	0	88	54.7	25.5	3.3
76	Tablespoon	1 tbs	15	58	52	<1	<1	0	6	3.4	1.6	.2
77	Whipped cream, pressurized:	1 c	60	61	154	2	7	0	13	8.3	3.8	.5
78	Tablespoon	1 tbs	4	61	10	<1	<1	0	1	.6	.3	t
79	Cream, sour, cultured:	1 c	230	71	492	7	10	0	48	29.9	13.9	1.8
80	Tablespoon	1 tbs	14	71	30	<1	1	0	3	1.8	.8	.1
	Cream products—imitation and part dairy:											
81	Coffee whitener, frozen or liquid	1 tbs	15	77	20	<1	2	0	1	1.4	t	0
82	Coffee whitener, powdered	1 tsp	2	2	11	<1	1	0	1	.6	t	t
83	Dessert topping, frozen, nondairy:	1 c	75	50	238	1	17	0	19	16.4	1.2	.4
84	Tablespoon	1 tbs	5	50	16	<1	1	0	1	1.1	.1	t
85	Dessert topping, mix with whole milk:	1 c	80	67	151	3	13	0	10	8.6	.7	.2
86	Tablespoon	1 tbs	5	67	9	<1	1	0	1	.5	t	t
88	Dessert topping, pressurized:	1 c	70	60	184	1	11	0	16	13.2	1.3	.2
87	Tablespoon	1 tbs	4	60	10	<1	1	0	1	.8	.1	t

(1) For whipped cream, (non-pressurized), double the liquid cream volume of codes 73, 74 or 75, 76. One tablespoon liquid cream becomes 2 tablespoons when "whipped."

(Computer code number is for West Diet Analysis program)

PAGE KEY: A–2 = BEV A–4 = DAIRY A–10 = EGGS A–12 = FAT/OIL A–14 = FRUIT A–24 = BAKERY A–34 = GRAIN A–40 = FISH A–44 = MEATS A–48 = POULTRY A–50 = SAUSAGE A–52 = MIXED/FAST A–60 = NUTS/SEEDS A–62 = SWEETS A–66 = VEG/LEG A–78 = MISC A–80 = SOUPS/SAUCES A–84 = FAST A–96 = FRZN ENTREE A–98 = BABY FOODS

Chol (mg)	Calc (mg)	Iron (mg)	Magn (mg)	Phos (mg)	Pota (mg)	Sodi (mg)	Zinc (mg)	VT-A (RE)	Thia (mg)	Ribo (mg)	Niac (mg)	V-B6 (mg)	Fola (μg)	VT-C (mg)
31	286	.05	10	171	23	95	1.11	85	.02	.08	.03	.02	3	0
25	149	.12	8	121	26	512	.57	103	.01	.09	.2	.04	9	0
21	110	.12	7	100	68	389	.7	91	.01	.18	.1	.04	34	0
26	141	.04	6	111	36	227	.6	90	.02	.14	.05	.02	16	0
25	211	.2	8	126	23	152	.85	72	<.01	.11	.03	.02	5	0
22	146	.05	5	105	19	105	.63	68	<.01	.07	.02	.02	2	0
15	207	.07	7	148	27	149	.89	54	.01	.1	.03	.02	3	0
27	203	.12	8	132	38	178	.8	90	<.01	.09	.03	.02	3	0
5	162	–	–	202	81	425	–	101	–	.14	–	–	–	0
79	1375	.95	51	807	107	1861	3.19	173	.04	.39	.31	.1	8	0
4	69	.05	3	40	5	93	.16	9	<.01	.02	.02	<.01	<1	0
22	390	.27	14	229	30	528	.9	49	.01	.11	.09	.03	2	0
20	214	.15	8	140	39	247	.92	75	<.01	.09	.04	.02	3	0
124	509	.93	28	389	256	206	2.85	330	.03	.48	.26	.11	30	0
76	669	1.08	36	450	308	305	3.3	278	.05	.45	.19	.05	32	0
29	300	.22	12	215	24	339	.73	40	.01	.1	.02	.02	2	0
26	272	.05	10	171	31	74	1.11	72	.01	.1	.03	.02	2	0
27	174	.11	6	211	46	405	.85	82	.01	.1	.02	.02	2	0
24	219	.17	8	216	61	388	1.03	65	<.01	.08	.01	.01	2	0
18	163	.24	9	130	79	336	.85	62	.01	.13	.04	.04	2	0
16	159	.09	8	202	69	380	.73	54	.01	.12	.04	.03	2	0
89	254	.17	25	230	312	98	1.23	259	.08	.36	.19	.09	6	2
6	16	.01	2	14	19	6	.08	16	<.01	.02	.01	.01	<1	<1
158	230	.1	21	191	293	95	.65	437	.08	.35	.14	.08	6	2
10	14	.01	1	12	18	6	.04	27	<.01	.02	.01	<.01	<1	<1
265	165	.07	17	146	231	82	.6	705	.06	.3	.1	.07	9	1
17	10	<.01	1	9	14	5	.04	44	<.01	.02	.01	<.01	1	<1
326	153	.07	17	148	179	89	.55	1001	.05	.26	.09	.06	9	1
21	10	<.01	1	9	11	6	.03	63	<.01	.02	.01	<.01	1	<1
46	61	.03	6	54	88	78	.22	124	.02	.04	.04	.02	2	0
3	4	<.01	<1	4	6	5	.01	8	<.01	<.01	<.01	<.01	<1	0
102	267	.14	26	195	331	122	.62	449	.08	.34	.15	.04	25	2
6	16	.01	2	12	20	7	.04	27	<.01	.02	.01	<.01	2	<1
0	1	<.01	<1	10	29	12	<.01	1	0	0	0	0	0	0
0	<1	.02	<1	8	16	4	.01	<1	0	<.01	0	0	0	0
0	5	.09	1	6	14	19	.02	64[2]	0	0	0	0	0	0
0	<1	.01	<1	<1	1	1	<.01	4[2]	0	0	0	0	0	0
8	72	.03	8	69	120	53	.22	39[2]	.02	.09	.05	.02	3	1
<1	5	<.01	<1	4	7	3	.01	2[2]	<.01	.01	<.01	<.01	<1	<1
0	4	.01	1	13	13	43	.01	33[2]	.0	0	0	0	0	0
0	<1	<.01	<1	1	1	2	0	2[2]	0	0	0	0	0	0

(2)Vitamin A value is from beta-carotene used for coloring.

(For purposes of calculations, use "0" for t, <1, <.1, <.01, etc.)

A

Table A–1
Food Composition

Computer Code Number	Food Description	Measure	Wt (g)	H_2O (%)	Ener (kcal)	Prot (g)	Carb (g)	Dietary Fiber (g)	Fat (g)	Fat Breakdown (g) Sat	Mono	Poly
	DAIRY—Cont.											
91	Sour cream, imitation:	1 c	230	71	478	6	15	<1	45	40.9	1.3	.1
92	Tablespoon	1 tbs	14	71	29	<1	1	<1	3	2.5	.1	t
89	Sour dressing, part dairy:	1 c	235	75	416	8	11	0	39	31.3	4.6	1.1
90	Tablespoon	1 tbs	15	75	27	<1	1	0	2	2	.3	.1
	Milk, fluid:											
93	Whole milk	1 c	244	88	149	8	11	0	8	5.1	2.3	.3
94	2% low-fat milk	1 c	244	89	121	8	12	0	5	2.9	1.3	.2
95	2% milk solids added[1]	1 c	245	89	124	9	12	0	5	2.9	1.4	.2
96	1% low-fat milk	1 c	244	90	102	8	12	–	3	1.6	.7	.1
97	1% milk solids added[1]	1 c	245	90	104	9	12	0	2	1.5	.7	.1
98	Nonfat milk, vitamin A added	1 c	245	91	85	8	12	0	<1	.3	.1	t
99	Nonfat milk solids added[1]	1 c	245	90	90	9	12	0	1	.4	.2	t
100	Buttermilk, nonfat	1 c	245	90	99	8	12	0	2	1.3	.6	.1
	Milk, canned:											
101	Sweetened condensed	1 c	306	27	982	24	166	0	27	16.8	7.4	1
102	Evaporated, whole	1 c	252	74	338	17	25	0	19	11.6	5.9	.6
103	Evaporated, nonfat	1 c	255	79	199	19	29	0	1	.3	.2	t
	Milk, dried:											
104	Buttermilk, sweet	1 c	120	3	464	41	59	0	7	4.3	2	.3
105	Instant, nonfat, envelope[2]	1 ea	91	4	325	32	47	0	1	.4	.2	t
106	Instant nonfat, cup	1 c	68	4	243	24	35	0	<1	.3	.1	t
107	Goat milk	1 c	244	87	167	9	11	0	10	6.5	2.7	.4
108	Kefir, 2% milkfat[3]	1 c	233	82	122	9	9	0	4	2.9	1.2	.1
	Milk beverages and powdered mixes:											
	Chocolate:											
109	Whole	1 c	250	82	208	8	26	4	8	5.2	2.5	.3
110	2% fat	1 c	250	84	178	8	26	4	5	3.1	1.5	.2
111	1% fat	1 c	250	84	157	8	26	4	2	1.5	.7	.1
	Chocolate-flavored beverages:											
112	Powder containing nonfat dry milk:	1 oz	28	1	102	3	22	<1	1	.7	.4	t
113	Prepared with water	¾ c	206	86	100	4	23	<1	1	.7	.4	t
114	Powder without nonfat dry milk:	¾ oz	22	1	77	1	20	1	1	.4	.2	t
115	Prepared with whole milk	1 c	266	81	226	9	31	<1	9	5.5	2.6	.3
116	Eggnog, commercial	1 c	254	74	340	10	34	0	19	11.3	5.7	.9
1027	Instant Breakfast, envelope, powder only:	1 ea	37	7	131	7	24	<1	1	.3	.1	t
1028	Prepared with whole milk	1 c	281	77	280	15	36	<1	9	5.4	2.5	.3
1029	Prepared with 2% milk	1 c	281	78	252	15	36	<1	5	3.3	1.5	.2
1283	Prepared with 1% milk	1 c	281	80	215	16	36	<1	1	.6	.3	t
1284	Prepared with nonfat milk	1 c	282	80	216	16	36	<1	1	.6	.3	t
117	Malted milk, chocolate, powder:[4]	¾ oz	21	1	79	1	18	<1	1	.5	.2	.1
118	Prepared with whole milk	1 c	265	81	228	9	30	1	9	5.5	2.6	.4
1661	Ovaltine with whole milk	1 c	265	81	225	9	29	1	9	5.5	2.6	.4
119	Malted milk, regular, powder:[4]	¾ oz	21	2	87	2	16	<1	2	.9	.4	.3
120	Prepared with whole milk	1 c	265	81	236	10	27	<1	10	5.9	2.8	.6
121	Milk shakes, chocolate (10 fl oz)	1¼ c	283	71	359	10	58	<1	10	6.5	3	.4
122	Milk shakes, vanilla (10 fl oz)	1¼ c	283	75	314	10	51	<1	8	5.3	2.4	.3

(1) Milk solids added, label claims less than 10 g protein per cup.

(2) Yields 1 qt fluid milk when reconstituted according to package directions.

(3) Most values provided by product labeling.

(4) The latest USDA data from *Handbook 8–14* on beverages updates previous USDA data.

(Computer code number is for West Diet Analysis program)

Chol (mg)	Calc (mg)	Iron (mg)	Magn (mg)	Phos (mg)	Pota (mg)	Sodi (mg)	Zinc (mg)	VT-A (RE)	Thia (mg)	Ribo (mg)	Niac (mg)	V-B6 (mg)	Fola (µg)	VT-C (mg)
0	6	.9	15	102	368	235	2.71	0	0	0	0	0	0	0
0	<1	.05	1	6	22	14	.16	0	0	0	0	0	0	0
13	266	.07	23	204	378	113	.87	5[5]	.09	.38	.17	.04	28	2
1	17	<.01	1	13	24	7	.06	<1[5]	.01	.02	.01	<.01	2	<1
33	290	.12	33	227	368	119	.93	76	.09	.39	.2	.1	12	2
18	295	.12	33	232	376	121	.95	139	.09	.4	.21	.1	12	2
18	311	.12	35	244	397	128	.98	140	.1	.42	.22	.11	13	2
10	300	.12	34	235	381	123	.95	144	.09	.41	.21	.1	12	2
10	311	.12	35	244	397	128	.98	145	.1	.42	.22	.11	13	2
4	301	.1	28	247	404	126	.98	149	.09	.34	.22	.1	13	2
5	316	.12	35	255	419	129	1	149	.1	.43	.22	.11	13	2
9	284	.12	27	218	370	257	1.03	20	.08	.38	.14	.08	12	2
103	866	.58	79	774	1135	389	2.88	248	.27	1.27	.64	.16	34	8
74	658	.48	61	512	764	267	1.94	136	.12	.8	.49	.13	20	5
9	737	.74	69	497	844	293	2.29	298	.11	.79	.44	.14	22	3
83	1419	.36	131	1119	1909	620	4.82	65	.47	1.9	1.05	.41	57	7
17	1118	.28	106	895	1550	500	4.01	646[6]	.38	1.59	.81	.31	45	5
12	836	.21	80	669	1158	373	3	483[6]	.28	1.19	.61	.23	34	4
28	325	.12	34	271	498	121	.73	137	.12	.34	.68	.11	1	3
10	350	.5	28	319	205	50	.9	155	.45	.44	.3	.09	20	1
30	280	.6	32	250	418	149	1.03	72	.09	.4	.31	.1	12	2
17	285	.6	33	255	423	150	1.03	143	.09	.41	.31	.1	12	2
7	285	.6	33	255	425	151	1.03	148	.09	.41	.32	.1	12	2
1	92	.34	23	89	202	143	.41	1	.03	.16	.17	.03	0	1
1	89	.29	23	88	223	139	1.26	1	.03	.17	.18	.04	3	1
0	8	.69	22	28	129	46	.34	<1	.01	.03	.11	<.01	1	<1
32	301	.8	53	255	497	164	1.28	77	.1	.43	.32	.1	12	2
149	330	.51	47	277	419	138	1.17	203	.09	.48	.27	.13	2	4
4	105	4.74	84	158	350	142	3.16	554	.31	.07	5.25	.42	105	28
38	396	4.86	117	385	719	262	4.09	630	.41	.47	5.46	.52	118	31
23	401	4.86	118	390	726	264	4.12	693	.41	.48	5.46	.53	118	31
9	405	4.82	112	404	752	267	4.13	701	.4	.42	5.45	.52	118	31
9	407	4.83	112	406	755	268	4.14	703	.4	.42	5.47	.52	118	31
1	13	.48	15	37	129	53	.17	4	.04	.04	.42	.03	4	<1
34	305	.61	48	265	498	172	1.09	79	.13	.44	.62	.13	16	3
35	385	3.79	53	313	621	244	1.17	902	.74	1.26	10.9	1.02	32	34
4	63	.15	19	75	159	104	.21	18	.11	.19	1.1	.09	10	1
37	355	.26	53	302	530	223	1.14	95	.2	.59	1.31	.19	22	3
37	320	.88	48	289	566	274	1.16	65	.16	.69	.46	.14	10	1
31	345	.25	34	289	492	232	1.02	91	.13	.51	.52	.15	9	2

(5)Vitamin A value is from beta-carotene used for coloring.

(6)With added vitamin A.

(For purposes of calculations, use "0" for t, <1, <.1, <.01, etc.)

A

Table A–1
Food Composition

Computer Code Number	Food Description	Measure	Wt (g)	H_2O (%)	Ener (kcal)	Prot (g)	Carb (g)	Dietary Fiber (g)	Fat (g)	Fat Breakdown (g) Sat	Mono	Poly
	DAIRY—Cont.											
	Milk desserts:											
134	Custard, baked	1 c	265	79	278	13	28	0	12	6.2	4	1
1548	Low-fat frozen dessert bars	1 ea	81	72	90	2	18	0	1	.2	.1	.4
	Ice cream, vanilla (about 10% fat):											
123	Hardened: ½ gallon	1 ea	1064	61	2138	37	251	0	117	72.4	33.8	4.4
124	Cup	1 c	133	61	267	5	31	0	15	9	4.2	.5
125	Fluid ounces	3 oz	50	61	101	2	12	0	5	3.4	1.6	.2
126	Soft serve	1 c	173	60	372	7	38	0	22	12.9	6	.8
	Ice cream, rich vanilla (16% fat):											
127	Hardened: ½ gallon	1 ea	1188	60	2554	49	264	0	154	88.9	41.5	5.5
128	Cup	1 c	148	57	357	5	33	0	24	14.8	6.9	.9
1724	Ben & Jerry's	½ c	106	64	230	4	21	0	17	11	–	–
	Ice milk, vanilla (about 4% fat):											
129	Hardened: ½ gallon	1 ea	1048	68	1456	40	238	0	45	27.7	12.9	1.7
130	Cup	1 c	131	68	182	5	30	0	6	3.5	1.6	.2
131	Soft serve (about 3% fat)	1 c	175	70	221	9	38	0	5	2.8	1.3	.2
	Pudding, canned (5-oz can = .55 cup):											
135	Chocolate	1 ea	142	69	189	4	32	<1	6	1	2.4	2
136	Tapioca	1 ea	142	74	169	3	27	<1	5	.9	2.2	1.9
137	Vanilla	1 ea	142	71	184	3	31	<1	5	.8	2.2	1.9
	Puddings, dry mix with whole milk:											
138	Chocolate, instant	1 c	260	74	289	8	49	<1	8	4.8	2.4	.5
139	Chocolate, regular, cooked	½ c	130	74	144	4	23	<1	4	2.7	1.3	.2
140	Rice, cooked	½ c	132	73	154	4	27	<1	4	2.3	1.1	.1
141	Tapioca, cooked	½ c	130	74	148	4	25	<1	4	2.3	1.1	.1
142	Vanilla, instant	½ c	130	73	148	4	26	<1	4	2.3	1.1	.2
143	Vanilla, regular, cooked	½ c	130	75	144	4	24	<1	4	2.4	1.1	.2
132	Sherbet (2% fat): ½ gallon	1 ea	1542	66	2127	17	469	<1	31	17.9	8.3	1.2
133	Cup	1 c	193	66	266	2	59	<1	4	2.2	1	.2
144	Soy milk	1 c	240	93	79	7	4	3	5	.5	.8	2
1584	Yogurt, frozen, low-fat[1]	½ c	87	65	138	3	21	–	5	3	1.4	.2
1512	Scoop	1 ea	79	74	78	4	15	0	<1	.1	t	t
	Yogurt, low-fat:											
1172	Fruit added with low-calorie sweetener	1 c	241	86	122	11	19	1	<1	.2	.1	t
145	Fruit added[2]	1 c	227	74	232	10	43	<1	2	1.6	.7	.1
146	Plain	1 c	227	85	143	12	16	0	4	2.3	1	.1
147	Vanilla or coffee flavor	1 c	227	79	193	11	31	0	3	1.8	.8	.1
148	Yogurt, made with nonfat milk	1 c	227	85	126	13	17	0	<1	.3	.1	t
149	Yogurt, made with whole milk	1 c	227	88	139	8	11	0	7	4.8	2	.2
	EGGS[3]											
	Raw, large:											
150	Whole, without shell	1 ea	50	75	74	6	1	0	5	1.5	1.9	.7
151	White	1 ea	33	88	17	4	<1	0	0	0	0	0
152	Yolk	1 ea	17	49	59	3	<1	0	5	1.6	1.9	.7

(1) Data is from 1992 USDA data on snacks and sweets.

(2) Carbohydrate and kcalories vary widely—consult label if more precise values are needed.

(3) This data is newest revised information from the USDA with 24% less cholesterol.

(Computer code number is for West Diet Analysis program)

Chol (mg)	Calc (mg)	Iron (mg)	Magn (mg)	Phos (mg)	Pota (mg)	Sodi (mg)	Zinc (mg)	VT-A (RE)	Thia (mg)	Ribo (mg)	Niac (mg)	V-B6 (mg)	Fola (μg)	VT-C (mg)
231	297	.79	37	299	405	204	1.4	255	.09	.6	.22	.13	26	1
1	81	.09	9	65	109	41	.26	38	.03	.11	.06	.03	3	1
468	1361	.96	149	1117	2117	851	7.34	1244	.44	2.55	1.23	.51	53	6
58	170	.12	19	140	265	106	.92	156	.05	.32	.15	.06	7	1
22	64	.04	7	52	99	40	.34	58	.02	.12	.06	.02	2	<1
157	227	.36	21	201	306	106	.9	266	.08	.31	.16	.08	16	1
1081	1556	2.49	143	1378	2102	725	6.18	1829	.58	2.16	1.13	.57	107	6
90	173	.07	16	141	235	83	.59	272	.06	.24	.12	.06	7	1
95	150	.36	–	–	–	55	–	225	–	–	–	–	–	0
147	1456	1.05	157	1142	2211	891	4.61	493	.61	2.78	.94	.68	63	6
18	182	.13	20	143	276	111	.58	62	.08	.35	.12	.08	8	1
21	275	.1	24	212	387	123	.93	51	.09	.35	.21	.08	10	1
4	128	.72	30	113	255	183	.6	31	.04	.22	.49	.04	4	<1
1	119	.33	11	112	147	167	.38	<1	.03	.14	.44	.14	6	<1
10	125	.18	11	96	160	191	.35	9	.03	.2	.36	.02	6	<1
29	265	.75	47	621	432	738	1.09	86	.09	.37	.25	.1	10	2
16	144	.47	19	121	212	134	.58	34	.04	.23	.13	.05	5	1
15	133	.5	16	110	165	140	.6	33	.1	.18	.6	.05	6	1
16	135	.08	16	107	172	157	.44	35	.04	.18	.09	.05	5	1
14	131	.09	16	256	166	372	.43	33	.04	.18	.1	.05	5	1
16	139	.06	17	107	177	208	.45	35	.04	.18	.1	.04	5	1
77	833	2.16	123	617	1480	709	7.4	310	.39	1.05	1.48	.52	62	31
10	104	.27	15	77	185	89	.93	39	.05	.13	.18	.07	8	4
0	10	1.39	46	117	338	29	.55	7	.39	.17	.35	.1	4	0
2	124	.26	12	112	184	76	.36	50	.03	.19	.25	.07	5	–
1	137	.07	13	108	176	53	.67	1	.03	.16	.08	.04	8	1
3	369	.61	41	291	550	139	1.83	6	.1	.45	.5	.11	32	26
10	345	.16	33	270	440	132	1.68	25	.08	.4	.22	.09	21	1
14	413	.18	39	325	529	159	2.02	36	.1	.49	.26	.11	25	2
11	388	.16	37	304	497	149	1.88	29	.09	.46	.24	.1	24	2
4	452	.2	43	354	579	173	2.2	5	.11	.53	.28	.12	28	2
29	272	.11	26	215	350	105	1.34	68	.07	.32	.17	.07	17	1
212	24	.72	5	89	60	63	.55	95	.03	.25	.04	.07	23	0
0	2	.01	4	4	48	55	<.01	0	<.01	.15	.03	<.01	1	0
212	23	.59	1	81	16	7	.52	97	.03	.11	<.01	.06	24	0

(For purposes of calculations, use "0" for t, <1, <.1, <.01, etc.)

Table A–1
Food Composition

Computer Code Number	Food Description	Measure	Wt (g)	H_2O (%)	Ener (kcal)	Prot (g)	Carb (g)	Dietary Fiber (g)	Fat (g)	Fat Breakdown (g) Sat	Mono	Poly
	EGGS—Cont.											
	Cooked:											
153	Fried in margarine	1 ea	46	69	91	6	1	0	7	1.9	2.8	1.3
154	Hard-cooked, shell removed	1 ea	50	75	77	6	1	0	5	1.6	2	.7
155	Hard-cooked, chopped	1 c	136	75	211	17	2	0	14	4.4	5.5	1.9
156	Poached, no added salt	1 ea	50	75	74	6	1	0	5	1.5	1.9	.7
157	Scrambled with milk & margarine	1 ea	61	73	101	7	1	0	7	2.2	2.9	1.3
1681	Egg substitute, liquid	½ c	126	82	106	15	1	0	4	.8	1.1	2
	FATS and OILS											
158	Butter: Stick	½ c	113	16	810	1	<1	0	92	56.7	26.4	3.4
159	Tablespoon	1 tbs	14	16	102	<1	<1	0	11	7.1	3.3	.4
160	Pat (about 1 tsp)[1]	1 ea	5	16	36	<1	<1	0	4	2.5	1.2	.2
1682	Whipped	1 tsp	3	16	23	<1	<1	0	3	1.6	.8	.1
	Fats, cooking:											
1363	Bacon fat	1 tbs	14	0	126	0	0	0	14	6.4	5.9	1.1
1362	Beef fat/tallow	1 c	205	0	1849	0	0	0	205	102	85.7	8.2
1364	Chicken fat	1 c	205	<1	1845	0	0	0	204	61.1	91.6	42.8
161	Vegetable shortening:	1 c	205	0	1812	0	0	0	205	51.5	91.2	53.5
162	Tablespoon	1 tbs	13	0	115	0	0	0	13	3.3	5.8	3.4
163	Lard:	1 c	205	0	1849	0	0	0	205	80.4	92.5	23
164	Tablespoon	1 tbs	13	0	117	0	0	0	13	5.1	5.9	1.5
	Margarine:											
165	Imitation (about 40% fat), soft:	1 c	227	58	783	1	1	0	88	17.5	35.6	31.3
166	Tablespoon	1 tbs	14	58	49	<1	<1	0	6	1.1	2.2	2
167	Regular, hard (about 80% fat):	½ c	113	16	812	1	1	0	91	17.9	40.5	28.7
168	Tablespoon	1 tbs	14	16	101	<1	<1	0	11	2.2	5	3.6
169	Pat	1 ea	5	16	36	<1	<1	0	4	.8	1.8	1.3
170	Regular, soft (about 80% fat):	1 c	227	16	1625	2	1	0	182	31.3	64.7	78.5
171	Tablespoon	1 tbs	14	16	100	<1	<1	0	11	1.9	4	4.8
172	Spread (about 60% fat), hard:	½ c	113	37	609	1	0	0	69	15.9	29.4	20.5
173	Tablespoon	1 tbs	14	37	75	<1	0	0	9	2	3.6	2.5
174	Pat[1]	1 ea	5	37	27	<1	0	0	3	.7	1.2	1
175	Spread (about 60% fat), soft:	1 c	227	37	1225	1	0	0	138	29.1	71.5	31.3
176	Tablespoon	1 tbs	14	37	76	<1	0	0	9	1.8	4.4	1.9
	Oils:											
1585	Canola:	1 c	218	0	1927	0	0	0	218	15.5	128	64.5
1586	Tablespoon	1 tbs	14	0	124	0	0	0	14	1	8.2	4.1
177	Corn:	1 c	218	0	1927	0	0	0	218	27.7	52.8	127
178	Tablespoon	1 tbs	14	0	124	0	0	0	14	1.8	3.4	8.2
179	Olive:	1 c	216	0	1909	0	0	0	216	29.2	159	18.4
180	Tablespoon	1 tbs	14	0	124	0	0	0	14	1.9	10.3	1.2
1683	Olive, extra virgin	1 tbs	14	<1	126	–	–	–	14	2	10.8	1.3
181	Peanut:	1 c	216	0	1909	0	0	0	216	36.5	99.8	69.1
182	Tablespoon	1 tbs	14	0	124	0	0	0	14	2.4	6.5	4.5

(1)Pat is 1" square, ⅓" thick; about 1 tsp; 90 per lb.

(Computer code number is for West Diet Analysis program)

PAGE KEY: A–2 = BEV A–4 = DAIRY A–10 = EGGS A–12 = FAT/OIL A–14 = FRUIT A–24 = BAKERY A–34 = GRAIN A–40 = FISH A–44 = MEATS A–48 = POULTRY A–50 = SAUSAGE A–52 = MIXED/FAST A–60 = NUTS/SEEDS A–62 = SWEETS A–66 = VEG/LEG A–78 = MISC A–80 = SOUPS/SAUCES A–84 = FAST A–96 = FRZN ENTREE A–98 = BABY FOODS

Chol (mg)	Calc (mg)	Iron (mg)	Magn (mg)	Phos (mg)	Pota (mg)	Sodi (mg)	Zinc (mg)	VT-A (RE)	Thia (mg)	Ribo (mg)	Niac (mg)	V-B6 (mg)	Fola (μg)	VT-C (mg)
211	25	.72	5	89	61	162	.55	114	.03	.24	.03	.07	17	0
212	25	.59	5	86	63	62	.52	84	.03	.26	.03	.06	22	0
577	68	1.62	14	234	171	169	1.43	228	.09	.7	.09	.17	60	0
211	24	.72	5	88	60	61	.55	95	.02	.21	.03	.06	17	0
214	43	.73	7	103	84	170	.61	119	.03	.27	.05	.07	18	<1
1	67	2.64	11	152	415	222	1.65	271	.14	.38	.14	<.01	19	0
247	27	.18	2	26	29	933[2]	.06	852[3]	.01	.04	.05	<.01	3	0
31	3	.02	<1	3	4	117[2]	.01	107[3]	<.01	<.01	.01	0	<1	0
11	1	.01	<1	1	1	41[2]	<.01	38[3]	0	<.01	<.01	0	<1	0
7	1	.01	<1	1	1	26[2]	<.01	24[3]	0	<.01	<.01	0	<1	0
14	<1	0	<1	0	<1	76	<.01	<1	0	0	0	0	0	0
223	0	0	0	27	<1	<1	0	0	0	0	0	0	0	0
174	0	0	0	0	0	0	0	351	0	0	0	0	0	0
0	0	0	0	0	0	0	0	0	0	0	0	0	0	0
0	0	0	0	0	0	0	0	0	0	0	0	0	0	0
194	<1	0	<1	6	<1	<1	.23	0	0	0	0	0	0	0
12	<1	0	<1	<1	<1	<1	.01	0	0	0	0	0	0	0
0	40	0	4	31	57	2176[4]	.23	2254[5]	.01	.05	.03	.01	2	<1
0	3	0	<1	2	4	136[4]	.01	141[5]	<.01	<.01	<.01	<.01	<1	<1
0	34	.07	3	26	48	1065[4]	.23	1122[5]	.01	.04	.03	.01	1	<1
0	4	.01	<1	3	6	132[4]	.03	139[5]	<.01	<.01	<.01	<.01	<1	<1
0	1	<.01	<1	1	2	47[4]	.01	50[5]	<.01	<.01	<.01	0	<1	<1
0	60	0	5	46	86	2444[4]	.46	2254[5]	.02	.07	.04	.02	2	<1
0	4	0	<1	3	5	151[4]	.03	139[5]	<.01	<.01	<.01	<.01	<1	<1
0	24	0	2	18	34	1122[4]	.17	1122[5]	.01	.03	.02	.01	1	<1
0	3	0	<1	2	4	139[4]	.02	139[5]	<.01	<.01	<.01	<.01	<1	<1
0	1	0	<1	1	1	50[4]	0	50[5]	0	<.01	<.01	0	<1	<1
0	47	0	4	36	68	2256[4]	0	2254[5]	.02	.06	.04	.01	2	<1
0	3	0	<1	2	4	139[4]	0	139[5]	<.01	<.01	<.01	<.01	<1	<1
0	0	0	0	0	0	0	0	0	0	0	0	0	0	0
0	0	0	0	0	0	0	0	0	0	0	0	0	0	0
0	0	.01	0	2	4	0	.02	0	0	0	0	0	0	0
0	0	<.01	0	<1	<1	0	<.01	0	0	0	0	0	0	0
0	<1	.82	<1	3	0	<1	.13	0	0	0	0	0	0	0
0	<1	.05	<1	<1	0	<1	.01	0	0	0	0	0	0	0
0	–	–	–	–	–	–	–	0	0	0	0	0	0	0
0	<1	.06	<1	0	<1	<1	.02	0	0	0	0	0	0	0
0	<1	<.01	<1	0	<1	<1	<.01	0	0	0	0	0	0	0

(2)For salted butter, unsalted butter contains 12 mg sodium per stick or ½ c, 1.5 mg/tbs, or .5 mg/pat.

(3)Values for vitamin A are a year-round average.

(4)For salted margarine.

(5)Based on average vitamin A content of fortified margarine. Federal specifications require a minimum of 15,000 IU/lb.

A

Table A–1
Food Composition

Computer Code Number	Food Description	Measure	Wt (g)	H_2O (%)	Ener (kcal)	Prot (g)	Carb (g)	Dietary Fiber (g)	Fat (g)	Fat Breakdown (g) Sat	Mono	Poly
	FATS and OILS—Cont.											
	Oils—Cont.											
183	Safflower:	1 c	218	0	1927	0	0	0	218	19.8	26.4	162
184	Tablespoon	1 tbs	14	0	124	0	0	0	14	1.3	1.7	10.4
185	Soybean:	1 c	218	0	1927	0	0	0	218	31.4	50.8	126
186	Tablespoon	1 tbs	14	0	124	0	0	0	14	2	3.3	8.1
187	Soybean/cottonseed:	1 c	218	0	1927	0	0	0	218	39.2	64.3	105
188	Tablespoon	1 tbs	14	0	124	0	0	0	14	2.5	4.1	6.7
189	Sunflower:	1 c	218	0	1927	0	0	0	218	22.7	42.5	143
190	Tablespoon	1 tbs	14	0	124	0	0	0	14	1.5	2.7	9.2
	Salad dressings/sandwich spreads:											
191	Blue cheese, regular	1 tbs	15	32	76	1	1	<1	8	1.5	1.9	4.4
1040	Low calorie	1 tbs	15	79	15	1	<1	<1	1	.2	.5	.4
1684	Caesar's	1 tbs	12	36	52	1	<1	<1	5	.9	3.5	.5
192	French, regular	1 tbs	16	38	67	<1	3	<1	9	1.5	1.2	3.4
193	Low calorie	1 tbs	16	69	21	<1	3	<1	1	.1	.2	.5
194	Italian, regular	1 tbs	15	38	69	<1	1	<1	9	1	1.6	4.1
195	Low calorie	1 tbs	15	82	8	<1	1	<1	1	t	.1	.2
199	Mayo type, regular	1 tbs	15	40	58	<1	3	0	5	.7	1.4	2.7
1030	Low calorie	1 tbs	15	81	20	<1	1	0	3	.3	.8	1.4
196	Mayonnaise:											
196	Regular (soybean)	1 tbs	14	15	99	<1	<1	0	11	1.6	3.1	5.7
197	Imitation, low calorie	1 tbs	15	63	35	<1	2	0	3	.5	.7	1.6
1488	Regular, low calorie, low sodium	1 tbs	14	63	32	<1	2	0	3	.5	.6	1.4
1493	Regular, low calorie	1 tbs	16	63	36	<1	2	0	3	.5	.7	1.6
198	Ranch, regular	½ c	119	35	436	4	5	0	45	6.7	19.4	17
1042	Low calorie	1 tbs	15	40	31	0	1	–	3	0	–	1
1685	Russian	1 tbs	15	34	76	<1	2	0	8	1.1	1.8	4.5
1502	Salad dressing, low calorie, oil free	1 tbs	15	88	4	<1	1	<1	<1	0	0	0
	Salad dressing, no cholesterol											
1605	(Miracle Whip)	1 tbs	15	57	48	0	2	0	4	1.1	1.1	2.1
203	Salad dressing, from recipe, cooked[1]	1 tbs	16	69	25	1	2	0	2	.5	.6	.3
200	Tartar sauce, regular	1 tbs	14	34	74	<1	1	<1	8	1.5	2.6	4.1
1503	Low calorie	1 tbs	14	63	31	<1	2	<1	2	.4	.6	1.3
201	Thousand island, regular	1 tbs	16	46	60	<1	2	<1	6	1	1.3	3.2
202	Low calorie	1 tbs	15	69	25	<1	2	<1	2	.2	.4	.9
204	Vinegar & oil	1 tbs	16	47	72	0	<1	0	8	1.5	2.4	3.9
	FRUITS and FRUIT JUICES											
	Apples:											
	Fresh, raw, with peel:											
205	2 ¾" diam (about 3 per lb w/cores)	1 ea	138	84	81	<1	21	3	<1	.1	t	.1
206	3 ¼" diam (about 2 per lb w/cores)	1 ea	212	84	125	<1	32	4	1	.1	t	.2
207	Raw, peeled slices	1 c	110	84	63	<1	16	2	<1	.1	t	.1
208	Dried, sulfured	10 ea	64	32	155	1	42	6	<1	t	t	.1

(1)Fatty acid values apply to product made with regular margarine.

Chol (mg)	Calc (mg)	Iron (mg)	Magn (mg)	Phos (mg)	Pota (mg)	Sodi (mg)	Zinc (mg)	VT-A (RE)	Thia (mg)	Ribo (mg)	Niac (mg)	V-B6 (mg)	Fola (µg)	VT-C (mg)
0	0	.01	0	0	0	0	.41	0	0	0	0	0	0	0
0	0	<.01	0	0	0	0	.03	0	0	0	0	0	0	0
0	<1	.04	<1	1	0	0	.4	0	0	0	0	0	0	0
0	<1	<.01	<1	<1	0	0	.03	0	0	0	0	0	0	0
0	0	.02	<1	0	0	0	.4	0	0	0	0	0	0	0
0	0	<.01	<1	0	0	0	.03	0	0	0	0	0	0	0
0	0	.06	<1	0	0	<1	0	0	0	0	0	0	0	0
0	0	<.01	<1	0	0	<1	0	0	0	0	0	0	0	0
3	12	.03	<1	11	6	167	.04	10	<.01	.02	.01	.01	3	<1
<1	14	.08	1	13	1	184	.04	<1	<.01	.01	.01	<.01	<1	<1
11	21	.19	3	18	19	194	.12	6	<.01	.02	.47	.01	2	<1
0	2	.06	2	1	2	188	.01	3	<.01	<.01	<.01	<.01	1	0
1	2	.06	0	2	13	126	.03	0	0	0	0	0	0	0
0	1	.03	<1	1	5	116	.02	3	<.01	<.01	0	<.01	1	0
0	<1	.03	<1	1	2	120	.02	0	0	0	0	0	0	0
4	2	.03	<1	4	1	105	0	13	<.01	<.01	<.01	<.01	1	0
7	3	.03	–	4	1	18	.02	10	<.01	<.01	0	–	0	0
8	2	.07	<1	4	5	78	.02	12	0	0	<.01	.08	1	0
4	<1	0	<1	<1	1	75	.02	0	0	0	0	0	0	0
3	0	0	0	0	1	15	.01	1	0	<.01	0	0	<1	0
4	<1	0	<1	<1	2	77	02	0	0	0	0	0	0	0
47	119	.31	12	100	158	522	.44	86	.04	.17	.08	.05	6	1
5	–	–	–	–	5	153	–	–	–	–	–	–	–	–
3	3	.09	<1	6	24	133	.07	32	.01	.01	.09	<.01	2	1
0	1	.04	2	1	7	256	<.01	<1	0	0	<.01	<.01	<1	<1
0	0	<.01	0	0	0	102	0	2	0	0	0	0	0	0
9	13	.08	0	14	19	117	0	20	.01	.02	.04	0	0	<1
7	3	.13	<1	4	11	99	.02	9	<.01	<.01	0	<.01	1	<1
3	2	.09	<1	1	6	82	.02	2	0	<.01	.01	<.01	<1	<1
4	2	.09	<1	3	18	110	.02	15	<.01	<.01	<.01	<.01	1	<1
2	2	.09	1	3	17	153	.02	14	<.01	<.01	.03	<.01	1	<1
0	0	0	0	0	1	<1	0	0	0	0	0	0	0	0
0	10	.25	7	10	157	0	.05	7	.02	.02	.11	.07	4	8
0	15	.38	11	15	242	0	.08	11	.04	.03	.16	.1	6	12
0	4	.08	3	8	124	0	.04	4	.02	.01	.1	.05	<1	4
0	9	.9	10	24	288	56[2]	.13	0	0	.1	.59	.08	0	2

(2)Sodium bisulfite used to preserve color; unsulfured product would contain lower levels of sodium.

(For purposes of calculations, use "0" for t, <1, <.1, <.01, etc.)

A

A

Table A–1
Food Composition

Computer Code Number	Food Description	Measure	Wt (g)	H_2O (%)	Ener (kcal)	Prot (g)	Carb (g)	Dietary Fiber (g)	Fat (g)	Fat Breakdown (g) Sat	Mono	Poly
	FRUITS and FRUIT JUICES—Cont.											
209	Apple juice, bottled or canned	1 c	248	88	116	<1	29	<1	<1	t	t	.1
210	Applesauce, sweetened	1 c	255	80	193	<1	51	3	<1	.1	t	.1
211	Applesauce, unsweetened	1 c	244	88	104	<1	28	4	<1	t	t	t
	Apricots:											
212	Raw, w/o pits (about 12 per lb w/ pits)	3 ea	106	86	51	1	12	2	<1	t	.2	.1
	Canned (fruit and liquid):											
213	Heavy syrup	1 c	258	78	214	1	55	3	<1	t	.1	t
214	Halves	3 ea	85	78	70	<1	18	1	<1	t	t	t
215	Juice pack	1 c	248	87	119	2	30	4	<1	t	t	t
216	Halves	3 ea	84	87	40	1	10	1	<1	t	t	t
217	Dried, halves	10 ea	35	31	83	1	22	3	<1	t	.1	t
218	Dried, cooked, unsweetened, w/liquid	1 c	250	76	212	3	55	8	<1	t	.2	.1
219	Apricot nectar, canned	1 c	251	85	140	1	36	2	<1	t	.1	t
	Avocados, raw, edible part only:											
220	California (2 lb with refuse)	1 ea	173	73	306	4	12	5	30	4.5	19.4	3.5
221	Florida (1 lb with refuse)	1 ea	304	80	340	5	27	18	27	5.3	14.8	4.5
222	Mashed, fresh, average	1 c	230	74	370	5	17	14	35	5.6	22.1	4.5
	Bananas, raw, without peel:											
223	Whole, 8¾" long (175 g w/peel)	1 ea	114	74	104	1	27	2	1	.2	t	.1
224	Slices	1 c	150	74	137	2	35	3	1	.3	.1	.1
1285	Bananas, dehydrated slices	1 oz	28	3	98	1	25	2	1	.2	t	.1
225	Blackberries, raw	1 c	144	86	75	1	18	7	1	.3	.1	.1
	Blueberries:											
226	Fresh	1 c	145	85	81	1	20	3	1	t	.2	.3
227	Frozen, sweetened	10 oz	284	77	230	1	62	7	<1	.1	.1	.2
228	Frozen, thawed	1 c	230	77	186	1	50	5	<1	.1	.1	.2
	Cherries:											
229	Sour, red pitted, canned water pack	1 c	244	90	88	2	22	2	<1	.1	.1	.1
230	Sweet, red pitted, raw	10 ea	68	81	49	1	11	1	1	.1	.2	.2
231	Cranberry juice cocktail[1]	1 c	253	85	144	0[2]	36	1	<1	.1	t	.1
1411	Cranberry juice, low calorie	¾ c	178	95	34	0	8	1	0	0	0	0
232	Cranberry-apple juice	1 c	253	83	169	<1	43	<1	<1[3]	t	t	.1
233	Cranberry sauce, canned, strained	1 c	277	61	418	1	107	6	<1	t	.1	.2
234	Dates, whole, without pits	10 ea	83	22	228	2	61	7	<1	.2	.1	t
235	Dates, chopped	1 c	178	22	490	4	130	15	1	.3	.2	t
236	Figs, dried	10 ea	187	28	477	6	122	17	2	.4	.5	1
	Fruit cocktail, canned, fruit and liq:											
237	Heavy syrup pack	1 c	255	80	186	1	48	3	<1	t	t	.1
238	Juice pack	1 c	248	87	114	1	29	3	<1	t	t	t
	Grapefruit:											
	Raw 3¾" diam (half w/rind = 241 g)											
239	Pink/red, half fruit, edible part	1 ea	123	91	37	1	9	1	<1	t	t	t
240	White, half fruit, edible part	1 ea	118	90	39	1	10	1	<1	t	t	t
241	Canned sections with light syrup	1 c	254	84	152	1	39	1	<1	t	t	.1

(1)Data here are from the newest USDA *Handbook 8–14* on beverages. These data are somewhat different from that presented in *Handbook 8–9* on fruits and fruit juices.

(2)The newest USDA *Handbook 8–14* data on beverages indicates "0" for protein.

(3)The newest USDA *Handbook 8–14* data on beverages indicates "0" for fat.

PAGE KEY: A–2 = BEV A–4 = DAIRY A–10 = EGGS A–12 = FAT/OIL A–14 = FRUIT A–24 = BAKERY A–34 = GRAIN A–40 = FISH A–44 = MEATS A–48 = POULTRY A–50 = SAUSAGE A–52 = MIXED/FAST A–60 = NUTS/SEEDS A–62 = SWEETS A–66 = VEG/LEG A–78 = MISC A–80 = SOUPS/SAUCES A–84 = FAST A–96 = FRZN ENTREE A–98 = BABY FOODS

Chol (mg)	Calc (mg)	Iron (mg)	Magn (mg)	Phos (mg)	Pota (mg)	Sodi (mg)	Zinc (mg)	VT-A (RE)	Thia (mg)	Ribo (mg)	Niac (mg)	V-B6 (mg)	Fola (μg)	VT-C (mg)
0	17	.92	7	17	295	7	.07	<1	.05	.04	.25	.07	<1	2
0	10	.89	8	18	155	8	.1	3	.03	.07	.48	.07	2	4[4]
0	7	.29	7	17	183	5	.07	7	.03	.06	.46	.06	1	3[4]
0	15	.57	8	20	313	1	.28	277	.03	.04	.64	.06	9	11
0	23	.77	18	31	361	10	.28	317	.05	.06	.97	.14	4	8
0	8	.25	6	10	119	3	.09	105	.02	.02	.32	.05	1	3
0	30	.74	25	50	409	10	.27	419	.04	.05	.85	.13	4	12
0	10	.25	8	17	139	3	.09	142	.01	.02	.29	.04	1	4
0	16	1.65	16	41	482	3	.26	253	<.01	.05	1.05	.05	4	1
0	40	4.18	42	102	1222	7	.66	590	.01	.07	2.36	.28	0	4
0	18	.95	13	23	286	8	.23	331	.02	.03	.65	.05	3	2[5]
0	19	2.04	71	73	1096	21	.73	106	.19	.21	3.32	.48	113	14
0	33	1.61	103	118	1483	15	1.28	185	.33	.37	5.84	.85	162	24
0	25	2.35	90	94	1377	23	.97	140	.25	.28	4.42	.64	142	18
0	7	.35	33	23	451	1	.18	9	.05	.11	.62	.66	22	10
0	9	.46	43	30	594	1	.24	12	.07	.15	.81	.87	29	14
0	6	.33	31	21	423	1	.17	9	.05	.07	.79	.15	11	2
0	46	.82	29	30	282	0	.39	23	.04	.06	.58	.08	49	30
0	9	.25	7	14	129	9	.16	14	.07	.07	.52	.05	9	19
0	17	1.11	6	20	170	3	.17	11	.06	.15	.72	.17	19	3
0	14	.9	5	16	138	2	.14	9	.05	.12	.58	.14	15	2
0	27	3.34	15	24	239	17	.17	183	.04	.1	.43	.11	19	5
0	10	.26	7	13	152	0	.04	14	.03	.04	.27	.02	3	5
0	8	.38	5	5	45	5	.18	1	.02	.02	.09	.05	1	90[6]
0	16	.07	4	2	39	5	.04	1	.02	.02	.06	.03	<1	57
0	18	.15	5	8	68	5	.1	1	.01	.05	.15	.05	1	81[6]
0	11	.61	8	17	72	80	.14	6	.04	.06	.28	.04	2	6
0	27	.95	29	33	541	2	.24	4	.07	.08	1.83	.16	10	0
0	57	2.05	62	71	1160	5	.52	9	.16	.18	3.92	.34	22	0
0	269	4.17	110	127	1331	21	.95	24	.13	.16	1.3	.42	14	1
0	15	.74	13	28	224	15	.2	51	.05	.05	.95	.13	7	5
0	20	.52	17	35	235	10	.22	77	.03	.04	1	.13	6	7
0	13	.15	10	11	157	0	.09	32[7]	.04	.02	.23	.05	15	47
0	14	.07	11	9	173	0	.08	1	.04	.02	.32	.05	12	39
0	36	1.02	25	25	328	5	.2	0	.1	.05	.62	.05	22	54

(4) Value based on products without added vitamin C. Bottled apple juice with added vitamin C usually contains 41.6 mg/100 g, or 103 mg per cup. Check label for specific vitamin C values.

(5) Without added vitamin C. Products with added vitamin C contain 136 mg per cup. Check label.

(6) Nutrient added.

(7) Vitamin A in Texas red grapefruit would be 74 RE.

(For purposes of calculations, use "0" for t, <1, <.1, <.01, etc.)

Table A–1
Food Composition

Computer Code Number	Food Description	Measure	Wt (g)	H_2O (%)	Ener (kcal)	Prot (g)	Carb (g)	Dietary Fiber (g)	Fat (g)	Fat Breakdown (g) Sat	Mono	Poly
	FRUITS and FRUIT JUICES—Cont.											
	Grapefruit juice:											
242	Fresh, raw	1 c	247	90	96	1	23	<1	<1	t	t	.1
243	Canned, unsweetened	1 c	247	90	94	1	22	<1	<1	t	t	.1
244	Sweetened	1 c	250	87	115	1	28	<1	<1	t	t	.1
	Frozen concentrate, unsweetened:											
245	Undiluted, 6-fl-oz can	¾ c	207	62	302	4	71	3	1	.1	.1	.2
246	Diluted with 3 cans water	1 c	247	89	101	1	24	<1	<1	t	t	.1
	Grapes, raw European (adherent skin):											
247	Thompson seedless	10 ea	50	81	35	<1	9	<1	<1	.1	t	.1
248	Tokay/Emperor, seeded types	10 ea	57	81	40	<1	10	<1	<1	.1	t	.1
	Grape juice:											
249	Bottled or canned	1 c	253	84	154	1	38	2	<1	.1	t	.1
	Frozen concentrate, sweetened:											
250	Undiluted, 6-fl-oz can	¾ c	216	54	387	1	96	5	1	.2	t	.2
251	Diluted with 3 cans water	1 c	250	87	127	<1	32	2	<1	.1	t	.1
1410	Low calorie	1 c	250	84	153	1	37	<1	<1	.1	t	.1
252	Kiwi fruit, raw, peeled (88 g with peel)	1 ea	76	83	46	1	11	3	<1	t	.1	.1
253	Lemons, raw, without peel and seeds (about 4 per lb whole)	1 ea	58	89	17	1	5	1	<1	t	t	.1
	Lemon juice:											
254	Fresh:	1 c	244	91	61	1	21	1	<1	.1	t	.2
255	Tablespoon	1 tbs	15	91	4	<1	1	<1	<1	t	t	t
256	Canned or bottled, unsweetened:	1 c	244	92	51	1	16	1	1	.1	t	.2
257	Tablespoon	1 tbs	15	92	3	<1	1	<1	<1	t	t	t
258	Frozen, single strength, unsweetened:	1 c	244	92	54	1	16	1	1	.1	t	.2
259	Tablespoon	1 tbs	15	92	3	<1	1	<1	<1	t	t	t
	Lime juice:											
260	Fresh:	1 c	246	90	66	1	22	1	<1	t	t	.1
261	Tablespoon	1 tbs	15	90	4	<1	1	<1	<1	t	t	t
262	Canned or bottled, unsweetened	1 c	246	92	52	1	16	1	1	.1	.1	.2
263	Mangoes, raw, edible part (300 g w/skin & seeds)	1 ea	207	82	134	1	35	4	1	.1	.2	.1
	Melons, raw, without rind and contents:											
264	Cantaloupe, 5" diam (2 ⅓ lb whole with refuse), orange flesh	½ ea	267	90	93	2	22	2	1	.1	.1	.2
265	Honeydew, 6½" diam (5¼ lb whole with refuse), slice = ⅒ melon	1 pce	129	90	45	1	12	1	<1	t	t	t
266	Nectarines, raw, w/o pits, 2½" diam	1 ea	136	86	67	1	16	3	1	.1	.2	.3
	Oranges, raw:											
267	Whole w/o peel and seeds, 2 ⅝" diam (180 g with peel and seeds)	1 ea	131	87	62	1	15	3	<1	t	t	t
268	Sections, without membranes	1 c	180	87	85	2	21	4	<1	t	t	t

(Computer code number is for West Diet Analysis program)

Chol (mg)	Calc (mg)	Iron (mg)	Magn (mg)	Phos (mg)	Pota (mg)	Sodi (mg)	Zinc (mg)	VT-A (RE)	Thia (mg)	Ribo (mg)	Niac (mg)	V-B6 (mg)	Fola (µg)	VT-C (mg)
0	22	.49	30	37	400	2	.12	2[1]	.1	.05	.49	.11	25	94
0	17	.49	25	27	378	2	.22	2	.1	.05	.57	.05	26	72
0	20	.9	25	27	405	5	.15	0	.1	.06	.8	.05	26	67
0	56	1.01	79	101	1001	6	.37	6	.3	.16	1.6	.32	26	246
0	20	.35	27	35	336	2	.12	2	.1	.05	.54	.11	9	83
0	5	.13	3	6	92	1	.02	3	.05	.03	.15	.05	2	5
0	6	.15	3	7	105	1	.03	4	.05	.03	.17	.06	2	6
0	23	.61	25	28	334	8	.13	3	.07	.09	.66	.16	7	<1
0	28	.78	32	32	159	15	.28	6	.11	.2	.93	.32	9	179[2]
0	10	.25	10	10	52	5	.1	2	.04	.06	.31	.1	3	60[2]
0	22	.6	25	27	330	7	.12	2	.06	.09	.65	.16	6	<1
0	20	.31	23	30	252	4	.08[3]	14	.01	.04	.38	.04	17	74
0	15	.35	5	9	80	1	.03	2	.02	.01	.06	.05	6	31
0	17	.07	15	15	303	2	.12	5	.07	.02	.24	.12	31	112
0	1	<.01	1	1	19	<1	.01	<1	<.01	<.01	.01	.01	2	7
0	27	.32	19	22	249	51	.15	5	.1	.02	.48	.1	25	60
0	2	.02	1	1	15	3	.01	<1	.01	<.01	.03	.01	2	4
0	19	.29	19	19	217	2	.12	2	.14	.03	.33	.15	23	77
0	1	.02	1	1	13	<1	.01	<1	.01	<.01	.02	.01	1	5
0	22	.07	15	17	268	2	.15	2	.05	.02	.25	.11	20	72
0	1	<.01	1	1	16	<1	.01	<1	<.01	<.01	.01	.01	1	4
0	29	.57	17	25	184	39[4]	.15	5	.08	.01	.4	.07	19	16
0	21	.27	19	23	323	4	.08	805	.12	.12	1.21	.28	39	57
0	29	.56	29	45	825	24	.43	860	.1	.06	1.53	.31	45	113
0	8	.09	9	13	350	13	.11	5	.1	.02	.77	.08	39	32
0	7	.2	11	22	288	0	.12	101	.02	.06	1.35	.03	5	7
0	52	.13	13	18	237	0	.09	27	.11	.05	.37	.08	40	70
0	72	.18	18	25	326	0	.13	38	.16	.07	.51	.11	54	96

(1)This is vitamin A for white grapefruit juice; pink or red grapefruit juice = 109 RE per cup.

(2)With added vitamin C (ascorbic acid).

(3)Data are estimated from other fruit data.

(4)Sodium benzoate and sodium bisulfite added as preservatives.

(For purposes of calculations, use "0" for t, <1, <.1, <.01, etc.)

Table A–1
Food Composition

Computer Code Number	Food Description	Measure	Wt (g)	H_2O (%)	Ener (kcal)	Prot (g)	Carb (g)	Dietary Fiber (g)	Fat (g)	Fat Breakdown (g) Sat	Mono	Poly
	FRUITS and FRUIT JUICES—Cont.											
	Orange juice:											
269	Fresh, all varieties	1 c	248	88	111	2	26	<1	<1	.1	.1	.1
270	Canned, unsweetened	1 c	249	89	104	1	24	<1	<1	t	.1	.1
271	Chilled	1 c	249	88	109	2	25	<1	1	.1	.1	.2
	Frozen concentrate:											
272	Undiluted (6-oz can)	¾ c	213	58	339	5	81	1	<1	.1	.1	.1
273	Diluted w/3 parts water by volume	1 c	249	88	112	2	27	<1	<1	t	t	t
1345	Orange juice, from dry crystals	1 c	248	88	114	0	29	0	<1	t	t	t
274	Orange and grapefruit juice, canned	1 c	247	89	106	1	25	<1	<1	t	t	t
	Papayas, raw:											
275	½" slices	1 c	140	89	54	1	14	2	<1	.1	.1	t
276	Whole, 3½" diam by 5⅛" w/o seeds and skin (1 lb w/refuse)	1 ea	304	89	118	2	30	5	<1	.1	.1	.1
1031	Papaya nectar, canned	1 c	250	85	142	<1	36	1	<1	.1	.1	.1
	Peaches:											
277	Raw, whole, 2½" diam, peeled, pitted (about 4 per lb whole)	1 ea	87	88	37	1	10	1	<1	t	t	t
278	Raw, sliced	1 c	170	88	73	1	19	3	<1	t	.1	.1
	Canned, fruit and liquid:											
279	Heavy syrup pack:	1 c	256	79	189	1	51	3	<1	t	.1	.1
280	Half	1 ea	81	79	60	<1	16	1	<1	t	t	t
281	Juice pack:	1 c	248	87	109	2	29	2	<1	t	t	t
282	Half	1 ea	77	87	34	<1	9	1	<1	t	t	t
283	Dried, uncooked	10 ea	130	32	309	5	80	11	1	.1	.4	.5
284	Dried, cooked, fruit and liquid	1 c	258	78	198	3	51	7	1	.1	.2	.3
	Frozen, slice, sweetened:											
285	10-oz package	1 ea	284	75	266	2	68	4	<1	t	.1	.2
286	Cup, thawed measure	1 c	250	75	235	2	60	4	<1	t	.1	.2
1032	Peach nectar, canned	1 c	249	86	134	1	35	1	<1	t	t	t
	Pears:											
	Fresh, with skin, cored:											
287	Bartlett, 2½" diam (about 2½ per lb)	1 ea	166	84	98	1	25	4[1]	1	t	.1	.2
288	Bosc, 2 1/5" diam (about 3 per lb)	1 ea	141	84	83	1	21	4[1]	1	t	.1	.1
289	D'Anjou, 3" diam (about 2 per lb)	1 ea	200	84	118	1	30	5[1]	1	t	.2	.2
	Canned, fruit and liquid:											
290	Heavy syrup pack:	1 c	255	80	188	1	49	5[1]	<1	t	.1	.1
291	Half	1 ea	79	80	58	<1	15	2[1]	<1	t	t	t
292	Juice pack:	1 c	248	86	124	1	32	5[1]	<1	t	t	t
293	Half	1 ea	77	86	38	<1	10	2[1]	<1	t	t	t
294	Dried halves	10 ea	175	27	459	3	121	23	1	.1	.2	.3
1033	Pear nectar, canned	1 c	250	84	150	<1	39	2	<1	t	t	t
	Pineapple:											
295	Fresh chunks, diced	1 c	155	86	76	1	19	2	1	t	.1	.2
	Canned, fruit and liquid:											
	Heavy syrup pack:											
296	Crushed, chunks, tidbits	⅓ c	84	79	65	<1	17	1	<1	t	t	t
297	Slices	1 ea	58	79	45	<1	12	<1	<1	t	t	t

[1]Dietary fiber data vary 2.4 to 3.4 g/100 g for fresh pears; 1.6 to 2.6 g/100 g for canned pears.

Chol (mg)	Calc (mg)	Iron (mg)	Magn (mg)	Phos (mg)	Pota (mg)	Sodi (mg)	Zinc (mg)	VT-A (RE)	Thia (mg)	Ribo (mg)	Niac (mg)	V-B6 (mg)	Fola (µg)	VT-C (mg)
0	27	.5	27	42	496	2	.12	50	.22	.07	.99	.1	75	124
0	20	1.1	27	35	436	5	.17	45	.15	.07	.78	.22	45	86
0	25	.42	27	27	473	2	.1	20[2]	.28	.05	.7	.13	45[2]	82[2]
0	68	.75	72	121	1435	6	.38	60	.6	.14	1.53	.33	330	294
0	22	.25	25	40	473	2	.12	20	.2	.04	.5	.11	109	97
0	62	.2	2	37	50	12	.1	551	<.01	.04	0	0	142	121
0	20	1.14	25	35	390	7	.17	30	.14	.07	.83	.06	35	72
0	34	.14	14	7	360	4	.1	39	.04	.04	.47	.03	53	86
0	73	.3	30	15	781	9	.21	85	.08	.1	1.03	.06	115	187
0	25	.85	7	0	77	12	.37	27	.01	.01	.37	.02	5	7
0	4	.1	6	10	171	0	.12	47	.01	.04	.86	.02	3	6
0	8	.19	12	20	335	0	.24	92	.03	.07	1.68	.03	6	11
0	8	.69	13	28	235	15	.23	84	.03	.06	1.57	.05	8	7
0	2	.22	4	9	74	5	.07	27	.01	.02	.5	.01	3	2
0	15	.67	17	42	317	10	.27	94	.02	.04	1.44	.05	8	9
0	5	.21	5	13	99	3	.08	29	.01	.01	.45	.01	3	3
0	36	5.28	55	153	1293	9	.74	281	<.01	.28	5.69	.09	<1	6
0	23	3.38	33	98	826	5	.46	52	.01	.05	3.92	.1	<1	10
0	9	1.05	14	31	369	17	.14	79	.04	.1	1.85	.05	9	267[3]
0	7	.92	12	27	325	15	.12	70	.03	.09	1.63	.04	8	236[3]
0	12	.47	10	15	100	17	.2	65	.01	.03	.72	.02	3	13
0	18	.41	10	18	208	0	.2	3	.03	.07	.17	.03	12	7
0	15	.35	8	15	176	0	.17	3	.03	.06	.14	.02	10	6
0	22	.5	12	22	250	0	.24	4	.04	.08	.2	.04	15	8
0	13	.56	10	18	165	13	.2	1	.03	.06	.62	.04	3	3
0	4	.17	3	6	51	4	.06	<1	.01	.02	.19	.01	1	1
0	22	.72	17	30	238	10	.22	2	.03	.03	.5	.03	3	4
0	7	.22	5	9	74	3	.07	1	.01	.01	.15	.01	1	1
0	59	3.68	58	103	933	10	.68	1	.01	.25	2.4	.13	0	12
0	12	.65	7	7	32	10	.17	<1	<.01	.03	.32	.03	3	3
0	11	.57	22	11	175	2	.12	3	.14	.06	.65	.13	16	24
0	12	.32	13	6	87	1	.1	1	.08	.02	.24	.06	4	6
0	8	.22	9	4	60	1	.07	1	.05	.01	.17	.04	3	4

(2) Values for juice from California oranges indicate the following values for 1 c: 36 RE of vitamin A, 72 µg of folate, and 106 mg of vitamin C.

(3) With added vitamin C (ascorbic acid).

A

Table A–1
Food Composition

Computer Code Number	Food Description	Measure	Wt (g)	H_2O (%)	Ener (kcal)	Prot (g)	Carb (g)	Dietary Fiber (g)	Fat (g)	Fat Breakdown (g)		
										Sat	Mono	Poly
	FRUITS and FRUIT JUICES—Cont.											
	Pineapple, canned—Cont.											
298	Juice pack, crushed, chunks, tidbits	1 c	250	83	150	1	39	2	<1	t	t	.1
299	Juice pack, slices	1 ea	58	83	35	<1	9	<1	<1	t	t	t
300	Pineapple juice, canned, unsweetened	1 c	250	85	140	1	34	<1	<1	t	t	.1
	Plantains, without peel:											
301	Raw slices (whole = 179 g w/o peel)	1 c	148	65	181	2	47	3[1]	1	.2	.1	.1
302	Cooked, boiled, sliced	1 c	154	67	179	1	48	4	<1	.1	t	.1
	Plums:											
303	Fresh, medium, 2⅛" diam	1 ea	66	85	36	1	9	1	<1	t	.3	.1
304	Fresh, small, 1½" diam	1 ea	28	85	15	<1	4	<1	<1	t	.1	t
	Canned, purple, with liquid:											
305	Heavy syrup pack:	1 c	258	76	229	1	60	3	<1	t	.2	.1
306	Plums	3 ea	110	76	98	<1	26	1	<1	t	.1	t
307	Juice pack:	1 c	252	84	146	1	38	3	<1	t	t	t
308	Plums	3 ea	95	84	55	<1	14	1	<1	t	t	t
1698	Pomegranate, fresh	1 ea	154	81	105	2	27	1	<1	–	–	–
	Prunes, dried, pitted:											
309	Uncooked (10 = 97 g w/pits, 84 g w/o pits)	10 ea	84	32	200	2	53	6[2]	<1	t	.3	.1
310	Cooked, unsweetened, fruit & liq (250 g w/pits)	1c	212	70	227	2	60	14	<1	t	.3	.1
311	Prune juice, bottled or canned	1c	256	81	182	2	45	3	1	t	.5	t
	Raisins, seedless:											
312	Cup, not pressed down	1 c	145	15	435	5	114	6	1	.2	t	.2
313	One packet, ½ oz	½ oz	14	15	42	<1	11	1	<1	t	t	t
	Raspberries:											
314	Fresh	1 c	123	87	60	1	14	5	1	t	.1	.4
315	Frozen, sweetened:	10 oz	284	73	293	2	74	12	<1	t	t	.3
316	Cup, thawed measure	1 c	250	73	258	2	65	11	<1	t	t	.2
317	Rhubarb, cooked, added sugar	1 c	240	68	278	1	75	5	<1	t	t	.1
	Strawberries:											
318	Fresh, whole, capped	1 c	149	92	45	1	10	3	1	t	.1	.3
	Frozen, sliced, sweetened:											
319	10-oz container	10 oz	284	73	272	2	74	5	<1	t	.1	.2
320	Cup, thawed measure	1 c	255	73	244	1	66	5	<1	t	t	.2
	Tangerines, without peel and seeds:											
321	Fresh (2⅜" whole) 116 g w/refuse	1 ea	84	88	37	1	9	1	<1	t	t	t
322	Canned, light syrup, fruit and liquid	1 c	252	83	153	1	41	2	<1	t	t	t
323	Tangerine juice, canned, sweetened	1 c	249	87	124	1	30	<1	<1	t	t	.1
	Watermelon, raw, without rind & seeds:											
324	Piece, 1" by 10" diam (2 lb w/refuse or 926 g)	1 pce	482	91	154	3	35	2	2	.3	.4	1.1
325	Diced	1 c	160	91	51	1	11	1	1	.1	.1	.3

(1)Dietary fiber value partially derived from data for bananas.

(2)Dietary fiber data can vary between 6 and 13 g for 10 prunes.

Chol (mg)	Calc (mg)	Iron (mg)	Magn (mg)	Phos (mg)	Pota (mg)	Sodi (mg)	Zinc (mg)	VT-A (RE)	Thia (mg)	Ribo (mg)	Niac (mg)	V-B6 (mg)	Fola (µg)	VT-C (mg)
0	35	.7	35	15	305	2	.25	10	.24	.05	.71	.18	12	24
0	8	.16	8	3	71	1	.06	2	.05	.01	.16	.04	3	6
0	42	.65	32	20	335	2	.27	1	.14	.05	.64	.24	58	27[3]
0	4	.89	55	50	739	6	.21	167[4]	.08	.08	1.02	.44	33	27
0	3	.89	49	43	716	8	.2	140	.07	.08	1.16	.37	40	17
0	3	.07	5	7	113	0	.07	21	.03	.06	.33	.05	1	6
0	1	.03	2	3	48	0	.03	9	.01	.03	.14	.02	1	3
0	23	2.17	13	33	234	49	.18	67	.04	.1	.75	.07	6	1
0	10	.92	5	14	100	21	.08	29	.02	.04	.32	.03	3	<1
0	25	.86	20	38	388	3	.28	255	.06	.15	1.19	.07	7	7
0	9	.32	8	14	146	1	.1	96	.02	.06	.45	.03	2	3
0	5	.46	5	12	399	5	–	0	.05	.05	.46	.16	–	9
0	43	2.08	38	66	625	3	.44	167	.07	.14	1.65	.22	3	3
0	49	2.35	42	74	708	4	.51	66	.05	.21	1.53	.46	<1	6
0	31	3	36	64	707	10	.54	8	.04	.18	2	.56	1	11
0	71	3.02	48	141	1088	17	.39	1	.23	.13	1.19	.36	5	5
0	7	.29	5	14	105	2	.04	<1	.02	.01	.11	.03	<1	<1
0	27	.7	22	15	186	0	.57	16	.04	.11	1.11	.07	32	31
0	43	1.85	37	48	324	3	.51	17	.05	.13	.65	.1	74	47
0	37	1.63	32	42	285	2	.45	15	.05	.11	.57	.08	65	41
0	348	.5	29	19	230	2	.19	17	.04	.05	.48	.05	13	8
0	21	.57	15	28	247	1	.19	4	.03	.1	.34	.09	26	84
0	31	1.68	20	37	278	9	.17	6	.04	.14	1.14	.08	42	117
0	28	1.51	18	33	250	8	.15	5	.04	.13	1.02	.08	38	105
0	12	.08	10	8	131	1	.2	77	.09	.02	.13	.06	17	26
0	18	.93	20	25	196	15	.6	212	.13	.11	1.12	.11	12	50
0	45	.5	20	35	443	2	.07	105	.15	.05	.25	.08	11	55
0	39	.82	53	43	559	10	.34	178	.39	.1	.96	.69	11	46
0	13	.27	18	14	186	3	.11	59	.13	.03	.32	.23	4	15

(3) If vitamin C is added, it contains 96 mg per cup.

(4) Vitamin A values range from 1.5 RE for white-fleshed varieties to 178 RE for yellow-fleshed varieties.

A

Table A–1
Food Composition

Computer Code Number	Food Description	Measure	Wt (g)	H_2O (%)	Ener (kcal)	Prot (g)	Carb (g)	Dietary Fiber (g)	Fat (g)	Fat Breakdown (g)		
										Sat	Mono	Poly
	BAKED GOODS: BREADS, CAKES, COOKIES, CRACKERS, PIES											
326	Bagels, plain, enriched, 3½" diam	1 ea	68	33	187	7	36	1	1	.1	.1	.5
1663	Bagel, oat bran	1 ea	68	33	173	7	36	9	1	.1	.2	.3
	Biscuits:											
327	From home recipe	1 ea	28	29	101	2	13	<1	5	1.2	2	1.2
328	From mix	1 ea	28	29	95	2	14	1	3	.8	1.2	1.2
329	From refrigerated dough	1 ea	20	27	75	1	9	<1	3	.7	1.6	.4
330	Bread crumbs, dry, grated (see #364, 365 for soft crumbs)	1 c	100	6	395	12	72	4	5	1.3	2.1	1.5
	Breads:											
331	Boston brown, canned, 3¼" slice	1 pce	45	47	88	2	19	2	1	.1	.1	.3
332	Cracked wheat (¼ cracked-wheat & ¾ enr wheat flour): 1-lb loaf	1 ea	454	36	1180	39	225	24	18	4.2	8.6	3.1
333	Slice (18 per loaf)	1 pce	25	36	65	2	12	1	1	.2	.5	.2
334	Slice, toasted	1 pce	21	30	59	2	11	1	1	.2	.4	.2
335	French/Vienna, enriched: 1-lb loaf	1 ea	454	34	1243	40	236	12	14	2.9	5.5	3.1
336	French, slice, 5 x 2½"	1 pce	35	34	96	3	18	1	1	.2	.4	.2
337	Vienna, slice, 4¾ x 4 x ½"	1 pce	25	34	68	2	13	1	1	.2	.3	.2
	French toast: see Mixed Dishes, and Fast Foods, #691											
338	Italian, enriched: 1-lb loaf	1 ea	454	36	1230	40	227	14	16	3.9	3.7	6.3
339	Slice, 4½ x 3¼ x ¾"	1 pce	30	36	81	3	15	1	1	.3	.2	.4
340	Mixed grain, enriched: 1-lb loaf	1 ea	454	38	1135	45	211	32	17	3.7	6.9	4.2
341	Slice (18 per loaf)	1 pce	25	38	62	2	12	2	1	.2	.4	.2
342	Slice, toasted	1 pce	23	32	63	3	12	2	1	.2	.4	.2
343	Oatmeal, enriched: 1-lb loaf	1 ea	454	37	1221	38	220	18	20	3.2	7.2	7.7
344	Slice (18 per loaf)	1 pce	25	37	67	2	12	1	1	.2	.4	.4
345	Slice, toasted	1 pce	23	31	67	2	12	1	1	.2	.4	.4
346	Pita pocket bread, enr, 6½" round	1 ea	60	32	165	5	33	1	1	.1	.1	.3
347	Pumpernickel (⅔ rye & ⅓ enr wheat flour): 1-lb loaf	1 ea	454	38	1135	39	216	27	14	2	4.2	5.6
348	Slice, 5 x 4 x ⅜"	1 pce	32	38	80	3	15	2	1	.1	.3	.4
349	Slice, toasted	1 pce	29	32	80	3	15	2	1	.1	.3	.4
350	Raisin, enriched: 1-lb loaf	1 ea	454	34	1243	36	237	12	20	4.9	10.4	3.1
351	Slice (18 per loaf)	1 pce	25	34	68	2	13	1	1	.3	.6	.2
352	Slice, toasted	1 pce	21	28	62	2	12	1	1	.2	.5	.2
353	Rye, light (⅓ rye & ⅔ enr wheat flour): 1-lb loaf	1 ea	454	37	1175	39	219	28	15	2.8	6	3.6
354	Slice, 4¾ x 3¾ x 7/16"	1 pce	25	37	65	2	12	2	1	.2	.3	.2
355	Slice, toasted	1 pce	22	31	62	2	12	2	1	.2	.3	.2
356	Wheat (enr wheat & whole-wheat flour):[1] 1-lb loaf	1 ea	454	37	1160	43	213	25	19	3.9	7.3	4.5
357	Slice (18 per loaf)	1 pce	25	37	64	2	12	1	1	.2	.4	.2
358	Slice, toasted	1 pce	23	32	65	2	12	1	1	.2	.4	.2
359	White, enriched: 1-lb loaf	1 ea	454	37	1210	38	222	12	18	5.6	6.5	4.2
360	Slice (18 per loaf)	1 pce	25	37	67	2	12	1	1	.2	.4	.2
361	Slice, toasted	1 pce	22	30	64	2	12	1	1	.2	.4	.2
362	Slice (22 per loaf)	1 pce	20	37	53	2	10	1	1	.2	.3	.2
363	Slice, toasted	1 pce	17	30	50	2	9	<1	1	.2	.3	.1

(1)A blend of white and whole-wheat flour—no official ratio specified.

Chol (mg)	Calc (mg)	Iron (mg)	Magn (mg)	Phos (mg)	Pota (mg)	Sodi (mg)	Zinc (mg)	VT-A (RE)	Thia (mg)	Ribo (mg)	Niac (mg)	V-B6 (mg)	Fola (µg)	VT-C (mg)
0	50	2.43	20	65	69	363	.6	0	.37	.21	3.1	.03	15	0
0	8	2.1	39	112	139	345	1.42	<1	.23	.23	2.01	.14	31	<1
1	67	.83	5	47	34	165	.15	7	.1	.09	.84	.01	3	<1
1	52	.58	7	133	53	271	.17	7	.1	.1	.86	.02	2	<1
1	24	.44	2	70	23	158	.08	7	.07	.05	.44	.01	2	0
0	227	6.13	46	147	221	862	1.23	0	.76	.43	6.85	.1	25	0
<1	31	.95	28	50	143	284	.22	6	.01	.05	.5	.04	3	0
0	195	12.8	236	695	804	2442	5.68	0	1.63	1.09	16.7	1.38	177	0
0	11	.7	13	38	44	135	.31	0	.09	.06	.92	.08	10	0
0	10	.64	12	35	40	123	.29	0	.07	.05	.75	.06	6	0
0	341	11.5	123	477	513	2764	3.95	0	2.36	1.49	21.6	.19	141	0
0	26	.89	9	37	40	213	.3	0	.18	.11	1.66	.01	11	0
0	19	.63	7	26	28	152	.22	0	.13	.08	1.19	.01	8	0
0	354	13.4	123	468	499	2651	3.9	0	2.15	1.33	19.9	.22	136	0
0	23	.88	8	31	33	175	.26	0	.14	.09	1.31	.01	9	0
0	413	15.8	241	799	926	2210	5.81	0	1.85	1.55	19.8	1.51	218	1
0	23	.87	13	44	51	122	.32	0	.1	.09	1.09	.08	12	<1
0	23	.87	13	44	51	122	.32	0	.08	.08	.98	.07	9	<1
0	300	12.3	168	572	645	2719	4.68	9	1.81	1.09	14.3	.31	123	2
0	16	.68	9	31	35	150	.26	<1	.1	.06	.78	.02	7	<1
0	17	.68	9	31	35	150	.26	<1	.08	.05	.71	.01	5	<1
0	52	1.58	16	58	72	322	.5	0	.36	.2	2.78	.02	14	0
0	309	13.1	245	808	944	3046	6.76	0	1.48	1.38	14	.57	154	0
0	22	.92	17	57	67	215	.48	0	.1	.1	.99	.04	11	0
0	21	.92	17	57	66	214	.47	0	.08	.09	.89	.04	8	0
0	300	13.2	118	495	1030	1770	3.27	0	1.54	1.81	15.8	.31	154	2
0	16	.73	6	27	57	97	.18	0	.08	.1	.87	.02	8	<1
0	15	.66	6	25	52	89	.16	0	.06	.08	.71	.01	5	<1
0	331	12.9	182	568	754	2996	5.22	0	1.97	1.52	17.3	.34	232	0
0	18	.71	10	31	41	165	.29	0	.11	.08	.95	.02	13	0
0	18	.68	9	30	40	160	.28	0	.08	.07	.83	.02	9	<1
0	572	15.8	209	835	627	2447	4.77	0	2.09	1.45	20.5	.49	204	0
0	21	.87	11	46	34	135	.26	0	.11	.08	1.13	.03	11	0
0	26	.83	11	37	50	132	.26	0	.08	.06	.93	.02	7	0
0	572	12.9	95	490	508	2334	2.81	0	2.13	1.41	17	.15	159	0
0	21	.71	5	27	28	129	.15	0	.12	.06	.83	.01	9	0
<1	26	.73	6	23	29	130	.15	0	.09	.07	.86	.01	6	0
0	25	.57	4	22	22	103	.12	0	.09	.06	.75	.01	7	0
<1	20	.57	4	17	22	101	.12	0	.07	.06	.67	.01	4	0

(For purposes of calculations, use "0" for t, <1, <.1, <.01, etc.)

Table A-1
Food Composition

Computer Code Number	Food Description	Measure	Wt (g)	H_2O (%)	Ener (kcal)	Prot (g)	Carb (g)	Dietary Fiber (g)	Fat (g)	Fat Breakdown (g) Sat	Mono	Poly
	BAKED GOODS: BREADS, CAKES, COOKIES, CRACKERS, PIES—Cont.											
364	White bread cubes, soft	1 c	30	37	80	2	15	1	1	.2	.5	.2
365	White bread crumbs, soft	1 c	45	37	120	4	22	1	2	.4	.7	.3
366	Whole-wheat: 1-lb loaf	1 ea	454	38	1116	44	209	31	19	4.2	7.6	4.5
367	Slice (16 per loaf)	1 pce	28	38	70	3	13	2	1	.3	.5	.3
368	Slice, toasted	1 pce	25	30	69	3	13	2	1	.3	.5	.3
	Bread stuffing, prepared from mix:											
369	Dry type	1 c	140	65	249	4	30	4	12	2.4	5.3	3.6
370	Moist type, with egg and margarine	1 c	203	65	341	8	45	4	15	3	6.5	4.3
	Cakes, prepared from mixes:[1]											
	Angel food:											
371	Whole cake, 9¾" diam tube	1 ea	635	33	1638	37	367	10	5	.8	.5	2.3
372	Piece, 1/12 of cake	1 pce	53	33	137	3	31	1	<1	.1	t	.2
373	Boston cream pie, 1/8 of cake	1 pce	120	45	302	3	51	2	10	3	5.3	1.2
	Coffee cake:											
374	Whole cake, 7¾ x 5⅝ x 1¼"	1 ea	430	30	1367	24	227	9	41	8	16.6	13.6
375	Piece, 1/6 of cake	1 pce	72	30	229	4	38	1	7	1.3	2.8	2.3
	Devil's food, chocolate frosting:											
376	Whole cake, 2 layer, 8 or 9" diam	1 ea	1107	23	4062	45	604	31	182	51.4	99.6	21.1
377	Piece, 1/16 of cake	1 pce	69	23	253	3	38	2	11	3.2	6.2	1.3
378	Cupcake, 2½" diam	1 ea	42	23	154	2	23	1	7	1.9	3.8	.8
	Gingerbread:											
379	Whole cake, 8" square	1 ea	570	33	1761	23	289	18	58	14.8	21.9	7.6
380	Piece, 1/9 of cake	1 pce	63	33	195	3	32	2	6	1.6	3.5	.8
	Yellow, chocolate frosting, 2 layer:											
381	Whole cake, 8 or 9" diam	1 ea	1108	22	4199	42	614	20	193	52.4	107	23.2
382	Piece, 1/16 of cake	1 pce	69	22	262	3	38	1	12	3.3	6.7	1.4
	Cakes from home recipes w/enr flour:											
	Carrot cake, cream cheese frosting:[2]											
383	Whole, 9 x 13" cake	1 ea	1536	21	6696	71	725	20	406	75.1	100	209
384	Piece, 1/16 of cake, 2¼ x 3¼" slice	1 pce	112	21	488	5	53	1	30	5.5	7.3	15.2
	Fruitcake, dark:											
385	Whole cake, 7½" diam tube, 2¼" high	1 ea	1361	25	4409	39	838	48	124	15.2	56.8	44.1
386	Piece, 1/32 of cake, ⅔" arc	1 pce	43	25	139	1	26	2	4	.5	1.8	1.4
	Sheet, plain, no frosting:[3]											
387	Whole cake, 9" square	1 ea	777	24	2828	35	434	3	108	30	45.1	25.6
388	Piece, 1/9 of cake	1 pce	86	24	313	4	48	<1	12	3.3	5	2.8
	Sheet, plain, uncooked white frosting:[4]											
389	Whole cake, 9" square	1 ea	1096	22	4088	38	644	3	159	26.1	67	56.1
390	Piece, 1/9 of cake	1 pce	121	22	451	4	71	<1	17	2.9	7.4	6.2
	Pound cake:											
391	Loaf, 8½ x 3½ x 3¼"	1 ea	478	26	1946	22	224	4	108	15.5	24.9	62
392	Piece, 1/17 of loaf, ½" slice	1 pce	28	26	114	1	13	<1	6	.9	1.5	3.6

(1)Excepting angel food cake, cakes were made from mixes containing vegetable shortening, and frostings were made with margarine. All mixes use enriched flour.

(2)Made with vegetable oil.

(3)Cake made with vegetable shortening.

(4)Made with margarine.

Chol (mg)	Calc (mg)	Iron (mg)	Magn (mg)	Phos (mg)	Pota (mg)	Sodi (mg)	Zinc (mg)	VT-A (RE)	Thia (mg)	Ribo (mg)	Niac (mg)	V-B6 (mg)	Fola (µg)	VT-C (mg)
<1	32	.91	7	28	36	161	.19	0	.14	.1	1.19	.02	10	0
<1	49	1.37	11	42	54	242	.28	0	.21	.15	1.79	.03	15	0
0	327	15	390	1039	1144	2392	8.85	0	1.59	.93	17.4	.81	227	0
0	20	.94	24	65	72	150	.55	0	.1	.06	1.09	.05	14	0
0	20	.93	24	64	71	148	.55	0	.08	.05	.97	.04	10	0
0	45	1.54	17	59	104	760	.39	273	.19	.15	2.07	.06	24	0
0	130	3.35	30	99	266	936	.65	256	.34	.29	3.23	.11	34	3
0	889	3.3	76	1473	591	4756	.44	0	.65	3.12	5.61	.2	19	0
0	74	.28	6	123	49	397	.04	0	.05	.26	.47	.02	2	0
44	28	.46	7	59	47	173	.19	70	.49	.32	.23	.03	10	<1
211	585	6.19	77	925	482	1810	1.94	207	.72	.75	6.54	.21	52	1
35	98	1.04	13	155	81	303	.32	35	.12	.13	1.09	.04	9	<1
509	476	24.5	376	1350	2214	3697	7.64	310	.3	1.47	6.39	.41	89	1
32	30	1.52	23	84	138	230	.48	19	.02	.09	.4	.03	6	<1
19	18	.93	14	51	84	140	.29	12	.01	.06	.24	.02	3	<1
200	393	18.9	91	958	1373	2610	2.34	91	1.08	1.06	8.89	.22	57	1
22	43	2.09	10	106	152	289	.26	10	.12	.12	.98	.02	6	<1
609	410	23.2	332	1783	1972	3733	6.87	450	1.33	1.74	13.9	.32	89	1
38	25	1.44	21	111	123	233	.43	28	.08	.11	.86	.02	6	<1
829	384	19.4	276	1090	1720	3778	7.53	9538	2.09	2.4	15.5	1.17	184	17
60	28	1.41	20	79	125	276	.55	696	.15	.17	1.13	.08	13	1
68	449	28.3	218	708	2082	3674	3.67	475	.68	1.35	10.8	.63	41	5
2	14	.89	7	22	66	116	.12	15	.02	.04	.34	.02	1	<1
505	497	11.7	108	793	613	2331	2.75	373	1.24	1.4	10.1	.26	54	2
56	55	1.3	12	88	68	258	.3	41	.14	.15	1.12	.03	6	<1
614	680	11.8	66	1567	581	3770	2.74	643	1.1	.77	5.48	.38	99	2
68	75	1.31	7	173	64	416	.3	71	.12	.08	.6	.04	11	<1
0	85	1.71	–	–	324	1502	–	137	0	.51	3.41	.07	–	0
0	5	.1	–	–	19	88	–	8	0	.03	.2	<.01	–	0

Table A-1
Food Composition

Computer Code Number	Food Description	Measure	Wt (g)	H_2O (%)	Ener (kcal)	Prot (g)	Carb (g)	Dietary Fiber (g)	Fat (g)	Fat Breakdown (g) Sat	Mono	Poly
	BAKED GOODS: BREADS, CAKES, COOKIES, CRACKERS, PIES—Cont.											
	Cakes, commercial:											
	Cheesecake:											
401	Whole cake, 9" diam	1 ea	1110	46	3563	61	283	23	250	128	86	15.3
402	Piece, 1/12 of cake	1 pce	92	46	295	5	23	2	21	10.6	7.1	1.3
	Pound cake:											
393	Loaf, 8½ x 3½ x 3"	1 ea	500	25	1940	27	244	3	99	55.5	27.9	5.4
394	Slice, 1/17 of loaf, 2" slice	1 pce	29	25	113	2	14	<1	6	3.2	1.6	.3
	Snack: 2 small cakes per package											
395	Chocolate w/creme filling (Ding Dong)	1 ea	28	20	107	1	17	<1	4	.9	1.5	1.2
396	Sponge w/creme filling (Twinkie)	1 ea	42	20	153	1	27	<1	5	1.1	1.9	1.5
1677	Sponge cake, 1/12 of 12" cake	1 pce	65	30	188	4	40	<1	2	.5	.6	.3
1678	Strawberry shortcake, fresh	1 ea	254	74	327	5	40	4	17	10.1	4.9	1
	White, white frosting, 2 layer:											
397	Whole cake, 8 or 9" diam	1 ea	1140	20	4275	38	718	15	154	45.7	68.1	39.8
398	Piece, 1/16 of cake	1 pce	71	20	266	2	45	1	10	2.8	4.2	2.5
	Yellow, chocolate frosting, 2 layer:											
399	Whole cake, 8 or 9" diam	1 ea	1108	22	4199	42	614	20	193	52.4	107	23.2
400	Piece, 1/16 of cake	1 pce	69	22	262	3	38	1	12	3.3	6.7	1.4
1332	Bagel chips	5 pce	70	4	300	6	52	3	7	1.2	1.9	3.3
1035	Cheese puffs/Cheetos	1 oz	28	1	157	2	15	<1	10	1.9	5.8	1.3
	Cookies made with enriched flour:											
	Brownies with nuts:											
403	Commercial w/frosting, 1½ x 1¾ x ⅞"	1 ea	25	14	101	1	16	1	4	1.1	2.1	.6
404	Home recipe, 1¾ x 1¾ x ⅞"[1]	1 ea	20	13	93	1	10	<1	6	1.5	2.2	1.9
	Chocolate chip:											
405	Commercial, 2¼" diam	4 ea	42	12	192	1	25	1	10	3.1	5.5	1.1
406	Home recipe, 2¼" diam	4 ea	40	6	195	2	23	1	11	3.2	4.2	3.4
407	From refrigerated dough, 2¼" diam	4 ea	48	13	213	2	29	1	10	3.3	4.8	1
408	Fig bars	4 ea	56	16	195	2	40	3	4	.7	2.2	.7
409	Oatmeal raisin, 2⅝" diam	4 ea	52	6	226	3	36	1	8	1.7	3.6	2.6
410	Peanut butter, home recipe, 2⅝" diam[2]	4 ea	48	6	228	4	28	1	11	2.1	5.2	3.5
411	Sandwich-type, all	4 ea	40	2	189	2	28	1	8	1.7	4.7	1.1
412	Shortbread, commercial, small	4 ea	32	4	161	2	21	1	8	2	4.3	1
413	Shortbread, home recipe, large[3]	2 ea	28	3	155	2	16	1	9	5.8	2.7	.4
414	Sugar, from refrigerated dough, 2" diam	4 ea	48	5	232	2	31	<1	11	2.8	6.2	1.4
415	Vanilla wafers	10 ea	40	5	176	2	29	8	6	1.4	2.4	1.5
416	Corn chips	1 oz	28	1	153	2	16	1	9	1.3	2.7	4.7
	Crackers:[4]											
1034	Armenian cracker bread	4 pce	28	4	117	5	19	4	2	.4	.7	1.1
417	Cheese	10 ea	10	3	50	1	6	<1	3	.9	.9	.5
418	Cheese with peanut butter	4 ea	30	4	145	4	17	<1	7	1.5	3.6	1.3
419	Graham	2 ea	14	4	59	1	11	<1	1	.4	.7	.2
420	Melba toast, plain	1 pce	5	5	19	1	4	<1	<1	t	t	.1

(1) Made with vegetable oil.

(2) Made with vegetable shortening.

(3) Made with margarine.

(4) Crackers made with enriched white (wheat) flour except for rye wafers and whole-wheat wafers.

Chol (mg)	Calc (mg)	Iron (mg)	Magn (mg)	Phos (mg)	Pota (mg)	Sodi (mg)	Zinc (mg)	VT-A (RE)	Thia (mg)	Ribo (mg)	Niac (mg)	V-B6 (mg)	Fola (µg)	VT-C (mg)
611	566	6.99	122	1032	999	2297	5.66	1787	.31	2.14	2.16	.58	167	7
51	47	.58	10	86	83	190	.47	148	.03	.18	.18	.05	14	1
1105	175	6.95	55	685	595	1990	2.3	1035	.68	1.15	6.55	.17	55	<1
64	10	.4	3	40	34	115	.13	60	.04	.07	.38	.01	3	<1
5	21	.96	12	26	35	121	.16	4	.06	.08	.69	.01	2	<1
7	19	.55	3	32	38	153	.13	9	.06	.06	.51	.01	2	<1
66	46	1.77	7	89	64	158	.33	30	.16	.18	1.25	.03	8	0
53	209	2.33	29	289	359	510	.57	172	.29	.33	2.26	.13	40	95
91	547	9.12	60	742	661	2667	1.77	369	1.14	1.48	10.3	.16	64	1
6	34	.57	4	46	41	166	.11	23	.07	.09	.64	.01	4	<1
609	410	23.2	332	1783	1972	3733	6.87	450	1.33	1.74	13.9	.32	89	1
38	25	1.44	21	111	123	233	.43	28	.08	.11	.86	.02	6	<1
0	9	1.07	41	103	137	418	.88	0	.1	.12	1.33	.1	56	0
1	16	.67	5	31	47	298	.11	26	.07	.1	.92	.04	34	<1
4	7	.56	8	25	37	78	.18	5	.06	.05	.43	.01	3	<1
15	11	.37	11	26	35	69	.19	42	.03	.04	.2	.02	3	<1
0	6	1.02	15	21	39	137	.19	15	.05	.08	.68	.07	2	0
13	16	.99	22	40	90	144	.37	66	.07	.07	.54	.03	5	<1
11	12	1.08	11	33	86	100	.24	8	.09	.09	.95	.02	4	0
0	36	1.63	15	35	116	196	.22	6	.09	.12	1.05	.04	6	<1
17	52	1.38	22	84	124	280	.45	85	.13	.09	.65	.04	6	<1
15	19	1.08	19	56	111	249	.39	75	.11	.1	1.68	.04	9	<1
0	10	1.56	18	39	70	242	.32	0	.03	.07	.83	.01	2	0
6	11	.88	5	35	32	146	.17	8	.11	.1	1.07	.01	3	0
25	5	.75	4	20	20	132	.12	89	.1	.07	.83	.01	3	0
15	43	.89	4	90	78	225	.13	11	.09	.06	1.16	.01	3	0
23	19	.96	6	42	39	125	.14	16	.11	.13	1.24	.03	4	0
0	36	.37	21	52	40	179	.36	11	.01	.04	.33	.07[5]	6[6]	<1
0	21	.45	41	1	77	–	.9	1	.06	.04	1.05	.02	12	2
1	15	.48	4	22	14	99	.11	9	.06	.04	.47	.05	2	0
1	24	.88	17	97	73	298	.33	3	.12	.1	1.96	.45	7	0
0	3	.52	4	15	19	85	.11	0	.03	.04	.58	.01	2	0
0	5	.19	3	10	10	41	.1	0	.02	.01	.21	<.01	1	0

(5) Vitamin B_6 values vary between brands. Check the label.

(6) Values from 1992 USDA data for snacks and sweets.

Table A–1
Food Composition

Computer Code Number	Food Description	Measure	Wt (g)	H_2O (%)	Ener (kcal)	Prot (g)	Carb (g)	Dietary Fiber (g)	Fat (g)	Fat Breakdown (g) Sat	Mono	Poly
	BAKED GOODS: BREADS, CAKES, COOKIES, CRACKERS, PIES—Cont.											
	Crackers—Cont.											
1514	Rice cakes, unsalted	2 ea	18	5	69	1	14	<1	1	.2	.2	.2
421	Rye wafer, whole grain	2 ea	14	5	47	1	11	2	<1	t	t	.1
422	Saltine®[1]	4 ea	12	4	52	1	9	<1	1	.3	.8	.2
423	Snack-type, round like Ritz	3 ea	9	4	45	1	5	<1	2	.4	1	.8
424	Wheat, thin	4 ea	8	3	35	1	5	1	1	.5	.5	.4
425	Whole-wheat wafers	2 ea	8	3	35	1	5	1	1	.2	.8	.2
426	Croissants, 4½ x 4 x 1¾"	1 ea	57	23	231	5	26	2	12	6.7	3.2	.7
1699	Croutons, seasoned	½ c	15	3	70	2	10	<1	3	.8	1.4	.4
	Danish pastry:											
427	Packaged ring, plain, 12 oz	1 ea	340	21	1349	19	181	1	65	13.5	40.8	6.4
428	Round piece, plain, 4¼" diam, 1" high	1 ea	57	21	226	3	30	<1	11	2.3	6.8	1.1
429	Ounce, plain	1 oz	28	21	113	2	15	<1	5	1.1	3.4	.5
430	Round piece with fruit	1 ea	65	29	231	3	31	–	11	2.3	7	1.1
	Desserts, 3 x 3" piece:											
1348	Apple crisp	1 pce	78	61	127	1	25	–	3	.6	1.2	.8
1353	Apple cobbler	1 pce	104	57	199	2	35	1	6	1.3	2.7	1.9
1349	Cherry crisp	1 pce	138	75	158	2	27	1	5	1	2.4	1.7
1352	Cherry cobbler	1 pce	129	66	198	2	34	1	6	1.3	2.7	1.9
1350	Peach crisp	1 pce	139	73	166	1	30	1	5	1	2.3	1.6
1351	Peach cobbler	1 pce	130	65	204	2	36	1	6	1.3	2.7	1.9
	Doughnuts:											
431	Cake type, plain, 3¼" diam	1 ea	50	21	211	2	25	1	11	1.9	4.8	4.1
432	Yeast-leavened, glazed, 3¾" diam	1 ea	60	25	242	4	27	1	14	3.5	7.7	1.7
	English muffins:											
433	Plain, enriched	1 ea	57	42	134	4	26	2	1	.1	.2	.5
434	Toasted	1 ea	50	37	128	4	25	2	1	.1	.2	5
1504	Whole wheat	1 ea	50	46	102	4	20	3	1	.2	.3	.4
1414	Granola bar, soft	1 ea	42	6	188	3	29	2	7	3.1	1.6	2.3
1415	Granola bar, hard	1 ea	28	4	134	3	18	2	6	.7	1.2	3.4
	Muffins, 2½" diam, 1½" high:											
	From home recipe											
435	Blueberry[2]	1 ea	45	39	131	3	18	2	5	1.1	1.2	2.4
436	Bran, wheat[3]	1 ea	45	35	130	3	19	3	6	1.2	1.4	2.8
437	Cornmeal	1 ea	45	32	144	3	20	2	6	1.2	1.4	2.8
	From commercial mix:											
438	Blueberry	1 ea	45	36	135	2	22	2	4	.7	1.6	1.4
439	Bran, wheat	1 ea	45	35	124	3	21	3	4	1.1	2.1	.6
440	Cornmeal	1 ea	45	30	144	3	22	2	5	1.3	2.4	.6
	Pancakes, 4" diam:											
441	Buckwheat, from mix w/ egg and milk	1 ea	27	54	56	2	8	1	2	.5	.5	.8
442	Plain, from home recipe	1 ea	27	53	61	2	8	<1	3	.6	.7	1.2
443	Plain, from mix; egg, milk, oil added	1 ea	27	53	52	1	10	<1	1	.1	.2	.2

(1) Made with lard.

(2) Made with vegetable shortening.

(3) Made with vegetable oil

(Computer code number is for West Diet Analysis program)

Chol (mg)	Calc (mg)	Iron (mg)	Magn (mg)	Phos (mg)	Pota (mg)	Sodi (mg)	Zinc (mg)	VT-A (RE)	Thia (mg)	Ribo (mg)	Niac (mg)	V-B6 (mg)	Fola (μg)	VT-C (mg)
0	3	.37	25	63	50	1	.54	1	0	<.01	.78	.02	3	0
0	6	.83	17	47	69	111	.39	<1	.06	.04	.22	.04	6	<1
0	14	.65	3	13	15	156	.09	0	.07	.05	.63	<.01	4	0
<1	11	.32	2	21	18	64	.06	0	.03	.03	.36	<.01	1	0
<1	3	.25	6[4]	15	17	69	.24[4]	0	.04	.03	.4	.01	3	0
0	4	.25	8[4]	24	24	53	.17	0	.02	.01	.36	.01	2	0
43	21	1.16	9	60	67	424	.43	78	.22	.14	1.25	.03	16	<1
<1	14	.42	6	21	27	186	.14	1	.08	.06	.7	.01	6	0
105	143	6.94	54	286	371	1261	1.87	20	.99	.75	8.5	.2	54	10
18	24	1.16	9	48	62	211	.31	3	.16	.12	1.43	.03	9	2
9	12	.58	5	24	31	105	.16	2	.08	.06	.71	.02	5	1
13	15	.97	10	47	76	230	.33	17	.2	.14	1.24	.04	10	1
0	22	.58	5	19	76	142	.12	24	.07	.06	.6	.03	4	–
1	31	.78	6	44	87	304	.16	76	.1	.09	.74	.04	3	<1
0	29	2.15	12	23	164	73	.15	145	.07	.08	.59	.06	10	3
1	37	1.81	10	48	114	311	.2	135	.1	.11	.85	.05	9	2
0	23	.95	13	31	198	69	.2	104	.05	.05	1.03	.03	6	5
1	33	.91	10	54	140	308	.23	105	.09	.09	1.18	.03	6	3
18	22	.98	10	135	63	273	.27	9	.11	.12	.92	.03	4	<1
4	26	1.23	13	56	65	205	.46	11	.22	.13	1.71	.03	13	0
0	99	1.43	12	76	75	264	.4	0	.25	.16	2.21	.02	21	<1
0	94	1.37	11	72	71	252	.38	0	.19	.14	1.9	.02	14	<1
0	133	1.23	35	141	105	319	.8	0	.15	.07	1.71	.08	24	0
<1	45	1.09	31	98	138	118	.64	0	.12	.07	.22	.04	10	0
0	17	.84	27	79	95	83	.58	4	.07	.03	.45	.02	7	<1
18	85	1.03	7	65	55	198	.24	13	.12	.13	.99	.02	5	1
16	84	1.89	35	128	143	265	1.24	108	.15	.2	1.81	.14	23	4
20	116	1.18	10	79	65	263	.27	18	.14	.14	1.07	.04	8	<1
21	11	.51	5	85	35	197	.17	11	.07	.14	1.01	.03	5	<1
31	14	1.14	26	150	66	210	.52	14	.09	.11	1.29	.08	7	0
28	34	.88	9	173	59	358	.29	20	.11	.12	.94	.05	5	<1
18	69	.51	15	110	63	144	.32	18	.05	.07	.36	.04	5	<1
16	59	.49	4	43	36	119	.15	15	.05	.08	.42	.01	3	<1
3	34	.42	5	90	47	170	.1	16	.06	.06	.46	.02	2	<1

[4] Values derived from whole-wheat recipes and retention values.

(For purposes of calculations, use "0" for t, <1, <.1, <.01, etc.)

Table A–1
Food Composition

Computer Code Number	Food Description	Measure	Wt (g)	H_2O (%)	Ener (kcal)	Prot (g)	Carb (g)	Dietary Fiber (g)	Fat (g)	Fat Breakdown (g) Sat	Mono	Poly
	BAKED GOODS: BREADS, CAKES, COOKIES, CRACKERS, PIES—Cont.											
	Piecrust, with enriched flour, vegetable shortening, baked:											
444	Home recipe, 9" shell	1 ea	180	10	949	11	85	3	62	15.5	27.4	16.4
	From mix:											
445	For 2-crust pie	1 ea	320	10	1686	20	152	6	111	27.6	48.6	29.2
446	1 pie shell	1 ea	180	11	902	12	91	3	55	13.9	31.1	6.9
	Pies, 9" diam; crust made with vegetable shortening, enriched flour:											
447	Apple:[1] Whole pie	1 ea	945	52	2239	18	321	16	104	19.9	56.1	19.8
448	Piece, ⅙ of pie	1 pce	158	52	374	3	54	3	17	3.3	9.4	3.3
449	Banana cream: Whole pie	1 ea	1188	48	3195	52	391	–	162	44.7	68	39.2
450	Piece, ⅙ of pie	1 pce	198	48	533	9	65	–	27	7.4	11.3	6.5
451	Blueberry:[1] Whole pie	1 ea	945	51	2315	25	317	13	112	27.6	48.4	29.1
452	Piece, ⅙ of pie	1 pce	158	51	387	4	53	2	19	4.6	8.1	4.9
453	Cherry:[1] Whole pie	1 ea	945	46	2551	26	364	14	115	28.3	50.2	30.7
454	Piece, ⅙ of pie	1 pce	158	46	427	4	61	2	19	4.7	8.4	5.1
455	Chocolate cream:[2] Whole pie	1 ea	1194	56	2704	53	320	6	139	44.3	57.1	30.7
456	Piece, ⅙ of pie	1 pce	199	56	451	9	53	1	23	7.4	9.5	5.1
457	Custard:[1] Whole pie	1 ea	910	61	1911	50	189	11	106	25.3	52.4	17.5
458	Piece, ⅙ of pie	1 pce	152	61	319	8	32	2	18	4.2	8.8	2.9
459	Lemon meringue:[1] Whole pie	1 ea	840	42	2251	13	396	10	73	13.1	30.5	24.3
460	Piece, ⅙ of pie	1 pce	140	42	375	2	66	2	12	2.2	5.1	4
461	Peach: Whole pie	1 ea	945	45	2546	22	377	13	111	26.4	47.4	31.8
462	Piece, ⅙ of pie	1 pce	158	45	426	4	63	2	18	4.4	7.9	5.3
463	Pecan:[1] Whole pie	1 ea	825	19	3300	33	472	29	153	31	89.1	24.5
464	Piece, ⅙ of pie	1 pce	138	19	552	6	79	5	25	5.2	14.9	4.1
465	Pumpkin:[1] Whole pie	1 ea	1240	58	2604	48	339	33	118	25	62.1	19.8
466	Piece, ⅙ of pie	1 pce	206	58	433	8	56	6	20	4.2	10.3	3.3
467	Pies, fried, commercial: Apple	1 ea	85	40	266	2	33	1	14	6.5	5.8	1.2
468	Pies, fried, commercial: Cherry	1 ea	85	40	266	2	33	1	14	6.5	5.8	1.2
	Pretzels, made with enriched flour:											
469	Thin sticks, 2¼" long	10 ea	3	3	11	<1	2	<1	<1	t	t	t
470	Dutch twists, 2¾ x 2⅝"	1 ea	16	3	61	1	13	<1	1	.1	.2	.2
471	Thin twists, 3¼ x 2¼ x ¼"	10 ea	60	3	229	5	47	2	2	.4	.8	.7
	Rolls & buns, enriched, commercial:											
472	Cloverleaf rolls, 2½" diam, 2" high	1 ea	28	32	85	2	14	1	2	.5	1.1	.3
473	Hot dog buns	1 ea	40	34	114	3	20	1	2	.5	1	.4
474	Hamburger buns	1 ea	45	34	129	4	23	1	2	.5	1.1	.4
475	Hard roll, white, 3¾" diam, 2" high	1 ea	50	31	147	5	26	1	2	.3	.6	.9
476	Submarine rolls/hoagies, 11½ x 3 x 2½"	1 ea	135	31	392	12	75	4	4	.9	1.3	1.4
	Rolls & buns, enriched, home recipe:											
477	Dinner rolls 2½" diam, 2" high	1 ea	35	29	112	3	19	1	3	.7	1.1	.7
478	Toaster pastries, fortified (Poptarts)	1 ea	54	12	212	3	38	1	6	.8	2.2	2.1

(1) Values from latest USDA data for Baked Goods.

(2) Values based on recipe: pie crust, cooked chocolate pudding, whipped cream topping.

(Computer code number is for West Diet Analysis program)

Chol (mg)	Calc (mg)	Iron (mg)	Magn (mg)	Phos (mg)	Pota (mg)	Sodi (mg)	Zinc (mg)	VT-A (RE)	Thia (mg)	Ribo (mg)	Niac (mg)	V-B6 (mg)	Fola (µg)	VT-C (mg)
0	18	5.22	25	121	121	976	.79	0	.7	.5	5.96	.04	20	0
0	32	9.28	45	214	214	1734	1.41	0	1.25	.89	10.6	.08	35	0
0	108	3.89	27	151	112	1312	.7	0	.54	.33	4.27	.1	22	0
0	104	4.25	66	227	614	2513	1.51	284	.26	.25	2.49	.36	38	30
0	17	.71	11	38	103	420	.25	47	.04	.04	.42	.06	6	5
606	891	12.5	190	1092	1960	2851	5.7	832	1.65	2.46	12.5	1.58	131	19
101	149	2.08	32	182	327	475	.95	139	.27	.41	2.08	.26	22	3
0	66	11.7	76	284	473	1748	1.89	38	1.45	1.25	11.2	.32	47	7
0	11	1.96	13	47	79	292	.32	6	.24	.21	1.88	.05	8	1
0	94	17.6	85	284	728	1804	1.89	454	1.4	1.18	12.1	.32	66	9
0	16	2.94	14	47	122	302	.32	76	.23	.2	2.02	.05	11	2
93	902	12.3	170	951	1582	2670	4.95	203	1.52	2.56	11.6	.36	69	5
16	150	2.04	28	159	264	445	.82	34	.25	.43	1.94	.06	11	1
300	728	5.28	100	1019	965	2184	4.73	575	.35	1.89	2.66	.44	182	3
50	122	.88	17	170	161	365	.79	96	.06	.32	.44	.07	30	<1
378	470	5.12	126	882	748	1226	4.12	462	.52	1.76	5.45	.25	67	27
63	78	.85	21	147	125	204	.69	77	.09	.29	.91	.04	11	4
0	50	10.3	68	256	891	1722	1.59	328	1.2	1.01	13	.17	49	501
0	8	1.73	11	43	149	288	.27	55	.2	.17	2.17	.03	8	84
264	140	8.66	149	635	611	3498	4.7	388	.75	1.01	2.05	.17	49	9
44	23	1.45	25	106	102	585	.79	65	.13	.17	.34	.03	8	2
248	744	9.8	186	880	1909	3496	5.58	11544[3]	.68	1.9	2.32	.71	186	19
41	124	1.63	31	146	317	581	.93	1917[3]	.11	.31	.38	.12	31	3
13	13	.88	8	37	51	325	.17	8	.1	.08	.98	.03	4	2
13	13	.88	8	37	51	325	.17	42	.1	.08	.98	.03	4	1
0	1	.13	1	3	4	51	.03	0	.01	.02	.16	<.01	2	0
0	6	.69	6	18	23	274	.14	0	.07	.1	.84	.02	13	0
0	22	2.59	21	68	88	1029	.51	0	.28	.37	3.15	.07	50	0
<1	34	.89	7	33	38	148	.22	0	.14	.09	1.14	.01	9	<1
0	56	1.27	8	35	56	224	.25	0	.19	.12	1.57	.02	11	0
0	63	1.43	9	40	63	252	.28	0	.22	.14	1.77	.02	12	0
0	47	1.65	13	50	54	272	.47	0	.24	.17	2.12	.03	7	0
0	122	3.78	27	115	122	783	.85	0	.54	.33	4.47	.05	40	0
13	21	1.04	7	44	53	145	.24	28	.14	.14	1.21	.02	15	<1
0	14	1.89	10	60	60	226	.36	150[4]	.16	.2	2.13	.21	43	<1

(3)Latest USDA values of vitamin A for canned pumpkin are almost 3.5 times greater than previously published values. Canned pumpkin is usually a blend of pumpkin and winter squash.

(4)Vitamin A values from label declarations vary.

Table A–1
Food Composition

Computer Code Number	Food Description	Measure	Wt (g)	H_2O (%)	Ener (kcal)	Prot (g)	Carb (g)	Dietary Fiber (g)	Fat (g)	Fat Breakdown (g) Sat	Mono	Poly
	BAKED GOODS: BREADS, CAKES, COOKIES, CRACKERS, PIES—Cont.											
	Tortilla chips:											
1271	Plain	1 oz	28	2	142	2	18	2	7	1.4	4.4	1
1036	Nacho flavor	1 oz	28	2	141	2	18	1	7	1.4	4.3	1
1037	Taco flavor	1 oz	28	2	136	2	18	–	7	1.3	4	1
	Tortillas:											
479	Corn, enriched, 6" diam	1 ea	30	44	67	2	14	2	1	.1	.2	.3
480	Flour, 8" diam	1 ea	35	27	115	3	20	1	3	.4	1	1
1301	Flour, 10" diam	1 ea	57	27	185	5	32	2	4	.6	1.6	1.6
481	Taco shells	1 ea	14	4	62	1	9	1	3	.4	1.5	.6
	Waffles, 7" diam:											
482	From home recipe	1 ea	75	42	218	6	25	1	11	2.1	2.6	5.1
483	From mix, egg/milk added	1 ea	75	42	218	5	26	1	10	1.7	2.7	5.2
1510	Whole grain, prepared from frozen	1 ea	39	44	106	4	12	1	5	1.6	1.9	1
	GRAIN PRODUCTS: CEREAL, FLOUR, GRAIN, PASTA and NOODLES, POPCORN											
484	Barley, pearled, dry, uncooked	1 c	200	10	704	20	155	31	2	.5	.3	1.1
485	Barley, pearled, cooked	1 c	157	69	193	4	44	9	1	.1	.1	.3
	Breakfast cereals, hot, cooked:											
	Corn grits (hominy) enriched:											
486	Regular and quick, prepared, yellow	1 c	242	85	145	3	31	4	<1	.1	.1	.2
487	Instant, prepared from packet, white	1 ea	137	85	82	2	18	<1	<1	t	t	.1
	Cream of wheat:											
488	Regular, quick, instant	1 c	244	87	131	4	27	3	<1	.1	.1	.2
489	Mix and eat, plain, packet	1 ea	142	82	102	3	21	<1	<1	t	t	.1
1664	Farina cereal, cooked	½ c	117	87	58	2	12	2	<1	t	t	t
490	Malt-O-Meal	1 c	240	88	122	4	26	3	<1	t	t	.1
494	Maypo	1 c	242	83	172	6	32	4	2	.1	.1	.3
	Oatmeal or rolled oats:											
491	Regular, quick, instant, nonfort	1 c	234	85	145	6	25	4	2	.4	.7	.9
	Instant, fortified:											
492	Plain, from packet	¾ c	177	85	104	4	18	2	2	.3	.6	.7
493	Flavored, from packet	¾ c	164	76	160	5	31	3	2	.3	.7	.8
	Breakfast cereals, ready to eat:											
495	All-Bran	⅓ c	28	3	71	4	21	10	1	.1	.1	.3
1306	Alpha Bits	1 c	28	1	111	2	25	1	1	.1	.2	.3
1307	Apple Jacks	1 c	28	2	109	2	26	1	<1	t	t	t
1308	Bran Buds	1 c	84	3	216	12	64	24	2	.4	.3	1.1
1305	Bran Chex	1 c	49	2	156	5	39	7	1	.2	.2	.8
1309	Honey BucWheat Crisp	¾ c	28	5	110	3	23	3	1	.2	.2	.4
1310	C. W. Post, plain	1 c	97	2	431	9	69	3	15	11.3	1.7	1.4
1311	C. W. Post, with raisins	1 c	103	4	445	9	74	2	15	11	1.7	1.4
496	Cap'n Crunch	1 c	37	2	156	2	30	1	3	2.2	.4	.5
1312	Cap'n Crunchberries	1 c	38	3	160	2	31	1	3	2.1	.4	.5

(Computer code number is for West Diet Analysis program)

PAGE KEY: A–2 = BEV A–4 = DAIRY A–10 = EGGS A–12 = FAT/OIL A–14 = FRUIT A–24 = BAKERY A–34 = GRAIN A–40 = FISH A–44 = MEATS A–48 = POULTRY A–50 = SAUSAGE A–52 = MIXED/FAST A–60 = NUTS/SEEDS A–62 = SWEETS A–66 = VEG/LEG A–78 = MISC A–80 = SOUPS/SAUCES A–84 = FAST A–96 = FRZN ENTREE A–98 = BABY FOODS

Chol (mg)	Calc (mg)	Iron (mg)	Magn (mg)	Phos (mg)	Pota (mg)	Sodi (mg)	Zinc (mg)	VT-A (RE)	Thia (mg)	Ribo (mg)	Niac (mg)	V-B6 (mg)	Fola (µg)	VT-C (mg)
0	44	.43	25	58	56	150	.43	6	.02	.05	.36	.08	3	<1
1	42	.4	23	69	61	201	.34	13	.04	.05	.4	.08	4	1
1	44	.57	25	68	61	223	.36	26	.07	.06	.57	.08	6	<1
0	52	.42	19	94	46	48	.28	8	.03	.02	.45	.07	4	0
0	44	1.17	9	44	46	169	.25	0	.19	.1	1.26	.02	4	0
0	71	1.88	15	70	74	272	.4	0	.3	.17	2.03	.03	7	0
0	34	.35	14	31	33	24	.18	6	.04	.02	.23	.04	4	0
52	191	1.74	14	143	119	383	.51	49	.2	.26	1.55	.04	11	<1
38	93	1.23	15	252	134	458	.35	50	.15	.19	1.23	.07	9	<1
39	85	.7	15	83	88	150	.41	25	.08	.12	.59	.04	7	<1
0	58	5	158	442	560	18	4.26	4	.38	.23	9.22	.52	46	0
0	17	2.09	34	85	146	5	1.29	2	.13	.1	3.23	.18	25	0
0	0	1.55[1]	10	29	53	0[2]	.17	14[3]	.24[1]	.14[1]	1.96[1]	.06	2	0
0	7	1.01[1]	5	16	29	343	.08	0	.18[1]	.08[1]	1.3[1]	.03	1	0
0	51[1]	10.5[1]	12	102[4]	46	141[4]	.34	0	.24[1]	0[1]	1.46[1]	.03	10	0
0	20[1]	8.09[1]	7	20[1]	38	241	.24	376[1]	.43[1]	.28[1]	4.97[1]	.57	100	0
0	2	.58	2	14	15	0[5]	.08	0	.09	.06	.64	.01	2	0
0	5	9.6[1]	5	24[1]	31	2[5]	.17	0	.48[1]	.24[1]	5.76[1]	.02	5	0
0	126	8.47	51	249	213	261	1.5	709	.73	.73	9.44	.97	10	29
0	19	1.59	56	177	131	2[5]	1.15	5	.26	.05	.3	.05	9	0
0	162[1]	6.3[1]	42	132	99	283[1]	.87	453[1]	.53[1]	.28[1]	5.47[1]	.74	150	0
0	168[1]	6.7[1]	51	148	137	254[1]	1	460[1]	.53[1]	.38[1]	5.9[1]	.76	150	<1
0	23	4.52[1]	105	264	350	320	3.75	376[1]	.37[1]	.43[1]	5[1]	.51	100	15[1]
0	8	2.7	17	51	110	180	1.51	376	.37	.43	5	.51	100	0
0	3	4.52	6	30	23	124	3.75	376	.37	.43	5	.51	100	15
0	56	13.4	267	729	1403	515	11.1	1111	1.09	1.26	14.8	1.51	296	44
0	29	7.79	125	326	393	454	2.14	11	.64	.26	8.62	.88	172	26
0	40	8.12	32	80	106	270	.51	682	.68	.77	9	1.4	9	27
<1	47	15.4	67	224	197	166	1.64	1283	1.26	1.46	17.1	1.75	342	0
<1	50	16.4	74	231	260	160	1.64	1362	1.34	1.55	18.1	1.85	363	0
0	6	9.81[1]	15	47	48	278	4	5[1]	.66[1]	.71[1]	8.62[1]	1	238	0
<1	12	9.92	15	51	54	268	3.88	5	.65	.74	8.92	1.02	140	0

(1)Nutrient added (values sometimes based on label declaration).

(2)Cooked without salt. If salt is added according to label recommendation, sodium content is 540 mg.

(3)Value for yellow corn grits; cooked white corn grits contain 0 RE of vitamin A.

(4)Values for quick cereal.

(5)Cooked without salt. If added according to label recommendations, sodium content is 390 mg for Cream of Wheat; 324 mg for Malt-O-Meal; 374 mg for oatmeal; 385 mg for Farina.

(For purposes of calculations, use "0" for t, <1, <.1, <.01, etc.)

A

Table A–1
Food Composition

Computer Code Number	Food Description	Measure	Wt (g)	H_2O (%)	Ener (kcal)	Prot (g)	Carb (g)	Dietary Fiber (g)	Fat (g)	Fat Breakdown (g) Sat	Mono	Poly
	GRAIN PRODUCTS: CEREAL, FLOUR, GRAIN, PASTA and NOODLES, POPCORN—Cont.											
	Breakfast cereals, ready to eat—Cont.											
1313	Cap'n Crunch, peanut butter	1 c	38	2	169	3	29	1	5	2.1	1.5	1.1
497	Cheerios	1 c	23	5	90	3	16	2	1	.3	.5	.6
1314	Cocoa Krispies	1 c	36	2	139	2	32	<1	1	.1	.1	.2
1316	Cocoa Pebbles	1 c	31	2	128	1	27	<1	2	t	t	t
1315	Corn Bran	1 c	36	2	124	2	30	7	1	.2	.3	.7
1317	Corn Chex	1 c	28	2	111	2	25	<1	1	.1	.2	.6
498	Corn Flakes, Kellogg's	1¼ c	28	3	108	2	24	1	<1	t	t	t
499	Corn Flakes, Post Toasties	1¼ c	28	3	108	2	24	1	<1	t	t	t
1340	Corn Pops	1 c	28	3	108	1	26	<1	<1	t	t	.1
1318	Cracklin' Oat Bran	1 c	60	4	229	6	41	8	9	2.1	2.3	3.5
1038	Crispy Wheat `N Raisins	1 c	43	7	150	3	35	3	1	.1	.1	.4
1319	Fortified Oat Flakes	1 c	48	3	177	9	35	3	1	.1	.3	.3
500	40% Bran Flakes, Kellogg's	1 c	39	3	127	5	30	7	1	.1	.1	.4
501	40% Bran Flakes, Post	1 c	47	3	152	5	37	9	1	.2	.2	.3
502	Froot Loops	1 c	28	2	111	2	25	1	1	.2	.1	.1
518	Frosted Flakes	1 c	35	2	133	2	32	1	<1	t	t	t
1320	Frosted Mini-Wheats	4 ea	31	5	111	3	26	3	<1	.1	t	.2
1321	Frosted Rice Krispies	1 c	28	3	108	1	26	<1	<1	t	t	t
1324	Fruit & Fibre w/dates	½ c	28	9	89	2	22	3	1	.2	.2	.5
1325	Fruitful Bran	¾ c	34	2	110	3	27	5	<1	.1	.1	.2
1322	Fruity Pebbles	1 c	32	3	131	1	28	1	2	.4	.3	.4
503	Golden Grahams	1 c	39	2	150	2	33	2	1	1	.1	.2
504	Granola, homemade	½ c	61	3	297	7	34	6	17	2.9	4.7	8.6
1670	Granola, low fat, commercial	½ c	47	3	182	5	38	3	3	0	–	–
505	Grape Nuts	½ c	57	3	203	7	47	6	<1	t	t	. 2
1326	Grape Nuts Flakes	1 c	32	3	116	3	26	3	<1	.1	t	.1
1665	Heartland Natural with raisins	1 c	101	5	430	10	70	6	14	–	–	–
1327	Honey & Nut Corn Flakes	1 c	38	4	151	2	31	1	2	.3	.7	1
506	Honey Nut Cheerios	1 c	33	3	126	4	27	2	1	.1	.3	.3
1328	HoneyBran	1 c	35	2	119	3	29	4	1	.1	.1	.4
1329	HoneyComb	1 c	22	1	86	1	20	<1	<1	.1	.1	.2
1330	King Vitaman	1 c	19	2	77	1	16	1	1	.7	.1	.2
1039	Kix	1 c	19	3	74	2	16	<1	<1	.1	.1	.2
1331	Life	1 c	43	4	158	8	31	3	1	.1	.2	.4
507	Lucky Charms	1 c	32	3	125	3	26	1	1	.2	.4	.5
1323	Mueslix Five Grain	1 c	82	5	279	7	63	7	3	.5	1	1.2
1416	Granola, low-fat	⅓ c	31	–	120	3	25	2	2	0	–	–
508	Nature Valley Granola	1 c	113	4	502	11	75	12	20	13	2.9	2.8
1666	Nutri Grain Almond Raisin	⅔ c	40	9	140	3	31	3	2	0	–	–
1333	Nutri-Grain—corn	1 c	42	3	160	3	35	4	1	.1	.2	.6
1335	Nutri-Grain—wheat	1 c	44	3	158	4	37	5	<1	.1	.1	.3
1336	100% Bran	1 c	66	3	177	8	48	23	3	.6	.6	1.9
509	100% Natural cereal, plain	½ c	57	2	267	7	36	4	12	8.2	2.3	1.1
1337	100% Natural with apples & cinnamon	1 c	104	2	478	11	70	6	20	15.4	1.8	1.3
1338	100% Natural with raisins & dates	1 c	110	3	496	11	72	7	20	13.6	3.7	1.7
510	Product 19	1 c	33	3	125	3	27	1	<1	t	t	.1
1339	Quisp	1 c	30	2	124	1	25	<1	2	1.5	.3	.3
511	Raisin Bran, Kellogg's	1 c	49	8	152	5	37	6	1	.2	.1	.4
512	Raisin Bran, Post	1 c	56	9	171	5	42	7	1	.2	.2	.4

(Computer code number is for West Diet Analysis program)

PAGE KEY: A–2 = BEV A–4 = DAIRY A–10 = EGGS A–12 = FAT/OIL A–14 = FRUIT A–24 = BAKERY A–34 = GRAIN A–40 = FISH A–44 = MEATS A–48 = POULTRY A–50 = SAUSAGE A–52 = MIXED/FAST A–60 = NUTS/SEEDS A–62 = SWEETS A–66 = VEG/LEG A–78 = MISC A–80 = SOUPS/SAUCES A–84 = FAST A–96 = FRZN ENTREE A–98 = BABY FOODS

Chol (mg)	Calc (mg)	Iron (mg)	Magn (mg)	Phos (mg)	Pota (mg)	Sodi (mg)	Zinc (mg)	VT-A (RE)	Thia (mg)	Ribo (mg)	Niac (mg)	V-B6 (mg)	Fola (μg)	VT-C (mg)
0	8	10	20	53	62	294	4.15	6	.66	.77	9.85	1.14	268	0
0	39	3.66[1]	32	109	82	249	.64	304[1]	.3[1]	.34[1]	4.05[1]	.41	5	12[1]
<1	6	2.27	12	47	53	275	1.91	476	.47	.54	6.34	.65	127	19
0	5	1.97	13	24	52	149	1.66	415	.41	.47	5.52	.56	111	0
0	41	12.2	18	52	70	309	4	8	.37	.7	10.9	.86	232	0
0	3	1.79	4	11	23	271	.1	14	.37	.07	5	.51	100	15
0	1	1.76[1]	3	18	26	286	.08	370[1]	.36[1]	.42[1]	4.93[1]	.5	99	15[1]
0	1	.74[1]	4	12	32	293	.08	370[1]	.36[1]	.42[1]	4.93[1]	.5	99	0
0	1	1.79	2	28	17	103	1.51	376	.37	.43	5	.51	100	15
0	40	3.78	116	241	355	487	3.18	794	.78	.9	10.6	1.08	212	32
0	71	6.84	34	117	173	204	.51	569	.56	.64	7.57	.77	15	0
0	68	13.7	58	176	343	429	1.5	635	.62	.72	8.45	.86	169	0
0	19	24.8[1]	71	191	247	302	5.15	516[1]	.51[1]	.58[1]	6.86[1]	.7	137	0
0	21	7.47[1]	101	296	250	430	2.49	622[1]	.61[1]	.7[1]	8.27[1]	.85	165	0
0	3	4.52[1]	7	24	26	144	3.75	376[1]	.37[1]	.43[1]	5[1]	.51	100	15[1]
0	1	2.21[1]	3	26	22	283	.05	463[1]	.45[1]	.52[1]	6.16[1]	.63	123	19[1]
0	10	1.95	25	81	105	9	1.64	410	.4	.46	5.46	.56	109	16
0	1	1.79	5	27	21	239	.31	376	.37	.43	5	.51	100	15
0	15	4.52	48	123	167	149	1.51	379	.37	.43	5	.5	100	0
0	<1	8.09	58	133	150	240	3.74	378	.38	.43	5	.5	100	<1
0	4	2.04	9	19	25	180	1.73	429	.42	.49	5.71	.58	114	0
<1	24	6.21[1]	16	56	86	386	.34	517[1]	.51[1]	.59[1]	6.87[1]	.7	6	21[1]
0	38	2.42	71	247	306	6	2.23	2	.37	.15	1.07	.21	49	1
0	–	2.72	36	121	143	91	5.66	227	.57	.64	7.55	.76	151	–
0	5	2.47[1]	38	143	190	396	1.25	755[1]	.74[1]	.85[1]	9.98[1]	1.03	201	0
0	13	9.28	36	97	113	183	.65	429	.42	.49	5.71	.58	114	0
0	61	3.7	130	346	382	207	2.61	6	.29	.13	1.43	.18	41	1
0	5	2.39	8	17	48	300	.14	501	.49	.57	6.67	.68	133	20
0	23	5.3[1]	39	124	116	302	.87	441[1]	.43[1]	.5[1]	5.87[1]	.6	22	18[1]
0	16	5.57	46	131	150	202	.9	463	.45	.52	6.16	.63	23	19
0	4	2.09	7	22	70	123	1.17	291	.29	.33	3.87	.4	78	0
0	2	11.4	6	24	23	145	.15	644	.83	.95	11.6	1.06	257	30
0	24	5.44	8	26	30	194	.16	252	.25	.28	3.35	.34	67	10
0	150	11.3	14	232	192	224	1.42	9	.93	.97	11.3	.08	36	0
0	36	5.09[1]	27	89	66	227	.56	424[1]	.42[1]	.48[1]	5.63[1]	.58	113	17[1]
0	38	8.94	82	215	369	107	7.46	747	.75	.84	9.84	.99	197	1
0	–	1.8	24	80	95	60	3.74	150	.37	.42	4.99	.5	100	–
0	71	3.77	115	353	388	232	2.19	7	.4	.19	.82	.09	85	0
0	16	.8	11	77	130	220	3.75	–	.38	.43	5	.5	100	–
0	1	.89	27	120	98	276	5.54	556	.55	.63	7.39	.76	148	22
0	12	1.24	34	164	119	299	5.81	583	.57	.66	7.74	.79	155	23
0	46	8.12	312	801	822	457	5.74	0	1.58	1.78	20.9	2.11	47	63
<1	99	1.68	68	209	281	24	1.28	3	.17	.31	1.3	.1	17	0
1	157	2.9	72	351	515	52	2	6	.33	.57	1.88	.11	17	1
1	159	3.12	124	347	537	47	2.11	6	.31	.65	2.09	.16	45	0
0	4	21[1]	12	46	51	378	.49	1746[1]	1.75[1]	1.98[1]	23.3[1]	2.34	465	70[1]
0	9	6.33	12	25	45	240	.18	5	.54	.76	5.79	.91	8	0
0	17	22.2[1]	63	182	254	271	5	498[1]	.49[1]	.59[1]	6.66[1]	.69	132	0
0	26	8.9[1]	95	234	344	365	2.97	741[1]	.73[1]	.84[1]	9.86[1]	1.01	197	0

(1)Nutrient added (values sometimes based on label declaration). (For purposes of calculations, use "0" for t, <1, <.1, <.01, etc.)

A

Table A-1
Food Composition

Computer Code Number	Food Description	Measure	Wt (g)	H_2O (%)	Ener (kcal)	Prot (g)	Carb (g)	Dietary Fiber (g)	Fat (g)	Fat Breakdown (g) Sat	Mono	Poly
	GRAIN PRODUCTS: CEREAL, FLOUR, GRAIN, PASTA and NOODLES, POPCORN—Cont.											
	Breakfast cereals, ready to eat—Cont.											
1667	Raisin Squares	½ c	28	8	90	2	23	2	0	0	0	0
1041	Rice Chex	¾ c	19	3	75	1	17	1	1	.2	.2	.3
513	Rice Krispies, Kellogg's	1 c	29	2	114	2	25	<1	<1	t	t	.1
514	Rice, puffed	1 c	14	3	56	1	13	<1	<1	t	t	t
515	Shredded Wheat	1 c	43	5	152	5	34	5	1	.2	.2	.5
516	Special K	1 c	21	2	83	4	16	1	<1	t	t	t
517	Super Golden Crisp	1 c	33	1	123	2	30	1	<1	t	t	.1
519	Honey Smacks	1 c	38	3	140	3	33	<1	1	.1	.1	.3
1341	Tasteeos	1 c	24	2	94	3	19	1	1	.2	.2	.3
1342	Team	1 c	42	4	164	3	36	<1	1	.2	.2	.3
520	Total, wheat, with added calcium	1 c	33	4	116	3	26	3	1	.1	.1	.3
521	Trix	1 c	28	2	109	2	25	<1	<1	.2	.1	.1
1344	Wheat Chex	1 c	46	2	168	5	38	3	1	.2	.2	.6
1043	Wheat cereal, puffed, fortified	1 c	12	3	44	2	10	1	<1	t	t	.1
522	Wheaties	1 c	29	5	101	3	23	3	<1	.1	t	.2
	Buckwheat flour:											
523	Dark	1 c	98	11	328	12	69	8	3	.7	.9	.9
524	Light	1 c	98	12	340	6	78	6	1	.2	.4	.4
525	Buckwheat, whole grain, dry	1 c	175	10	600	23	125	16	6	1.3	1.8	1.8
526	Bulgar, dry, uncooked	1 c	140	9	477	17	106	31	2	.3	.2	.8
527	Bulgar, cooked	1 c	182	78	151	6	34	11	<1	.1	.1	.2
	Cornmeal:											
528	Whole-ground, unbolted, dry	1 c	122	10	440	10	94	13	4	.6	1.2	2
529	Bolted, nearly whole, dry	1 c	122	10	441	10	94	12	4	.6	1.2	2
530	Degermed, enriched, dry	1 c	138	12	505	12	107	10	2	.3	.6	1
531	Degermed, enriched, cooked	1 c	240	78	209	5	44	4	1	.1	.2	.4
	Macaroni, cooked:											
532	Enriched	1 c	140	66	197	7	40	2	1	.1	.1	.4
533	Whole wheat	1 c	140	67	174	7	37	5	1	.1	.1	.3
534	Vegetable, enriched	1 c	134	68	172	6	36	6	<1	t	t	.1
535	Millet, cooked	½ c	120	71	142	4	28	1	1	.2	.2	.6
	Noodles (see also Pasta and Spaghetti)											
1507	Cellophane noodles	1 c	190	79	160	<1	39	<1	<1	t	t	t
537	Chow mein, dry	1 c	45	1	237	4	26	2	14	2	3.5	7.8
536	Egg noodles, cooked, enriched	1 c	160	69	213	8	40	4	2	.5	.7	.7
538	Spinach noodles, dry	3½ oz	100	8	372	13	75	7	2	.2	.2	.6
1343	Oat bran, dry	¼ c	23	7	58	4	16	4	2	.3	.6	.7
	Pasta, cooked (see also #953–956):											
1418	Fresh	2 oz	57	69	74	3	14	1	1	.1	.1	.2
1417	Linguini	1 c	140	66	197	7	40	2	1	.1	.1	.4
1598	Rotini	1 c	140	66	197	7	40	2	1	.1	.1	.4

(Computer code number is for West Diet Analysis program)

PAGE KEY: A–2 = BEV A–4 = DAIRY A–10 = EGGS A–12 = FAT/OIL A–14 = FRUIT A–24 = BAKERY A–34 = GRAIN A–40 = FISH A–44 = MEATS A–48 = POULTRY A–50 = SAUSAGE A–52 = MIXED/FAST A–60 = NUTS/SEEDS A–62 = SWEETS A–66 = VEG/LEG A–78 = MISC A–80 = SOUPS/SAUCES A–84 = FAST A–96 = FRZN ENTREE A–98 = BABY FOODS

Chol (mg)	Calc (mg)	Iron (mg)	Magn (mg)	Phos (mg)	Pota (mg)	Sodi (mg)	Zinc (mg)	VT-A (RE)	Thia (mg)	Ribo (mg)	Niac (mg)	V-B6 (mg)	Fola (µg)	VT-C (mg)
0	10	8.1	26	84	110	0	1.5	0	.38	.43	5	.5	100	–
0	3	1.2	5	19	22	158	.26	1	.25	.01	3.34	.34	67	10
0	4	1.83[1]	10	35	30	348	.49	384[1]	.38[1]	.43[1]	5.1[1]	.52	102	15[1]
0	1	.15[1]	3	14	16	<1	.14	0	.01[1]	.01[1]	.42[1]	.01	3	0
0	16	1.8	56	149	153	4	1.41	0	.11	.12	2.24	.11	21	0
<1	6	3.39[1]	12	41	37	199	2.82	282[1]	.28[1]	.32[1]	3.75[1]	.38	75	11[1]
0	7	2.08[1]	20	60	123	29	1.75	437[1]	.43[1]	.49[1]	5.81[1]	.59	116	0
0	4	2.39[1]	18	41	56	100	.38	501[1]	.49[1]	.57[1]	6.67[1]	.68	133	20[1]
0	11	3.82	26	96	71	182	.69	318	.31	.36	4.22	.43	9	13
0	6	2.57	18	65	71	259	.58	556	.55	.63	7.39	.76	7	22
0	281	21[1]	37	136	123	326	.78	1746[1]	1.75[1]	1.98[1]	23.3[1]	2.34	465	70[1]
0	6	4.52[1]	6	19	27	181	.13	376[1]	.37[1]	.43[1]	5[1]	.51	3	15[1]
0	18	7.31	58	181	173	308	1.23	0	.6	.17	8.1	.83	162	24
0	3	.57	17	43	42	<1	.28	0	.02	.03	1.3	.02	4	0
0	44	4.61[1]	32	100	108	276	.65	384[1]	.38[1]	.43[1]	5.1[1]	.52	102	15[1]
0	40	3.98	246	330	565	11	3.06	0	.41	.19	6.03	.57	53	0
0	11	1	47	86	314	1	2.56	0	.09	.05	.47	.09	100	0
0	31	3.85	404	606	805	2	4.2	0	.18	.74	12.3	.37	52	0
0	49	3.44	230	420	574	24	2.7	0	.32	.16	7.15	.48	38	0
0	18	1.75	58	73	123	9	1.04	0	.1	.05	1.82	.15	33	0
0	7	4.21	154	294	350	43	2.22	57	.47	.24	4.43	.37	31	0
0	7	4.21	154	294	350	43	2.22	57	.37	.1	2.3	.37	31	0
0	7	5.7	55	115	224	4	.99	57	.99	.56	6.96	.35	66	0
0	3	2.35	22	48	91	1	.41	23	.3	.21	2.42	.12	22	0
0	10	1.96	25	76	43	1	.74	0	.29	.14	2.34	.05	10	0
0	21	1.48	42	124	62	4	1.13	0	.15	.06	.99	.11	7	0
0	15	.66	25	67	41	8	.59	7	.15	.08	1.43	.03	8	0
0	4	.76	53	120	74	2	1.09	0	.13	.1	1.6	.13	23	0
0	14	1	3	15	5	9	.23	0	.07	0	.09	.02	1	0
0	9	2.13	23	72	54	197	.63	4	.26	.19	2.68	.05	10	0
53	19	2.54	30	110	45	11	.99	10	.3	.13	2.38	.06	11	0
0	58	2.13	174	332	376	36	2.76	46	.37	.2	4.55	.32	48	0
0	14	1.27	55	172	133	1	.73	0	.27	.05	.22	.04	12	0
19	3	.65	10	36	14	3	.32	3	.12	.09	.56	.02	4	0
0	10	1.96	25	76	43	1	.74	0	.29	.14	2.34	.05	10	0
0	10	1.96	25	76	43	1	.74	0	.29	.14	2.34	.05	10	0

[1]Nutrient added (values sometimes based on label declaration).

(For purposes of calculations, use "0" for t, <1, <.1, <.01, etc.)

Table A–1
Food Composition

Computer Code Number	Food Description	Measure	Wt (g)	H_2O (%)	Ener (kcal)	Prot (g)	Carb (g)	Dietary Fiber (g)	Fat (g)	Fat Breakdown (g) Sat	Fat Breakdown (g) Mono	Fat Breakdown (g) Poly
	GRAIN PRODUCTS: CEREAL, FLOUR, GRAIN, PASTA and NOODLES, POPCORN—Cont.											
	Popcorn:											
539	Air popped, plain	1 c	8	4	31	1	6	1	<1	t	.1	.2
540	Popped in vegetable oil/salted	1 c	11	3	55	1	6	1	3	.5	.9	1.5
541	Sugar-syrup coated	1 c	35	3	151	1	28	2	4	1.3	1	1.6
	Rice:											
542	Brown rice, cooked	1 c	195	73	216	5	45	3	2	.4	.6	.6
	White, enriched, all types:											
543	Regular/long grain, dry	1 c	185	12	675	13	147	3	1	.3	.4	.3
544	Regular/long grain, cooked	1 c	205	68	267	6	58	1	1	.2	.2	.2
545	Instant, prepared without salt	1 c	165	76	161	3	35	1	<1	.1	.1	.1
	Parboiled/converted rice:											
546	Raw, dry	1 c	185	10	686	13	151	3	1	.3	.3	.3
547	Cooked	1 c	175	72	200	4	43	1	<1	.1	.1	.1
1486	Sticky rice (glutinous), cooked	1 c	241	77	233	5	51	2	<1	.1	.2	.2
548	Wild rice, cooked	1 c	164	74	166	7	35	4	1	.1	.1	.4
1700	Rice and pasta (Rice-a-Roni), cooked	½ c	109	72	133	3	23	4	3	.6	1.2	1
549	Rye flour, medium	1 c	102	10	361	10	79	15	2	.2	.2	.8
1044	Soy flour, low-fat	1 c	88	3	324	45	30	1	6	.9	1.3	3.3
	Spaghetti pasta:											
550	Without salt, enriched	1 c	140	66	197	7	40	2	1	.1	.1	.4
551	With salt, enriched	1 c	140	66	197	7	40	2	1	.1	.1	.4
552	Whole-wheat spaghetti, cooked	1 c	140	67	174	7	37	5	1	.1	.1	.3
1302	Tapioca, pearl, dry	1 c	152	11	518	<1	134	2	<1	t	t	t
553	Wheat bran, crude	½ c	30	10	65	5	19	8	1	.2	.2	.7
554	Wheat germ, raw	1 c	100	11	360	23	52	15	10	1.7	1.4	6
555	Wheat germ, toasted	1 c	113	6	432	33	56	16	12	2.1	1.7	7.5
1669	Wheat germ, with brown sugar & honey	½ c	57	6	213	12	34	3	5	.8	.7	2.8
556	Rolled wheat, cooked	1 c	240	84	149	5	33	9	1	.2	.2	.4
557	Whole-grain wheat, cooked	⅓ c	50	86	28	1	7	1	<1	t	t	.1
	Wheat flour (unbleached):											
	All-purpose white, enriched:											
558	Sifted	1 c	115	12	419	12	88	3	1	.2	.1	.5
559	Unsifted	1 c	125	12	455	13	95	3	1	.2	.1	.5
560	Cake or pastry, enriched, sifted	1 c	96	23	343	5	55	–	12	3.1	5.1	3
561	Self-rising, enriched, unsifted	1 c	125	11	443	12	93	3	1	.2	.1	.5
562	Whole wheat, from hard wheats	1 c	120	10	406	16	87	15	2	.4	.3	.9
	MEATS: FISH and SHELLFISH											
1045	Bass, baked or broiled	4 oz	113	69	166	27	0	0	5	1.1	2.1	1.5
1046	Bluefish, baked or broiled	4 oz	113	63	180	29	0	0	6	1.3	2.6	1.5
1047	Bluefish, fried in bread crumbs	4 oz	113	61	232	26	5	<1	11	2.4	4.9	2.8
1686	Catfish, breaded/flour fried	4 oz	113	56	304	24	14	1	17	4	7	4
	Clams:											
563	Raw meat only	4 oz	113	82	84	14	3	0	1	.1	.1	.3
564	Canned, drained	4 oz	113	64	168	29	6	<1	2	.2	.2	.6
1290	Steamed, meat only	20 ea	90	64	133	23	5	<1	2	.2	.2	.5
	Cod:											
565	Baked with butter	4 oz	113	75	150	26	0	0	4	.4	.3	.6
566	Batter fried	4 oz	113	67	196	20	8	<1	9	2.2	3.6	2.6
567	Poached, no added fat	4 oz	113	76	117	25	0	0	1	.2	.1	.3

(Computer code number is for West Diet Analysis program)

PAGE KEY: A–2 = BEV A–4 = DAIRY A–10 = EGGS A–12 = FAT/OIL A–14 = FRUIT A–24 = BAKERY A–34 = GRAIN A–40 = FISH A–44 = MEATS A–48 = POULTRY A–50 = SAUSAGE A–52 = MIXED/FAST A–60 = NUTS/SEEDS A–62 = SWEETS A–66 = VEG/LEG A–78 = MISC A–80 = SOUPS/SAUCES A–84 = FAST A–96 = FRZN ENTREE A–98 = BABY FOODS

Chol (mg)	Calc (mg)	Iron (mg)	Magn (mg)	Phos (mg)	Pota (mg)	Sodi (mg)	Zinc (mg)	VT-A (RE)	Thia (mg)	Ribo (mg)	Niac (mg)	V-B6 (mg)	Fola (μg)	VT-C (mg)
0	1	.21	10	24	24	<1	.27	2	.02	.02	.15	.02	2	0
0	1	.31	12	27	25	97	.29	2	.01	.01	.17	.02	2	<1
2	15	.61	12	29	38	72	.2	3	.02	.02	.77	.01	1	0
0	19	.82	84	161	84	10	1.23	0	.19	.05	2.98	.28	8	0
0	52	7.97	46	213	213	9	2.02	0	1.07	.09	7.75	.3	15	0
0	20	2.48	25	88	72	2	1	0	.33	.03	3.03	.19	6	0
0	13	1.04	8	23	7	5[1]	.4	0	.12	.08	1.45	.02	7	0
0	111	6.6	57	252	222	9	1.78	0	1.1	.13	6.72	.65	31	0
0	33	1.98	21	73	65	5	.54	0	.44	.03	2.45	.03	7	0
0	5	.34	12	19	24	12	.99	0	.05	.03	.7	.06	2	0
0	5	.98	52	134	166	5	2.2	0	.08	.14	2.12	.22	43	0
1	9	1.02	13	40	46	619	.31	0	.13	.08	1.94	.11	8	<1
0	24	2.16	76	211	346	3	2.03	0	.29	.12	1.76	.27	38	0
0	165	5.27	201	521	2260	16	1.04	4	.33	.25	1.9	.46	360	0
0	10	1.96	25	76	43	1	.74	0	.29	.14	2.34	.05	10	0
0	10	1.96	25	76	43	140	.74	0	.29	.14	2.34	.05	10	0
0	21	1.48	42	124	62	4	1.13	0	.15	.06	.99	.11	7	0
0	30	2.4	2	11	17	2	.18	0	.01	0	0	.01	6	0
0	22	3.18	183	303	354	1	2.18	0	.16	.17	4.08	.39	24	0
0	39	6.26	239	842	892	12	12.3	0	1.88	.5	6.81	1.3	281	0
0	51	10.3	362	1294	1070	5	18.8	0	1.89	.93	6.32	1.11	398	7
0	19	3.86	136	485	401	2	7.06	0	.71	.35	2.37	.42	149	7
0	17	1.49	53	166	170	0	1.15	0	.17	.12	2.14	.17	26	0
0	3	.29	12	26	33	<1	.24	0	.04	.01	.5	.03	4	0
0	17	5.34	25	124	122	2	.8	0	.9	.57	6.79	.05	30	0
0	19	5.8	27	135	133	2	.87	0	.98	.62	7.38	.05	32	0
2	125	1.47	11	89	91	314	.31	15	.18	.23	1.47	.02	7	<1
0	423	5.84	24	743	155	1586	.77	0	.84	.52	7.29	.06	52	0
0	41	4.66	166	415	486	6	3.52	0	.54	.26	7.64	.41	53	0
99	117	2.17	43	290	517	102	.94	40	.1	.1	1.72	.16	19	2
86	10	.7	48	330	541	87	1.19	156	.08	.11	8.22	.53	2	0
68	9	.6	42	323	468	76	1.02	136	.07	.09	6.24	.41	2	<1
104	76	2	36	283	434	611	1.03	36	.1	.22	3.2	.22	24	<1
39	52	15.9	10	191	355	63	1.54	102	.09	.24	2	.07	18	15
76	104	31.6	20	383	712	127	3.1	194	.17	.48	3.81	.12	33	25
60	83	25.2	16	304	565	100	2.46	154	.13	.38	3.02	.1	26	20
68	23	.56	48	159	278	254	.66	34	.1	.09	2.85	.32	11	<1
64	43	.9	36	230	443	124	.61	17	.12	.12	2.54	.23	10	1
61	23	.54	41	259	498	69	.64	14	.09	.08	2.48	.28	8	1

(1) If prepared with salt according to label recommendation, sodium would be 608 mg.

(Computer code number is for West Diet Analysis program)

Table A–1
Food Composition

Computer Code Number	Food Description	Measure	Wt (g)	H_2O (%)	Ener (kcal)	Prot (g)	Carb (g)	Dietary Fiber (g)	Fat (g)	Fat Breakdown (g) Sat	Mono	Poly
	MEATS: FISH and SHELLFISH—Cont.											
	Crab, meat only:											
1048	Blue crab, cooked	4 oz	113	77	115	23	0	0	2	.3	.3	.8
1049	Dungeness crab, cooked	4 oz	113	73	125	25	1	0	1	.2	.2	.5
568	Blue crab, canned	4 oz	113	76	112	23	0	0	1	.3	.2	.5
1587	Crab, imitation, from surimi	4 oz	113	74	116	14	12	0	1	.3	.2	.8
569	Fish sticks, breaded pollock	2 ea	57	46	155	9	13	<1	7	1.8	2.9	1.8
	Flounder/sole, baked w/lemon juice:											
570	With butter	4 oz	113	73	160	21	<1	0	8	4.3	2	.7
571	With margarine	4 oz	113	73	160	21	<1	0	8	1.6	3.1	2.5
572	Without added fat	4 oz	113	73	133	27	0	0	2	.4	.3	.7
1599	Grouper, baked or broiled	4 oz	113	73	134	28	0	0	1	.3	.3	.5
573	Haddoc, breaded, fried[1]	4 oz	113	55	265	22	14	1	13	3.2	5.4	3.3
1050	Haddock, smoked	4 oz	113	71	132	29	0	0	1	.2	.2	.4
	Halibut:											
1600	Baked or broiled	4 oz	113	72	159	30	0	0	3	.5	1.1	1.1
574	Baked with butter & lemon juice	4 oz	113	69	186	29	0	0	7	2.7	2.1	1.1
1051	Smoked	1 oz	28	49	63	6	0	0	4	.7	1.3	1.9
1054	Raw	4 oz	113	78	125	24	0	0	3	.4	.9	.9
575	Herring, pickled	3 oz	85	55	223	12	8	0	15	2	10.1	1.4
1052	Lobster meat, cooked w/moist heat	1 c	145	76	142	30	2	0	1	.2	.2	.1
1687	Ocean perch, baked/broiled	4 oz	113	82	137	27	0	0	2	.4	.9	.6
576	Ocean perch, breaded/fried	4 oz	113	59	249	22	9	1	13	3.2	5.7	3.4
1056	Octopus, raw	4 oz	113	80	93	17	2	0	1	.3	.2	.3
	Oysters:											
577	Raw, Eastern	1 c	248	85	169	17	10	0	6	1.9	.8	2.4
578	Raw, Pacific	1 c	248	82	201	23	12	0	6	1.3	.9	2.2
	Cooked:											
579	Eastern, breaded, fried, medium	6 ea	88	65	173	8	10	<1	11	2.8	4.1	2.9
580	Western, simmered	4 oz	113	64	185	21	11	0	5	1.2	2.8	2
581	Pollock, baked or broiled	4 oz	113	74	128	27	0	0	1	.3	.2	.6
1055	Pollock, moist heat, poached	4 oz	113	74	128	27	0	0	1	.3	.2	.6
	Salmon:											
582	Canned pink, solids and liquid	4 oz	113	69	158	22	0	0	7	1.7	2.1	2.3
583	Broiled or baked	4 oz	113	62	245	31	0	0	12	2.2	6	2.7
584	Smoked	4 oz	113	72	133	21	0	0	5	1	2.3	1.1
585	Atlantic sardines, canned, drained, 2 = 24 g	4 oz	113	60	236	28	0	0	13	1.7	4.4	5.8
586	Scallops, breaded, cooked from frozen	6 ea	93	58	199	17	9	<1	10	2.5	4.2	2.7
1588	Scallops, imitation, from surimi	4 oz	113	74	112	14	12	0	<1	.1	.1	.2
1688	Scallops, steamed/boiled	½ c	60	81	64	10	1	0	2	.3	.7	.6
	Shrimp:											
587	Cooked, boiled, 2 large = 14 g	6 ea	86	77	85	18	0	0	1	.2	.2	.4
588	Canned, drained	½ c	64	73	76	15	1	0	1	.2	.2	.5
589	Fried, 2 large = 15 g[1]	12 ea	90	53	217	19	10	<1	11	1.9	3.6	4.6
1057	Raw, large, about 7 g each	14 ea	100	76	106	20	1	0	2	.3	.3	.7
1589	Shrimp, imitation, from surimi	4 oz	113	75	115	14	10	0	2	.3	.2	.9
1053	Snapper, baked or broiled	4 oz	113	70	145	30	0	0	2	.4	.4	.7
1060	Squid, fried in flour[2]	4 oz	113	64	197	20	9	<1	8	2.1	3.1	2.4

(1)Dipped in egg, bread crumbs, and flour; fried in vegetable shortening. (2)Recipe is 94.6% squid, 4.9% flour, and 0.6% salt.

(Computer code number is for West Diet Analysis program)

Chol (mg)	Calc (mg)	Iron (mg)	Magn (mg)	Phos (mg)	Pota (mg)	Sodi (mg)	Zinc (mg)	VT-A (RE)	Thia (mg)	Ribo (mg)	Niac (mg)	V-B6 (mg)	Fola (μg)	VT-C (mg)
113	118	1.03	37	234	367	316	4.79	2	.11	.06	3.74	.2	58	4
86	67	.49	66	198	463	429	6.21	35	.06	.23	4.11	.2	48	4
101	115	.95	44	295	423	378	4.56	2	.09	.09	1.55	.17	48	3
23	15	.44	49	320	102	954	.37	23	.04	.03	.2	.03	2	0
64	11	.42	14	103	148	331	.38	18	.07	.1	1.21	.03	10	0
91	21	.37	67	249	363	193	.71	72	.09	.13	2.47	.27	13	1
73	21	.37	67	249	364	201	.71	92	.09	.13	2.47	.27	13	1
77	20	.39	66	327	390	119	.72	12	.09	.13	2.47	.27	10	0
53	24	1.29	42	162	539	60	.58	57	.09	.01	.43	.4	12	0
96	63	1.93	46	228	346	524	.59	33	.08	.14	4.51	.28	19	<1
87	56	1.59	61	285	471	865	.57	25	.05	.06	5.75	.45	17	0
47	68	1.21	121	323	652	78	.6	61	.08	.1	8.07	.45	16	0
54	66	1.17	116	308	636	112	.57	93	.08	.1	7.69	.43	16	5
28	14	.24	23	63	128	136	.12	13	.01	.02	1.64	.09	1	<1
36	53	.95	94	252	510	61	.48	53	.07	.08	6.62	.39	14	0
11	65	1.04	7	76	59	740	.45	219	.03	.12	2.81	.14	2	0
104	88	.57	51	268	510	551	4.23	38	.01	.1	1.55	.11	16	0
61	155	1	44	314	397	109	.7	16	.15	.15	2.77	.31	12	1
71	136	1.58	38	263	324	432	.67	23	.14	.18	2.69	.24	15	1
54	60	6.01	34	211	397	261	1.91	51	.03	.04	2.38	.41	18	6
131	112	16.5	117	335	387	523	225	74	.25	.24	3.42	.15	25	9
124	20	12.6	55	402	417	263	41.2	201	.17	.58	4.98	.12	25	20
71	55	6.12	51	139	214	366	76.7	79	.13	.18	1.45	.06	12	3
113	18	10.4	50	276	342	240	37.6	166	.14	.5	4.11	.1	17	14
109	7	.32	83	547	439	132	.68	26	.08	.09	1.87	.08	4	0
109	7	.32	83	547	439	132	.68	26	.08	.09	1.87	.08	4	0
62	242[3]	.95	38	373	370	628	1.04	19	.03	.21	7.42	.34	17	0
99	8	.62	35	313	425	75	.58	71	.24	.19	7.56	.25	6	0
26	12	.96	20	186	197	889	.35	29	.03	.11	5.35	.31	2	0
160	433[3]	3.31	44	555	450	572	1.5	76	.09	.26	5.95	.19	13	0
57	39	.76	55	219	309	431	.99	20	.04	.1	1.4	.13	17	2
25	9	.35	49	320	117	902	.37	23	.01	.02	.35	.03	2	0
19	15	.15	33	95	168	111	.55	31	.01	.04	.6	.08	7	1
167	33	2.65	29	117	156	192	1.34	57	.03	.03	2.22	.11	3	2
110	38	1.75	26	148	133	108	.8	11	.02	.02	1.76	.07	1	1
159	60	1.13	36	196	202	309	1.24	50	.12	.12	2.76	.09	7	1
152	52	2.41	37	205	185	148	1.11	54	.03	.03	2.55	.1	3	2
41	21	.68	49	320	101	799	.37	23	.03	.04	.19	.03	2	0
53	45	.27	42	228	592	65	.5	40	.06	<.01	.39	.52	7	2
295	44	1.15	43	285	316	347	1.97	12	.06	.52	2.95	.07	6	5

[3]If bones are discarded, calcium value is greatly reduced.

(For purposes of calculations, use "0" for t, <1, <.1, <.01, etc.)

Table A–1
Food Composition

Computer Code Number	Food Description	Measure	Wt (g)	H_2O (%)	Ener (kcal)	Prot (g)	Carb (g)	Dietary Fiber (g)	Fat (g)	Fat Breakdown (g) Sat	Mono	Poly
	MEATS: FISH and SHELLFISH—Cont.											
1590	Surimi[1]	4 oz	113	76	112	17	8	0	1	.2	.2	.5
1058	Swordfish, raw	4 oz	113	76	137	22	0	0	5	1.2	1.8	1
1059	Swordfish, baked or broiled	4 oz	113	69	176	29	0	0	6	1.6	2.2	1.3
590	Trout, baked or broiled	4 oz	113	70	170	26	0	0	7	1.8	2	2.1
	Tuna, light, canned, drained solids:											
591	Oil pack	3 oz	85	60	168	25	0	0	7	1.3	2.5	2.4
592	Water pack	3 oz	85	74	99	22	0	0	1	.2	.1	.3
1061	Bluefin tuna, fresh	4 oz	113	68	163	26	0	0	6	1.4	1.8	1.9
	MEATS: BEEF, LAMB, PORK, and others											
	BEEF, cooked:[2]											
	Braised, simmered, pot roasted:											
	Relatively fat, choice chuck blade:											
593	Lean and fat, piece 2½ x 2½ x ¾"	4 oz	113	47	393	30	0	0	29	11.6	12.6	1.1
594	Lean only	4 oz	113	55	297	35	0	0	16	6.3	7	.5
	Relatively lean, like choice round:											
595	Lean and fat, pce 4⅛ x 2¼ x ¾"	4 oz	113	52	311	32	0	0	19	7.2	8.3	.7
596	Lean only	4 oz	113	57	249	36	0	0	11	3.6	4.7	.4
	Ground beef, broiled, patty 3 x ⅝":											
597	Extra lean, about 16% fat	4 oz	113	54	301	32	0	0	18	7	7.8	.7
598	Lean, 21% fat	4 oz	113	53	318	32	0	0	20	7.9	8.7	.7
	Roasts, oven cooked, no added liquid:											
	Relatively fat, prime rib:											
601	Lean and fat, pce 4⅛ x 2¼ x ½"	4 oz	113	46	425	25	0	0	35	14.3	15.2	1.3
602	Lean only	4 oz	113	58	272	31	0	0	16	6.6	6.8	.5
	Relatively lean, choice round:											
603	Lean and fat, pce 2½ x 2½ x ¾"	4 oz	113	59	272	30	0	0	16	6.2	6.9	.6
604	Lean only	4 oz	113	65	197	33	0	0	6	2.3	2.7	.2
1701	Steak, rib, broiled, lean	4 oz	113	65	250	32	0	0	13	5	5	.4
	Steak, broiled, relatively lean, choice sirloin:											
605	Lean and fat, pce 2½ x 2½ x ¾"	4 oz	113	52	320	31	0	0	21	8.7	9.3	.8
606	Lean only	4 oz	113	62	228	34	0	0	9	3.5	3.9	.4
	Steak, broiled, relatively fat, choice T-bone:											
1063	Lean and fat	4 oz	113	53	338	28	0	0	24	9.7	10.1	.9
1064	Lean only	4 oz	113	60	242	32	0	0	12	4.7	4.7	.4
	Variety meats:											
1086	Brains, panfried	4 oz	113	71	221	14	0	0	18	4.2	4.5	2.6
599	Heart, simmered	4 oz	113	64	197	33	<1	0	6	1.9	1.4	1.5
600	Liver, fried	4 oz	113	56	245	30	9	0	9	3	1.8	1.9
1062	Tongue, cooked	4 oz	113	56	320	25	<1	0	23	10.3	11	.9
607	Beef, canned, corned	4 oz	113	58	282	31	0	0	17	7	6.8	.7
608	Beef, dried, cured	1 oz	28	56	47	8	<1	0	1	.5	.5	.1

(1)Surimi is processed from Walleye (Alaska) pollock. Also see Imitation crab, shrimp, scallops.

(2)Outer layer of fat removed to about ½" of the lean. Deposits of fat within the cut remain.

PAGE KEY: A–2 = BEV A–4 = DAIRY A–10 = EGGS A–12 = FAT/OIL A–14 = FRUIT A–24 = BAKERY A–34 = GRAIN A–40 = FISH A–44 = MEATS A–48 = POULTRY A–50 = SAUSAGE A–52 = MIXED/FAST A–60 = NUTS/SEEDS A–62 = SWEETS A–66 = VEG/LEG A–78 = MISC A–80 = SOUPS/SAUCES A–84 = FAST A–96 = FRZN ENTREE A–98 = BABY FOODS

Chol (mg)	Calc (mg)	Iron (mg)	Magn (mg)	Phos (mg)	Pota (mg)	Sodi (mg)	Zinc (mg)	VT-A (RE)	Thia (mg)	Ribo (mg)	Niac (mg)	V-B6 (mg)	Fola (µg)	VT-C (mg)
34	10	.29	49	320	127	162	.37	23	.02	.02	.25	.03	2	0
44	5	.92	31	298	327	102	1.3	41	.04	.11	11	.37	2	1
57	7	1.18	39	382	418	130	1.67	46	.05	.13	13.3	.43	3	1
78	97	.43	35	305	508	63	.58	17	.17	.11	6.54	.39	21	2
15	11	1.18	26	264	175	301	.77	20	.03	.1	10.5	.09	5	0
25	9	1.3	23	139	201	287	.65	14	.03	.06	11.3	.3	3	0
43	9	1.16	57	288	286	44	.68	743	.27	.28	9.81	.52	2	0
112	11	3.46	22	244	274	67	7.61	0	.08	.27	3.55	.32	10	0
120	15	4.17	26	265	297	81	11.7	0	.09	.32	3.03	.33	7	0
109	7	3.54	25	278	319	57	5.57	0	.08	.27	4.23	.37	11	0
109	6	3.92	28	308	348	58	6.21	0	.08	.29	4.63	.41	12	0
112	10	3.14	28	215	418	93	7.29	0	.08	.36	6.63	.36	12	0
115	14	2.78	27	206	396	101	7.03	0	.07	.27	6.77	.34	12	0
96	12	2.62	22	195	335	72	5.94	0	.08	.19	3.81	.26	8	0
92	11	2.96	28	242	425	84	7.87	0	.09	.24	4.67	.34	9	0
82	7	2.09	27	234	407	67	4.89	0	.09	.18	3.93	.4	7	0
78	6	2.21	31	256	447	70	5.38	0	.1	.19	4.25	.43	8	0
90	15	3	31	235	445	78	8	0	.11	.25	5.92	.45	9	0
102	12	3.4	32	247	407	70	6.5	0	.13	.3	4.38	.45	10	0
101	12	3.81	36	277	456	75	7.39	0	.15	.33	4.85	.51	11	0
94	9	3.01	28	209	401	69	5.31	0	.11	.25	4.63	.39	8	0
91	8	3.4	33	235	460	75	6.12	0	.13	.28	5.26	.44	9	0
2261	10	2.52	17	438	400	179	1.53	0	.15	.29	4.29	.44	7	4
219	7	8.52	28	282	264	72	3.55	0	.16	1.75	4.62	.24	2	2
545	12	7.12	26	522	413	120	6.18	12165[3]	.24	4.69	16.4	1.63	249	26
121	8	3.84	19	160	204	68	5.44	0	.03	.4	2.44	.18	6	1
97	14	2.36	16	126	153	1139	4.04	0	.02	.17	2.77	.15	10	2
12	2	1.28	9	49	126	983	1.49	0	.02	.06	1.55	.1	3	4

(3) Value varies widely.

(For purposes of calculations, use "0" for t, <1, <.1, <.01, etc.)

A

A

Table A–1
Food Composition

Computer Code Number	Food Description	Measure	Wt (g)	H_2O (%)	Ener (kcal)	Prot (g)	Carb (g)	Dietary Fiber (g)	Fat (g)	Fat Breakdown (g) Sat	Mono	Poly
	MEATS: BEEF, LAMB, PORK, and others—Cont.											
	LAMB, domestic, cooked:											
	Chop, arm, braised (5.6 oz raw w/bone):											
609	Lean and fat	1 ea	70	44	241	21	0	0	17	6.9	7.1	1.2
610	Lean only	1 ea	55	49	152	20	0	0	8	2.8	3.4	.5
	Chop, loin, broiled (4.2 oz. raw w/bone):											
611	Lean and fat	1 ea	64	52	202	16	0	0	15	6.3	6.2	1.1
612	Lean only	1 ea	46	61	99	14	0	0	4	1.6	2	.3
1067	Cutlet, avg of lean cuts, cooked	4 oz	113	54	331	28	0	0	23	9.9	9.9	1.7
	Leg, roasted, 3 oz = 4⅛ x 2¼ x ½":											
613	Lean and fat	4 oz	113	57	293	29	0	0	19	7.8	7.9	1.3
614	Lean only	4 oz	113	64	217	32	0	0	9	3.1	3.8	.6
615	Rib, roasted, lean and fat	4 oz	113	48	407	24	0	0	34	14.5	14.2	2.5
616	Rib, roasted, lean only	4 oz	113	60	263	30	0	0	15	5.4	6.6	1
1065	Shoulder, roasted, lean and fat	4 oz	113	56	312	25	0	0	23	9.6	9.2	1.8
1066	Shoulder, roasted, lean only	4 oz	113	63	231	28	0	0	12	4.6	4.9	1.1
	Variety meats:											
1069	Brains, panfried	4 oz	113	76	164	14	0	0	11	2.9	2.1	1.2
1068	Heart, braised	4 oz	113	64	210	28	2	0	9	3.6	2.5	.9
1070	Sweetbreads, cooked	4 oz	113	60	265	26	0	0	17	7.8	6.2	.8
1071	Tongue, cooked	4 oz	113	58	311	24	0	0	23	8.9	11.3	1.4
	PORK, cured, cooked (see also #669–672):											
617	Bacon, medium slices	3 pce	19	13	109	6	<1	0	9	3.3	4.5	1.1
1087	Breakfast strips, cooked	2 pce	23	27	104	7	<1	0	8	2.9	3.7	1.3
618	Canadian-style bacon	2 pce	47	62	87	11	1	0	4	1.3	1.9	.4
	Ham, roasted:											
619	Lean and fat, 2 pces 4⅛ x 2¼ x ¼"	4 oz	113	65	202	26	0	0	10	3.5	5	1.6
620	Lean only	4 oz	113	68	164	24	2	0	6	2	3	.6
621	Ham, canned, roasted, 8% fat	4 oz	113	69	154	24	1	0	6	1.8	2.8	.5
	PORK, fresh, cooked:											
	Chops, loin (cut 3 per lb with bone):											
1291	Braised, lean and fat	1 ea	71	44	261	19	0	0	20	7.2	9.1	2.2
1292	Braised, lean only	1 ea	55	51	150	18	0	0	8	2.8	3.6	1
622	Broiled, lean and fat	1 ea	87	50	275	24	0	0	19	7	8.9	2.2
623	Broiled, lean only	1 ea	72	57	166	23	0	0	8	2.6	3.4	.9
624	Panfried, lean and fat	1 ea	89	45	333	21	0	0	27	9.8	12.5	3.1
625	Panfried, lean only	1 ea	67	53	189	16	0	0	13	4.6	6	1.7
626	Leg, roasted, lean and fat	4 oz	113	53	308	30	0	0	20	7	9	2
627	Leg, roasted, lean only	4 oz	113	59	233	35	0	0	9	3	4	1
628	Rib, roasted, lean and fat	4 oz	113	51	361	28	0	0	27	9.7	12.2	1
629	Rib, roasted, lean only	4 oz	113	57	277	32	0	0	16	5.4	7	1.9
630	Shoulder, braised, lean and fat	4 oz	113	47	391	30	0	0	29	10.5	13.4	3.2
631	Shoulder, braised, lean only	4 oz	113	54	281	36	0	0	14	4.8	6.2	1.7
1088	Spareribs, cooked, yield from 1 lb raw with bone	4 oz	113	40	450	33	0	0	34	13.4	16.1	4
1095	Rabbit, roasted (1 cup meat = 140 g)	4 oz	113	61	223	33	0	0	9	2.7	2.5	1.8

(Computer code number is for West Diet Analysis program)

PAGE KEY: A–2 = BEV A–4 = DAIRY A–10 = EGGS A–12 = FAT/OIL A–14 = FRUIT A–24 = BAKERY A–34 = GRAIN A–40 = FISH A–44 = MEATS A–48 = POULTRY A–50 = SAUSAGE A–52 = MIXED/FAST A–60 = NUTS/SEEDS A–62 = SWEETS A–66 = VEG/LEG A–78 = MISC A–80 = SOUPS/SAUCES A–84 = FAST A–96 = FRZN ENTREE A–98 = BABY FOODS

Chol (mg)	Calc (mg)	Iron (mg)	Magn (mg)	Phos (mg)	Pota (mg)	Sodi (mg)	Zinc (mg)	VT-A (RE)	Thia (mg)	Ribo (mg)	Niac (mg)	V-B6 (mg)	Fola (μg)	VT-C (mg)
84	18	1.68	18	144	214	50	4.26	0	.05	.18	4.67	.08	12	0
67	14	1.49	16	127	186	42	4.01	0	.04	.15	3.48	.07	12	0
64	13	1.16	15	125	209	49	2.23	0	.06	.16	4.54	.08	11	0
44	9	.92	13	104	173	39	1.9	0	.05	.13	3.15	.07	11	0
110	12	2.27	25	206	340	77	4.68	0	.13	.32	7.51	.16	19	0
106	12	2.25	27	217	355	75	4.99	0	.11	.31	7.47	.17	23	0
101	9	2.4	29	234	383	77	5.6	0	.13	.33	7.19	.19	26	0
110	25	1.81	23	188	307	83	3.96	0	.1	.24	7.65	.13	17	0
100	24	2.01	26	221	356	92	5.07	0	.1	.26	6.99	.17	25	0
104	23	2.22	26	209	285	75	5.94	0	.1	.27	6.97	.15	24	0
99	22	2.42	28	227	301	77	6.85	0	.1	.29	6.53	.17	28	0
2316	14	1.91	16	382	232	152	1.54	0	.12	.27	2.8	.12	6	14
282	16	6.26	27	288	213	71	4.17	0	.19	1.35	4.94	.34	2	8
454	14	2.4	21	489	330	59	3.04	<1	.02	.24	2.9	.06	15	23
213	11	2.99	18	151	179	76	3.39	0	.09	.48	4.18	.19	3	8
16	2	.31	5	64	92	303	.62	0	.13	.05	1.39	.05	1	6[1]
24	3	.45	6	60	105	475	.83	0	.17	.08	1.72	.08	1	10
27	5	.38	10	139	183	726	.8	0	.39	.09	3.25	.21	2	10[1]
67	9	1.52	25	319	464	1701	2.8	0	.83	.37	6.97	.35	3	26
60	9	1.68	16	222	325	1364	3.27	0	.85	.23	4.56	.45	3	24
34	7	1.04	24	237	395	1287	2.53	0	1.18	.28	5.55	.51	6	31[1]
72	6	.82	14	141	244	46	2.15	2	.43	.21	4.24	.26	3	<1
58	5	.77	13	131	230	41	2.05	1	.38	.2	3.82	.25	3	<1
85	3	.71	22	184	313	61	1.69	3	.87	.24	4.37	.35	4	<1
71	4	.66	22	175	302	56	1.61	1	.83	.22	3.99	.34	4	<1
92	4	.75	23	190	323	64	1.74	3	.91	.24	4.58	.35	4	<1
65	9	.7	16	157	264	50	2.47	1	.49	.25	3.03	.27	3	<1
106	16	1.15	25	297	398	68	3.36	3	.72	.35	5.16	.45	11	<1
108	8	1.29	33	322	442	73	3.41	3	.91	.4	5.56	.38	3	<1
92	11	1.01	21	253	416	50	2.22	3	.67	.31	5.56	.34	9	<1
89	12	1.13	24	289	480	52	2.53	3	.72	.35	6.07	.45	10	<1
124	8	1.83	20	217	380	100	4.58	3	.61	.35	5.91	.31	5	<1
129	9	2.22	25	255	458	116	5.64	2	.68	.41	6.74	.46	6	<1
137	53	2.1	27	295	363	105	5.22	3	.46	.43	6.2	.4	5	0
93	21	2.57	24	298	434	53	2.59	0	.1	.24	9.56	.53	12	0

(1) Values based on products containing added ascorbic acid or sodium ascorbate. If none added, ascorbic acid content would be negligible.

(For purposes of calculations, use "0" for t, <1, <.1, <.01, etc.)

Table A–1
Food Composition

Computer Code Number	Food Description	Measure	Wt (g)	H_2O (%)	Ener (kcal)	Prot (g)	Carb (g)	Dietary Fiber (g)	Fat (g)	Fat Breakdown (g) Sat	Mono	Poly
MEATS:	BEEF, LAMB, PORK, and others—Cont.											
	VEAL, cooked:											
632	Cutlet, braised or broiled, 4⅛ x 2¼ x ½"	4 oz	113	52	322	34	0	0	19	7.6	7.6	1.3
633	Rib roasted, lean, 2 pieces 4⅛ x 2¼ x ¼"	4 oz	113	60	257	27	0	0	16	6.1	6.2	1.1
634	Liver, panfried	4 oz	113	67	187	24	3	0	8	2.9	1.7	1.2
1096	Venison (deer meat), roasted	4 oz	113	65	179	34	0	0	4	1.4	1	.7
MEATS:	POULTRY and POULTRY PRODUCTS											
	CHICKEN, cooked:											
	Fried, batter dipped:[1]											
635	Breast (5.6 oz with bones)	1 ea	140	52	364	35	13	<1	18	4.9	7.6	4.3
636	Drumstick (3.4 oz with bones)	1 ea	72	53	192	16	6	<1	11	3	4.6	2.7
637	Thigh	1 ea	86	51	238	19	8	<1	14	3.8	5.8	3.3
638	Wing	1 ea	49	46	158	10	5	<1	11	2.9	4.4	2.5
	Fried, flour coated:[1]											
639	Breast (4.2 oz with bones)	1 ea	98	57	217	31	2	<1	9	2.4	3.4	1.9
1212	Breast, without skin	1 ea	86	60	160	29	<1	0	4	1.1	1.5	.9
640	Drumstick (2.6 oz with bones)	1 ea	49	57	120	13	1	<1	7	1.8	2.7	1.6
641	Thigh	1 ea	62	54	162	17	2	<1	9	2.5	3.6	2.1
1099	Thigh, without skin	1 ea	52	59	113	15	1	<1	5	1.4	2	1.3
642	Wing	1 ea	32	49	102	8	1	<1	7	1.9	2.8	1.6
	Roasted:											
643	All types of meat	1 c	140	64	266	40	0	0	10	2.9	3.7	2.4
644	Dark meat	1 c	140	63	287	38	0	0	14	3.7	5	3.2
645	Light meat	1 c	140	65	242	43	0	0	6	1.8	2.2	1.4
646	Breast, without skin	1 ea	86	65	141	27	0	0	3	.9	1.1	.7
647	Drumstick	1 ea	44	67	76	12	0	0	2	.7	.8	.6
1703	Leg, without skin	1 ea	95	65	182	26	0	0	8	2.2	2.9	1.9
648	Thigh	1 ea	62	59	153	15	0	0	10	2.7	3.8	2.1
1100	Thigh, without skin	1 ea	52	63	108	13	0	0	6	1.6	2.2	1.3
649	Stewed, all types:	1 c	140	67	246	38	0	0	9	2.6	3.3	2.2
656	Canned, boneless chicken	4 oz	113	69	187	25	0	0	9	2.5	3.6	2
1102	Gizzards, simmered	3 ea	66	67	101	18	1	0	2	.7	.6	.7
1101	Hearts, simmered	8 ea	25	65	45	6	<1	0	2	.6	.5	.6
650	Liver, simmered: Ounce	3 oz	85	68	128	21	7	0	5	1.6	1.1	.8
1098	Liver, simmered: Piece = 20 g	6 ea	120	68	187	29	1	0	7	2.2	1.6	1.1
	DUCK, roasted:											
1293	Meat with skin, about 2.7 cups	½ ea	382	52	1287	73	0	0	108	36.9	49.3	13.9
651	Meat only, about 1.5 cups	½ ea	221	64	444	52	0	0	25	9.2	8.2	3.2
	GOOSE, domesticated, roasted:											
1294	Meat only, 4.2 cups	½ ea	591	57	1406	171	0	0	75	26.9	25.6	9.1
1295	Meat with skin, about 5.5 cups	½ ea	774	52	2360	194	0	0	169	53.2	78.9	19.5
	TURKEY:											
	Roasted, meat only:											
652	Dark meat	4 oz	113	63	212	32	0	0	8	2.7	1.9	2.4
653	Light meat	4 oz	113	66	177	34	0	0	4	1.2	.6	1

[(1)] Fried in vegetable shortening.

(Computer code number is for West Diet Analysis program)

PAGE KEY: A–2 = BEV A–4 = DAIRY A–10 = EGGS A–12 = FAT/OIL A–14 = FRUIT A–24 = BAKERY A–34 = GRAIN A–40 = FISH A–44 = MEATS A–48 = POULTRY A–50 = SAUSAGE A–52 = MIXED/FAST A–60 = NUTS/SEEDS A–62 = SWEETS A–66 = VEG/LEG A–78 = MISC A–80 = SOUPS/SAUCES A–84 = FAST A–96 = FRZN ENTREE A–98 = BABY FOODS

Chol (mg)	Calc (mg)	Iron (mg)	Magn (mg)	Phos (mg)	Pota (mg)	Sodi (mg)	Zinc (mg)	VT-A (RE)	Thia (mg)	Ribo (mg)	Niac (mg)	V-B6 (mg)	Fola (μg)	VT-C (mg)
134	32	1.24	27	249	318	91	4.13	0	.04	.34	10.3	.29	16	0
125	12	1.1	25	222	333	104	4.64	0	.06	.31	7.92	.28	15	0
635	8	2.97	22	362	232	60	10.8	9126[2]	.15	2.2	9.62	.56	861	35
127	8	5.07	27	256	379	61	3.12	0	.2	.68	7.61	.43[3]	5[3]	0
119	28	1.75	34	259	281	385	1.33	28	.16	.2	14.7	.6	8	0
62	12	.97	14	105	133	193	1.68	19	.08	.15	3.67	.19	6	0
80	15	1.25	18	133	165	247	1.75	25	.1	.19	4.91	.22	8	0
39	10	.63	8	59	68	156	.68	17	.05	.07	2.58	.15	3	0
87	16	1.17	29	228	253	74	1.08	15	.08	.13	13.5	.57	4	0
78	14	.98	27	211	237	68	.93	6	.07	.11	12.7	.55	3	0
44	6	.66	11	86	112	44	1.42	12	.04	.11	2.96	.17	4	0
60	9	.92	15	115	146	55	1.56	18	.06	.15	4.31	.2	5	0
53	7	.76	13	103	134	49	1.45	11	.05	.13	3.7	.2	5	0
26	5	.4	6	48	57	25	.56	12	.02	.04	2.14	.13	1	0
124	21	1.69	35	273	340	120	2.94	22	.1	.25	12.8	.66	8	0
130	21	1.86	32	251	336	130	3.92	31	.1	.32	9.17	.5	11	0
119	21	1.48	38	302	344	107	1.72	13	.09	.16	17.4	.84	6	0
73	13	.89	25	196	220	64	.86	5	.06	.1	11.8	.52	3	0
41	5	.57	11	81	108	42	1.4	8	.03	.1	2.67	.17	4	0
90	11	1.26	23	174	230	87	2.73	18	.07	.22	6.02	.35	8	0
58	7	.83	14	107	137	52	1.46	30	.04	.13	3.95	.19	4	0
49	6	.68	12	95	123	46	1.34	10	.04	.12	3.39	.18	4	0
116	20	1.64	29	210	252	98	2.79	21	.07	.23	8.55	.36	8	0
70	16	1.79	14	126	155	570	1.6	39	.02	.15	7.18	.4	5	2
128	7	2.74	13	102	118	44	2.89	37	.02	.16	2.63	.08	35	1
59	5	2.22	5	49	32	12	1.8	2	.01	.18	.69	.08	20	<1
536	12	7.23	7	264	119	42	3.68	4177	.13	1.49	3.78	.5	655	14
757	17	10.2	25	373	168	61	5.21	5894	.18	2.1	5.34	.7	924	19
320	42	10.3	61	596	779	225	7.11	241	.66	1.03	18.4	.69	23	0
196	26	5.97	44	449	557	143	5.75	51	.57	1.04	11.3	.55	22	0
567	83	17	147	1826	2293	449	18.7	71	.54	2.3	24.1	2.78	71	0
704	100	21.9	170	2089	2546	541	20.3	163	.6	2.5	32.3	2.86	15	0
96	36	2.64	27	231	329	90	5.06	0	.07	.28	4.14	.41	10	0
78	22	1.53	32	248	346	73	2.31	0	.07	.15	7.76	.61	7	0

(2)Value varies widely.

(3)Values estimated from other game meat.

Table A–1
Food Composition

Computer Code Number	Food Description	Measure	Wt (g)	H_2O (%)	Ener (kcal)	Prot (g)	Carb (g)	Dietary Fiber (g)	Fat (g)	Fat Breakdown (g) Sat	Mono	Poly
	MEATS: POULTRY and POULTRY PRODUCTS—Cont.											
	TURKEY—Cont.											
	Roasted, meat only—Cont.											
654	All types, chopped or diced	1 c	140	65	238	41	0	0	7	2.3	1.5	2
655	All types, sliced	4 oz	113	65	193	33	0	0	6	1.9	1.2	1.6
1103	Ground, cooked	4 oz	113	59	266	31	0	0	15	3.8	5.5	3.7
1104	Breast, barbecued	2 oz	57	69	72	11	2	0	2	.6	.6	.4
1105	Breast, hickory smoked	2 oz	57	72	62	13	1	0	1	.3	.3	.2
1106	Gizzard, cooked	2 ea	134	65	218	39	1	0	5	1.5	1	1.5
1107	Heart, cooked	4 ea	64	64	113	17	1	0	4	1.1	.8	1.1
1108	Liver, cooked	1 ea	75	66	126	18	3	0	4	1.4	1.1	.8
	POULTRY FOOD PRODUCTS (see also items in Sausages and Lunchmeats section):											
658	Chicken roll, light meat	2 pce	57	69	91	11	1	0	4	1.1	1.7	.9
1567	Chicken patty, breaded, cooked	1 ea	75	49	222	13	9	<1	15	3.9	6	3.5
659	Turkey and gravy, frozen package	3 oz	85	85	57	5	4	<1	2	.7	.8	.4
660	Turkey loaf, breast meat	4 oz	113	72	125	25	0	0	2	.5	.5	.3
661	Turkey patty, breaded, fried	2 oz	57	50	160	8	9	<1	10	2.7	4.2	2.7
662	Turkey, frozen, roasted, seasoned	4 oz	113	68	175	24	3	0	7	2.2	1.4	1.9
1704	Turkey roll, light meat	1 pce	28	72	42	5	<1	0	2	.6	.7	.5
	MEATS: SAUSAGES and LUNCHMEATS (see also Poultry Food Products)											
1072	Beerwurst/beer salami, beef	1 oz	28	53	93	4	<1	0	8	3.7	4	.3
1074	Beerwurst/beer salami, pork	1 oz	28	61	67	4	1	0	5	1.8	2.5	.7
1075	Berliner sausage	1 oz	28	61	65	4	1	0	5	1.7	2.3	.4
	Bologna:											
1297	Beef	1 pce	23	55	72	3	<1	0	7	2.8	3.2	.3
663	Beef & pork	1 pce	28	54	90	3	1	0	8	3	3.8	.7
1298	Pork	1 pce	23	61	57	4	<1	0	5	1.6	2.2	.5
664	Turkey	1 pce	28	65	56	4	<1	0	4	1.4	1.4	1.2
665	Braunschweiger sausage	2 pce	57	48	205	8	2	0	18	6.2	8.5	2.1
1073	Bratwurst, link	1 ea	70	51	226	10	2	0	19	6.9	9.3	2
666	Brown & serve sausage links, cooked	2 ea	26	45	102	4	1	0	10	3.4	4.4	1
1089	Cheesefurter/cheese smokie	2 ea	86	52	280	12	1	0	25	9	11.8	2.6
1556	Chorizo, pork & beef	3 oz	85	32	387	20	2	0	33	12.2	15.6	2.9
1090	Corned beef loaf, jellied	1 pce	28	69	43	6	0	0	2	.7	.8	.1
	Frankfurters (see also #657):											
1077	Beef, large link, 8/package	1 ea	57	55	180	7	1	0	16	6.9	7.7	.8
1078	Beef and pork, large link, 8/package	1 ea	57	54	182	6	1	0	17	6.2	7.8	1.6
667	Beef and pork, small link, 10/pkg	1 ea	45	54	144	5	1	0	13	4.9	6.2	1.2
657	Chicken frankfurter, 10/package	1 ea	45	57	115	6	3	0	9	2.5	3.8	1.8
668	Turkey frankfurter, 10/package	1 ea	45	63	101	6	1	0	8	2.7	2.5	2.2
	Ham:											
669	Ham lunchmeat, canned, 3 x 2 x ½"	1 pce	21	52	70	3	<1	0	6	2.3	3	.7
670	Chopped ham, packaged	2 pce	42	64	96	7	0	0	7	2.4	3.4	.9
671	Ham lunchmeat, regular	2 pce	57	65	103	10	2	0	6	1.9	2.8	.7
672	Ham lunchmeat, extra lean	2 pce	57	71	74	11	1	0	3	.9	1.3	.3

(Computer code number is for West Diet Analysis program)

Chol (mg)	Calc (mg)	Iron (mg)	Magn (mg)	Phos (mg)	Pota (mg)	Sodi (mg)	Zinc (mg)	VT-A (RE)	Thia (mg)	Ribo (mg)	Niac (mg)	V-B6 (mg)	Fola (µg)	VT-C (mg)
106	35	2.49	36	298	417	98	4.34	0	.09	.25	7.62	.64	10	0
86	28	2.02	29	242	338	79	3.52	0	.07	.21	6.17	.52	8	0
116	28	2.2	27	222	306	121	3.25	0	.06	.19	5.47	.44	8	0
22	10	.4	12	184	166	609	.5	0	.02	.06	5.45	.22	2	<1
23	4	.23	11	130	158	811	.64	0	.02	.06	4.72	.2	2	0
310	20	7.28	25	172	281	72	5.57	74	.04	.44	4.11	.16	69	2
145	8	4.4	14	131	117	35	3.37	5	.04	.56	2.08	.2	50	1
469	8	5.85	11	204	145	48	2.32	2805	.04	1.07	4.46	.39	499	1
28	24	.55	11	89	129	332	.41	14	.04	.07	3.02	.12	1	0
50	7	.86	18	195	208	352	.61	21	.11	.1	5.18	.26	7	0
15	12	.79	7	69	52	471	.59	11	.02	.11	1.53	.08	3	0
46	8	.45	23	260	315	1621	1.28	0	.04	.12	9.45	.41	5	0[1]
35	8	1.25	9	153	156	454	.82	6	.06	.11	1.3	.11	5	0
60	6	1.86	25	277	338	771	2.88	0	.05	.19	7.11	.31	6	0
12	11	.37	5	52	71	139	.45	0	.03	.06	1.98	.09	1	0
17	3	.43	3	27	49	291	.69	0	.02	.03	.96	.05	1	5
17	2	.22	4	29	72	351	.49	0	.16	.05	.92	.1	1	8
13	3	.33	4	37	80	367	.7	0	.11	.06	.88	.06	1	2
13	3	.38	3	20	36	226	.5	0	.01	.02	.55	.03	1	5
16	3	.43	3	26	51	288	.55	0	.05	.04	.73	.05	1	6[2]
14	3	.18	3	32	65	272	.47	0	.12	.04	.9	.06	1	8
28	24	.43	4	37	56	249	.49	0	.02	.05	1	.06	2	<1
89	5	5.34	6	96	113	652	1.6	2405	.14	.87	4.77	.19	25	6[2]
44	34	.72	11	94	196	778	1.47	0	.17	.16	2.31	.09	3	20
16	2	.62	4	42	70	248	.3	0	.21	.09	.96	.06	1	0
58	50	.93	11	153	177	930	1.94	33	.21	.14	2.5	.11	3	17
75	7	1.35	15	128	338	1049	2.9	0	.54	.25	4.36	.45	2	0
13	3	.58	3	21	29	271	1.16	0	0	.03	.5	.03	2	2
35	11	.81	2	50	95	585	1.24	0	.03	.06	1.38	.07	2	14
28	6	.66	6	49	95	638	1.05	0	.11	.07	1.5	.07	2	15
22	5	.52	4	39	75	504	.83	0	.09	.05	1.18	.06	2	12[2]
45	43	.9	6	48	38	616	.47	17	.03	.05	1.39	.14	2	0
39	48	.83	6	60	81	641	1.4	0	.02	.08	1.86	.1	4	0
13	1	.15	2	17	45	270	.31	0	.08	.04	.65	.04	1	<1
21	3	.35	7	65	134	576	.81	0	.26	.09	1.63	.15	<1	8[2]
32	4	.56	11	140	188	746	1.21	0	.49	.14	2.98	.19	2	16[2]
27	4	.43	10	124	198	810	1.09	0	.53	.13	2.74	.26	2	15[2]

(1)If sodium ascorbate is added, product contains 11 mg ascorbic acid.

(2)Values based on products containing added ascorbic acid or sodium ascorbate. If none added, ascorbic acid content would be negligible.

(For purposes of calculations, use "0" for t, <1, <.1, <.01, etc.)

A

Table A–1
Food Composition

Computer Code Number	Food Description	Measure	Wt (g)	H_2O (%)	Ener (kcal)	Prot (g)	Carb (g)	Dietary Fiber (g)	Fat (g)	Fat Breakdown (g) Sat	Mono	Poly
	MEATS: SAUSAGES and LUNCHMEATS (see also Poultry Food Products)—Cont.											
	Ham—Cont.											
673	Turkey ham lunchmeat	2 pce	57	71	73	11	<1	0	3	1	.7	.9
1091	Kielbasa sausage	1 pce	26	54	81	3	1	0	7	2.6	3.4	.8
1092	Knockwurst sausage, link	1 ea	68	55	209	8	1	0	19	6.9	8.7	2
1093	Mortadella lunchmeat	2 pce	30	52	93	5	1	0	8	2.9	3.4	.9
1097	Olive loaf lunchmeat	2 pce	57	58	134	7	5	<1	9	3.3	4.5	1.1
1080	Turkey pastrami	2 pce	57	71	80	10	1	0	4	1	1.2	.9
1081	Pepperoni sausage	2 pce	11	27	54	2	<1	0	5	1.8	2.3	.5
1094	Pickle & pimento loaf	2 pce	57	57	149	7	3	<1	12	4.5	5.5	1.5
1082	Polish sausage	1 oz	28	53	92	4	<1	0	8	2.9	3.9	.9
674	Pork sausage, cooked,[1] link, small	2 ea	26	45	96	5	<1	0	8	2.8	3.6	1
1079	Pork sausage, cooked, patty	4 oz	113	45	418	22	1	0	35	12.2	15.8	4.3
675	Salami, pork and beef	2 pce	57	60	141	8	1	0	11	4.6	5.2	1.1
676	Salami, turkey	2 pce	57	66	111	9	<1	0	8	2.3	2.6	2
677	Beef & pork, dry	3 pce	30	35	125	7	1	0	10	3.7	5.1	1
	Sandwich spreads:											
1300	Ham salad spread	1 c	240	63	518	21	26	0	37	12.2	17.3	6.5
678	Pork and beef	2 tbs	30	60	70	2	4	<1	5	1.8	2.3	.8
1296	Chicken/turkey	2 tbs	26	66	52	3	2	0	4	.9	.8	1.6
1084	Smoked link sausage, beef and pork	1 ea	68	52	228	9	1	0	21	7.2	9.7	2.2
1083	Smoked link sausage, pork	1 ea	68	39	265	15	1	0	22	7.7	9.9	2.6
1085	Summer sausage	2 pce	46	51	154	7	<1	0	14	5.5	6	.6
1076	Turkey breakfast sausage	1 pce	28	60	65	6	0	0	5	1.6	1.8	1.2
679	Vienna sausage, canned	2 ea	32	60	89	3	1	0	8	3	4	.5
	MIXED DISHES and FAST FOODS											
	MIXED DISHES:											
1445	Almond chicken	1 c	242	77	273	20	18	4	14	2	5.3	5.8
1454	Bean cake	1 ea	32	23	130	2	16	1	7	1	2.9	2.6
680	Beef stew w/ vegetables, homemade	1 c	245	82	218	16	15	2	10	4.9	4.5	.5
1109	Beef stew w/ vegetables, canned	1 c	245	82	194	14	17	3	8	2.4	3.1	.3
1116	Beef, macaroni, tomato sauce casserole	1 c	226	73	284	21	25	3	11	4.2	4.7	.6
1452	Beef fajita	1 ea	189	67	250	15	32	2	7	2	3	1
681	Beef pot pie, homemade[2]	1 pce	210	55	517	21	39	1	31	8.4	14.9	7.4
1462	Buffalo wings/spicy chicken wings	2 ea	32	53	98	8	<1	<1	7	1.8	2.8	1.6
1675	Carrot raisin salad	½ c	88	58	202	1	21	3	14	2.1	3.9	7.1
682	Chicken à la king, homemade	1 c	245	68	468	27	12	1	34	12.7	14.3	6.2
683	Chicken & noodles, homemade	1 c	240	71	367	22	26	2	18	5.9	7.1	3.5
684	Chicken chow mein, canned	1 c	250	89	95	6	18	5	1	0	.1	.8
685	Chicken chow mein, homemade	1 c	250	78	255	31	10	4	10	2.4	4.3	3.1
1451	Chicken fajitas	1 ea	189	68	230	17	30	3	5	2	2	1
686	Chicken pot pie, homemade (⅓)	1 pce	232	57	545	23	42	3	33	10.9	15.5	6.6
1672	Chili con carne	½ c	127	77	128	12	11	2	4	1.7	1.7	.3
1112	Chicken salad with celery	2 c	78	53	268	11	1	<1	25	4	7.2	12.1
687	Chili with beans, canned	1 c	255	76	286	15	30	8	14	6	5.9	.9
1479	Chinese pastry	1 oz	28	46	67	1	13	<1	1	.2	.4	.8
688	Chop suey with beef & pork	1 c	250	63	465	26	35	4	25	5.7	13.3	3.9

(1)Cooked weight is half the weight of raw sausage.

(2)Crust made with vegetable shortening and enriched flour.

(Computer code number is for West Diet Analysis program)

Chol (mg)	Calc (mg)	Iron (mg)	Magn (mg)	Phos (mg)	Pota (mg)	Sodi (mg)	Zinc (mg)	VT-A (RE)	Thia (mg)	Ribo (mg)	Niac (mg)	V-B6 (mg)	Fola (μg)	VT-C (mg)
32	6	1.57	9	108	185	567	1.68	0	.03	.14	2.01	.14	3	0
17	11	.38	4	38	70	279	.52	0	.06	.06	.75	.05	1	5
39	7	.62	7	67	135	685	1.13	0	.23	.09	1.86	.12	1	18
17	5	.42	3	29	49	372	.63	0	.04	.05	.8	.04	1	8
22	62	.31	11	72	169	846	.79	11	.17	.15	1.05	.13	1	5
31	5	.95	8	114	148	595	1.23	0	.03	.14	2.01	.15	3	0
9	1	.15	2	13	38	224	.27	0	.03	.03	.54	.03	<1	0
21	54	.58	10	80	194	792	.8	4	.17	.14	1.17	.11	3	8
20	3	.41	4	39	67	247	.55	0	.14	.04	.97	.05	1	<1
22	8	.32	4	48	94	336	.65	0	.19	.07	1.18	.09	1	<1
94	36	1.42	19	209	409	1467	2.84	0	.84	.29	5.13	.37	2	2
37	7	1.51	9	65	112	603	1.21	0	.14	.21	2.01	.12	1	7[3]
47	11	.92	9	60	139	572	1.03	0	.04	.1	2.01	.14	2	0
24	2	.45	5	43	113	558	.97	0	.18	.09	1.46	.15	1	8[3]
89	19	1.42	24	288	360	2188	2.64	0	1.04	.29	5.04	.36	2	14
11	4	.24	2	18	33	302	.31	3	.05	.04	.52	.04	1	0
8	3	.16	3	9	48	98	.27	11	.01	.02	.43	.03	1	<1
48	7	.99	8	73	128	642	1.43	0	.18	.12	2.19	.12	1	13
46	20	.79	13	110	228	1020	1.92	0	.48	.17	3.08	.24	3	1
34	6	1.17	6	51	125	571	1.18	0	.07	.15	1.98	.12	1	9
23	5	.52	6	52	76	191	.97	0	.03	.08	1.42	.08	1	–
17	3	.28	2	16	32	304	.51	0	.03	.03	.51	.04	1	0
35	79	2.12	59	238	550	617	1.56	75	.08	.19	8.59	.4	27	10
0	3	.65	6	19	56	55	.15	0	.06	.04	.49	.02	8	0
64	29	2.94	40	184	613	292	5.29	568	.15	.17	4.66	.28	37	17
34	29	2.21	39	110	426	1006	4.24	262	.07	.12	2.45	.2	31	7
57	28	3.11	42	161	559	841	4.3	93	.23	.25	5.22	.33	22	13
20	100	1.8	–	–	350	630	–	20	.3	.51	5	.35	–	2
44	29	3.78	6	149	334	596	3.17	519	.29	.29	4.83	.24	29	6
26	5	.4	6	47	59	61	.56	17	.01	.04	2.06	.13	1	<1
10	26	.74	14	46	315	117	.18	1453	.08	.05	.63	.22	9	5
186	127	2.45	20	358	404	760	1.8	272	.1	.42	5.39	.23	11	12
96	26	2.16	26	247	149	600	1.53	10	.05	.17	4.32	.19	10	0
7	45	1.25	14	85	418	725	1.3	28	.05	.1	1	.09	12	12
77	57	2.5	28	293	473	718	2.12	50	.07	.22	4.25	.41	19	10
30	40	1.1	–	–	300	590	–	40	.23	.34	4	.03	–	2
72	70	3.02	25	232	343	594	2	735	.32	.32	4.87	.46	29	5
67	34	2.62	23	99	347	506	1.8	84	.06	.57	1.25	.17	15	<1
47	16	.62	11	80	138	201	.8	31	.03	.07	3.27	.34	8	1
43	120	8.75	115	393	931	1331	5.1	87	.12	.27	.91	.34	58	4
0	7	.55	6	14	26	3	.2	<1	.04	<.01	.35	.02	1	0
57	48	4.45	69	255	568	1027	3.9	147	.21	.26	4.45	.47	37	3

(3)Values based on products containing added ascorbic acid or sodium ascorbate. If none added, ascorbic acid content would be negligible.

(For purposes of calculations, use "0" for t, <1, <.1, <.01, etc.)

A

Table A–1
Food Composition

Computer Code Number	Food Description	Measure	Wt (g)	H_2O (%)	Ener (kcal)	Prot (g)	Carb (g)	Dietary Fiber (g)	Fat (g)	Fat Breakdown (g) Sat	Mono	Poly
	MIXED DISHES and FAST FOOD—Cont.											
	MIXED DISHES—Cont.											
690	Coleslaw[1]	1 c	120	74	178	2	15	2	13	2	2.9	7.7
689	Corn pudding[2]	1 c	250	76	273	11	32	9	13	6.3	4.3	1.7
1110	Corned beef hash, canned	1 c	220	67	398	19	23	1	25	11.9	10.9	.9
	Egg foo yung patty:											
1467	Meatless	1 ea	86	94	26	3	<1	0	1	.4	.5	.2
1458	With beef	1 ea	86	75	127	9	3	<1	9	2.2	3.2	2.4
1465	With chicken	1 ea	86	75	128	9	3	<1	9	2.1	3.1	2.5
1602	Egg roll, meatless	1 ea	64	70	101	3	10	1	6	1.2	2.5	1.6
1550	Egg roll, with meat	1 ea	64	66	117	5	9	1	7	1.6	2.9	1.6
1113	Egg salad	1 c	183	57	586	17	3	0	56	10.6	17.5	24.2
691	French toast w/wheat bread, homemade[3]	1 pce	65	54	151	5	16	<1	7	2	3	1.7
1355	Green pepper, stuffed	1 ea	172	74	236	11	20	2	12	5.3	5.3	.6
1487	Hot & sour soup (Chinese)	1 c	244	88	130	12	5	<1	7	2.2	2.9	1.2
	Lasagna:											
1346	With meat, homemade	1 pce	245	66	390	23	41	3	15	7.7	5	.8
1111	Without meat, homemade	1 pce	218	68	305	16	40	3	9	5.4	2.4	.6
1117	Frozen entree	1 pce	205	74	238	15	26	2	9	4	3.3	.5
1606	Lo mein, meatless	1 c	200	83	123	6	23	3	1	.3	.3	.4
1607	Lo mein, with meat	1 c	200	71	284	16	27	3	13	2.9	4.2	4.7
692	Macaroni & cheese, canned[4]	1 c	240	80	228	9	26	1	10	4.2	3.1	1.4
693	Macaroni & cheese, homemade[5]	1 c	200	58	430	17	40	1	22	8.9	8.8	3.6
1115	Macaroni salad, no cheese	1 c	141	60	363	3	21	3	30	4.4	8.5	15.5
1120	Meat loaf, beef	1 pce	87	58	206	19	4	<1	12	4.7	5.2	.6
1119	Meat loaf, beef and pork (⅓)	1 pce	87	57	221	17	4	<1	15	5.4	6.4	1.2
1303	Moussaka (lamb & eggplant)	1 c	250	83	209	18	14	3	9	2.7	3.7	1.5
715	Potato salad with mayonnaise and eggs[6]	½ c	125	76	179	3	14	2	10	1.8	3.1	4.7
1674	Pizza, combination, 1/12 of 12" round	1 pce	53	48	123	9	14	–	4	1	1.7	.6
1673	Pizza, pepperoni, 1/12 of 12" round	1 pce	47	46	121	7	13	–	5	1.5	2.1	.8
694	Quiche Lorraine, ⅛ of 8" quiche[7]	1 pce	176	52	540	15	23	1	43	20.1	15.6	5.3
1449	Ramen noodles, cooked	1 c	227	83	147	5	27	3	2	.4	.4	.4
1671	Ravioli, meat	½ c	125	68	194	11	18	1	9	3	3.6	1
1597	Fried rice (meatless)	1 c	166	71	241	5	30	1	11	1.7	2.9	6.2
	Spaghetti (enriched) in tomato sauce:											
	With cheese:											
695	Canned	1 c	250	80	190	5	38	2	1	0	.4	.5
696	Homemade	1 c	250	77	260	9	37	2	9	2	5.4	1.2
	With meatballs:											
697	Canned	1 c	250	78	258	12	28	6	10	2.1	3.9	3.9
698	Homemade	1 c	248	70	332	19	39	8	12	3.3	6.3	2.2
716	Spinach soufflé[8]	1 c	136	74	219	11	3	4	18	7.1	6.8	3.1
1553	Sweet & sour pork	1 c	226	76	247	14	25	1	10	2.8	3.8	2.9

(1)Recipe: 41% cabbage; 12% celery; 12% table cream; 12% sugar; 7% green pepper; 6% lemon juice; 4% onion; 3% pimento; 3% vinegar; 2% each for salt, dry mustard, and white pepper.

(2)Recipe: 55% yellow corn, 23% whole milk, 14% egg, 4% sugar, 3% salt, and 1% pepper.

(3)Recipe: 35% whole milk, 32% white bread, 29% egg, and cooked in 4% margarine.

(4)Made with corn oil.

(5)Made with margarine.

(6)Recipe: 62% potatoes; 12% egg; 8% mayonnaise; 7% celery; 6% sweet pickle relish; 2% onion; 1% each for green pepper, pimento, salt, and dry mustard.

(7)Crust made with vegetable shortening and enriched flour.

(8)Recipe: 29% whole milk, 26% spinach, 13% egg white, 13% cheddar cheese, 7% egg yolk, 7% butter, 4% flour, 1% salt and pepper.

(Computer code number is for West Diet Analysis program)

PAGE KEY: A–2 = BEV A–4 = DAIRY A–10 = EGGS A–12 = FAT/OIL A–14 = FRUIT A–24 = BAKERY A–34 = GRAIN A–40 = FISH A–44 = MEATS A–48 = POULTRY A–50 = SAUSAGE A–52 = MIXED/FAST A–60 = NUTS/SEEDS A–62 = SWEETS A–66 = VEG/LEG A–78 = MISC A–80 = SOUPS/SAUCES A–84 = FAST A–96 = FRZN ENTREE A–98 = BABY FOODS

Chol (mg)	Calc (mg)	Iron (mg)	Magn (mg)	Phos (mg)	Pota (mg)	Sodi (mg)	Zinc (mg)	VT-A (RE)	Thia (mg)	Ribo (mg)	Niac (mg)	V-B6 (mg)	Fola (μg)	VT-C (mg)
6[9]	41	.88	11	43	215	324	.24	60	.05	.04	.1	.13	47	10
250	100	1.4	37	143	403	138	1.25	90	1.03	.32	2.47	.29	63	7
73	29	4.4	36	147	440	1188	3.3	0	.02	.2	4.62	.43	20	0
37	7	.26	2	38	77	257	.17	14	.01	.07	1.07	.02	5	0
180	26	1.1	11	110	143	185	1.16	92	.05	.24	.73	.16	22	3
182	28	.85	11	102	143	188	.81	95	.05	.24	.95	.13	22	3
30	12	.74	9	36	97	307	.25	15	.07	.1	.75	.05	11	3
38	12	.77	9	56	117	305	.5	14	.13	.12	1.26	.09	8	2
578	74	1.8	13	236	180	666	1.44	262	.08	.66	.08	.47	61	0
76	64	1.09	11	76	86	311	.44	81	.13	.21	1.06	.05	15	<1
38	17	1.88	20	89	230	203	2.2	44	.14	.09	2.91	.31	17	55
22	27	1.87	27	156	345	1562	1.15	2	.19	.22	4.56	.15	12	1
56	262	3.43	45	301	510	745	3.19	158	.21	.33	3.72	.26	19	16
31	256	2.73	38	250	424	714	1.7	156	.2	.28	2.25	.22	17	15
33	160	2.17	36	190	478	496	2.19	149	.16	.24	2.93	.21	17	25
22	48	2.18	30	115	396	624	.91	163	.18	.23	2.48	.18	41	13
61	25	2.2	34	177	260	276	1.85	38	.42	.27	3.4	.26	39	9
24	199	.96	31	182	139	730	1.2	73	.12	.24	.96	.02	8	<1
42	362	1.8	37	322	240	1086	1.2	234	.2	.4	1.8	.05	10	1
22	27	.67	16	51	137	289	.38	39	.08	.05	.75	.26	16	3
94	32	1.82	17	126	222	158	3.89	23	.07	.22	3.36	.17	13	1
91	35	1.55	16	129	236	389	3.12	23	.2	.22	3.18	.19	11	1
101	104	2.2	38	204	578	400	2.84	105	.21	.31	4.01	.26	45	6
85	24	.81	19	65	318	661	.39	41	.1	.07	1.11	.18	8	12
14	68	1.03	12	88	119	255	.75	68	.14	.12	1.31	.06	18	1
10	43	.63	6	50	102	178	.35	36	.09	.16	2.04	.04	35	1
218	229	1.71	23	253	236	567	1.48	276	.22	.45	1.81	.1	17	3
36	17	1.78	17	70	69	1343	.61	221	.16	.09	1.42	.07	8	<1
84	33	1.99	20	105	256	619	1.67	94	.13	.20	2.85	.15	13	11
42	27	2.22	22	72	119	281	.84	62	.15	.11	1.69	.1	17	6
7	40	2.75	21	87	303	955	1.12	120	.35	.27	4.5	.13	6	10
7	80	2.25	26	135	408	955	1.3	140	.25	.17	2.25	.2	8	12
22	52	3.25	20	113	245	1220	2.39	100	.15	.17	2.25	.12	5	5
74	124	3.72	40	236	665	1009	2.45	159	.25	.3	3.97	.2	10	22
184	230	1.35	38	231	201	763	1.29	676	.09	.3	.48	.12	62	3
43	25	1.49	31	151	380	1203	1.7	27	.45	.22	3.62	.35	10	23

(9) From dairy cream in recipe.

(For purposes of calculations, use "0" for t, <1, <.1, <.01, etc.)

Table A–1
Food Composition

Computer Code Number	Food Description	Measure	Wt (g)	H_2O (%)	Ener (kcal)	Prot (g)	Carb (g)	Dietary Fiber (g)	Fat (g)	Fat Breakdown (g) Sat	Mono	Poly
	MIXED DISHES and FAST FOODS—Cont.											
	MIXED DISHES—Cont.											
1515	Three bean salad	1 ea	340	82	316	9	30	7	19	2.8	4.3	11.1
717	Tuna salad[1]	1 c	205	63	383	33	19	1	19	3.2	5.9	8.4
1121	Tuna noodle casserole, homemade	1 c	202	75	238	17	25	2	7	1.9	1.5	3.2
1270	Waldorf salad	1 c	142	59	411	3	13	2	41	5.4	10.9	22.2
	FAST FOODS and SANDWICHES (see end of this appendix for additional Fast Foods):											
699	Burrito,[2] beef & bean	1 ea	175	52	385	17	50	4	13	6.3	5.3	.9
700	Burrito, bean	1 ea	174	53	358	11	57	7	11	5.5	3.8	1
701	Cheeseburger with bun, regular	1 ea	112	55	261	13	20	–	14	6.7	5.2	1.1
702	Cheeseburger with bun, 4-oz patty	1 ea	194	51	487	25	41	–	25	10.2	9.1	3.1
703	Chicken patty sandwich	1 ea	157	47	444	21	33	1	25	7.4	9	7.2
704	Corndog	1 ea	111	47	292	11	35	–	12	3.3	5.8	2.2
705	Enchilada	1 ea	230	63	451	14	40	–	27	15	8.9	1.1
706	English muffin with egg, cheese, bacon	1 ea	138	49	362	19	30	<1	19	8.6	6.4	1.9
	Fish sandwich:											
707	Regular, with cheese	1 ea	140	45	400	16	36	<1	22	6.2	6.8	7.2
708	Large, no cheese	1 ea	170	47	464	18	44	<1	24	5.6	8.3	8.9
709	Hamburger with bun, regular	1 ea	98	46	252	12	30	–	9	3.2	3.4	1.6
710	Hamburger with bun, 4-oz patty	1 ea	174	51	466	26	31	–	26	9.7	11.4	2.2
711	Hot dog/frankfurter with bun	1 ea	85	54	210	9	16	–	13	4.4	5.9	1.5
712	Pizza, cheese, ⅛ of 15" round[3]	1 pce	120	48	268	15	39	2	6	2.9	1.9	.9
	SANDWICHES:											
	Avocado, cheese, tomato, & lettuce:											
1276	On white bread, firm	1 ea	205	58	467	15	40	4	29	8.7	11.9	6
1278	On part whole wheat	1 ea	195	59	432	14	33	5	28	8.6	11.9	5.9
1277	On whole wheat	1 ea	209	58	458	16	39	7	29	8.7	12.1	6.1
	Bacon, lettuce & tomato:											
1137	On white bread, soft	1 ea	135	46	404	12	34	2	24	6	9	8
1139	On part whole wheat	1 ea	136	47	398	13	32	3	25	6	9.5	8
1138	On whole wheat	1 ea	149	47	421	14	37	6	26	6	9.6	8
	Cheese, grilled:											
1140	On white bread, soft	1 ea	117	37	393	17	29	1	23	12.2	7.6	2.1
1142	On part whole wheat	1 ea	117	37	389	18	27	2	24	12.3	7.7	2.2
1141	On whole wheat	1 ea	131	38	416	19	33	5	24	12.5	8	2.4
1596	Chicken fillet	1 ea	182	47	515	24	39	1	29	8.5	10.4	8.4
	Chicken salad:											
1143	On white bread, soft	1 ea	105	39	371	10	28	1	24	4	7.3	12
1145	On part whole wheat	1 ea	105	40	366	10	27	2	25	4	7	12
1144	On whole wheat	1 ea	118	40	389	12	32	5	25	4	7.6	12
1146	Corned beef & swiss on rye	1 ea	147	45	439	28	25	3	25	9.8	8.3	4.8

(1)Made with drained chunk light tuna, celery, onion, pickle relish, and mayonnaise-type salad dressing.

(2)Made with a 10½"-diameter flour tortilla.

(3)Crust made with vegetable shortening and enriched flour.

Chol (mg)	Calc (mg)	Iron (mg)	Magn (mg)	Phos (mg)	Pota (mg)	Sodi (mg)	Zinc (mg)	VT-A (RE)	Thia (mg)	Ribo (mg)	Niac (mg)	V-B6 (mg)	Fola (µg)	VT-C (mg)
0	80	3.21	57	147	508	1164	1.22	52	.16	.21	.91	.1	120	10
27	35	2.05	39	365	365	824	1.15	55	.06	.14	13.7	.17	15	5
41	34	2.3	31	156	182	775	1.21	13	.18	.15	7.81	.2	10	1
22	42	.85	36	78	268	250	.59	41	.09	.05	.35	.37	27	6
37	80	3.71	63	107	497	1011	2.91	49	.4	.63	4.1	.28	56	1
3	90	3.62	70	78	524	790	1.22	26	.5	.49	3.25	.24	94	2
38	132	1.93	19	157	167	710	1.9	51	.23	.17	4.64	.11	16	2
70	200	4	35	283	392	1228	4.07	76	.41	.33	9.41	.21	27	2
52	52	4.03	30	201	305	826	1.62	27	.28	.2	5.87	.17	25	8
50	64	3.92	11	105	167	617	.83	23	.18	.44	2.64	.06	38	0
62	458	1.86	71	189	338	1106	3.54	262	.11	.6	2.69	.55	48	1
221	196	3.11	32	302	201	741	1.71	149	.45	.5	3.71	.15	41	1
52	141	2.67	28	238	270	718	.9	74	.35	.32	3.23	.08	24	2
59	90	2.81	36	228	366	661	1.07	32	.36	.24	3.66	.12	48	3
39	47	2.25	21	101	197	516	1.88	12	.23	.29	4.3	.12	16	2
83	75	4.49	36	230	426	600	4.7	3	.28	.33	5.45	.3	36	1
38	20	2.01	11	84	124	581	1.72	0	.2	.24	3.16	.04	25	<1
18	222	1.1	30	215	209	640	1.56	140	.35	.31	4.73	.08	112	2
33	287	2.98	53	236	565	538	1.67	146	.36	.38	3.68	.3	77	11
30	283	3.01	65	253	596	511	1.85	136	.33	.37	3.82	.34	77	11
31	275	3.45	99	329	661	581	2.63	137	.34	.36	4.18	.41	89	11
29	60	2.33	22	144	254	737	1.16	35	.4	.23	3.8	.19	31	14
27	73	2.6	38	177	313	753	1.43	35	.4	.25	4.3	.23	35	14
26	62	3.18	75	257	378	818	2.29	35	.4	.23	4.6	.29	47	14
54	406	1.93	26	471	160	1148	2.03	209	.28	.39	2.27	.08	23	<1
53	405	2.08	38	502	206	1143	2.27	209	.25	.36	2.35	.09	27	<1
53	398	2.53	73	581	269	1219	3.05	211	.26	.34	2.72	.16	39	<1
60	60	4.68	35	233	353	957	1.87	31	.33	.24	6.81	.2	29	9
32	56	1.98	17	95	129	447	.73	26	.23	.17	3.69	.25	24	<1
31	67	2.13	30	124	181	461	.98	26	.24	.18	3.78	.29	27	<1
30	58	2.58	63	196	240	526	1.72	26	.25	.17	4.17	.34	39	<1
79	316	2.75	40	298	198	1070	3.69	78	.23	.35	3.26	.19	33	1

(For purposes of calculations, use "0" for t, <1, <.1, <.01, etc.)

Table A–1
Food Composition

Computer Code Number	Food Description	Measure	Wt (g)	H_2O (%)	Ener (kcal)	Prot (g)	Carb (g)	Dietary Fiber (g)	Fat (g)	Fat Breakdown (g) Sat	Mono	Poly
	FAST FOODS and SANDWICHES (see end of this appendix for additional Fast Foods)—Cont.											
	SANDWICHES—Cont.											
	Egg salad:											
1147	On white bread, soft	1 ea	111	43	383	9	29	1	26	4.5	8	11.8
1149	On part whole wheat	1 ea	111	43	378	9	27	2	26	4.5	8	11.8
1148	On whole wheat	1 ea	125	43	401	11	33	5	27	4.7	8	12
	Ham:											
1279	On rye bread	1 ea	116	56	241	16	20	3	10	2.2	3.8	3.6
1151	On white bread, soft	1 ea	122	55	260	17	23	1	11	2.3	4.1	3.6
1153	On part whole wheat	1 ea	122	55	257	17	22	2	11	2.3	4.1	3.7
1152	On whole wheat	1 ea	136	54	284	19	27	4	12	2.5	4.4	3.9
	Ham & cheese:											
1280	On white bread, soft	1 ea	151	50	388	21	29	1	21	7.8	6.8	4.6
1282	On part whole wheat	1 ea	151	50	384	22	27	2	21	7.8	6.9	4.7
1281	On whole wheat	1 ea	165	49	411	24	33	5	22	8	7.1	4.9
1150	Ham & swiss on rye	1 ea	145	50	368	23	25	3	19	7.2	6.2	4.6
	Ham salad:											
1154	On white bread, soft	1 ea	125	47	344	10	34	1	18	4.5	7.3	5.8
1156	On part whole wheat	1 ea	125	48	340	10	33	2	19	4.6	7.3	5.9
1155	On whole wheat	1 ea	139	47	367	12	39	5	19	4.8	7.6	6.1
1157	Patty melt: Ground beef & cheese on rye	1 ea	177	43	583	36	25	3	37	13.8	13.8	6.2
	Peanut butter & jelly:											
1158	On white bread, soft	1 ea	100	27	345	10	47	3	14	2.7	6.6	3.9
1160	On part whole wheat	1 ea	100	27	341	11	46	4	14	2.8	6.6	4
1159	On whole wheat	1 ea	114	28	368	13	51	7	15	2.9	6.9	4.2
1161	Reuben, grilled: Corned beef, swiss cheese, sauerkraut on rye	1 ea	233	61	496	29	29	5	29	10.7	10.2	6.1
	Roast beef:											
713	On a bun	1 ea	150	49	374	23	36	–	15	3.9	7.3	1.8
1162	On white bread, soft	1 ea	122	47	314	22	26	1	13	2.7	4.3	4.9
1164	On part whole wheat	1 ea	122	47	311	23	25	2	13	2.8	4.3	5
1163	On whole wheat	1 ea	136	46	339	25	30	4	14	3	4.6	5.3
	Tuna salad:											
1165	On white bread, soft	1 ea	116	47	310	13	33	2	14	2.3	4.4	6.3
1167	On part whole wheat	1 ea	116	47	306	13	32	3	14	2.4	4.5	6.4
1166	On whole wheat	1 ea	130	46	333	15	37	5	15	2.5	4.7	6.6
	Turkey:											
1168	On white bread, soft	1 ea	122	54	270	19	22	1	11	2	3.5	5
1170	On part whole wheat	1 ea	122	54	267	19	21	2	11	2	3.5	5
1169	On whole wheat	1 ea	136	53	294	21	26	4	12	2.2	3.8	5.3
	Turkey ham:											
1272	On rye bread	1 ea	116	57	239	16	19	3	10	2.2	3	4.3
1273	On white bread, soft	1 ea	122	56	258	16	23	1	11	2.3	3.3	4.3
1275	On part whole wheat	1 ea	122	56	255	17	22	2	11	2.4	3.3	4.4
1274	On whole wheat	1 ea	136	55	282	19	27	4	12	2.6	3.6	4.7

PAGE KEY: A–2 = BEV A–4 = DAIRY A–10 = EGGS A–12 = FAT/OIL A–14 = FRUIT A–24 = BAKERY A–34 = GRAIN A–40 = FISH A–44 = MEATS A–48 = POULTRY A–50 = SAUSAGE A–52 = MIXED/FAST A–60 = NUTS/SEEDS A–62 = SWEETS A–66 = VEG/LEG A–78 = MISC A–80 = SOUPS/SAUCES A–84 = FAST A–96 = FRZN ENTREE A–98 = BABY FOODS

Chol (mg)	Calc (mg)	Iron (mg)	Magn (mg)	Phos (mg)	Pota (mg)	Sodi (mg)	Zinc (mg)	VT-A (RE)	Thia (mg)	Ribo (mg)	Niac (mg)	V-B6 (mg)	Fola (μg)	VT-C (mg)
150	66	2.21	15	114	106	511	.72	73	.24	.29	1.82	.2	35	0
149	79	2.36	29	146	161	525	.96	73	.26	.32	2.35	.24	39	0
147	67	2.81	61	215	217	590	1.74	73	.27	.31	2.71	.3	49	0
35	38	1.72	29	197	303	1289	1.76	6	.78	.28	4.66	.38	23	17
36	57	1.97	24	191	293	1277	1.59	6	.83	.3	4.96	.38	18	17
35	56	2.09	34	216	329	1274	1.79	6	.8	.27	5.03	.39	21	17
36	50	2.5	62	283	389	1364	2.45	6	.83	.27	5.45	.46	31	18
57	237	2.34	31	381	311	1582	2.26	87	.78	.4	4.84	.36	24	14
57	236	2.49	43	412	356	1578	2.5	87	.75	.37	4.92	.38	27	14
57	228	2.93	77	488	419	1655	3.27	88	.76	.36	5.29	.45	39	14
56	309	1.99	41	353	313	1289	2.74	77	.73	.38	4.52	.37	29	14
28	67	2.11	20	127	159	898	1.02	8	.52	.26	3.49	.18	20	4
27	66	2.27	32	158	206	893	1.26	8	.49	.23	3.57	.2	24	4
28	57	2.71	66	234	269	967	2.04	8	.51	.21	3.94	.27	36	4
116	224	3.83	44	416	377	892	6.96	137	.28	.47	6.56	.33	39	<1
1	74	2.36	52	130	263	309	1.02	<1	.3	.22	5.55	.15	43	<1
0	73	2.52	65	162	309	305	1.26	<1	.27	.19	5.63	.17	47	<1
0	64	2.97	99	238	374	375	2.04	<1	.28	.18	6.03	.24	59	<1
80	347	3.96	51	320	337	1655	3.91	128	.25	.37	3.43	.3	52	12
55	58	4.56	33	258	341	855	3.66	22	.4	.33	6.33	.28	43	2
34	57	3.21	23	157	341	1257	2.95	9	.26	.28	5.29	.32	23	10
34	56	3.33	33	182	377	1254	3.14	9	.24	.25	5.36	.33	26	10
34	50	3.77	61	247	438	1343	3.85	9	.25	.25	5.78	.4	36	10
12	71	2.26	23	146	160	558	.65	21	.28	.23	5.63	.13	23	1
12	69	2.42	36	177	206	553	.89	21	.25	.19	5.71	.15	27	1
12	60	2.86	70	253	270	625	1.66	21	.26	.18	6.1	.22	39	1
34	55	1.67	24	198	242	1252	1.05	9	.24	.22	7.32	.33	19	0
34	53	1.8	34	223	279	1249	1.24	9	.21	.19	7.39	.35	22	0
35	47	2.19	62	289	336	1339	1.89	9	.22	.19	7.88	.41	32	0
41	40	3.03	28	178	287	1004	2.43	6	.2	.29	3.81	.23	24	0
42	59	3.29	23	172	276	991	2.27	6	.24	.31	4.11	.23	20	0
41	58	3.42	33	197	313	987	2.46	6	.22	.29	4.17	.25	23	0
43	52	3.86	61	263	371	1069	3.15	6	.23	.28	4.57	.31	33	0

(For purposes of calculations, use "0" for t, <1, <.1, <.01, etc.)

Table A–1
Food Composition

Computer Code Number	Food Description	Measure	Wt (g)	H_2O (%)	Ener (kcal)	Prot (g)	Carb (g)	Dietary Fiber (g)	Fat (g)	Fat Breakdown (g) Sat	Mono	Poly
	FAST FOODS and SANDWICHES (see end of this appendix for additional Fast Foods)—Cont.											
714	Taco	1 ea	78	58	168	9	12	–	9	5.2	3	4
	Tostada:											
1114	With refried beans	1 ea	157	66	243	10	29	8	11	5.9	3.3	.8
1118	With beans & beef	1 ea	192	70	284	14	25	3	14	9.8	3	.5
1354	With beans & chicken	1 ea	157	67	253	19	19	3	11	4.5	4.4	1.6
	Vegetarian foods:											
1511	Baked beans, canned	½ c	127	73	118	6	26	10	1	.1	t	.2
1175	Breakfast links	1 ea	34	52	89	7	3	1	6	–	–	–
1171	Nuteena	1 pce	67	58	160	8	5	2	12	1.7	4.6	3.7
1173	Redi-burger	1 pce	68	57	130	14	5	1	6	.7	1.3	3.3
1174	Vege-burger	½ c	108	73	110	22	4	1	1	.1	.1	.4
	NUTS, SEEDS, and PRODUCTS											
	Almonds:											
1365	Dry roasted, salted	1 c	138	3	810	22	33	18	71	6.7	46.2	14.9
718	Slivered, packed, unsalted	1 c	135	4	795	27	27	15[1]	70	6.7	45.8	14.9
719	Whole, dried, unsalted:	1 c	142	4	836	28	29	16[1]	74	7	48.1	15.6
720	Ounce	1 oz	28	4	167	6	6	3[1]	15	1.4	9.6	3.1
721	Almond butter	1 tbs	16	1	101	2	3	1	9	.9	6.1	2
722	Brazil nuts, dry (about 7)	1 oz	28	3	186	4	4	2	19	4.6	6.5	6.8
	Cashew nuts, salted:											
723	Dry roasted:	1 c	137	2	786	21	45	9	64	12.5	37.4	10.7
724	Ounce	1 oz	28	2	163	4	9	2	13	2.6	7.7	2.2
725	Oil roasted:	1 c	130	4	748	21	37	8	63	12.4	36.9	10.6
726	Ounce	1 oz	28	4	163	5	8	2	14	2.7	8	2.3
1366	Cashew nuts, unsalted, dry roasted	1 c	137	2	786	21	45	8	64	12.5	37.4	10.7
1367	Cashew nuts, unsalted, oil roasted	1 c	130	4	748	21	37	8	63	12.4	36.9	10.6
727	Cashew butter, unsalted	1 tbs	16	3	94	3	4	1	8	1.6	4.7	1.3
728	Chestnuts, European, roasted (1 cup = approx 17 kernels)	1 c	143	40	350	5	76	18	3	.6	1.1	1.2
	Coconut, raw:											
729	Piece 2 x 2 x ½"	1 pce	45	47	159	1	7	4	15	13.4	.6	.2
730	Shredded/grated, unpacked[2]	½ c	40	47	142	1	6	4	13	11.9	.6	.1
	Coconut, dried, shredded/grated:											
731	Unsweetened	1 c	78	3	514	5	19	10	50	44.6	2.1	.6
732	Sweetened	1 c	93	13	465	3	44	7	33	29.3	1.4	.4
733	Filberts/hazelnuts, chopped:	1 c	115	5	726	15	18	7	72	5.3	56.4	6.9
734	Ounce	1 oz	28	5	179	4	4	2	18	1.3	13.9	1.7
735	Macadamias, oil roasted, salted:	1 c	134	2	962	10	17	8	102	15.3	80.9	1.8
736	Ounce	1 oz	28	2	201	2	4	2	21	3.2	16.9	.4
1368	Macadamias, oil roasted, unsalted	1 c	134	2	962	10	17	7	102	15.3	80.9	1.8
	NUTS, SEEDS, and PRODUCTS—Cont.											

(1) Values reported for dietary fiber in almonds vary from 7.0 to 14.3 g/100 g.

(2) ½ cup packed = 65 g.

(Computer code number is for West Diet Analysis program)

PAGE KEY: A–2 = BEV A–4 = DAIRY A–10 = EGGS A–12 = FAT/OIL A–14 = FRUIT A–24 = BAKERY A–34 = GRAIN A–40 = FISH A–44 = MEATS A–48 = POULTRY A–50 = SAUSAGE A–52 = MIXED/FAST A–60 = NUTS/SEEDS A–62 = SWEETS A–66 = VEG/LEG A–78 = MISC A–80 = SOUPS/SAUCES A–84 = FAST A–96 = FRZN ENTREE A–98 = BABY FOODS

Chol (mg)	Calc (mg)	Iron (mg)	Magn (mg)	Phos (mg)	Pota (mg)	Sodi (mg)	Zinc (mg)	VT-A (RE)	Thia (mg)	Ribo (mg)	Niac (mg)	V-B6 (mg)	Fola (µg)	VT-C (mg)
26	101	1.1	32	93	216	366	1.79	67	.07	.2	1.47	.11	11	1
33	229	2.06	64	127	440	592	2.07	93	.11	.36	1.44	.17	82	1
63	161	2.09	58	148	419	743	2.71	148	.08	.42	2.44	.21	83	3
53	171	1.81	49	240	367	435	2.29	87	.11	.2	4.49	.32	54	3
0	63	.37	41	132	376	504	1.78	22	.19	.08	.54	.17	30	4
<1	11	1.96	–	–	43	203	–	<1	1.65	.17	3.77	.2	–	<1
0	21	1.2	40	111	200	120	.87	10	.47	.58	.14	.45	60	<1
0	19	1.4	13	56	120	370	1.2	10	.6	.4	6.7	.8	17	<1
0	32	2.7	24	105	110	190	1.1	10	.53	.68	5	.56	27	<1
0	389	5.24	420	756	1062	1076	6.76	0	.18	.83	3.89	.1	88	1
0	359	4.94	400	702	988	15	3.94	0	.28	1.05	4.54	.15	79	1
0	378	5.2	420	738	1039	16[3]	4.15	0	.3	1.11	4.77	.16	83	1
0	75	1.04	84	147	208	3[3]	.83	0	.06	.22	.95	.03	17	<1
0	43	.59	48	84	121	2[4]	.49	0	.02	.1	.46	.01	10	<1
0	50	.96	64	170	170	1	1.3	0	.28	.03	.46	.07	1	<1
0	62	8.22	356	671	774	875[5]	7.67	0	.27	.27	1.92	.35	95	0
0	13	1.7	74	139	160	181[5]	1.59	0	.06	.06	.4	.07	20	0
0	53	5.33	332	553	689	813[6]	6.18	0	.55	.23	2.34	.32	88	0
0	12	1.16	72	120	150	177[6]	1.35	0	.12	.05	.51	.07	19	0
0	62	8.22	356	671	774	22	7.67	0	.27	.27	1.92	.35	95	0
0	53	5.33	332	553	689	22	6.18	0	.55	.23	2.34	.32	88	0
0	7	.8	41	73	87	2[7]	.83	0	.05	.03	.26	.04	11	0
0	41	1.3	47	153	847	3	.81	3	.35	.25	1.92	.71	100	37
0	6	1.09	14	51	160	9	.49	0	.03	.01	.24	.02	12	1
0	6	.97	13	45	142	8	.44	0	.03	.01	.22	.02	11	1
0	20	2.59	70	160	423	29	1.57	0	.05	.08	.47	.23	7	1
0	14	1.79	46	99	313	243	1.69	0	.03	.02	.44	.25	8	1
0	216	3.76	327	358	511	3	2.76	8	.57	.13	1.31	.7	83	1
0	53	.93	80	88	126	1	.68	2	.14	.03	.32	.17	20	<1
0	60	2.41	155	268	440	348[8]	1.47	1	.28	.15	2.71	.26	50	0
0	13	.5	32	56	92	73[8]	.31	<1	.06	.03	.57	.05	10	0
0	60	2.41	155	268	440	9	1.47	1	.28	.15	2.71	.26	21	0

(3) Salted almonds contain 1108 mg sodium per cup, 221 mg per ounce.

(4) Salted almond butter contains 72 mg sodium per tablespoon.

(5) Dry-roasted cashews without salt contain 21 mg sodium per cup, or 4 mg per ounce.

(6) Oil-roasted cashews without salt contain 22 mg sodium per cup, or 5 mg per ounce.

(7) Salted cashew butter contains 98 mg sodium per tablespoon.

(8) Macadamia nuts without salt contain 9 mg sodium per cup, or 2 mg per ounce.

(For purposes of calculations, use "0" for t, <1, <.1, <.01, etc.)

Table A–1
Food Composition

Computer Code Number	Food Description	Measure	Wt (g)	H_2O (%)	Ener (kcal)	Prot (g)	Carb (g)	Dietary Fiber (g)	Fat (g)	Fat Breakdown (g) Sat	Mono	Poly
	Mixed nuts:											
737	Dry roasted, salted	1 c	137	2	812	24	35	12	71	9.4	43	14.7
738	Oil roasted, salted	1 c	142	2	876	24	30	13	80	12.4	45	18.9
1369	Oil roasted, unsalted	1 c	142	2	876	24	30	13	80	12.4	45	18.9
	Peanuts:											
739	Oil roasted, salted:	1 c	144	2	837	38	27	13	71	9.8	35.3	22.5
740	Ounce	1 oz	28	2	165	7	5	2	14	1.9	6.9	4.4
1370	Oil roasted, unsalted	1 c	144	2	837	38	27	13	71	9.8	35.3	22.5
741	Dried, unsalted:	1 c	146	2	854	35	31	12	73	10.1	36.1	22.9
742	Ounce	1 oz	28	2	166	7	6	2	14	2	7	4.4
743	Peanut butter:	½ c	129	1	759	32	27	8	64	12.3	30.4	18.6
1371	Tablespoon	2 tbs	32	1	190	8	7	2	16	3.1	7.6	4.6
744	Pecan halves, dried, unsalted:	1 c	108	5	720	8	20	7[1]	73	5.8	45.5	18.1
745	Ounce	1 oz	28	5	189	2	5	2[1]	19	1.5	11.9	4.8
1372	Pecan halves, dry roasted, salted	¼ c	28	1	187	2	6	2	18	1.5	11.4	4.5
746	Pine nuts/piñons, dried	1 oz	28	6	161	3	5	2	17	2.7	6.5	7.3
747	Pistachios, dried, shelled	1 oz	28	4	164	6	7	3	14	1.7	9.3	2.1
1373	Pistachios, dry roasted, salted, shelled	1 c	128	2	774	19	35	15	68	8.6	45.6	10.2
748	Pumpkin kernels, dried, unsalted	1 oz	28	7	154	7	5	2	13	2.5	4	5.9
1374	Pumpkin kernels, roasted, salted	1 c	227	7	1184	75	30	24	96	18.1	29.7	43.6
749	Sesame seeds, hulled, dried	¼ c	38	5	223	10	4	3	21	2.9	7.9	9.1
	Sunflower seed kernels:											
750	Dry	¼ c	36	5	205	8	7	2	18	1.9	3.4	11.8
751	Oil roasted	¼ c	34	3	209	7	5	2	19	2	3.7	12.9
752	Tahini (sesame butter)	1 tbs	15	3	91	3	3	1	8	1.2	3.2	3.7
1334	Trail Mix w/chocolate chips	1 c	146	7	707	21	66	–	47	8.9	19.8	16.5
753	Black walnuts, chopped:	1 c	125	4	758	30	15	6	71	4.5	15.9	46.9
754	Ounce	1 oz	28	4	172	7	3	1	16	1	3.6	10.6
755	English walnuts, chopped:	1 c	120	4	770	17	22	6	74	6.7	17	47
756	Ounce	1 oz	28	4	182	4	5	1	17	1.6	4	11.1
	SWEETENERS and SWEETS (see also Dairy [milk desserts] and Baked Goods)											
757	Apple butter	2 tbs	35	52	64	<1	17	<1	<1	t	t	.1
1124	Butterscotch topping	2 tbs	41	32	103	<1	27	<1	<1	t	t	0
1125	Caramel topping	2 tbs	41	32	103	<1	27	<1	<1	t	t	0
	Cake frosting, creamy vanilla:											
1127	Canned	2 tbs	31	13	131	<1	22	0	5	1.5	2.7	.7
1123	From mix	2 tbs	31	12	132	<1	22	0	5	1	2.1	1.8

(1)Dietary fiber data calculated/derived from data on other nuts.

Chol (mg)	Calc (mg)	Iron (mg)	Magn (mg)	Phos (mg)	Pota (mg)	Sodi (mg)	Zinc (mg)	VT-A (RE)	Thia (mg)	Ribo (mg)	Niac (mg)	V-B6 (mg)	Fola (µg)	VT-C (mg)
0	96	5.07	308	595	817	917[2]	5.21	1	.27	.27	6.44	.41	69	1
0	153	4.56	334	657	825	924[2]	7.21	3	.71	.31	7.19	.34	117	1
0	153	4.56	334	657	825	16	7.21	3	.71	.31	7.19	.34	117	1
0	126	2.64	266	744	982	624[3]	9.55	0	.36	.16	20.4	.37	181	0
0	25	.52	52	147	193	123[3]	1.88	0	.07	.03	4.03	.07	36	0
0	126	2.64	266	744	982	9	9.55	0	.36	.16	20.4	.37	181	0
0	79	3.3	256	523	961	9	4.83	0	.64	.14	19.7	.37	212	0
0	15	.64	50	101	187	2	.94	0	.12	.03	3.83	.07	41	0
0	44	2.15	203	417	928	617[4]	3.24	0	.18	.13	16.9	.48	101	0
0	11	.54	51	104	232	153[4]	.81	0	.04	.03	4.22	.12	25	0
0	39	2.3	138	314	423	1[5]	5.91	14	.92	.14	.96	.2	42	2
0	10	.6	36	82	111	<1[5]	1.55	4	.24	.04	.25	.05	11	1
0	10	.62	38	86	105	221	1.61	4	.09	.03	.26	.05	12	1
0	2	.87	66	10	178	20	1.22	1	.35	.06	1.24	.03	16	1
0	38	1.92	45	142	310	2[6]	.38	7	.23	.05	.31	.07	16	2
0	90	4.06	166	609	1241	998	1.74	31	.54	.31	1.8	.33	76	9
0	12	4.24	152	332	229	5[7]	2.12	11	.06	.09	.49	.06	26	<1
0	98	33.8	1212	2658	1829	1305	16.9	86	.48	.72	3.95	.2	130	4
0	50	2.96	132	295	155	15	3.91	3	.27	.03	1.78	.05	36	0
0	42	2.44	127	253	248	1[8]	1.82	2	.82	.09	1.62	.28	82	1
0	19	2.28	43	387	164	1[8]	1.77	2	.11	.09	1.4	.27	80	<1
0	21	.95	53	118	69	<1	1.58	1	.24	.02	.85	.02	15	0
0	72	3.84	253	580	655	1	4.28	37	.27	.14	.86	.69	82	4
0	73	4.95	235	565	946	2	4.58	37	.6	.33	.8	.38	82	4
0	16	.87	57	132	149	<1	.97	9	.06	.03	.2	.16	19	1
0	113	2.93	203	380	602	12	3.28	15	.46	.18	1.25	.67	79	4
0	27	.69	48	90	142	3	.77	4	.11	.04	.29	.16	19	1
0	2	.05	1	2	32	<1	.02	0	<.01	<.01	.03	.01	<1	1
<1	22	.07	3	19	34	143	.08	11	.01	.04	.02	.01	1	<1
<1	22	.07	3	19	34	143	.08	11	.01	.04	.02	.01	1	<1
0	1	.03	<1	12	11	28	0	70	0	<.01	<.01	0	0	0
0	3	.07	1	8	7	69	.03	33	.01	.01	.11	<.01	0	0

(2)Mixed nuts without salt contain about 15 mg sodium per cup.

(3)Peanuts without salt contain 22 mg sodium per cup, or 4 mg per ounce.

(4)Peanut butter without added salt contains 3 mg sodium per tablespoon.

(5)Salted pecans contain 816 mg sodium per cup, or 214 mg per ounce.

(6)Salted pistachios contain approx 221 mg sodium per ounce.

(7)Salted pumpkin/squash kernels contain approximately 163 mg sodium per ounce.

(8)Unsalted sunflower seeds contain 1 mg sodium per ¼ cup.

(For purposes of calculations, use "0" for t, <1, <.1, <.01, etc.)

Table A–1
Food Composition

Computer Code Number	Food Description	Measure	Wt (g)	H_2O (%)	Ener (kcal)	Prot (g)	Carb (g)	Dietary Fiber (g)	Fat (g)	Fat Breakdown (g) Sat	Mono	Poly
	SWEETENERS and SWEETS (see also Dairy [milk desserts] and Baked Goods)—Cont.											
	Candy:											
1128	Almond Joy candy bar	1 oz	28	8	132	1	17	2	8	4.7	1.5	.7
758	Caramel, plain or chocolate	1 oz	28	8	108	1	22	<1	2	1.9	.2	.1
	Chocolate (see also #784, 785, 971):											
	Milk chocolate:											
759	Plain	1 oz	28	1	145	2	17	1	9	5.2	2.8	.3
760	With almonds	1 oz	28	1	149	3	15	2	10	4.8	3.8	.6
761	With peanuts	1 oz	28	1	157	5	11	2	12	3.4	5.1	2.6
762	With rice cereal	1 oz	28	2	141	2	18	6	8	4.5	2.4	.2
763	Semisweet chocolate chips	1 c	170	1	811	7	108	11	50	29.8	16.9	1.6
764	Sweet dark chocolate (candy bar)	1 oz	28	1	135	1	17	1	9	5.9	3.3	.3
1133	SKOR English toffee candy bar	1 ea	32	4	169	1	18	<1	16	7	6.9	2
765	Fondant candy, uncoated (mints, candy corn, other)	1 oz	28	7	101	0	26	0	<1	.1	–	–
1697	Fruit Roll-up (small)	1 ea	14	21	41	<1	11	<1	<1	t	t	.1
766	Fudge, chocolate	1 oz	28	10	108	<1	22	1	2	1.5	.7	.1
767	Gumdrops	1 oz	28	1	109	<1	28	0	<1	0	t	.1
768	Hard candy, all flavors	1 oz	28	1	106	0	28	0	0	0	0	0
769	Jellybeans	1 oz	28	6	104	0	26	0	<1	0	t	.1
1134	M&M's plain chocolate candy	1 pkg	48	1	228	3	33	1	11	5	3	.3
1135	M&M's peanut chocolate candy	1 pkg	47	1	234	5	28	1	13	5	5.1	2
1130	Mars almond bar	1 ea	50	4	234	4	31	1	11	4.8	4.4	.8
1129	Milky Way candy bar	1 ea	60	6	251	3	43	<1	9	4.7	3.3	.3
1708	Milk chocolate-coated peanuts	½ c	85	4	441	11	42	4	29	12.4	11	3.7
1709	Peanut brittle, recipe	½ c	74	3	333	6	51	1	14	3.7	6.2	3.5
1132	Reese's peanut butter cup	2 ea	45	8	218	5	21	2	14	10.4	.9	.9
1131	Snickers candy bar (2.2oz)	1 ea	61	6	278	6	37	2	14	7.3	4.1	.5
1482	Fruit juice bar (2.5 fl oz)	1 ea	77	78	63	1	16	–	<1	–	–	–
771	Gelatin dessert/Jello, prepared	½ c	120	85	71	1	17	<1	0	0	0	0
1702	SugarFree	½ c	113	98	8	1	1	0	0	0	0	0
772	Honey:	1 c	339	17	1030	1	279	0	0	0	0	0
773	Tablespoon	1 tbs	21	17	64	<1	17	0	0	0	0	0
774	Jams or preserves:	1 tbs	20	29	54	<1	14	<1	<1	0	t	t
775	Packet	1 ea	14	34	34	<1	9	<1	<1	t	t	0
776	Jellies:	1 tbs	18	28	49	<1	13	<1	<1	t	t	t
777	Packet	1 ea	14	28	38	<1	10	<1	<1	t	t	t
1136	Marmalade	2 tbs	40	33	98	<1	26	<1	0	0	0	0
770	Marshmallows	4 ea	28	16	90	1	23	0	<1	0	0	0
1126	Marshmallow creme topping	3 tbs	50	18	155	1	40	0	<1	0	0	0
778	Popsicle/ice pops	1 ea	95	80	68	0	18	0	0	0	0	0
	Sugars:											
779	Brown sugar	1 c	220	2	827	0	214	0	0	0	0	0
780	White sugar, granulated:	1 c	200	<1	774	0	200	0	0	0	0	0
781	Tablespoon	1 tbs	12	<1	46	0	12	0	0	0	0	0
782	Packet	1 ea	6	<1	23	0	6	0	0	0	0	0
783	White sugar, powdered, sifted	1 c	100	<1	389	0	99	0	<1	0	0	0

(Computer code number is for West Diet Analysis program)

Chol (mg)	Calc (mg)	Iron (mg)	Magn (mg)	Phos (mg)	Pota (mg)	Sodi (mg)	Zinc (mg)	VT-A (RE)	Thia (mg)	Ribo (mg)	Niac (mg)	V-B6 (mg)	Fola (µg)	VT-C (mg)
1	22	.34	19	40	105	38	.23	3	.01	.04	.13	.02	2	<1
2	39	.04	5	32	61	69	.12	2	<.01	.05	.07	.01	1	0
6	54	.39	17	61	109	23	.39	14	.02	.08	.09	.01	2	0
5	63	.46	25	75	126	21	.38	17	.02	.12	.21	.01	3	<1
3	33	.53	35	83	152	11	.69	6	.08	.05	2.14	.04	23	0
5	48	.21	14	55	97	41	.32	93	.02	.08	.13	.02	3	3
0	54	5.32	196	224	621	19	2.75	3	.09	.15	.73	.08	5	<1
0	5	.59	33	45	96	3	.42	1	.01	.07	.19	.01	1	<1
19	36	.13	11	48	76	74	.24	22	.01	.11	.03	.01	2	0
0	1	.02	<1	1	5	11	.01	0	0	<.01	<.01	0	0	0
0	6	.55	13	6	12	2	.01	<1	<.01	.01	.2	.03	0	<1
4	12	.14	7	16	29	18	.11	13	<.01	.02	.03	<.01	1	0
0	1	.11	<1	<1	1	12	0	0	0	<.01	<.01	0	0	0
0	1	.08	1	1	1	11	<.01	0	<.01	<.01	<.01	<.01	0	0
0	1	.31	1	1	10	7	.01	0	0	0	0	0	0	0
0	81	.73	32	94	188	49	.61	12	.03	.12	.26	.03	4	0
0	63	.7	39	130	184	44	.72	2	.03	.1	1.51	.08	26	0
4	84	.55	36	114	163	85	.55	22	.02	.16	.47	.03	7	<1
12	78	.46	20	98	145	144	.43	28	.02	.13	.21	.03	5	1
8	88	1.12	77	180	427	35	1.61	0	.1	.15	3.61	.18	7	0
10	22	1.02	37	82	153	332	.71	35	.14	.04	2.57	.08	52	0
7	35	.49	38	108	180	131	.63	9	.02	.09	1.79	.04	13	0
7	70	.48	37	129	200	164	.7	19	.03	.11	1.83	.11	24	<1
0	4	.15	3	5	41	3	.04	2	.01	.01	.12	.02	5	–
0	2	.04	1	26	1	50	.04	0	<.01	<.01	<.01	<.01	0	0
0	2	.01	1	31	0	54	.03	0	0	<.01	<.01	<.01	0	0
0	20	1.42	7	14	176	14	.75	0	0	.13	.41	.08	7	3
0	1	.09	<1	1	11	1	.05	0	0	.01	.02	<.01	<1	<1
0	4	.2	1	2	18	2	.01	<1	<.01	.01	.04	<.01	2	<1
0	3	.07	1	2	11	6	.01	<1	0	<.01	<.01	<.01	5	<1
0	1	.04	1	1	11	6	.01	<1	0	<.01	.01	<.01	<1	1
0	1	.03	1	1	9	5	.01	<1	0	<.01	<.01	<.01	<1	1
0	15	.06	1	2	15	22	.02	2	<.01	<.01	.02	.01	14	2
0	1	.06	1	2	1	13	.01	0	0	0	.02	<.01	<1	0
0	1	.11	1	4	2	23	.02	0	<.01	<.01	.04	<.01	<1	2
0	0	<.01	1	0	4	11	.02	0	0	0	0	0	0	0
0	187	4.2	64	48	761	86	.4	0	.02	.01	.18	.06	2	0
0	2	.13	0	4	4	2	.07	0	0	.04	0	0	0	0
0	<1	.01	<1	<1	<1	<1	<.01	0	0	<.01	0	0	0	0
0	<1	<.01	<1	<1	<1	<1	<.01	0	0	<.01	0	0	0	0
0	1	.06	1	2	2	1	.03	0	0	0	0	0	0	0

(For purposes of calculations, use "0" for t, <1, <.1, <.01, etc.)

Table A–1
Food Composition

Computer Code Number	Food Description	Measure	Wt (g)	H_2O (%)	Ener (kcal)	Prot (g)	Carb (g)	Dietary Fiber (g)	Fat (g)	Fat Breakdown (g)		
										Sat	Mono	Poly
	SWEETENERS and SWEETS (see also Dairy [milk desserts] and Baked Goods)—Cont.											
	Sweeteners:											
1711	Equal, packet	1 ea	1	<1	4	0	1	0	0	0	0	0
1712	Sweet 'N Low, packet	1 ea	1	<1	4	0	1	0	0	0	0	0
	Syrups:											
	Chocolate:											
785	Hot fudge type	2 tbs	38	22	131	2	22	1	5	2.1	1.4	1.2
784	Thin type	2 tbs	38	37	85	1	22	1	1	.3	.2	.1
786	Molasses, blackstrap[1]	2 tbs	40	29	94	0	24	0	0	0	0	0
1710	Light cane	1 tbs	21	24	52	0	13	0	0	0	0	0
787	Pancake table syrup (corn and maple)	¼ c	79	24	226	0	60	0	0	0	0	0
	VEGETABLES and LEGUMES											
788	Alfalfa sprouts	1 c	33	91	10	1	1	1	<1	t	t	.1
789	Artichokes, cooked globe (300 g w/refuse)	1 ea	120	84	60	4	13	10	<1	t	t	.1
1177	Artichoke hearts, cooked from frozen	9 oz	240	86	108	7	22	13	1	.3	t	.5
1176	Artichoke hearts, marinated	6 oz	170	59	168	4	13	7	13	2	3	7.7
	Asparagus, green, cooked:											
	From fresh:											
790	Cuts and tips	½ c	90	92	22	2	4	1	<1	.1	t	.1
791	Spears, ½" diam at base	6 ea	90	92	22	2	4	1	<1	.1	t	.1
	From frozen:											
792	Cuts and tips	½ c	90	91	25	3	4	2	<1	.1	t	.2
793	Spears, ½" diam at base	6 ea	90	91	25	3	4	2	<1	.1	t	.2
794	Canned, spears, ½" diam at base	6 ea	120	94	23	3	3	1	1	.2	t	.3
795	Bamboo shoots, canned, drained slices	1 c	131	94	25	2	4	3	1	.1	t	.2
	Beans (see also alphabetical listing in this section):											
796	Black beans, cooked	½ c	86	66	114	8	20	8	<1	.1	t	.2
	Canned beans (white/navy):											
803	With pork and tomato sauce	½ c	126	73	123	7	24	7	1	.5	.6	.2
804	With sweet sauce	1 c	253	71	281	13	53	14	4	1.4	1.6	.5
805	With frankfurters	1 c	257	69	365	17	40	18	17	6	7.3	2.1
	Lima beans:											
797	Thick seeded (Fordhooks), cooked from frozen	½ c	85	73	85	5	16	5	<1	.1	t	.1
798	Thin seeded (Baby), cooked from frozen	½ c	90	72	94	6	17	6	<1	.1	t	.1
799	Cooked from dry, drained	½ c	94	70	108	7	20	8	<1	.1	t	.2
	Snap bean/green string beans cuts and french style:											
800	Cooked from fresh	½ c	62	89	22	1	5	2	<1	t	t	.1
801	Cooked from frozen	½ c	67	92	18	1	4	2	<1	t	t	t
802	Canned, drained	½ c	67	93	13	1	3	1	<1	t	t	t
1713	Snap bean, yellow, cooked f/fresh	½ c	63	89	22	1	5	1	<1	t	t	t

(1)Light molasses would contain about 66 mg calcium, 2.1 mg iron, 18 mg magnesium, and 366 mg potassium for 2 tbsp.

(Computer code number is for West Diet Analysis program)

Chol (mg)	Calc (mg)	Iron (mg)	Magn (mg)	Phos (mg)	Pota (mg)	Sodi (mg)	Zinc (mg)	VT-A (RE)	Thia (mg)	Ribo (mg)	Niac (mg)	V-B6 (mg)	Fola (µg)	VT-C (mg)
0	–	–	–	–	–	0	–	–	–	–	–	–	–	–
0	<1	–	<1	–	1	1	–	–	–	–	–	–	–	–
5	38	.46	18	65	82	49	.3	13	.01	.08	.08	.01	2	0
0	6	.75	26	49	85	36	.39	1	.01	.02	.11	<.01	3	0
0	344[1]	7[1]	86[1]	16	997[1]	22	.4	0	.01	.02	.43	.28	<1	0
0	34	.88	–	9	188	3	–	0	.01	.01	.04	–	–	0
0	1	.08	2	7	2	65	.03	0	.01	.01	.02	0	<1	0
0	11	.32	9	23	26	2	.3	5	.02	.04	.16	.01	12	3
0	54	1.55	72	103	424	114	.59	22	.08	.08	1.2	.13	61	12
0	50	1.34	74	146	634	127	.86	39	.15	.38	2.2	.21	286	12
0	39	1.62	48	102	439	899	.54	28	.06	.17	1.38	.15	149	52
0	18	.66	9	49	144	10	.38	49	.11	.11	.97	.11	131	10
0	18	.66	9	49	144	10	.38	49	.11	.11	.97	.11	131	10
0	21	.57	12	49	196	4	.5	74	.06	.09	.94	.02	121	22
0	21	.57	12	49	196	4	.5	74	.06	.09	.94	.02	121	22
0	19	2.2	12	52	205	468[2]	.48	64	.07	.12	1.14	.13	115	22
0	10	.42	5	33	104	9	.85	1	.03	.03	.18	.18	4	1
0	23	1.81	60	120	305	1	.96	1	.21	.05	.43	.06	127	0
9	70	4.15	44	148	380	557	7.4	15	.07	.06	.63	.09	28	4
18	154	4.2	86	266	673	850	3.8	28	.12	.15	.89	.21	95	8
15	123	4.45	72	267	604	1105	4.81	39	.15	.14	2.32	.12	77	6
0	19	1.16	29	54	347	45	.37	16	.06	.05	.91	.1	55	11
0	25	1.76	50	100	369	26	.49	15	.06	.05	.69	.1	58	5
0	16	2.25	40	104	478	2	.89	0	.15	.05	.4	.15	78	0
0	29	.8	16	24	186	2	.22	42[3]	.05	.06	.38	.03	21	6
0	30	.55	14	16	76	9	.42	36[4]	.03	.05	.28	.04	6	6
0	18	.61	9	13	74	169[5]	.2	24[6]	.01	.04	.14	.02	21	3
0	29	.8	16	24	187	2	.23	5	.05	.06	.38	.04	21	6

(2)Low sodium pack contains 3 mg sodium.

(3)Data is for green varieties; yellow beans contain 10 RE per cup.

(4)Data is for green varieties; yellow beans contain 15 RE per cup.

(5)Low sodium pack contains 3 mg sodium per cup.

(6)For green varieties; yellow beans contain 14 RE per cup.

(For purposes of calculations, use "0" for t, <1, <.1, <.01, etc.)

A

Table A–1
Food Composition

Computer Code Number	Food Description	Measure	Wt (g)	H_2O (%)	Ener (kcal)	Prot (g)	Carb (g)	Dietary Fiber (g)	Fat (g)	Fat Breakdown (g) Sat	Mono	Poly
	VEGETABLES AND LEGUMES—Cont.											
	Bean sprouts (mung):											
806	Raw	1 c	104	90	31	3	6	3	<1	t	t	.1
807	Cooked, stir-fried	1 c	124	84	62	5	13	4	<1	t	.1	.1
808	Cooked, boiled, drained	1 c	124	93	26	3	5	2	<1	t	t	t
	Beets, cooked from fresh:											
809	Sliced or diced	½ c	85	87	37	1	8	1	<1	t	t	.1
810	Whole beets, 2" diam	2 ea	100	87	44	2	10	1	<1	t	t	.1
	Beets, canned:											
811	Sliced or diced	½ c	85	91	26	1	6	1	<1	t	t	t
812	Pickled slices	½ c	114	82	74	1	19	2	<1	t	t	t
813	Beet greens, cooked, drained	½ c	72	89	19	2	4	1	<1	t	t	.1
	Broccoli, raw:											
817	Chopped	1 c	88	91	25	3	5	2	<1	t	t	.1
818	Spears	1 ea	151	91	42	4	8	4	1	.1	t	.3
	Broccoli, cooked from fresh:											
819	Spears	1 ea	180	91	50	5	9	5	1	.1	t	.3
820	Chopped	1 c	156	91	44	5	8	4	1	.1	t	.3
	Broccoli, cooked from frozen:											
821	Spear, small piece	3 ea	90	91	25	3	5	3	<1	t	t	.1
822	Chopped	1 c	184	91	51	6	10	5	<1	t	t	.1
1603	Broccoflower, steamed	3½ oz	100	90	32	3	6	3	<1	–	–	–
823	Brussels sprouts, cooked from fresh	½ c	78	87	30	2	7	3	<1	.1	t	.2
824	Brussels sprouts, cooked from frozen	½ c	77	87	33	3	6	3	<1	.1	t	.2
	Cabbage, common varieties:											
825	Raw, shredded or chopped	1 c	70	92	17	1	4	1	<1	t	t	.1
826	Cooked, drained	1 c	150	94	33	2	7	4	1	.1	t	.3
	Cabbage, Chinese:											
1178	Bok choy, raw, shredded	1 c	70	95	9	1	2	1	<1	t	t	.1
827	Bok choy, cooked, drained	1 c	170	96	20	3	3	3	<1	t	t	.1
828	Pe tsai, raw, chopped	1 c	76	94	12	1	2	1	<1	t	t	.1
	Cabbage, red, coarsely chopped:											
829	Raw	1 c	70	92	19	1	4	1	<1	t	t	.1
830	Cooked, drained	½ c	75	94	16	1	3	1	<1	t	t	.1
831	Cabbage, savoy, coarsely chopped, raw	1 c	70	91	19	1	4	2	<1	t	t	t
	Carrots, raw:											
832	Whole, 7 ½ x 1 ⅛"	1 ea	72	88	31	1	7	2	<1	t	t	.1
833	Grated	½ c	55	88	24	1	6	2	<1	t	t	t
	Carrots, cooked, sliced, drained:											
834	From fresh	½ c	78	87	35	1	8	3	<1	t	t	.1
835	From frozen	½ c	73	90	26	1	6	3	<1	t	t	t
836	Carrots, canned, sliced, drained	½ c	73	93	17	<1	4	1	<1	t	t	.1
837	Carrot juice, canned	½ c	123	89	49	1	11	2	<1	t	t	.1
	Cauliflower, flowerets:											
838	Raw	½ c	50	92	12	1	3	1	<1	t	t	t
839	Cooked from fresh, drained	½ c	62	93	14	1	3	1	<1	t	t	.1
840	Cooked, from frozen, drained	½ c	90	94	17	1	3	2	<1	t	t	.1

(Computer code number is for West Diet Analysis program)

Chol (mg)	Calc (mg)	Iron (mg)	Magn (mg)	Phos (mg)	Pota (mg)	Sodi (mg)	Zinc (mg)	VT-A (RE)	Thia (mg)	Ribo (mg)	Niac (mg)	V-B6 (mg)	Fola (µg)	VT-C (mg)
0	13	.95	22	56	154	6	.43	2	.09	.13	.78	.09	63	14
0	16	2.36	41	98	272	11	1.12	4	.17	.22	1.49	.16	86	20
0	15	.81	17	35	125	12	.58	1	.06	.13	1.01	.07	36	14
0	14	.67	20	32	259	65	.3	3	.02	.03	.28	.06	68	3
0	16	.79	23	38	305	77	.35	4	.03	.04	.33	.07	80	4
0	13	1.55	14	14	125	232[1]	.18	1	.01	.03	.13	.05	26	3
0	12	.47	17	19	168	300	.3	1	.01	.05	.29	.06	30	3
0	82	1.37	49	29	654	174	.36	367	.08	.21	.36	.09	10	18
0	42	.77	22	58	286	24	.35	136[2]	.06	.1	.56	.14	62	82
0	72	1.33	38	100	491	41	.6	233[2]	.1	.18	.96	.24	107	141
0	83	1.51	43	106	526	47	.68	250[2]	.1	.2	1.03	.26	90	134
0	72	1.31	37	92	456	41	.59	217[2]	.09	.18	.89	.22	78	116
0	46	.55	18	49	162	22	.27	170[2]	.05	.07	.41	.12	27	36
0	94	1.12	37	101	331	44	.55	348[2]	.1	.15	.84	.24	103	74
0	32	.7	20	64	322	23	.5	67	.07	.09	.76	.18	48	63
0	28	.94	16	44	247	16	.26	56	.08	.06	.47	.14	47	48
0	19	.57	19	42	252	18	.28	46	.08	.09	.42	.22	78	35
0	33	.41	10	16	172	13	.13	9	.03	.03	.21	.07	30	22
0	46	.25	12	22	146	12	.13	19	.09	.08	.42	.17	30	30
0	73	.56	13	26	176	45	.13	210	.03	.05	.35	.14	46	31
0	158	1.77	19	49	631	58	.29	437	.05	.11	.73	.28	69	44
0	58	.24	10	22	180	7	.17	91	.03	.04	.3	.18	60	20
0	36	.34	10	29	144	8	.15	3	.03	.02	.21	.15	14	40
0	28	.26	8	22	105	6	.11	2	.03	.01	.15	.1	9	26
0	24	.28	20	29	161	20	.19	70	.05	.02	.21	.13	56	22
0	19	.36	11	32	232	25	.14	2024	.07	.04	.67	.11	10	7
0	15	.27	8	24	177	19	.11	1546	.05	.03	.51	.08	8	5
0	24	.48	10	23	177	51	.23	1913	.03	.04	.39	.19	11	2
0	20	.34	7	19	115	43	.17	1291	.02	.03	.32	.09	8	2
0	18	.47	6	17	130	175[3]	.19	1004	.01	.02	.4	.08	7	2
0	29	.57	17	52	359	36	.22	3166	.11	.07	.47	.27	5	10
0	11	.22	7	22	152	15	.14	1	.03	.03	.26	.11	28	23
0	10	.2	6	20	88	9	.11	1	.03	.03	.25	.11	27	27
0	15	.37	8	22	125	16	.12	2	.03	.05	.28	.08	37	28

(1)Low sodium pack contains 39 mg sodium.

(2)Vitamin A for whole plant: leaves are 1600 RE/100 g raw; flower clusters are 300/100 g raw; stalks are 40 RE/100 g raw.

(3)Low sodium pack contains 31 mg sodium.

(For purposes of calculations, use "0" for t, <1, <.1, <.01, etc.)

Table A–1
Food Composition

Computer Code Number	Food Description	Measure	Wt (g)	H_2O (%)	Ener (kcal)	Prot (g)	Carb (g)	Dietary Fiber (g)	Fat (g)	Fat Breakdown (g) Sat	Mono	Poly
	VEGETABLES AND LEGUMES—Cont.											
	Celery, pascal type, raw:											
841	Large outer stalk, 8 x 1½" (root end)	1 ea	40	95	6	<1	1	1	<1	t	t	t
842	Diced	1 c	120	95	19	1	4	2	<1	t	t	.1
1179	Chard, swiss, raw, chopped	1 c	36	93	7	1	1	1	<1	t	t	t
1180	Chard, swiss, cooked	1 c	175	93	35	3	7	4	<1	t	t	.1
	Chickpeas (see Garbanzo Beans #854)											
	Collards, cooked, drained:											
843	From fresh	½ c	64	92	17	1	4	2	<1	t	t	.1
844	From frozen	½ c	85	88	31	3	6	3	<1	.1	t	.1
	Corn, cooked, drained:											
845	From fresh, on cob, 5" long	1 ea	77	73	72	2	17	3	1	.1	.2	.3
846	From frozen, on cob, 3½" long	1 ea	63	73	59	2	14	3	<1	.1	.1	.2
847	Kernels, cooked from frozen	½ c	82	76	66	2	17	3	<1	t	t	t
	Corn, canned:											
848	Cream style	½ c	128	79	92	2	23	2	1	.1	.2	.3
849	Whole kernel, vacuum pack	½ c	105	77	82	3	20	1	1	.1	.2	.2
	Cowpeas (see Black-eyed peas #814–816)											
850	Cucumber slices with peel	7 pce	28	96	4	<1	1	<1	<1	t	t	t
	Dandelion greens:											
851	Raw	1 c	55	86	25	1	5	1	<1	t	t	.2
852	Chopped, cooked, drained	1 c	105	90	35	2	7	1	1	.1	.1	.4
853	Eggplant, cooked	1 c	160	92	45	1	11	5	<1	.1	t	.1
1714	Endive, fresh, chopped	¼ c	13	94	2	<1	<1	<1	<1	t	t	t
856	Escarole/curly endive, chopped	1 c	50	94	8	1	2	1	<1	t	t	t
854	Garbanzo beans (chickpeas), cooked	1 c	164	60	267	14	45	10	4	.4	1	1.9
855	Great northern beans, cooked	1 c	177	69	209	15	37	11	1	.2	t	.3
857	Jerusalem artichoke, raw slices	1 c	150	78	114	3	26	2	<1	0	t	t
	Kale, cooked, drained:											
858	From fresh	½ c	65	91	21	1	4	2	<1	t	t	.1
859	From frozen	½ c	65	90	19	2	3	2	<1	t	t	.2
860	Kidney beans, canned	1 c	256	77	217	13	40	15	1	.1	.1	.5
1181	Kohlrabi, raw slices	1 c	140	91	38	2	9	2	<1	t	t	.1
861	Kohlrabi, cooked	1 c	165	90	48	3	11	2	<1	t	t	.1
1183	Leeks, raw, chopped	1 c	104	83	63	2	15	2	<1	t	t	.2
1182	Leeks, cooked, chopped	½ c	52	91	16	<1	4	2	<1	t	t	.1
862	Lentils, cooked from dry	½ c	99	70	115	9	20	5	<1	.1	.1	.2
1288	Lentils, sprouted, stir-fried	4 oz	113	69	115	10	24	4	1	.1	.1	.2
1289	Lentils, sprouted, raw	1 c	77	67	82	7	17	3	<1	t	.1	.2
	Lettuce:											
	Butterhead/Boston types:											
863	Head, 5" diameter	¼ ea	41	96	5	1	1	<1	<1	t	t	t
864	Leaves, inner or outer	4 ea	30	96	4	<1	1	<1	<1	t	t	t
	Iceberg/crisphead:											
865	Head, 6" diameter	¼ ea	135	96	17	1	3	1	<1	t	t	.1
866	Wedge, ¼ head	1 ea	135	96	18	1	3	1	<1	t	t	.1
867	Chopped or shredded	1 c	56	96	7	1	1	<1	<1	t	t	.1

(Computer code number is for West Diet Analysis program)

PAGE KEY: A–2 = BEV A–4 = DAIRY A–10 = EGGS A–12 = FAT/OIL A–14 = FRUIT A–24 = BAKERY A–34 = GRAIN A–40 = FISH A–44 = MEATS A–48 = POULTRY A–50 = SAUSAGE A–52 = MIXED/FAST A–60 = NUTS/SEEDS A–62 = SWEETS A–66 = VEG/LEG A–78 = MISC A–80 = SOUPS/SAUCES A–84 = FAST A–96 = FRZN ENTREE A–98 = BABY FOODS

Chol (mg)	Calc (mg)	Iron (mg)	Magn (mg)	Phos (mg)	Pota (mg)	Sodi (mg)	Zinc (mg)	VT-A (RE)	Thia (mg)	Ribo (mg)	Niac (mg)	V-B6 (mg)	Fola (μg)	VT-C (mg)
0	16	.16	4	10	115	35	.05	5	.02	.02	.13	.03	11	3
0	48	.48	13	30	344	104	.16	16	.06	.05	.39	.1	34	8
0	18	.65	29	17	136	77	.13	119	.01	.03	.14	.04	5	11
0	101	3.96	150	58	961	313	.58	550	.06	.15	.63	.15	15	31
0	15	.1	4	5	83	10	.07	175	.01	.03	.19	.03	4	8
0	179	.95	25	23	213	42	.23	508	.04	.1	.54	.1	64	22
0	2	.47	22	58	193	3	.48	16[1]	.13	.05	1.17	.17	23	4
0	2	.38	18	47	158	3	.4	13[1]	.11	.04	.96	.14	19	3
0	2	.25	15	38	113	4	.29	20[1]	.06	.06	1.05	.08	19	2
0	4	.49	22	65	172	364[2]	.68	13[1]	.03	.07	1.23	.08	57	6
0	5	.44	24	67	195	286[3]	.48	25[1]	.04	.08	1.23	.06	51	9
0	4	.07	3	6	41	1	.06	6	.01	.01	.06	.01	4	2
0	102	1.71	20	36	218	42	.23	770	.1	.14	.44	.14	15	19
0	147	1.89	25	44	243	46	.29	1227	.14	.18	.54	.17	13	19
0	10	.56	21	35	397	5	.24	10	.12	.03	.96	.14	23	2
0	7	.10	2	4	39	3	.1	26	.01	.01	.05	<.01	18	1
0	26	.41	7	14	157	11	.39	103	.04	.04	.2	.01	71	3
0	80	4.74	79	276	477	11	2.51	5	.19	.1	.86	.23	282	2
0	120	3.77	88	292	692	4	1.56	<1	.28	.1	1.21	.21	181	2
0	21	5.1	25	117	644	6	.18	3	.3	.09	1.95	.12	20	6
0	47	.58	12	18	148	15	.16	481	.03	.05	.32	.09	9	27
0	90	.61	12	18	209	10	.12	413	.03	.07	.44	.06	9	16
0	61	3.23	72	240	658	873	1.41	0	.27	.22	1.17	.06	129	3
0	34	.56	27	64	490	28	.04	6	.07	.03	.56	.21	22	87
0	41	.66	31	74	561	35	.51	7	.07	.03	.64	.25	20	89
0	61	2.18	29	36	187	21	.12	10	.06	.03	.42	.24	67	12
0	16	.57	7	9	45	5	.03	2	.01	.01	.1	.06	13	2
0	19	3.3	36	178	365	2	1.26	1	.17	.07	1.05	.18	178	1
0	16	3.52	40	174	322	11	1.81	5	.25	.1	1.36	.19	76	14
0	19	2.47	28	133	247	8	1.16	4	.18	.1	.87	.15	77	13
0	13	.12	5	9	104	2	.07	39	.02	.02	.12	.02	30	3
0	10	.09	4	7	76	1	.05	29	.02	.02	.09	.01	22	2
0	25	.67	12	27	213	12	.3	44	.06	.04	.25	.05	76	5
0	25	.67	12	27	213	12	.3	45	.06	.04	.25	.05	76	5
0	11	.28	5	11	88	5	.12	18	.03	.02	.1	.02	31	2

(1)For yellow varieties; white varieties contain only a trace of vitamin A.

(2)Low sodium pack contains 4 mg sodium per ½ cup.

(3)Low sodium pack contains 6 mg sodium per cup.

(For purposes of calculations, use "0" for t, <1, <.1, <.01, etc.)

A

Table A–1
Food Composition

Computer Code Number	Food Description	Measure	Wt (g)	H_2O (%)	Ener (kcal)	Prot (g)	Carb (g)	Dietary Fiber (g)	Fat (g)	Fat Breakdown (g) Sat	Mono	Poly
	VEGETABLES AND LEGUMES—Cont.											
	Lettuce—Cont.											
868	Looseleaf, chopped	½ c	28	94	5	<1	1	<1	<1	t	t	t
869	Romaine, chopped	½ c	28	95	4	<1	1	<1	<1	t	t	t
870	Romaine, inner leaf	3 ea	30	95	5	<1	1	<1	<1	t	t	t
	Mushrooms:											
871	Raw, sliced	½ c	35	92	9	1	2	<1	<1	t	t	.1
872	Cooked from fresh, pieces	½ c	78	91	21	2	4	2	<1	t	t	.1
873	Canned, drained	½ c	78	91	19	1	4	2	<1	t	t	.1
	Mustard greens:											
874	Cooked from fresh	½ c	70	94	10	2	1	1	<1	t	.1	t
875	Cooked from frozen	½c	75	94	14	2	2	1	<1	t	.1	t
876	Navy beans, cooked from dry	1 c	182	63	258	16	48	16	1	.3	.1	.4
	Okra, cooked:											
877	From fresh pods	8 ea	85	90	27	2	6	2	<1	t	t	t
878	From frozen slices	½ c	92	91	34	2	8	2	<1	.1	t	.1
1236	Batter fried from fresh	1 c	92	69	175	3	11	2	13	2.1	3.4	7.1
	Onions:											
879	Raw, chopped	1 c	160	90	61	2	14	3	<1	t	t	.1
880	Raw, sliced	1 c	115	90	44	1	10	2	<1	t	t	.1
881	Cooked, drained, chopped	½ c	105	88	46	1	11	1	<1	t	t	.1
882	Dehydrated flakes	¼ c	14	4	45	1	12	1	<1	t	t	t
	Spring/green onions, chopped:											
883	Bulb and top	½ c	50	90	16	1	4	1	<1	t	t	t
1185	Green tops only	1 c	100	92	34	2	5	2	<1	.1	.1	.2
1184	White part only	½ c	50	92	25	<1	5	1	<1	t	t	t
884	Onion rings, breaded, heated f/frozen	2 ea	20	28	81	1	8	<1	5	1.7	2.2	1
	Parsley:											
885	Raw, chopped	½ c	30	88	11	1	2	1	<1	t	.1	t
886	Raw, sprigs	5 ea	5	88	2	<1	<1	<1	<1	t	t	t
887	Freeze dried	¼ c	1	2	4	<1	1	1	<1	t	t	t
888	Parsnips, sliced, cooked	½ c	78	78	63	1	15	3	<1	t	.1	t
	Peas:											
	Black-eyed, cooked:											
814	From dry, drained	½ c	85	70	99	7	18	8	<1	.1	t	.2
815	From fresh, drained	½ c	82	75	80	3	17	6	<1	.1	t	.1
816	From frozen, drained	½ c	85	66	112	7	20	7	1	.1	.1	.2
889	Edible pod peas, cooked	1 c	160	89	67	5	11	4	<1	.1	t	.2
890	Green, canned, drained	½ c	85	82	59	4	11	3	<1	.1	t	.1
891	Green, cooked from frozen	½ c	80	79	62	4	11	4	<1	t	t	.1
892	Split, green, cooked from dry	½ c	98	69	116	8	21	5	<1	.1	.1	.2
1187	Peas & carrots, cooked from frozen	½ c	80	86	38	2	8	3	<1	.1	t	.2
1186	Peas & carrots, canned w/liquid	½ c	128	88	49	3	11	4	<1	.1	t	.2
	Peppers, hot:											
893	Hot green chili, canned	½ c	68	92	17	1	4	1	<1	t	t	t
894	Hot green chili, raw	1 ea	45	88	18	1	4	1	<1	t	t	t
1715	Hot red chili, raw, diced	1 tbs	9	88	4	<1	1	<1	<1	t	t	t
895	Jalapeno, chopped, canned	½ c	68	90	16	1	3	2	<1	t	t	.2

(Computer code number is for West Diet Analysis program)

Chol (mg)	Calc (mg)	Iron (mg)	Magn (mg)	Phos (mg)	Pota (mg)	Sodi (mg)	Zinc (mg)	VT-A (RE)	Thia (mg)	Ribo (mg)	Niac (mg)	V-B6 (mg)	Fola (μg)	VT-C (mg)
0	19	.39	3	7	74	3	.08	53	.01	.02	.11	.01	14	5
0	10	.31	2	13	81	2	.07	73	.03	.03	.14	.01	38	7
0	11	.33	2	13	87	2	.07	78	.03	.03	.15	.01	41	7
0	2	.43	3	36	129	1	.26	0	.04	.16	1.44	.03	7	1
0	5	1.36	9	68	277	2	.68	0	.06	.23	3.48	.07	14	3
0	9	.62	12	51	100	331	.56	0	.07	.02	1.24	.05	10	0
0	51	.49	10	29	141	11	.08	212	.03	.04	.3	.07	51	18
0	76	.84	10	18	104	19	.15	335	.03	.04	.19	.08	52	10
0	127	4.51	107	286	670	2	1.93	<1	.37	.11	.97	.3	255	2
0	54	.38	48	48	273	4	.47	49	.11	.05	.74	.16	39	14
0	88	.62	47	42	215	3	.57	47	.09	.11	.72	.04	133	11
15	104	.77	37	106	214	137	.5	43	.13	.1	.75	.13	37	10
0	32	.35	16	53	251	5	.3	0	.07	.03	.24	.19	30	10
0	23	.25	11	38	181	3	.22	0	.05	.02	.17	.13	22	7
0	23	.25	12	37	174	3	.22	0	.04	.02	.17	.13	16	5
0	36	.22	13	42	227	3	.26	0	.07	.01	.14	.22	23	10
0	36	.74	10	18	138	8	.19	19	.03	.04	.26	.03	32	9
0	56	2.2	21	39	260	7	.22	40	.07	.1	.6	0	80	51
0	20	.44	8	20	115	3	.12	<1	.03	.02	.17	.05	18	13
0	6	.34	4	16	26	75	.08	5	.06	.03	.72	.01	3	<1
0	41	1.86	15	17	166	17	.32	156	.03	.03	.39	.03	46	40
0	6	.31	2	2	27	2	.04	26	<.01	.01	.03	.01	9	4
0	2	.75	5	8	88	5	.09	88	.01	.03	.15	.02	21	2
0	29	.45	23	53	286	8	.2	0	.06	.04	.56	.07	45	10[1]
0	20	2.15	45	133	238	3	1.1	2	.17	.05	.42	.09	178	<1
0	106	.92	43	42	345	3	.85	65	.08	.12	1.16	.05	105	2
0	20	1.8	42	104	319	4	1.21	7	.22	.05	.62	.08	120	2
0	67	3.15	42	88	384	6	.59	21	.2	.12	.86	.23	47	77
0	17	.81	14	57	147	186[2]	.6	65	.1	.07	.62	.05	38	8
0	19	1.26	23	72	134	70	.75	54	.23	.08	1.18	.09	47	8
0	14	1.26	35	97	355	2	.98	1	.19	.05	.87	.05	63	<1
0	18	.75	13	39	126	54	.36	621	.18	.05	.92	.07	21	6
0	29	.96	18	59	128	332	.74	739	.09	.07	.74	.11	23	8
0	5	.34	10	12	127	797	.12	41[3]	.01	.03	.54	.1	7	46
0	8	.54	11	21	153	3	.13	35[3]	.04	.04	.43	.13	11	108
0	2	.11	2	4	32	1	.03	101	.01	.01	.09	.03	2	23
0	18	1.9	8	12	92	993	.13	116	.02	.03	.34	.14	9	9

(1)Value for Vitamin C is highest right after harvest and drops after that.

(2)Low sodium pack contains 1.7 mg sodium.

(3)Data is for green chili peppers; red varieties contain 809 RE vitamin A per ½ cup; 484 RE per whole pepper.

(For purposes of calculations, use "0" for t, <1, <.1, <.01, etc.)

Table A–1
Food Composition

Computer Code Number	Food Description	Measure	Wt (g)	H_2O (%)	Ener (kcal)	Prot (g)	Carb (g)	Dietary Fiber (g)	Fat (g)	Fat Breakdown (g) Sat	Mono	Poly
	VEGETABLES AND LEGUMES—Cont.											
	Peppers, sweet, green:											
896	Whole pod (90 g with refuse), raw	1 ea	74	92	20	1	5	1	<1	t	t	.1
897	Cooked, chopped (1 pod cooked = 73 g)	½ c	68	92	19	1	5	2	<1	t	t	.1
	Peppers, sweet, red:											
1286	Raw, chopped	1 c	100	92	27	1	6	2	<1	t	t	.1
1287	Cooked, chopped	½ c	68	92	19	1	5	1	<1	t	t	.1
898	Pinto beans, cooked from dry	½ c	85	64	117	7	22	10	<1	.1	.1	.2
1191	Poi, two finger	¼ c	60	72	67	<1	16	<1	<1	t	t	t
	Potatoes:[1]											
	Baked in oven, 4¾" x 2⅓" diam:											
899	With skin	1 ea	202	71	220	5	51	4	<1	.1	t	.1
900	Flesh only	1 ea	156	75	145	3	33	2	<1	t	t	.1
901	Skin only	1 ea	58	47	114	2	27	2	<1	t	t	t
	Baked in microwave, 4¾" x 2⅓" diam:											
902	With skin	1 ea	202	72	212	5	49	5	<1	.1	t	.1
903	Flesh only	1 ea	156	74	156	3	36	2	<1	t	t	.1
904	Skin only	1 ea	58	63	77	3	17	2	<1	t	t	t
	Boiled, about 2½" diam:											
905	Peeled after boiling	1 ea	136	77	118	3	27	2	<1	t	t	.1
906	Peeled before boiling	1 ea	135	77	116	2	27	2	<1	t	t	.1
	French fried, strips 2–3½" long:											
907	Oven heated	10 pce	50	35	163	2	19	1	12	3.8	7.2	.9
908	Fried in vegetable oil	10 ea	50	38	157	2	20	1	8	2.5	1.6	3.8
1188	Fried in veg and animal oil	10 ea	50	38	157	2	20	1	8	3.4	4	.5
909	Hashed browns from frozen	1 c	156	56	340	5	44	3	18	7	8	2.1
	Mashed:											
910	Home recipe with whole milk[2]	½ c	105	78	81	2	18	2	1	.3	.2	.1
911	Home recipe with milk and marg	½ c	105	76	111	2	17	1	4	1.1	1.9	1.3
912	Prepared from flakes; water, milk, margarine, salt added	½ c	110	76	124	2	16	1	6	1.6	2.5	1.7
	Potato products, prepared:											
	Au gratin:											
913	From dry mix	½ c	122	79	114	3	16	2	5	3.2	1.4	.2
914	From home recipe[3]	½ c	122	74	162	6	14	2	9	4.3	3.2	1.3
	Scalloped:											
915	From dry mix	½ c	122	79	114	3	16	1	5	3.2	1.5	.2
916	From home recipe[4]	½ c	122	81	105	4	13	1	5	1.7	1.6	.9
	Potato salad (see Mixed Dishes #715)											
1192	Potato puffs, cooked from frozen	½ c	62	53	137	2	19	2	7	3.2	2.7	.5
917	Potato chips	14 ea	28	2	152	2	15	1	10	3.1	2.8	3.5
918	Pumpkin, cooked from fresh, mashed	1 c	245	94	49	2	12	4	<1	.1	t	t
919	Pumpkin, canned	½ c	123	90	42	1	10	3	<1	.2	t	t
920	Red radishes	10 ea	45	95	8	<1	2	1	<1	t	t	t

(1)Vitamin C varies with length of storage. After 3 months of storage approximately two-thirds of the ascorbic acid remains; after 6 to 7 months, about one-third remains.

(2)Recipe: 84% potatoes, 15% whole milk, 1% salt.

(3)Recipe: 55% potatoes, 30% whole milk, 9% cheddar cheese, 3% butter, 2% flour, 1% salt.

(4)Recipe: 59% potatoes, 36% whole milk, 2% butter, 2% flour, 1% salt.

(Computer code number is for West Diet Analysis program)

Chol (mg)	Calc (mg)	Iron (mg)	Magn (mg)	Phos (mg)	Pota (mg)	Sodi (mg)	Zinc (mg)	VT-A (RE)	Thia (mg)	Ribo (mg)	Niac (mg)	V-B6 (mg)	Fola (μg)	VT-C (mg)
0	7	.34	7	14	131	1	.09	47	.05	.02	.38	.18	16	66
0	6	.31	7	12	112	1	.08	40	.04	.02	.32	.16	11	51
0	9	.46	10	19	177	2	.12	570	.07	.03	.51	.25	22	190
0	6	.31	7	12	112	1	.08	256	.04	.02	.32	.16	11	116
0	41	2.23	47	137	400	2	.92	<1	.16	.08	.34	.13	147	2
0	10	.53	14	23	110	7	.13	1	.08	.02	.66	.16	13	2
0	20	2.75	54	115	844	16	.65	0	.22	.07	3.31	.7	22	26[1]
0	8	.55	39	78	608	8	.45	0	.16	.03	2.18	.47	14	20[1]
0	20	4.08	25	59	332	12	.28	0	.07	.06	1.78	.36	12	8[1]
0	22	2.5	54	212	903	16	.73	0	.24	.06	3.45	.69	24	30[1]
0	8	.64	39	170	641	11	.51	0	.2	.04	2.54	.5	19	24[1]
0	27	3.45	21	48	377	9	.3	0	.04	.04	1.29	.28	10	9[1]
0	7	.42	30	60	515	5	.41	0	.14	.03	1.96	.41	14	18[1]
0	11	.42	27	54	441	7	.36	0	.13	.03	1.77	.36	12	10[1]
0	6	.83	11	48	269	306	.2	0	.04	.02	1.33	.11	11	3
0	9	.38	17	46	366	108	.19	0	.09	.01	1.63	.12	14	5
6	9	.38	17	46	366	108	.19	0	.09	.01	1.63	.12	14	5
0	23	2.36	26	112	680	53	.5	0	.17	.03	3.78	.2	10	10
2	27	.28	19	50	314	318	.3	20	.09	.04	1.18	.24	9	7[1]
2[5]	27	.27	19	48	303	310	.28	21	.09	.04	1.13	.23	8	6[1]
4[5]	53	.24	20	61	256	365	.2	23	.12	.05	.73	.01	8	11
6	102	.39	18	116	268	538	.29	38	.02	.1	1.15	.05	8	4
18[6]	146	.78	24	138	485	530	.84	47	.08	.14	1.22	.21	10	12
13	44	.47	17	68	249	418	.31	26	.02	.07	1.26	.05	12	4
7[7]	70	.7	23	77	463	410	.49	23	.08	.11	1.29	.22	11	13
0	19	.97	12	30	235	462	.19	1	.12	.04	1.34	.14	10	4
0	7	.46	19	47	362	169[8]	.31	0	.05	.06	1.09	.19	13	9
0	37	1.4	22	73	564	2	.56	265	.08	.19	1.01	.11	21	11
0	32	1.71	28	43	253	6	.21	2712	.03	.07	.45	.07	15	5
0	9	.13	4	8	104	11	.13	<1	<.01	.02	.13	.03	12	10

(5)Data is for margarine; if butter is used, cholesterol = 25 mg for 29 total mg.

(6)Data is for butter; if margarine is used, cholesterol = 37 mg.

(7)Data is for butter; if margarine is used cholesterol = 15 mg.

(8)If no salt added, sodium = 2 mg.

Table A–1
Food Composition

Computer Code Number	Food Description	Measure	Wt (g)	H_2O (%)	Ener (kcal)	Prot (g)	Carb (g)	Dietary Fiber (g)	Fat (g)	Fat Breakdown (g) Sat	Mono	Poly
	VEGETABLES AND LEGUMES—Cont.											
921	Refried beans, canned	½ c	126	72	135	8	23	9	1	.5	.6	.2
1375	Rutabaga, cooked cubes	½ c	85	89	33	1	7	1	<1	t	t	.1
922	Sauerkraut, canned with liquid	½ c	118	92	22	1	5	3	<1	t	t	.1
923	Seaweed, kelp, raw	1 oz	28	82	12	<1	3	<1	<1	.1	t	t
924	Seaweed, spirulina, dried	1 oz	28	5	82	16	7	1	2	.8	.2	.6
1557	Snow peas, stir-fried	1 c	165	89	69	5	12	4	<1	.1	t	.1
925	Soybeans, cooked from dry	½ c	86	63	149	14	9	3	8	1.1	1.7	4.4
	Soybean products:											
926	Miso	½ c	138	46	282	16	38	7	8	1.2	1.8	4.7
927	Tofu (soybean curd, regular)	½ c	124	85	94	10	2	1	6	.9	1.3	3.3
	Spinach:											
928	Raw, chopped	1 c	56	92	12	2	2	1	<1	t	t	.1
929	Cooked, from fresh, drained	½ c	90	91	21	3	3	2	<1	t	t	.1
930	Cooked from frozen (leaf)	½ c	95	90	27	3	5	2	<1	t	t	.1
931	Canned, drained solids	½ c	107	92	25	3	4	3	1	.1	t	.2
	Spinach soufflé (see Mixed Dishes)											
	Squash, summer varieties, cooked:											
932	Varieties averaged	½ c	90	94	18	1	4	1	<1	.1	t	.1
933	Crookneck	½ c	90	94	18	1	4	1	<1	.1	t	.1
934	Zucchini	½ c	90	95	14	1	4	1	<1	t	t	t
	Squash, winter varieties, cooked:											
	Average of all varieties, baked:											
935	Mashed	1 c	245	89	96	2	21	7	2	.3	.1	.6
936	Cubes	1 c	205	89	80	2	18	6	1	.3	.1	.5
937	Acorn, baked, mashed	½ c	122	83	68	1	18	5	<1	t	t	.1
1218	Acorn, boiled, mashed	½ c	122	90	42	1	11	3	<1	t	t	t
	Butternut:											
938	Baked cubes	1 c	205	88	82	2	21	6	<1	t	t	.1
1219	Baked, mashed	½ c	122	88	49	1	13	3	<1	t	t	t
1193	Cooked from frozen	½ c	120	88	47	1	12	3	<1	t	t	t
1194	Hubbard, baked, mashed	½ c	120	85	60	3	13	3	1	.2	.1	.3
1195	Hubbard, boiled, mashed	½ c	118	91	35	2	8	3	<1	.1	t	.2
1196	Spaghetti, baked or boiled	½ c	77	92	22	1	5	2	<1	t	t	.1
1189	Succotash, cooked from frozen	½ c	85	74	79	4	17	4	1	.1	.1	.4
	Sweet potatoes:											
939	Baked in skin, peeled, 5 x 2" diam	1 ea	114	73	117	2	28	3	<1	t	t	.1
940	Boiled without skin, 5 x 2" diam	1 ea	151	73	159	2	37	5	<1	.1	t	.2
941	Candied, 2½ x 2"	1 pce	105	67	143	1	29	2	3	1.4	.7	.2
	Canned:											
942	Solid pack	½ c	128	74	129	3	30	3	<1	.1	t	.1
943	Vacuum pack, mashed	½ c	127	76	116	2	27	3	<1	.1	t	.1
944	Vacuum pack, 3¾ x 1"	2 pce	80	76	73	1	17	2	<1	t	t	.1

(Computer code number is for West Diet Analysis program)

Chol (mg)	Calc (mg)	Iron (mg)	Magn (mg)	Phos (mg)	Pota (mg)	Sodi (mg)	Zinc (mg)	VT-A (RE)	Thia (mg)	Ribo (mg)	Niac (mg)	V-B6 (mg)	Fola (μg)	VT-C (mg)
0	58	2.24	49	106	497	536	1.73	<1	.06	.07	.61	.13	106	8
0	41	.45	20	48	277	17	.3	48	.07	.03	.61	.09	13	16
0	35	1.73	15	24	201	780	.22	2	.02	.03	.17	.15	28	17
0	48	.81	34	12	25	66	.35	3	.01	.04	.13	<.01	51	<1
0	34	8.08	55	33	386	296	.57	16	.67	1.04	3.63	.1	27	3
0	71	3.43	40	87	330	7	.45	21	.22	.12	.94	.25	55	84
0	88	4.42	73	211	443	1	.99	1	.13	.24	.34	.2	46	1
0	92	3.76	58	210	226	5014	4.57	12	.13	.34	1.19	.3	45	0
0	130	6.65	126	120	150	9	.99	11	.1	.06	.24	.06	19	<1
0	55	1.52	44	27	312	44	.3	376	.04	.11	.4	.11	108	16
0	122	3.21	78	50	419	63	.68	737	.09	.21	.44	.22	131	9
0	139	1.44	65	46	283	81	.66	739	.06	.16	.4	.14	102	12
0	136	2.46	81	47	370	159[1]	.49	939	.02	.15	.41	.11	105	15
0	24	.32	22	35	173	1	.35	26[2]	.04	.04	.46	.06	18	5
0	24	.32	22	35	173	1	.35	26[2]	.04	.04	.46	.08	18	5
0	12	.31	20	36	228	3	.16	22[2]	.04	.04	.38	.07	15	4
0	34	.81	20	49	1070	2	.64	872	.21	.06	1.72	.18	69	23
0	29	.68	16	41	896	2	.53	730	.17	.05	1.44	.15	57	20
0	54	1.14	53	55	535	5	.21	53	.2	.02	1.08	.24	23	13
0	32	.68	32	33	322	4	.13	32	.12	.01	.65	.14	14	8
0	84	1.23	59	55	582	8	.27	1435	.15	.03	1.99	.25	39	31
0	50	.73	35	33	348	5	.16	858	.09	.02	1.19	.15	23	18
0	23	.69	11	17	160	2	.14	401	.06	.05	.56	.08	20	4
0	20	.56	26	28	430	10	.18	725	.09	.06	.67	.21	19	11
0	12	.33	15	16	253	6	.12	473	.05	.03	.39	.12	11	8
0	16	.26	9	11	91	14	.15	9	.03	.02	.63	.08	6	3
0	13	.75	20	59	225	38	.38	20	.06	.06	1.11	.08	28	5
0	32	.51	23	63	396	11	.33	2486	.08	.14	.69	.27	26	28
0	32	.85	15	41	276	20	.41	2573	.08	.21	.97	.37	17	26
8[3]	27	1.19	12	27	198	73	.16	440	.02	.04	.41	.04	12	7
0	38	1.7	31	67	268	96	.27	1935	.03	.11	1.22	.3	14	7
0	28	1.13	28	62	398	67	.23	1017	.05	.07	.94	.24	21	34
0	18	.71	18	39	250	42	.14	638	.03	.05	.59	.15	13	21

(1) Dietary pack contains 58 mg sodium.

(2) Applies to squash including skin; flesh has no appreciable vitamin A value.

(3) For recipe using butter.

(For purposes of calculations, use "0" for t, <1, <.1, <.01, etc.)

Table A–1
Food Composition

Computer Code Number	Food Description	Measure	Wt (g)	H_2O (%)	Ener (kcal)	Prot (g)	Carb (g)	Dietary Fiber (g)	Fat (g)	Fat Breakdown (g) Sat	Mono	Poly
	VEGETABLES AND LEGUMES—Cont.											
	Tomatoes:											
945	Raw, whole, 2⅗" diam	1 ea	123	94	26	1	6	2	<1	.1	.1	.2
946	Raw, chopped	1 c	180	94	38	2	8	2	1	.1	.1	.2
947	Cooked from raw	1 c	240	92	65	3	14	4	1	.1	.2	.4
948	Canned, solids and liquid	1 c	240	94	48	2	10	4	1	.1	.1	.2
949	Tomato juice, canned	1 c	244	94	41	2	10	2	<1	t	t	.1
	Tomato products, canned:											
950	Paste	1 c	262	74	220	10	49	11	2	.3	.4	.9
951	Puree	1 c	250	87	102	4	25	6	<1	t	t	.1
952	Sauce	1 c	245	89	73	3	18	4	<1	.1	.1	.2
953	Turnips, cubes, cooked from fresh	½ c	78	94	14	1	4	2	<1	t	t	t
	Turnip greens, cooked:											
954	From fresh, leaves and stems	1 c	144	93	29	2	6	4	<1	.1	t	.1
955	From frozen, chopped	1 c	164	90	49	5	8	7	1	.2	t	.3
956	Vegetable juice cocktail, canned	½ c	121	93	23	1	6	1	<1	t	t	t
	Vegetables, mixed:											
957	Canned, drained	½ c	81	87	38	2	8	3	<1	t	t	.1
958	Frozen, cooked, drained	½ c	91	83	53	3	12	3	<1	t	t	.1
959	Water chestnuts, canned, slices	½ c	70	86	35	1	9	2	<1	t	t	t
960	Water chestnuts, canned, whole	4 ea	28	86	14	<1	4	1	<1	t	t	t
1190	Watercress, fresh, chopped	½ c	17	95	2	<1	<1	<1	<1	t	t	t
	MISCELLANEOUS											
	Baking powders for home use:											
	Sodium aluminum sulfate:											
962	With monocalcium phosphate monohydrate	1 tsp	3	2	4	<1	1	0	0	0	0	0
963	With monocalcium phosphate monohydrate, calcium sulfate	1 tsp	3	5	2	0	1	0	0	0	0	0
964	Straight phosphate	1 tsp	4	4	2	<1	1	0	0	0	0	0
965	Low sodium	1 tsp	4	6	4	<1	2	0	<1	0	0	0
1204	Baking soda	1 tsp	3	<1	0	0	0	0	0	0	0	0
966	Basil, dried	1 tbs	4	6	11	1	3	1	<1	–	–	–
961	Carob flour	1 c	103	4	394	5	92	13	1	.1	.2	.2
967	Catsup:	¼ c	61	67	64	1	17	1	<1	t	t	.1
968	Tablespoon	1 tbs	15	67	16	<1	4	<1	<1	t	t	t
1200	Cayenne/red pepper	1 tbs	5	8	16	1	3	2	1	.2	.1	.4
969	Celery seed	1 tsp	2	6	8	<1	1	<1	1	t	.3	.1
1203	Chili powder:	1 tbs	8	8	25	1	4	3	1	.3	.3	.6
970	Teaspoon	1 tsp	3	8	8	<1	1	1	<1	.1	.1	.2

Chol (mg)	Calc (mg)	Iron (mg)	Magn (mg)	Phos (mg)	Pota (mg)	Sodi (mg)	Zinc (mg)	VT-A (RE)	Thia (mg)	Ribo (mg)	Niac (mg)	V-B6 (mg)	Fola (μg)	VT-C (mg)
0	6	.55	13	29	273	11	.11	76	.07	.06	.77	.1	18	23[1]
0	9	.81	20	43	400	16	.16	112	.11	.09	1.13	.14	27	34[1]
0	14	1.34	34	74	670	26	.26	178	.17	.14	1.8	.23	31	55
0	62[2]	1.46	29	46	530	391[3]	.38	144	.11	.07	1.76	.22	19	36
0	22	1.42	27	46	537	881[4]	.34	137	.11	.08	1.64	.27	49	45
0	92	7.83	133	206	2441	170[5]	2.1	647	.41	.5	8.44	1	59	110
0	37	2.33	60	100	1050	50[6]	.55	340	.18	.13	4.3	.38	27	88
0	34	1.89	47	78	909	1482[7]	.61	240	.16	.14	2.82	.38	23	32
0	17	.17	6	15	105	39	.16	0	.02	.02	.23	.05	7	9
0	197	1.15	32	42	292	42	.2	792	.06	.1	.59	.26	170	39
0	248	3.18	43	56	366	25	.67	1308	.09	.12	.77	.11	65	36
0	13	.51	13	21	234	442	.24	142	.05	.03	.88	.17	25	33
0	22	.86	13	34	237	121	.33	949	.04	.04	.47	.06	19	4
0	23	.74	20	46	154	32	.45	389	.06	.11	.77	.07	17	3
0	3	.61	3	13	83	6	.27	<1	.01	.02	.25	.11	4	1
0	1	.25	1	5	33	2	.11	<1	<.01	.01	.1	.04	2	<1
0	20	.03	4	10	56	7	.02	80	.01	.02	.03	.02	2	7
0	58	0	<1	87	4	328	0	0	0	0	0	0	0	0
0	170	.32	1	63	1	307	0	0	0	0	0	0	0	0
0	280	.43	1	377	<1	300	<.01	0	0	0	0	0	0	0
0	186	.35	1	295	434	4	.03	0	0	0	0	0	0	0
0	0	0	0	0	0	821	0	0	0	0	0	0	0	0
0	95	1.89	19	22	154	2	.26	42	.01	.01	.31	–	–	3
0	358	3.04	56	81	852	36	.95	1	.05	.47	1.96	.38	30	<1
0	12	.43	13	24	295	726	.14	62	.05	.04	.84	.11	9	9
0	3	.1	3	6	72	178	.03	15	.01	.01	.21	.03	2	2
0	8	.41	8	15	106	2	.13	220	.02	.05	.46	–	–	4
0	35	.9	9	11	28	3	.14	<1	.01	.01	.1	–	–	<1
0	22	1.12	13	24	149	79	.21	272	.03	.06	.61	–	4	5
0	7	.37	4	8	50	26	.07	91	.01	.02	.2	–	1	2

[1] Year-round average. From June through October, ascorbic acid is approximately 32 mg and 47 mg, respectively, for one tomato and 1 c chopped tomato. From November through May, market samples average around 12 and 18 mg, respectively.

[2] Calcium is added as a firming agent.

[3] Dietary pack contains 31 mg sodium.

[4] If no salt is added, sodium content is 24 mg.

[5] If salt is added, sodium content is 2070 mg.

[6] If salt is added, sodium content is 998 mg.

[7] With salt added.

(For purposes of calculations, use "0" for t, <1, <.1, <.01, etc.)

Table A–1
Food Composition

Computer Code Number	Food Description	Measure	Wt (g)	H_2O (%)	Ener (kcal)	Prot (g)	Carb (g)	Dietary Fiber (g)	Fat (g)	Fat Breakdown (g) Sat	Mono	Poly
	MISCELLANEOUS—Cont.											
	Chocolate:											
971	Baking, unsweetened, square	1 oz	28	1	148	3	8	4	16	9.2	5.2	.5
	For other chocolate items, see Sweeteners & Sweets											
972	Cilantro/coriander, fresh	1 tbs	1	93	<1	<1	<1	<1	<1	t	t	t
1197	Cornstarch	1 tbs	8	8	30	<1	7	<1	<1	t	t	t
973	Cinnamon	1 tsp	2	9	6	<1	2	1	<1	t	t	t
974	Curry powder	1 tsp	2	9	6	<1	1	<1	<1	t	.2	t
1202	Dill weed, dried	1 tbs	3	7	8	1	2	<1	<1	–	–	–
1705	Dip, french onion	1 tbs	14	70	31	<1	<1	<1	3	1.9	.9	.1
975	Garlic cloves	1 ea	3	59	4	<1	1	<1	<1	t	0	t
976	Garlic powder	1 tsp	3	6	9	<1	2	<1	<1	t	t	t
977	Gelatin, dry, unsweetened: Envelope	1 ea	7	13	23	6	0	0	<1	t	t	t
978	Ginger root, slices, raw	2 pce	4	82	3	<1	1	<1	<1	t	t	t
1198	Horseradish, prepared	1 tbs	15	87	6	<1	1	<1	<1	t	t	t
1199	Hummous/hummus	1 c	246	35	420	12	50	10	21	3	9	8
979	Mustard, prepared (1 packet = 1 tsp)	1 tsp	5	80	4	<1	<1	<1	<1	t	.2	t
	Miso (see #926 under Vegetables and Legumes, Soybean products)											
980	Olives, green	5 ea	19	78	23	<1	<1	<1	2	.3	1.9	.2
981	Olives, ripe, pitted	5 ea	22	80	26	<1	1	1	2	.3	1.8	.2
982	Onion powder	1 tsp	2	5	5	<1	2	<1	<1	t	t	t
983	Oregano, ground	1 tsp	1	7	5	<1	1	<1	<1	t	t	.1
984	Paprika	1 tsp	2	9	6	<1	1	<1	<1	t	t	.2
985	Black pepper	1 tsp	2	10	5	<1	1	<1	<1	t	t	t
	Pickles:											
986	Dill, medium, 3¾ x 1¼" diam	1 ea	65	92	12	<1	3	1	<1	t	t	t
987	Fresh pack, slices, 1½" diam x ¼"	2 pce	15	79	11	<1	3	<1	<1	0	0	t
988	Sweet, medium	1 ea	35	65	41	<1	11	<1	<1	t	t	t
989	Pickle relish, sweet	2 tbs	30	63	41	<1	10	1	<1	t	t	.1
	Popcorn (see Grain Products #539–541)											
1201	Sage, ground	1 tsp	1	8	2	<1	<1	<1	<1	t	t	t
1347	Salsa, from recipe	1 tbs	14	94	2	<1	1	<1	<1	t	t	t
990	Salt	1 tsp	5	0	0	0	0	0	0	0	0	0
	Salt substitutes:											
1205	Morton, salt substitute	1 tsp	2	0	0	0	<1	0	0	0	0	0
1207	Morton, Light Salt	1 tsp	6	0	0	0	0	0	0	0	0	0
1206	Norcliff Thayer, No Salt, packet	1 ea	1	0	0	0	0	0	0	0	0	0
991	Vinegar, cider	½ c	120	94	14	0	7	0	0	0	0	0
	Yeast:											
992	Baker's, dry, active, package	1 ea	7	8	21	3	3	2	<1	t	.2	t
993	Brewer's, dry	1 tbs	8	5	23	3	3	3	<1	t	t	0
	SOUPS, SAUCES, AND GRAVIES											
	SOUPS, canned, condensed:											
	Unprepared, condensed:											
1210	Cream of celery	1 c	251	85	180	3	18	2	11	2.8	2.6	5
1215	Cream of chicken	1 c	251	82	233	7	18	1	15	4.2	6.5	3
1216	Cream of mushroom	1 c	251	81	259	4	19	1	19	5.1	3.6	8.9
1220	Onion	1 c	246	86	113	8	16	1	3	.5	1.5	1.3

(Computer code number is for West Diet Analysis program)

Chol (mg)	Calc (mg)	Iron (mg)	Magn (mg)	Phos (mg)	Pota (mg)	Sodi (mg)	Zinc (mg)	VT-A (RE)	Thia (mg)	Ribo (mg)	Niac (mg)	V-B6 (mg)	Fola (μg)	VT-C (mg)
0	21	1.79	88	118	236	4	1.14	3	.02	.05	.31	.03	2	0
0	1	.02	<1	<1	5	<1	<.01	3	<.01	<.01	.01	<.01	<1	<1
0	<1	.04	<1	1	<1	1	<.01	0	0	0	0	0	0	0
0	28	.86	1	1	11	1	.04	1	<.01	<.01	.03	.02	–	1
0	10	.59	5	7	31	1	.08	2	<.01	.01	.07	–	–	<1
0	55	1.51	14	17	102	6	.1	0	.01	.01	.09	.04	–	–
6	17	.01	2	13	22	27	.04	28	.01	.02	.02	<.01	2	<1
0	5	.05	1	5	12	1	.03	0	.01	<.01	.02	.04	<1	1
0	2	.08	2	12	31	1	.07	0	.01	<.01	.02	.57	2	<1
0	4	.08	2	3	1	14	.01	0	<.01	.02	.01	0	2	0
0	1	.02	2	1	18	1	.01	0	<.01	<.01	.03	.01	<1	<1
0	9	.13	4	5	43	14	.18	0	0	0	0	.01	2	0
0	123	4	71	275	428	600	2.7	6	.26	.13	1	.98	146	19
0	4	.1	2	4	6	63	.03	0	0	0	0	<.01	0	0
0	12	.31	4	3	11	468	.01	6	0	0	0	<.01	<1	0
0	20	.74	1	1	2	146	.05	9	0	0	.01	<.01	0	<1
0	8	.06	3	7	20	1	.05	0	.01	<.01	.01	.03	3	<1
0	24	.66	4	3	25	<1	.07	10	<.01	<.01	.09	–	–	1
0	4	.5	4	7	49	1	.08	127	.01	.04	.32	–	–	1
0	9	.61	4	4	26	1	.03	<1	<.01	<.01	.02	0	–	0
0	6	.34	7	14	75	833	.09	21	.01	.02	.04	.01	1	1
0	5	.27	1	4	30	101	0	2	0	<.01	0	<.01	0	1
0	1	.21	1	4	11	328	.03	5	<.01	.01	.06	<.01	<1	<1
0	6	.24	1	4	60	214	.02	3	0	.01	0	0	0	2
0	11	.19	3	1	7	<1	.03	4	<.01	<.01	.04	–	–	<1
0	1	.06	1	3	21	53	.02	23	.01	<.01	.05	.01	1	5
0	14	.01	2	3	<1	2132	.02	0	0	0	0	0	0	0
0	10	0	0	9	933	0	0	0	0	0	0	0	0	0
0	3	0	4	0	1500	1099	0	0	0	0	0	0	0	0
0	–	–	–	–	385	0	–	0	0	0	0	0	0	0
0	7	.7	1	8	120	1	.14	0	0	0	0	0	0	0
0	4	1.16	7	90	140	3	.45	0	.16	.38	2.79	.11	164	<1
0	17[1]	1.38	18	140	151	10	.63	0	1.25	.34	3.03	.4	313	0
28	80	1.26	13	75	245	1900	.3	60	.06	.1	.66	.02	5	1
20	68	1.2	5	75	175	1972	1.26	113	.06	.12	1.64	.03	3	<1
3	65	1.05	10	85	168	2033	1.19	0	.06	.17	1.62	.02	8	2
0	54	1.35	5	22	137	2115	1.23	0	.07	.05	1.21	.1	30	2

(1)Value varies from 6 to 60 mg.

(For purposes of calculations, use "0" for t, <1, <.1, <.01, etc.)

Table A–1
Food Composition

Computer Code Number	Food Description	Measure	Wt (g)	H_2O (%)	Ener (kcal)	Prot (g)	Carb (g)	Dietary Fiber (g)	Fat (g)	Fat Breakdown (g) Sat	Mono	Poly
	SOUPS, SAUCES, AND GRAVIES—Cont.											
	SOUPS, canned, condensed—Cont.											
	Prepared w/equal volume whole milk:											
994	Clam chowder, New England	1 c	248	85	163	9	17	1	7	2.9	2.3	1.1
1209	Cream of celery	1 c	248	86	163	6	14	<1	10	3.9	2.5	2.6
995	Cream of chicken	1 c	248	85	190	7	15	<1	11	4.6	4.5	1.6
996	Cream of mushroom	1 c	248	85	203	6	15	<1	14	5.1	3	4.6
1214	Cream of potato	1 c	248	87	148	6	17	<1	6	3.8	1.7	.6
1213	Oyster stew	1 c	245	89	134	6	10	0	8	5	2.1	.3
997	Tomato	1 c	248	85	161	6	22	–	6	2.9	1.6	1.1
	Prepared with equal volume of water:											
998	Bean with bacon	1 c	253	84	172	8	23	9	6	1.5	2.2	1.8
999	Beef broth/bouillon/consommé	1 c	240	98	17	3	<1	0	1	.3	.2	t
1000	Beef noodle	1 c	244	92	83	5	9	1	3	1.1	1.2	.5
1001	Chicken noodle	1 c	241	92	75	4	9	1	2	.7	1.1	.6
1002	Chicken rice	1 c	241	94	60	4	7	1	2	.5	.9	.4
1208	Chili beef	1 c	250	85	170	7	21	9	7	3.3	2.8	.3
1003	Clam chowder, Manhatten	1 c	244	92	78	2	12	1	2	.4	.4	1.3
1004	Cream of chicken	1 c	244	91	117	3	9	<1	7	2.1	3.3	1.5
1005	Cream of mushroom	1 c	244	90	129	2	9	<1	9	2.4	1.7	4.2
1006	Minestrone	1 c	241	91	82	4	11	1	3	.6	.7	1.1
1211	Onion	1 c	241	93	58	4	8	1	2	.3	.7	.7
1007	Split pea & ham	1 c	253	82	189	10	28	5	4	1.8	1.8	.6
1008	Tomato	1 c	244	90	85	2	17	<1	2	.4	.4	1
1009	Vegetable beef	1 c	244	92	78	6	10	<1	2	.9	.8	.1
1010	Vegetarian vegetable	1 c	241	92	72	2	12	<1	2	.3	.8	.7
1707	Ready to serve											
	Chunky chicken soup	½ c	126	84	89	6	9	<1	3	1	1.5	.7
	SOUPS, dehydrated:											
	Unprepared, dry products:											
1011	Beef bouillon, packet	1 ea	6	3	14	1	1	<1	1	.3	.2	t
1012	Onion soup, packet	1 ea	34	4	100	4	18	4	2	.5	1.2	.2
	Prepared with water:											
1299	Beef broth/bouillon	1 c	244	97	19	1	2	0	1	.3	.3	t
1376	Chicken broth	1 c	244	97	22	1	1	0	1	.3	.4	.4
1013	Chicken noodle	1 c	251	94	53	3	8	<1	1	.3	.5	.3
1122	Cream of chicken	1 c	261	91	107	2	13	1	5	3.4	1.2	.4
1014	Onion	1 c	246	96	27	1	5	<1	1	.1	.3	.1
1217	Split pea	1 c	255	87	124	7	21	3	1	.4	.7	.3
1015	Tomato vegetable	1 c	252	93	55	2	10	1	1	.4	.3	.1
	SAUCES											
	From dry mixes, prepared with milk:											
1016	Cheese sauce	1 c	279	77	307	16	23	1	17	9.3	5.3	1.6
1017	Hollandaise	1 c	259	84	240	5	14	<1	20	11.6	5.9	.9
1018	White sauce	1 c	264	81	240	10	21	<1	13	6.4	4.7	1.7
	From home recipe:											
1019	White sauce, medium[1]	1 c	250	77	355	9	20	<1	27	7.8	9.1	8.8
	Ready to serve:											
1020	Barbeque sauce	1 tbs	16	81	10	<1	1	<1	<1	t	.1	.1
1706	Chili sauce, tomato base	1 tbs	17	68	18	<1	4	<1	<1	t	t	t
1021	Soy sauce	1 tbs	18	71	10	1	2	0	<1	t	t	t
1380	Teriyaki sauce	1 tbs	18	68	15	1	3	0	0	0	0	0

(1)Made with enriched flour, margarine, and whole milk.

(Computer code number is for West Diet Analysis program)

Chol (mg)	Calc (mg)	Iron (mg)	Magn (mg)	Phos (mg)	Pota (mg)	Sodi (mg)	Zinc (mg)	VT-A (RE)	Thia (mg)	Ribo (mg)	Niac (mg)	V-B6 (mg)	Fola (µg)	VT-C (mg)
22	186	1.49	22	156	300	992	.8	40	.07	.24	1.03	.13	10	3
32	186	.69	22	151	310	1009	.2	67	.07	.25	.44	.06	8	1
27	181	.67	17	151	273	1046	.67	94	.07	.26	.92	.07	8	1
20	178	.59	20	156	270	1076	.64	37	.08	.28	.91	.06	10	2
22	166	.55	17	161	322	1061	.67	67	.08	.24	.64	.09	9	1
32	166	1.05	20	161	235	1041	10.3	44	.07	.23	.34	.06	10	4
17	158	1.81	22	148	449	932	.29	109	.13	.25	1.52	.16	21	68
3	81	2.05	45	131	402	951	1.03	89	.09	.03	.57	.04	32	2
0	14	.41	5	31	129	782	0	0	<.01	.05	1.87	.02	5	0
5	15	1.1	5	46	100	952	1.54	63	.07	.06	1.07	.04	4	<1
7	17	.77	5	36	55	1106	.39	72	.05	.06	1.39	.03	2	<1
7	17	.75	1	22	101	815	.26	65	.02	.02	1.13	.02	1	<1
12	42	2.13	30	147	525	1035	1.4	150	.06	.07	1.07	.16	17	4
2	27	1.63	12	41	187	578	.98	98	.03	.04	.82	.1	10	4
10	34	.61	2	37	88	986	.63	56	.03	.06	.82	.02	2	<1
2	46	.51	5	49	100	1032	.59	0	.05	.09	.72	.01	5	1
2	34	.92	7	55	313	911	.73	234	.05	.04	.94	.1	16	1
0	26	.67	2	12	67	1053	.61	0	.03	.02	.6	.05	15	1
8	23	2.28	48	212	400	1006	1.32	45	.15	.08	1.47	.07	3	2
0	12	1.76	7	34	264	871	.24	68	.09	.05	1.42	.11	15	66
5	17	1.12	5	41	173	956	1.54	190	.04	.05	1.03	.08	10	2
0	22	1.08	7	34	209	822	.46	301	.05	.05	.92	.05	11	1
15	13	.87	4	57	88	445	.5	65	.04	.09	2.21	.03	2	1
1	4	.06	3	19	27	1018	0	<1	<.01	.01	.27	.01	2	0
2	48	.51	22	110	226	3044	.2	1	.1	.21	1.73	.03	6	1
0	10	.02	7	24	37	1361	.07	1	<.01	.02	.36	0	0	0
0	15	.07	5	12	24	1483	.01	12	.01	.03	.19	0	2	0
3	32	.5	7	32	31	1276	.2	5	.07	.06	.88	.01	1	<1
3	76	.26	5	97	214	1184	1.57	123	.1	.2	2.61	.05	5	1
0	12	.15	5	29	64	849	.06	1	.03	.06	.48	0	1	<1
3	20	.94	43	124	224	1147	.56	5	.21	.14	1.26	.05	39	0
0	8	.63	20	31	104	1141	.17	20	.06	.04	.79	.05	10	7
53	569	.28	47	438	552	1565	.97	117	.15	.56	.32	.14	13	2
52	124	.9	8	127	124	1564	.7	220	.04	.18	.06	.5	22	<1
34	425	.26	264	256	444	797	.55	92	.08	.45	.53	.07	16	3
29	263	.73	32	217	345	370	.94	310	.19	.42	.98	.1	14	2
0	3	.12	1	3	27	128	.03	14	<.01	<.01	.06	.01	1	1
0	3	.14	2	9	63	228	.05	24	.02	.01	.27	.02	1	3
0	3	.36	6	20	32	1027	.07	0	.01	.02	.6	.03	3	0
0	4	.31	11	28	40	689	.02	0	<.01	.01	.23	.02	4	0

(For purposes of calculations, use "0" for t, <1, <.1, <.01, etc.)

Table A–1
Food Composition

Computer Code Number	Food Description	Measure	Wt (g)	H_2O (%)	Ener (kcal)	Prot (g)	Carb (g)	Dietary Fiber (g)	Fat (g)	Fat Breakdown (g) Sat	Mono	Poly
	SOUPS, SAUCES, AND GRAVIES—Cont.											
	SAUCES—Cont.											
	Spaghetti sauce, canned:											
1377	Plain	1 c	249	75	271	5	40	3	12	1.7	6.1	3.3
1378	With meat	1 c	257	74	309	9	39	8	14	2.8	7.2	3.3
1379	With mushrooms	½ c	123	75	108	2	13	1	3	.4	1.5	.8
	GRAVIES											
	Canned:											
1022	Beef	1 c	233	87	123	9	11	1	5	2.7	1.2	.2
1023	Chicken	1 c	238	85	188	5	13	<1	14	3.4	6.1	3.5
1024	Mushroom	1 c	238	89	119	3	13	<1	6	1	2.8	2.4
1025	From dry mix, brown	1 c	258	92	75	2	13	<1	2	.8	.7	.1
1026	From dry mix, chicken	1 c	260	91	83	3	14	<1	2	.5	.9	.4
	FAST FOOD RESTAURANTS											
	ARBY'S											
1402	Bac'n cheddar deluxe	1 ea	226	56	526	27	33	<1	36	9.7	15.6	11.2
	Roast beef sandwiches:											
1403	Regular	1 ea	147	51	353	22	32	1	15	7.3	5.1	2.4
1404	Junior	1 ea	86	48	218	12	22	<1	8	3.9	2.9	1.7
1405	Super	1 ea	234	58	501	25	50	1	22	8.5	8.2	5.4
1407	Beef 'n cheddar	1 ea	197	57	455	26	28	1	27	7.6	12.1	7.1
1408	Chicken breast sandwich	1 ea	184	52	493	23	48	1	25	5.1	9.6	10.3
1412	Ham'n cheese sandwich	1 ea	156	62	292	23	19	<1	14	4.7	6.3	2.7
1413	Turkey sandwich, deluxe	1 ea	197	61	375	24	32	<1	17	4.1	4.7	7.8
	Milk shakes:											
1419	Chocolate	1 ea	340	74	451	10	76	<1	12	2.8	7	1.7
1420	Jamocha	1 ea	326	75	368	9	59	0	10	2.5	6.4	1.6
1421	Vanilla	1 ea	312	75	330	10	46	0	11	3.9	5.3	2.3
	Source: Arby's Inc. for the basic nutrients. Values for some nutrients from known values of major ingredients.											
	BURGER KING											
	Croissant sandwiches:											
1422	Egg, bacon, & cheese	1 ea	119	49	364	15	19	<1	24	8.1	12.1	3
1423	Egg, sausage, & cheese	1 ea	163	46	547	21	23	1	41	13.3	20.5	5.1
1424	Egg, ham, & cheese	1 ea	145	57	348	19	19	<1	21	7	11.1	2
	Whopper sandwiches:											
1425	Whopper	1 ea	265	59	603	26	44	<1	35	11.8	10.8	12.8
1426	Whopper with cheese	1 ea	289	57	694	31	46	<1	43	15.7	12.8	12.8
1427	Double beef	1 ea	351	58	844	46	45	<1	53	19	19	13
1428	Double beef & cheese	1 ea	374	57	933	51	47	<1	61	23.9	21.9	14
1429	Hamburger deluxe	1 ea	136	53	339	15	28	<1	19	5.9	5.9	6.9
1430	Cheeseburger deluxe	1 ea	158	52	408	19	30	<1	24	8.4	7.3	7.3
1431	Hamburger	1 ea	109	48	275	15	28	<1	11	4	5	1
1432	Cheeseburger	1 ea	120	50	315	17	28	<1	15	6.9	5.9	1
1433	Double cheeseburger with bacon	1 ea	159	43	512	32	26	<1	31	13.9	12.9	2
1434	Chicken sandwich	1 ea	230	46	688	26	56	<1	40	8	11	20.1
1435	Chicken tenders	1 ea	95	50	249	17	15	0	14	3.2	5.3	3.2
1436	Ham & cheese sandwich	1 ea	230	59	471	24	44	<1	23	10	8	4
1437	Ocean catch fish fillet	1 ea	189	50	482	19	48	<1	24	3.9	5.8	12.7

(Computer code number is for West Diet Analysis program)

Chol (mg)	Calc (mg)	Iron (mg)	Magn (mg)	Phos (mg)	Pota (mg)	Sodi (mg)	Zinc (mg)	VT-A (RE)	Thia (mg)	Ribo (mg)	Niac (mg)	V-B6 (mg)	Fola (µg)	VT-C (mg)
0	70	1.62	60	90	956	1235	.52	306	.14	.15	3.76	.88	54	28
16	69	2	61	117	981	1215	1.41	299	.14	.17	4.64	.9	54	27
0	15	1	15	30	333	496	.34	242	.08	.08	.93	.16	13	9
7	14	1.63	5	70	188	1304	2.33	0	.07	.08	1.54	.02	5	0
5	48	1.12	5	69	259	1373	1.9	264	.04	.1	1.05	.02	5	0
0	17	1.57	5	36	252	1356	1.67	0	.08	.15	1.6	.05	29	0
3	67	.23	10	44	57	1075	.31	0	.04	.08	.81	0	0	0
3	39	.26	10	47	62	1133	.32	0	.05	.15	.78	.03	3	3
83	150	4.5	–	–	422	1672	3	100	.38	.51	8	–	–	9
39	80	3.6	16	120	368	588	3.75	1	.23	.43	7	.2	14	1
20	40	1.8	8	60	197	345	1.5	–	.15	.25	4	.1	7	–
40	100	4.5	25	190	503	798	3.75	150	.38	.6	9	.3	21	4
63	60	3.6	24	260	335	955	3.75	80	.38	.51	8	.22	19	0
91	80	3.6	30	180	330	1019	.15	–	.23	.51	8	.38	18	5
45	200	2.7	31	405	312	1350	.9	50	.15	.26	6	.31	26	24
39	80	2.7	30	250	346	1047	1.5	60	.23	.43	12	.52	20	5
36	250	2.7	48	350	410	341	1.5	40	.06	.85	.8	.14	14	5
35	250	2.7	36	350	525	262	1.5	60	.06	.77	5	.14	14	2
32	300	2.7	36	350	686	281	1.5	100	.23	.85	4	.14	37	2
229	137	2.02	–	–	–	725	–	151	.32	.3	2.02	.11	–	2
275	149	2.97	–	–	–	1009	–	154	.37	.33	4.1	.12	–	<1
243	137	2.22	–	–	–	969	–	151	.49	.32	3.02	.22	–	10
88	78	4.81	–	–	–	849	–	59	.32	.4	6.87	.34	–	14
113	206	4.82	–	–	–	1156	–	84	.33	.47	6.88	.32	–	14
169	91	7.3	–	–	–	933	–	60	.34	.56	10	–	–	14
193	221	7.28	–	–	–	1241	–	85	.35	.63	9.97	–	–	14
42	39	2.76	–	–	–	489	–	30	.23	.25	3.94	.14	–	6
59	110	2.93	–	–	–	682	–	89	.24	.3	4.19	–	–	6
37	37	2.73	–	–	–	510	–	15	.23	.25	4.04	–	–	3
50	101	3.77	–	–	–	656	–	69	.23	.29	3.97	–	–	3
104	167	3.78	–	–	–	743	–	84	.31	.42	5.96	–	–	1
82	79	3.31	–	–	–	1423	–	13	.45	.31	10	–	–	1
49	19	.74	–	–	–	571	–	5	.08	.08	7.39	–	–	<1
70	195	3.2	–	–	–	1534	–	85	.87	.42	6	–	–	7
55	82	2.14	–	–	–	856	–	19	.27	.2	3.9	–	–	2

(For purposes of calculations, use "0" for t, <1, <.1, <.01, etc.)

Table A–1
Food Composition

Computer Code Number	Food Description	Measure	Wt (g)	H_2O (%)	Ener (kcal)	Prot (g)	Carb (g)	Dietary Fiber (g)	Fat (g)	Fat Breakdown (g) Sat	Mono	Poly
	BURGER KING—Cont.											
1439	French fries (salted)	1 ea	74	42	227	3	24	1	13	6.7	6	14
1440	Onion rings	1 ea	79	33	277	4	31	<1	16	3.7	7.3	3.7
1441	Milk shakes, chocolate	1 ea	273	75	313	9	47	<1	10	5.8	3.8	0
1442	Milk shakes, vanilla	1 ea	273	75	321	9	49	<1	10	5.8	2.9	0
1443	Fried apple pie	1 ea	125	49	311	3	44	1	14	4	8	1
	Source: Burger King Corporation.											
	DAIRY QUEEN											
	Ice cream cones:											
1446	Small vanilla	1 ea	85	63	140	4	22	0	4	3	1	–
1447	Regular vanilla	1 ea	142	65	230	6	36	0	7	5	1	1
1448	Large vanilla	1 ea	213	66	340	9	53	0	10	7	1	1
1450	Chocolate dipped	1 ea	156	60	330	6	40	<1	16	8	4	3
1453	Chocolate sundae	1 ea	177	62	300	6	54	<1	7	5	1	1
1455	Banana split	1 ea	383	68	529	9	96	2	11	8.3	3.1	.4
1456	Peanut Buster Parfait	1 ea	305	52	710	16	94	1	32	10	10	9
1457	Hot Fudge Brownie Delight	1 ea	266	52	619	10	89	1	25	12.2	10.5	1.7
1459	Buster bar	1 ea	149	45	450	11	40	<1	29	9	10	8
1460	Dilly bar	1 ea	85	55	210	3	21	<1	13	6	3	3
1461	DQ ice cream sandwich	1 ea	60	47	138	3	24	<1	4	2	1	1
1463	Milk shakes, regular	1 ea	418	71	548	13	93	<1	15	8.4	2.1	2.1
1464	Milk shakes, large	1 ea	489	71	636	14	107	<1	17	10.6	2.1	2.1
1466	Malted milkshake	1 ea	418	68	610	13	106	<1	14	8	2	2
1468	Float	1 ea	397	76	410	5	82	0	7	5	1	1
1469	Freeze	1 ea	397	72	500	9	89	0	12	7.5	3.4	.4
	Mr. Misty:											
1470	Regular	1 ea	330	81	250	0	63	0	0	0	0	0
1471	Kiss	1 ea	89	81	70	0	17	0	0	0	0	0
1472	Freeze	1 ea	411	72	500	9	91	0	12	7.4	3.4	.4
1473	Float	1 ea	411	78	390	5	74	0	7	4.3	2	.3
	Sandwiches:											
1474	Chicken	1 ea	202	56	455	25	39	<1	21	4.2	7.4	8.5
1475	Fish fillet	1 ea	177	57	385	17	41	<1	17	3.1	5.2	8.3
1476	Fish fillet with cheese	1 ea	191	56	436	20	41	<1	22	6.2	7.3	8.3
1477	Hamburger, single	1 ea	148	55	323	18	30	<1	17	6.2	6.2	1
1478	Hamburger, double	1 ea	210	57	488	33	31	<1	26	12.7	11.7	2.1
1480	Cheeseburger, single	1 ea	162	55	379	21	31	<1	19	9.3	7.3	1
1481	Cheeseburger, double	1 ea	239	54	603	39	33	<1	36	19	13.7	2.1
	Hot dog:											
1483	Regular	1 ea	100	51	283	9	23	<1	16	6.1	7.1	2
1484	With cheese	1 ea	114	49	333	12	24	<1	21	9.1	8.1	2
1485	With chili	1 ea	128	52	323	11	26	2	19	7.1	8.1	2
1489	French fries, small	1 ea	71	38	210	3	29	1	10	2	5	3
1490	French fries, large	1 ea	113	49	344	4	46	2	16	3.5	7.1	5.3
1491	Onion rings	1 ea	85	46	240	4	29	<1	12	3	5	4
	Source: International Dairy Queen.											

(Computer code number is for West Diet Analysis program)

Chol (mg)	Calc (mg)	Iron (mg)	Magn (mg)	Phos (mg)	Pota (mg)	Sodi (mg)	Zinc (mg)	VT-A (RE)	Thia (mg)	Ribo (mg)	Niac (mg)	V-B6 (mg)	Fola (μg)	VT-C (mg)
14	6	.33	–	–	–	161	–	0	.07	.2	5	–	–	3
3	114	.73	–	–	–	514	–	0	.05	.03	.66	–	–	<1
30	250	1.54	–	–	–	190	–	58	.12	.53	.12	–	–	0
32	284	–	–	–	–	205	–	77	.11	.55	.12	–	–	0
4	15	1.2	–	–	–	412	–	4	.27	.16	.6	–	–	5
15	100	.4	–	100	150	60	–	25	.03	.17	.06	–	–	<1
20	150	.7	–	200	260	95	–	49	.06	.34	.11	.09	–	<1
30	250	1.4	–	300	380	140	–	98	.12	.51	.17	–	–	<1
20	150	.7	–	200	290	100	–	49	.06	.34	.11	.09	–	<1
20	200	1.1	–	200	290	140	–	49	.06	.34	.3	.14	–	<1
31	259	1.87	–	363	893	259	–	166	.16	.53	.41	.21	–	16
30	250	1.8	–	450	660	410	–	74	.15	.43	2	.22	–	2
30	174	1.57	–	262	445	297	–	64	.1	.3	.26	.16	–	1
15	100	1.1	–	250	400	220	–	25	.12	.17	2	.08	–	1
10	100	.4	–	100	170	50	–	25	.03	.17	–	.06	–	<1
5	59	.04	–	59	103	133	–	15	.03	.07	.39	.05	–	<1
47	474	2.84	–	526	600	242	–	194	.24	.81	.42	.2	–	<1
53	583	3.82	–	636	700	276	–	212	.32	1	.42	–	–	<1
45	450	4.5	–	600	570	230	–	184	.3	.85	.8	.19	–	<1
20	200	1.1	–	200	–	85	–	40	.06	.26	.05	.09	–	<1
30	300	1.8	–	350	–	180	–	98	.15	.51	–	.15	–	2
0	0	0	–	–	–	10	–	0	0	0	–	0	–	2
0	0	0	–	–	–	10	–	0	0	0	–	0	–	0
30	300	1.4	–	200	–	140	–	98	.12	.51	–	.18	–	2
20	200	.7	–	200	–	95	–	49	.06	.26	–	.09	–	1
58	159	5.71	–	264	370	804	–	21	.63	.62	8.46	–	–	3
47	156	3.75	–	156	292	656	–	16	.62	.44	8.33	–	–	–
62	260	3.74	–	208	301	882	–	62	.69	.53	8.3	–	–	–
47	104	3.75	–	156	271	605	–	10	.31	.18	5.21	–	–	1
101	106	6.68	–	318	440	668	–	21	.48	.36	9.55	–	–	1
62	208	3.74	–	260	280	831	–	114	.31	.18	5.19	–	–	1
127	370	6.66	–	529	465	1131	–	169	.48	.45	9.52	–	–	1
25	81	1.41	–	101	172	707	–	0	.12	.14	3.03	–	–	<1
35	151	1.41	–	202	182	928	–	86	.12	.17	3.03	–	–	<1
30	81	1.81	–	151	262	726	–	60	.15	.26	4.03	–	–	<1
0	10	.34	–	60	430	115	–	0	.06	.02	.8	–	–	9
0	13	.95	–	88	689	177	–	0	.08	.03	1.06	–	–	13
0	20	.72	–	60	90	135	–	15	.09	.05	.4	–	–	2

(For purposes of calculations, use "0" for t, <1, <.1, <.01, etc.)

Table A–1
Food Composition

Computer Code Number	Food Description	Measure	Wt (g)	H_2O (%)	Ener (kcal)	Prot (g)	Carb (g)	Dietary Fiber (g)	Fat (g)	Fat Breakdown (g)		
										Sat	Mono	Poly
	JACK IN THE BOX											
	Breakfast items:											
1492	Breakfast Jack sandwich	1 ea	126	50	307	18	30	–	13	5.2	5	2.5
1494	Sausage crescent	1 ea	156	39	584	22	28	–	43	15.5	21.5	5.7
1495	Supreme crescent	1 ea	146	39	547	20	27	–	40	13.2	18.9	7.8
1496	Pancake platter	1 ea	231	45	612	15	87	–	22	8.6	7.6	3.5
1497	Scrambled egg platter	1 ea	249	52	653	21	58	–	37	10.2	19.4	5.1
	Sandwiches:											
1498	Hamburger	1 ea	98	43	267	13	28	1	11	4.1	4.9	2
1499	Cheeseburger	1 ea	113	46	318	16	33	1	14	5.7	5.9	2.3
1500	Jumbo Jack burger	1 ea	205	52	539	24	39	1	31	10.2	12	7.4
1501	Jumbo Jack burger with cheese	1 ea	246	50	688	32	47	1	41	14.2	15.2	9.1
1505	Chicken supreme	1 ea	228	53	597	25	44	–	36	9.3	13.8	10.6
1583	Double cheeseburger	1 ea	149	50	467	21	33	–	27	12.3	11.6	3.1
1508	Tacos, regular	1 ea	81	57	191	8	16	–	11	–	–	–
1509	Tacos, super	1 ea	135	63	288	12	21	–	17	–	–	–
1513	Taco salad	1 ea	402	76	503	34	28	–	31	13.4	11.9	1.6
1516	French fries	1 ea	109	38	351	4	45	–	17	4	.7	.6
1517	Hash browns	1 ea	62	51	170	1	15	–	12	2.8	7.4	.3
1518	Onion rings	1 ea	108	34	398	5	40	–	24	5.8	15.9	.9
	Milk shakes:											
1519	Chocolate	1 ea	322	77	330	11	55	0	7	4.3	2.1	–
1520	Strawberry	1 ea	328	77	320	10	55	0	7	4.3	2	–
1521	Vanilla	1 ea	317	76	320	10	57	0	6	3.6	1.8	–
1522	Apple turnover	1 ea	119	35	410	4	49	–	22	6.6	12.5	1.8
	Source: Jack in the Box Restaurant, Inc.											
	KENTUCKY FRIED CHICKEN											
	Original recipe:											
1253	Center breast	1 ea	95	53	234	23	7	<1	13	3.1	6.4	1.6
1251	Side breast	1 ea	69	46	205	14	8	<1	13	3.2	6.7	1.7
1250	Drumstick	1 ea	47	51	120	11	3	<1	7	1.8	3.4	1.1
1252	Thigh	1 ea	88	51	249	15	9	<1	17	4.5	7.9	2.6
1249	Wing	1 ea	42	41	136	9	5	<1	9	2.3	4.6	1.4
	Dinners:											
1254	2-pce dinner, white	1 ea	322	59	702	32	56	2	39	9.5	18.4	7.9
1255	2-pce dinner, dark	1 ea	346	71	721	33	57	1	40	10.1	17.9	8.5
1256	2-pce dinner, combo	1 ea	341	47	741	32	58	1	42	10.7	19.3	8.8
	Extra crispy recipe:											
1261	Center breast	1 ea	104	51	263	25	9	<1	15	3.7	8.3	1.6
1259	Side breast	1 ea	84	45	262	17	11	<1	17	4.2	9.8	1.8
1258	Drumstick	1 ea	58	48	171	11	5	<1	12	2.9	6.5	1.4
1260	Thigh	1 ea	107	44	365	18	13	<1	27	6.9	14.4	3.8
1257	Wing	1 ea	53	35	207	10	8	<1	15	3.6	8.7	2
	Dinners:											
1262	2-pce dinner, white	1 ea	348	57	829	34	62	1	49	11.8	25.6	8.6
1263	2-pce dinner, dark	1 ea	375	59	878	36	62	1	54	13.3	26.9	9.9
1264	2-pce dinner, combo	1 ea	371	57	919	35	65	1	58	14.1	29.4	10.6
1265	Mashed potatoes	⅓ c	80	81	60	2	12	1	1	.2	.4	t
1268	Corn-on-the-cob	1 ea	143	70	176	5	32	1	3	.5	1	1.5

(Computer code number is for West Diet Analysis program)

PAGE KEY: A–2 = BEV A–4 = DAIRY A–10 = EGGS A–12 = FAT/OIL A–14 = FRUIT A–24 = BAKERY A–34 = GRAIN A–40 = FISH A–44 = MEATS A–48 = POULTRY A–50 = SAUSAGE A–52 = MIXED/FAST A–60 = NUTS/SEEDS A–62 = SWEETS A–66 = VEG/LEG A–78 = MISC A–80 = SOUPS/SAUCES A–84 = FAST A–96 = FRZN ENTREE A–98 = BABY FOODS

Chol (mg)	Calc (mg)	Iron (mg)	Magn (mg)	Phos (mg)	Pota (mg)	Sodi (mg)	Zinc (mg)	VT-A (RE)	Thia (mg)	Ribo (mg)	Niac (mg)	V-B6 (mg)	Fola (µg)	VT-C (mg)
203	170	3.1	–	–	–	871	–	90	.47	.41	3	–	–	–
187	170	2.9	–	–	–	1012	–	110	.6	.51	4.6	–	–	–
178	150	2.7	–	–	–	1053	–	110	.65	.54	4.2	–	–	–
99	100	1.8	–	–	–	888	–	80	.03	.85	7	–	–	6
442	175	5.73	–	–	–	1239	–	164	–	.77	5.85	–	–	11
26	150	1.8	–	–	–	556	–	–	.15	.26	2	–	–	–
41	252	2.72	–	–	–	753	–	40	.23	.23	3.03	–	–	–
67	129	2.86	–	–	–	677	–	–	.33	.27	1.66	–	–	–
104	274	3.86	–	–	–	1108	–	–	.37	.45	1.63	–	–	–
79	223	2.7	–	–	–	1368	–	74	.36	.3	10.2	–	–	6
72	400	2.7	–	–	–	842	–	200	.15	.34	6	–	–	–
21	100	1.1	35	146	257	460	1.2	57	.07	.17	1	.13	–	<1
37	150	1.6	45	198	347	765	1.8	85	.12	.08	1.4	.18	–	2
92	410	3.8	–	–	–	1600	–	270	.29	.53	5.8	–	–	9
0	–	1.3	–	–	–	194	–	–	.18	.03	3.8	–	–	26
0	–	.39	–	–	–	339	–	0	.05	–	1.09	–	–	8
0	31	2.31	–	–	–	473	–	–	.3	.18	2.73	–	–	3
25	350	.72	–	–	–	270	–	–	.15	.6	.4	–	–	–
25	350	.36	–	–	–	240	–	–	.15	.43	.4	–	–	–
25	350	–	–	–	–	230	–	–	.15	.34	.4	–	–	–
8	–	2.12	–	–	–	372	–	–	.24	.14	2.12	–	–	3
76	30	.83	–	–	–	555	–	6	.07	.14	9.5	–	–	–
59	52	.92	–	–	–	564	–	4	.05	.1	5.29	–	–	–
55	17	.91	–	–	–	227	–	3	.04	.1	2.64	–	–	–
104	55	1.1	–	–	–	524	–	26	.07	.25	4.65	–	–	–
49	37	.92	–	–	–	284	–	3	.02	.06	2.83	–	–	–
119	215	3.71	–	–	–	1854	–	76	.22	.38	11.8	.5	–	36
164	197	3.84	–	–	–	1738	–	76	.25	.57	10.6	.46	–	37
160	217	3.88	–	–	–	1801	–	57	.24	.53	10.9	.47	–	38
88	26	.62	–	–	–	609	–	6	.08	.1	10.1	–	–	–
62	23	.61	–	–	–	571	–	5	.07	.08	6.49	–	–	–
60	11	.59	–	–	–	272	–	4	.05	.1	3.11	–	–	–
116	44	1.08	–	–	–	619	–	35	.09	.19	5.84	–	–	–
55	14	.05	–	–	–	344	–	3	–	.03	.05	2.69	–	–
125	161	2.51	–	–	–	1915	–	76	.31	.34	12.8	.56	–	36
176	180	3.48	–	–	–	1869	–	77	.32	.5	12	.53	–	36
172	183	2.96	–	–	–	1949	–	76	.31	.45	11.7	.49	–	36
<1	21	.28	14	41	218	228	.16	5	.01	.04	.96	.11	7	4
–	7	.8	–	–	–	–	–	27	.14	.11	1.8	–	–	2

(For purposes of calculations, use "0" for t, <1, <.1, <.01, etc.)

A

Table A–1
Food Composition

Computer Code Number	Food Description	Measure	Wt (g)	H_2O (%)	Ener (kcal)	Prot (g)	Carb (g)	Dietary Fiber (g)	Fat (g)	Fat Breakdown (g) Sat	Mono	Poly
	KENTUCKY FRIED CHICKEN—Cont.											
1269	Coleslaw	⅓ c	79	75	103	1	11	<1	6	.9	1.5	2.9
1381	Kentucky nuggets	6 ea	96	44	276	17	13	<1	17	5.5	8.7	2.2
	Kentucky nugget sauce:											
1382	Barbeque	2 tsp	30	68	37	<1	8	–	1	.1	–	.3
1383	Sweet & sour	2 tbs	30	48	61	<1	14	–	1	.1	–	.3
1384	Honey	2 tbs	30	8	104	0	26	–	–	–	–	–
1385	Mustard	2 tbs	30	69	38	1	6	–	1	.1	–	1.2
1386	Kentucky fries	1 ea	119	37	377	5	48	1	18	4	12.5	1.1
1387	Mashed potatoes & gravy	⅓ c	86	82	62	2	10	<1	1	.4	.4	.2
1388	Buttermilk biscuit	1 ea	75	30	271	5	32	<1	13	3.7	6.7	2.5
1389	Potato salad	⅓ c	90	76	141	2	13	1	9	1.4	2.8	4.8
1390	Baked beans	⅓ c	89	71	105	5	18	6	1	.4	.5	.2
1391	Chicken Little sandwich	1 ea	57	32	204	7	17	1	12	2.4	–	4.1
	Source: Kentucky Fried Chicken Corporation.											
	LONG JOHN SILVER'S											
	Fish, batter fried:											
1523	Fish & Fryes (fries), 3 piece	1 ea	350	55	853	43	64	–	48	–	–	–
1524	Fish & Fryes, 2 piece	1 ea	260	53	651	30	53	–	36	–	–	–
1525	Fish dinner, 3 piece	1 ea	540	60	1180	47	93	–	70	–	–	–
	Fish, breaded & fried:											
1526	Fish dinner, 3 piece	1 ea	450	60	940	35	84	–	52	–	–	–
1527	Fish dinner, 2 piece	1 ea	400	60	818	26	76	–	46	–	–	–
	Chicken:											
1528	Chicken Plank dinner, 3 piece	1 ea	370	60	885	32	72	–	51	–	–	–
1529	Chicken Plank dinner, 4 piece	1 ea	440	60	1037	41	82	–	59	–	–	–
1530	Chicken Nugget dinner, 6 piece	1 ea	300	60	699	23	54	–	45	–	–	–
1531	Clam chowder	1 ea	185	85	128	7	15	1	5	–	–	–
1532	Clam dinner	1 ea	460	60	955	22	100	–	58	–	–	–
1533	Fish & chicken dinner	1 ea	460	60	935	36	73	–	55	–	–	–
1534	Oyster dinner	1 ea	360	60	789	17	78	–	45	–	–	–
1535	Scallop dinner	1 ea	320	60	747	17	66	–	45	–	–	–
1536	Seafood platter	1 ea	410	60	976	29	85	–	58	–	–	–
1537	Shrimp dinner, batter fried	1 ea	300	60	711	17	60	–	45	–	–	–
1538	Fish sandwich platter	1 ea	400	59	835	30	84	–	42	–	–	–
	Salads:											
1539	Ocean chef salad	1 ea	320	85	229	27	13	2	8	–	–	–
1540	Seafood salad	1 ea	480	85	426	19	22	2	30	–	–	–
1541	Coleslaw	1 ea	98	70	182	1	11	1	15	–	–	–
1542	Fryes (fries) serving	1 ea	85	42	247	4	31	1	12	–	–	–
1543	Hush puppies	1 ea	47	37	145	3	18	<1	7	–	–	–
	Source: Long John Silver's, Lexington, KY.											
	McDONALD'S											
	Sandwiches:											
1221	Big Mac	1 ea	215	55	500	25	42	1	26	16	1	9
1444	McChicken	1 ea	187	58	415	19	39	–	19	9	7	4
1591	McLean Deluxe	1 ea	206	66	320	22	35	–	10	5	1	4

Chol (mg)	Calc (mg)	Iron (mg)	Magn (mg)	Phos (mg)	Pota (mg)	Sodi (mg)	Zinc (mg)	VT-A (RE)	Thia (mg)	Ribo (mg)	Niac (mg)	V-B6 (mg)	Fola (μg)	VT-C (mg)
4	28	.17	–	–	–	171	–	28	.03	.03	.17	–	–	19
71	14	.6	–	–		840	–	180	.11	.12	6	.28	–	1
–	6	.21	–	–	–	477	–	39	–	.01	.2	–	–	–
–	5	.21	–	–	–	157	–	60	–	.02	.04	–	–	–
–	1	.21	–	–	–	–	–	0	–	.01	.08	–	–	–
–	11	.32	–	–	–	367	–	1	–	.01	.17	–	–	–
2	19	.93	–	–	–	215	–	0	.23	.08	3.09	–	–	24
–	19	.35	–	–	–	297	–	5	–	.03	1.05	–	–	–
1	110	1.85	–	–	–	756	–	30	.28	.22	3	–	–	–
11	10	.32	15	32	256	396	.29	27	.07	.02	.6	.19	7	3
1	54	1.43	29	90	229	387	1.29	10	.06	.04	.5	.07	32	2
21	27	2.05	–	–	–	399	–	6	.19	.14	2.65	–	–	–
106	–	–	–	–	–	2025	–	–	–	–	–	–	–	–
75	–	–	–	–	–	1352	–	–	–	–	–	–	–	–
119	–	–	–	–	–	2797	–	–	–	–	–	–	–	–
101	–	–	–	–	–	1900	–	–	–	–	–	–	–	–
76	–	–	–	–	–	1526	–	–	–	–	–	–	–	–
25	–	–	–	–	–	1918	–	–	–	–	–	–	–	
25	–	–	–	–	–	2433	–	–	–	–	–	–	–	–
25	–	–	–	–	–	853	–	–	–	–	–	–	–	–
17	–	–	–	–	–	611	–	–	–	–	–	–	–	–
27	–	–	–	–	–	1543	–	–	–	–	–	–	–	–
56	–	–	–	–	–	2076	–	–	–	–	–	–	–	–
55	–	–	–	–	–	763	–	–	–	–	–	–	–	–
37	–	–	–	–	–	1579	–	–	–	–	–	–	–	–
95	–	–	–	–	–	2161	–	–	–	–	–	–	–	–
127	–	–	–	–	–	1297	–	–	–	–	–	–	–	–
75	–	–	–	–	–	1402	–	–	–	–	–	–	–	–
64	–	–	–	–	–	986	–	–	–	–	–	–	–	–
113	–	–	–	–	–	1086	–	–	–	–	–	–	–	–
12	–	–	–	–	–	367	–	–	–	–	–	–	–	–
13	–	–	–	–	–	1	–	–	–	–	–	–	–	–
–	–	–	–	–	–	405	–	–	–	–	–	–	–	–
100	250	3.6	–	–	–	890	–	60	.45	.43	7	.22	–	1
50	150	2.7	–	–	–	83	–	20	.9	.17	9	–	–	2
60	150	3.6	–	–	–	670	–	100	.38	.34	7	–	–	6

(For purposes of calculations, use "0" for t, <1, <.1, <.01, etc.)

Table A–1
Food Composition

Computer Code Number	Food Description	Measure	Wt (g)	H_2O (%)	Ener (kcal)	Prot (g)	Carb (g)	Dietary Fiber (g)	Fat (g)	Fat Breakdown (g)		
										Sat	Mono	Poly
	McDONALD'S—Cont.											
	Sandwiches—Cont.											
1438	McLean Deluxe with Cheese	1 ea	219	66	370	24	35	–	14	8	1	5
1222	Quarter-Pounder	1 ea	166	52	410	23	34	1	20	11	1	8
1223	Quarter-Pounder with Cheese	1 ea	194	52	510	28	34	1	28	16	1	11
1224	Filet-O-Fish	1 ea	142	49	373	14	38	<1	18	8.1	6	4
1225	Hamburger	1 ea	102	48	255	12	30	<1	9	5	1	3
1226	Cheeseburger	1 ea	116	48	305	15	30	<1	13	7	1	5
1227	French fries, small serving	1 ea	68	36	220	3	26	1	12	2.5	8	1
1228	Chicken McNuggets	6 ea	112	52	270	20	17	<1	15	10	1.5	3.5
	Sauces (packet):											
1229	Hot mustard	1 ea	30	57	70	0	8	<1	4	1.2	1.9	.5
1230	Barbecue	1 ea	32	57	50	0	12	<1	<1	.2	.2	.1
1231	Sweet & sour	1 ea	32	52	60	0	14	<1	<1	.1	.1	0
	Low-fat (frozen yogurt) milk shakes:											
1232	Chocolate	1 ea	293	71	324	12	66	<1	2	.9	.1	.7
1233	Strawberry	1 ea	293	72	320	11	67	<1	1	.6	.1	.6
1234	Vanilla	1 ea	293	75	291	11	60	<1	1	.6	.1	.6
	Low-fat (frozen yogurt) sundaes:											
1237	Hot caramel	1 ea	168	56	270	7	59	<1	3	1	.5	1.5
1235	Hot fudge	1 ea	168	60	240	7	50	<1	3	.5	.5	2
1267	Strawberry	1 ea	168	61	210	6	49	<1	1	.3	.2	.5
1238	Vanilla	1 ea	80	65	100	4	21	<1	1	.3	.2	.5
1239	Pie, apple	1 ea	83	47	220	2	31	–	10	2.5	4.5	2.8
	Muffins (fat-free)											
1266	Blueberry	1 ea	75	41	170	3	40	–	0	0	0	0
1240	Apple bran	1 ea	85	39	204	6	45	3	0	0	0	0
1241	Cookies, McDonaldland	1 ea	56	2	262	4	42	<1	8	6.3	.9	.9
1242	Cookies, Chocolaty chip	1 ea	56	2	293	4	37	2	13	8.9	.9	3.6
	Breakfast items:											
1243	English muffin with spread	1 ea	59	33	177	5	28	–	5	2.3	1.4	1.3
1244	Egg McMuffin	1 ea	138	56	286	18	29	<1	11	6.1	1	4.1
1245	Hotcakes with marg & syrup	1 ea	176	45	445	8	75	<1	12	5	5	2
1246	Scrambled eggs	1 ea	100	75	140	12	1	<1	10	5	2	3
1247	Pork sausage	1 ea	48	46	179	8	0	<1	17	8.9	2.2	5.6
1248	Hashbrown potatoes	1 ea	53	53	130	1	15	1	7	4	2	1
1392	Sausage McMuffin	1 ea	117	49	299	13	23	<1	17	9.5	1.7	6.1
1393	Sausage McMuffin with egg	1 ea	167	53	452	22	28	<1	26	14.7	3.1	8.4
1394	Biscuit with biscuit spread	1 ea	75	31	260	5	32	<1	13	9	1	3
1395	Biscuit with sausage	1 ea	123	37	438	12	33	<1	29	17.7	3.1	8.3
1396	Biscuit with sausage & egg	1 ea	180	50	519	19	34	<1	34	20.6	3.1	10.3
1397	Biscuit with bacon, egg, cheese	1 ea	156	50	449	15	34	<1	26	16.3	2	8.2
	Salads:											
1398	Chef salad	1 ea	283	86	182	18	9	2	10	4.3	1.1	4.3
1400	Garden salad	1 ea	213	92	56	5	7	2	2	1.1	.5	.7
1401	Chunky chicken salad	1 ea	250	85	147	24	7	–	4	2	1	1

Source: McDonald's Corporation.

Chol (mg)	Calc (mg)	Iron (mg)	Magn (mg)	Phos (mg)	Pota (mg)	Sodi (mg)	Zinc (mg)	VT-A (RE)	Thia (mg)	Ribo (mg)	Niac (mg)	V-B6 (mg)	Fola (μg)	VT-C (mg)
75	200	3.6	–	–	–	890	–	150	.38	.34	7	–	–	6
85	150	3.6	–	–	–	645	–	40	.38	.26	7	.32	–	4
115	300	3.6	–	–	–	1110	–	150	.38	.34	7	.32	–	4
50	151	1.81	–	–	–	735	–	20	.3	.14	9.06	.1	–	<1
37	100	2.7	–	–	–	490	–	40	.3	.17	4	–	–	2
50	200	2.7	–	–	–	725	–	80	.3	.26	4	–	–	2
0	10	.36	–	–	–	110	–	0	.15	0	2	.18	–	9
55	13	1.08	–	–	–	580	–	0	.12	.14	8	.36	–	0
5	20	.22	–	–	–	250	–	2	.01	.01	.15	–	–	<1
0	13	.36	–	–	–	340	–	40	.01	.01	.17	–	–	2
0	11	.17	–	–	–	190	–	60	0	.01	.08	–	–	1
10	352	.84	–	–	–	242	–	60	.12	.51	.4	.1	–	0
10	352	.09	–	–	–	171	–	60	.12	.51	.4	.11	–	0
10	352	.1	–	–	–	171	–	60	.12	.51	.31	–	–	0
13	200	.08	–	–	–	180	–	60	.09	.34	.27	–	–	0
6	250	.36	–	–	–	170	–	40	.09	.34	.29	–	–	0
5	200	.16	–	–	–	95	–	40	.06	.34	.25	–	–	1
3	95	.23	–	–	–	76	–	19	.03	.16	.38	–	–	0
0	6	.94	6	23	66	175	.16	10	.12	.09	1.02	.03	3	1
0	80	.72	–	–	–	220	–	–	.12	.14	.8	–	–	1
0	45	1.22	–	–	–	227	–	1	.17	.19	2.27	–	–	1
0	18	1.63	–	–	–	271	–	0	.13	.15	1.81	.03	–	0
4	18	1.6	–	–	–	249	–	0	.13	.15	1.78	–	–	0
12	96	1.49	12	80	65	362	.39	31	.24	.29	2.45	.03	16	1
240	256	2.76	–	–	–	726	–	102	.48	.34	3.79	.08	–	0
8	101	1.81	–	–	–	693	–	40	.3	.34	3.03	.11	–	0
425	60	1.8	–	–	–	290	–	100	.07	.26	.05	–	–	0
48	8	.8	–	–	–	346	–	0	.26	.11	2.23	–	–	0
0	6	.27	–	–	–	330	–	0	.06	.02	.8	–	–	1
49	173	2.34	–	–	–	667	–	35	.46	.22	4.33	.13	–	0
284	263	3.78	–	–	–	966	–	105	.56	.45	5.25	.21	–	0
1	80	1.44	–	–	–	730	–	0	.23	.1	1.65	.03	–	0
46	83	1.88	–	–	–	1084	–	0	.47	.18	4.17	.21	–	0
267	103	3.7	–	–	–	1244	–	62	.46	.36	4.1	.21	–	0
24	204	2.75	–	–	–	1238	–	102	.39	.35	2.04	.13	–	0
119	160	1.54	–	–	–	427	–	1067	.32	.28	4.27	–	–	22
73	45	1.62	–	–	–	79	–	1014	.1	.11	.45	–	–	24
76	39	1.06	–	–	–	225	–	1666	.22	.17	8.82	–	–	26

(For purposes of calculations, use "0" for t, <1, <.1, <.01, etc.)

A

Table A–1
Food Composition

Computer Code Number	Food Description	Measure	Wt (g)	H_2O (%)	Ener (kcal)	Prot (g)	Carb (g)	Dietary Fiber (g)	Fat (g)	Fat Breakdown (g) Sat	Mono	Poly
	PIZZA HUT											
	Pan Pizza:											
1657	Cheese	2 pce	205	48	492	30	57	5	18	8.6	5.5	2.7
1658	Pepperoni	2 pce	211	45	540	29	62	5	22	9.2	9.3	3.4
1659	Supreme	2 pce	255	54	589	32	53	7	30	13.8	11.9	4.3
1660	Super Supreme	2 pce	257	55	563	33	53	6	26	12	–	–
	Thin 'N Crispy:											
1649	Cheese Pizza	2 pce	148	43	398	28	37	4	17	10	4.6	2.3
1623	Pepperoni Pizza	2 pce	146	42	413	26	36	4	20	11	–	–
1622	Supreme Pizza	2 pce	200	53	459	28	41	5	22	11	–	–
1620	Super Supreme Pizza	2 pce	203	52	463	29	44	5	21	10	–	–
	Hand Tossed:											
1619	Cheese Pizza	2 pce	220	50	518	34	55	7	20	13.6	–	–
1618	Pepperoni Pizza	2 pce	197	47	500	28	50	6	23	12.9	–	–
1648	Supreme Pizza	2 pce	239	54	540	32	50	7	26	13.8	–	–
1617	Super Supreme Pizza	2 pce	243	53	556	33	54	7	25	13	–	–
	Personal Pan Pizza:											
1610	Pepperoni	1 ea	256	43	675	37	76	8	29	12.5	12.1	4.5
1609	Supreme	1 ea	264	47	647	33	76	9	28	11.2	12.4	4.4
	Source: Pizza Hut.											
	TACO BELL											
	Burritos:											
1544	Bean with red sauce	1 ea	191	54	414	14	58	11	13	6.4	4.4	1.1
1545	Beef with red sauce	1 ea	191	53	457	23	44	4	19	9.7	6.9	.8
1546	Beef & bean with red sauce	1 ea	191	59	393	17	44	5	15	4.8	5.8	1.9
1547	Supreme with red sauce	1 ea	241	61	475	19	52	5	21	7.3	7.5	1.9
1549	Enchirito with red sauce	1 ea	213	62	382	20	31	5	20	9.3	4.9	1.5
	Tacos:											
1551	Taco	1 ea	78	59	183	10	11	1	11	4.6	4.5	.8
1552	Taco Bellgrande	1 ea	163	63	355	18	18	1	23	10.9	9	1.3
1554	Soft taco	1 ea	92	54	225	12	18	1	12	5.4	4.3	1.2
1555	Tostada with red sauce	1 ea	156	69	243	9	27	5	11	4.1	5.5	.8
1558	Mexican pizza	1 ea	223	55	575	21	40	2	37	11.4	14	9.7
1559	Taco salad with salsa	1 ea	595	73	939	36	60	8	62	19	26.6	12.3
1560	Nachos, regular	1 ea	107	39	349	8	38	3	19	6.1	7.6	2.1
1561	Nachos, Bellgrande	1 ea	287	58	649	22	61	–	35	12.3	–	2.6
1562	Pintos & cheese with red sauce	1 ea	128	69	190	9	19	7	9	3.6	4	.8
1563	Taco sauce, packet	1 ea	4	96	1	<1	<1	<1	<1	0	0	0
1564	Salsa	1 ea	10	42	18	1	4	–	<1	0	0	0
1565	Cinnamon twists	1 ea	47	3	231	3	32	1	11	5.4	3.5	1.2
	Source: Taco Bell Corporation.											
	WENDY'S											
	Hamburgers:											
1566	Single on white bun, no toppings	1 ea	119	44	350	21	29	<1	16	–	–	–
1568	Double on white bun, no toppings	1 ea	197	44	560	41	32	<1	34	7.4	12.5	8
1569	Big Classic	1 ea	241	63	470	26	36	–	25	–	–	–

PAGE KEY: A–2 = BEV A–4 = DAIRY A–10 = EGGS A–12 = FAT/OIL A–14 = FRUIT A–24 = BAKERY A–34 = GRAIN A–40 = FISH A–44 = MEATS A–48 = POULTRY A–50 = SAUSAGE A–52 = MIXED/FAST A–60 = NUTS/SEEDS A–62 = SWEETS A–66 = VEG/LEG A–78 = MISC A–80 = SOUPS/SAUCES A–84 = FAST A–96 = FRZN ENTREE A–98 = BABY FOODS

Chol (mg)	Calc (mg)	Iron (mg)	Magn (mg)	Phos (mg)	Pota (mg)	Sodi (mg)	Zinc (mg)	VT-A (RE)	Thia (mg)	Ribo (mg)	Niac (mg)	V-B6 (mg)	Fola (µg)	VT-C (mg)
34	630	5.4	60	470	320	940	4.1	90	.56	.6	5.2	.17	–	7
42	520	6.3	56	440	405	1127	4.2	100	.63	.49	5.4	.17	0	8
48	500	5	76	460	580	1363	5.6	120	.81	.8	6	.31	–	10
55	540	6.7	72	470	532	1447	5.4	120	.75	.66	6.4	–	–	11
33	660	3.2	48	470	261	867	3.6	70	.39	.39	4.8	.16	–	5
46	450	3.2	44	370	287	986	3.5	70	.42	.43	5.2	–	–	6
42	430	5.9	68	400	544	1328	4.7	100	.6	.49	5.4	–	–	10
56	460	4.9	60	420	463	1336	4.5	100	.59	.44	5.4	–	–	8
55	750	5.4	72	550	396	1276	4.7	100	.48	.49	5.4	–	–	10
50	440	5	60	390	415	1267	3.8	100	.54	.53	5.6	–	–	7
55	480	8.1	80	460	578	1470	5.7	110	.69	.53	7.2	–	–	12
54	440	6.8	76	420	516	1648	4.8	110	.71	.58	7.4	–	–	12
53	730	5.8	60	450	408	1335	3.8	120	.56	.66	8.2	.2	–	10
49	520	6.7	60	400	487	1313	3.8	120	.59	.66	8	.32	–	11
9	136	3.22	–	–	459	1064	–	46	.03	1.87	1.84	.29	–	49
53	106	3.46	–	–	352	1215	–	67	.37	1.98	3.19	.3	–	2
32	107	2.07	48	212	426	1095	2.58	77	.47	.4	2.98	.57	37	2
31	145	3.4	47	215	473	1116	–	118	.39	2	2.73	.33	–	24
54	269	2.84	–	–	423	1243	–	100	.26	.42	2.3	1	–	28
32	84	1.07	–	–	159	276	–	24	.05	.14	1.2	.12	–	1
56	182	1.9	–	–	334	472	–	40	.11	.29	2.02	.21	–	5
32	116	2.27	–	–	196	554	–	30	.39	.22	2.74	.1	–	1
16	179	1.53	–	–	401	596	–	95	.06	.17	.63	.26	–	45
52	257	3.74	80	400	408	1031	5.4	215	.32	.33	2.96	1.11	60	31
82	405	7.22	–	–	1066	1307	–	407	.52	.77	4.88	.57	–	78
9	193	.91	52	262	161	403	1.7	88	.17	.16	.69	.19	10	2
36	297	3.48	–	–	674	997	–	40	.1	.34	2.17	–	–	58
16	156	1.42	110	156	384	642	2.17	87	.05	.15	.4	.21	68	52
0	1	.02	–	–	4	42	–	6	0	<.01	.02	<.01	–	<1
0	36	.6	–	–	376	376	–	7	.02	.14	0	–	–	2
1	37	.49	–	–	36	316	–	0	.14	.05	.96	.05	–	1
65	100	4.5	–	–	265	420	–	0	.38	.34	6	–	–	–
125	48	6.3	42	339	431	575	8.35	0	.22	.43	9	.47	29	<1
80	40	4.5	–	–	470	900	–	60	.3	.25	5	–	–	12

(For purposes of calculations, use "0" for t, <1, <.1, <.01, etc.)

Table A–1
Food Composition

Computer Code Number	Food Description	Measure	Wt (g)	H_2O (%)	Ener (kcal)	Prot (g)	Carb (g)	Dietary Fiber (g)	Fat (g)	Fat Breakdown (g)		
										Sat	Mono	Poly
	WENDY'S—Cont.											
	Cheeseburgers:											
1570	Bacon cheeseburger	1 ea	147	46	460	29	23	<1	28	13	13	2
1571	Double with lettuce & tomato	1 ea	215	50	548	30	32	2	33	12.9	11.8	5.4
1572	Double with all toppings	1 ea	291	50	735	48	27	2	47	18.4	18	5.9
	Baked potatoes:											
1573	Plain	1 ea	250	75	250	6	52	4	<1	t	t	.1
1574	With bacon & cheese	1 ea	350	71	570	19	57	4	30	11.8	11.4	5.6
1575	With broccoli & cheese	1 ea	365	74	500	13	54	5	25	9.2	8.3	4.5
1576	With cheese	1 ea	350	71	590	16	55	4	34	12.5	12.7	7.1
1577	With chili & cheese	1 ea	400	72	510	22	63	8	20	13	6.8	.9
1578	With sour cream & chives	1 ea	310	71	460	6	53	4	24	10	7.9	3.3
1579	Chili	1ea	256	81	230	21	16	–	9	–	–	–
1580	French fries	1 ea	106	43	306	4	38	1	15	7	5	2
1581	Frosty dairy dessert	1 c	216	35	354	7	53	0	13	5	3	2
1582	Chocolate chip cookies	1 ea	64	4	320	3	40	1	17	5.5	5.8	4.9
	Source: Wendy's International.											
	FROZEN CONVENIENCE FOODS & MEALS											
	BUDGET GOURMET											
1695	Chicken cacciatore	1 ea	312	80	300	20	27	–	13	–	–	–
1694	Sweet & sour chicken with rice	1 ea	284	72	350	18	53	–	7	–	–	–
1689	Teriyaki chicken	1 ea	340	77	360	20	44	–	12	–	–	–
1692	Linguini & shrimp	1 ea	284	77	330	15	33	–	15	–	–	–
1691	Scallops & shrimp	1 ea	326	79	320	16	43	–	9	–	–	–
1693	Sirloin tips with country gravy	1 ea	284	80	310	16	21	–	18	–	–	–
1690	Veal parmigiana	1 ea	340	75	440	26	39	–	20	–	–	–
1696	Yankee pot roast	1 ea	312	77	380	27	22	–	21	–	–	–
	Source: The All American Gourmet Company.											
	HEALTHY CHOICE											
	Entrees:											
1628	Chicken Chow Mein	1 ea	241	78	220	18	31	–	3	.8	–	.8
1630	Fillet of Fish Florentine	1 ea	273	80	220	26	13	–	7	3	–	2
1624	Lasagna	1 ea	284	78	260	18	37	–	5	–	–	–
1629	Seafood Newburg	1 ea	227	80	200	13	30	–	3	.8	–	.8
1625	Spaghetti	1 ea	284	77	280	14	42	–	6	–	–	–
	Dinners:											
1627	Sirloin Tips	1 ea	334	81	280	23	30	–	8	–	–	–
1626	Sole Au Gratin	1 ea	312	80	270	16	40	–	5	–	–	–
	Low-fat ice milk:											
1601	Berry	½ c	113	–	120	3	23	–	2	1	–	0
1604	Chocolate	½ c	113	–	130	3	24	–	2	1	–	0
1608	Cookie & Cream	½ c	113	–	130	4	24	–	2	–	–	0
1621	Vanilla	½ c	113	–	120	4	21	–	2	1	–	0
	Source: ConAgra Frozen Foods, Omaha, NE.											

(Computer code number is for West Diet Analysis program)

PAGE KEY: A–2 = BEV A–4 = DAIRY A–10 = EGGS A–12 = FAT/OIL A–14 = FRUIT A–24 = BAKERY A–34 = GRAIN A–40 = FISH A–44 = MEATS A–48 = POULTRY A–50 = SAUSAGE A–52 = MIXED/FAST A–60 = NUTS/SEEDS A–62 = SWEETS A–66 = VEG/LEG A–78 = MISC A–80 = SOUPS/SAUCES A–84 = FAST A–96 = FRZN ENTREE A–98 = BABY FOODS

Chol (mg)	Calc (mg)	Iron (mg)	Magn (mg)	Phos (mg)	Pota (mg)	Sodi (mg)	Zinc (mg)	VT-A (RE)	Thia (mg)	Ribo (mg)	Niac (mg)	V-B6 (mg)	Fola (μg)	VT-C (mg)
65	136	3.6	33	296	332	860	5.14	82	.26	.28	5.7	.23	25	1
84	177	4	33	339	430	864	4.41	111	.34	.35	5.29	.25	28	5
165	180	5.4	50	470	620	883	8.8	112	.36	.53	10	.46	31	5
0	40	2.7	66	169	1360	60	.65	0	.27	.1	3.82	.7	67	36
22	200	3.7	80	406	1380	180	2.53	150	.22	.17	4.64	.87	33	36
22	250	3.6	83	373	1550	2	.86	350	.3	.25	4	.86	66	90
22	350	3.6	78	50	1380	2	.61	200	.22	.25	3.3	.8	33	36
22	250	6.13	111	498	1590	810	3.78	172	.3	.26	4.1	.9	50	36
15	40	2.7	70	185	1420	230	.9	100	.22	.14	3	.79	32	36
–	60	4.5	–	–	565	960	–	200	.12	.17	3	–	–	9
15	13	1.02	45	197	689	105	.51	0	.15	.04	2.96	.26	33	12
44	257	.86	43	238	518	194	.92	143	.11	.45	.31	.12	17	<1
5	10	1.09	15	62	100	235	.46	0	.06	.07	.4	.03	6	0
60	150	1.8	–	–	–	810	–	40	.23	.51	5	–	–	21
40	60	.72	–	–	–	640	–	80	.12	.34	3	–	–	2
55	80	1.4	–	–	–	610	–	300	.15	.34	6	–	–	12
75	10	3.6	–	–	–	1250	–	1000	.3	.17	3	–	–	2
70	150	.72	–	–	–	690	–	150	–	.26	3	–	–	12
40	60	.36	–	–	–	570	–	150	.15	.17	4	–	–	2
165	30	4.5	–	–	–	1160	–	1000	.45	.6	6	–	–	6
70	150	1.8	–	–	–	690	–	600	.15	.43	7	–	–	6
45	20	1.4	–	290	290	440	–	81	.15	.14	4	–	–	4
65	150	.72	58	–	780	590	1.2	500	.15	.34	2	.14	<1	1
20	100	2.7	–	210	500	420	–	150	.3	.26	2	–	–	2
55	60	1.1	–	160	270	440	–	3	.12	.14	1.2	–	–	4
20	6	3.6	–	160	540	480	–	250	.38	.26	2	–	–	5
65	20	2.7	–	190	540	370	–	700	.15	.17	5	.35	–	42
55	80	1.1	–	260	430	470	–	–	.23	.17	1.6	–	–	6
5	100	–	–	10	160	60	–	–	.03	.17	–	–	–	–
5	100	–	–	10	191	70	–	–	.03	.17	–	–	–	–
5	150	–	–	10	180	80	–	–	.03	.17	–	–	–	–
5	150	–	–	10	180	60	–	–	.06	.25	–	–	–	–

(For purposes of calculations, use "0" for t, <1, <.1, <.01, etc.)

A

Table A–1
Food Composition

Computer Code Number	Food Description	Measure	Wt (g)	H_2O (%)	Ener (kcal)	Prot (g)	Carb (g)	Dietary Fiber (g)	Fat (g)	Fat Breakdown (g)		
										Sat	Mono	Poly
	LEAN CUISINE											
	Dinners:											
1639	Baked Cheese Ravioli	1 ea	241	77	240	13	30	3	8	3	3	.5
1640	Chicken Cacciatore	1 ea	308	80	280	22	31	4	7	2	–	1
1632	Chicken Chow Mein	1 ea	255	78	240	14	34	–	5	1	–	1
1633	Lasagna	1 ea	291	79	260	19	34	2	5	2	2	.5
1634	Macaroni & Cheese	1 ea	255	74	290	15	37	–	9	4	–	.5
1631	Spaghetti w/Meatballs	1 ea	269	75	280	19	35	11	7	2	2.6	1
	Pizza:											
1635	French Bread Cheese Pizza	1 ea	145	52	300	17	38	<1	9	3	5	.5
1638	French Bread Deluxe Pizza	1 ea	174	56	320	22	39	2	8	3	3	.5
1637	French Bread Pepperoni Pizza	1 ea	149	51	330	19	38	2	11	3	5.4	1
1636	French Bread Sausage Pizza	1 ea	170	55	330	22	40	2	9	3	4.3	.5
	Source: Stouffer's Foods Corp, Solon, OH.											
	WEIGHT WATCHERS											
	Dinners:											
1641	Beef Stroganoff	1 ea	238	73	290	22	26	3	9	4	3	2
1646	Oven Fried Fish	1 ea	198	79	240	20	23	–	7	–	5	2
1647	Fried Chicken Patty	1 pce	184	73	270	16	14	–	16	8	6	2
1654	Chicken Burrito w/Vegetable	1 ea	216	68	330	15	36	–	14	4	6	3
1656	Pasta Primavera	1 ea	238	75	260	15	22	2	11	.8	8	3
	Pizza:											
1653	Cheese Pizza	1 ea	164	56	300	22	37	2	7	3	3	1
1650	Deluxe Combination Pizza	1 ea	200	64	330	26	35	3	10	3	5	2
1651	Sausage Pizza	1 ea	175	60	320	24	35	2	10	2	6	2
1652	Pepperoni Pizza	1 ea	171	56	320	26	31	–	10	3	5	2
	Desserts:											
1645	Apple pie	1 ea	98	49	200	2	39	–	5	1	2	2
1643	Boston cream pie	1 ea	85	48	170	4	35	1	4	1	1	2
1644	Chocolate brownie	1 ea	35	29	100	3	17	<1	4	1	2	1
1642	Strawberry cheesecake	1 ea	109	62	180	7	28	–	5	1	1	2
1655	Chocolate mousse	1 ea	70	46	170	6	24	<1	6	–	4	2
	Source: Foodway National Inc., Boise, ID.											
	BABY FOODS											
1720	Apple juice	4 fl oz	125	88	59	0	15	–	<1	–	–	–
1721	Applesauce, strained	1 tbs	14	89	6	<1	2	–	<1	–	–	–
1716	Carrots, strained	1 tbs	14	92	4	<1	1	–	<1	–	–	–
1718	Cereal, mixed, millk added	1 tbs	14	75	16	1	2	–	<1	–	–	–
1719	Cereal, rice, milk added	1 tbs	14	75	16	1	2	–	<1	–	–	–
1723	Chicken and noodles, strained	1 tbs	14	88	7	<1	1	–	<1	–	–	–
1722	Peas, strained	1 tbs	14	88	6	1	1	–	<1	–	–	–
1717	Teething biscuits	1 ea	11	6	43	1	8	–	<1	–	–	–

Chol (mg)	Calc (mg)	Iron (mg)	Magn (mg)	Phos (mg)	Pota (mg)	Sodi (mg)	Zinc (mg)	VT-A (RE)	Thia (mg)	Ribo (mg)	Niac (mg)	V-B6 (mg)	Fola (μg)	VT-C (mg)
55	200	1.44	42	168	380	590	1.5	60	.06	.25	1.2	.2	48	36
45	40	1.44	47	–	560	570	.97	100	.22	.17	6	–	–	9
30	40	1.08	30	–	350	530	1.1	60	.15	.17	5	–	–	6
25	150	1.8	44	–	700	590	2.9	100	.15	.25	3	.32		6
30	250	.72	–	–	160	550	–	20	.12	.25	1.2	–	–	0
35	100	1.8	47	–	500	490	2.5	60	.15	.25	3	.2	–	4
15	250	2.7	34	–	320	590	1.6	60	.37	.34	4	.1	–	6
40	200	1.44	38	–	440	860	2.08	150	.45	.51	5	.16	–	6
25	200	3.6	34	–	390	790	1.8	100	.45	.42	5	.07	–	6
40	250	2.7	39	–	440	860	2.2	80	.45	.51	5	.07	–	6
25	80	2.7	–	–	350	600	–	60	.23	.26	4	.32	–	4
15	20	.72	–	–	340	380	–	100	.09	.14	1.6	–	–	5
70	39	1.7	–	–	350	610	–	75	.19	.18	4	–	–	6
65	56	2.3	–	–	390	800	–	38	.52	.39	5.9	–	–	3
5	300	1.8	–	–	260	800	–	350	.23	.26	3	.18	–	18
35	450	1.4	–	–	420	630	–	200	.3	.51	3	.06	–	12
25	350	1.8	–	–	490	650	–	350	.3	.51	3	.2	–	21
35	300	1.8	–	–	470	630	–	250	.3	.51	3	.06	–	18
35	400	1.8	–	–	420	710	–	200	.23	.51	3	–	–	15
5	20	1.1	–	–	80	280	–	–	.06	.07	.4	–	–	1
5	65	.6	–	–	120	290	–	14	.03	.02	.3	.08	–	1
10	19	.9	–	–	120	150	–	14	.06	.03	.2	.03	–	1
20	80	.36	–	–	140	210	–	40	.06	.07	1.6	–	–	2
5	60	1.1	–	–	210	190	–	–	.03	.03	.4	.06	–	5
–	5	.71	4	6	114	4	.04	3	.01	.02	.1	.04	<1	72
–	1	.03	<1	1	10	<1	<.01	<1	<.01	<.01	.01	<.01	<1	6
–	3	.05	1	3	28	5	.02	164	<.01	.01	.07	.01	2	1
–	31	1.49	4	20	28	7	.1	3	.06	.08	.82	.01	2	–
–	34	1.73	6	25	27	7	.09	4	.07	.07	.74	.02	1	–
–	3	.06	1	3	6	2	.04	16	<.01	.01	.07	.01	1	<1
–	3	.14	2	6	16	<1	.05	8	.01	.01	.14	.01	4	1
–	29	.39	4	18	36	40	.1	1	.03	.06	.48	.01	2	1

(For purposes of calculations, use "0" for t, <1, <.1, <.01, etc.)

Contents

RECOMMENDED NUTRIENT INTAKES AND OTHER NUTRITION RECOMMENDATIONS

U.S. RECOMMENDATIONS

Some of the U.S. recommendations for nutrient intakes appear in the RDA table on the inside front cover, left. The remaining RDA are here, in Tables B–1, B–2, and B–3.

Food labels use another set of standards that derive from the RDA. From the late 1960s to the early 1990s, the set of standards used on food labels was called the U.S. RDA. The U.S. RDA were derived from the 1968 RDA and were established by the Food and Drug Administration (FDA) so that labels could express the nutrient contents of foods as percentages of those standards. The intent was to help consumers evaluate the nutrient contents of foods for themselves and at the same time to spare them the burden of learning the different units in which nutrient amounts are expressed. Thus all nutrient amounts in a food, whether originally measured in micrograms, milligrams, grams, or RE, could be expressed as "percent of U.S. RDA."

Table B–1
Estimated Safe and Adequate Daily Dietary Intakes of Additional Selected Vitamins and Minerals (United States)[a]

	Vitamins		Trace Elements[b]				
Age (yr)	Biotin (μg)	Pantothenic Acid (mg)	Chromium (μg)	Molybdenum (μg)	Copper (mg)	Manganese (mg)	Fluoride (mg)
Infants							
0–0.5	10	2	10–40	15–30	0.4–0.6	0.3–0.6	0.1–0.5
0.5–1	15	3	20–60	20–40	0.6–0.7	0.6–1.0	0.2–1.0
Children							
1–3	20	3	20–80	25–50	0.7–1.0	1.0–1.5	0.5–1.5
4–6	25	3–4	30–120	30–75	1.0–1.5	1.5–2.0	1.0–2.5
7–10	30	4–5	50–200	50–150	1.0–2.0	2.0–3.0	1.5–2.5
11+	30–100	4–7	50–200	75–250	1.5–2.5	2.0–5.0	1.5–2.5
Adults	30–100	4–7	50–200	75–250	1.5–3.0	2.0–5.0	1.5–4.0

[a]Less information is available on which to base allowances for these nutrients. Therefore, they are not included in the main table of the RDA, and the figures provided here are in the form of ranges of recommended intakes.

[b]The toxic levels for many trace elements may be only several times usual intakes, so the upper levels for the trace elements given in this table should not be habitually exceeded.

Source: Recommended Dietary Allowances, © 1989 by the National Academy of Sciences, National Academy Press, Washington, D.C.

Table B–2
Estimated Minimum Requirements of Sodium, Chloride, and Potassium

Age (yr)	Weight (kg)	Sodium[a] (mg)	Chloride (mg)	Potassium[b] (mg)
Infants				
0.0–0.5	4.5	120	180	500
0.5–1.0	8.9	200	300	700
Children				
1	11.0	225	350	1000
2–5	16.0	300	500	1400
6–9	25.0	400	600	1600
Adolescents	50.0	500	750	2000
Adults	70.0	500	750	2000

[a]Sodium requirements are based on estimates of needs for growth and for replacement of obligatory losses. They cover a wide variation of physical activity patterns and climatic exposure but do not provide for large, prolonged losses from the skin through sweat.

[b]Dietary potassium may benefit the prevention and treatment of hypertension, and recommendations to include many servings of fruits and vegetables would raise potassium intakes to about 3500 milligrams per day.

Source: Recommended Dietary Allowances, © 1989 by the National Academy of Sciences, National Academy Press, Washington, D.C.

Table B–3
Median Heights and Weights and Recommended Energy Intakes (United States)

Age (yr)	Weight		Height		Average Energy Allowance			
	kg	lb	cm	in	REE[a] (kcal/day)	MULTIPLES OF REE[b]	kcal/kg	kcal/day[c]
Infants								
0.0–0.5	6	13	60	24	320		108	650
0.5–1.0	9	20	71	28	500		98	850
Children								
1–3	13	29	90	35	740		102	1300
4–6	20	44	112	44	950		90	1800
7–10	28	62	132	52	1130		70	2000
Males								
11–14	45	99	157	62	1440	1.70	55	2500
15–18	66	145	176	69	1760	1.67	45	3000
19–24	72	160	177	70	1780	1.67	40	2900
25–50	79	174	176	70	1800	1.60	37	2900
51+	77	170	173	68	1530	1.50	30	2300
Females								
11–14	46	101	157	62	1310	1.67	47	2200
15–18	55	120	163	64	1370	1.60	40	2200
19–24	58	128	164	65	1350	1.60	38	2200
25–50	63	138	163	64	1380	1.55	36	2200
51+	65	143	160	63	1280	1.50	30	1900
Pregnant (2nd and 3rd trimesters)								+300
Lactating								+500

[a]REE (resting energy expenditure) represents the energy expended by a person at rest under normal conditions.

[b]Recommended energy allowances assume light-to-moderate activity and were calculated by multiplying the REE by an activity factor.

[c]Average energy allowances have been rounded.

Source: Recommended Dietary Allowances, © 1989 by the National Academy of Sciences, National Academy Press, Washington, D.C.

Four sets of U.S. RDA were developed for different groups of people—infants, children, adults, and pregnant and lactating women. The most commonly used set was the U.S. RDA for adults. The one for infants was used for formulas. Supplements designed for children and for pregnant and lactating women used the U.S. RDA for these groups on their labels. The complete U.S. RDA are in Table B–4.

With the new labeling regulations came a name change. The revised set of standards used on food labels—the Daily Values—are discussed fully in Chapter 1. The Daily Values derive from two sets of standards—the Reference Daily Intakes (RDI) and the Daily Reference Values (DRV). The current RDI continue to use the same values as the old U.S. RDA for now (see inside front cover, right).

CANADIAN RECOMMENDATIONS

The Canadian equivalent of the RDA is the Recommended Nutrient Intakes (RNI). The Canadian RNI are presented in Tables B–5 and B–6.

Like the *Diet and Health* report, the *Nutrition Recommendations for Canadians* examines the relationships linking nutrition and disease. The intent is to make recommendations that will supply enough nutrients, while reducing the risk of chronic disease. The Scientific Review Committee adopted the following key statements as the Nutrition Recommendations for Canadians:[1]

Table B–4
U.S. Recommended Daily Allowances (U.S. RDA)

Nutrient	Adults and Children over 4 Years	Infants	Children under 4 Years	Pregnant or Lactating Women
Protein (g)	45[a]	18[a]	20[a]	
Vitamin A (RE)	1000	300	500	1600
Vitamin D[b] (IU)	400	400	400	400
Vitamin E[b] (IU)	30	5.0	10	30
Vitamin C (mg)	60	35	40	60
Folate (mg)	0.4	0.1	0.2	0.8
Thiamin (mg)	1.5	0.5	0.7	1.7
Riboflavin (mg)	1.7	0.6	0.8	2.0
Niacin (mg)	20	8	9	20
Vitamin B_6[b] (mg)	2.0	0.4	0.7	2.5
Vitamin B_{12}[b] (μg)	6.0	2.0	3.0	8.0
Biotin[b] (mg)	0.3	0.5	0.15	0.3
Pantothenic acid[b] (mg)	10	3	5	10
Calcium (g)	1.0	0.6	0.8	1.3
Phosphorus[b] (g)	1.0	0.5	0.8	1.3
Iodine[b] (μg)	150	45	70	150
Iron (mg)	18	15	10	18
Magnesium[b] (mg)	400	70	200	450
Copper[b] (mg)	2.0	0.6	1.0	2.0
Zinc[b] (mg)	15	5	8	15

Note: The values for adults and children over 4 years are the ones most commonly used on food labels.

[a]If protein efficiency ratio of protein is equal to or better than that of casein.

[b]Optional for adults and children 4 years or over in vitamin and mineral supplements.

Source: U.S. Department of Health and Human Services, Public Health Service, Food and Drug Administration, Office of Public Affairs, 5600 Fishers Lane, Rockville, Maryland 20857, HHS publication no. (FDA) 81–2146, revised March 1981.

Table B-5
Average Energy Requirements for Canadians

Age	Sex	Average Height (cm)	Average Weight (kg)	Requirements[a]					
				(kcal/kg)[b]	(MJ/kg)[b]	(kcal/day)	(MJ/day)	(kcal/cm)	(MJ/cm)
Infants (months)									
0–2	Both	55	4.5	120–100	0.50–0.42	500	2.0	9	0.04
3–5	Both	63	7.0	100–95	0.42–0.40	700	2.8	11	0.05
6–8	Both	69	8.5	95–97	0.40–0.41	800	3.4	11.5	0.05
9–11	Both	73	9.5	97–99	0.41	950	3.8	12.5	0.05
Children and Adults (years)									
1	Both	82	11	101	0.42	1100	4.8	13.5	0.06
2–3	Both	95	14	94	0.39	1300	5.6	13.5	0.06
4–6	Both	107	18	100	0.42	1800	7.6	17	0.07
7–9	M	126	25	88	0.37	2200	9.2	17.5	0.07
	F	125	25	76	0.32	1900	8.0	15	0.06
10–12	M	141	34	73	0.30	2500	10.4	17.5	0.07
	F	143	36	61	0.25	2200	9.2	15.5	0.06
13–15	M	159	50	57	0.24	2800	12.0	17.5	0.07
	F	157	48	46	0.19	2200	9.2	14	0.06
16–18	M	172	62	51	0.21	3200	13.2	18.5	0.08
	F	160	53	40	0.17	2100	8.8	13	0.05
19–24	M	175	71	42	0.18	3000	12.6		
	F	160	58	36	0.15	2100	8.8		
25–49	M	172	74	36	0.15	2700	11.3		
	F	160	59	32	0.13	1900	8.0		
50–74	M	170	73	31	0.13	2300	9.7		
	F	158	63	29	0.12	1800	7.6		
75+	M	168	69	29	0.12	2000	8.4		
	F	155	64	23	0.10	1500	6.3		

[a]Requirements can be expected to vary within a range of ±30 percent.

[b]First and last figures are averages at the beginning and end of the three-month period.

Source: Health and Welfare Canada, *Nutrition Recommendations: The Report of the Scientific Review Committee* (Ottawa: Canadian Government Publishing Centre, 1990), Tables 5 and 6, pp. 25, 27.

B

Table B-6
Recommended Nutrient Intakes for Canadians, 1990

Age	Sex	Weight (kg)	Protein (g/day)[a]	Fat-Soluble Vitamins: VITAMIN A (RE/day)[b]	VITAMIN D (μg/day)[c]	VITAMIN E (mg/day)[d]
Infants (months)						
0–4	Both	6	12[f]	400	10	3
5–12	Both	9	12	400	10	3
Children and Adults (years)						
1	Both	11	13	400	10	3
2–3	Both	14	16	400	5	4
4–6	Both	18	19	500	5	5
7–9	M	25	26	700	2.5	7
	F	25	26	700	2.5	6
10–12	M	34	34	800	2.5	8
	F	36	36	800	5	7
13–15	M	50	49	900	5	9
	F	48	46	800	5	7
16–18	M	62	58	1000	5	10
	F	53	47	800	2.5	7
19–24	M	71	61	1000	2.5	10
	F	58	50	800	2.5	7
25–49	M	74	64	1000	2.5	9
	F	59	51	800	2.5	6
50–74	M	73	63	1000	5	7
	F	63	54	800	5	6
75+	M	69	59	1000	5	6
	F	64	55	800	5	5
Pregnancy (additional amount needed)						
1st trimester			5	0	2.5	2
2nd trimester			20	0	2.5	2
3rd trimester			24	0	2.5	2
Lactation (additional amount needed)			20	400	2.5	3

Note: Recommended intakes of energy and of certain nutrients are not listed in this table because of the nature of the variables upon which they are based. The figures for energy are estimates of average requirements for expected patterns of activity (see Table B–5). For nutrients not shown, the following amounts are recommended based on at least 2000 kcalories per day and body weights as given: thiamin, 0.4 milligrams per 1000 kcalories (0.48 milligrams/5000 kilojoules); riboflavin, 0.5 milligrams per 1000 kcalories (0.6 milligrams/5000 kilojoules); niacin, 7.2 niacin equivalents per 1000 kcalories (8.6 niacin equivalents/5000 kilojoules); vitamin B_6, 15 micrograms, as pyridoxine, per gram of protein. Recommended intakes during periods of growth are taken as appropriate for individuals representative of the midpoint in each age group. All recommended intakes are designed to cover individual variations in essentially all of a healthy population subsisting upon a variety of common foods available in Canada.

Source: Health and Welfare Canada, *Nutrition Recommendations: The Report of the Scientific Review Committee* (Ottawa: Canadian Government Publishing Centre, 1990), Table 20, p. 204.

Table B–6 (*continued*)

Water-Soluble Vitamins			Minerals					
VITAMIN C (mg/day)[e]	FOLATE (µg/day)	VITAMIN B_{12} (µg/day)	CALCIUM (mg/day)	PHOSPHORUS (mg/day)	MAGNESIUM (mg/day)	IRON (mg/day)	IODINE (µg/day)	ZINC (mg/day)
20	25	0.3	250	150	20	0.3[g]	30	2[h]
20	40	0.4	400	200	32	7	40	3
20	40	0.5	500	300	40	6	55	4
20	50	0.6	550	350	50	6	65	4
25	70	0.8	600	400	65	8	85	5
25	90	1.0	700	500	100	8	110	7
25	90	1.0	700	500	100	8	95	7
25	120	1.0	900	700	130	8	125	9
25	130	1.0	1100	800	135	8	110	9
30	175	1.0	1100	900	185	10	160	12
30	170	1.0	1000	850	180	13	160	9
40	220	1.0	900	1000	230	10	160	12
30	190	1.0	700	850	200	12	160	9
40	220	1.0	800	1000	240	9	160	12
30	180	1.0	700	850	200	13	160	9
40	230	1.0	800	1000	250	9	160	12
30	185	1.0	700	850	200	13[i]	160	9
40	230	1.0	800	1000	250	9	160	12
30	195	1.0	800	850	210	8	160	9
40	215	1.0	800	1000	230	9	160	12
30	200	1.0	800	850	210	8	160	9
0	200	0.2	500	200	15	0	25	6
10	200	0.2	500	200	45	5	25	6
10	200	0.2	500	200	45	10	25	6
25	100	0.2	500	200	65	0	50	6

[a]The primary units are expressed per kilogram of body weight. The figures shown here are examples.

[b]One retinol equivalent (RE) corresponds to the biological activity of 1 microgram of retinol, 6 micrograms of beta-carotene, or 12 micrograms of other carotenes.

[c]Expressed as cholecalciferol or ergocalciferol.

[d]Expressed as δ-α-tocopherol equivalents, relative to which β- and γ-tocopherol and α-tocotrienol have activities of 0.5, 0.1, and 0.3, respectively.

[e]Cigarette smokers should increase intake by 50 percent.

[f]The assumption is made that the protein is from breast milk or has the same biological value as breast milk and that, between 3 and 9 months, adjustment for the quality of the protein is made.

[g]Based on the assumption that breast milk is the source of iron.

[h]Based on the assumption that breast milk is the source of zinc.

[i]After menopause, the recommended intake is 8 milligrams per day.

- The Canadian diet should provide energy consistent with the maintenance of body weight within the recommended range.
- The Canadian diet should include essential nutrients in amounts recommended.
- The Canadian diet should include no more than 30 percent of energy as fat (33 grams/1000 kcalories or 39 grams/5000 kilojoules) and no more than 10 percent as saturated fat (11 grams/1000 kcalories or 13 grams/5000 kilojoules).
- The Canadian diet should provide 55 percent of energy as carbohydrate (138 grams/1000 kcalories or 165 grams/5000 kilojoules) from a variety of sources.
- The sodium content of the Canadian diet should be reduced.
- The Canadian diet should include no more than 5 percent of total energy as alcohol, or two drinks daily, whichever is less.
- The Canadian diet should contain no more caffeine than the equivalent of four regular cups of coffee per day.
- Community water supplies containing less than 1 milligram per liter should be fluoridated to that level.

NUTRITION RECOMMENDATIONS FROM WHO

The World Health Organization (WHO) has also assessed the relationships between diet and the development of chronic diseases.[2] Their recommendations are expressed in average daily ranges that represent the lower and upper limits:

- Total energy: sufficient to support normal growth, physical activity, and body weight (body mass index = 20–22).
- Total fat: 15 to 30 percent of total energy.
  - Saturated fatty acids: 0 to 10 percent total energy.
  - Polyunsaturated fatty acids: 3 to 7 percent total energy.
  - Dietary cholesterol: 0 to 300 milligrams per day.
- Total carbohydrate: 55 to 75 percent total energy.
  - Complex carbohydrates: 50 to 75 percent total energy.
  - Dietary fiber: 27 to 40 grams per day.
  - Refined sugars: 0 to 10 percent total energy.
- Protein: 10 to 15 percent total energy.
- Salt: upper limit of 6 grams/day (no lower limit set).

NOTES

1. *Nutrition Recommendations: The Report of the Scientific Review Committee* is sold for $18.95, plus postage and handling, by the Canadian Government Publishing Centre, Ottawa, Ontario K1A 0S9.
2. Diet, nutrition and the prevention of chronic diseases: A report of the WHO Study Group on Diet, Nutrition and Prevention of Noncommunicable Diseases, *Nutrition Reviews* 49 (1991): 291–301.

APPENDIX C

Contents

DIETARY GUIDELINES AND FOOD EXCHANGE SYSTEMS

Chapter 1 introduced dietary guidelines and food group plans, and Nutrition in Practice 6 explained the U.S. food exchange system. This appendix provides details of the U.S. exchange system and then presents the Canadian exchange system, guidelines, and food group plan.

THE U.S. EXCHANGE SYSTEM

The U.S. exchange system divides the foods suitable for use in planning a healthy diet into six lists—the starch/bread, meat/meat alternate, vegetable, fruit, milk, and fat lists.[1] These lists are shown in Tables C–1 through C–6. Following these lists are three other sets of foods: free foods, combination foods, and foods for occasional use (Tables C–7, C–8, and C–9).

Table C-1
The U.S. Exchange System: Starch/Bread List

15 g carbohydrate, 3 g protein, trace fat, 80 kcal

Amount	Food
Cereals/Grains/Pasta	
1/3 c	Bran cereals, concentrated
1/2 c	Bran cereals, flaked
1/2 c	Bulgur, cooked
1/2 c	Cooked cereals
2 1/2 tbs	Cornmeal, dry
3 tbs	Grapenuts
1/2 c	Grits, cooked
3/4 c	Other ready-to-eat unsweetened cereals
1/2 c	Pasta, cooked
1 1/2 c	Puffed cereals
1/3 c	Rice, white or brown, cooked
1/2 c	Shredded wheat
3 tbs	Wheat germ
Dried Beans/Peas/Lentils	
1/4 c	Baked beans
1/3 c	Beans and peas, cooked, such as kidney, white, split, black-eyed
1/3 c	Lentils, cooked
Starchy Vegetables	
1/2 c	Corn
1 cob	Corn on the cob, 6" long
1/2 c	Lima beans
1/2 c	Peas, green, canned or frozen
1/2 c	Plantains
1 small (3 oz)	Potatoes, baked
1/2 c	Potatoes, mashed
3/4 c	Squash, winter (acorn, butternut)
1/3 c	Yams, sweet potatoes, plain
Bread	
1/2 (1 oz)	Bagels
2 (2/3 oz)	Bread sticks, crisp, 4" × 1/2"
1 c	Croutons, low-fat
1/2	English muffins
1/2 (1 oz)	Frankfurter or hamburger buns
1/2 loaf	Pita, 6" across
1 (1 oz)	Plain rolls, small
1 slice (1 oz)	Raisin, unfrosted
1 slice (1 oz)	Rye, pumpernickel
1	Tortillas, 6" across
1 slice (1 oz)	White (including French, Italian)
1 slice (1 oz)	Whole-wheat
Crackers/Snacks	
8	Animal crackers
3	Graham crackers, 2 1/2" square
3/4 oz	Matzoth
5 slices	Melba toast
24	Oyster crackers
3 c	Popcorn, popped, no fat added
3/4 oz	Pretzels
4	Rye crisp, 2" × 3 1/2"
6	Saltine-type crackers
2 to 4 (3/4 oz)	Whole-wheat crackers, no fat added (crisp breads)
Starch Foods Prepared with Fat (Count as 1 starch/bread serving, plus 1 fat serving.)	
1	Biscuits, 2 1/2" across
1/2 c	Chow mein noodles
1 (2 oz)	Cornbread, 2" cube
6	Crackers, round butter type
10 (1 1/2 oz)	French fries, 2" to 3 1/2" long
1	Muffins, plain, small
2	Pancakes, 4" across
1/4 c	Stuffing, bread, prepared
2	Taco shells, 6" across
1	Waffles, 4 1/2" square
4 to 6 (1 oz)	Whole-wheat crackers, fat added

3 grams or more dietary fiber per serving. Average fiber content of whole-grain products is 2 grams per serving. For starch foods not on this list, the general rule is that 1/2 cup cereal, grain, or pasta is 1 serving: 1 ounce of a bread product is 1 serving.

C

Table C–2
U.S. Exchange System: Meat/Meat Alternate Lists

Lean meat = 7 g protein, 3 g fat, 55 kcal; medium-fat meat = 7 g protein, 5 g fat, 75 kcal; high-fat meat = 7 g protein, 8 g fat, 100 kcal.

Category	Amount	Food
Lean Meat and Alternates		
Beef	1 oz	USDA Good or Choice grades of lean beef, such as round, sirloin, and flank steak; tenderloin; chipped beef
Pork	1 oz	Lean pork, such as fresh ham; canned, cured, or boiled ham, Canadian bacon, tenderloin
Veal	1 oz	All cuts are lean except veal cutlets (ground or cubed); examples of lean veal: chops and roasts
Poultry	1 oz	Chicken, turkey, Cornish hen (without skin)
Fish	1 oz	All fresh and frozen fish
	2 oz	Crab, lobster, scallops, shrimp, clams (fresh or canned in water)
	6 medium	Oysters
	1/4 c	Tuna, canned in water
	1 oz	Herring, uncreamed or smoked
	2 medium	Sardines, canned
Wild game	1 oz	Venison, rabbit, squirrel
	1 oz	Pheasant, duck, goose (without skin)
Cheese	1/4 c	Any cottage cheese
	2 tbs	Grated parmesan
	1 oz	Diet cheeses (with less than 55 cal/oz)
Other	1 oz	95% fat-free lunch meats
	3 whites	Egg whites
	1/4 c	Egg substitutes with less than 55 cal per 1/4 c
Medium-Fat Meat and Alternates		
Beef	1 oz	Most beef products fall into this category; examples: all ground beef, roasts (rib, chuck, rump), steak (cubed, porterhouse, T-bone), meatloaf
Pork	1 oz	Most pork products fall into this category; examples: chops, loin roast, Boston butt, cutlets
Lamb	1 oz	Most lamb products fall into this category; examples: chops, leg, roast
Veal	1 oz	Cutlet, ground or cubed, unbreaded
Poultry	1 oz	Chicken (with skin), domestic duck or goose (well drained of fat), ground turkey
Fish	1/4 c	Tuna, canned in oil and drained
	1/4 c	Salmon, canned
Cheese		Skim or part-skim milk cheeses, such as:
	1/4 c	Ricotta
	1 oz	Mozzarella
	1 oz	Diet cheeses (with 56 to 80 kcal/oz)
Other	1 oz	86% fat-free lunch meat
	1	Eggs (high in cholesterol, limit to 3 per week)
	1/4 c	Egg substitutes with 56 to 80 kcal per 1/4 c
	4 oz	Tofu, 2 1/2" × 2 3/4" × 1"
	1 oz	Liver, hearts, kidneys, sweetbreads (high in cholesterol)

400 milligrams or more sodium per exchange. Meats contribute no fiber to the diet.

(continued)

Table C-2 (*continued*)

Lean meat = 7 g protein, 3 g fat, 55 kcal; medium-fat meat = 7 g protein, 5 g fat, 75 kcal; high-fat meat = 7 g protein, 8 g fat, 100 kcal.

Category	Amount	Food
High-Fat Meat and Alternates[a]		
Beef	1 oz	Most USDA Prime cuts of beef, such as ribs, corned beef 🧂
Pork	1 oz	Spareribs, ground pork, pork sausages 🧂 (patties or links)
Lamb	1 oz	Patties, ground lamb
Fish	1 oz	Any fried fish product
Cheese	1 oz	All regular cheeses 🧂, such as American, blue, Cheddar, Monterey, Swiss
Other	1 oz	Lunch meats 🧂 such as bologna, salami, pimento loaf
	1 oz	Sausage 🧂 such as Polish, Italian
	1 oz	Knockwurst, smoked
	1 oz	Bratwurst 🧂
	1 (10/lb)	Frankfurters 🧂 (turkey or chicken)
	1 tbs	Peanut butter (contains unsaturated fat)
Count as 1 high-fat meat plus 1 fat exchange:		
1 frank	(10/lb)	Frankfurters 🧂 (beef, pork, or combination)

🧂 400 milligrams or more sodium per exchange. Meats contribute no fiber to the diet.

[a]These items are high in saturated fat, cholesterol, and kcalories and should be used no more than three times per week.

Table C-3
U.S. Exchange System: Vegetable List

5 g carbohydrate, 2 g protein, 25 kcal
All portion sizes, except as otherwise noted, are 1/2 c of any cooked vegetable or vegetable juice, 1 c of any raw vegetable.

Artichokes, 1/2 medium	Mushrooms, cooked
Asparagus	Okra
Bean sprouts	Onions
Beans (green, wax, Italian)	Pea pods
Beets	Rutabagas
Broccoli	Sauerkraut 🧂
Brussels sprouts	Spinach, cooked
Cabbage, cooked	Summer squash (crookneck)
Carrots	Tomatoes, 1 large
Cauliflower	Tomato/vegetable juice 🧂
Eggplant	Turnips
Green peppers	Water chestnuts
Greens (collard, mustard, turnip)	Zucchini, cooked
Kohlrabi	
Leeks	

Starchy vegetables such as corn, peas, and potatoes are found on the Starch/Bread List.
For free vegetables, see the Free Food List (Table C-7).

🧂 400 milligrams or more sodium per serving. Most vegetable servings contain 2 to 3 grams dietary fiber.

Table C-4
U.S. Exchange System: Fruit List

15 g carbohydrate, 60 kcal
All portion sizes, unless otherwise noted, are 1/2 c fresh fruit or fruit juice, 1/4 c dried fruit.

Amount	Food
Fresh, Frozen, and Unsweetened Canned Fruit	
1	Apples, raw, 2" across
1/2 c	Applesauce, unsweetened
4	Apricots, medium, raw
1/2 c (4 halves)	Apricots, canned
1/2	Bananas, 9" long
3/4 c	Blackberries, raw *
3/4 c	Blueberries, raw *
1/3	Cantaloupe, 5" across
1 c	Cantaloupe, cubes
12	Cherries, large, raw
1/2 c	Cherries, canned
2	Figs, raw, 2" across
1/2 c	Fruit cocktail, canned
1/2	Grapefruit, medium
3/4 c	Grapefruit, segments
15	Grapes, small
1/8	Honeydew melon, medium
1 c	Honeydew melon, cubes
1	Kiwis, large
3/4 c	Mandarin oranges
1/2	Mangoes, small
1	Nectarines, 1 1/2" across *
1	Oranges, 2 1/2" across
1 c	Papayas
1 (3/4 c)	Peaches, 2 3/4" across
1/2 c (2 halves)	Peaches, canned
1/2 large or 1 small	Pears
1/2 c (2 halves)	Pears, canned
2	Persimmons, medium, native
3/4 c	Pineapple, raw
1/3 c	Pineapple, canned
2	Plums, raw, 2" across
1/2	Pomegranates *
1 c	Raspberries, raw *
1 1/4 c	Strawberries, raw, whole *
2	Tangerines, 2 1/2" across
1 1/4 c	Watermelon, cubes

Amount	Food
Dried Fruit	
4 rings	Apples *
7 halves	Apricots *
2 1/2 medium	Dates
1 1/2	Figs *
3 medium	Prunes *
2 tbs	Raisins
Fruit Juice	
1/2 c	Apple juice/cider
1/3 c	Cranberry juice cocktail
1/3 c	Grape juice
1/2 c	Grapefruit juice
1/2 c	Orange juice
1/2 c	Pineapple juice
1/3 c	Prune juice

* 3 grams or more dietary fiber per serving. Average fiber contents of fresh, frozen, and dry fruits: 2 grams per serving.

Table C-5
U.S. Exchange System: Milk List

Nonfat and very low-fat milk = 12 g carbohydrate, 8 g protein, trace fat, 90 kcal; low-fat milk = 12 g carbohydrate, 8 g protein, 5 g fat, 120 kcal; whole milk = 12 g carbohydrate, 8 g protein, 8 g fat, 150 kcal.

Amount	Food
Nonfat and Very Low-Fat Milk	
1 c	Nonfat milk
1 c	1/2% milk
1 c	1% milk
1/3 c	Dry nonfat milk
1/2 c	Evaporated nonfat milk
1 c	Low-fat buttermilk
8 oz	Plain nonfat yogurt
Low-Fat Milk	
1 c fluid	2% milk
8 oz	Plain low-fat yogurt, with added nonfat milk solids
Whole Milk	
1 c	Whole milk
1/2 c	Evaporated whole milk
8 oz	Whole plain yogurt

Table C-6
U.S. Exchange System: Fat List

5 g fat, 45 kcal

Amount	Food
Unsaturated Fats	
1/8 medium	Avocados
1 tsp	Margarine
1 tbs	Margarine, diet[a]
1 tsp	Mayonnaise
1 tbs	Mayonnaise, reduced calorie[a]
	Nuts and seeds:
6 whole	Almonds, dry roasted
1 tbs	Cashews, dry roasted
20 small or 10 large	Peanuts
2 whole	Pecans
2 tsp	Pumpkin seeds
1 tbs	Other nuts
1 tbs	Seeds, pine nuts, sunflower seeds (without shells)
2 whole	Walnuts
1 tsp	Oil (corn, cottonseed, safflower, soybean, sunflower, olive, peanut)
10 small or 5 large	Olives[a]
1 tbs	Salad dressing, all varieties[a]
2 tsp	Salad dressing, mayonnaise type
1 tbs	Salad dressing, mayonnaise type, reduced calorie
2 tbs	Salad dressing, reduced calorie (salt shaker symbol)
Saturated Fats	
1 slice	Bacon[a]
1 tsp	Butter
1/2 oz	Chitterlings
2 tbs	Coconut, shredded
2 tbs	Coffee whitener, liquid
4 tsp	Coffee whitener, powder
1 tbs	Cream (heavy, whipping)
2 tbs	Cream (light, coffee, table)
2 tbs	Cream (sour)
1 tbs	Cream cheese
1/4 oz	Salt pork[a]

Two tablespoons of low-kcalorie salad dressing is a free food.

[a]If more than one or two servings are eaten, these foods provide 400 milligrams or more sodium.

(salt shaker symbol) 400 milligrams or more sodium per serving.

C

Table C-7
U.S. Exchange System: Free Foods

A free food is any food or drink that contains less than 20 kcal/serving. People with diabetes are advised to eat as much as they want of those items that have no serving size specified. They may eat two or three servings per day of those items that have a specific serving size. It is suggested that they spread the servings out through the day.

Amount	Food
Drinks	Bouillon, low-sodium
	Bouillon or broth without fat
	Carbonated drinks, sugar-free
	Carbonated water
	Club soda
1 tbs	Cocoa powder, unsweetened
	Coffee/tea
	Drink mixes, sugar-free
	Tonic water, sugar-free
Nonstick Pan Spray	
Fruit	
1/2 c	Cranberries, unsweetened
1/2 c	Rhubarb, unsweetened
Vegetables (raw, 1 c)	Cabbage
	Celery
	Chinese cabbage
	Cucumbers
	Green onions
	Hot peppers
	Mushrooms
	Radishes
	Zucchini
Salad Greens	Endive
	Escarole
	Lettuce
	Romaine
	Spinach
Sweet Substitutes	Candy, hard, sugar-free
	Gelatin, sugar-free
	Gum, sugar-free
2 tsp	Jam/jelly, sugar-free
1 to 2 tbs	Pancake syrup, sugar-free
	Sugar substitutes (saccharin, aspartame, acesulfame-K)
2 tbs	Whipped topping

Amount	Food
Condiments	
1 tbs	Catsup
	Horseradish
	Mustard
	Pickles, dill, unsweetened
2 tbs	Salad dressing, low-calorie
1 tbs	Taco sauce
	Vinegar
Seasonings	Basil, fresh
	Celery seeds
	Chili powder
	Chives
	Cinnamon
	Curry
	Dill
	Flavoring extracts (almond, butter, lemon, peppermint, vanilla, walnut, etc.)
	Garlic
	Garlic powder
	Herbs
	Hot pepper sauce
	Lemon
	Lemon juice
	Lemon pepper
	Lime
	Lime juice
	Mint
	Onion powder
	Oregano
	Paprika
	Pepper
	Pimento
	Soy sauce
	Soy sauce, low-sodium ("lite")
	Spices
1/4 c	Wine, used in cooking
	Worcestershire sauce

3 grams or more dietary fiber per serving.

400 milligrams or more sodium per serving.

Table C-8
U.S. Exchange System: Combination Foods

Much of the food we eat is mixed together in various combinations. These combination foods do not fit into only one exchange list. It can be quite hard to tell what is in a certain casserole dish or baked food item. This is a list of average values for some typical combination foods. This list will help you fit these foods into your meal plan. Ask your dietitian for information about any other foods you'd like to eat. The *American Diabetes Association/American Dietetic Association Family Cookbooks* and the *American Diabetes Associates Holiday Cookbook* have many recipes and further information about many foods, including combination foods. Check your library or local bookstore.

Food	Amount	Exchanges
Casseroles, homemade	1 c (8 oz)	2 starch, 2 medium-fat meat, 1 fat
Cheese pizza, thin crust	1/4 of 15 oz or 1/4 of 10"	2 starch, 1 medium-fat meat, 1 fat
Chili with beans, commercial	1 c (8 oz)	2 starch, 2 medium-fat meat, 2 fat
Chow mein, without noodles or rice	2 c (16 oz)	1 starch, 2 vegetable, 2 lean meat
Macaroni and cheese	1 c (8 oz)	2 starch, 1 medium-fat meat, 2 fat
Soups:		
Bean	1 c (8 oz)	1 starch, 1 vegetable, 1 lean meat
Chunky, all varieties	10 3/4-oz can	1 starch, 1 vegetable, 1 medium-fat meat
Cream, made with water	1 c (8 oz)	1 starch, 1 fat
Vegetable or broth	1 c (8 oz)	1 starch
Spaghetti and meatballs, canned	1 c (8 oz)	2 starch, 1 medium-fat meat, 1 fat
Sugar-free pudding, made with nonfat milk	1/2 c	1 starch
If beans are used as a meat substitute:		
Dried beans, peas, lentils	1 c (cooked)	2 starch, 1 lean meat

400 milligrams or more sodium per serving.

3 grams or more dietary fiber per serving

Table C-9
U.S. Exchange System: Foods for Occasional Use

The following list includes average exchange values for some foods high in sugar and fat. People are advised to use them only occasionally and in moderate amounts.

Food	Amount	Exchanges
Angel food cake	1/12 cake	2 starch
Cake, no icing	1/12 cake or a 3" square	2 starch, 2 fat
Cookies	2 small, 1 3/4" across	1 starch, 1 fat
Frozen fruit yogurt	1/3 c	1 starch
Gingersnaps	3	1 starch
Granola	1/4 c	1 starch, 1 fat
Granola bars	1 small	1 starch, 1 fat
Ice cream, any flavor	1/2 c	1 starch, 2 fat
Ice milk, any flavor	1/2 c	1 starch, 1 fat
Sherbet, any flavor	1/4 c	1 starch
Snack chips, all varieties	1 oz	1 starch, 2 fat
Vanilla wafers	6 small	1 starch, 1 fat

If more than one serving is eaten, these foods have 400 milligrams or more sodium.

THE CANADIAN EXCHANGE SYSTEM

The *Good Health Eating Guide* is the Canadian exchange system of meal planning.[2] It contains several features similar to those of the U.S. exchange system including the following:

- Foods are divided into six groups according to carbohydrate, protein, and fat content.
- Foods are interchangeable within a group.
- Most foods are eaten in measured amounts.
- An energy value is given for each food group.

Tables C–10 through C–16 present the Canadian exchange system.

CANADA'S GUIDELINES FOR HEALTHY EATING

Canada's Guidelines for Healthy Eating were developed by the Communications/Implementation Committee as the key messages to be communicated to healthy Canadians over two years of age.[3] The guidelines encourage people to:

- Enjoy a variety of foods.
- Emphasize cereals, breads, other grain products, vegetables, and fruits.
- Choose lower-fat dairy products, leaner meats, and foods prepared with little or no fat.
- Achieve and maintain a healthy body weight by enjoying regular physical activity and healthy eating.
- Limit salt, alcohol, and caffeine.

Table C–10
Canadian Exchange System: Protein Foods Group

7 g protein, 3 g fat, 230 kJ (55 kcal)

Food	Measure	Mass (Weight)
Cheese		
All types, made from partly skim milk (e.g., mozzarella, part-skim)	1 piece, 5 cm × 2 cm × 2 cm (2" × 3/4" × 3/4")	25 g
Cottage cheese, all types	50 mL (1/4 c)	55 g
Fish		
Anchovies (see "Extras," Table C–16)		
Canned, drained (e.g., chicken haddie, mackerel, salmon, tuna)	50 mL (1/4 c)	30 g
Cod tongues/cheeks	75 mL (1/3 c)	50 g
Fillet or steak (e.g., Boston blue, cod, flounder, haddock, halibut, perch, pickerel, pike, salmon, shad, sole, trout, whitefish)	1 piece, 6 cm × 2 cm × 2 cm (2 1/2" × 3/4" × 3/4")	30 g
Herring	1/3 fish	30 g
Octopus	50 mL (1/4 c)	40 g
Sardines	2 medium or 3 small	30 g
Seal, walrus	1 slice, 6 cm × 4 cm × 1 cm (2 1/2" × 1 1/2" × 1/2")	25 g
Smelts	2 medium	30 g
Squid	50 mL (1/4 c)	40 g
Shellfish		
Clams, mussels, oysters, scallops, snails	3 medium	30 g
Crab, lobster, flaked	50 mL (1/4 c)	30 g
Shrimp, fresh	5 large	30 g
Frozen	10 medium	30 g
Canned	18 small	30 g
Dry pack	50 mL (1/4 c)	30 g

(continued)

Table C–10 (*continued*)

7 g protein, 3 g fat, 230 kJ (55 kcal)		
Food	**Measure**	**Mass (Weight)**
Meat and Poultry (e.g., beef, chicken, ham, lamb, pork, turkey, veal, wild game)		
Back bacon	3 slices, thin	25 g
Chop	1/2 chop, with bone	35 g
Minced or ground, lean	30 mL (2 tbs)	25 g
Sliced, lean	1 slice, 10 cm × 5 cm × 5 mm (4" × 2" × 1/4")	25 g
Steak, lean	1 piece, 4 cm × 3 cm × 2 cm (1 1/2" × 1 1/4" × 3/4")	25 g
Organ Meats		
Hearts, liver	1 slice, 5 cm × 5 cm × 1 cm (2" × 2" × 1/2")	25 g
Kidneys, sweetbreads, chopped	50 mL (1/4 c)	25 g
Tongue	1 slice, 80 cm × 6 cm × 5 mm (3 1/4" × 2 1/2" × 1/4")	25 g
Tripe, 1 piece = 4 cm × 4 cm × 8 mm (1 1/2" × 1 1/2" × 3/8")	5 pieces	50 g
Soyabean		
Bean curd or tofu, 1 block = 6 cm × 6 cm × 4 cm (2 1/2" × 2 1/2" × 1 1/2")	1/2 block	70 g
Note: The following choices contain extra fat, so use them less often.		
Cheese		
Cheeses, all types made from whole milk (e.g., brick, Brie, Camembert, Cheddar, Edam, Tilsit)	1 piece, 5 cm × 2 cm × 2 cm (2" × 3/4" × 3/4")	25 g
Cheese, coarsely grated (e.g., Cheddar)	75 mL (1/3 c)	25 g
Cheese, dry, finely grated (e.g., parmesan)	45 mL (3 tbs)	15 g
Cheese, ricotta	50 mL (1/4 c)	55 g
Eggs		
In shell, raw or cooked	1 medium	50 g
Without shell, cooked or poached in water	1 medium	45 g
Scrambled	50 mL (1/4 c)	55 g
Fish		
Eel	5 cm, 4 cm diameter (2", 1 1/2" diameter)	50 g
Meat		
Bologna	1 slice, 5 mm, 10 cm diameter (1/4", 4" diameter)	40 g
Canned lunch meats	1 slice, 85 mm × 45 mm × 10 mm (3 1/2" × 1 3/4" × 1/2")	40 g
Corned beef, canned	1 slice, 75 mm × 55 mm × 5 mm (3" × 2 1/4" × 1/4")	25 g
Corned beef, fresh	1 slice, 10 cm × 5 cm × 5 mm (4" × 2" × 1/4")	25 g
Ground beef, medium-fat	30 mL (2 tbs)	25 g
Meat spreads, canned	45 mL (3 tbs)	35 g
Pâté (see "Fats and Oils Group," Table C–15)		
Sausages, garlic, Polish or knockwurst	1 slice, 1 cm, 5 cm diameter (1/2", 2" diameter)	50 g
Sausages, pork, links	1 link	25 g
Spareribs or shortribs, with bone	10 cm × 6 cm (4" × 2 1/2")	65 g
Stewing beef	1 cube, 25 mm (1")	25 g
Summer sausage or salami	1 slice, 5 mm, 10-cm diameter (1/4", 4" diameter)	40 g
Weiners	1/2 medium	25 g
Miscellaneous		
Blood pudding	1 slice, 5 cm × 1 cm (2" × 1/2")	25 g
Peanut butter, all kinds	15 mL (1 tbs)	15 g

Table C-11 (*continued*)

15 g carbohydrate [starch], 2 g protein, 290 kJ (68 kcal)

Food	Measure	Mass (Weight)
Breads		
Bagels	1/2	25 g
Bread crumbs	50 mL (1/4 c)	25 g
Bread cubes	250 mL (1 c)	25 g
Bread sticks, 11 cm × 1 cm (4 1/2" × 1/2")	2	20 g
Brewis, cooked	50 mL (1/4 c)	45 g
English muffins, crumpets	1/2	25 g
Flour	40 mL (2 1/2 tbs)	20 g
Hamburger buns	1/2	30 g
Hot dog buns	1/2	30 g
Kaiser rolls	1/2	25 g
Matzoh, 15 cm (6") square	1	20 g
Melba toast, rectangular	4	15 g
Pita, 20-cm (8") diameter	1/4	25 g
Plain rolls	1 small	25 g
Raisin	1 slice	25 g
Rusks	2	20 g
Rye, coarse or pumpernickel, 10 cm × 10 cm × 8 mm (4" × 4" × 3/8")	1/2 slice	25 g
Tortillas, 15 cm (6")	1	20 g
White (French and Italian)	1 slice	25 g
Whole-wheat, cracked wheat, rye, white enriched	1 slice	25 g
Cereals		
Bran flakes, 40% bran	125 mL (1/2 c)	20 g
Cooked cereals, cooked	125 mL (1/2 c)	125 g
Dry	30 mL (2 tbs)	20 g
Cornmeal, cooked	125 mL (1/2 c)	125 g
Dry	30 mL (2 tbs)	20 g
Ready-to-eat unsweetened cereals	125 mL (1/2 c)	20 g
Shredded wheat, bite size	125 mL (1/2 c)	20 g
Shredded wheat biscuits, rectangular or round	1	20 g
Wheat germ	75 mL (1/3 c)	30 g
Cookies and Biscuits		
See "Prepared Foods" below.		
Grains		
Barley, cooked	125 mL (1/2 c)	120 g
Dry	30 mL (2 tbs)	20 g
Bulgur, kasha, cooked, moist	125 mL (1/2 c)	70 g
Cooked, crumbly	75 mL (1/3 c)	40 g
Dry	30 mL (2 tbs)	20 g
Rice, cooked, loosely packed	125 mL (1/2 c)	105 g
Cooked, tightly packed	75 mL (1/3 c)	70 g
Tapioca, pearl and granulated, quick cooking, dry	30 mL (2 tbs)	15 g
Pastas		
Macaroni, cooked	125 mL (1/2 c)	70 g
Noodles, cooked	125 mL (1/2 c)	80 g
Spaghetti, cooked	125 mL (1/2 c)	70 g

(continued)

Table C-11 (*continued*)

15 g carbohydrate [starch], 2 g protein, 290 kJ (68 kcal)

Food	Measure	Mass (Weight)
Starchy Vegetables		
Beans and peas, dried, cooked	125 mL (1/2 c)	80 g
Breadfruit	1 slice	75 g
Corn, canned, whole kernel	125 mL (1/2 c)	85 g
Canned, creamed	75 mL (1/3 c)	60 g
Corn on the cob, 13 cm, 4 cm diameter (5", 1 1/2" diameter)	1 small cob	140 g
Cornstarch	30 mL (2 tbs)	15 g
Plantains	1/3 small	50 g
Popcorn, unbuttered, large kernel	750 mL (3 c)	20 g
Potatoes, whipped	125 mL (1/2 c)	105 g
Potatoes, whole, 13 cm, 5 cm diameter (5", 2" diameter)	1/2	95 g
Yams, sweet potatoes, 13 cm, 5 cm diameter (5", 2" diameter)	1/2	75 g
Food items found in this category contain an additional 5 g fat and consequently an extra 190 kJ (45 kcal) = 1 Fats and Oils Choice		
Prepared Foods		
Baking powder biscuits, 5 cm diameter (2" diameter)	1	30 g
Cookies, plain (e.g., digestive, oatmeal)	2	20 g
Cupcake, uniced, 5 cm diameter (2" diameter)	1 small	35 g
Doughnuts, cake type, plain, 7 cm diameter (2 3/4" diameter)	1	30 g
Muffins, plain, 6 cm diameter (2 1/2" diameter)	1 small	40 g
Pancakes, homemade using 50 mL (1/4 c) batter	1 small	50 g
Potatoes, french fried, 5 cm × 1 cm × 1 cm (2" × 1/2" × 1/2")	10	65 g
Soup, canned, prepared with equal volume of water	250 mL (1 c)	260 g
Waffles, homemade, using 50 mL (1/4 c) batter	1 small	35 g

Table C-12
Canadian Exchange System: Milk Group

Type of Milk	Carbohydrate	Protein	Fat	Energy
Nonfat	6 g	4 g	0 g	170 kJ (40 kcal)
2%	6 g	4 g	2 g	240 kJ (58 kcal)
Whole	6 g	4 g	4 g	320 kJ (76 kcal)

Food	Measure	Mass (Weight)
Buttermilk	125 mL (1/2 c)	125 g
Evaporated milk	50 mL (1/4 c)	50 g
Milk	125 mL (1/2 c)	125 g
Powdered milk, regular	30 mL (2 tbs)	15 g
Instant	50 mL (1/4 c)	15 g
Unflavoured yogurt	125 mL (1/2 c)	125 g

Table C-13
Canadian Exchange System: Fruits and Vegetables Group

10 g carbohydrate [simple sugar], 1 g protein, 190 kJ, (44 kcal)

Food	Measure	Mass (Weight)
Fruits (fresh, frozen without sugar, canned in water)		
Apples, raw	1/2 medium	75 g
Raw, without skin and core	1/2 medium	65 g
Sauce	125 mL (1/2 c)	120 g
Apricots, raw	2 medium	115 g
Canned, in water	4 halves, plus 30 mL (2 tbs) liquid	110 g
Bake-apples (cloudberries), raw	125 mL (1/2 c)	120 g
Bananas, 15 cm (6"), with peel	1/2 small	75 g
Peeled	1/2 small	50 g
Blackberries, raw	125 mL (1/2 c)	70 g
Canned, in water	125 mL (1/2 c), includes 30 mL (2 tbs) liquid	100 g
Blueberries, raw	125 mL (1/2 c)	70 g
Boysenberries, raw	125 mL (1/2 c)	70 g
Canned, in water	125 mL (1/2 c), includes 30 mL (2 tbs) liquid	100 g
Cantaloupe, wedge with rind, 13-cm (5") diameter	1/4	240 g
Cubed or diced	250 mL (1 c)	160 g
Cherries, raw, with pits	10	75 g
Raw, without pits	10	70 g
Canned, in water, with pits	75 mL (1/3 c), includes 30 mL (2 tbs) liquid	90 g
Canned, in water, without pits	75 mL (1/3 c), includes 30 mL (2 tbs) liquid	85 g
Crabapples, raw	1 small	55 g
Cranberries, raw	250 mL (1 c)	100 g
Figs, raw	1 medium	50 g
Canned, in water	3 medium, plus 30 mL (2 tbs) liquid	100 g
Foxberries, raw	250 mL (1 c)	100 g
Fruit, mixed, cut up	125 mL (1/2 c)	120 g
Fruit cocktail, canned, in water	125 mL (1/2 c), includes 30 mL (2 tbs) liquid	120 g
Gooseberries, raw	250 mL (1 c)	150 g
Canned, in water	250 mL (1 c), includes 30 mL (2 tbs) liquid	230 g
Grapefruit, raw, with rind	1/2 small	185 g
Raw, sectioned	125 mL (1/2 c)	100 g
Canned, in water	125 mL (1/2 c), includes 30 mL (2 tbs) liquid	120 g
Grapes, raw, slip skin	125 mL (1/2 c)	75 g
Raw, seedless	125 mL (1/2 c)	75 g
Canned, in water	75 mL (1/3 c), includes 30 mL (2 tbs) liquid	115 g
Guavas, raw	1/2	50 g
Honeydew melon, raw, with rind	1/10	225 g
Cubed or diced	250 mL (1 c)	170 g
Huckleberries, raw	125 mL (1/2 c)	70 g

(continued)

Table C-13 (*continued*)

10 g carbohydrate [simple sugar], 1 g protein, 190 kJ, (44 kcal)

Food	Measure	Mass (Weight)
Kiwis, raw, with skin	2	155 g
Kumquats, raw	3	60 g
Loganberries, raw	125 mL (1/2 c)	70 g
Loquats, raw	8	130 g
Lychee fruit, raw	8	120 g
Mandarin oranges, raw, with rind	1	135 g
Raw, sectioned	125 mL (1/2 c)	100 g
Canned, in water	125 mL (1/2 c), includes 30 mL (2 tbs) liquid	100 g
Mangoes, raw, without skin and seed	1/3	65 g
Diced	75 mL (1/3 c)	65 g
Nectarines	1/2 medium	75 g
Oranges, raw, with rind	1 small	130 g
Raw, sectioned	125 mL (1/2 c)	95 g
Papayas, raw, with skin and seeds	1/4 medium	150 g
Raw, without skin and seeds	1/4 medium	100 g
Cubed or diced	125 mL (1/2 c)	100 g
Peaches, raw, with seed and skin, 6 cm (2 1/2") diameter	1 large	130 g
Raw, sliced, diced	125 mL (1/2 c)	100 g
Canned in water, halves or slices	125 mL (1/2 c), includes 30 mL (2 tbs) liquid	120 g
Pears, raw, with skin and core	1/2	90 g
Raw, without skin and core	1/2	85 g
Canned, in water, halves	2 halves, plus 30 mL (2 tbs) liquid	90 g
Persimmons, raw, native	1	30 g
Raw, Japanese	1/4	50 g
Pineapple, raw, sliced	1 slice, 8 cm diameter, 2 cm thick (3 1/3" diameter, 3/4" thick)	75 g
Raw, diced	125 mL (1/2 c)	75 g
Canned, in juice, diced	75 mL (1/3 c), includes 15 mL (1 tbs) liquid	55 g
Canned, in juice, sliced	1 slice, plus 15 mL (1 tbs) liquid	55 g
Canned, in water, diced	125 mL (1/2 c), includes 30 mL (2 tbs) liquid	100 g
Canned, in water, sliced	2 slices, plus 15 mL (1 tbs) liquid	100 g
Plums, raw, prune type	2	60 g
Damson	6	65 g
Japanese	1	70 g
Canned, in apple juice	2, plus 30 mL (2 tbs) liquid	70 g
Canned, in water	3, plus 30 mL (2 tbs) liquid	100 g
Pomegranates, raw	1/2	140 g
Raspberries, raw, black or red	125 mL (1/2 c)	65 g
Canned, in water	125 mL (1/2 c), includes 30 mL (2 tbs) liquid	100 g
Saskatoons (see Blueberries)	250 mL (1 c)	150 g
Strawberries, raw	250 mL (1 c)	150 g
Canned, in water	250 mL (1 c), includes 30 mL (2 tbs) liquid	240 g

(continued)

C

Table C-13 (*continued*)

10 g carbohydrate [simple sugar], 1 g protein, 190 kJ, (44 kcal)

Food	Measure	Mass (Weight)
Tangelos, raw	1	205 g
Tangerines, raw	1	115 g
Raw, sectioned	125 mL (1/2 c)	100 g
Watermelon, raw, with rind	1 wedge, 125-mm triangle, 22 mm thick (5" triangle, 1" thick)	310 g
Cubed or diced	250 mL (1 c)	160 g
Dried Fruit		
Apples	5 pieces	15 g
Apricots	4 halves	15 g
Banana flakes	30 mL (2 tbs)	15 g
Currants	30 mL (2 tbs)	15 g
Dates, without pits	2	15 g
Peaches	1/2	15 g
Pears	1/2	15 g
Prunes, raw, with pits	2	15 g
Raw, without pits	2	10 g
Stewed, no liquid	2	20 g
Stewed, with liquid	2, plus 15 mL (1 tbs) liquid	35 g
Raisins	30 mL (2 tbs)	15 g
Juices (no sugar added or unsweetened)		
Apricot, grape, guava, mango, prune	50 mL (1/4 c)	55 g
Apple, carrot, papaya, pear, pineapple, pomegranate	75 mL (1/3 c)	80 g
Grapefruit, loganberry, orange, raspberry, tangelo, tangerine	125 mL (1/2 c)	130 g
Tomato, tomato-based mixed vegetables	250 mL (1 c)	255 g
Vegetables (fresh, frozen, or canned)		
Artichokes, Jerusalem, mature or late season[a]	2 small	50 g
Beets, diced or sliced	125 mL (1/2 c)	85 g
Carrots, diced	125 mL (1/2 c)	75 g
Parsnips, mashed	125 mL (1/2 c)	80 g
Peas, fresh or frozen	125 mL (1/2 c)	80 g
Canned	75 mL (1/3 c)	55 g
Pumpkin, mashed	125 mL (1/2 c)	45 g
Rutabagas, mashed	125 mL (1/2 c)	85 g
Sauerkraut	250 mL (1 c)	235 g
Snow peas	10 pods	100 g
Squash, yellow or winter, mashed	125 mL (1/2 c)	115 g
Succotash	75 mL (1/3 c)	55 g
Tomatoes, canned	250 mL (1 c)	240 g
Turnips, mashed	125 mL (1/2 c)	115 g
Vegetables, mixed	125 mL (1/2 c)	90 g
Water chestnuts	8 medium	50 g

[a]Jerusalem artichokes contain inulin, which converts to carbohydrate during storage in or out of the ground. Jerusalem artichokes in early season (autumn) are low in carbohydrate, but in late season (winter/spring) they become a fruits and vegetables choice.

Table C-14
Canadian Exchange System: Extra Vegetables Group

125 mL (1/2 c) = 3.5 g carbohydrate, 60 kJ (14 kcal).

Artichokes, globe or French
Artichokes, Jerusalem, early season[a]
Asparagus
Bamboo shoots
Bean sprouts, mung or soya
Beans, string, green, or yellow
Bitter melon (balsam pear)
Bok choy
Broccoli
Brussels sprouts
Cabbage
Cauliflower
Celery
Chard
Cucumbers
Eggplant
Endive
Fiddleheads
Greens: beet, collard, dandelion, mustard, turnip, etc.
Kale
Kohlrabi
Leeks
Lettuce
Mushrooms
Okra
Onions, green or mature
Parsley
Peppers, green or red
Radishes
Rhubarb
Shallots
Spinach
Sprouts: alfalfa, radish, etc.
Tomatoes, raw
Vegetable marrow
Watercress
Zucchini

If eaten in large amounts, the following foods must be counted as 1 fruits and vegetables choice:

Brussels sprouts, cooked, 250 mL (1 c)	155 g
Eggplant, cooked, diced, 250 mL (1 c)	200 g
Kohlrabi, cooked, diced, 250 mL (1 c)	140 g
Leeks, cooked, edible parts of 4 leeks	100 g
Okra, cooked, sliced, 250 mL (1 c)	160 g
Onion, mature, cooked, 250 mL (1 c)	210 g
Rhubarb, cooked, no sugar added, 250 mL (1 c)	244 g
Tomatoes, raw, 2 medium (6 cm, or 2 1/2", diameter) *or* 1 large (13 cm, or 5", diameter)	270 g

[a]Jerusalem artichokes contain inulin, which converts to carbohydrate during storage in or out of the ground. Jerusalem artichokes in early season (autumn) are low in carbohydrate, but in late season (winter/spring) they become a fruits and vegetables choice.

Table C–15
Canadian Exchange System: Fats and Oils Group

5 g fat, 190 kJ (45 kcal)

Food	Measure	Mass (Weight)
Avocado pears	1/8	30 g
Bacon, side, crisp	1 slice	5 g
Butter	5 mL (1 tsp)	5 g
Cheese spread	15 mL (1 tsp)	15 g
Coconut, fresh	45 mL (3 tbs)	15 g
Dried	15 mL (1 tbs)	10 g
Cream, half and half (cereal), 10%	30 mL (2 tbs)	30 g
Light (coffee), 20%	15 mL (1 tbs)	15 g
Sour, 12 to 14%	45 mL (3 tbs)	35 g
Whipping, 32 to 37%	15 mL (1 tbs)	15 g
Cream cheese	15 mL (1 tbs)	15 g
Gravy	30 mL (2 tbs)	30 g
Lard	5 mL (1 tsp)	5 g
Margarine	5 mL (1 tsp)	5 g
Nuts, shelled:		
Almonds	8	20 g
Brazil nuts	2	5 g
Cashews	5	10 g
Filberts, hazelnuts	5	10 g
Macadamia	3	5 g
Peanuts	10	10 g
Pecans	5 halves	5 g
Nuts, shelled (continued):		
Pignolias, pine nuts	25 mL (5 tsp)	10 g
Pistachios, shelled	20	10 g
In shell	20	20 g
Pumpkin and squash seeds	20 mL (4 tsp)	10 g
Seasame seeds	15 mL (1 tbs)	10 g
Sunflower seeds, shelled	15 mL (1 tbs)	10 g
In shell	45 mL (3 tbs)	15 g
Walnuts	4 halves	10 g
Oil, cooking and salad	5 mL	5 g
Olives, green	10	45 g
Ripe	7	40 g
Pâté, liverwurst, meat spreads	15 mL (1 tbs)	15 g
Salad dressing: blue, French, Italian, mayonnaise, Thousand Island	5 mL (1 tsp)	5 g
Salt pork, raw or cooked	5 mL	5 g
Sesame oil	5 mL	5 g

Table C-16
Canadian Exchange System: Extras

May be used without measuring

Beverages

Bouillon from cube, powder, or liquid
Bouillon or clear broth
Coffee, clear
Consommé
Herbal teas, unsweetened
Mineral water
Soda water, club soda
Sugar-free soft drinks
Tea, clear
Water

Condiments

Chowchow, unsweetened tomato pickles
Garlic
Gelatin, unsweetened
Ginger root
Horseradish, uncreamed
Lemon juice or lemon wedges
Lime juice or lime wedges

Condiments (continued)

Mustard
Parsley
Pickles, unsweetened dill pickles or sour cucumber pickles
Pimentos
Soya sauce
Vinegar
Worcestershire sauce

Herbs and Spices

Cinnamon, marjoram, pepper, salt, thyme, etc.

Miscellaneous

Artificial sweetener, such as cyclamate or saccharin
Baking powder, baking soda
Dulse
Flavorings and extracts (e.g., vanilla)
Rennet

2.5 g carbohydrate, 60 kJ (15 kcal), limited to amount indicated

Food	Measure	Food	Measure
Anchovies	2 fillets	Dietetic fruit spreads	5 mL (1 tsp)
Barbecue sauce	15 mL (1 tbs)	Maraschino cherries	1
Bran, natural	30 mL (2 tbs)	Nondairy coffee whitener	5 mL (1 tsp)
Brewer's yeast	5 mL (1 tsp)	Nuts, chopped pieces	5 mL (1 tsp)
Carob powder	5 mL (1 tsp)	Relishes	5 mL (1 tsp)
Catsup	5 mL (1 tsp)	Sugar substitutes, granular	5 mL (1 tsp) (3 to 4 packages)
Chili sauce	5 mL (1 tsp)	Whipped toppings	15 mL (1 tbs)
Cocoa powder	5 mL (1 tsp)	Yogurt, plain	30 mL (2 tbs)
Cranberry sauce, unsweetened	15 mL (1 tbs)		

CANADA'S FOOD GUIDE FOR HEALTHY EATING

The 1992 Canada's Food Guide to Healthy Eating gives consumers detailed information for selecting foods to meet Canada's Guidelines for Healthy Eating (1990). The Food Guide was designed to meet the nutritional needs of all Canadians four years of age and older and takes a total diet approach, rather than emphasizing a single food, meal, or day's meals and snacks.

The rainbow side of the Food Guide shows the four food groups with their revised names and pictorial examples of foods in each group. Key statements direct consumers about selecting foods generally from all the groups, and more specifically within each group. The bar side shows the number of servings recommended for each group, using a range of servings instead of a single minimum number. Other notable changes include the number of servings for some food groups and the size of servings for some foods.

Healthy Canada

Health and Welfare Canada | Santé et Bien-être social Canada

CANADA'S
Food Guide
TO HEALTHY EATING

Enjoy a variety of foods from each group every day.

Choose lower-fat foods more often.

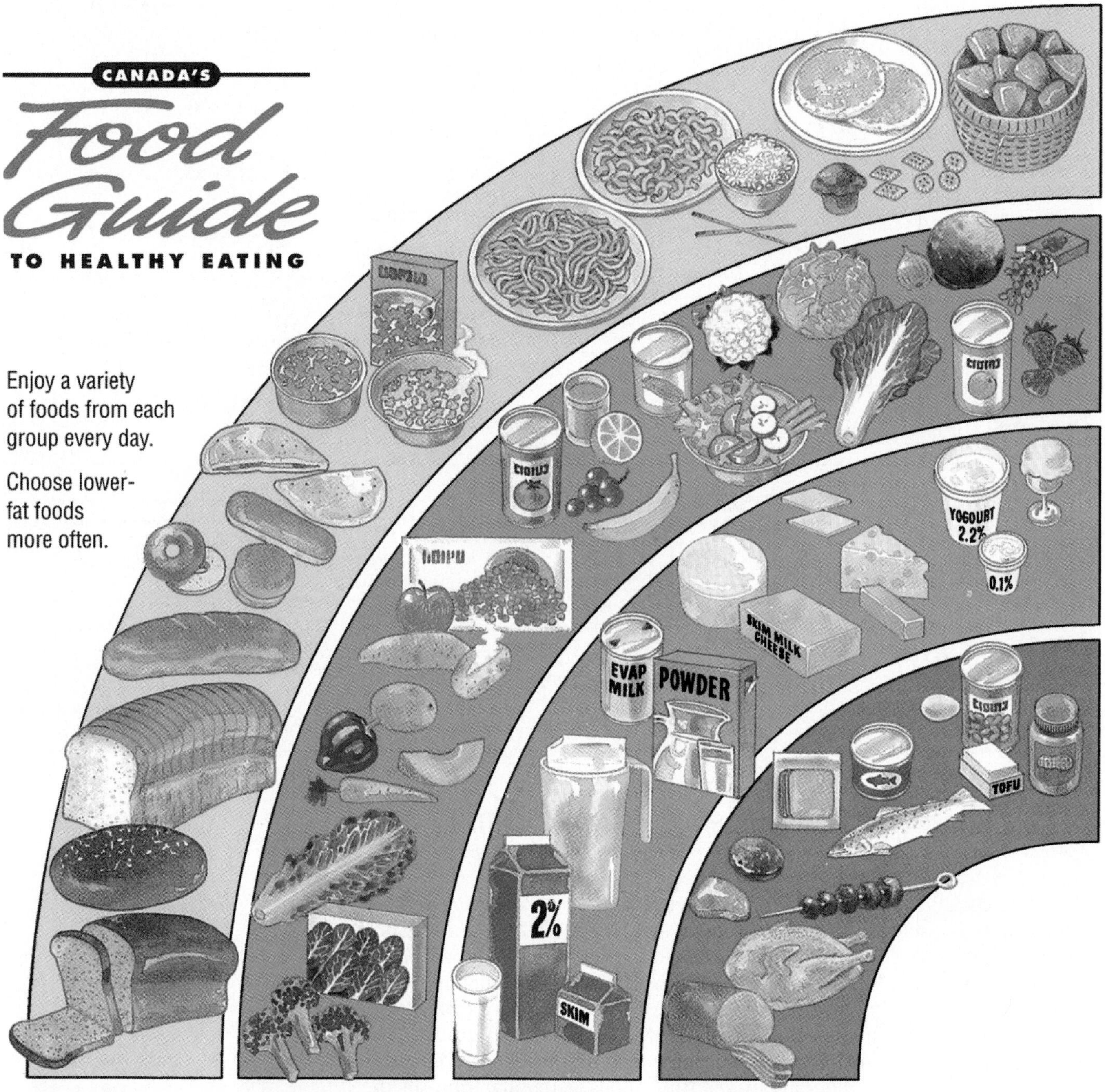

Grain Products
Choose whole grain and enriched products more often.

Vegetables & Fruit
Choose dark green and orange vegetables and orange fruit more often.

Milk Products
Choose lower-fat milk products more often.

Meat & Alternatives
Choose leaner meats, poultry and fish, as well as dried peas, beans and lentils more often.

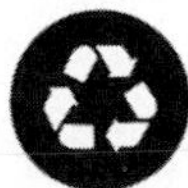

CANADA'S

Food Guide TO HEALTHY EATING

FOR PEOPLE FOUR YEARS AND OVER

Different People Need Different Amounts of Food

The amount of food you need every day from the 4 food groups and other foods depends on your age, body size, activity level, whether you are male or female and if you are pregnant or breast-feeding. That's why the Food Guide gives a lower and higher number of servings for each food group. For example, young children can choose the lower number of servings, while male teenagers can go to the higher number. Most other people can choose servings somewhere in between.

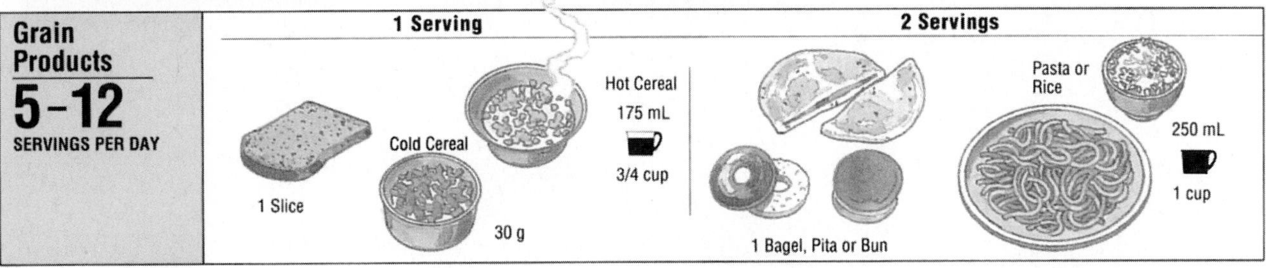

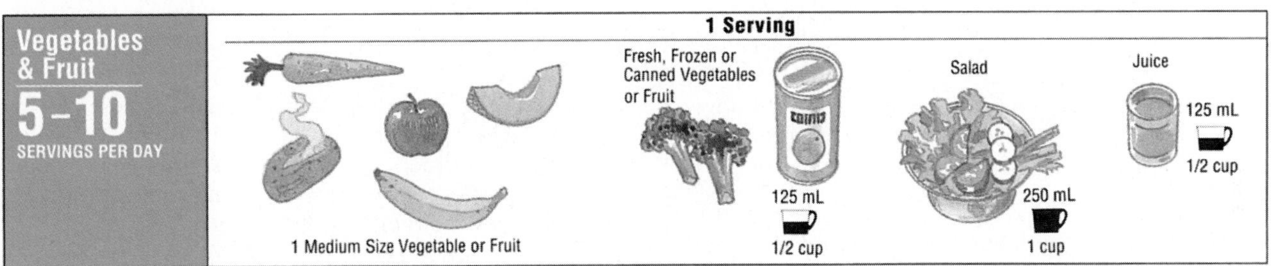

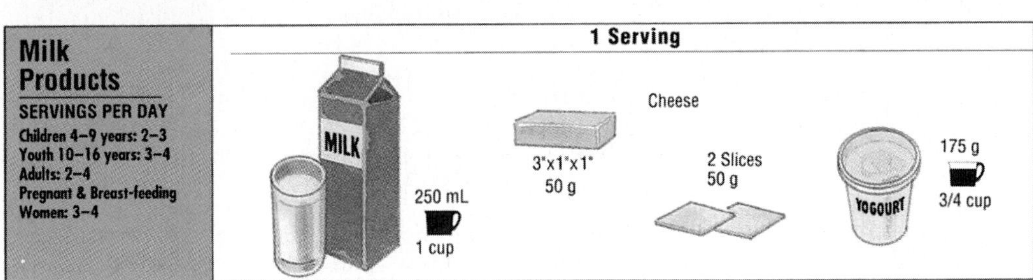

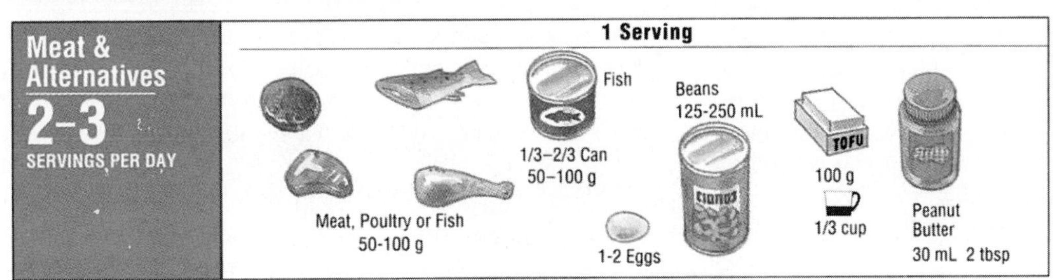

Other Foods

Taste and enjoyment can also come from other foods and beverages that are not part of the 4 food groups. Some of these foods are higher in fat or Calories, so use these foods in moderation.

Enjoy eating well, being active and feeling good about yourself. That's VITALIT*E*

ISBN 0-662-19648-1

C

APPENDIX D

NUTRITION RESOURCES

Contents

People interested in nutrition often want to know where they can find reliable nutrition information. Wherever you live, there are several sources you can turn to:

- The Department of Health may have a nutrition expert.
- The local extension agent is often an expert.
- The food editor of your local paper may be well informed.
- The dietitian at the local hospital had to fulfill a set of qualifications before he or she became an RD (see Nutrition in Practice 1).
- There may be knowledgeable professors of nutrition or biochemistry at a nearby college or university.

The syndicated column on nutrition by J. Mayer and J. Dwyer, which appears in many newspapers, presents well-researched, reliable answers to current questions. The column by R. Alfin-Slater and D. B. Jelliffe is also accurate and trustworthy. In addition, you may be interested in building a nutrition library of your own. Books you can buy, journals you can subscribe to, and addresses you can write to for general information are given below.

BOOKS

For students seeking to establish a personal library of nutrition references, the authors of this text recommend the following books:

- *Present Knowledge in Nutrition,* 6th ed. (Washington, D.C.: International Life Sciences Institute—Nutrition Foundation, 1990).

This 532-page paperback has a chapter on each of 59 topics, including energy, obesity, each of the nutrients, several diseases, malnutrition, growth and its assessment, immunity, alcohol, fiber, exercise, drugs, and toxins. Watch for an update; new editions come out every few years.

- M. E. Shils, J. A. Olson, and M. Shike, eds., *Modern Nutrition in Health and Disease,* 8th ed. (Philadelphia: Lea & Febiger, 1994).

This two-volume set is a major technical reference on nutrition topics. It contains encyclopedic articles on the nutrients, foods, the diet, metabolism, malnutrition, age-related needs, and nutrition in disease.

- Food and Nutrition Board, *Recommended Dietary Allowances,* 10th ed. (Washington, D.C.: National Academy Press, 1989).

This book reviews the function of each nutrient, dietary sources, and deficiency and toxicity symptoms as well as recommendations for intakes. The Canadian equivalent is *Nutrition Recommendations,* available by mail from the Canadian Government Publishing Centre, Supply and Services Canada, Ottawa, Ontario K1A OS9, Canada.

- Food and Nutrition Board, *Diet and Health: Implications for Reducing Chronic Disease Risk* (Washington, D.C.: National Academy Press, 1989).

This 749-page book presents the integral relationship between diet and chronic disease prevention. Its nutrient chapters provide evidence on how diet influences disease development, and its disease chapters review the dietary patterns implicated in each chronic disease.

- E. M. N. Hamilton and S. A. S. Gropper, *The Biochemistry of Human Nutrition: A Desk Reference* (St. Paul, Minn.: West, 1987).

This 324-page paperback presents the biochemical concepts necessary for an understanding of nutrition. It is a handy reference book for those who have forgotten the basics of biochemistry or for those who are learning biochemistry for the first time.

We also recommend three of our own books that explore current topics in nutrition, fitness, and the life span:

- F. S. Sizer and E. N. Whitney, *Nutrition: Concepts and Controversies,* 6th ed. (St. Paul, Minn.: West, 1994).
- L. K. DeBruyne, F. S. Sizer, and E. N. Whitney, *The Fitness Triad: Motivation, Nutrition, and Training* (St. Paul, Minn.: West, 1991).
- E. N. Whitney and S. R. Rolfes, *Understanding Nutrition,* 6th ed. (St. Paul, Minn.: West, 1993).

JOURNALS

Nutrition Today is an excellent magazine for the interested layperson. It makes a point of raising controversial issues and providing a forum for conflicting opinions. Six issues per year are published. Order from Williams and Wilkins, 428 East Preston Street, Baltimore, MD 21202.

The *Journal of the American Dietetic Association,* the official publication of the ADA, contains articles of interest to dietitians and nutritionists, news of legislative action on food and nutrition, and a very useful section of abstracts of articles from many other journals of nutrition and related areas. There are twelve issues per year, available from the American Dietetic Association (see "Addresses," next).

Nutrition Reviews, a publication of the International Life Sciences Institute, does much of the work for the library researcher, compiling recent evidence on current topics and presenting extensive bibliographies. Twelve issues per year are available from Springer-Verlag New York, 175 Fifth Avenue, New York, NY 10010.

Nutrition and the M.D. is a monthly newsletter that provides up-to-date, easy-to-read, practical information on nutrition for health care providers. It is available from PM, Inc., 7100 Hayven Hurst Avenue, Suite 107, Van Nuys, CA 91406.

Other journals that deserve mention here are *Food Technology, Journal of Nutrition, American Journal of Clinical Nutrition,* and *Journal of Nutrition Education. FDA Consumer,* a government publication with many articles of interest to the consumer, is available from the Food and Drug Administration (see "Addresses," next). Many other journals of value are referred to throughout this book.

Many of the organizations listed next will also provide publication lists free on request.

ADDRESSES

U.S. GOVERNMENT

- Federal Trade Commission (FTC)
  Public Reference Branch
  (202) 326-2222
- Food and Drug Administration (FDA)
  Office of Consumer Affairs
  HFE 881 Room 16–63
  5600 Fishers Lane
  Rockville, MD 20857
  (301) 443-3170
- FDA Office of Nutrition and Food Sciences
  200 C Street SW
  Washington, DC 20204
  (202) 205-4561
- Superintendent of Documents
  U.S. Government Printing Office
  Washington, DC 20402
- U.S. Department of Agriculture (USDA)
  14th Street SW and Independence Avenue
  Washington, DC 20250
  (202) 720-2791
- USDA Food Safety and Inspection Service
  Publications Office
  Room 1165–S
  Washington, DC 20250
- USDA Human Nutrition Information Service
  6505 Belcrest Road
  Federal Building One, Room 325–A
  Hyattsville, MD 20782
- USDA Meat and Poultry Hotline
  (800) 535-4555
- U.S. Department of Education (DOE)
  Accreditation Agency Evaluation Branch
  7th and D Street SW
  Building 3, Room 336
  Washington, DC 20202
  (202) 708-7417
- U.S. Environmental Protection Agency (EPA)
  401 M Street NW
  Washington, DC 20460
  (202) 382-3535
- U.S. EPA Safe Drinking Water Hotline
  (800) 426-4791
- U.S. Public Health Service Public Affairs Office
  Hubert H. Humphrey Building
  Room 725–H
  200 Independence Avenue SW
  Washington, DC 20201
  (202) 245-6867

CANADIAN GOVERNMENT

- Department of Community Health
  1075 Ste-Foy Road, 10th Floor
  Quebec, Quebec G1S 2M1, Canada
- Home Economics Section,
  Manitoba Agriculture
  Room 908 Norquay Building
  401 York Avenue
  Winnipeg, Manitoba R3C 0P8, Canada
- Nutrition Programs Unit, Health Promotion Directorate
  Health and Welfare Canada
  Room 448 Jeanne Mance Building
  Tunney's Pasture
  Ottawa, Ontario K1A 1B4, Canada
- Nutrition Services
  P.O. Box 5100
  Fredericton, New Brunswick E3B 5G8, Canada

INTERNATIONAL AGENCIES

- Food and Agriculture Organization of the United Nations (FAO)
  Liaison Office for North America
  1001 22nd Street NW
  Washington, DC 20437
  (202) 653-2400
- World Health Organization (WHO)
  Regional Office
  525 23rd Street NW
  Washington, DC 20037
  (202) 861-3200

CONSUMER ORGANIZATIONS

- Center for Science in the Public Interest (CSPI)
  1875 Connecticut Avenue NW, Suite 300
  Washington, DC 20009
- Choice in Dying
  200 Varick Street
  New York, NY 10014
  (212) 366-5540
- Consumer Information Center
  Department 609K
  Pueblo, CO 81009
- Consumer's Union
  101 Truman Avenue
  Yonkers, NY 10703–1057
  (914) 378-2000
- National Council Against Health Fraud, Inc.
  P.O. Box 1276
  Loma Linda, CA 92354

FOOD SAFETY

- Alliance for Food & Fiber
  Food Safety Hotline
  (800) 266-0200
- National Pesticide Telecommunications Network
  Texas Tech University
  Thompson Hall, Room S129
  Lubbock, TX 79430
  NPTN Hotline (800) 858-PEST

INFANCY AND CHILDHOOD

- Action for Children's Television
  Department A, 20 University Road
  Cambridge, MA 02138
- American Academy of Pediatrics
  P.O. Box 927
  141 Northwest Point Boulevard
  Elk Grove Village, IL 60009–0927
- Children's Foundation
  815 15th Street NW
  Washington, DC 20012

PROFESSIONAL NUTRITION ORGANIZATIONS

- American Dietetic Association
  216 West Jackson Boulevard, Suite 800
  Chicago, IL 60606–6995
  (312) 899-0040
- American Institute of Nutrition
  American Society for Clinical Nutrition
  9650 Rockville Pike
  Bethesda, MD 20814–3998
- Canadian Dietetic Association
  480 University Avenue, Suite 601
  Toronto, Ontario M5G 1V2, Canada
  (416) 596-0857
- Community Nutrition Institute
  2001 S Street NW, Suite 530
  Washington, DC 20009
  (202) 462-4700
- National Academy of Sciences/National Research Council (NAS/NRC)
  2101 Constitution Avenue NW
  Washington, DC 20418
- Nutrition Foundation, Inc. (INACG)
  1126 Sixteenth Street NW, Suite 111
  Washington, DC 20036

- Nutrition Information Service
University of Alabama at Birmingham
Room 447 Webb Building
UAB Station
Birmingham, AL 35294–3360
- Nutrition Today Society
428 East Preston Street
Baltimore, MD 21202

ALCOHOL AND DRUG ABUSE

- Al-Anon Family Group Headquarters
P.O. Box 862
Midtown Station
New York, NY 10018–0862
(800) 356-9996
- Alateen
1372 Broadway
New York, NY 10018
(800) 356-9996
- Alcohol & Drug Abuse Information Line
(800) 252-6465
- Alcoholics Anonymous (AA)
General Service Office
475 Riverside Drive
New York, NY 10115
(212) 870-3400
- Narcotics Anonymous (NA)
P.O. Box 9999
Van Nuys, CA 91409
(818) 780-3951
- National Council on Alcoholism and Drug Dependence
12 West 21st Street
New York, NY 10010
(800) NCA-CALL
- OSAP's National Clearinghouse for Alcohol and Drug Information (ONCADI)
P.O. Box 2345
Rockville, MD 20847–2345
(800) 729-6686

WEIGHT CONTROL AND EATING DISORDERS

- American Anorexia & Bulimia Association, Inc.
418 East 76th Street
New York, NY 10021
(212) 734-1114
- Anorexia Nervosa and Related Eating Disorders (ANRED)
P.O. Box 5102
Eugene, OR 97405
(503) 344-1144
- Bulimia Anorexia Self-Help Crisis Line
(800) 227-4785
(800) 762-3347
- National Association of Anorexia Nervosa and Associated Disorders, Inc. (ANAD)
P.O. Box 7
Highland Park, IL 60035
(708) 831-3438
- Overeaters Anonymous (OA)
383 Van Ness Avenue, Suite 1601
Torrace, CA 90501
- T.O.P.S. (Take Off Pounds Sensibly)
P.O. Box 07360
Milwaukee, WI 53207
- Weight Watchers
Consumer Affairs Department A
500 North Broadway
Jericho, NY 11753–2196
(800) 874-4170

FITNESS

- American College of Sports Medicine
P.O. Box 1440
Indianapolis, IN 46204
(317) 637-9200

PREGNANCY

- American College of Obstetricians and Gynecologists
Resource Center
409 12th Street SW
Washington, DC 20024–2188
- March of Dimes Birth Defects Foundation
(National Headquarters)
1275 Mamaroneck Avenue
White Plains, NY 10605

TRADE ORGANIZATIONS AND MANUFACTURERS

- Beech-Nut
Checkerboard Square, 1B
St. Louis, MO 63164
(800) 523-6633
- Borden Farm Products
Product Publicity
180 East Broad Street
Columbus, OH 43215
- Campbell Soup Company
Food Service Division
Campbell Place
Camden, NJ 08103–1799

D

- Clintec Nutrition Company
  Three Parkway North, Suite 500
  P.O. Box 760
  Deerfield, IL 60015–0760
- Elan Pharma
  Nutrition Division
  320 Charles Street
  Cambridge, MA 02141
- General Foods Consumer Center
  250 North Street
  White Plains, NY 10625
- General Mills, Inc.
  Nutrition Department
  Number One General Mills Boulevard
  Minneapolis, MN 55426
- Kellogg Company
  P.O. Box CAMB
  Battle Creek, MI 49016–1986
- McGaw, Inc.
  2525 McGaw Avenue
  Irvine, CA 92714
- Mead Johnson Enteral Nutritionals
  2400 West Lloyd Expressway
  Evansville, IN 47721
- Nabisco Consumer Affairs
  100 DeForest Avenue
  East Hanover, NJ 07936
  (800) 932-7800
  (800) NABISCO
- National Dairy Council
  O'Hare International Center
  10255 West Higgins Road, Suite 900
  Rosemond, IL 60018
- NutraSweet Simplesse Company
  P.O. Box 830
  Deerfield, IL 60015
  (800) 321-7254
- Pillsbury Company
  Consumer Relations
  P.O. Box 550
  Minneapolis, MN 55440–9843
- Procter and Gamble Company
  One Procter and Gamble Plaza
  Cincinnati, OH 45202
- Ross Laboratories
  625 Cleveland Avenue
  Columbus, OH 43216
- Sandoz Nutrition
  5320 W. 23rd Street
  P.O. Box 370
  Minneapolis, MN 55440
- Sherwood Medical
  1915 Olive Street
  St. Louis, MO 63103
- Sunkist Growers, Inc.
  Consumer Affairs Department
  P.O. Box 7888
  Van Nuys, CA 91409–7888
- United Fresh Fruit and Vegetable Association
  727 North Washington Street
  Alexandria, VA 22314
  (800) 336-3065
- USA Rice Council
  P.O. Box 740123
  Houston, TX 77274
- Vitamin Nutrition Information Service (VNIS)
  Hoffmann-LaRoche, Inc.
  340 Kingsland Street
  Nutley, NJ 07110
- Weight Watchers Food Company
  Consumer Affairs Department
  P.O. Box 10
  Boise, ID 83707–0010

WORLD HUNGER

- Bread for the World
  802 Rhode Island Avenue NE
  Washington, DC 20018
- Center on Hunger, Poverty, and Nutrition Policy
  Tufts University School of Nutrition
  11 Curtis Avenue
  Medford, MA 02155
  (617) 627-3956
- End Hunger Network
  365 Sycamore Road
  Santa Monica, CA 80402
  (310) 454-3716
- Food Research and Action Center
  1875 Connecticut Avenue NW, Suite 540
  Washington, DC 20009
  (202) 986-2200
- Freedom from Hunger
  P.O. Box 2000
  1644 DaVinci Court
  Davis, CA 95617
  (916) 758-6200
- The Hunger Project
  One Madison Avenue
  New York, NY 10010
- Institute for Food and Development Policy
  398 60th Street
  Oakland, CA 94618

♦ Interfaith Impact for Justice and Peace
110 Maryland Avenue NE
Box 63, Suite 509
Washington, DC 20002

♦ Oxfam America
115 Broadway
Boston, MA 02116

♦ Seeds
P.O. Box 6170
Waco, TX 76706
(817) 775-7745

♦ World Hunger Year
505 8th Avenue #21FL
New York, NY 10018–6582
(212) 629-8850

♦ Worldwatch Institute
1776 Massachusetts Avenue NW
Washington, DC 20036

HEALTH AND DISEASE

♦ AIDS Referral
1620 Eye Street NW
Washington, DC 20006
(202) 293-7330

♦ Alzheimer's Disease Information and Referral Service
919 North Michigan Avenue
Chicago, IL 60611
(800) 272-3900

♦ American Cancer Society
Cancer Information Center
1701 Rickenbacker Drive, Suite 5B
Sun City Center, FL 33573–5361
(800) ACS-2345

♦ American Council on Science and Health
1995 Broadway, 16th Floor
New York, NY 10023–5860

♦ American Dental Association
Division of Communications
211 East Chicago Avenue
Chicago, IL 60611–2678

♦ American Diabetes Association
1660 Duke Street
Alexandria, VA 22314
(703) 549-1500
(800) 232-3472

♦ American Heart Association
Box BHG, National Center
7320 Greenville Avenue
Dallas, TX 75231
(800) 242-8721

♦ American Institute for Cancer Research
1759 R Street NW
Washington, DC 20009

♦ American Medical Association
515 North State Street
Chicago, IL 60610
(312) 464-5000

♦ American Public Health Association
1015 Fifteenth Street NW
Washington, DC 20005

♦ American Red Cross AIDS Education Office
1730 D Street NW
Washington, DC 20006
(202) 737-8300

♦ American Red Cross National Headquarters
17th and D Streets NW
Washington, DC 20006

♦ Canadian Diabetes Association
78 Bond Street
Toronto, Canada M5B 2J8
(416) 362-4440

♦ Centers for Disease Control (CDC)
Information Hotline
(404) 332-4555

♦ Disease Prevention and Health Promotion's National Health Information Center, Office of
(800) 336-4797

♦ National AIDS Hotline (CDC)
(800) 342-AIDS (English)
(800) 344-SIDA (Spanish)
(800) 2437-TTY (Deaf)
(900) 820-2437

♦ National Cancer Institute
Office of Cancer Communications
Building 31, Room 10824
Bethesda, MD 20892
(800) 4–CANCER

♦ National Heart, Lung, and Blood Institute
National High Blood Pressure Education Program
Information Center
P.O. Box 30105
Bethesda, MD 20824–0105
(301) 951-3260

♦ National Osteoporosis Foundation
2100 M Street NW, Suite 602
Washington, DC 20037
(202) 223-2226

♦ Smoking and Health Office (CDC)
Technical Information Center
Mail Stop K-12
1600 Clifton Road NE
Atlanta, GA 30333

D

NUTRITION ASSESSMENT: SUPPLEMENTAL INFORMATION

Contents

APPENDIX E

Chapter 9 offers some ways to determine body weights appropriate for height, and Chapters 12 and 13 describe the nutrition assessment techniques health care professionals commonly use to determine clients' nutrition status. These assessments lay the groundwork for identifying clients' nutrition needs and developing care plans to meet those needs. This appendix provides additional details and alternative methods of assessing nutrition status to support a complete nutrition assessment.

DRUG HISTORY: NUTRITION AND DRUG INTERACTIONS

Chapter 12 described nutrient-drug interactions, and the chapters on diseases provided a series of "prescription pads," listing drugs used in the treatment of the specific diseases being discussed. Table E–1 (A and B) presents information on how the drugs are administered with respect to timing of food intake and on common side effects that may influence nutrition status.

E

Table E-1A
Alphabetical Listing of Selected Drugs and Their Classifications

The left column of this table lists drugs alphabetically. The right column indicates the class to which each drug belongs. To find out how to administer a drug and to learn of its nutrition-related side effects, look it up under its class in Table E-1B.

Drug Name	Drug Classification in Table E-1B
Acebutolol	Antihypertensive Agents
Acetaminophen	Analgesic Agents
Acetylsalicylic acid	Analgesic Agents
Acyclovir	Anti-Infective Agents
Adrenocorticosteroids	Antineoplastic Agents
Aluminum hydroxide	Phosphate Binders
Amiloride HCl	Diuretics
Amoxicillin	Anti-Infective Agents
Amphetamine sulfate	Miscellaneous
Amphotericin B	Anti-Infective Agents
Ampicillin	Anti-Infective Agents
Asparaginase	Antineoplastic Agents
Astemizole	Miscellaneous
Atenolol	Antihypertensive Agents
Azathioprine	Immunosuppressive Agents
Azidothymidine (AZT)	Anti-Infective Agents
Belladonna	Antidiarrheal Agents
Bisacodyl	Laxatives
Bleomycin	Antineoplastic Agents
Buspirone HCl	Antianxiety Agents
Busulfan	Antineoplastic Agents
Calcium acetate	Phosphate Binders
Calcium carbonate	Phosphate Binders
Calcitriol	Miscellaneous
Captopril	Antihypertensive Agents
Carmustine	Antineoplastic Agents
Castor oil	Laxatives
Chloramphenicol	Anti-Infective Agents
Chlorothiazide	Diuretics
Chlorpromazine HCl	Antipsychotic Agents
Chlorpropamide	Antidiabetic Agents
Chlorthalidone	Diuretics
Cholestyramine	Antilipemic Agents
Cimetidine	Antiulcer Agents
Cisplatin	Antineoplastic Agents
Clofibrate	Antilipemic Agents
Clonidine HCl	Antihypertensive Agents
Clotrimazole	Anti-Infective Agents
Colchicine	Miscellaneous
Colestipol	Antilipemic Agents
Cyclophosphamide	Antineoplastic Agents
Cyclosporine	Immunosuppressive Agents
Dactinomycin	Antineoplastic Agents
Deserpidine/methyclothiazide	Antihypertensive Agents
Dicumarol	Anticoagulants
Digitalis	Antihypertensive Agents
Digitoxin	Antihypertensive Agents
Digoxin	Antihypertensive Agents
Dihydroxyaluminum sodium carbonate	Antacids

Table E-1A (*continued*)

Drug Name	Drug Classification in Table E-1B
Diphenoxylate HCl	Antidiarrheal Agents
Doxepin HCl	Antidepressant Agents—Other
Doxorubicin	Antineoplastic Agents
Enalapril maleate	Antihypertensive Agents
Erythromycin	Anti-Infective Agents
Erythropoietin	Miscellaneous
Estrogen	Antineoplastic Agents
Ethambutol HCl	Anti-Infective Agents
Famotidine	Antiulcer Agents
Fluconazole	Anti-Infective Agents
Fluorouracil	Antineoplastic Agents
Ganciclovir	Anti-Infective Agents
Gemfibrozil	Antilipemic Agents
Glipizide	Antidiabetic Agents
Glyburide	Antidiabetic Agents
Guanethidine sulfate	Antihypertensive Agents
Guanfacine HCl	Antihypertensive Agents
Hydralazine HCl	Antihypertensive Agents
Hydrochlorothiazide	Diuretics
Hydroxyurea	Antineoplastic Agents
Ibuprofen	Analgesic Agents
Indapamide	Diuretics
Isocarboxide	Antidepressant Agents—MAO Inhibitors
Isoniazid (INH)	Anti-Infective Agents
Kaolin	Antidiarrheal Agents
Ketoconazole	Anti-Infective Agents
Labetalol HCl	Antihypertensive Agents
Lactulose	Laxatives
Levodopa	Miscellaneous
Lisinopril	Antihypertensive Agents
Lithium carbonate	Miscellaneous
Loperamide	Antidiarrheal Agents
Lovastatin	Antilipemic Agents
Loxapine HCl	Antipsychotic Agents
Magaldrate	Antacids
Magnesium hydroxide	Antacids
Meprobamate	Antianxiety Agents
Mercaptopurine	Antineoplastic Agents
Methotrexate	Antineoplastic Agents
Methyldopa	Antihypertensive Agents
Metoprolol tartrate	Antihypertensive Agents
Metronidazole	Anti-Infective Agents
Mineral oil	Laxatives
Minoxidil	Antihypertensive Agents
Mithramycin	Antineoplastic Agents
Nadolol	Antihypertensive Agents
Neomycin	Anti-Infective Agents
Nicotinic acid	Antilipemic Agents
Nifedipine	Antihypertensive Agents

(continued)

E

E

Table E-1A (*continued*)

Drug Name	Drug Classification in Table E-1B
Nystatin	Anti-Infective Agents
Omeprazole	Antilipemic Agents
Opium	Antidiarrheal Agents
Oral contraceptives	Miscellaneous; see also estrogen
Paregoric	Antidiarrheal Agents
Pectin	Antidiarrheal Agents
Penicillin	Anti-Infective Agents
Pentamidine isethionate	Anti-Infective Agents
Perphenazine	Antipsychotic Agents
Phenelzine sulfate	Antidepressant Agents—MAO Inhibitors
Phenytoin	Anticonvulsants
Pindolol	Antihypertensive Agents
Pravastatin	Antiulcer Agents
Prazosin HCl	Antihypertensive Agents
Prednisone	Immunosuppressive Agents
Probucol	Antilipemic Agents
Procarbazine	Antineoplastic Agents
Propranolol HCl	Antihypertensive Agents
Pyrimethamine	Anti-Infective Agents
Ranitidine	Antiulcer Agents
Rauwolfia serpentina	Antihypertensive Agents
Rifampin	Anti-Infective Agents
Simvastatin	Antilipemic Agents
Sodium bicarbonate	Antacids
Spironolactone	Diuretics
Sucralfate	Antiulcer Agents
Sulfadiazine	Anti-Infective Agents
Sulfasalazine	Anti-Infective Agents
Terazosin HCl	Antihypertensive Agents
Tetracycline	Anti-Infective Agents
Thioridazine HCl	Antipsychotic Agents
Timolol maleate	Antihypertensive Agents
Tolazamide	Antidiabetic Agents
Tolbutamide	Antidiabetic Agents
Tranylcypromine sulfate	Antidepressant Agents—MAO Inhibitors
Trazodone HCl	Antidepressant Agents—Other
Triamterene	Diuretics
Trimethoprim	Anti-Infective Agents
Valproic acid	Anticonvulsants
Vinblastine	Antineoplastic Agents
Vincristine	Antineoplastic Agents
Warfarin	Anticoagulants

Note: The drug classifications shown here have been adapted for use in this text and are not always the formal drug classification. For example, lithium carbonate, listed here as "Miscellaneous," is formally a "Miscellaneous Psychotherapeutic Agent." Also, many drugs actually have more than one classification. For example, corticosteroid hormones can be classified as both "Immunosuppressive Agents" and "Antineoplastic Agents." Only one classification is shown in this table for each drug.

Table E–1B
Administration and Common Nutrition-Related Side Effects of Selected Drugs

Drug Classification and Name	Administration	Common Side Effects That May Influence Nutrition Status
Analgesic Agents		
Acetaminophen	Give with food to reduce GI distress.	Side effects rarely occur.
Acetylsalicylic acid	Give with water, or with food to reduce GI distress.	Stomach upset, vomiting, nausea, GI bleeding, irritation of ulcers. May induce iron deficiency by causing GI bleeding. May enhance effects of anticlotting and antidiabetic medicine. Severe allergic reaction in some people.
Ibuprofen	Give on empty stomach, or with food to reduce GI distress.	Nausea, stomach pain, heartburn, anorexia, dry mouth, diarrhea, vomiting, indigestion, constipation, abdominal cramps or pain, bloating, gas. May induce iron deficiency by causing GI bleeding.
Antacids		
Dihydroxyaluminum sodium carbonate	Give 1 to 3 hr after meals.	Constipation, diarrhea, anorexia, weight loss.
Magaldrate	Give on empty stomach.	Chalky taste. May decrease absorption of fat-soluble vitamins, especially vitamin A.
Magnesium hydroxide	Give 1 hr after meals.	Constipation. May decrease absorption of vitamin A, phosphorus, and calcium; inactivates thiamin.
Sodium bicarbonate	Give 1 to 3 hr after meals.	Belching, gas, bloating, weight gain. Decreases iron absorption.
Antianxiety Agents		
Buspirone HCl	Give with food.	Nausea, vomiting, diarrhea, dry mouth.
Meprobamate	Give with food to reduce GI distress.	Anorexia, nausea, vomiting.
Anticoagulant Agents		
Dicumarol	Avoid excessive amounts of foods containing vitamin K.	Anorexia, nausea, vomiting, diarrhea, abdominal pain, mouth ulcers.
Warfarin	Avoid excessive amounts of foods containing vitamin K.	Nausea, vomiting, diarrhea, abdominal pain.
Anticonvulsants		
Phenytoin	Give with food to reduce GI distress. Tube feedings may reduce drug absorption and should be stopped for 2 hr before and after giving the drug, if possible.	Nausea, vomiting, swollen gums. May cause folate and vitamin B_{12} deficiencies.
Valproic acid	Give with food to reduce GI distress. Do not mix liquid form with carbonated beverages.	Anorexia, nausea, vomiting, abdominal pain.

(continued)

E

Table E-1B (*continued*)

Drug Classification and Name	Administration	Common Side Effects That May Influence Nutrition Status
Antidepressant Agents—MAO Inhibitors		
Isocarboxide	Avoid foods containing tyramine and tryptophan. Avoid alcohol and caffeine.	Anorexia, constipation.
Phenelzine sulfate	Avoid foods containing tyramine and tryptophan. Avoid alcohol and caffeine.	Anorexia, constipation.
Tranylcypromine sulfate	Avoid foods containing tyramine and tryptophan. Avoid alcohol and caffeine.	Anorexia.
Antidepressant Agents—Other		
Doxepin HCl	Dilute oral concentrate with water, milk, or juice. Do not mix with carbonated beverages. Avoid alcohol and caffeine.	Dry mouth, constipation.
Trazodone HCl	Give with food.	Nausea, dry mouth, constipation.
Antidiabetic Agents		
Chlorpropamide	Give with breakfast. Avoid alcohol.	Dyspepsia, nausea, vomiting, metallic taste, anorexia. Water intoxication, edema.
Glipizide	Give 30 min before breakfast. Limit alcohol.	GI distress, nausea, diarrhea, constipation, heartburn, altered taste perceptions.
Glyburide	Give before breakfast. Limit alcohol.	GI distress, nausea, diarrhea, constipation, heartburn.
Tolazamide	Give in morning or divided during day with meals. Limit alcohol.	Diarrhea, GI distress, nausea, vomiting, dyspepsia, heartburn, altered taste perceptions, anorexia.
Tolbutamide	(same as Tolazamide)	(same as Tolazamide)
Antidiarrheal Agents		
Diphenoxylate HCl	May give with food to reduce GI distress.	Nausea, vomiting, bloating, anorexia, dry mouth, sore or swollen gums.
Kaolin, pectin	Mix at room temperature with milk or juice.	Constipation, dry mouth, altered taste perception.
Loperamide	Give without regard to food.	Abdominal pain, constipation, bloating, dry mouth, vomiting, nausea.
Opium, belladonna, and paregoric	Give without regard to food.	Nausea, vomiting, constipation. Sedation.
Antihypertensive Agents		
Acebutolol	Give without regard to food.	Constipation, gas, abdominal pain. May mask the signs of hypoglycemia. May induce electrolyte imbalance and anemias.
Atenolol	Give without regard to food.	Dry mouth, diarrhea, nausea. May mask signs of hypoglycemia.

Table E–1B (*continued*)

Drug Classification and Name	Administration	Common Side Effects That May Influence Nutrition Status
Antihypertensive Agents (*continued*)		
Captopril	Give on empty stomach 1 hr before meals.	Altered taste perception, weight loss, sore mouth. May induce hypokalemia, anemias.
Clonidine HCl	Limit alcohol.	Dry mouth, weight gain, nausea, vomiting, constipation. May induce edema.
Deserpidine/methyclothiazide	Give with food 6 or more hr before bedtime. Avoid natural licorice.	Dry mouth, weight gain, anorexia, nausea, vomiting, diarrhea, cramps.
Digitalis, digitoxin, digoxin	Give with water 1/2 hr before or 2 hr after food. Avoid natural licorice.	May inhibit glucose absorption. Nausea, vomiting.
Enalapril maleate	Give without regard to food.	Altered taste perceptions. Diarrhea, nausea, vomiting, abdominal pain.
Guanethidine sulfate	Give at same time each day. Avoid natural licorice.	Dry mouth, weight gain, diarrhea, nausea. May induce edema.
Guanfacine HCl	Avoid alcohol.	Constipation, nausea, vomiting, stomach cramps.
Hydralazine HCl	Give with food at the same time each day. Avoid natural licorice.	Anorexia, GI distress, constipation.
Labetalol HCl	Give with food.	Altered taste perception, nausea, vomiting, indigestion. May mask signs of hypoglycemia.
Lisinopril	Give without regard to food. Limit alcohol.	Diarrhea, vomiting.
Methyldopa	Avoid natural licorice.	Dry mouth, weight gain, diarrhea, nausea. May induce edema.
Metoprolol tartrate	Give with food.	Dry mouth, diarrhea, GI pain, gas, constipation, heartburn. May mask the signs of hypoglycemia.
Minoxidil	Give at same time each day.	May induce edema.
Nadolol	Give without regard to food. Avoid natural licorice.	Dry mouth, constipation, GI distress, nausea, gas. May mask the signs of hypoglycemia.
Nifedipine	Give with food or milk.	Altered taste perception, nausea, diarrhea, constipation, cramps, gas. May induce edema.
Pindolol	Give without regard to food.	Diarrhea, vomiting. May mask the signs of hypoglycemia. May alter glucose tolerance. May induce edema.
Prazosin HCl	Limit alcohol. Avoid natural licorice.	Dry mouth, nausea, diarrhea, constipation, GI distress. May induce edema.
Propranolol HCl	Give with food. Avoid natural licorice.	Dry mouth, constipation, GI distress, nausea. May mask the signs of hypoglycemia.

(continued)

E

Table E–1B (*continued*)

Drug Classification and Name	Administration	Common Side Effects That May Influence Nutrition Status
Antihypertensive Agents (*continued*)		
Rauwolfia serpentina	Give with food or milk to reduce GI irritation.	Anorexia, weight gain, dry mouth, diarrhea, nausea, vomiting, raises GI motility and gastric secretion. May lower glucose tolerance.
Terazosin HCl	Avoid salt substitutes. Give without regard to food at the same time each day.	May alter serum glocose. Sore throat. Nausea. May induce edema.
Timolol maleate	Give with food at the same time each day.	Weight loss, nausea. May mask signs of hypoglycemia. May induce edema.
Anti-Infective Agents		
Acyclovir	Give parenterally or orally with food.	Nausea, diarrhea, vomiting, anorexia.
Amoxicillin	Give with food to reduce GI distress.	Nausea, vomiting, diarrhea; stomatitis, oral infections.
Amphotericin B	Give parenterally.	Nausea, vomiting, fever, anemia, kidney dysfunction.
Ampicillin	Give with water 1 hr before or 2 hr after meals; do not give with fruit juice, beer, wine.	Nausea, vomiting, diarrhea, steatorrhea, anemia, inflammation of the mouth and tongue; stomatitis, altered taste perceptions, hypokalemia.
Azidothymidine (AZT)	Give without regard to food.	Anorexia, nausea, vomiting, diarrhea, constipation, altered taste perceptions, mouth ulcers, edema of tongue and lips, abdominal pain, anemia.
Chloramphenicol	Give with water 1 hr before or 2 hr after meals.	Diarrhea, nausea, vomiting, irritation of mouth or tongue. May enhance effects of antidiabetic medicine. May raise requirements of riboflavin, vitamin B_6, and vitamin B_{12}.
Clotrimazole	Dissolve slowly in mouth and swallow saliva.	Nausea, vomiting.
Erythromycin	Give on empty stomach 1 hr before or 2 hr after meals; if GI distress, give with meals, not milk, fruit juice, beer, or wine.	Nausea, vomiting, cramps, abdominal pain, diarrhea, inflammation of the mouth.
Ethambutol HCl	Give with food to reduce GI distress.	Anorexia, nausea, vomiting, abdominal pain.
Fluconazole	Give orally or parenterally.	Nausea, vomiting, diarrhea, intestinal inflammation.
Ganciclovir	Give parenterally.	Anorexia, nausea, vomiting.
Isoniazid (INH)	Give 1 hr before or 2 hr after meals; may give with food to reduce GI distress.	Anorexia, nausea, vomiting, dry mouth, diarrhea, anemia, cracked lips.
Ketoconazole	Give with food to reduce GI distress.	Nausea, vomiting, abdominal pain, diarrhea, anemia. Renal and liver dysfunction.

Table E–1B (*continued*)

Drug Classification and Name	Administration	Common Side Effects That May Influence Nutrition Status
Anti-Infective Agents (*continued*)		
Metronidazole	Give with food.	Anorexia, nausea, vomiting, diarrhea, altered taste perceptions, dry mouth, constipation, stomatitis, abdominal discomfort.
Neomycin	Give without regard to food. Encourage fluids.	Nausea, vomiting, diarrhea, sore mouth. Decreases absorption of fats, nitrogen, carbohydrates, folate, vitamin B_6, vitamin B_{12}, fat-soluble vitamins, calcium, and iron.
Nystatin	Give orally as directed; retain drug in mouth as long as possible.	Diarrhea, nausea, and vomiting, GI pain (occasionally).
Penicillin	Give penicillin G on an empty stomach; penicillin K with or without meals.	Nausea, vomiting, diarrhea, gas, anemia, sore mouth, altered taste perceptions, anorexia.
Pentamidine isethionate	Give parenterally or as an inhalant.	Nausea, vomiting, taste alterations. Hypoglycemia or hyperglycemia, diabetes, kidney dysfunction.
Pyrimethamine	Give with food.	Anorexia, nausea, vomiting, diarrhea, and anemia.
Rifampin	Give with water on empty stomach.	Anorexia, nausea, vomiting, cramps, diarrhea, altered taste perceptions, abdominal distress.
Sulfadiazine	Give with full glass of water and encourage fluids.	Anorexia, nausea, vomiting, and diarrhea.
Sulfasalazine	Give with food or milk.	May cause anorexia, nausea, GI distress.
Tetracycline	Give on an empty stomach; don't give with milk or dairy products. Give iron-containing supplements 3 hr before or after use.	Anorexia, nausea, vomiting, diarrhea, altered taste perceptions, sore mouth. Decreases absorption of fat, amino acids, calcium, iron, magnesium, and zinc. Decreases bacterial synthesis of vitamin K in intestines.
Trimethoprim	Give with water on empty stomach.	Nausea, vomiting, anorexia, anemia, diarrhea, stomatitis, GI distress.
Antilipemic Agents		
Cholestyramine	Give with water or other fluids; never give dry or with carbonated beverages.	Nausea, vomiting, abdominal discomfort, gas, diarrhea, constipation, heartburn, steatorrhea, anorexia, altered taste perception. May decrease absorption of calcium, fat, vitamins A, D, K, B_{12}, folate, and glucose. Depletes iron stores.
Colestipol	(same as Cholestyramine)	(same as Cholestyramine)

(continued)

E

Table E–1B (*continued*)

Drug Classification and Name	Administration	Common Side Effects That May Influence Nutrition Status
Antilipemic Agents (*continued*)		
Clofibrate	Give with food.	Nausea, vomiting, abdominal discomfort, loose stools, gas, aftertaste, altered taste perception, increased appetite. May decrease absorption of glucose, iron, and vitamin B_{12}. May induce anemia.
Gemfibrozil	Give 1/2 hr before meals.	Nausea, vomiting, abdominal discomfort, gas, constipation. May induce anemia.
Lovastatin	Give with food.	Diarrhea, gas, constipation, abdominal pain, heartburn, nausea, indigestion, altered taste perception.
Nicotinic acid	Give with food.	Nausea, vomiting, abdominal discomfort, diarrhea. Flushing. Decreased glucose tolerance.
Pravastatin	Give without regard to food. Limit alcohol.	Nausea, vomiting, upset stomach, diarrhea.
Probucol	Give with food.	Nausea, vomiting, gas, abdominal discomfort, diarrhea, anorexia, altered taste and smell perceptions.
Simvastatin	Give without regard to food. Limit alcohol.	Upset stomach, constipation.
Antineoplastic Agents		
Adrenocorticosteroids	Give with food.	Increased appetite, GI upset. Glucose intolerance, negative nitrogen and calcium balances.
Asparaginase	Give parenterally.	Anorexia, nausea, vomiting. Pancreatitis, hepatitis, glucose intolerance.
Bleomycin	Give parenterally, intramuscularly, or subcutaneously.	Anorexia, nausea, vomiting, mouth ulcers, stomatitis, weight loss, altered taste perceptions.
Busulfan	Give with food.	Nausea, vomiting, diarrhea, cracking at corners of mouth, inflammation of the tongue, anemia, weight loss, dry mouth.
Carmustine	Give parenterally.	Anorexia, nausea, vomiting, esophagitis, diarrhea. Impaired liver function.
Cisplatin	Give parenterally.	Anorexia, nausea, vomiting, altered taste perceptions.
Cyclophosphamide	Give during or after meals.	Anorexia, nausea, vomiting, mouth ulcers, inflammation of the colon, anemia.
Dactinomycin	Give parenterally.	Anorexia, nausea, vomiting, mouth ulcers, heartburn, anemia.

Table E–1B (*continued*)

Drug Classification and Name	Administration	Common Side Effects That May Influence Nutrition Status
Antineoplastic Agents (*continued*)		
Doxorubicin	Give parenterally.	Anorexia, nausea, vomiting, diarrhea, stomach pain, sore throat, mouth ulcers, mouth blindness, esophagitis.
Estrogen	Give with food at same time each day.	Anorexia, nausea, vomiting, edema, weight changes. Alters glucose tolerance.
Fluorouracil	Give parenterally. If given orally, give with water, not acidic beverages.	Anorexia, nausea, vomiting, stomatitis, diarrhea, heartburn, sore mouth, altered taste perceptions, GI bleeding, esophagitis.
Hydroxyurea	Give with food.	Anorexia, nausea, vomiting, mouth ulcers.
Mercaptopurine	Give with food.	Anorexia, nausea, vomiting, stomatitis, stomach pain, diarrhea, anemia, vitamin B_6 depletion.
Methotrexate	Give on an empty stomach; may give with food to reduce GI distress. Do not give with milk.	Anorexia, nausea, vomiting, diarrhea, GI ulcers, GI inflammation, anemia, stomatitis, steatorrhea, mouth ulcers.
Mithramycin	Give parenterally; slow infusion reduces nausea.	Anorexia, nausea, vomiting, diarrhea, inflammation of the tongue, metallic taste.
Procarbazine	Give with food. Avoid foods containing tyramine (see Table 12–5).	Anorexia, nausea, vomiting, diarrhea, constipation, anemia, sore throat, dry mouth, difficulty swallowing.
Vinblastine	Give parenterally.	Anorexia, nausea, vomiting, diarrhea, constipation, stomatitis, sore throat, reduced bowel activity, abdominal pain, bowel inflammation.
Vincristine	Give parenterally.	Anorexia, nausea, vomiting, diarrhea, constipation, abdominal pain, mouth ulcers, anemia, thirst, weight loss, altered taste perceptions.
Antipsychotic Agents		
Chlorpromazine HCl	Give with food. Dilute liquid concentrate with milk, fruit juice, or semisolid foods.	Dry mouth, constipation.
Loxapine HCl	Give with food or water. Dilute liquid concentrate with orange or grapefruit juice.	Dry mouth, constipation.

(continued)

Table E-1B (*continued*)

Drug Classification and Name	Administration	Common Side Effects That May Influence Nutrition Status
Antipsychotic Agents (*continued*)		
Perphenazine	Give with food. Dilute liquid concentrate with milk, fruit juice, carbonated beverages, or semisolid foods; do not dilute with caffeine-containing beverages, tea, or grape or apple juice.	Dry mouth, constipation.
Thioridazine HCl	Give with food. Dilute liquid concentrate with fruit juice or water.	Dry mouth, constipation.
Antiulcer Agents		
Cimetidine	Give with meals. Limit caffeine and avoid alcohol.	Diarrhea. Reduced gastric secretion. May induce hyperglycemia.
Famotidine		Nausea, diarrhea, constipation, flatulence.
Omeprazole	Give just before meals. Do not open, chew, or crush. Take iron supplements separately.	Abdominal pain, constipation, diarrhea. Decreases absorption of iron.
Ranitidine	Give with meals. Limit caffeine and avoid alcohol.	Constipation, nausea, abdominal discomfort. (Fewer reported side effects and interactions than with cimetidine.)
Sucralfate	Give with water on empty stomach 1 hr before meals and at bedtime. Avoid or limit alcohol. Give calcium or magnesium supplements 30 minutes before or after use.	Constipation, diarrhea, nausea, cramps, dry mouth. Interferes with absoprtion of fat-soluble vitamins.
Diuretics		
Amiloride HCl with hydrochlorothiazide	Give with food at the same time each day.	Anorexia, dry mouth, appetite changes, nausea, diarrhea, GI pain, constipation.
Chlorothiazide	Give with food 6 or more hr before bedtime. Avoid natural licorice.	Nausea, vomiting, diarrhea, constipation, anorexia, dry mouth.
Chlorthalidone	Give with food 6 or more hr before bedtime. Avoid natural licorice.	Anorexia, dry mouth, GI irritation, nausea, vomiting, diarrhea, constipation.
Hydrochlorothiazide	Give with food 6 or more hr before bedtime. Avoid natural licorice.	Anorexia, dry mouth, nausea, vomiting, diarrhea, constipation. May alter insulin requirements in diabetes. May induce hypokalemia.
Indapamide	Give with food to reduce GI distress. Avoid natural licorice. Limit alcohol.	Dry mouth, weight loss, anorexia, constipation, GI distress. May alter glucose tolerance.
Spironolactone with hydrochlorothiazide	Give with food 6 or more hr before bedtime. Avoid natural licorice.	Anorexia, cramps, diarrhea, nausea, vomiting.

E

Table E-1B (*continued*)

Drug Classification and Name	Administration	Common Side Effects That May Influence Nutrition Status
Diuretics (*continued*)		
Triamterene with hydrochlorothiazide	Give with food or milk 6 or more hr before bedtime.	Dry mouth, thirst, dehydration, nausea, vomiting, diarrhea, constipation. May alter glucose levels.
Immunosuppressive Agents		
Azathioprine	Give with food.	Nausea, vomiting, diarrhea, stomach pain, anorexia, sore throat, altered taste perceptions.
Cyclosporine	Give with water, juice, or milk at the same time each day.	Raises blood pressure. Nausea, vomiting, diarrhea, inflamed gums, anorexia. May induce anemia and hyperglycemia.
Prednisone	Give with food or milk.	Fluid retention, stomach upset, peptic ulcers, blood glucose abnormalities, growth inhibition in children, decreased resistance to infection, weight gain. May decrease effects of insulin or antidiabetic medicine. May induce edema. Alters protein and carbohydrate metabolism. Decreases absorption of calcium and phosphorus.
Laxatives		
Bisacodyl	Do not give with milk or antacids.	Nausea, vomiting, abdominal cramps.
Castor oil	Give with juice or carbonated beverages to mask taste.	Nausea, abdominal cramps. May reduce absorption of fat-soluble vitamins.
Lactulose	May be mixed with fruit juice, milk, water, or citrus-flavored carbonated beverage.	Nausea, constipation, abdominal cramps.
Mineral oil	Give with juice or carbonated beverages to mask taste. Do not give with food.	Nausea, abdominal cramps. May reduce absorption of fat-soluble vitamins.
Phosphate Binders		
Aluminum hydroxide	Give 1 to 3 hr after meals.	Constipation, cramps, bloating, nausea, vomiting, anorexia, chalky taste. Inactivates thiamin; decreases absorption of vitamin A, phosphorous, and calcium.
Calcium acetate	Give with meals. Avoid calcium supplements.	Anorexia, nausea, vomiting, constipation. Decreased iron absorption, increased blood calcium levels.
Calcium carbonate	Give 1 to 3 hr after meals. Give iron supplements 1 to 2 hr before or after use. Do not take with large amounts of dairy products.	Belching, nausea, constipation, steatorrhea, chalky taste. May decrease iron absorption.

(continued)

E

Table E–1B (*continued*)

Drug Classification and Name	Administration	Common Side Effects That May Influence Nutrition Status
Miscellaneous		
Amphetamine sulfate	Give 1/2 to 1 hr before meals. Avoid caffeine.	Anorexia, nausea, vomiting, cramps, dry mouth, diarrhea, constipation, weight loss.
Astemizole	Give 1 to 3 hr after meals.	Increased appetite, weight gain, nausea, dry mouth, diarrhea, abdominal pain.
Calcitriol	Do not give with vitamin D or magnesium supplements. Avoid high-phosphorus foods if on dialysis.	Anorexia, nausea, vomiting, dry mouth, taste alterations, constipation. Increases blood calcium, phosphorus, magnesium, and cholesterol levels. Increased urinary excretion of calcium and phosphorus.
Colchicine	Give with food to reduce GI distress.	Nausea, vomiting, diarrhea, abdominal pain.
Erythropoietin	Give parenterally. Give only if iron, folate, and vitamin B_{12} status is adequate.	Nausea, vomiting, diarrhea.
Lithium carbonate	Give with food. Maintain consistent sodium intake daily.	Thirst, metallic taste.
Oral contraceptives	Give with food.	Nausea, edema, weight changes. May cause hyperglycemia, hypercalcemia, or folate deficiency.

Note: The multitude of drugs and nutrients that interact are far too numerous to list in a nutrition textbook like this one. Indeed, whole books are available to cover the subject. The side effects shown in this table are common side effects. Other side effects can and do occur. This table provides only a sampling of interactions. More detailed texts should be consulted for the drugs you encounter in clinical practice.

Source: Nursing 94 Drug Handbook (Springhouse, Pa.: Springhouse Corporation, 1994), and D. E. Powers and A. O. Moore, *Food Medication Interaction*, 8th ed. (Phoenix, Ariz.: Food Medication Interactions, 1993).

GROWTH CHARTS AND ANTHROPOMETRIC DATA

♦

Growth charts, shown in Figures E–1 through E–6, allow health care professionals to evaluate the growth and development of children from birth to 18 years of age. The assessor follows these steps to plot a weight measurement on a percentile graph:

- Select the appropriate chart based on age and gender. (When length is measured, use the chart for birth to 36 months; when height is measured, use the chart for 2 to 18 years.)
- Locate the child's age along the horizontal axis on the bottom or top of the chart.
- Locate the child's weight in pounds or kilograms along the vertical axis on the lower left or right side of the chart.

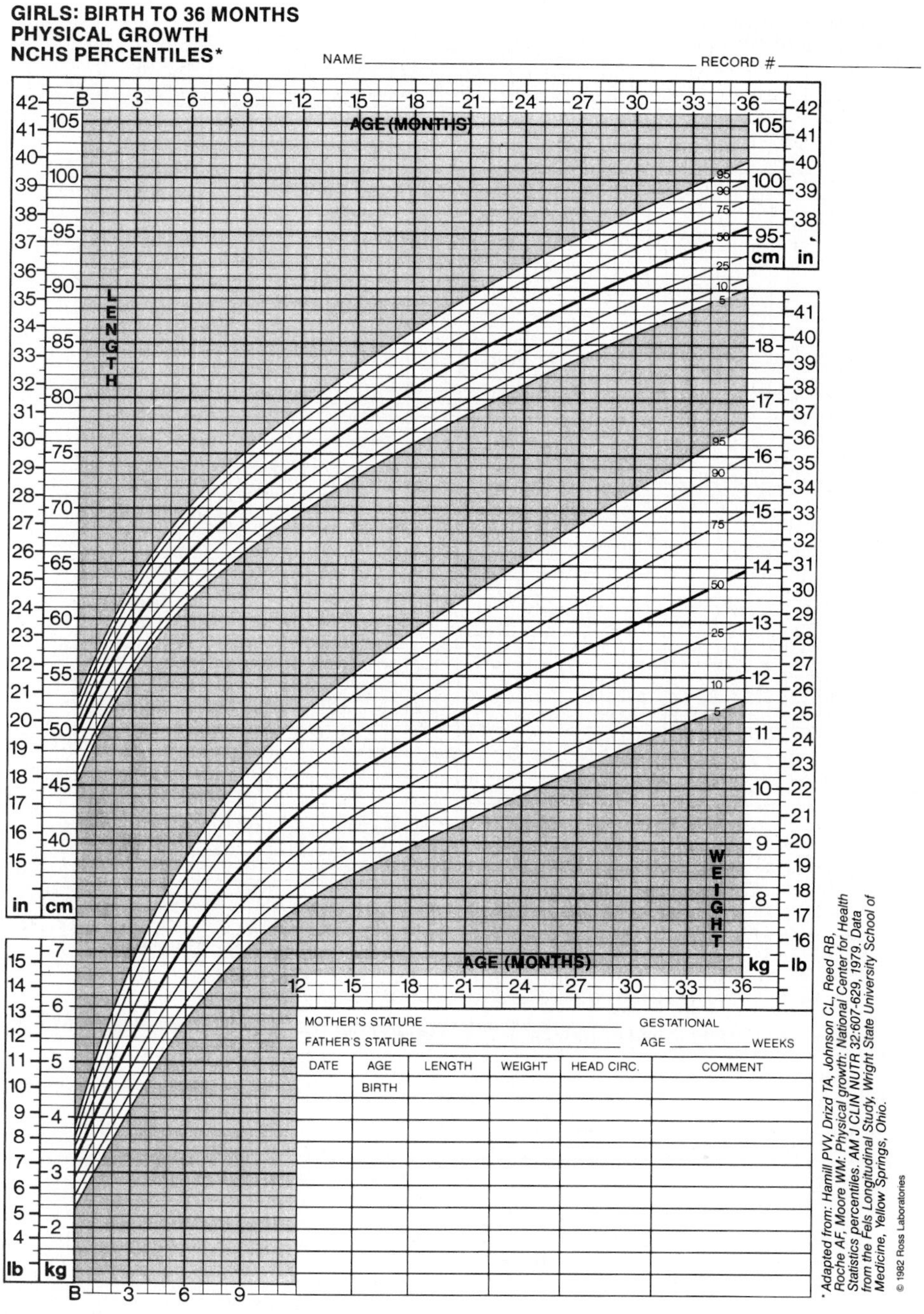

GIRLS: BIRTH TO 36 MONTHS
PHYSICAL GROWTH
NCHS PERCENTILES*
NAME
RECORD #
AGE (MONTHS)
LENGTH
WEIGHT
in
cm
lb
kg
MOTHER'S STATURE
FATHER'S STATURE
GESTATIONAL AGE WEEKS
DATE
AGE
LENGTH
WEIGHT
HEAD CIRC.
COMMENT
BIRTH
*Adapted from: Hamill PVV, Drizd TA, Johnson CL, Reed RB, Roche AF, Moore WM: Physical growth: National Center for Health Statistics percentiles. AM J CLIN NUTR 32:607-629, 1979. Data from the Fels Longitudinal Study, Wright State University School of Medicine, Yellow Springs, Ohio.
© 1982 Ross Laboratories

Figure E-1A
Girls: Birth to 36 Months Physical Growth NCHS Percentiles—Length and Weight for Age

- ♦ Mark the chart where the age and weight lines intersect, and read off the percentile.

To assess length, height, or head circumference, the assessor follows the same procedure, using the appropriate chart. Head circumference percentile should be similar to the child's height and weight percentiles.

Figure E–1B
Girls: Birth to 36 Months Physical Growth NCHS Percentiles—Head Circumference for Age and Weight for Length

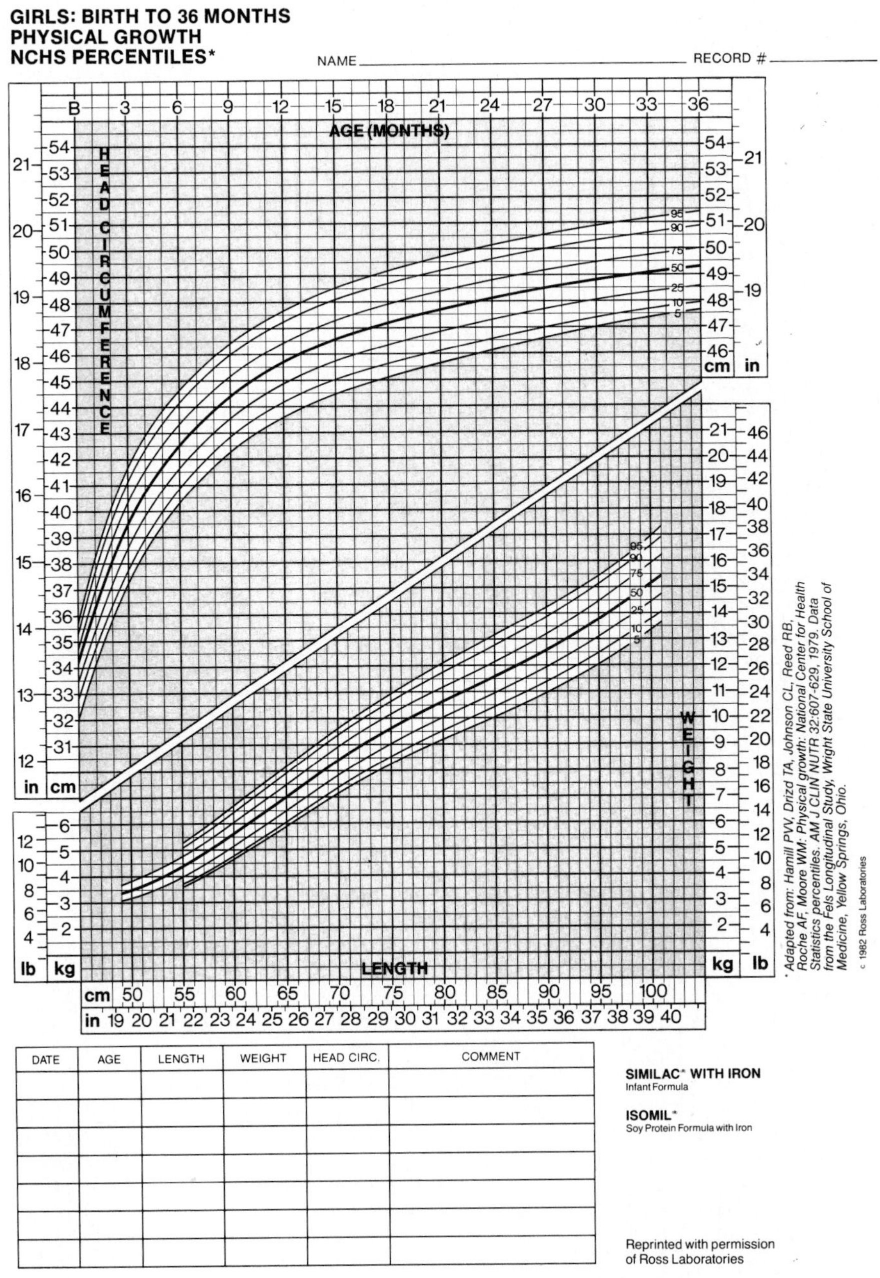

With height, weight, and head circumference measures plotted on growth percentile charts, a skilled clinician can begin to interpret the data. Percentile charts divide the measures of a population into 100 equal divisions. Thus half of the population falls above the 50th percentile, and half

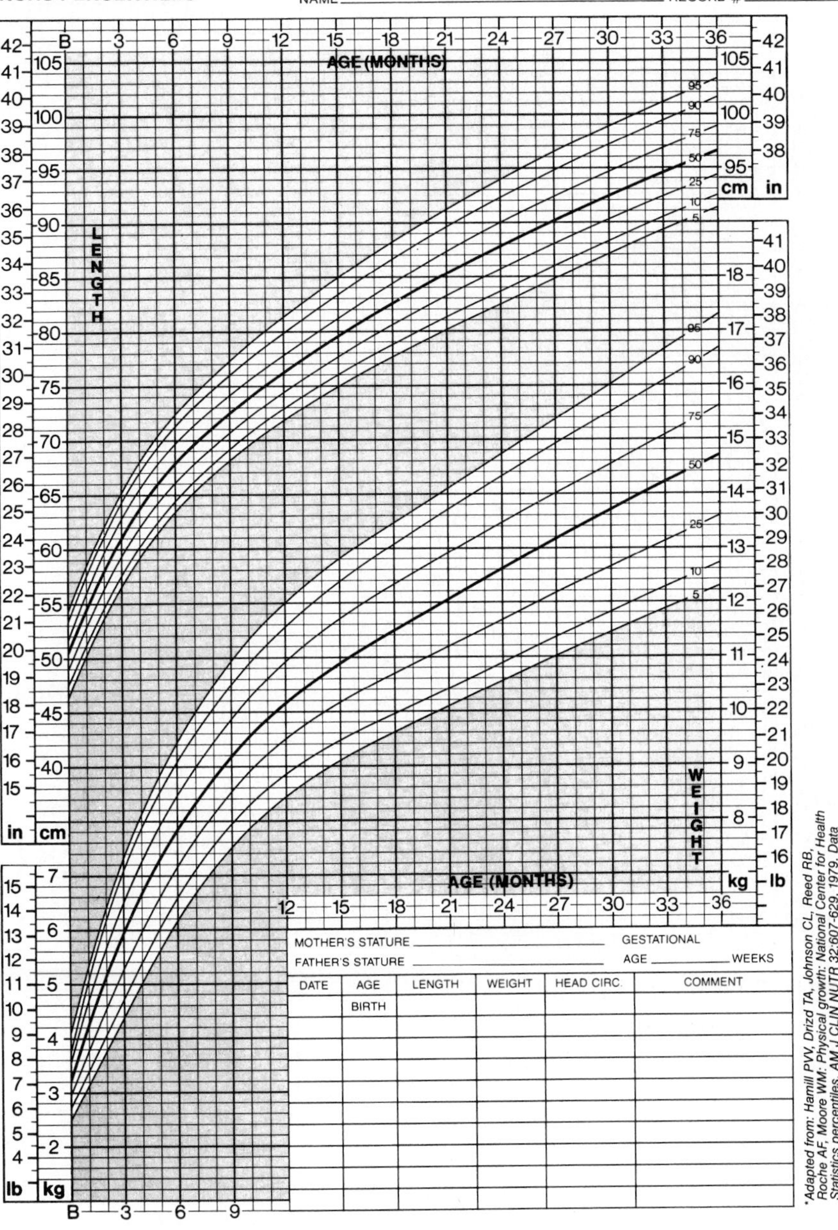

Figure E-2A
Boys: Birth to 36 Months Physical Growth NCHS Percentiles—Length and Weight for Age

falls below. The use of percentile measures allows for comparisons among people of the same age and gender. For example, a six-month-old female infant whose weight is at the 75th percentile weighs more than 75 percent of the female infants her age.

Figure E-2B
Boys: Birth to 36 Months Physical Growth NCHS Percentiles—Head Circumference for Age and Weight for Length

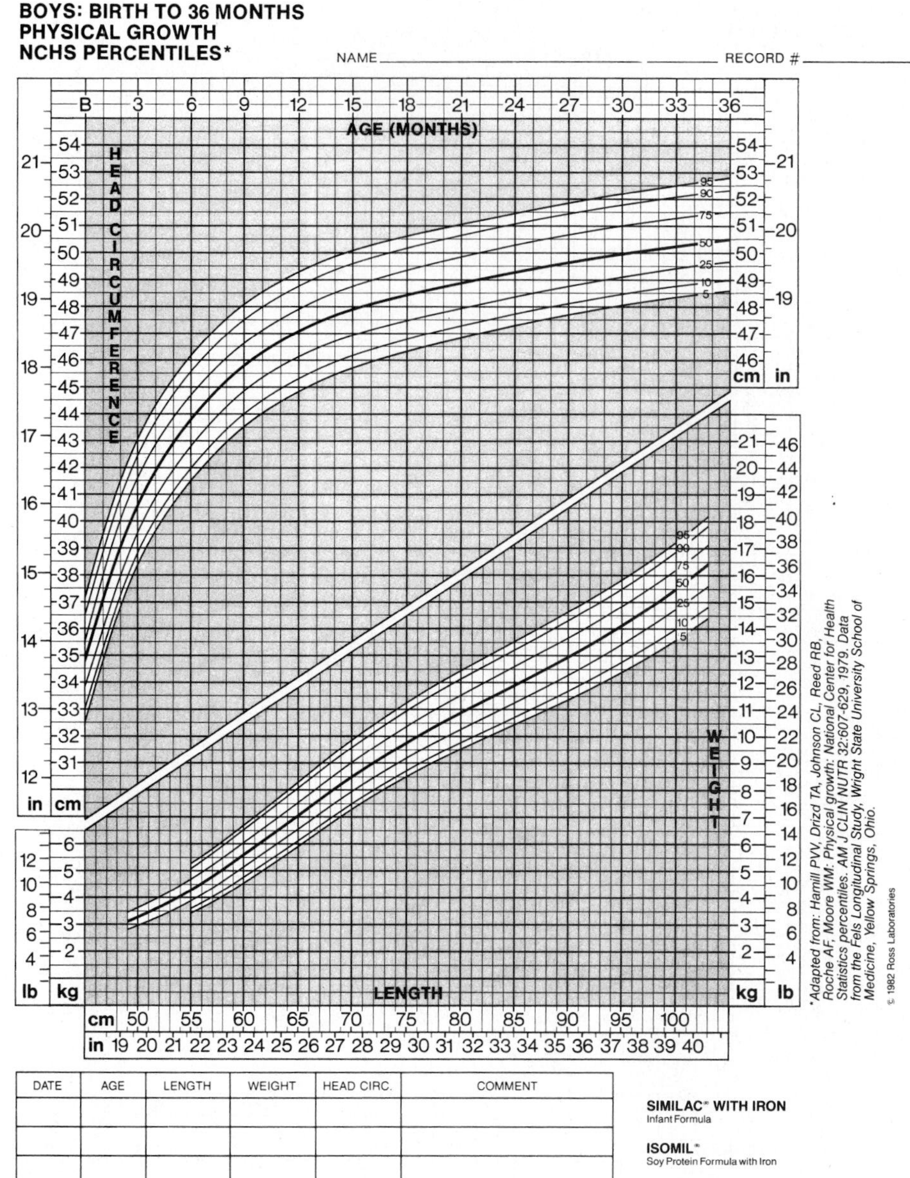

DATE	AGE	LENGTH	WEIGHT	HEAD CIRC.	COMMENT

GIRLS: 2 TO 18 YEARS
PHYSICAL GROWTH
NCHS PERCENTILES*

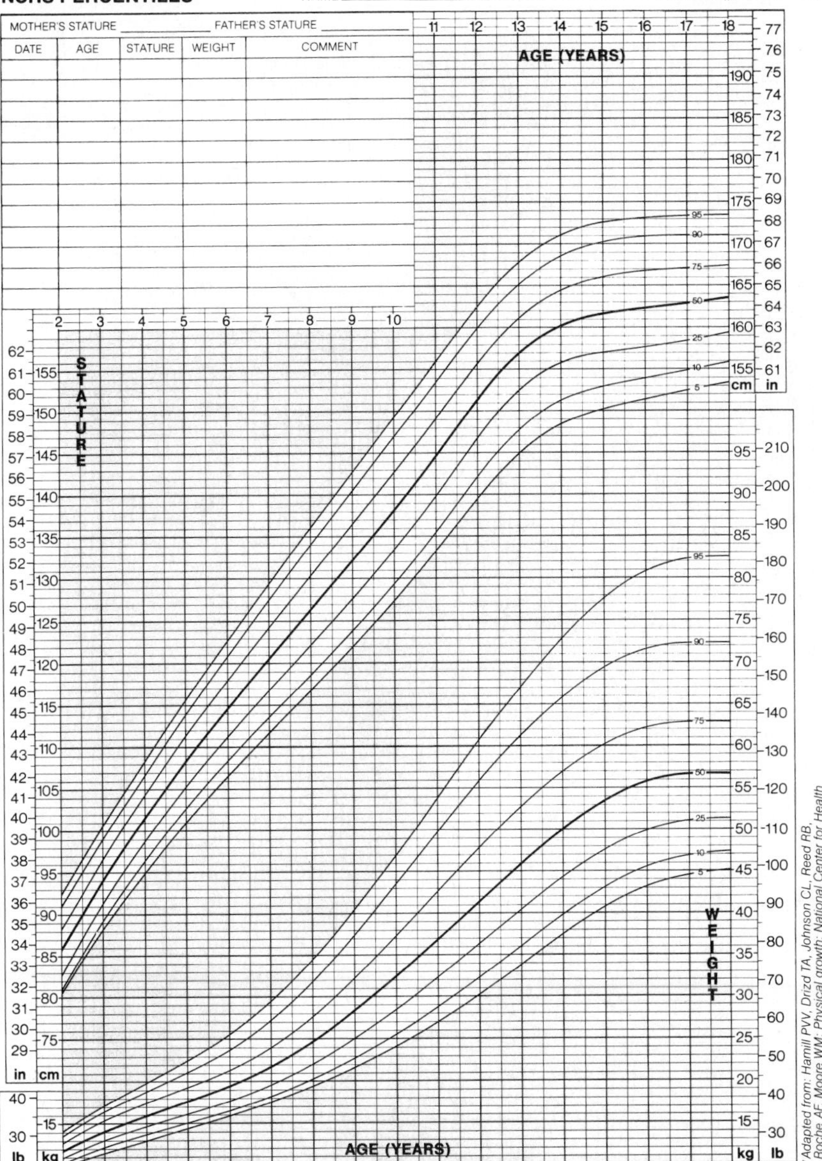

*Adapted from: Hamill PVV, Drizd TA, Johnson CL, Reed RB, Roche AF, Moore WM: Physical growth: National Center for Health Statistics percentiles. AM J CLIN NUTR 32:607-629, 1979. Data from the National Center for Health Statistics (NCHS), Hyattsville, Maryland.

Figure E-3
Girls: 2 to 18 Years Physical Growth NCHS Percentiles—Height and Weight for Age

Figure E–4
Boys: 2 to 18 Years Physical Growth NCHS Percentiles—Height and Weight for Age

BOYS: 2 TO 18 YEARS
PHYSICAL GROWTH
NCHS PERCENTILES*

NAME ______ RECORD # ______

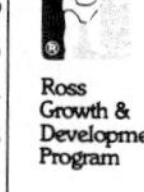

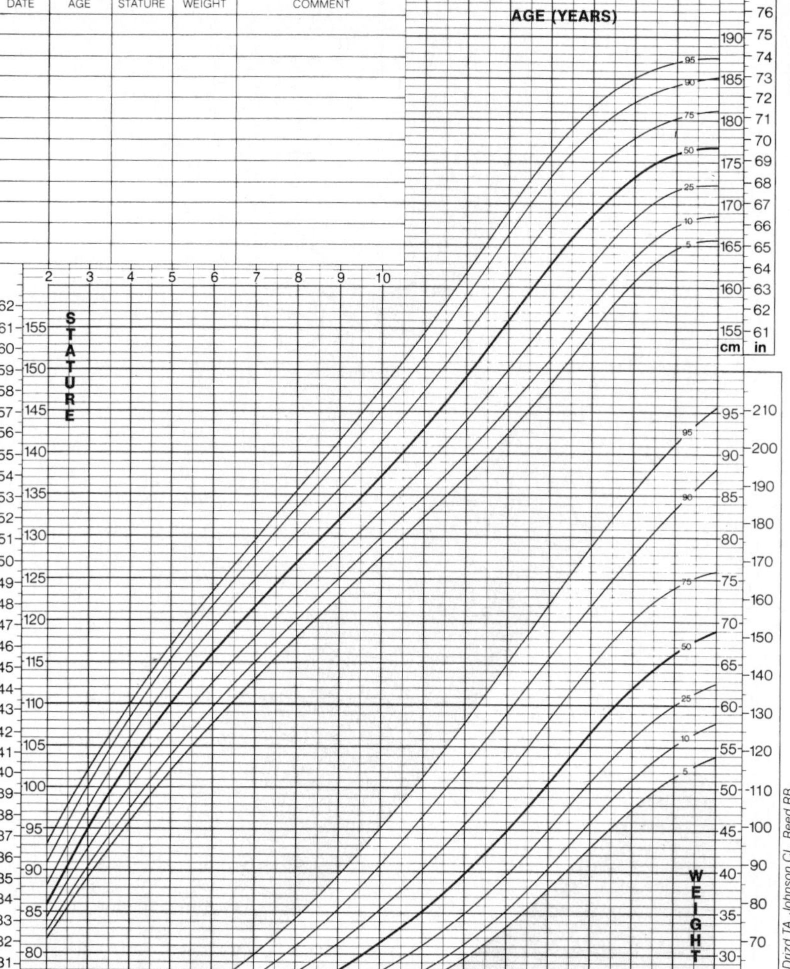

*Adapted from: Hamill PVV, Drizd TA, Johnson CL, Reed RB, Roche AF, Moore WM: Physical growth: National Center for Health Statistics percentiles. AM J CLIN NUTR 32:607-629, 1979. Data from the National Center for Health Statistics (NCHS), Hyattsville, Maryland.

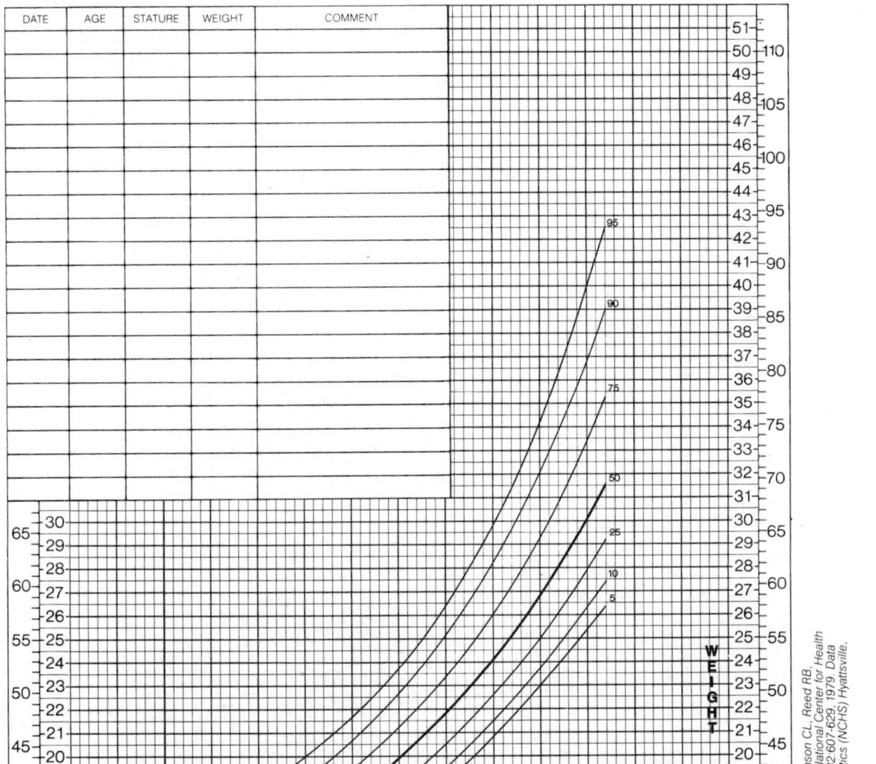

Figure E–5
Girls: Prepubescent Physical Growth NCHS Percentiles—Weight for Height

E

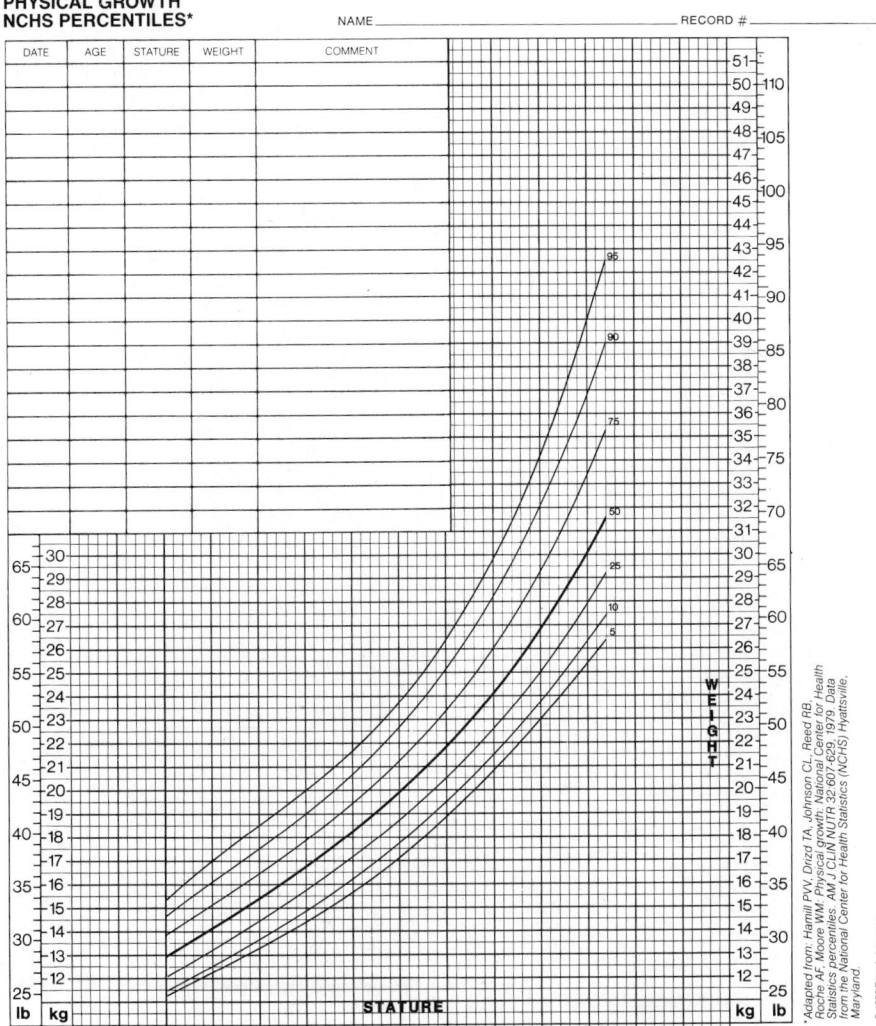

Figure E-6
Boys: Prepubescent Physical Growth NCHS Percentiles—Weight for Height

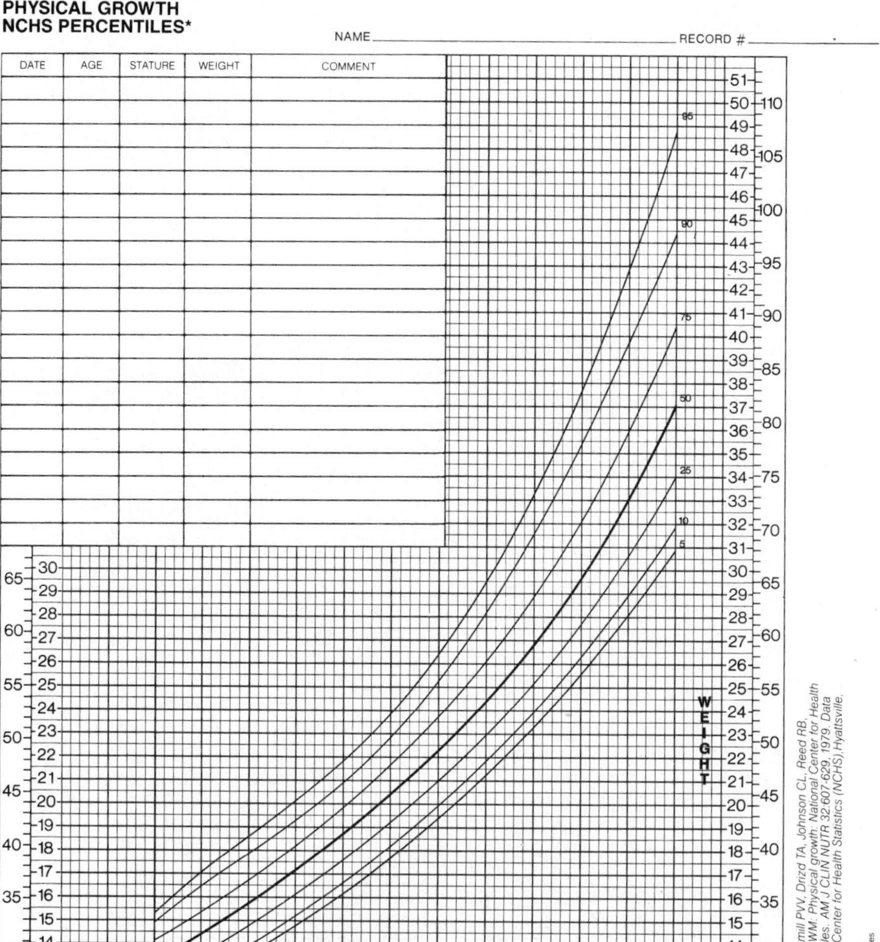

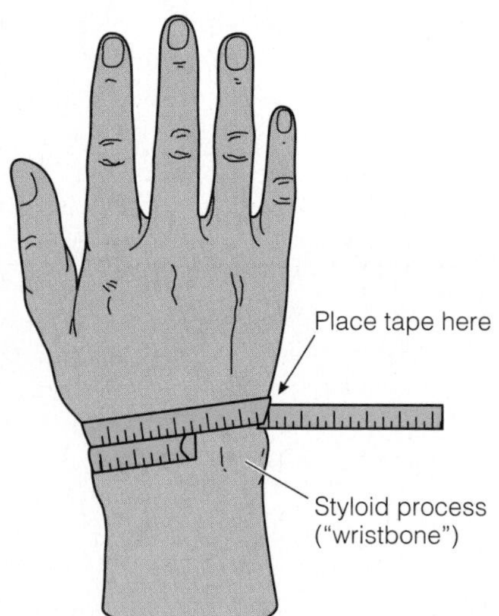

Figure E-7
Wrist Circumference

In adults, assessors evaluate weight for height by comparing measures with population standards. Table E–2 presents the Metropolitan Height-Weight tables, which have been used for years, but which are now somewhat out of date (see discussion in Chapter 9). Table 9–1 in Chapter 9 is more current: it presents suggested weights for adults adjusted for age. To use some height-weight tables, the assessor must determine the client's frame size. Tables E–3 and E–4 present two methods of determining frame size, and Figure E–7 shows how to measure the wrist when it is used to determine frame size. Another method of assessing body weight in adults is the body mass index (BMI). Figure E–8 (p. E–24) presents a nomogram for BMI. Figure E–9 (p. E–25) shows normal weight gains related to duration of pregnancy in weeks for women who start their pregnancies at normal weight, underweight, or overweight.

Fatfold measurements assist health care professionals in evaluating the composition of body weight. As already explained in Chapter 13, a *lean* tissue measure can be computed from the triceps fatfold measurement together with the midarm circumference measurement: the midarm muscle circumference (see p. 326). Table E-5 (p. E-26) gives triceps fatfold percentile standards. Table E-6 shows the midarm muscle circumference percentile standards, and Figure E-10 (p. E-27) illustrates a nomogram method for determining midarm muscle circumference from these two measures.

Table E-2
1983 Metropolitan Height and Weight Tables

Men					Women				
Height		Frame			Height		Frame		
FEET	INCHES	SMALL	MEDIUM	LARGE	FEET	INCHES	SMALL	MEDIUM	LARGE
5	2	128–134	131–141	138–150	4	10	102–111	109–121	118–131
5	3	130–136	133–143	140–153	4	11	103–113	111–123	120–134
5	4	132–138	135–145	142–156	5	0	104–115	113–126	122–137
5	5	134–140	137–148	144–160	5	1	106–118	115–129	125–140
5	6	136–142	139–151	146–164	5	2	108–121	118–132	128–143
5	7	138–145	142–154	149–168	5	3	111–124	121–135	131–147
5	8	140–148	145–157	152–172	5	4	114–127	124–138	134–151
5	9	142–151	148–160	155–176	5	5	117–130	127–141	137–155
5	10	144–154	151–163	158–180	5	6	120–133	130–144	140–159
5	11	146–157	154–166	161–184	5	7	123–136	133–147	143–163
6	0	149–160	157–170	164–188	5	8	126–139	136–150	146–167
6	1	152–164	160–174	168–192	5	9	129–142	139–153	149–170
6	2	155–168	164–178	172–197	5	10	132–145	142–156	152–173
6	3	158–172	167–182	176–202	5	11	135–148	145–159	155–176
6	4	162–176	171–187	181–207	6	0	138–151	148–162	158–179

Note: To use the table, add an inch to your barefoot height (you are assumed to be wearing shoes with 1-inch heels), and adjust for clothing (the tables assume 5 pounds for clothes for men and 3 pounds for women). Weights are at age 25 to 29 based on lowest mortality, in pounds according to frame size.

Source: Reproduced courtesy of Metropolitan Life Insurance Company *STATISTICAL BULLETIN.* Source of basic data: Society of Actuaries and Association of Life Insurance Medical Directors of America, *1979 Build Study,* 1980.

Table E-3
How to Determine Body Frame by Elbow Breadth

To make a simple approximation of frame size, do the following: Extend the arm, and bend the forearm upward at a 90° angle. Keep the fingers straight, and turn the inside of the wrist away from the body. Place the thumb and index finger on the two prominent bones on *either side* of the elbow. Measure the space between the fingers against a ruler or a tape measure.[a] Compare the measurements with the following standards.

These standards represent the elbow measurements for medium-framed men and women of various heights. Measurements smaller than those listed indicate a small frame, and larger measurements indicate a large frame.

Men		Women	
HEIGHT IN 1-INCH HEELS	ELBOW BREADTH	HEIGHT IN 1-INCH HEELS	ELBOW BREADTH
5 ft 2 in to 5 ft 3 in	2½ to 2⅞ in	4 ft 10 in to 4 ft 11 in	2¼ to 2½ in
5 ft 4 in to 5 ft 7 in	2⅝ to 2⅞ in	5 ft 0 in to 5 ft 3 in	2¼ to 2½ in
5 ft 8 in to 5 ft 11 in	2¾ to 3 in	5 ft 4 in to 5 ft 7 in	2⅜ to 2⅝ in
6 ft 0 in to 6 ft 3 in	2¾ to 3⅛ in	5 ft 8 in to 5 ft 11 in	2⅜ to 2⅝ in
6 ft 4 in and over	2⅞ to 3¼ in	6 ft 0 in and over	2½ to 2¾ in

[a]For the most accurate measurement, measure elbow breadth with a caliper.

Source: Metropolitan Life Insurance Company.

E

Table E-4
Frame Size from Height-Wrist Circumference Ratios (r)[a]

Frame Size	Male r Values	Female r Values
Small	>10.4	>11.0
Medium	9.6–10.4	10.1–11.0
Large	<9.6	<10.1

[a] $r = \frac{\text{height (cm)}}{\text{wrist circumference (cm)}}$. The wrist is measured where it bends (distal to the styloid process), on the right arm (see Figure E-7).

Figure E-8
Nomogram for Body Mass Index (BMI)

Weights and heights are without clothing. With clothes, add 5 pounds for men or 3 pounds for women, and 1 inch in height for shoes. Draw a straight line, or place a ruler, from your height (left) to your weight (right). At the point where it crosses the BMI line, read your BMI. The accompanying table indicates the BMI used to define cutoff points, and the inside back covers present this information graphically.

Source: Courtesy of Metropolitan Life Insurance Company, *STATISTICAL BULLETIN* and NIH Consensus Development Conference, Copyright The American Dietetic Association. Reprinted by permission from JOURNAL OF THE AMERICAN DIETETIC ASSOCIATION, Vol. 85 (1985): 1117–1121.

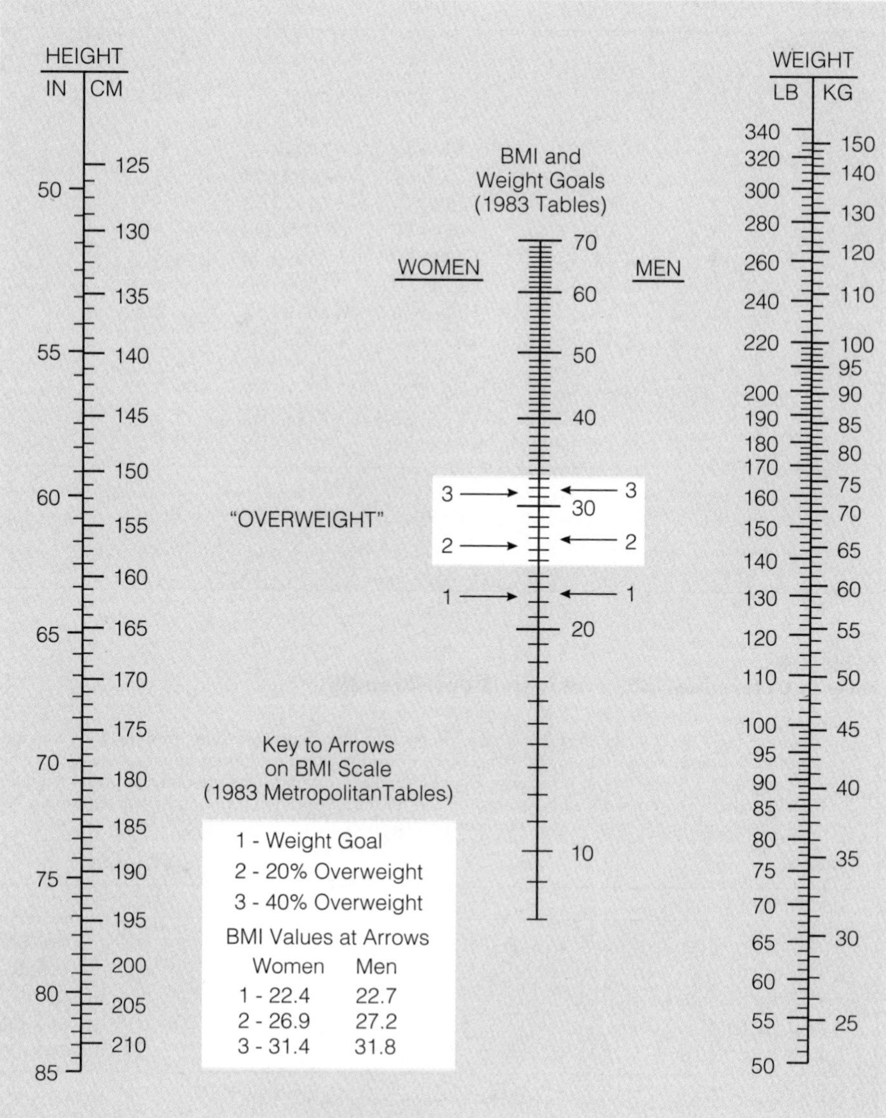

	Men	Women
Underweight	<20.7	<19.1
Acceptable weight	20.7 to 27.8	19.1 to 27.3
Overweight	≥27.8	≥27.3
Severe overweight	≥31.1	≥32.3
Morbid obesity	≥45.4	≥44.8

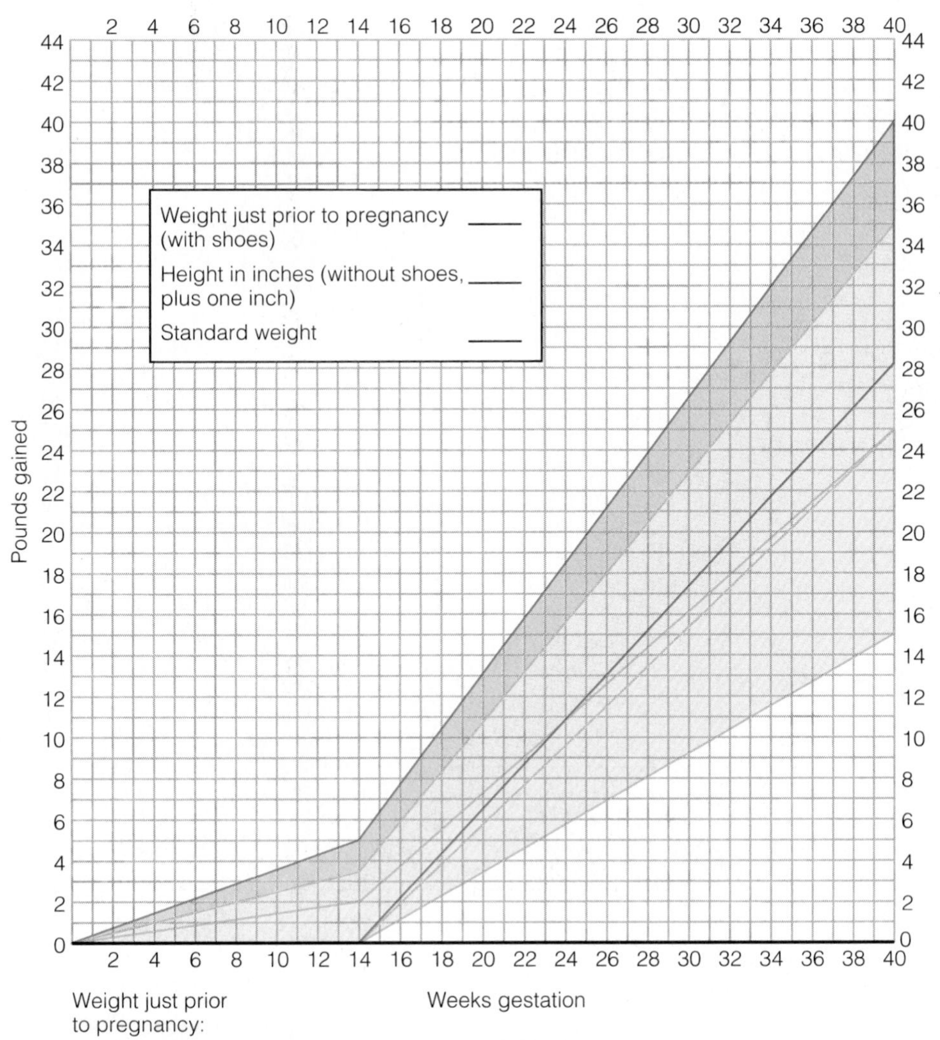

Figure E–9
Prenatal Weight Gain Grid

A prenatal weight gain grid plots the rate of weight gain during pregnancy. Normal-weight women should gain about 3½ pounds in the first trimester and just under 1 pound per week thereafter, achieving a total gain of 25 to 35 pounds by term; underweight women should gain about 5 pounds in the first trimester and just over 1 pound per week thereafter, achieving a total gain of 28 to 40 pounds by term; and overweight women should gain about 2 pounds in the first trimester and ⅔ pound per week thereafter, achieving a total gain of 15 to 25 pounds.

E

Table E–5
Triceps Fatfold Percentiles (millimeters)

Age	Male 5TH	Male 25TH	Male 50TH	Male 75TH	Male 95TH	Female 5TH	Female 25TH	Female 50TH	Female 75TH	Female 95TH
1–1.9	6	8	10	12	16	6	8	10	12	16
2–2.9	6	8	10	12	15	6	9	10	12	16
3–3.9	6	8	10	11	15	7	9	11	12	15
4–4.9	6	8	9	11	14	7	8	10	12	16
5–5.9	6	8	9	11	15	6	8	10	12	18
6–6.9	5	7	8	10	16	6	8	10	12	16
7–7.9	5	7	9	12	17	6	9	11	13	18
8–8.9	5	7	8	10	16	6	9	12	15	24
9–9.9	6	7	10	13	18	8	10	13	16	22
10–10.9	6	8	10	14	21	7	10	12	17	27
11–11.9	6	8	11	16	24	7	10	13	18	28
12–12.9	6	8	11	14	28	8	11	14	18	27
13–13.9	5	7	10	14	26	8	12	15	21	30
14–14.9	4	7	9	14	24	9	13	16	21	28
15–15.9	4	6	8	11	24	8	12	17	21	32
16–16.9	4	6	8	12	22	10	15	18	22	31
17–17.9	5	6	8	12	19	10	13	19	24	37
18–18.9	4	6	9	13	24	10	15	18	22	30
19–24.9	4	7	10	15	22	10	14	18	24	34
25–34.9	5	8	12	16	24	10	16	21	27	37
35–44.9	5	8	12	16	23	12	18	23	29	38
45–54.9	6	8	12	15	25	12	20	25	30	40
55–64.9	5	8	11	14	22	12	20	25	31	38
65–74.9	4	8	11	15	22	12	18	24	29	36

Note: If measurements fall between the percentiles shown here, the percentile can be estimated from the information in this table. For example, a measurement of 7 millimeters for a 27-year-old male would be about the 20th percentile.

Source: Adapted from A. R. Frisancho, New norms of upper limb fat and muscle areas for assessment of nutritional status. *American Journal of Clinical Nutrition* 34 (1981): 2540–2545.

Table E–6
Midarm Muscle Circumference Percentiles (centimeters)

Age	Male 5TH	Male 25TH	Male 50TH	Male 75TH	Male 95TH	Female 5TH	Female 25TH	Female 50TH	Female 75TH	Female 95TH
1–1.9	11.0	11.9	12.7	13.5	14.7	10.5	11.7	12.4	13.9	14.3
2–2.9	11.1	12.2	13.0	14.0	15.0	11.1	11.9	12.6	13.3	14.7
3–3.9	11.7	13.1	13.7	14.3	15.3	11.3	12.4	13.2	14.0	15.2
4–4.9	12.3	13.3	14.1	14.8	15.9	11.5	12.8	13.6	14.4	15.7
5–5.9	12.8	14.0	14.7	15.4	16.9	12.5	13.4	14.2	15.1	16.5
6–6.9	13.1	14.2	15.1	16.1	17.7	13.0	13.8	14.5	15.4	17.1
7–7.9	13.7	15.1	16.0	16.8	19.0	12.9	14.2	15.1	16.0	17.6
8–8.9	14.0	15.4	16.2	17.0	18.7	13.8	15.1	16.0	17.1	19.4
9–9.9	15.1	16.1	17.0	18.3	20.2	14.7	15.8	16.7	18.0	19.8
10–10.9	15.6	16.6	18.0	19.1	22.1	14.8	15.9	17.0	18.0	19.7
11–11.9	15.9	17.3	18.3	19.5	23.0	15.0	17.1	18.1	19.6	22.3
12–12.9	16.7	18.2	19.5	21.0	24.1	16.2	18.0	19.1	20.1	22.0
13–13.9	17.2	19.6	21.1	22.6	24.5	16.9	18.3	19.8	21.1	24.0
14–14.9	18.9	21.2	22.3	24.0	26.4	17.4	19.0	20.1	21.6	24.7
15–15.9	19.9	21.8	23.7	25.4	27.2	17.5	18.9	20.2	21.5	24.4
16–16.9	21.3	23.4	24.9	26.9	29.6	17.0	19.0	20.2	21.6	24.9
17–17.9	22.4	24.5	25.8	27.3	31.2	17.5	19.4	20.5	22.1	25.7
18–18.9	22.6	25.2	26.4	28.3	32.4	17.4	19.1	20.2	21.5	24.5
19–24.9	23.8	25.7	27.3	28.9	32.1	17.9	19.5	20.7	22.1	24.9
25–34.9	24.3	26.4	27.9	29.8	32.6	18.3	19.9	21.2	22.8	26.4
35–44.9	24.7	26.9	28.6	30.2	32.7	18.6	20.5	21.8	23.6	27.2
45–54.9	23.9	26.5	28.1	30.0	32.6	18.7	20.6	22.0	23.8	27.4
55–64.9	23.6	26.0	27.8	29.5	32.0	18.7	20.9	22.5	24.4	28.0
65–74.9	22.3	25.1	26.8	28.4	30.6	18.5	20.8	22.5	24.4	27.9

Source: Adapted from A. R. Frisancho, New norms of upper limb fat and muscle areas for assessment of nutritional status, *American Journal of Clinical Nutrition* 34 (1981): 2540–2545.

Figure E–10
Nomograms for Determination of Midarm Muscle Circumference

To obtain arm muscle circumference using either nomogram, lay a ruler between the arm circumference and fatfold values, and read off the arm muscle circumference.

Source: Reproduced with permission from J. Gurney and D. Jelliffe, Arm anthropometry in nutritional assessment; nomogram for rapid calculation of muscle circumference and cross-sectional muscle and fat areas. *American Journal of Clinical Nutrition* 26 (1973): 912, as adapted by A. Grant, *Nutritional Assessment Guidelines,* 2nd ed., 1979 (available from Anne Grant, Box 25057, Northgate Station, Seattle, WA 98125).

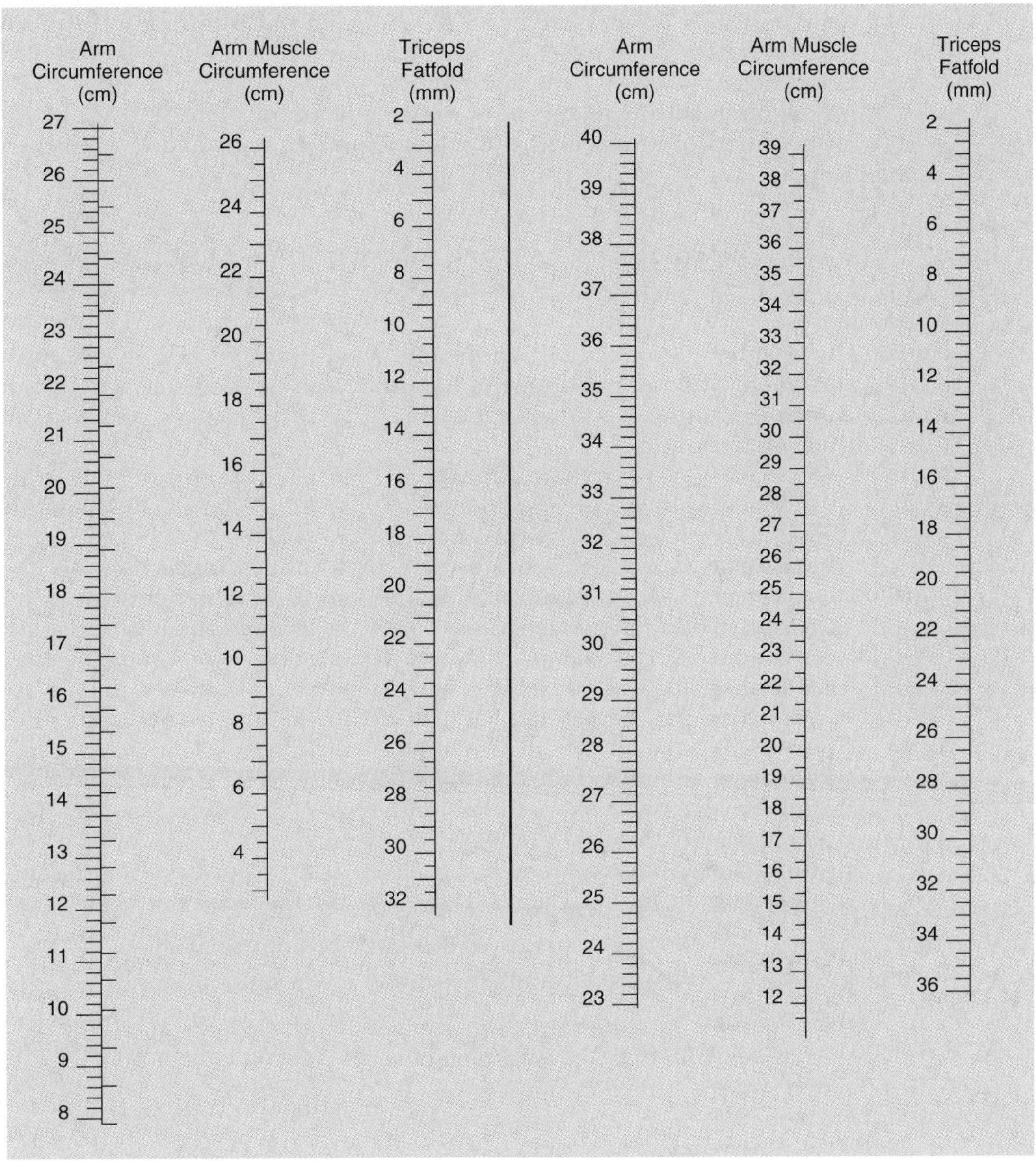

Arm Circumference (cm): 27 26 25 24 23 22 21 20 19 18 17 16 15 14 13 12 11 10 9 8

Arm Muscle Circumference (cm): 26 24 22 20 18 16 14 12 10 8 6 4

Triceps Fatfold (mm): 2 4 6 8 10 12 14 16 18 20 22 24 26 28 30 32

Arm Circumference (cm): 40 39 38 37 36 35 34 33 32 31 30 29 28 27 26 25 24 23

Arm Muscle Circumference (cm): 39 38 37 36 35 34 33 32 31 30 29 28 27 26 25 24 23 22 21 20 19 18 17 16 15 14 13 12

Triceps Fatfold (mm): 2 4 6 8 10 12 14 16 18 20 22 24 26 28 30 32 34 36

E

Table E–7
Lower Limits of Acceptable Grip Strength

Age	Female Grip Strength (kg)	Male Grip Strength (kg)
15	28	42
20	29	43
25	30	44
30	30	45
35	30	45
40	30	45
45	30	45
50	29	45
55	28	44
60	27	43
65	25	41
70	23	39
75	20	37
80	18	35
85	15	32
90	11	29
95	8	26

Note: The figures shown in this table represent 85% of the standard for each age and gender category.

Source: Reprinted by permission of the American Society of Parenteral and Enteral Nutrition, Silver Spring, MD 20879, from A. R. Webb, L. A. Newman, M. Taylor, and J. B. Keogh, Hand grip dynamometry as a predictor of postoperative complications: Reappraisal using age standardized grip strength, *Journal of Parenteral and Enteral Nutrition* 13 (1989): 30–33.

FUNCTIONAL TESTS OF NUTRITION STATUS

♦

Nutrition assessors sometimes use functional tests of nutrition status to identify nutrient deficiencies. One such test uses a dynamometer (described in Chapter 13) to measure hand grip strength (see p. 327). As with all assessment methods, following instructions carefully helps to ensure accurate measures. To measure hand grip strength, the assessor asks the client to squeeze the dynamometer as tightly as possible, takes three or four measurements, and records the highest value measured. Measurements can be taken on either the dominant or nondominant arm. Table E–7 shows the lower limits of acceptable hand grip strength in males and females based on age.

LABORATORY TESTS OF NUTRITION STATUS

♦

As Chapter 13 pointed out, urine and blood tests provide valuable information in a nutrition assessment. Two urine tests—creatinine excretion and urine urea nitrogen—require a 24-hour urine collection and, therefore, are not routinely used.

Collecting a 24-hour urine sample presents many problems. Much effort is wasted if everyone involved does not conscientiously follow proper techniques. The collection of urine and recording of food intake data require client cooperation. The client must receive thorough instructions on how to collect and save all urine samples and must be advised to call for help if needed. Each urine sample is added to the collection container and refrigerated until the collection is complete. If even one urine sample is spilled or discarded, the test is invalid.

Most hospitals have a standard time for beginning urinary collections (often, between 6:00 A.M. and 6:00 P.M.). For nitrogen balance studies, food intake must also be recorded during the exact same time period. All nurses caring for the client on all shifts must record, or ensure that the client records, food intake data carefully.

To calculate the creatinine-height index (CHI) from the measured urinary creatinine and the client's height, use the following equation:

$$\text{CHI} = \frac{\text{Measured urinary creatinine (24-hour sample)}}{\text{Standard creatinine excretion for height and sex}} \times 100.$$

For example, to calculate the CHI in a man of medium frame, 5 feet 8 inches tall, who excretes 1090 milligrams of creatinine in 24 hours, follow these steps:

Table E-8
Creatinine-Height Index Standards for Men

Height		Small Frame			Medium Frame			Large Frame		
		Ideal Weight	Creatinine		Ideal Weight	Creatinine		Ideal Weight	Creatinine	
in	cm	(kg)	(g/24 h)	(mmol/d)	(kg)	(g/24 h)	(mmol/d)	(kg)	(g/24 h)	(mmol/d)
61	154.9	52.7	1.21	10.7	56.1	1.29	11.4	60.7	1.40	12.4
62	157.5	54.1	1.24	11.0	57.7	1.33	11.8	62.0	1.43	12.6
63	160.0	55.4	1.27	11.2	59.1	1.36	12.0	63.6	1.46	12.9
64	162.5	56.8	1.31	11.6	60.4	1.39	12.3	65.2	1.50	13.3
65	165.1	58.4	1.34	11.8	62.0	1.43	12.6	66.8	1.54	13.6
66	167.6	60.2	1.39	12.3	63.9	1.47	13.0	68.9	1.59	14.1
67	170.2	62.0	1.43	12.6	65.9	1.52	13.4	71.1	1.64	14.5
68	172.7	63.9	1.47	13.0	67.7	1.56	13.8	72.9	1.68	14.9
69	175.3	65.9	1.52	13.4	69.5	1.60	14.1	74.8	1.72	15.2
70	177.8	67.7	1.56	13.8	71.6	1.65	14.6	76.8	1.77	15.6
71	180.3	69.5	1.60	14.1	73.6	1.69	14.9	79.1	1.82	16.1
72	182.9	71.4	1.64	14.5	75.7	1.74	15.4	81.1	1.87	16.5
73	185.4	73.4	1.69	14.9	77.7	1.79	15.8	83.4	1.92	17.0
74	187.9	75.2	1.73	15.3	80.0	1.85	16.4	85.7	1.97	17.4
75	190.5	77.0	1.77	15.6	82.3	1.89	16.7	87.7	2.02	17.9

Note: To convert urinary creatinine measures (g/24 h) to standard international units (mmol/d) multiply by 8.840.

Source: Courtesy of Metropolitan Life Insurance Company, *STATISTICAL BULLETIN.*

◆ Look up the standard creatinine excretion (Table E–8).

In this example, the standard creatinine excretion is 1.56 gram or 1560 milligrams.

◆ Use this information to complete the CHI equation:

$$\text{CHI} = \frac{1090 \text{ mg}}{1560 \text{ mg}} \times 100 = 70\%.$$

Based on the CHI, the man in this example has a skeletal muscle mass 70 percent of that considered typical for a man of his height. Table E–9 (p. E–30) shows the standard creatinine excretions for women.

Other laboratory tests help detect anemias. Chapter 13 (pp. 333–336) describes the tests used in assessing iron status and provides standard values for hemoglobin and hematocrit. Tables E–10 through E–13 (pp. E-30 and E–31) provide standards for other measures of iron status: serum ferritin, serum iron, transferrin saturation, erythrocyte protoporphyrin, and mean corpuscular volume. Table E–14 (p. E–31) provides standards for measures of folate status.

Table E-9
Creatinine-Height Index Standards for Women

Height		Small Frame			Medium Frame			Large Frame		
		Ideal Weight	Creatinine		Ideal Weight	Creatinine		Ideal Weight	Creatinine	
in	cm	(kg)	(g/24 h)	(mmol/d)	(kg)	(g/24 h)	(mmol/d)	(kg)	(g/24 h)	(mmol/d)
56	142.2	43.2	0.79	7.0	46.1	0.83	7.3	50.7	0.91	8.0
57	144.8	44.3	0.80	7.1	47.3	0.85	7.5	51.8	0.93	8.2
58	147.3	45.4	0.82	7.2	48.6	0.88	7.8	53.2	0.96	8.5
59	149.8	46.8	0.84	7.4	50.0	0.90	8.0	54.5	0.98	8.7
60	152.4	48.2	0.87	7.7	51.4	0.93	8.2	55.9	1.01	8.9
61	154.9	49.5	0.89	7.9	52.7	0.95	8.4	57.3	1.03	9.1
62	157.5	50.9	0.92	8.1	54.3	0.98	8.7	58.9	1.06	9.4
63	160.0	52.3	0.94	8.3	55.9	1.01	8.9	60.6	1.09	9.6
64	162.5	53.9	0.97	8.6	57.9	1.04	9.2	62.5	1.13	10.0
65	165.1	55.7	1.00	8.8	59.8	1.08	9.5	64.3	1.16	10.3
66	167.6	57.5	1.04	9.2	61.6	1.11	9.8	66.1	1.19	10.5
67	170.2	59.3	1.07	9.5	63.4	1.14	10.1	67.9	1.22	10.8
68	172.7	61.4	1.11	9.8	65.2	1.17	10.3	70.0	1.26	11.1
69	175.2	63.2	1.14	10.1	67.0	1.21	10.7	72.0	1.30	11.5
70	177.8	65.0	1.17	10.3	68.9	1.24	11.0	74.1	1.33	11.8

Note: To convert urinary creatinine measures (g/24 h) to standard international units (mmol/d) multiply by 8.840.

Source: A. Grant and S. DeHoog, *Nutritional Assessment and Support*, 3rd ed., 1985 (available from Anne Grant and Susan DeHoog, P.O. Box 25057, Northgate Station, Seattle, WA 98125).

Table E-10
Standards for Serum Ferritin

Group	Deficient (ng/ml)
Children (3–14 years of age)	<10
Adolescents and adults	<12
Pregnant women	<10

Table E-11
Standards for Serum Iron

Age (yr)	Sex	Deficient (μg/100 ml)	Deficient (μmol/L)	Acceptable (μg/100ml)	Acceptable (μmol/L)
<2	M–F	<30	<5.3	30 or >	5.3 or >
2–5	M–F	<40	<7.1	40 or >	7.1 or >
6–12	M–F	<50	<8.9	50 or >	8.9 or >
>12	M	<60	<10.7	60 or >	10.7 or >
	F	<40	<7.1	40 or >	7.1 or >

Note: To convert (μg/100 ml) to international standard units, multiply by 0.1791.

Table E-12
Standards for Percent Transferrin Saturation

Age (yr)	Sex	Deficient	Acceptable
<2	M–F	<15%	15% or >
2–12	M–F	<20%	20% or >
≥13	M	<20%	20% or >
	F	<15%	15% or >

Table E-13
Standards for Erythrocyte Protoporphyrin and Mean Corpuscular Volume

Age (yr)	Erythrocyte Protoporphyrin (μg/dl RBC)	MCV (fL)
1–2	>80	<73
3–4	>75	<75
5–10	>70	<76
11–14	>70	<78
15–74	>70	<80

Note: The abbreviation fL stands for femtoliter, the standard international unit equivalent to a cubic micrometer (μm^3).

Table E-14
Standards for Folate Concentrations

	Deficient (ng/ml)	Borderline (ng/ml)	Acceptable (ng/ml)
Serum folate	<3.0	3.0–6.0	>6.0
Erythrocyte folate	<140	140–160	>160

Note: To convert folate values (ng/ml) to international standard units (nmol/L), multiply by 2.266.

APPENDIX F

HOSPITAL MENUS

Contents

The menus shown in the clinical chapters of this book provide examples of how modified diets translate into meals. People who create hospital menus and meals follow the same principles, but they face added challenges. They must prepare hundreds of meals designed to accommodate dozens of special diets, and they must ensure that each client receives the correct diet. This appendix uses the lunch meal to show how hospital menus are modified to meet each client's needs. The menus on the following pages, which are typical of those in most hospitals, were provided courtesy of the Nutrition and Food Services Department at Kennestone Hospital in Marietta, Georgia.

GENERAL MENU FEATURES

In a typical hospital setting, each client receives a menu every day and can choose among its various options. Each menu shows the day of the week, the type of diet, and the client's name and room number. The client marks food choices on the menu and sends it back to the kitchen. The dietary department uses the menu in preparing the tray to make sure the appropriate foods are provided. The menu goes with the tray to the client's room. The nursing or dietary personnel use the menu to check the tray before it goes to the client's room. If a client has not marked a menu, or if a menu has been lost, the client will receive meals selected by the dietary department.

FOOD PREPARATION

Foods prepared for regular and soft/bland/low-residue diets are prepared with some fat and salt, because these dietary components are not restricted on such diets. Note that menus for the other diets often list low-fat (LF) or low-sodium, low-fat (LSLF) foods. The logistics of preparing foods tailored to each special diet can be overwhelming. For this reason, foodservice departments use special systems designed to keep errors to a minimum. Take baked chicken, for example. If the dietary depart-

Lunch

REGULAR **SUNDAY**

Meats

Baked chicken❤ Fried fish
Hamburger on bun with chips (with lettuce and tomato)

Starchy Vegetables

Cornbread dressing Parsleyed potatoes❤

Vegetables

Baby carrots❤ Stewed tomatoes

Soup/Salad/Juice

Coleslaw
Clam chowder
Gelatin
Tossed salad❤

Dressings

French
Thousand Island
Italian
Diet Thousand Island❤

Desserts

Apple pie Butterscotch pudding
Fresh fruit❤

Breads

Dinner roll Bran bread❤
White bread Crackers
Wheat bread

Beverages & Condiments

Coffee Sugar
Decaf. coffee Sugar substitute
Hot tea Herb seasoning
Decaf. hot tea Creamer
Iced tea Lemon
Whole milk Mustard
Buttermilk Mayonnaise
2% milk Catsup
Skim milk❤ Margarine
Chocolate milk

PLEASE DO NOT LEAVE MENU ON THE TRAY

NAME ______________ **ROOM** ________

People on regular diets select the foods of their choice. The regular menu may also be used for high-kcalorie, high-protein diets. The menu items marked with a heart guide people in selecting foods that are lower in fat, cholesterol, sodium, and caffeine or higher in fiber than other menu choices.

Lunch

SOFT/BLAND/LOW RESIDUE **SUNDAY**

Meats

Baked chicken Baked fish(cod)
Hamburger on bun

Starchy Vegetables

Rice Boiled potatoes

Vegetables

Baby carrots Green beans

Soup/Salad/Juice

Gelatin
Lemonade
Tomato soup

Dressings

Mayonnaise
Catsup

Desserts

Apple pie Pears

Breads

Dinner roll Crackers
White bread

Beverages & Condiments

Decaf. coffee Sugar
Decaf. hot tea Sugar substitute
Decaf. iced tea Creamer
Hot chocolate Lemon
Whole milk Margarine
2% milk
Buttermilk
Skim milk

NO PEPPER

PLEASE DO NOT LEAVE MENU ON THE TRAY

NAME ______________ **ROOM** ________

Foods for soft/bland/low-residue diets are similar to those for regular diets. Foods from the regular menu that are not appropriate have been eliminated from the menu, and substitutions have been made.

Lunch

KCALORIE RESTRICTED, DIABETIC
1200 CALORIES **SUNDAY**

LF = Low Fat LSLF = Low Sodium, Low Fat

Meat Exchange (Select 1)

LSLF Baked chicken (2oz) LSLF Baked fish (2oz)
LSLF Hamburger on bun (with lettuce and tomato, 2oz meat) omit 2 starches

Vegetable Exchange (Select 2)

LSLF Baby carrots (1/2 c) LSLF Green beans (1/2 c)

Starch Exchange (Select 1)

Clam chowder (1 c) LF Dinner roll (1)
LSLF Rice (1/3 c) White bread (1 slice)
LSLF Boiled potatoes (1/2 c) Wheat bread (1 slice)
Angel food cake (1" slice) Bran bread (1 slice)
Crackers (6)

Fat Exchange (Select 1)

Margarine (1 tsp) Creamer (1 = 1/2 fat)
Diet mayonnaise (1/2 oz)

Fruit Exchange (Select 1)

Diet pears (1/2 c) Fresh fruit

Milk Exchange (Select 1)

Whole milk (1 c) omit 2 fats Buttermilk (1 c)
2% Milk (1 c) omit 1 fat Skim milk (1 c)

Calorie-free Foods

Coffee LSLF Coleslaw (1/2 c)
Decaf. coffee Tossed salad (1 c)
Hot tea Diet gelatin (1/2 c)
Decaf. hot tea Diet French
Iced tea Diet Thousand Island
Sugar substitute Diet Italian
Lemon Mustard
Herb seasoning Diet catsup

PLEASE DO NOT LEAVE MENU ON THE TRAY

NAME ______________ **ROOM** ________

For kcalorie-restricted and diabetic diets, the number of exchanges allowed is written on the menu beforehand. (This example uses a 1200-kcalorie diet.) Note that the meat exchange is written in 2-ounce portions so that 1 serving = 2 exchanges.

---

ment were to prepare baked chicken for each different diet, it would have to prepare regular baked chicken, low-fat baked chicken, low-sodium baked chicken, and low-sodium, low-fat baked chicken. Instead, only two types of baked chicken need be prepared, one with some fat and salt, the other without fat or salt. Not only is this easier for the dietary department, but it often is best for client care as well. People on special diets are often advised to limit fat, salt, and kcalories.

Keep in mind that baked chicken is only one of many menu items in a day, and you can see why preparing individual foods for each diet is not feasible. Instead, clients can add allowed items to their foods. For example, the person on a low-sodium diet could add margarine to a serving of vegetables; the person on a low-fat diet (not restricted in sodium) could add salt to a serving of rice.

Lunch

LOW-FAT/LOW CHOLESTEROL/ CARDIAC **SUNDAY**

LF = Low Fat LSLF = Low Sodium, Low Fat

Meats

LSLF Baked chicken
LSLF Baked fish (cod)
LSLF Hamburger on bun (with lettuce and tomato)

Starchy Vegetables

LSLF Rice
LSLF Boiled potatoes

Vegetables

LSLF Baby carrots
LSLF Green beans

Soup/Salad/Juice

LSLF Coleslaw
Gelatin
Tomato soup
LS Chicken broth
Tossed salad

Dressings

Diet French
Diet Thousand Island
Diet Italian

Desserts

Pears
Angel food cake
Fresh fruit

Breads

LF Dinner roll
White bread
Wheat bread
Bran bread
Crackers
LS Crackers

Beverages & Condiments

Coffee
Decaf. coffee
Hot tea
Decaf. hot tea
Iced tea
Buttermilk
Skim milk
Creamer
Sugar
Sugar substitute
Herb seasoning
Lemon
Margarine
Mustard
Diet mayonnaise
Catsup

'LEASE DO NOT LEAVE MENU ON THE TRAY

NAME ________________ **ROOM** ______

People on low-fat, low-cholesterol diets who also need kcalorie restriction receive a kcalorie-restricted menu to control portion sizes and number of servings. Both menus provide low-fat, low-cholesterol foods. Foods not appropriate for a low-fat, low-cholesterol diet, such as whole milk, would be crossed off the menu beforehand.

Lunch

LOW SODIUM **SUNDAY**

LF = Low Fat LSLF = Low Sodium, Low Fat

Meats

LSLF Baked chicken
LSLF Baked fish (cod)
LSLF Hamburger on bun (with lettuce and tomato)

Starchy Vegetables

LSLF Rice
LSLF Boiled potatoes

Vegetables

LSLF Baby carrots
LSLF Green beans

Soup/Salad/Juice

LSLF Coleslaw
LS Chicken broth
Apple juice
Tossed salad

Dressings

Diet French
Diet Thousand Island
Diet Italian

Desserts

Angel food cake
Pears
Fresh fruit

Breads

Dinner roll
White bread
Wheat bread
Bran bread
LS Crackers

Beverages & Condiments

Coffee
Decaf. coffee
Hot tea
Decaf. hot tea
Iced tea
Whole milk
2% Milk
Skim milk
Sugar
Sugar substitute
Creamer
Lemon
Herb seasoning
Margarine
Diet mustard
Diet mayonnaise
Diet catsup

NO SALT

PLEASE DO NOT LEAVE MENU ON TRAY

NAME ________________ **ROOM** ______

Low-sodium menus are similar to those provided for low-fat, low-cholesterol diets, but they eliminate high-sodium foods, such as tomato soup. The person on a low-sodium, low-fat, low-cholesterol diet selects foods from a low-fat menu with high-sodium foods crossed off beforehand. If the person is also on a low-kcalorie diet, foods would be selected from a low-kcalorie menu with high-sodium foods crossed off the menu beforehand.

Lunch

RENAL **SUNDAY**

LF = Low Fat LSLF = Low Sodium, Low Fat

Meats (2 oz)

LSLF Baked chicken
LSLF Baked fish
LSLF Hamburger on bun (with lettuce)

Starchy Vegetables

LSLF Rice
LSLF Dialyzed potatoes

Vegetables

LSLF Baby carrots
LSLF Green beans

Soup/Salad/Juice

Lemonade
LSLF Coleslaw
Tossed salad (no tomato)

Dressings

Diet French
Diet Thousand Island
Diet Italian

Desserts

Pears
Apple pie

Breads

Dinner roll
White bread
Wheat bread
Bran bread
LS Crackers

Beverages & Condiments

Coffee
Decaf. coffee
Hot tea
Decaf. hot tea
Iced tea
Sugar
Sugar substitute
Creamer
Lemon
Margarine
Diet mustard
Mayonnaise

NO SALT

PLEASE DO NOT LEAVE MENU ON THE TRAY

NAME ________________ **ROOM** ______

Renal diets must be highly individualized, and the person checking the menu has to carefully consider the client's selections and make appropriate changes when necessary.

SPECIAL MENU USES

♦

In addition to food selection, completed menus can provide valuable clues about a client's food habits. Menus (especially those of individuals on special diets) are checked by dietary personnel (often a registered dietary technician) to ensure that clients are selecting appropriate foods to meet their needs. In checking menus, the technician may notice that one person on a regular diet is selecting very little or that another is selecting too much. In another case, the technician may see that a person on a low-kcalorie diet did not omit one fat exchange when selecting 2% milk. Such problems suggest the need for intervention by a dietitian.

APPENDIX G

AIDS TO CALCULATION

Contents

Many mathematical problems have been worked out as examples at appropriate places in the text. This appendix aims to help with the use of the metric system and with problems not fully explained elsewhere.

CONVERSION FACTORS

Conversion factors are useful mathematical tools in everyday calculations, including those encountered in the study of nutrition. Skill in the use of conversion factors is especially desirable as the United States "goes metric."

A conversion factor is a fraction in which the numerator (top) and the denominator (bottom) express the same quantity in different units. For example, 2.2 pounds (lb) and 1 kilogram (kg) are equivalent; they express the same weight. The conversion factor used to change pounds to kilograms or vice versa is:

$$\frac{2.2 \text{ lb}}{1 \text{ kg}} \text{ or } \frac{1 \text{ kg}}{2.2 \text{ lb}}.$$

Because both factors equal 1, measurements can be multiplied by the factor without changing the value of the measurement. Thus the units can be changed.

To perform a conversion, use the factor with the unit you are seeking in the numerator (top) of the fraction. Following are two examples of problems commonly encountered in nutrition study; they illustrate the usefulness of conversion factors.

Example 1 Convert the weight of 130 pounds to kilograms.

1. Choose the conversion factor in which *the unit you are seeking is on top:*

$$\frac{1 \text{ kg}}{2.2 \text{ lb}}.$$

2. Multiply 130 pounds by the factor:

$$130 \not{\text{lb}} \times \frac{1 \text{ kg}}{2.2 \not{\text{lb}}} = \frac{130 \text{ kg}}{2.2} =$$

59 kg (rounded off to the nearest whole number).

Example 2 How many grams (g) of saturated fat are contained in a 3-ounce (oz) hamburger?

1. Consider a 4-ounce hamburger that contains 7 grams of saturated fat. You are seeking grams of saturated fat; therefore, the conversion factor is:

$$\frac{7 \text{ g saturated fat}}{4 \text{ oz hamburger}}.$$

2. Multiply 3 ounces of hamburger by the conversion factor:

$$3 \not{\text{oz}} \text{ hamburger} \times \frac{7 \text{ g saturated fat}}{4 \not{\text{oz}} \text{ hamburger}} =$$

$$\frac{3 \times 7}{4} = \frac{21}{4}$$

= 5 g saturated fat (rounded off to the nearest whole number).

PERCENTAGES

◆

A percentage is a comparison between a number of items (perhaps your intake of energy) and a standard number (perhaps the number of kcalories recommended for your age and sex—your energy RDA). *The standard number is the number you divide by.* The answer you get after the division must be multiplied by 100 to be stated as a percentage (*percent* means "per 100").

Example 3 What percentage of the RDA for energy is your energy intake?

1. Find your energy RDA (inside front cover, left). We'll use 2200 kcalories to demonstrate.
2. Total your energy intake for a day—for example, 1500 kcalories.
3. Divide your kcalorie intake by the RDA kcalories:

$$1500 \text{ kcal (your intake)} \div 2200 \text{ kcal (RDA)} = 0.68.$$

4. Multiply your answer by 100 to state it as a percentage:

$$0.68 \times 100 = 68 = 68\%.$$

In some problems in nutrition, the percentage may be more than 100. For example, suppose your daily intake of vitamin A is 3200 RE and your RDA (male) is 1000 RE. Your intake as a percentage of the RDA is more than 100 percent (that is, you consume more than 100 percent of your vitamin A RDA). The following calculations show your vitamin A intake as a percentage of the RDA:

$$3200 \div 1000 = 3.2.$$

$$3.2 \times 100 = 320\% \text{ of RDA}.$$

Sometimes the comparison is between a part of a whole (for example, your kcalories from protein) and the total amount (your total kcalories). In this case, *the total number is the one you divide by.*

Example 4 What percentages of your total kcalories for the day come from protein, fat, and carbohydrate?

1. Using Appendix A and your diet record, find the total grams of protein, fat, and carbohydrate you consumed—for example, 60 grams protein, 80 grams fat, and 310 grams carbohydrate.
2. Multiply the number of grams by the number of kcalories from 1 gram of each energy nutrient (conversion factors):

$$60 \text{ g protein} \times \frac{4 \text{ kcal}}{1 \text{ g protein}} = 240 \text{ kcal}.$$

$$80 \text{ g fat} \times \frac{9 \text{ kcal}}{1 \text{ g fat}} = 720 \text{ kcal}.$$

$$310 \text{ g carbohydrate} \times \frac{4 \text{ kcal}}{1 \text{ g carbohydrate}} = 1240 \text{ kcal}.$$

$$240 + 720 + 1240 = 2200 \text{ kcal}.$$

3. Find the percentage of total kcalories from each energy nutrient (see Example 3):

- Protein: $240 \div 2200 = 0.109 \times 100 = 10.9 = 11\%$ of kcal.
- Fat: $720 \div 2200 = 0.327 \times 100 = 32.7 = 33\%$ of kcal.
- Carbohydrate: $1240 \div 2200 = 0.563 \times 100 = 56.3 = 56\%$ of kcal.
- $11\% + 33\% + 56\% = 100\%$ of kcal (total).

The percentages total 100 percent, but sometimes they total 99 or 101 because of rounding off. This is a reasonable error.

G

RATIOS

◆

A ratio is a comparison of two or three values in which one of the values is reduced to 1. A ratio compares identical units and so is expressed without units. For example, Figure 8–2 in Chapter 8 compares the milligrams of potassium to the milligrams of sodium in selected foods.

Example 5 Find the potassium-to-sodium ratio of your diet.

1. Using Appendix A and your diet record, find how many milligrams of potassium and sodium you consumed, say, 3000 milligrams potassium and 2500 milligrams sodium.
2. Divide the potassium milligrams by the sodium milligrams:

$$3000 \text{ mg potassium} \div 2500 \text{ mg sodium} = 1.2.$$

3. The potassium-to-sodium ratio is usually expressed as correct to one decimal point: 1.2.

The potassium-to-sodium ratio of your diet is 1.2:1 (read as "one point two to one" or simply "one point two"). A ratio greater than 1 means that the first value (in this case, milligrams of potassium) is greater than the second (sodium). When the second value is larger, the ratio is less than 1.

WEIGHTS AND MEASURES

♦

Length

1 inch (in) = 2.54 centimeters.
1 foot (ft) = 30.48 centimeters.
1 meter (m) = 39.37 inches.

Temperature

Celsius*		Fahrenheit	
Steam	100°C	212°F	Steam
Body temperature	37°C	98.6°F	Body temperature
Ice	0°C	32°F	Ice

To find degrees Fahrenheit (t_F) when you know degrees Celsius (t_C), multiply by 9/5 and then add 32:

$$9/5\ t_C + 32 = t_F.$$

To find degrees Celcius (t_C) when you know degrees Fahrenheit (t_F), multiply by 5/9 after subtracting 32:

$$5/9\ (t_F - 32) = t_C.$$

Volume

1 liter (L) = 1.06 quarts (qt) or 0.85 imperial quart.
1 liter = 1000 milliliters (ml).
1 milliliter = 0.03 fluid ounces.
1 gallon = 3.79 liters.
1 quart = 0.95 liter or 32 fluid ounces.
1 cup (c) = 8 fluid ounces.
1 tablespoon (tbs) = 15 milliliters.
3 teaspoons (tsp) = 1 tablespoon.
1 teaspoon = about 5 grams or 5 milliliters.
16 tablespoons = 1 cup.
4 cups = 1 quart.

Weight

1 ounce (oz) = approximately 28 grams (g).
16 ounces = 1 pound (lb).
1 pound = 454 grams.
1 kilogram (kg) = 1000 grams or 2.2 pounds.
1 gram = 1000 milligrams (mg).
1 milligram = 1000 micrograms (μg).

Energy units

1 kcalorie (kcal) = 4.2 kilojoules (kJ).
1 millijoule (mJ) = 240 kcalories.
1 kilojoule = 0.24 kcalories.
1 g carbohydrate = 4 kcal = 17 kJ.
1 g fat = 9 kcal = 37 kJ.
1 g protein = 4 kcal = 17 kJ.
1 g alcohol = 7 kcal = 29 kJ.

*Also known as *centigrade.*

G

ENTERAL FORMULAS

The staggering number of enteral formulas available allows health care professionals to meet a variety of their clients' medical needs, but also complicates the process of selecting an appropriate formula. This appendix provides some examples of enteral formulas, but the list is by no means complete. Each formula is listed only once, although the formula may have more than one use. A high-protein or high-fiber formula, for example, may also be isotonic. The information provided reflects the manufacturers' literature and does not suggest endorsement by the authors. Be aware that the composition of formulas changes periodically. Health care professionals (most frequently registered dietitians) must consult manufacturers' current literature before selecting a formula. Addresses of formula manufacturers listed in this appendix can be found in Appendix D (see Trade Organizations). The following products are listed in this appendix with permission from the manufacturers:

- Clintec Nutrition Company[a]
  - Entrition HN®
  - Nutren® 1.0
  - Nutren® 1.0 with Fiber
  - Nutren® 1.5
  - Nutren® 2.0
  - NutriHep™
  - NutriVent®
  - Peptamen®
  - Replete®
  - Replete® with Fiber
  - Travasorb HN®
  - Travasorb® MCT
  - Travasorb Renal®
  - Travasorb Standard®
- Elan Pharma[b]
  - Fiberlan®
  - Isolan®
  - Nitrolan®
  - Reabilan® HN
  - Ultralan®
- McGaw, Inc.[c]
  - Amin-Aid®
  - Hepatic-Aid II®
  - Immun-Aid®
- Mead Johnson Enteral Nutritionals[d]
  - Casec®
  - Criticare HN®
  - Isocal®
  - Isocal HCN®
  - Isocal® HN
  - Lipisorb®
  - MCT Oil®
  - Moducal®
  - Respalor™
  - Sustacal Liquid®
  - Sustacal HC®
  - TraumaCal®
  - Ultracal®
- Ross Laboratories[e]
  - Advera™
  - Allitraq®
  - Ensure®
  - Ensure® with Fiber
  - Ensure Plus HN®
  - Ensure Plus®
  - Glucerna®
  - Jevity®
  - Nepro™
  - Osmolite®
  - Osmolite® HN
  - Polycose Liquid®
  - Polycose Powder®
  - PediaSure®
  - Perative®
  - Pro Mod®
  - Pulmocare®
  - Suplena®
  - TwoCal HN®
  - Vital HN®
- Sandoz Nutrition[f]
  - Compleat® Modified
  - Compleat® Regular
  - Fibersource®
  - Fibersource® HN
  - Impact®
  - Impact® with Fiber
  - Isosource®
  - Isosource® HN
  - Isotein® HN
  - Resource Plus®
  - Tolerex®
  - Vivonex Plus®
- Sherwood Medical[g]
  - Accupep HPF®
  - Attain®
  - Comply®
  - Magnacal®
  - Microlipid®
  - Profiber®
  - Propac®
  - Protain XL®
  - Sumacal®

---

[a]*Enteral Product Guide* (December 1992) and *Nutrihep™ Information and Usage Guide* (September 1993), Clintec Nutrition Company, Deerfield, IL 60015.

[b]*Innovative Enteral Formulas* (1992), Elan Pharma, Cambridge, MA 02141.

[c]*Enteral Nutrition Products Ready Reference* (provided November 1993), McGaw Inc., Irvine, CA 92714.

[d]*Product Handbook* (1992), *A Lower Fat Alternate for Respiratory Patients* (1993), and *Lipisorb Ready-to-Use* (1992), Mead Johnson Enteral Nutritionals, Evansville, IN 47721.

[e]*Product Handbook* (July 1993) and *Features of Advera™ Specialized Complete Nutrition,* Ross Products Division, Abbott Laboratories, Columbus, OH 43216.

[f]*Enteral Products and Services Guide* (1992) and *Vivonex Plus®* (1993), Sandoz Nutrition, Minneapolis, MN 55440.

[g]*Enteral Formulas* (1991) and *Enteral Formula Comparison Chart* (1993), Sherwood Medical, St. Louis, MO 63103.

Table H–1
Enteral Formulas

Product	Form	Volume to Meet 100% RDI (ml)	Energy (kcal/ml)	Protein or Amino Acids (g/L)	Carbohydrate (g/L)	Fat (g/L)	Osmolality (mOsm/kg)	Notes
Intact Formulas: Isotonic or Near-Isotonic Formulas								
Attain®	liquid	1250	1.00	40	135	35	300	Lactose-free, low-residue, 50% fat from MCT
Compleat® Modified	liquid	1500	1.07	43	140	37	300	Lactose-free
Isocal®	liquid	1890	1.06	34	135	44	270	Lactose-free, low-residue, 20% fat from MCT
Isolan®	liquid	1250	1.06	40	144	36	300	Lactose-free
Isosource®	liquid	1500	1.20	43	170	41	360	Lactose-free, low-residue, 50% fat from MCT
Nutren® 1.0	liquid	1500	1.00	40	127	38	300	Lactose-free, low-residue, 24% fat from MCT
Osmolite®	liquid	1887	1.06	37	145	38	300	Lactose-free, low-residue, 20% fat from MCT
Intact Formulas: Standard, Low- to Moderate-Residue Formulas[a]								
Ensure®	liquid	1887	1.06	37	145	37	470	Lactose-free, low-residue
Sustacal®	liquid	1080	1.01	61	140	23	650	Lactose-free, low-residue
Intact Formulas: Standard, Fiber-Containing Formulas								
Compleat® Regular	liquid	1500	1.07	43	130	43	450	Blenderized formula, contains lactose, 4.3 g fiber/1000 ml
Ensure® with Fiber	liquid	1530	1.10	40	162	37	480	Lactose-free, 14 g fiber/1000 ml
Fiberlan®	liquid	1250	1.20	50	160	40	310	Near-isotonic, lactose-free, 14 g fiber/1000 ml
Fibersource®	liquid	1500	1.20	43	170	41	390	Lactose-free, 10 g fiber/1000 ml
Impact® with Fiber	liquid	1500	1.00	56	140	28	375	Lactose-free, 10 g fiber/1000 ml
Jevity®	liquid	1325	1.06	44	152	36	300	Isotonic, lactose-free, 14 g fiber/1000 ml
Nutren® 1.0 with Fiber	liquid	1500	1.00	40	127	38	303	Near-isotonic, lactose-free, 14 g fiber/1000 ml
Profiber®	liquid	1500	1.00	40	132	40	300	Isotonic, lactose-free, 12 g fiber/1000 ml
Replete® with Fiber	liquid	1000	1.00	63	113	34	300	Isotonic, lactose-free, 14 g fiber/1000 ml
Ultracal®	liquid	1250	1.06	44	123	45	310	Lactose-free, 14.4 g fiber/1000 ml

[a]All formulas listed under "Intact Formulas: Isotonic or Near-Isotonic Formulas" can be used as a standard, low- to moderate-residue formula.

Table H–1 (*continued*)

Product	Form	Volume to Meet 100% RDI (ml)	Energy (kcal/ml)	Protein or Amino Acids (g/L)	Carbohydrate (g/L)	Fat (g/L)	Osmolality (mOsm/kg)	Notes
Hydrolyzed Formulas								
Accupep HPF®	powder	1600	1.00	40	188	10	490	Lactose-free, low-residue
Criticare HN®	liquid	1890	1.06	38	220	5	650	Lactose-free, low-residue
Peptamen®	liquid	1500	1.00	40	127	39	270	Near-isotonic, lactose-free, low-residue
Tolerex®	powder	3160	1.00	21	230	1.5	550	Lactose-free, low-residue, contains arginine and glutamine
Travasorb Standard®	liquid	1900	1.06	35	136	35	488	Lactose-free, low-residue
Vital HN®	powder	1500	1.00	42	185	11	500	Lactose-free, low-residue
Vivonex Plus®	powder	1800	1.00	45	190	7	650	Lactose-free, low-residue, 100% free amino acids, contains arginine and glutamine
Special-Use Formulas: High-kCalorie, High-Protein Formulas								
Comply®	liquid	1000	1.50	60	180	60	410	Lactose-free
Ensure Plus HN®	liquid	1136	1.50	63	200	50	650	Lactose-free
Ensure Plus®	liquid	1704	1.50	55	200	53	690	Lactose-free
Isocal HCN®	liquid	1000	2.00	75	200	102	640	Lactose-free, 30% fat from MCT
Magnacal®	liquid	1000	2.00	70	250	80	590	Lactose-free
Nutren® 1.5	liquid	1000	1.50	60	170	68	410	Lactose-free, 48% fat from MCT
Nutren® 2.0	liquid	750	2.00	80	196	106	710	Lactose-free, 73% fat from MCT
Reabilan® HN	liquid	2222	1.33	58	158	52	490	Partially hydrolyzed formula, lactose-free
Resource Plus®	liquid	1600	1.50	55	200	53	600	Lactose-free
Sustacal HC®	liquid	1800	1.50	61	190	58	650	Lactose-free
TraumaCal®	liquid	1500	1.50	82	142	68	490	Lactose-free, 30% fat from MCT
TwoCal HN®	liquid	947	2.00	84	217	91	690	Lactose-free, 20% fat form MCT
Ultralan®	liquid	1000	1.50	60	202	20	540	Lactose-free, 50% fat from MCT
Special-Use Formulas: High-Nitrogen (Protein) Formulas								
Entrition HN®	liquid	1300	1.00	44	114	41	300	Isotonic, lactose-free, low-residue
Fibersource HN®	liquid	1500	1.20	53	160	41	390	Lactose-free, 7 g fiber/1000 ml
Isocal HN®	liquid	1250	1.06	44	124	45	270	Near-isotonic, lactose-free, low residue
Isosource HN®	liquid	1500	1.20	53	160	41	330	Near-isotonic, lactose-free, low residue
Isotein® HN	powder	1770	1.20	68	160	34	300	Isotonic, lactose-free
Nitrolan®	liquid	1250	1.24	60	160	40	310	Near-isotonic, lactose-free
Osmolite® HN	liquid	1321	1.06	44	141	36	300	Lactose-free, low-residue
Replete®	liquid	1500	1.00	63	113	33	350	Near-isotonic, lactose-free, low-residue
Travasorb HN®	powder	2000	1.00	45	175	14	560	Hydrolyzed formula, lactose-free, low-residue

Table H-1 (*continued*)

Product	Form	Volume to Meet 100% RDI (ml)	Energy (kcal/ml)	Protein or Amino Acids (g/L)	Carbohydrate (g/L)	Fat (g/L)	Osmolality (mOsm/kg)	Notes
Special-Use Formulas: Hepatic Insufficiency Formulas								
Hepatic-Aid II®	powder	—	1.20	44	169	36	560	Free amino acids with 46% protein as branched-chain amino acids, lactose-free, no added vitamins or electrolytes
NutriHep™	liquid	1000	1.50	40	290	21	690	Partially hydrolyzed formula with 50% protein as branched-chain amino acids, 66% fat from MCT, contains vitamins and electrolytes
Special-Use Formulas: Renal Insufficiency Formulas								
Amin-Aid®	powder	—	2.00	19	366	46	700	Free amino acids, lactose-free, no added vitamins, minimal electrolytes; intended for use in renal failure
Nepro™	liquid	—	2.00	70	215	96	635	Lactose-free, low in electrolytes; intended for use once dialysis has been instituted
Suplena®	liquid	—	2.00	30	255	96	600	Lactose-free, low in electrolytes; intended for use in renal disease before dialysis is instituted
Travasorb Renal®	powder	—	1.35	23	271	18	590	Free amino acids, lactose-free, does not contain fat-soluble vitamins or electrolytes
Special-Use Formulas: Respiratory Insufficiency Formulas								
NutriVent®	liquid	1000	1.50	68	101	95	450	Lactose-free, 55% kcal from fat, 40% fat from MCT
Pulmocare®	liquid	947	1.50	63	106	93	490	Lactose-free, 55% kcal from fat, 20% fat from MCT
Respalor™	liquid	1520	1.52	76	148	71	580	Lactose-free, 41% kcal from fat, 30% fat from MCT

Table H–1 (*continued*)

Product	Form	Volume to Meet 100% RDI (ml)	Energy (kcal/ml)	Protein or Amino Acids (g/L)	Carbohydrate (g/L)	Fat (g/L)	Osmolality (mOsm/kg)	Notes
Special-Use Formulas: Severe Stress Formulas								
Allitraq®	powder	1500	1.00	53	165	16	575	Partially hydrolyzed formula with some free amino acids, contains glutamine and arginine; intended to protect immunocompetence during metabolic stress
Immun-Aid®	powder	2000	1.00	80	120	22	460	Enriched with arginine, glutamine, branched-chain amino acids, nucleic acids, and omega-3 fatty acids; intended to protect immunocompetence during metabolic stress
Impact®	liquid	1500	1.00	56	130	28	375	Lactose-free, enriched with arginine, nucleic acids, and omega-3 fatty acids; intended to protect immunocompetence during metabolic stress
Perative®	liquid	1155	1.30	67	177	37	385	Partially hydrolyzed, low-lactose, contains arginine, enriched with nutrients associated with wound healing
Protain XL®	liquid	1250	1.00	55	138	30	340	Enriched with nutrients associated with wound healing, 8 g fiber/1000 ml
Special-Use Formulas: Other								
Advera™	liquid	1184	1.28	60	216	23	680	Lactose-free, partially hydrolyzed; intended for use in HIV infection or AIDS
Glucerna®	liquid	1422	1.00	42	94	56	375	Low-carbohydrate, 14 g fiber/1000 ml; intended for use in glucose intolerance
Lipisorb®	liquid powder[b]	1600	1.35	43	42	119	630	Lactose-free, 85% fat from MCT; intended for use in severe fat malabsorption
PediaSure®	liquid	1000	1.00	30	110	50	310	Virtually lactose-free; intended for use with children ages 1 to 6
Travasorb® MCT	powder	2000	1.00	50	123	33	250	Lactose-free, 80% fat from MCT; intended for use in severe fat malabsorption

[b]Information for liquid preparation.

Table H-2
Enteral Formulas—Protein Modules

Product	Form	Major Protein Source	Energy (kcal/g)	Protein (g/100 g)
Casec®	powder	Calcium caseinate	3.7	88
Pro Mod®	powder	Whey protein	5.6	100
Propac®	powder	Whey protein	4.0	395

Table H-3
Enteral Formulas—Carbohydrate Modules

Product	Form	Major Carbohydrate Source	Energy (kcal/ml or g)	Carbohydrate (g/100 kcal)
Moducal®	powder	Hydrolyzed corn starch	3.8 kcal/g	25
Polycose Liquid®	liquid	Hydrolyzed corn starch	2.0 kcal/ml	25
Polycose Powder®	powder	Hydrolyzed corn starch	3.8 kcal/g	25
Sumacal®	powder	Maltodextrin	3.8 kcal/g	25

Table H-4
Enteral Formulas—Fat Modules

Product	Form	Major Fat Source	Energy (kcal/ml)	Fat (g/100 ml)	Notes
MCT Oil®	liquid	Coconut oil	7.7	87	84% fat from MCT
Microlipid®	liquid	Safflower oil	4.5	50	

GLOSSARY

Where these terms are defined in the margins of the chapters, their pronunciations are also given. The alphabetical order followed here ignores hyphens (for example, *iron-deficiency anemia* falls between *iron deficiency* and *iron overload*).

1,25-dihydroxycholecalciferol: active vitamin D, also known as dihydroxy vitamin D.

22 oxa calcitriol: an experimental form of active vitamin D used in the treatment of renal disease.

24-hour recall: a record of foods eaten by a person for one 24-hour period, used in nutrition status assessment.

7-dehydrocholesterol: the precursor of vitamin D made in the liver.

abscess: an accumulation of pus, caused by a local infection, that builds up and may eventually burst.

accidental additives: see *incidental additives.*

acesulfame potassium: a low-kcalorie sweetener; also known as *acesulfame-K.*

acetone breath: the distinctive, fruity odor of acetone, which can be detected on the breath of a person who is experiencing ketosis.

acetyl CoA: a nickname for a molecule of acetate attached to coenzyme A, a common intermediate in many metabolic reactions.

acid-base balance: the balance maintained between acid and base concentrations in the blood and body fluids.

acidosis: too much acid in the blood and body fluids.

acids: compounds that release hydrogen ions in a solution.

acquired immune deficiency syndrome (AIDS): the end stage of HIV infection, in which severe complications are manifested.

acquired immunity: immunity directed at specific organisms, also called *specific immunity.*

acute malnutrition: severe, rapid-onset protein-energy malnutrition; hypoalbuminemic PEM; kwashiorkor.

acute phase (of the stress response, also called *flow phase*): the catabolic period immediately following the onset of stress.

adaptive phase (of the stress response): the period during which the body adjusts to the stress to minimize losses.

adaptogens: see *plant sterols.*

additives: substances that are not normally consumed as foods by themselves, but are added to foods.

adequacy (dietary): the characteristic of a diet that provides all the essential nutrients, fiber, and energy necessary to maintain health and body weight.

ADH (antidiuretic hormone): a hormone released by the pituitary gland in response to high osmotic pressure of the blood, which prompts the kidneys to reabsorb water.

adipose tissue: the body's fat, which consists of masses of fat-storing cells called *adipose cells.*

administrative dietitian: a dietitian whose primary duty is to manage a foodservice system.

adult bone loss: see *osteoporosis.*

adult-onset diabetes: see *noninsulin-dependent diabetes mellitus.*

adult rickets: see *osteomalacia.*

aerobic: involving oxygen; in describing metabolism this term refers to energy-producing processes that require the immediate use of oxygen.

aerobic training: physical training designed to condition the body to perform oxygen-demanding activities; endurance training: see also *cardiorespiratory conditioning.*

afebrile: without fever.

AGA: see *appropriate for gestational age.*

agility: a skill-related component of fitness, the ability to move the entire body quickly.

AIDS: see *acquired immune deficiency syndrome.*

AIDS enteropathies: the diarrhea and malabsorption symptoms associated with AIDS.

AIDS-related complex (ARC): the cluster of mild symptoms that sometimes occurs early in the course of the disease AIDS.

albuminuria: albumin in the urine: see also *microalbuminuria.*

alimentary hypoglycemia: the type of hypoglycemia that occurs following gastric surgery; also called *postgastrectomy hypoglycemia.*

alitame: a compound of two amino acids (alanine and aspartic acid) that is used as an artificial sweetener.

alkalosis: the condition in which the blood and body fluids are too basic.

all-in-one admixture: a TPN solution that contains all nutrients, including fat.

alpha-lactalbumin: the chief protein in human breast milk.

alpha TE (alpha tocopherol equivalents): the units in which vitamin E is measured.

alveoli: air sacs in the lungs; one sac is an *alveolus.*

Alzheimer's disease: a degenerative disease of the brain involving memory loss and major structural changes in the brain's nerve cells.

amino acids: the building blocks of protein.

amniotic sac: the "bag of waters" in the uterus, in which the fetus floats.

amylase: an enzyme that splits amylose (a form of starch).

anabolism: those metabolic reactions in which small molecules are put together to build larger ones; energy-consuming reactions.

anemia: a condition in which the blood is unable to carry oxygen normally.

anemia of infection: the type of anemia caused by infection, in which iron moves from the blood to the liver, becoming unavailable to infective microorganisms and resulting in a decline in hemoglobin synthesis.

anorexia nervosa: an eating disorder involving a marked fear of fatness, self-starvation to the extreme, and a disturbed perception of body image.

anthropometric: relating to measurement of the physical characteristics of the body, such as height and weight.

antibiotics: anti-infective agents that kill bacteria.

antibodies: large proteins of the blood and body fluids, produced by the immune system in response to invasion by unfamiliar molecules (mostly proteins).

antidiuretic hormone: see *ADH.*

antifungal agents: anti-infective agents that kill fungi.

anti-infective (or antimicrobial) agents: drugs that kill microorganisms or interfere with their growth; also, substances used as food additives to prevent growth of illness-causing microorganisms in foods.

antioxidants: compounds that protect other compounds from oxygen by themselves reacting with oxygen.

antipromoters: factors (found in foods) that oppose the development of cancer.

antiviral agents: anti-infective agents that kill viruses.

anuria: no urine excretion.

anus: the terminal sphincter muscle of the GI tract.

appendix: a narrow blind sac extending from the beginning of the colon; a vestigial organ with no known function.

appetite: the psychological desire to eat, a learned reaction to the sight, smell, or thought of appealing foods, a pleasant sensation.

appropriate for gestational age (AGA): description of the weight of an infant born early but of normal size for age: see also *small for gestational age.*

ARC: see *AIDS-related complex.*

arginine: a nonessential amino acid, promoted as an ergogenic aid because it is a precursor of the high-energy compound phosphocreatine.

arteriosclerosis: a general term for all conditions in which the arteries lose elasticity; atherosclerosis is the most common of these conditions.

artery: a vessel that carries blood from the heart to body tissues.

arthritis: inflammation (usually painful) and often altered structure of a joint caused by many conditions, including infections, metabolic disturbances, or injury.

artificial colors: certified food colors, added to enhance appearance (*certified* means approved by the Food and Drug Administration).

artificial feeding: parenteral or enteral nutrition; feeding by a route other than normal eating.

artificial flavors: food additives that mimic natural flavors.

artificial sweeteners: alternative sweeteners that are noncarbohydrate, noncaloric, and synthetic; also called *nonnutritive sweeteners.*

ascites: edema in the abdominal cavity.

ascorbic acid: one of two active forms of vitamin C; the other is *dehydroascorbic acid.*

aspartame: an artificial sweetener; a compound of two amino acids (phenylalanine and aspartic acid).

aspiration: the inhaling of food or liquid into the lungs.

asterixis: uncontrolled movement of the muscle group that causes the outstretched arm and hand to flap like a wing, which occurs in hepatic coma and other diseases that cause encephalopathy; also called *flapping tremor.*

atheromatous plaques: see *plaques.*

atherosclerosis: the main form of cardiovascular disease, characterized by arterial blockages caused by plaques.

attention deficit hyperactivity disorder: see *hyperactivity.*

azotemia: excess nitrogen-containing substances in the blood (blood urea nitrogen).

B-cells: lymphocytes that produce antibodies.

balance (dietary): providing foods of a number of types in balance with one another such that foods rich in one nutrient do not crowd out foods that are rich in another nutrient; also (in fitness), the ability to maintain equilibrium in a fixed position or in motion.

basal metabolism: the energy needed to maintain life when a person is at complete rest after a 12-hour fast; sometimes called *basal metabolic rate (BMR).*

bases: compounds that accept hydrogen ions in a solution.

bedsores: see *decubitus ulcers.*

bee pollen: a product consisting of bee saliva, plant nectar, and pollen falsely promoted as of benefit to athletes.

behavior modification: the changing of behavior by the manipulation of *antecedents* (cues or environmental factors that trigger behavior), the behavior itself, and *consequences* (the penalties or rewards attached to behavior).

benign: causing no harm, used to describe tumors that pose no threat to life.

beriberi: the thiamin-deficiency disease.

beta-carotene: a vitamin A precursor made by plants and stored in human fat tissue; an orange pigment.

bicarbonate: an alkaline secretion of the pancreas; part of the pancreatic juice. (Bicarbonate also occurs widely in all cell fluids.)

bifidus factors: factors in colostrum and breast milk that favor the growth of the "friendly" bacteria *Lactobacillus bifidus* in the infant's intestinal tract and so help prevent other less desirable intestinal inhabitants from flourishing.

bile: an emulsifier that prepares fats and oils for digestion; made by the liver, stored in the gallbladder, and released into the small intestine when needed.

bile duct: the duct through which the gallbladder squirts bile into the duodenum.

bilirubin: a bile pigment.

bioaccumulation: the accumulation of toxins in living tissues at concentrations that increase at higher levels of the food chain.

bioelectrical impedance: a method for estimating body fat using low-intensity electrical current.

bland diet: a diet that excludes gastric irritants (such as alcohol and caffeine) and foods according to individual tolerances.

blind loop syndrome: the cluster of symptoms that results from the overgrowth of bacteria in a surgically bypassed segment of the intestine—notably, fat malabsorption and vitamin B_{12} and folate deficiencies.

blood doping: the process of harvesting, storing, and later reinjecting a person's own red blood cells to enhance the blood's oxygen-carrying ability in an athletic event; a dangerous and illegal procedure.

BMI: see *body mass index.*

BMR: see *basal metabolism.*

body composition: the proportions of muscle, bone, fat, and other tissue that make up a person's total body weight.

body mass index (BMI): an index of a person's weight, used in assessment of nutrition status, determined by dividing the weight (in kilograms) by the square of the height (in meters).

bolus: the portion of food swallowed at one time.

bolus feeding: delivery of up to 400 milliliters of an enteral formula within 10 minutes or less.

bone marrow transplant: the replacement of a person's diseased bone marrow with healthy bone marrow from a donor; used as a treatment for breast cancer and for leukemia and other blood disorders.

botulism: food poisoning caused by botulin toxin, a toxin produced by bacteria that grow without oxygen in nonacidic canned foods.

branched-chain amino acids: the amino acids leucine, isoleucine, and valine, which are present in large amounts in skeletal muscle tissue; also a product falsely promoted as of benefit to athletes.

bronchioles: the small air passages from the trachea to the lungs.

bronchitis: inflammation of the lungs' air passages.

brown sugar: refined white sugar crystals to which manufacturers have added molasses syrup.

buffers: compounds that can reversibly combine with hydrogen ions to help keep a solution's acidity or alkalinity constant.

bulimia nervosa: an eating disorder characterized by recurring binge eating combined with a morbid fear of becoming fat, and sometimes followed by self-induced vomiting or purging.

bypass surgery: see *intestinal bypass surgery.*

cachectin: a cytokine that induces anorexia.

caffeine: a stimulant that occurs naturally in many plants, including coffee and tea; falsely promoted as of benefit to athletes.

calcitriol: active vitamin D.

calcium pangamate: a salt of calcium, once thought to enhance aerobic metabolism, now known to have no such effect but falsely promoted as of benefit to athletes.

calcium rigor: hardness or stiffness of the muscles caused by high blood calcium.

calcium tetany: intermittent spasms of the extremities due to nervous and muscular excitability caused by low blood calcium.

calorie: see *kcalorie.*

calorie-free: as used on labels, a term that means a food contains fewer than 5 kcalories per serving.

cancer: a disease in which abnormal cells multiply out of control and disrupt the normal functioning of the body's organs.

cancer cachexia: a syndrome that accompanies many types of cancer, characterized by anorexia, inadequate food intake, malnutrition, accelerated metabolism, wasting, and general ill health.

candidiasis: a fungal infection of the mouth caused by *Candida albicans,* sometimes called *thrush.*

capillary: a small vessel that branches from an artery and connects to a vein.

carbohydrates: energy nutrients and fibers composed of monosaccharides—notably, sugars, starch, glycogen, and cellulose.

carcinogen: a cancer-initiating substance or type of radiation.

cardiac: pertaining to the heart.

cardiac cachexia: chronic protein-energy malnutrition that develops as a consequence of heart disease, in which peripheral tissues fail to receive enough nutrients.

cardiac sphincter: the sphincter muscle that controls the junction between the esophagus and the stomach.

cardiomegaly: enlargement of the heart.

cardiorespiratory conditioning: the strong heart and lung function and large blood volume brought about by aerobic training.

cardiorespiratory endurance: the ability to perform large-muscle, dynamic exercise of moderate to high intensity exercise for prolonged periods.

cardiovascular disease (CVD): a general term for all diseases of the heart and blood vessels. Common forms of CVD are *atherosclerosis, hypertension,* and *coronary heart disease.*

carnitine: an organic compound found in most body cells that serves as a carrier of unoxidized fatty acids, falsely promoted as of benefit to athletes.

carrier: in genetics, a term that refers to an individual who possesses one dominant and one recessive gene for a recessive trait, such as an inborn error of metabolism. Such a person may show no signs of the trait but can pass it on.

casein: the chief protein in cow's milk.

catabolism: those metabolic reactions in which large molecules are broken down to smaller ones; energy-releasing reactions.

catalyst: a compound that facilitates chemical reactions without itself being changed in the process.

cathartic: a strong laxative.

celiac disease: a sensitivity to gliadin that causes flattening of the intestinal villi and generalized malabsorption; also called *gluten-sensitive enteropathy* or *celiac sprue.*

celiac sprue: see *celiac disease.*

cell-mediated immunity: immunity that is conferred by the T-cells, which attack antigens directly.

cell salts: a preparation of minerals supposedly harvested from living cells, sold as a health-promoting supplement and falsely promoted as of benefit to athletes.

central obesity: excess fat on the abdomen and around the trunk of the body.

central total parenteral nutrition (central TPN): a method of meeting all nutrient needs by infusing formulas into large-diameter central veins.

central veins: the large-diameter veins located close to the heart.

cerebral thrombosis: blockage by a growing clot of a vessel that feeds the brain: see also *embolism, thrombosis.*

CHD: see *coronary heart disease.*

cheilosis: cracks at the corners of the mouth, which can be a symptom of malnutrition.

chemotherapy: the use of drugs (chemotherapeutic or antineoplastic agents) to arrest or destroy cancer cells.

CHF: see *congestive heart failure.*

chronic malnutrition: long-term malnutrition; marasmus.

chronic obstructive pulmonary diseases (COPD): disorders that cause blockage of the lungs' air passages and thus interfere with the exchange of gases between the air and the body.

chylomicrons: the lipoproteins that transport lipids from the intestinal cells into the body.

chyme: the semiliquid mass of partly digested food expelled by the stomach into the duodenum.

cirrhosis: advanced liver disease, in which liver cells turn orange, die, and harden, permanently losing their function.

clinical dietitian: a dietitian responsible for direct client care—assessing nutrition needs, developing and implementing nutrition care plans, and evaluating and reporting the results.

clinically severe obesity: obesity defined by a BMI of 40 or greater or 100 pounds or more overweight for an average adult; formerly called *morbid obesity.*

CoA: a nickname for coenzyme A, a small molecule that serves as a coenzyme in metabolism.

coenzyme: a small molecule that works with an enzyme to promote the enzyme's activity. Many coenzymes have B vitamins as part of their structure.

coenzyme Q10: a lipid found in cells (mitochondria) shown to improve exercise performance in heart disease patients, but not effective in improving performance of healthy athletes.

cofactor: a mineral element that, like a coenzyme, works with an enzyme to facilitate a chemical reaction.

collaterals: small blood vessels that develop to carry blood flow around an obstructed organ; also called *shunts.*

colostrum: a milklike fluid produced by the breast during the first day or so after delivery, before milk appears; it is rich in protective factors.

collagen: the predominant structural protein of connective tissue.

colon or large intestine: the last portion of the intestine, which absorbs water.

colostomy: a surgical procedure in which part of the colon is removed and the remaining part is joined to the abdominal wall via a stoma.

coma: a state of deep unconsciousness from which a person cannot be aroused.

comatose: in a coma.

competent: having sufficient mental

ability to understand a treatment, to weigh its risks and benefits, and to comprehend the consequences of refusing or accepting the treatment.

complementary proteins: two or more proteins whose amino acid assortments complement each other in such a way that the essential amino acids missing from each are supplied by the other.

complete formula: a liquid formula that, when given in sufficient volume, supplies all the nutrients a person needs.

complete protein: a protein that contains all the amino acids essential in human nutrition in proportions suitable for human use.

complex carbohydrates: long chains of monosaccharides arranged as starch or fiber; also called *polysaccharides.*

compulsive overeating: an eating disorder characterized by repeated episodes of uncontrolled overeating without other symptoms of eating disorders.

conditionally essential amino acid: a normally nonessential amino acid that must be supplied by the diet when the need for it becomes greater than the body's ability to produce it.

conditioning: the physical effect of training; improved flexibility, strength, and endurance.

confectioners' sugar: finely powdered sucrose; 99.9 percent pure.

congestive heart failure (CHF): a form of cardiovascular disease in which the heart can no longer adequately pump blood through the circulatory system.

continuous feeding: delivery of an enteral formula continuously over a period of 8 to 24 hours.

contracture: tightening of the skin at the scarred site of a burn wound, which may pull the area surrounding a joint into a nonfunctional position.

cool-down: five to ten minutes of light exercise used following a vigorous workout to allow the body's core to gradually cool to near-normal temperature.

coordination: a skill-related component of fitness, the harmonious functioning of the senses and the muscles to accurately perform complex movements, such as hitting a baseball or juggling.

COPD: see *chronic obstructive pulmonary diseases.*

corn sweeteners: corn syrup and sugars derived from corn.

corn syrup: a syrup produced by the action of enzymes on cornstarch, containing mostly glucose: see also *high-fructose corn syrup.*

cornea: the hard, transparent membrane covering the outside of the eye.

coronary embolism: sudden blockage by an embolus of an artery that feeds the heart muscle.

coronary heart disease (CHD): that form of cardiovascular disease that is characterized by atherosclerosis in the arteries that feed the heart muscle.

coronary thrombosis: blockage by a growing clot of a vessel that feeds the heart muscle: see also *thrombosis.*

cretinism: an iodine-deficiency disease characterized by mental and physical retardation.

crib death: see *sudden infant death syndrome.*

Crohn's disease: inflammation and ulceration along the length of the GI tract, often with granulomas; also called *regional ileitis.*

cruciferous vegetables: a group of vegetables that includes cauliflower, broccoli, and brussels sprouts, named for their cross-shaped blossoms. They have been shown to protect against cancer in laboratory animals.

CVD: see *cardiovascular disease.*

cyclamate: an artificial sweetener.

cyclic parenteral nutrition: the periodic administration of standard TPN solution.

cystic fibrosis: a hereditary disorder characterized by the production of thick mucus that affects many organs, including the pancreas, lungs, liver, heart, gallbladder, and small intestine.

cystinuria: cystine in the urine, the symptom of an inherited metabolic disorder.

cytokines: proteins secreted by phagocytes that activate metabolic and immune responses to infections and tumors and may also lead to the development of cancer cachexia.

Daily Food Guide: a plan for ensuring dietary adequacy that offers five categories of foods to choose from: grains, fruits, vegetables, milk and milk products, and meat and meat alternates.

Daily Reference Values (DRV): suggested daily intakes developed for food labels for nutrients and food components (such as fat and fiber) that have important relationships with health, but do not have RDA values; used in turn to develop the *Daily Values.*

Daily Values: reference values developed specifically for food labels. The Daily Values consist of two sets of standards: the Daily Reference Values (DRV) and the Reference Daily Intakes (RDI).

dawn phenomenon: early-morning hyperglycemia that develops in IDDM in response to the release of glucose by the liver after an overnight fast.

deamination: in metabolism, the removal of the amino (NH_2) group from a compound such as an amino acid.

death: permanent cessation of vital functions.

debridement: a medical procedure used to remove the eschar from a burn wound so that the wound can close as quickly as possible.

decubitus ulcers: ulcers caused by the breakdown of skin and underlying tissues where pressure and lack of oxygen have affected an area of skin; often called *pressure sores* or *bedsores.*

dehydration: body water depletion, which occurs whenever when water output exceeds water input.

Dehydroascorbic acid: see *ascorbic acid.*

DEJ: see *direct endoscopic jejunostomy.*

delusions: inappropriate beliefs not consistent with an individual's own knowledge and experience.

dementia: irreversible loss of mental function.

denaturation: the change in a protein's shape brought about by heat, acid, or other agents.

dental caries: the gradual decay and disintegration of a tooth.

dental soft diet: see *mechanical soft diet.*

dextrins: short chains of glucose units that result during digestion from the breakdown of starch; also, additives used as thickening agents in foods.

dextrose: a form of glucose that is especially soluble in water (and is, therefore, used in IV solutions).

DHA: a 20-carbon omega-3 fatty acid derived from linolenic acid. The full name for DHA is *docosahexaenoic acid.*

diabetes mellitus: a metabolic disorder characterized by altered blood glucose regulation and utilization usually caused by insufficient or relatively ineffective insulin: see also *insulin-dependent diabetes mellitus* and *noninsulin-dependent diabetes mellitus.*

diabetic coma: unconsciousness precipitated by ketosis in uncontrolled diabetes.

dialysis: a medical procedure used to filter wastes out of the blood using the principles of simple diffusion and osmosis through a semipermeable membrane: see also *hemodialysis* and *peritoneal dialysis.*

diet, dietetic: as used on labels, terms that indicate that a food is either a *low-calorie* or a *reduced-calorie* food.

diet history: a record of the foods a person eats, taken using a 24-hour recall form, a food frequency checklist, a food record, or a food diary; and used in nutrition status assessment.

diet manual: a book that describes the foods allowed and restricted on different diets, the rationale and indications for use of each diet, and sample menus.

diet order: a physician's written statement in the medical record of what diet a client should receive.

diet pills: pills used to depress the appetite temporarily.

dietetic technician registered (DTR): a technically skilled person with an associate's degree who meets the American Dietetic Association's (ADA's) educational standards, and who assists a registered dietitian.

dietetics: the practical application of nutrition, including the assessment of nutrition status, recommendation of appropriate diets, nutrition education, and the planning and serving of meals.

digitalis glycosides: drugs used to increase the strength of the heart's contractions.

dihydroxy vitamin D: active vitamin D, also known as *1,25-dihydroxycholecalciferol.*

dioxins: toxic organic compounds containing chlorine, arising in industry as (among other things) by-products of the bleaching process.

dipeptide: two amino acids bonded together.

direct calorimetry: an estimation of energy output based on measures of heat output.

direct endoscopic jejunostomy (DEJ): a surgical technique used to create an opening for a feeding tube directly into the jejunum.

disaccharide: a pair of monosaccharides bonded together.

dithiolthiones: a class of nonnutrient compounds important in connection with diet and cancer because some are found in plant foods and seem to exhibit anticancer activity.

diuretic: a drug that promotes renal water excretion.

diuretic abuse: use of diuretics not to promote water excretion but to promote weight loss.

diuretic phase (in renal failure): the late phase of acute renal failure, which is characterized by large fluid and electrolyte losses in the urine.

diverticula: out-pocketings of the intestinal wall that balloon out through weakened areas of the intestinal wall (the singular is *diverticulum*).

diverticulitis: the condition of having infected diverticula.

diverticulosis: the condition of having diverticula.

docosahexaenoic acid: see *DHA.*

DNA and RNA: the genetic materials of cells necessary in protein synthesis, falsely promoted as ergogenic aids.

dominant gene: a gene that has an observable effect on an organism even when it is paired with another gene that codes for a different trait: see also *recessive gene.*

DRV: see *Daily Reference Values.*

drug history: a record of all the drugs, over-the-counter and prescribed, that a person takes routinely, used in nutrition status assessment.

dumping syndrome: the cluster of symptoms that results from the rapid emptying of undigested food into the jejunum: sweating, weakness, and diarrhea shortly after eating and hypoglycemia later.

duodenal ulcer: see *ulcer.*

duodenum: the first one-fifth of the small intestine.

durable power of attorney: a legal document in which one competent adult authorizes another competent adult to make decisions for her or him in the event of incapacitation.

duration: as used in fitness training, a term that refers to the length of time that an activity is performed (for example, the length of time spent in each exercise session).

dysentery: an infection of the gastrointestinal tract caused by an amoeba or bacterium that gives rise to severe diarrhea.

dyspepsia: vague abdominal discomfort; a symptom, not a disease.

dysphagia: difficulty in swallowing.

dysuria: painful or difficult urination.

eating disorder: a disturbance in eating behavior that jeopardizes a person's physical or psychological health.

eclampsia: a severe stage that follows preeclampsia in which convulsions occur.

edema: abnormal accumulation of fluid in the interstitial spaces.

eicosapentaenoic acid: see *EPA.*

electrolyte solutions: solutions of water with dissolved electrolytes that can conduct electricity.

electrolytes: salts that dissolve in water and dissociate into ions.

embolism: the obstruction of a blood vessel by a traveling clot (an embolus), which causes the sudden death of tissue.

embolus: a clot that forms within the circulatory system, then breaks loose and travels until it either dissolves or lodges in a narrow-bore artery or capillary.

emphysema: a type of chronic obstructive pulmonary disease in which the lungs lose their elasticity and the victim has difficulty breathing.

emulsifier: a substance that mixes with both fat and water, that can permanently disperse fat in water, forming an emulsion.

end-stage renal disease (ESRD): the severe stage of renal disease in which diet alone is no longer effective in maintaining normal kidney functions.

endocrine glands: glands that release their secretions into the blood.

endurance: the ability to keep going: see also *cardiorespiratory endurance, muscle endurance.*

energy metabolism: all the chemical reactions by which the body obtains, stores, and spends energy.

energy-yielding nutrients: the fuel nutrients, those that yield energy the body can use—carbohydrate, fat, and protein.

engorgement: filling or overfilling; in lactation, overfilling of the breasts with milk.

enrichment: now considered synonymous with fortification; previously, the addition of four specific nutrients—iron, thiamin, riboflavin, and niacin—to refined breads and cereals.

enteral: into the stomach or intestine, a term used to describe tube feedings.

enteral formulas: liquid formulas intended for oral use or for tube feedings.

enteral nutrition: feeding into the intestine; this term technically refers to the regular eating of food by mouth or to feeding by tube, but is often used synonymously with *tube feeding.*

enteric hyperoxaluria: see *hyperoxaluria.*

enterostomal therapist (E.T.): a health care professional specially educated to assist ostomates in learning the proper methods of adjusting to and caring for ostomies.

enterotoxins: see *toxins.*

enzyme: a protein catalyst.

enzyme replacements: extracts of pork or beef pancreatic enzymes that can be taken as supplements to help with digestion.

EPA: a 22-carbon omega-3 fatty acid derived from linolenic acid. The full name for EPA is *eicosapentaenoic acid.*

epinephrine: one of the so-called stress hormones, secreted whenever emergency action is called for; it readies body systems for fast action and mobilizes fuel to support that action.

epiglottis: a cartilage structure in the throat that prevents fluid or food from entering the trachea when a person swallows.

epithelial cells: cells that line the surfaces of the skin and mucous membranes.

ergogenic aids: products falsely claimed to enhance athletic performance.

erythrocyte: an oxygen-carrying cell of the blood, red because it contains hemoglobin.

erythrocyte hemolysis: rupture of the red blood cells, caused by vitamin E deficiency.

erythropoietin: a hormone that stimulates red blood cell production.

eschar: dead, burned skin.

esophageal hiatus: the opening in the diaphragm through which the esophagus passes.

esophageal stricture: scarring of the esophageal mucosa, which narrows the diameter of the esophagus.

esophageal varices: tangles of distended blood vessels that protrude into the esophagus.

esophagus: the food pipe; the conduit from the mouth to the stomach.

ESRD: see *end-stage renal disease.*

essential: in nutrition, a term that refers to compounds that the body cannot synthesize in amounts sufficient to meet physiological need.

E.T.: See *enterostomal therapist.*

ethical: in accordance with moral principles or professional standards.

ethnic diets: foodways and cuisines typical of national origins, races, cultural heritages, or geographic locations.

exocrine glands: glands that release their secretions "out" of the body, i.e., into the digestive tract or onto the surface of the skin.

extra lean: as used on labels, a term that means a food contains less than 5 g of fat, less than 2 g of saturated fat, and less than 95 mg of cholesterol per serving.

exudate: the fluid, containing plasma proteins and electrolytes, that leaks out through the capillaries at the site of a burn or injury.

fad diets: diets based on exaggerated or false theories of weight loss.

FAS: see *fetal alcohol syndrome.*

fasting hypoglycemia: hypoglycemia that occurs after 8 to 14 hours of fasting.

fat: a term that may be used to refer to all lipids; or specifically to triglycerides, the principal component of both food fat and body fat; or just to those triglycerides that are solid at room temperature (as opposed to oils).

fat-free: as used on labels, a term that means a food contains less than 0.5 g of fat per serving.

fatty acids: organic compounds composed of a chain of carbon atoms with hydrogens attached and an acid group at one end.

fatty liver: accumulation of fat in the liver cells, an early sign of liver deterioration seen in several diseases, including kwashiorkor and alcoholic liver disease; also called *hepatic steatosis.*

febrile: having a fever.

feeding gastrostomy: a surgical opening through which a feeding tube can be passed into the stomach.

feeding jejunostomy: a surgical opening through which a feeding tube can be passed into the jejunum.

ferritin: one of the body's iron-storage proteins.

ferulic-acid: see *plant sterols.*

fetal alcohol syndrome (FAS): the cluster of symptoms seen in a person whose mother consumed excess alcohol during her pregnancy; includes mental and physical retardation with facial and other body deformities.

fetus: the developing infant from eight weeks after conception until its birth.

fever: an increase of body temperature of more than 1°F above normal.

fewer: as used on labels, a term that means a food provides 25% less of a nutrient or kcalories than a reference food either naturally or as a result of altering the food.

fibers: a general term denoting the polysaccharides and the nonpolysaccharide lignins of plant foods; the constituents of foods that humans cannot digest.

fibrocystic breast disease: a disease in which nonmalignant lumps or cysts form the breast, which may in some cases be associated with vitamin E deficiency.

filtrate (in the kidney): the fluid that passes from the blood through the capillary walls of the glomeruli, to eventually form urine.

fistula: an abnormal opening between two organs or from an organ to the skin.

fitness: the characteristics of the body that enable it to perform physical activity; more broadly, the ability to meet routine physical demands with enough reserve energy to rise to a sudden challenge; or the body's ability to withstand stress of all kinds.

flapping tremor: see *asterixis.*

flavor enhancers: food additives that enhance flavor.

flexibility: in fitness, the capacity of the joints to move through a full range of motion; the ability to bend and recover without injury.

flow phase (of the stress response): see *acute phase.*

fluorapatite: the stabilized form of bone and tooth crystal, in which fluoride has replaced the hydroxy portion of hydroxyapatite.

fluorosis: mottling of the tooth enamel from ingestion of too much fluoride during tooth development.

follicle: a group of cells in the skin from which a hair grows.

follicular hyperkeratosis: the accumulation of the hard material keratin around each hair follicle.

food allergy: an adverse reaction to a food that involves an immune response; also called a *food-hypersensitivity reaction.*

food aversion: a strong desire to avoid a particular food.

food craving: a deep longing for a particular food.

food diary: a food record that includes associated information such as when, where, and with whom each food is eaten.

food frequency checklist: a checklist of foods on which a person can record the frequency with which he or she eats each food.

food-hypersensitivity reaction: see *food allergy.*

food intolerance: an adverse response to a food or food additive that does not involve the immune system.

food poisoning: illness transmitted to human beings through food, caused by infectious agents or by toxins that they produce.

food record: an extensive, accurate log of all foods eaten over a period of several days or weeks, used in assessing nutrition status.

fortification (of food): the addition of nutrients to a food to correct or prevent a widespread nutrient deficiency or to balance or enhance the nutrient profile of a food.

Four Food Group Plan: the original and widely taught eating plan, developed to ensure dietary adequacy, now supplanted by the *Daily Food Guide.*

frame size: an estimate of the size of a person's bones and musculature, used in some assessments of body weight.

free: as used on labels, a term that means a food contains no amount or a trivial amount of a substance.

free radical: a highly reactive chemical form that can cause destructive changes in nearby compounds, sometimes setting up a chain reaction.

frequency: as used in fitness training, a term that refers to the number of occurrences per unit of time (for example, the number of exercise sessions per week).

fresh: as used on labels, a term that means a food is raw, unprocessed or minimally processed (blanched or irradiated) with no added preservatives.

fructose: a monosaccharide; fruit sugar.

galactose: a monosaccharide; part of the disaccharide lactose.

galactosemia: an inborn error of metabolism in which galactose cannot be metabolized normally to compounds the body can handle and an alternative metabolite accumulates in the tissues, causing damage.

gallbladder: the organ embedded in the liver that collects, stores, and concentrates bile.

gamma-interferon: one of the cytokines; the one that induces the fever and malaise that frequently occur during an infection.

gastric: pertaining to the stomach.

gastric glands: exocrine glands in the stomach wall that secrete gastric juice into the stomach.

gastric juice: the digestive secretion of the gastric glands containing a mixture of water, hydrochloric acid, and enzymes.

gastric motility: the spontaneous motions of the digestive tract accomplished by involuntary muscular contractions; peristalsis and segmentation.

gastric partitioning: a surgical procedure that limits the size of the stomach and delays gastric emptying by restricting the outlet, used to treat clinically severe obesity.

gastric residual: formula left in the stomach from a previous feeding.

gastric ulcer: see *ulcer.*

gastritis: inflammation of the stomach lining.

gastroparesis: delayed gastric emptying.

gastrostomy: a surgical technique used to create an opening through which a feeding tube can be passed into the stomach.

gatekeeper: with respect to nutrition, a key person who controls other people's access to foods and thereby exerts a profound impact on their nutritional health.

genes: the basic units of hereditary information, made of DNA, that are passed from parent to offspring in the chromosomes. Each gene codes for a protein.

geophagia: clay-eating behavior.

gestational diabetes: the appearance of abnormal glucose tolerance during pregnancy, with subsequent return to normal postpartum.

GFR: see *glomerular filtration rate.*

GI tract: the gastrointestinal tract or digestive tract; the principal organs are the stomach and intestines.

gland: a cell or group of cells that secretes materials for special uses in the body.

gliadin: a fraction of the gluten protein, the fraction to which people with celiac disease are sensitive.

glomerular filtration rate (GFR): the rate at which the kidney glomeruli form filtrate, an index of the kidneys' health.

glomeruli (singular, *glomerulus*): the units in the kidneys that filter the blood.

glossitis: smooth tongue, which can be a symptom of malnutrition.

gluconeogenesis: the metabolic pathway that produces glucose from protein or fat.

glucose: a monosaccharide, the sugar common to all disaccharides and polysaccharides; blood sugar; dextrose.

glucose tolerance: the ability of the body to restore its blood glucose to normal after receiving doses of dietary carbohydrate.

glucose tolerance factor (GTF): a small organic compound containing chromium, which enhances insulin's action.

glucosuria (or glycosuria): glucose in the urine.

gluten: a vegetable protein found in wheat, oats, rye, and barley.

gluten-sensitive enteropathy: see *celiac disease.*

glycated hemoglobin: a form of hemoglobin that contains glucose molecules; used in a test that monitors blood glucose control.

glycerol: a 3-carbon alcohol, the alcohol that forms the "backbone" of triglycerides and phospholipids.

glycine: a nonessential amino acid, falsely promoted to athletes as an ergogenic aid.

glycogen: a polysaccharide composed of glucose, made and stored by liver and muscle tissues of human beings and animals as a storage form of glucose.

glycolysis: the metabolic breakdown of glucose to pyruvate.

glycosuria (or glucosuria): glucose in the urine.

goiter: an enlargement of the thyroid gland due to an iodine deficiency *(simple goiter),* malfunction of the gland, or overconsumption of a goitrogen *(toxic goiter).*

goitrogen: a thyroid antagonist found in food, which can cause toxic goiter.

good source: as used on labels, a term that means a food provides 10 to 19% of the Daily Value of a given nutrient per serving.

gout: a metabolic disorder that results in high body (and sometimes urinary) uric acid; crystals of uric acid precipitate in the joints and produce inflammation and pain.

graft-versus-host disease: the destruction of healthy donor cells by the recipient of a graft.

granulated sugar: common table sugar, crystalline sucrose; 99.9 percent pure.

GRAS (generally recognized as safe) list: a list of food additives, established by the FDA in 1958, that had long been in use and were known or believed safe at that time.

growth hormone releasers: herbs or pills falsely promoted for enhancing athletic performance.

GTF (glucose tolerance factor): hazard: the ability of a substance to produce injury under the conditions of its use.

HCG: see *human chorionic gonadotropin.*

HDL (high-density lipoprotein): the type of lipoprotein that transports cholesterol back to the liver from peripheral cells.

health history: a record of a person's past health and medical events, used in nutrition status assessment. Traditionally, the health history has been called the *medical history.*

heart attack: blockage of a vessel that feeds the heart muscle, which causes sudden tissue death; also called a *myocardial infarction (MI).*

heartburn: a burning sensation felt behind the sternum, caused by stomach acid splashing back up into the esophagus (reflux esophagitis).

hematuria: blood in the urine.

heme: the iron-holding part of the hemoglobin and myoglobin proteins.

hemochromatosis: a hereditary condition of iron overload characterized by deposits of iron-containing pigment in many tissues, with tissue damage.

hemodialysis: the method of dialysis in which a blood vessel is tapped and the blood is routed through a dialysis machine and then returned to the body; inside the machine, the blood flows within a semipermeable membrane that is surrounded by dialysis fluid so that exchange can take place.

hemoglobin: the oxygen-carrying protein of the red blood cells.

hemorrhagic disease: the vitamin K-deficiency disease in which blood fails to clot.

hemosiderin: one of the body's iron-storage proteins.

hemosiderosis: iron overload characterized by excessive iron deposits in hemosiderin.

hepatic artery: the blood vessel that carries oxygen-rich blood from the heart to the liver.

hepatic coma: a state of unconsciousness that occurs in severe liver disease; also called *hepatic encephalopathy* or *portal systemic encephalopathy.*

hepatic encephalopathy: see *hepatic coma.*

hepatic steatosis: see *fatty liver.*

hepatic vein: the vein that returns blood from the liver to the heart.

hepatic: of, like, or pertaining to the liver.

hepatitis: inflammation of the liver caused by a virus, alcohol, drug, or other toxin.

herpes virus: a virus that can lead to mouth lesions and may also affect the lower GI tract, causing diarrhea. (Another herpes strain causes sexually transmitted disease.)

HFCS: see *high-fructose corn syrup.*

hiatal hernia: protrusion of a portion of the stomach through the esophageal hiatus of the diaphragm.

high: as used on labels, a term that means a food provides 20% or more of the Daily Value per serving.

high-density lipoprotein: see *HDL.*

high-fructose corn syrup (HFCS): a sweetener made by concentrating corn syrup, the predominant sweetener used in processed foods today; mostly fructose; glucose makes up the balance.

high-quality protein: a complete protein that is also easy to digest.

HIV: see *human immunodeficiency virus.*

homeostasis: the maintenance of constant internal conditions (such as chemistry, temperature, and blood pressure) by the body's control systems.

hormones: chemical messengers, secreted by glands in response to altered conditions; each travels to target tissues and elicits specific responses to restore normal conditions.

honey: sugar formed from nectar gathered by bees, composed mostly of sucrose, fructose, and glucose.

human chorionic gonadotropin (HCG): a hormone excreted in the urine of pregnant women, which, given by injection, is incorrectly believed to enhance weight loss and reduce hunger.

human immunodeficiency virus (HIV): the virus that causes AIDS.

humoral immunity: immunity conferred by antibodies secreted by B-cells and carried to the invaded area by way of body fluids.

hunger: the physiological need to eat, experienced as a drive for obtaining food; an unpleasant sensation that demands relief.

hydrochloric acid (HCl): an acid composed of hydrogen and chloride atoms; the gastric glands produce this acid to aid in digestion, especially of proteins.

hydrodensitometry: measurement of body density by submerging a person underwater to obtain volume, also obtaining the person's weight, and then computing weight per unit volume.

hydrogenation: the process of adding hydrogen to unsaturated fat to make it more solid and resistant to chemical change.

hydrolyzed formula: a liquid diet that contains broken down molecules of protein such as amino acids and short peptide chains; also called a *monomeric formula.*

hydrophilic colloid: a substance that attracts water; a type of laxative that attracts water in the intestine to form a bulky stool, which then stimulates peristalsis.

hydrotherapy: a procedure in which a person with burn wounds is placed in a large whirlpool tub, where the wounds are gently cleansed with a special soap that helps prevent infections. Also called *tanking.*

hyperactivity: a disturbed behavior syndrome seen in children and adults in which the essential features are signs of developmentally inappropriate inattention, impulsivity, and high levels of motor activity; of interest in nutrition because foods, additives, or nutrient deficiencies have been (probably wrongly) suspected of causing it. Also called *attention deficit hyperactivity disorder.*

hyperammonemia: elevated blood ammonia.

hyperbilirubinemia: see *jaundice.*

hypercalciuria: excess urinary calcium.

hyperglycemia: abnormally high blood glucose.

hyperinsulinemia: abnormally high blood insulin.

hyperkalemia: abnormally high blood potassium.

hyperkeratosis: the progression of keratinization to the extreme: see also *follicular hyperkeratosis.*

hypermetabolism: accelerated metabolism, a part of the body's response to stress.

hyperosmolar hyperglycemic nonketotic coma: a complication of uncontrolled NIDDM precipitated by the presence of hypertonic blood and dehydration.

hyperoxaluria: high urinary oxalate. When caused by excessive oxalate absorption, it is known as *enteric hyperoxaluria.*

hypertension: high blood pressure.

hypertonic formula: a formula whose osmolality is higher than that of blood serum.

hypoalbuminemic PEM: protein-energy malnutrition characterized by low blood albumin; a term that some clinicians prefer to *kwashiorkor.*

hypochromic: pale or colorless, a description of the appearance of the red blood cells in some anemias.

hypoglycemia: abnormally low blood glucose.

hypothalamus: a part of the brain that helps regulate many body balances, including fluid balance.

IDDM: see *insulin-dependent diabetes mellitus.*

ideopathic: of unknown cause.

ileocecal valve: the sphincter muscle separating the small and large intestines.

ileostomy: a surgical procedure in which the colon is removed and the ileum is joined to the abdominal wall via a stoma.

ileum: the last two-fifths of the small intestine.

illness: as used in this book, any medical condition that alters nutrition status.

imitation food: a term that must be used on labels to describe a food intended to replace a standard food, if the replacement food lacks one or more nutrients found in the standard food.

immune system: the body's natural defense system against foreign materials that have penetrated the skin or mucous membranes.

immunity: the body's ability to recognize and eliminate tumors, foreign organisms, toxins, and the like.

immunoglobulin: a protein capable of acting as an antibody.

immunonutrition formula: see *stress formula.*

immunosuppressants: drugs that suppress the immune response.

inborn error of metabolism: an inherited flaw evident as a metabolic disorder or disease present from birth.

incidental food additives: substances that can get into food not through intentional introduction but as a result of contact with the food during growing, processing, packaging, storing, or some other stage before the food is consumed. The terms *accidental additives* and *indirect additives* mean the same thing.

indirect additives: see *incidental additives.*

indirect calorimetry: an estimation of energy output based on measures of oxygen consumption and carbon dioxide output.

individual approach (to diet advice): the approach that aims to identify and treat only people who are at the greatest risk of disease development: see also *population approach.*

indoles: a family of compounds with a structure resembling that of the amino acid tryptophan; of interest in nutrition because some are found in cruciferous vegetables and have anticancer activity.

infection: invasion of the body by a disease-causing organism.

inosine: an organic chemical that is falsely said to "activate cells, produce energy, and facilitate exercise," but which has been shown actually to reduce the endurance of runners.

insoluble fibers: plant food fibers that do not dissolve in water.

insulin: a hormone secreted by the pancreas in response to high blood glucose that promotes cellular glucose uptake and use or storage.

insulin-dependent diabetes mellitus (IDDM): the type of diabetes in which the person produces no insulin at all; also known as type I diabetes or juvenile-onset diabetes.

insulin reaction: hypoglycemia that results from an overdose of insulin, strenuous physical activity, skipped meals, or inadequate intake of food; also called *insulin shock.*

insulin resistance: the condition in which a normal amount of insulin produces a subnormal effect.

insulin shock: see *insulin resistance.*

intact formula: a liquid diet that contains complete molecules of protein; also called a *polymeric formula.*

intensity: as used in fitness training, a term that refers to the degree of exertion while exercising (for example, the amount of weight lifted or the speed of running).

interleukin-1: a cytokine that activates lymphocytes and is also partly responsible for the fever-induced anorexia that commonly accompanies stress.

intermittent claudication: a disorder characterized by cramps in the legs, which may be associated with vitamin E deficiency.

intermittent feeding by slow drip: delivery of no more than 250 milliliters of an enteral formula over 20 to 30 minutes.

international units: see *IU.*

intestinal bypass surgery: surgery that involves removing or disconnecting a portion of the small intestine to reduce absorption of energy nutrients, used to treat morbid obesity.

intestinal flora: the bacterial inhabitants of the digestive tract.

intestinal juice: the secretion of the intestinal glands which contains enzymes for the digestion of carbohydrate and protein and a minor enzyme for fat digestion.

intra-abdominal fat: fat stored within the abdominal cavity in association with the internal abdominal organs.

intractable: not responsive to treatment attempts.

intravenous nutrition: see *parenteral nutrition.*

intrinsic: inside the system.

intrinsic factor: a factor made in the stomach that aids in the absorption of vitamin B_{12}, necessary to prevent pernicious anemia.

invert sugar: a mixture of glucose and fructose formed by chemically splitting sucrose; sold in liquid form for use as an additive in foods.

ions: charged atomic particles.

iron deficiency: having depleted iron stores.

iron-deficiency anemia: anemia resulting from an iron deficiency severe enough to curtail hemoglobin production and cause synthesis of small, pale, red blood cells.

iron overload: toxicity from iron overdose. There are two types, hemochromatosis and hemosiderosis.

isotonic: having the same concentration of solute and therefore the same osmotic pressure, as human body fluid.

isotonic formula: a formula with an osmolality similar to that of blood serum (300 mOsm/L).

IU (international units): units used to express many vitamin amounts. Each can be converted to some other common unit; e.g., 1 IU of vitamin E is 1 mg of d-alpha-tocopherol.

IV catheter: a thin tube inserted into a vein through which nutrient solutions or medications can be given directly.

jaundice: yellowing of the skin caused by bile pigments (bilirubin) from the liver spilling into the bloodstream; also known as *hyperbilirubinemia.*

jejunostomy: a surgical technique used to create an opening through which a feeding tube can be passed into the jejunum.

jejunum: the two-fifths of the small intestine beyond the duodenum.

juvenile-onset diabetes: see *insulin-dependent diabetes mellitus.*

Kaposi's sarcoma: a type of cancer rare in the general population but common in people with HIV infections.

kcalorie (kilocalorie): a unit by which energy is measured; technically, the amount of heat energy necessary to raise the temperature of 1 kilogram of water 1 degree Centigrade under standard conditions. Most people speak of these units simply as calories, but actually, there are 1000 calories in a kcalorie. The abbreviation is *kcal.*

kcalorie control: management of food energy intake.

keratin: a water-insoluble protein; the normal protein of hair and nails. Keratin-producing cells may replace mucus-producing cells in vitamin A deficiency.

keratinization: accumulation of keratin in the skin's hair follicles, the cornea, or elsewhere, causing malfunction.

keratomalacia: total blindness caused by corneal keratinization, the last and most severe stage of vitamin A deficiency.

ketonemia: high blood ketones.

ketones: acidic, fat-related compounds formed from the incomplete breakdown of fat when carbohydrate is not available; technically known as *ketone bodies.*

ketonuria: ketones in the urine.

ketosis: the combination of high blood ketones (ketonemia) and ketones in the urine (ketonuria).

kilocalorie: see *kcalorie.*

kilojoule: the international unit of energy, equal to approximately 0.24 kcalories.

Krebs cycle: see *TCA cycle.*

kwashiorkor: a disease related to PEM, but of uncertain cause; possibly the same as acute or hypoalbuminemic PEM.

lactic acid: an organic acid, a common intermediate in metabolism; an incompletely oxidized product of metabolism produced in muscles when they break down glucose anaerobically.

lactoferrin: a factor in breast milk that binds iron and keeps it from supporting the growth of the infant's intestinal bacteria.

lactose: a disaccharide composed of glucose and galactose; commonly known as milk sugar.

lacto-ovo vegetarian diets: diets that include animal products but exclude animal flesh.

lacto-vegetarian diets: diets that include milk or milk products, but exclude eggs and animal flesh.

Laennec's cirrhosis: the type of cirrhosis associated with alcohol abuse and malnutrition.

large intestine: see *colon.*

latent period (in the course of a disease): the period in which the conditions are present but the symptoms have not begun to appear.

LDL (low-density lipoprotein): the type of lipoprotein derived from VLDL as cells remove triglycerides from them.

lean: as used on labels, a term that means a food contains less than 10 g of fat and less than 4.5 g of saturated fat and less than 95 mg of cholesterol per serving.

lecithin: a type of phospholipid.

less: as used on labels, a term that means a food provides 25% less of a nutrient or kcalories than a reference food, either naturally or as a result of altering the food.

letdown reflex: the reflex that forces milk to the front of the breast when the infant begins to nurse.

leucocytes: white blood cells; phagocytes and lymphocytes.

leukemia: cancer of the white blood cells.

life expectancy: the average number of years lived by people in a given society.

life span: the maximum number of years of life attainable by a member of a species.

light: as used on labels, a term that means (1) that a serving provides one-third fewer kcalories or half the fat of the regular product; or (2) that a serving of a low-kcalorie, low-fat product provides half the sodium normally present; or (3) that the product is light in color and texture (the label must make this intent clear; as in "light brown sugar").

limiting amino acid: the essential amino acid found in the shortest supply in a food protein relative to the amounts needed for protein synthesis in the body.

linoleic acid: an omega-6 polyunsaturated fatty acid, 18 carbons long with 2 double bonds, essential in human nutrition.

linolenic acid: an omega-3 polyunsaturated fatty acid, 18 carbons long with 3 double bonds, essential in human nutrition.

lipase: an enzyme that splits fats.

lipids: a family of compounds that includes triglycerides (fats and oils), phospholipids, and sterols.

lipoprotein lipase (LPL): an enzyme mounted on the surface of fat cells (and other cells), which promotes fat storage.

living will: a document signed by a competent adult that specifically states whether the person wishes any heroic measures to be taken in the event of terminal illness or irreversible coma from which the person is not expected to recover.

longevity: long duration of life.

low birthweight (LBW): a birthweight less than 5 1/2 lb (2500 g), which indicates probable poor health in the newborn and poor nutrition status of the mother during pregnancy.

low calorie: as used on labels, a term that means a food contains 40 kcalories or less per serving.

low-carbohydrate diets: diets designed to bring about metabolic responses such as ketosis, similar to those of fasting.

low-density lipoprotein: see *LDL.*

low cholesterol: as used on labels, a term that means a food contains 20 mg or less of cholesterol per serving and 2 g or less of saturated fat per serving.

low fat: as used on labels, a term that means a food contains 3 g or less fat per serving.

low-fiber diet: a diet that consists of foods that are low in fiber, also called a *soft diet.*

low saturated fat: as used on labels, a term that means a food contains 1 g or less saturated fat per serving.

low sodium: as used on labels, a term that means a food contains 140 mg or less sodium per serving.

lumen: the inner open space of a tube or hollow organ.

lymph: the body fluid found in lymphatic vessels, which consists of all the constituents of blood except the red blood cells.

lymphatic system: the system of vessels and ducts that carries lymph around the body and conveys the larger fat-soluble products of digestion toward the heart.

lymphocytes: white blood cells that participate in acquired immunity, B-cells and T-cells.

lysine: a nonessential amino acid, promoted as an ergogenic aid because it is a precursor of the high-energy compound phosphocreatine.

macrocytic: large-celled, a description of some anemias.

malignant: causing harm, a term used to describe tumors that pose a threat to life.

malnutrition: any condition caused by deficient or excess energy or nutrient intake or by an imbalance of nutrients.

maltitol: a sugar alcohol.

maltose: a disaccharide composed of two glucose units; malt sugar.

mannitol: a sugar alcohol.

maple sugar: a sugar (mostly sucrose) purified from concentrated sap of the sugar maple tree.

marasmus: a form of protein-energy malnutrition resulting from severe, chronic deprivation or impaired absorption of protein, energy, vitamins, and minerals; chronic malnutrition.

margin of safety: as used when speaking of food additives, a zone between the concentration normally used and that at which a hazard exists.

mastication: chewing.

mastitis: infection of a breast.

maturity-onset diabetes in the young (MODY): a type of noninsulin-dependent diabetes mellitus that develops during the teen years.

MCT: see *medium-chain triglycerides.*

mechanical soft diet: a diet in which all foods are easy to chew and swallow, also called a *dental soft diet.*

mechanical ventilator: see *ventilator.*

medical history: see *health history.*

medical record: the continuous written account of a client's health history, diagnosis, therapy, and prognosis, kept by the physician and other health care professionals.

medium-chain triglycerides (MCT): fats (such as coconut oil) that contain fatty acids only 6 to 12 carbon atoms long.

megadose: a dose much higher (eg., 100 times larger) than the physiological or RDA dose (eg., of a nutrient); a pharmacological dose.

megaloblastic: large-celled, a description of some anemias.

menadione: the synthetic substitute usually given for vitamin K.

mesentery (mesenteric membrane): the strong, flexible membrane that surrounds and supports the abdominal organs.

metabolism: the sum total of all the chemical reactions that go on in the body.

metastasize: to spread from one part of the body to another, a term used to describe malignant tumors.

MI: see *heart attack.*

microalbuminuria: small excesses of albumin in the urine, an early sign of renal disease.

microangiopathies: disorders of the capillaries, often seen in diabetes, including retinopathy, nephropathy, and neuropathy.

microcytic: small-celled, a description of some anemias.

microvilli: tiny, hairlike projections on each cell of every villus that can trap nutrients and transport them into the cells. The singular is *microvillus.*

milk anemia: iron-deficiency anemia caused by overconsumption of milk, which displaces iron-rich foods.

moderate exercise: exercise that can be sustained comfortably for 60 minutes or so.

moderation (dietary): providing enough, but not too much, of a dietary constituent.

modified or therapeutic diet: a regular diet that is adjusted to meet special nutrition needs by changing the consistency, level of energy and nutrients, amount of fluid, or number of meals, or by adding or eliminating certain foods.

modular formula: a formula made by combining several prepared mixtures or modules.

MODY: see *maturity-onset diabetes in the young.*

molasses: a thick brown syrup, left over from sugarcane juice during sugar refining.

molybdenum: a trace element.

monomeric formula: see *hydrolyzed formula.*

monosaccharide: a single sugar unit.

monounsaturated fatty acid: a fatty acid that has one point of unsaturation where hydrogens are missing, for example, oleic acid.

mood disorders: mental illnesses characterized by episodes of severe depression or excessive excitement (mania) or both.

morbid obesity: see *clinically severe obesity.*

more: as used on labels, a term that means a food contains at least 10% more of the Daily Value for a given nutrient than a comparable food. The nutrient may be added or may occur naturally.

mouth ulcers: lesions or sores in the lining of the mouth.

mucopolysaccharide: a polysaccharide with nitrogen-containing side groups.

mucous membrane: the cellular lining of a body organ with its coat of mucus. (The noun is *mucus;* the adjective is *mucous.*)

mucus: the smooth, slippery substance secreted by the cells of mucous membranes.

muscle endurance: the ability of a muscle to contract repeatedly within a given time without becoming exhausted.

muscle strength: the ability of a muscle to work against resistance.

muscular dystrophy: a hereditary disease in which the muscles gradually weaken; its most debilitating effects arise in the lungs.

mutation: an alteration in a gene such that it produces an altered protein.

mutual supplementation: the strategy of combining two protein foods in a meal so that each food provides the essential amino acid(s) lacking in the other.

myocardial infarction: see *heart attack.*

myoglobin: the oxygen-carrying protein of the muscle cells.

nasoduodenal (ND): from the nose to the duodenum.

nasoenteric: from the nose to the stomach or intestine. (Nasoenteric feedings include nasogastric, nasoduodenal, and nasojejunal feedings; or nasoduodenal and nasojejunal feedings only.)

nasogastric (NG): from the nose to the stomach.

nasojejunal (NJ): from the nose to the jejunum.

natural sweeteners: a term used freely, without legal definition, to refer to any sugar or sweetener except refined sucrose.

nausea: the inclination to vomit.

ND: see *nasoduodenal.*

neoplasm: see *tumor.*

nephritis: inflammation of the kidney.

nephrotic syndrome: the complex of symptoms, including proteinuria and albuminuria, that appears when glomerular function fails.

nephropathy: a type of microangiopathy affecting the capillaries of the kidney.

neuropathy: any disease of the nerves.

neurotoxins: see *toxins.*

NG: see *nasogastric.*

niacin equivalents: the units that describe the amount of niacin present in food, including the niacin that can theoretically be made from its precursor tryptophan present in the food.

NIDDM: see *noninsulin-dependent diabetes mellitus.*

nidus, or nucleus: a small bit of crystallized mineral or other material that serves as a matrix for crystallization.

night blindness: slow recovery of vision after exposure to flashes of bright light at night; an early symptom of vitamin A deficiency.

nitrites: salts containing the nitrite ion; used as additives in foods to prevent botulism.

nitrogen balance: the amount of nitrogen consumed (N in) as compared with the amount of nitrogen excreted (N out) in a given period of time.

nitrosamines: derivatives of nitrites that may form when nitrites combine with amines.

NJ: see *nasojejunal.*

nocturnal hypoglycemia: hypoglycemia that occurs while a person is sleeping.

noninsulin-dependent diabetes mellitus (NIDDM): the type of diabetes in which the fat cells resist insulin; also called type II diabetes or adult-onset diabetes.

nonhypoglycemia: a term used when people think they have hypoglycemia but don't.

nonnutritive sweeteners: see *artificial sweeteners.*

nonspecific immunity: immunity conferred by phagocytosis, the skin, and mucous membranes, which can be directed at many kinds of organisms.

NPO: *nil per os,* or "nothing by mouth."

nucleotides: nitrogen-containing components of RNA and DNA.

nursing bottle tooth decay: extensive tooth decay due to prolonged tooth contact with formula, milk, fruit juice, or other carbohydrate-rich liquid offered to an infant in a bottle.

nutritive sweeteners: sweeteners that yield energy, including both the sugars and the sugar alcohols.

nutrient: a substance obtained from food and used in the body to promote growth, maintenance, or repair of body tissues.

nutrient density: a measure of the nutrients a food provides relative to the energy it provides. The more nutrients and the fewer kcalories, the higher the nutrient density.

nutrition: see *science of nutrition.*

nutrition assessment: evaluation of the factors that influence or reflect nutrition status; its tools include histories, physical examinations, anthropometric measures, and biochemical analyses.

nutrition care plan: a plan that translates nutrition assessment data into a strategy for meeting a client's nutrient and nutrition education needs.

nutrition care process: an organized approach to nutrition intervention that consists of five steps (assessing, analyzing, planning, implementing, and evaluating).

nutrition screening: the use of preliminary nutrition assessment techniques to identify people who are malnourished or are at risk for malnutrition.

nutritionist: a person who specializes in the study of nutrition.

obesity: a chronic disease characterized by excessive body fat in relation to lean body tissue.

octacosanol: an alcohol extracted from wheat germ, often falsely promoted as of benefit to athletes.

oil: lipids (especially triglycerides) that are liquid at room temperature.

oligopeptide: a strand of between four and ten amino acids.

oliguria: minimal urine volume.

oliguric phase (in renal failure): the early phase of acute renal failure, in which urine volume is reduced.

omega: the last letter of the Greek alphabet (Ω, sometimes replaced by the letter *n*), used by chemists to refer to the position of the last double bond in a fatty acid.

omega-3 fatty acid: a polyunsaturated fatty acid in which the endmost double bond is three carbons from the non-acid end of the carbon chain.

omega-6 fatty acid: a polyunsaturated fatty acid in which the endmost double bond is six carbons from the non-acid end of the carbon chain.

opportunistic infections: infections caused by microorganisms that normally do not cause disease in the general population but can infect people once their immune systems are compromised (as in HIV infection).

oral hypoglycemic agents: drugs that can be taken by mouth to lower blood glucose in NIDDM.

oral rehydration therapy (ORT): a mixture of water, glucose, and sodium and potassium salts used to prevent or treat dehydration associated with diarrhea.

organic: carbon containing.

organic nutrients: carbohydrate, fat, protein, and vitamins.

ornithine: a nonessential amino acid, promoted as an ergogenic aid because it is a precursor of the high-energy compound phosphocreatine.

orogastric: from the mouth to the stomach.

ORT: see *oral rehydration therapy.*

ORT formulas: formulas that contain oral rehydration therapy ingredients already mixed.

oryzanol: see *plant sterols.*

osmolality: the number of molecular and ionic particles (measured in osmoles) per kilogram of water in a solution.

osmosis: the force that makes water follow salt; the force that causes a solute to move across a semipermeable membrane in the direction of the higher concentration of solute.

osmotic diarrhea: diarrhea that results from unabsorbed water and electrolytes which attract water into the intestinal contents.

osteomalacia: a bone disease characterized by softening of the bones; caused by vitamin D deficiency or renal osteodystrophy; sometimes known as *adult rickets.*

osteoporosis: literally, porous bones; reduced density of the bones, also known as *adult bone loss.*

ostomate: a person who has an ostomy.

ostomy: a surgically formed opening (ileostomy or colostomy) from the intestine to the outside of the body, bypassing the anus.

overload: an extra physical demand placed on the body; an increase in the frequency, duration, or intensity of exercise: see also *progressive overload principle.*

overnutrition: overconsumption of food energy or nutrients sufficient to cause disease or increased susceptibility to disease; a form of malnutrition.

overt period (in the course of a disease): the period in which the disease symptoms are obvious.

overweight: body weight above some standard of acceptable weight that is usually defined in relation to height (such as the weight-for-height tables).

oxidation: a reaction in which electrons are removed from a molecule. Often, this occurs when a molecule reacts with oxygen; it results in the release of energy.

oxidative phosphorylation: the series of metabolic reactions that completes oxidation of the products of the TCA cycle, with the release of energy.

PO: *per os,* or "by mouth," "orally."

pancreas: a gland that secretes enzymes and digestive juices into the duodenum and insulin and other hormones into the blood.

pancreatic juice: the exocrine secretion of the pancreas, containing enzymes for the digestion of carbohydrate, fat, and protein.

pancreatitis: inflammation of the pancreas.

paranoia: mental illness characterized by delusions of persecution.

parenteral: not into the intestine, a term that describes nutrition given by vein.

parenteral nutrition: the delivery of nutrients directly through a vein, bypassing the intestines; also called *intravenous nutrition.*

partial vegetarian diets: see *semivegetarian diets.*

pasteurization: the treatment of milk with heat sufficient to kill pathogens commonly transmitted through milk.

pathological stress: severe stress imposed by disease or by a bodily insult, such as an infection, surgery, or a burn.

PEG: see *percutaneous endoscopic gastrostomy.*

PEJ: see *percutaneous endoscopic jejunostomy.*

pellagra: the niacin-deficiency disease.

PEM: see *protein-energy malnutrition.*

pepsin: a protein-digesting enzyme (gastric protease) in the stomach.

peptic ulcer: an erosion of the top layer of cells from the mucosa of the stomach *(gastric ulcer)* or duodenum *(duodenal ulcer).*

percent fat free: as used on labels, a term that may be used only if the product meets the definition of *low fat* or *fat-free.* Requires disclosure of grams fat per 100 g of food.

percutaneous endoscopic gastrostomy (PEG): the technique for creating an opening for a tube feeding into the stomach without surgery.

percutaneous endoscopic jejunostomy (PEJ): a technique of creating an opening for a feeding tube from the stomach to the jejunum.

peripheral total parenteral nutrition (peripheral TPN): the provision by peripheral vein of a nutrient solution that meets all nutrient needs.

peripheral veins: the small-diameter veins that carry blood to the extremities (arms and legs).

peristalsis: successive waves of involuntary muscular contraction passing along the walls of the GI tract that push the contents along.

peritoneal dialysis: the method of dialysis in which the dialysis fluid is infused into the person's abdomen outside the peritoneal membrane; exchange takes place across the membrane, and the dialysis fluid is then withdrawn.

pernicious anemia: the name given to the anemia caused by vitamin B_{12} deficiency that is due to a lack of intrinsic factor (as opposed to dietary vitamin B_{12} deficiency).

persistent: of a stubborn or enduring nature; with respect to food contaminants, the quality of persisting and accumulating, rather than breaking down, in the bodies of animals and human beings.

persistent vegetative state: exhibiting motor reflexes but without the ability to regain cognitive behavior, to communicate, or to interact purposefully with the environment.

pH: an index of the concentration of hydrogen ions in a solution. The lower the pH, the stronger the acid.

phagocytes: white blood cells that have the ability to ingest and destroy foreign substances.

phagocytosis: the process by which phagocytes engulf and destroy foreign materials.

pharmacological dose: a high dose (eg., of a nutrient); a dose higher than the body normally handles, and one that may alter metabolism as a drug does.

phenylketonuria (PKU): an inborn error of metabolism in which phenylalanine, an essential amino acid, cannot be converted to tyrosine and abnormal phenylalanine metabolites (phenylketones) appear in the urine.

phosphate salts: salts containing phosphorus, falsely promoted as of benefit to athletes.

phospholipids: lipids similar in structure to triglycerides, but with choline (or a relative) and a phosphorus-containing acid in place of one of the fatty acids.

photophobia: hypersensitivity to light, which can be a symptom of malnutrition.

physiological dose: a normal dose (eg., of a nutrient); a dose the body normally handles.

physiological stress: a stress that the body's normal and healthy functioning can accommodate.

phytosterols: see *plant sterols.*

pica: a craving for nonfood substances; also known as geophagia when it refers to clay-eating behavior.

PIH: see *pregnancy-induced hypertension.*

pituitary gland: in the brain, the "king gland" that regulates the operation of many other glands.

placebo: an inert, harmless substance that resembles medicine; used in research to distinguish the effects of faith and hope from the effects of the medicine.

placenta: the organ that develops inside the uterus early in pregnancy in which maternal and fetal blood circulate in close proximity and exchange materials.

plant sterols: lipid extracts from plants, called *ferulic-acid, oryzanol, phytosterols,* or *adaptogens,* marketed with false claims that they contain hormones or balance hormonal activity.

plaques: mounds of lipid material, mixed with smooth muscle cells and calcium, which develop in the artery walls in atherosclerosis; also known as *atheromatous plaques.*

plasma: the fluid that remains when unclotted blood is centrifuged; unlike serum it contains some clotting factors.

platelets: tiny, disc-shaped bodies in the blood, important in blood clot formation.

PMS: see *premenstrual syndrome.*

polydipsia: excessive thirst.

polymeric formula: see *intact formula.*

polypeptide: a string of ten or more amino acids bonded together.

polyphagia: excessive eating.

polysaccharides: long chains of monosaccharides, including both the digestible complex carbohydrates and the fibers.

polyunsaturated fat: a triglyceride that contains mostly unsaturated fatty acids; or, a mixture of triglycerides that are mostly unsaturated.

polyunsaturated fatty acid (PUFA): a fatty acid with two or more points of unsaturation. For example, linoleic acid has two such points, and linolenic acid has three.

polyuria: excessive urine production.

population approach (to diet advice): the approach that aims to reduce disease risks among all people through population-wide changes in eating patterns: see also *individual approach.*

portal hypertension: elevated blood pressure in the portal vein caused by obstructed blood flow through the liver.

portal systemic encephalopathy: see *hepatic coma.*

portal vein: the vein that collects blood from the mesentery and conducts it to capillaries in the liver.

postgastrectomy diet: a carbohydrate-controlled diet given to prevent the symptoms of dumping syndrome and hypoglycemia that sometimes follow gastric surgery.

postgastrectomy hypoglycemia: see *alimentary hypoglycemia.*

postprandial hypoglycemia: see *reactive hypoglycemia.*

potassium-sparing diuretic: a diuretic that does not promote the excretion of potassium along with water.

power: a skill-related component of fitness, the combination of strength and speed that allows a person to move quickly and forcefully, such as in jumping, shot-putting, or spiking a ball.

precursor: a compound that can be converted into another compound.

preeclampsia: a disorder seen in pregnancy, characterized by hypertension, fluid retention, and protein in the urine.

preformed vitamin A: vitamin A found in foods in its active form.

pregnancy-induced hypertension (PIH): high blood pressure that develops in the second half of pregnancy.

premature infant: an infant born early and therefore of low birthweight, but with weight appropriate for gestational age (AGA).

premenstrual syndrome (PMS): a cluster of uncomfortable physical, psychological, and behavioral symptoms that arise in some women prior to menstruation and diminish during or after menstruation.

preservatives: antimicrobial agents, antioxidants, chelating agents, radiation, and other additives that retard spoilage or preserve desired qualities, such as softness in baked goods.

pressure sores: see *decubitus ulcers.*

progressive diet: the series of diets that progresses from clear liquids to full liquids to low-fiber foods to regular foods.

progressive overload principle: the training principle that a body system, in order to improve, must be worked at frequencies, durations, or intensities that gradually increase physical demand.

promoters: factors (found in foods) that favor the development of cancer once the initiating event has taken place.

protease: an enzyme that splits proteins.

protein-energy malnutrition (PEM): a deficiency of protein and food energy; the world's most widespread malnutrition problem.

protein isolate: a protein that has been separated from a food such as milk (for example, casein).

protein-losing enteropathy: the intestinal loss of serum proteins.

protein-sparing effect: the effect of carbohydrate (and to a limited extent, fat) in providing energy that allows protein to be used for other purposes.

protein-sparing fast: a variant on fasting and low-carbohydrate diets; the technique of eating only protein to lose weight.

proteins: compounds composed of carbon, hydrogen, oxygen, and nitrogen, and sometimes sulfur atoms arranged into strands of amino acids.

proteinuria: protein in the urine: see also *albuminuria.*

prothrombin time: the time it takes for blood to clot; also a test of the same.

PUFA: see *polyunsaturated fatty acid.*

pulmonary: concerning or involving the lungs.

pulmonary edema: fluid in the lungs.

pure vegetarian diets: see *vegan diets.*

pyloric sphincter: the sphincter muscle separating the stomach from the small intestine (also called *pylorus* or *pyloric valve*).

pyruvate: a salt of pyruvic acid, a 3-carbon compound derived from glucose, glycerol, and certain amino acids in metabolism.

R.D.: see *registered dietitian.*

radiation enteritis: changes in the structure of the small intestine caused by radiation therapy.

radiation therapy: the use of radiation to arrest or destroy cancer cells.

ratchet effect: see *weight cycling.*

raw sugar: technically, the first crop of crystals harvested during sugar processing. The so-called raw sugar sold in the United States has gone through several more processing steps.

RBP: see *retinol-binding protein.*

RDA: see *Recommended Dietary Allowances.*

RDI: see *Reference Daily Intakes.*

RE (retinol equivalents): the units in which vitamin A amounts in foods are expressed.

reaction time: a skill-related component of fitness, the amount of time between a stimulus and a response to the stimulus, such as when starting a race.

reactive hypoglycemia: hypoglycemia experienced simultaneously with epinephrine-release symptoms one to three hours after a meal; also called *postprandial hypoglycemia.*

rebound hyperglycemia: hyperglycemia that results from excessive secretion of counterregulatory hormones in response to excessive administration of insulin; also called the *Somogyi effect.*

recessive gene: a gene for an abnormal trait that has little or no observable effect on an organism as long as it is paired with a normal gene that can produce a normal product.

Recommended Dietary Allowances (RDA): daily recommended intakes of selected nutrients considered adequate to meet the nutrient needs of practically all healthy people in the United States.

Recommended Nutrient Intakes (RNI): daily recommended intakes of selected nutrients considered adequate to meet the nutrient needs of practically all healthy people in Canada.

rectum: the muscular terminal part of the GI tract extending from the sigmoid colon to the anus, which stores waste prior to elimination.

reduced calorie: as used on labels, a term that means a food contains at least 25% fewer kcalories per serving than a "regular" product.

reduced or less saturated fat: as used on labels, a term that means a food contains 25% or less saturated fat than the comparison food and is reduced by more than 1 g saturated fat per serving.

reduced: as used on labels, a term that means a food has been altered to provide 25% less per serving of something such as kcalories, fat, or sugar as compared to a "regular" product.

refeeding syndrome: a set of physiological and metabolic complications associated with reintroducing adequate nutrition too rapidly for a person with severe PEM.

Reference Daily Intakes (RDI): suggested daily intakes developed for food labels from the RDA for protein, vitamins, and minerals; previously known as the U.S. RDA: see also *Daily Values.*

reflux esophagitis: the backflow or regurgitation of gastric contents from the stomach into the esophagus, which causes inflammation of the esophagus (heartburn).

regional ileitis: see *Crohn's disease.*

registered dietitian (R.D.): a professional in dietetics with a bachelor's (B.S.) degree in nutrition or food science, a year's internship or the equivalent, and a passing score on the four-hour qualifying exam administered by the ADA or the Canadian Dietetic Association (CDA).

regular diet: see *standard diet.*

renal: pertaining to the kidneys.

renal colic: the severe pain that accompanies the movement of a kidney stone from the kidney through the ureter to the bladder.

renal failure: failure of the kidneys to maintain normal function.

renal osteodystrophy: a bone disorder resulting from calcium and phosphorus imbalances in renal disease. One type of renal osteodystrophy that leads to a softening of the bones is *osteomalacia.*

renal reserve: the capacity of the kidneys to function despite loss of some functioning tissue.

renin: an enzyme released by the kidneys in response to low blood pressure, which aids the kidneys in retaining water through a series of events known as the *renin-angiotensin mechanism.*

requirement: the amount of a nutrient that will just prevent the development of specific deficiency signs; a theoretical value impossible to state for everyone.

residue: the total amount of material in the colon; it includes dietary fiber and also undigested food, intestinal secretions, bacterial cell bodies, and cells shed from the intestinal mucosa.

respirator: see *ventilator.*

respiratory acidosis: a condition of having too much acid in the blood caused by failure of the lungs to ventilate properly.

respiratory distress: a disorder of the lung membranes that results in delayed onset of respiration at birth and difficulty in breathing after birth.

respiratory failure: failure of the lungs to exchange gases.

respiratory quotient (RQ): the ratio of carbon dioxide produced to oxygen consumed, an index of the relative amounts of carbohydrate and fat being metabolized for energy.

retina: the layer of light-sensitive nerve cells lining the back of the inside of the eye; consists of rods and cones.

retinal. the aldehyde form of vitamin A.

retinoic acid: the acid form of vitamin A.

retinol. the alcohol form of vitamin A.

retinol-binding protein (RBP): the protein made in the liver that carries vitamin A through the blood to the tissues that need it.

retinol equivalents: see *RE.*

retinopathy: a type of microangiopathy affecting the capillaries of the eye.

rickets: the vitamin D-deficiency disease in children.

rooting reflex: a reflex that causes an infant to turn toward whichever cheek is touched, in search of a nipple.

royal jelly: a substance produced by worker bees and fed to the queen bees, often falsely promoted as enhancing athletic performance.

RQ: see *respiratory quotient.*

saccharin: an artificial sweetener.

saliva: the secretion of the salivary glands that moistens food for chewing and swallowing.

salivary amylase: the principal enzyme in saliva, which initiates digestion of starch to maltose.

salivary glands: the exocrine glands that secrete saliva into the mouth.

salts: compounds composed of charged particles, or ions (except for acids and bases). An example is potassium chloride (K^+Cl^-).

satiety: the feeling of fullness or satisfaction that people feel after meals.

saturated fat: a triglyceride that contains three saturated fatty acids; or, a mixture of triglycerides that are mostly saturated.

saturated fat free: as used on labels, a term that means a food contains less than 0.5 g of saturated fat and less than 0.5 g of *trans*-fatty acids.

saturated fatty acid: a fatty acid carrying the maximum possible number of hydrogen atoms (having no points of unsaturation).

schizophrenia: mental illness characterized by an altered concept of reality and, in some cases, delusions and hallucinations.

science of nutrition: the study of nutrients in foods and of their ingestion, digestion, absorption, transport, metabolism, interaction, storage, and excretion. A broader definition includes the study of the environment and of human behavior as it relates to these processes.

scurvy: the vitamin C-deficiency disease.

secretory diarrhea: diarrhea that results from accelerated secretion of fluids and electrolytes by the intestinal capillaries into the lumen of the intestine.

sedentary: physically inactive (literally, "sitting down a lot").

segmentation: a periodic squeezing or partitioning of the intestine by its circular muscles that both mixes and slowly pushes the contents along.

selective menu: a menu from which clients can select the foods they will receive while hospitalized.

semivegetarian diets: diets that partake of some aspects of vegetarianism but include some animal flesh (such as fish or chicken). Also called *partial vegetarian diets.*

sepsis or septicemia: the presence of disease-causing microorganisms or their toxins within the bloodstream.

serum: the watery portion of the blood that remains after removal of the cells and clot-forming material: see also *plasma.*

set-point theory: as related to obesity, the theory that the body tends to maintain a certain weight by means of its own internal controls.

severe stress: see *pathological stress.*

SGA: see *small for gestational age.*

short bowel syndrome (short gut syndrome): a complex of symptoms that may arise whenever the absorptive surface of the small bowel is reduced; it includes diarrhea, weight loss, malabsorption, hypocalcemia, hypomagnesemia, and anemia.

shunts: see *collaterals.*

SIDS: see *sudden infant death syndrome.*

silent heart attack: a heart attack that goes unnoticed.

simple carbohydrates: the monosaccharides (glucose, fructose, and galactose) and the disaccharides (sucrose, lactose, and maltose); also called sugars.

simple goiter: see *goiter.*

simultaneous multiple analysis (SMA): the taking of several measurements during a single blood test.

small for gestational age (SGA): description of a low-birthweight infant whose low weight reflects inadequate growth during gestation: see also *appropriate for gestational age.*

small intestine: the 20-foot length of small-diameter (1-inch) intestine that is the major site of digestion of food and absorption of nutrients.

socioeconomic history: a record of a person's social and economic background, including such factors as education, income, and ethnic identity, used in nutrition status assessment.

sodium bicarbonate: an alkaline salt falsely promoted to athletes with the claim that it neutralizes blood lactic acid and thereby reduces pain. Actually, "soda loading" may cause intestinal bloating and diarrhea.

soft diet: see *low-fiber diet.*

soluble fibers: plant fibers that readily dissolve in water.

Somogyi effect: see *rebound hyperglycemia.*

sorbitol: a sugar alcohol.

specific immunity: see *acquired immunity.*

speed: a skill-related component of fitness, the ability to move fast, as in running or swimming.

sphincter: a circular muscle surrounding, and able to close, a body opening.

standard diet: a *regular diet*—that is, one that includes all foods and meets the nutrient needs of a normal, healthy person.

starch: a plant polysaccharide composed of glucose, digestible by human beings; the chief source of human food energy worldwide.

stasis: standing still. Normal intestinal motility keeps the intestinal contents flowing steadily; stasis allows bacteria to flourish.

steatorrhea: the fatty diarrhea characteristic of fat malabsorption.

sterile: free of microorganisms, such as bacteria.

steroid: a compound having the same basic ring structure as the sterols.

steroid drug: a drug used to reduce tissue inflammation, to suppress the immune response, or to replace certain steroid hormones in people who cannot synthesize them.

sterols: the family of lipids with a multiple-ring structure that includes cholesterol, vitamin D, testosterone, and others.

stoma: a surgically formed opening, as in an ileostomy or colostomy.

stress: any threat to a person's physical well-being.

stress formula: an enteral formula intended to meet the nutrient needs imposed by severe stress; may be called an *immunonutrition formula.*

strict vegetarian diets: see *vegan diets.*

stroke volume: the amount of oxygenated blood the heart ejects toward the tissues at each beat.

strokes: events in which the blood flow to a part of the brain is suddenly cut off.

struvite: crystals of magnesium ammonium phosphate.

subcutaneous fat: fat stored directly under the abdominal skin.

sucralose: an artificial sweetener.

sucrose: a disaccharide composed of glucose and fructose; commonly known as table sugar, beet sugar, or cane sugar.

sudden infant death syndrome (SIDS): the unexpected and unexplained death of an apparently well infant; also called *crib death.*

sugar alcohols: sugarlike alcohols that, like sugars, are sweet to taste and yield 4 calories per gram. Examples are maltitol, mannitol, sorbitol, and xylitol.

sugar free: as used on labels, a term that means a food contains less than half a gram of sugar per serving.

sulfites: salts containing sulfur; used as additives in fresh and frozen fruits and vegetables to prevent changes in color and texture due to oxidation.

supersaturation: a term that describes the concentration of a substance in a liquid at the point where it is too concentrated to stay in solution and begins to precipitate.

supplemental nutrition: foods or oral formulas used to augment nutrient intake.

synergism: an interaction between two or more factors that leads to effects greater than expected ("the whole is greater than the sum of the parts").

systemic: affecting the whole body rather than one part or organ system.

T-cells: lymphocytes that attack antigens.

tachycardia: a rapid heart rate.

tanking: see *hydrotherapy.*

TCA cycle: the series of metabolic reactions in which acetyl CoA is oxidized to two molecules of carbon dioxide and a free CoA, with the release of energy; also called the *Krebs cycle.*

tension-fatigue syndrome: apparent hyperactivity produced in a child by the combination of lack of sleep, overstimulation, and anxiety.

terminal illness: a progressive, irreversible disease that will lead to death in the near future.

therapeutic diet: see *modified diet.*

thermal injury: a burn.

thermic effect of food: an estimation of the energy the body uses to process food (digest, absorb, transport, metabolize, and store ingested nutrients).

three-in-one admixture: a TPN solution that contains all nutrients, including fat.

thrombosis: the growth of a *thrombus,* or blood clot that obstructs a blood vessel or the heart cavity, causing gradual death of tissue.

thrombus: a blood clot that forms in the circulatory system.

thrush: see *candidiasis.*

total parenteral nutrition (TPN): the delivery of all needed nutrients by vein.

toxic goiter: see *goiter.*

toxicity: the ability of a substance to harm living organisms. All substances are toxic if used in high enough concentrations.

toxins: poisons. Toxins produced by bacteria come in two varieties: *enterotoxins,* which act in the GI tract, and *neurotoxins,* which act on the nervous system.

TPN: see *total parenteral nutrition.*

trabeculae: the lacy networks of calcium crystals inside of the long bones, which provide structural support and serve as a storage depot for calcium.

trachea: the windpipe; the passageway from the mouth and nose to the lungs.

training: practicing an activity, which leads to conditioning.

***trans*-fatty acids:** Unsaturated fatty acids with a rare or unatural configuration of hydrogen atoms around a double bond, often a product of the hydrogenation process.

transferrin: the body's iron-carrying protein.

translocation: the passage of microorganisms from the interior of the intestines to the inside of the body.

transnasal: through the nose.

trauma: physical injury to the body, such as a broken bone, a gunshot wound, or surgery.

triglycerides: compounds composed of glycerol with three fatty acids attached; the principal component of both food fat and body fat.

tripeptide: three amino acids bonded together.

tube feeding: feeding a nutrient solution via a tube into the stomach or intestine; enteral nutrition.

tumor: an unchecked new growth of tissue forming an abnormal mass with no function; also called a *neoplasm.*

turbinado sugar: raw (brown) sugar from which the filth has been washed; legal to sell in the United States.

type I diabetes: see *insulin-dependent diabetes mellitus.*

type II diabetes: see *noninsulin-dependent diabetes mellitus.*

ulcerative colitis: inflammation and ulceration of the colon.

umbilical cord: the ropelike structure consisting of the fetus's veins and arteries, which ramify into the placenta; the route of nourishment and oxygen into the fetus and the route of waste disposal from the fetus.

undernutrition: underconsumption of food energy or nutrients severe enough to cause disease or increased susceptibility to disease; a form of malnutrition.

unsaturated fatty acid: a fatty acid in which one or more points of unsaturation occur (includes monounsaturated and polyunsaturated fatty acids).

unspecified eating disorders: eating disorders that do not meet the criteria for specific eating disorders such as anorexia nervosa and bulimia nervosa.

urea: the principal nitrogen-excretion product of metabolism.

uremia: the buildup of toxic waste products in the blood associated with renal insufficiency.

uremic frost: crystals of urea secreted onto the skin in renal disease.

uremic syndrome: the complex of symptoms seen late in renal failure, caused by uremia.

uterus: the womb, the muscular organ within which the infant develops before birth.

variety (dietary): using different foods to obtain the same nutrients on different occasions.

vegan diets: diets that exclude all animal products and include only plant foods; also known as *strict* or *pure vegetarian diets.*

vegetarian diets: a general term used to describe diets that exclude some or all animal-derived foods. See *lacto-ovo vegetarian diets, lacto-vegetarian diets, semi-vegetarian diets,* and *vegan diets.*

vein: a vessel that carries blood back to the heart.

ventilator: a machine that "breathes" for the person who can't; a respirator.

very-low-density lipoprotein: see *VLDL.*

very-low-kcalorie diets (VLCD): diets that provide from 400 to 800 kcalories per day to promote weight loss.

very low sodium: as used on labels, a term that means a food contains 35 mg or less sodium per serving.

villi: fingerlike projections of the cellular membrane that lines the small intestine. The singular is villus.

vitamin A: a fat-soluble vitamin. Its three chemical forms are *retinol, retinal,* and *retinoic acid.*

vitamin C dependency: the temporary condition manifested by withdrawal symptoms, experienced by the person who stops overdosing with vitamin C.

vitamins: essential, noncaloric, organic nutrients needed in tiny amounts in the diet.

VLCD: see *very-low-kcalorie diets.*

VLDL (very-low-density lipoprotein): the type of lipoprotein made primarily by liver cells to transport lipids to various tissues in the body; composed primarily of triglycerides.

voluntary activities: the component of a person's daily energy expenditure that involves conscious and deliberate muscular work—walking, lifting, climbing, and the like.

waist-to-hip ratio: an indicator of fat distribution; waist circumference divided by hip circumference.

warm-up: five to ten minutes of light exercise, such as easy jogging or cycling, to warm up the body in preparation for vigorous exercise.

water balance: the balance between water intake and water excretion, which keeps the body's water constant.

water intoxication: the condition in which body water contents are too high.

water-miscible vitamins: fat-soluble vitamins that readily mix with water and can be absorbed without fat.

weight cycling: repeated cycles of weight loss and subsequent regain, popularly called the *ratchet effect* or *yo-yo effect* of dieting.

white sugar: pure sucrose, produced by dissolving, concentrating, and recrystallizing raw sugar.

withdrawal reaction: a reaction to the withdrawal of a drug, revealing in most cases that the user has become dependent.

without: as used on labels, a term that means a food contains no amount or a trivial amount of a substance.

xerophthalmia: the end stage of the blindness caused by vitamin A deficiency.

xerosis: drying of the cornea, an early sign of vitamin A deficiency.

xylitol: a sugar alcohol.

yo-yo effect: see *weight cycling*.

zero: as used on labels, a term that means a food contains no amount or a trivial amount of a substance.

Zollinger-Ellison syndrome: a condition caused by pancreatic tumors secreting excess gastrin, which stimulates the stomach to release large amounts of hydrochloric acid and pepsin.

INDEX

Numbers in bold face (such as **123**) indicates pages on which definitions appear. Numbers in italics *(123)* indicate figures; numbers followed by the letter *t* (123t) refer to tables. Numbers followed by the letter *n* (123*n*) refer to footnotes on the page. Letters and numbers (such as D-1 to D-3) refer to Appendix pages.

F

Q

R

W

Photo Credits (continued)

33 Shirley Engen; **34** Ray Stanyard; **35, 36** Thomas Harm and Tom Peterson/Quest Photographic Inc.; **39** Ray Stanyard; **42** © Felicia Martinez/PhotoEdit; **43** © Tony Freeman/PhotoEdit; **47** Thomas Harm and Tom Peterson/Quest Photographic Inc.; **55** Shirley Engen; **67, 68** Thomas Harm and Tom Peterson/Quest Photographic Inc.; **76** Shirley Engen; **79** © Irving Geis/Science Photo Researchers; **85** © Steve Maines/Stock Boston; **92** Thomas Harm and Tom Peterson/Quest Photographic Inc.; **95, 116** Shirley Engen; **134, 135** Thomas Harm and Tom Peterson/Quest Photographic Inc.; **138** Shirley Engen; **144** Thomas Harm and Tom Peterson/Quest Photographic Inc.; **145** © Camerique/H. Armstrong Roberts; **149** Thomas Harm and Tom Peterson/Quest Photographic Inc.; **155 (top)** © Rosemary Weller/Tony Stone Worldwide; **(bottom)** © L. Fritz/H. Armstrong Roberts; **159, 164** Thomas Harm and Tom Peterson/Quest Photographic Inc.; **176** Shirley Engen; **183** Courtesy of Gjon Mill; **186, 188** Thomas Harm and Tom Peterson/Quest Photographic Inc.; **191** © Martin Rotker; **193 (margin)** Ray Stanyard; **193 194 196** Thomas Harm and Tom Peterson/Quest Photographic Inc.; **211** Shirley Engen; **213 (left)** © Tony Freeman/PhotoEdit; **(right)** © James Foote/Photo Researchers Inc.; **218** Courtesy of Andreas Cahling; **223** © Nathan Benn/Stock Boston; **224** © David Lissy/The Picture Cube; **230** © Ken Kaminsky/The Picture Cube; **234** © Tony Freeman/PhotoEdit; **237** © Michael Newman/PhotoEdit; **242** Shirley Engen; **252** © David Frazier; **255** © Michael Medford/Image Bank; **256** © Gray Mortimore/Tony Stone Worldwide; **257** © Greg Vaughn/Pacific Stock; **259** Felicia Martinez/PhotoEdit; **269** Shirley Engen; **270** © Charles Gupton/Tony Stone Worldwide; **272** © Michael Grecco/Stock Boston; **273, 274** Thomas Harm and Tom Peterson/Quest Photographic Inc.; **278** © Amanda Merullo/Stock Boston; **286 (top)** © Michael Newman/PhotoEdit; **(bottom)** © Robert Brenner/PhotoEdit; **287** © Robert Finken/The Picture Cube; **290** Thomas Harm and Tom Peterson/Quest Photographic Inc.; **291** © Susan Van Etten/PhotoEdit; **294, 296** © David Young-Wolff/PhotoEdit; **297** © Elizabeth Zuckerman/PhotoEdit; **299** Shirley Engen; **300** © David Joel/Tony Stone Worldwide; **303** © Joseph Nettis/Tony Stone Worldwide; **311** © Frank Siteman/Stock Boston; **314** © Blair Seitz/Photo Researchers Inc.; **317 (top)** © Mary Kate Denny/PhotoEdit; **(bottom)** © Tom McCarthy/PhotoEdit; **320** Shirley Engen; **322 (top)** © Mary Kate Denny/PhotoEdit; **(bottom)** © Tony Freeman/PhotoEdit; **323 (top)** © Michael Newman/PhotoEdit; **(bottom)** © John Coletti/The Picture Cube; **327** © David Young-Wolff/PhotoEdit; **328** © W & D McIntyre/Photo Researchers Inc.; **339 (top)** © Paul Conklin/PhotoEdit; **339 340** © Bob Daemmrich/Stock Boston; **343** Shirley Engen; **348** © Mary Kate Denny/PhotoEdit; **349** © Jeff Dunn/The Picture Cube; **351** © David Young-Wolff/PhotoEdit; **353** © Charles Gupton/Stock Boston; **355 (top)** © Don and Pat Valenti/Tony

Stone Worldwide; **(bottom)** © David Young-Wolff/ PhotoEdit; **356** © William Thompson/The Picture Cube; **358** © Charles Gupton/Stock Boston; **361** Shirley Engen; **368** © David J. Sams/Stock Boston; **372** © Jones, K. L., Smith, D. W., Ulleland, C. N., & Streissguth, A. P. *The Lancet*, June 9, 1973, pp. 1267–1271; **374** © Myrleen Ferguson Cate/PhotoEdit; **376** © C. J. Allen/Stock Boston; **379** © J. Gerard Smith/Photo Researchers Inc.; **384** © Felicia Martinez/PhotoEdit; **392** Shirley Engen; **393** © Anthony Vannelli; **398, 404, 408** © Tony Freeman/PhotoEdit; **417** Shirley Engen; **424 (top)** © Bill Bachmann/PhotoEdit; **(bottom)** © Michael Newman/PhotoEdit; **430** © Elena Rooraid/PhotoEdit; **431** © David Young-Wolff/PhotoEdit; **437** Shirley Engen; **448 (top)** © Rick Friedman/The Picture Cube; **(bottom)** © David Young-Wolff/PhotoEdit; **460** Shirley Engen; **461** © Charles Gupton/Tony Stone Worldwide; **462** © Bob Kramer/The Picture Cube; **471** © Bruce Ayers/Tony Stone Worldwide; **474** © Scott Berner/The Picture Cube; **478** Shirley Engen; **480** © Felicia Martinez/PhotoEdit; **484** © Roger Miller/The Image Bank; **489** © Robert Brenner/PhotoEdit; **500** © Caroline/H. Armstrong Roberts; **502** Shirley Engen; **506** © Felicia Martinez/PhotoEdit; **512** © Science Photo Library/Custom Medical Stock Photo; **519** © David Young-Wolff/PhotoEdit; **529** Shirley Engen; **535** © Mary Kate Denny/PhotoEdit; **538** © David Young-Wolff/PhotoEdit; **543** © Tony Freeman/PhotoEdit; **550** © David Young-Wolff/PhotoEdit; **554** Shirley Engen; **555** © Mary Kate-Denny/PhotoEdit; **557** © David Young-Wolff/PhotoEdit; **566 (left)** Courtesy of Abbott Laboratories; **(right)** Pharmacia Deltec Inc. St. Paul, Minnesota; **567, 582** Shirley Engen; **594** © Camerique/H. Armstrong Roberts; **595** © Tony Freeman/PhotoEdit; **598** © John Colletti/The Picture Cube; **613** Shirley Engen; **615** Reproduced by permission of ICI Pharmaceuticals Division Cheshire, England; **620** © Jerry Wachter/Photo Researchers Inc.; **621** © Rick Scott/The Picture Cube; **635** © Robert E. Daemmrich/Tony Stone Worldwide; **640** Shirley Engen; **649** © Felicia Martinez/PhotoEdit; **662** Shirley Engen; **663** © Amy C. Etra/PhotoEdit; **665** © H. Abernathy/H. Armstrong Roberts; **666, 668** © Martin Rotker; **682** © Camerique/H. Armstrong Roberts; **688** Shirley Engen; **690** © Marlene Karas/Atlanta Constitution; **693** © Gary A. Conner/PhotoEdit; **703** Shirley Engen.

"How to" Features appear on the following pages:

Acceptable Weight for Height Based on Body Mass Index (BMI)

To determine your acceptable weight range, find your height in the top line. Look down the column below it and find the range represented by the color blue. Look to the left column to see what weights are acceptable for you.

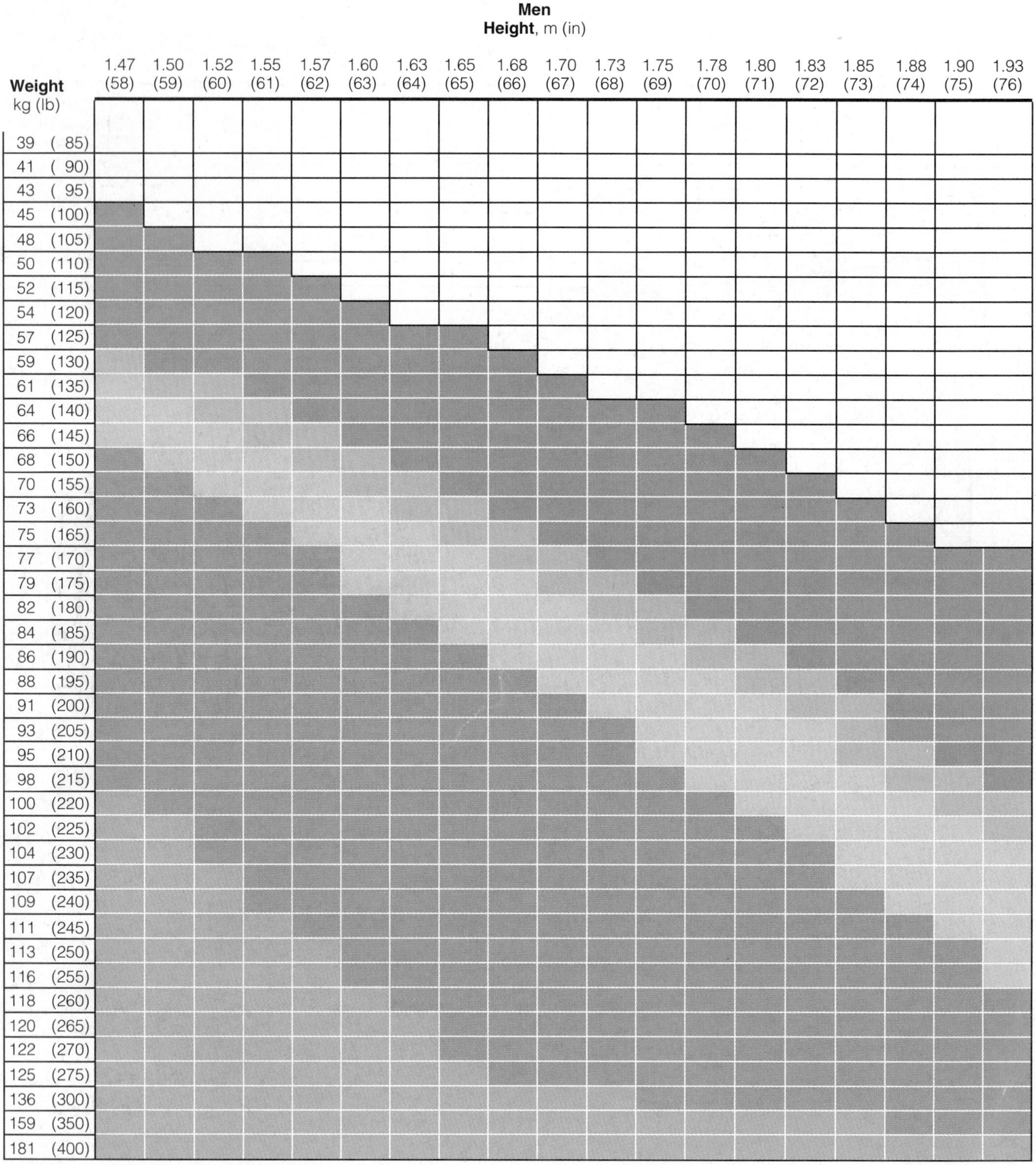

Men

Height, m (in)

Weight kg (lb)	1.47 (58)	1.50 (59)	1.52 (60)	1.55 (61)	1.57 (62)	1.60 (63)	1.63 (64)	1.65 (65)	1.68 (66)	1.70 (67)	1.73 (68)	1.75 (69)	1.78 (70)	1.80 (71)	1.83 (72)	1.85 (73)	1.88 (74)	1.90 (75)	1.93 (76)
39 (85)																			
41 (90)																			
43 (95)																			
45 (100)																			
48 (105)																			
50 (110)																			
52 (115)																			
54 (120)																			
57 (125)																			
59 (130)																			
61 (135)																			
64 (140)																			
66 (145)																			
68 (150)																			
70 (155)																			
73 (160)																			
75 (165)																			
77 (170)																			
79 (175)																			
82 (180)																			
84 (185)																			
86 (190)																			
88 (195)																			
91 (200)																			
93 (205)																			
95 (210)																			
98 (215)																			
100 (220)																			
102 (225)																			
104 (230)																			
107 (235)																			
109 (240)																			
111 (245)																			
113 (250)																			
116 (255)																			
118 (260)																			
120 (265)																			
122 (270)																			
125 (275)																			
136 (300)																			
159 (350)																			
181 (400)																			

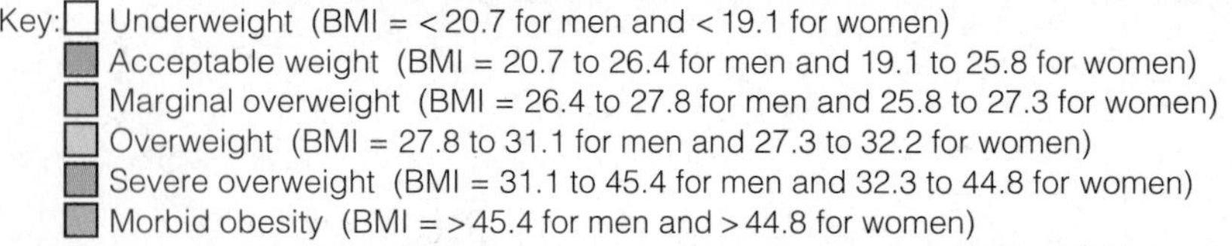
Key:
- Underweight (BMI = < 20.7 for men and < 19.1 for women)
- Acceptable weight (BMI = 20.7 to 26.4 for men and 19.1 to 25.8 for women)
- Marginal overweight (BMI = 26.4 to 27.8 for men and 25.8 to 27.3 for women)
- Overweight (BMI = 27.8 to 31.1 for men and 27.3 to 32.2 for women)
- Severe overweight (BMI = 31.1 to 45.4 for men and 32.3 to 44.8 for women)
- Morbid obesity (BMI = > 45.4 for men and > 44.8 for women)

Note: For more information on the body mass index, see Chapter 9 and Appendix E.

Source: Used with permission of Ross Products Division, Abbott Laboratories, Columbus, Ohio, from M.L. Rowland, A Nomogram for Computing Body Mass Index, *Dietetic Currents*, 1989; 16(2): 8-9.